AMERICAN
...CIATION
...CARE
...ES

T0092119

AACN
Core Curriculum
for Progressive
and Critical Care
Nursing

TONJA M. HARTJES, Editor
DNP, APRN, CNS, CCRN, CNEcl, FAANP

Owner, Nurse Practitioner and Consultant
Nursing Department
Coastal Consultants and Education LLC
St. Augustine Beach, Florida

Edition 8

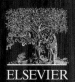

ELSEVIER

Elsevier
3251 Riverport Lane
St. Louis, Missouri 63043

AACN CORE CURRICULUM FOR PROGRESSIVE AND CRITICAL CARE NURSING, EIGHTH EDITION

ISBN: 978-0-323-77808-4

Previous editions copyrighted 2018, 2006, 1998, 1991, 1985, 1981, 1975.

Executive Content Strategist: Lee Henderson
Senior Content Development Manager: Lisa Newton
Senior Content Development Specialist: Laura Selkirk
Publishing Services Manager: Deepthi Unni
Senior Book Production Executive: Manchu Mohan
Senior Book Designer: Amy Buxton

Printed in India.

Last digit is the print number: 9   8   7   6   5   4   3   2

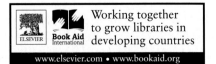

Working together
to grow libraries in
developing countries

www.elsevier.com • www.bookaid.org

Contributors

Bimbola Fola Akintade, PhD, MBA, MHA, ACNP-BC, NEA-BC, FAANP
Associate Professor and Associate Dean for the MSN Program
Organizational Systems and Adult Health
University of Maryland, School of Nursing;
Acute Care Nurse Practitioner
Surgical Intensive Care Unit
University of Maryland Medical Center
Baltimore, Maryland
Chapter 2: Psychosocial Aspects of Critical Care

Jenny G. Alderden, PhD, APRN, CCRN, CCNS
Associate Professor
Boise State University, School of Nursing
Boise, Idaho
Chapter 16: Older Adult Patients

Angela Benefield, DNP, RN, AGCNS-BC, CCRN-CSC-CMC
Clinical Education Specialist/Clinical Consultant
Education and Professional Development
Independent Clinical Education Consultant
Temecula, California
Chapter 15: Bariatric Patients

Patricia A. Blissitt, PhD, ARNP-CNS, CCRN, CNRN, SCRN, CCNS, CCM, ACNS-BC
Neuroscience Clinical Nurse Specialist
Professional Development and Nursing Excellence
Harborview Medical Center;
Associate Professor, Clinical Faculty
University of Washington, School of Nursing;
Neuroscience Clinical Nurse Specialist
Clinical Education and Practice
Swedish Medical Center
Seattle, Washington
Chapter 5: Neurologic System

Bryan Boling, DNP, AG-ACNP, CCRN-CSC, CEN
Advanced Practice Provider
Anesthesiology, Critical Care Medicine
University of Kentucky
Lexington, Kentucky
Adjunct Faculty
AGACNP Program
Georgetown University
Washington, District of Columbia
Chapter 4: Cardiovascular System
Chapter 6: Renal System

Nicole Brumfield, DNP, APRN, FNP-BC, AG-ACNP-BC
Anesthesiology, Critical Care Medicine
University of Kentucky
Lexington, Kentucky
Chapter 8: Hematologic and Immunologic Systems

Deborah Chapa, PhD, ACNP-BC, FAANP, ACHPN
Associate Professor, Nursing
Marshall University
Huntington, West Virginia
Chapter 2: Psychosocial Aspects of Critical Care

Catrina Cullen, RN, BSN, CCRN
University of Colorado, College of Nursing
Denver, Colorado
Chapter 19: Sedation

Anna Dermenchyan, MSN, RN, CCRN-K, CPHQ
Director of Quality
Department of Medicine
University of California – Los Angeles Health
Los Angeles, California
Chapter 1: Professional Caring and Ethical Practice

Andrea Efre, DNP, ARNP, ANP, FNP
Owner, Nurse Practitioner and Consultant
Healthcare Education Consultants
Tampa, Florida
Chapter 4: Cardiovascular System

Carrol Graves, MSN, RN, CCRN, CNL
Clinical Nurse Leader
Critical Care
North Florida/South Georgia Veterans Health System
Gainesville, Florida
Chapter 13: Hypothermia

Renee M. Holleran, FNP-BC, PhD, CCRN (Alumnus), CEN, CFRN, CTRN (Retired), FAEN
Nurse Practitioner
Anesthesia Chronic Pain
Veterans Health Administration;
Former Manager of Adult Transport
Intermountain Life Flight
Intermountain Health Care
Salt Lake City, Utah;
Former Chief Flight Nurse
University Air Care
University Hospital
Cincinnati, Ohio;
Family Nurse Practitioner
Hope Free Clinic
Midvale, Utah
Chapter 11: Multisystem Trauma

Jennifer MacDermott, MS, RN, ACNS-BC, NP-C, CCRN
Nurse Practitioner
Hospital Medicine
St. Luke's Health System
Boise, Idaho
Chapter 7: Endocrine System

Mary Beth Flynn Makic, PhD, RN, CCNS, CCRN-K, FAAN, FNAP, FCNS
Professor
University of Colorado, College of Nursing
Aurora, Colorado;
Research Scientist
Denver Health
Denver, Colorado
Chapter 19: Sedation

Diane McLaughlin, DNP, AGACNP-BC, CCRN
Acute Care Nurse Practitioner
Neurocritical Care
University of Florida Health - Jacksonville;
Acute Care Nurse Practitioner
Critical Care Medicine
Mayo Clinic
Jacksonville, Florida;
Lecturer
Case Western Reserve University, School of Nursing
Cleveland, Ohio
Chapter 10: Sepsis and Septic Shock

Shana Metzger, MS, FNP-BC, AG-ACNP-BC
Adjunct Instructor
School of Nursing and Health Studies
Georgetown University
Washington, District of Columbia
Chapter 14: Toxin Exposure

Denise O'Brien, DNP, RN, ACNS-BC, CPAN, CAPA, FASPAN, FCNS, FAAN
Perianesthesia Clinical Nurse Specialist
Consultant
Self-Employed
Ypsilanti, Michigan
Chapter 22 Perioperative Care

Jan Odom-Forren, PhD, RN, CPAN, FASPAN, FAAN
Associate Professor
University of Kentucky, College of Nursing
Lexington, Kentucky;
Perianesthesia Nursing Consultant
Louisville, Kentucky
Chapter 22 Perioperative Care

Patricia Radovich, PhD, CNS, FCCM
Director
Nursing Research
Loma Linda University Health Hospitals;
Assistant Professor
Loma Linda University, School of Nursing
Loma Linda, California;
Assistant Professor
California State University – Fullerton, School of Nursing
Fullerton, California;
Adjunct Professor
California State University - San Bernardino, School of Nursing
San Bernardino, California
Chapter 9: Gastrointestinal System

Tonya Sawyer-McGee, DNP, MBA, MSN, BSN, RN, ACNP-BC
Dean of Nursing
College of Nursing and Advanced Health Professions
The Chicago School of Professional Psychology
Richardson, Texas;
Adjunct Professor
Abilene Christian University, College of Nursing
Abilene, Texas
Chapter 20: Pain

Karah Cripe Sickler, RN, DNP, AG-ACNP-BC
Nurse Practitioner
Surgical Critical Care
University of Florida Health
Gainesville, Florida
Chapter 12: Burns

Daniel N. Storzer, DNP, ACNPC, ACNP-BC, CNRN, CCRN, CCEMT-P, FCCP, FCCM
Acute Care Nurse Practitioner
Pulmonary/Critical Care
Fox Valley Pulmonary Medicine
Neenah, Wisconsin;
Clinical Instructor
Acute Care Nurse Practitioner Program
Walden University;
Critical Care Paramedic
Waushara County EMS
Wautoma, Wisconsin
Chapter 3: Pulmonary System

Jennifer T.N. Treacy, MSN, APRN, FNP
Women, Infant, & Children Unit
Riverside Regional Medical Center
Newport News, Virginia
Chapter 17: High-Risk Obstetric Patients

Clareen Wiencek, PhD, RN, ACNP, ACHPN, FAAN
Associate Professor
Director of Advanced Practice
University of Virginia, School of Nursing
Charlottesville, Virginia
Chapter 21: Palliative and End-of-Life Care

Reviewers

Staccie Anne Allen, DNP, BSBA, APRN, AGACNP-BC, FNP-C, CFRN, EMT-P
Nurse Practitioner/Paramedic
ShandsCair Critical Care Transport Program
University of Florida Department of Emergency Medicine
University of Florida Health Shands Hospital
Gainesville, Florida

Angie Atwood, PhD, RN
Assistant Professor of Nursing
Campbellsville University
Campbellsville, Kentucky

Michele Beatty Bachmann, MSN, RN
Instructor
Department of Primary Care
Southern Illinois University – Edwardsville
Edwardsville, Illinois

Beverly L. Banks, BSN, MSN, RN
Senior Full-Time Faculty
Nursing
Alpena Community College
Alpena, Michigan

Debra J. Behr, DNP, RN, CCRN-K
Director of Professional Development and Magnet Program
Lutheran Medical Center
Wheat Ridge, Colorado

Collin Bowman-Woodall, MSN, RN
Assistant Professor
Samuel Merritt University, School of Nursing
San Mateo, California

Mary Ann "Cammy" Christie, APRN, MSN, CCRN, CMC-CSC, PCCN
Acute Care Nurse Practitioner
Department of Critical Care Medicine and Surgery
University of Florida
Gainesville, Florida

Judy E. Davidson, DNP, RN, MCCM, FAAN
Nurse Scientist
University of California – San Diego Health Sciences;
Scientist
Department of Psychiatry
University of California – San Diego, School of Medicine
La Jolla, California;
Associate Editor
Journal of Nursing Management

Tina Deatherage, DNP, RN, CCNS, CCRN, CNRN, NEA-BC
Hospital Accreditation Program Surveyor
The Joint Commission;
Adjunct Faculty, Nursing
Queens University
Charlotte, North Carolina

Christina Flint, MSN, MBA, RN
Assistant Professor
University of Indianapolis, School of Nursing
Indianapolis, Indiana

Matthew J. Fox, MSN, RN-BC
Assistant Professor
Nursing
Ohio University
Zanesville, Ohio

Keble Frazer, BSN, RN-BC, CCRN, PCCN
Registered Nurse
Medical and Surgical Intensive Care Units
Orange Regional Medical Center
Middletown, New York;
Montefiore Medical Center
Bronx, New York

Kelly A. Gaiolini, RN
Staff Nurse, Neuro/Surgical Intensive Care Unit
Lawnwood Regional Medical Center
Fort Pierce, Florida

Charles R. Gold, BSN, RN, CCRN
Registered Nurse
Neurosurgical Intensive Care Unit
Atrium Health's Carolinas Medical Center
Charlotte, North Carolina

Ami Grek, DNP, APRN, ACNP-BC
Lead Advanced Practice Provider
Department of Critical Care
Associate Director
NP/PA Critical Care Fellowship Program
Assistant Professor of Medicine
Mayo Clinic School of Medicine
Jacksonville, Florida

Christopher Guelbert, DNP, RN, CCRN, CNML
Assistant Professor
Nursing
Barnes Jewish College
St. Louis, Missouri

Stephanie A. Gustman, BSN, MSN, DNP, RN
Associate Professor
Ferris State University
Big Rapids, Michigan

Christian Guzman, MS, CCRN, ACNPC-AG, APRN
Facility Director, Advanced Practice Providers
Intensivist Nurse Practitioner
Intensive Care Consortium
Gainesville, Florida

Jillian Hamel, MS, RN, ACNP-BC
Acute Care Nurse Practitioner
Emergency Department Observation Unit
Providence Regional Medical Center
Everett, Washington

Sonya Renae Hardin, PhD, MBA/MHA, CCRN, ACNS-BC, NP-C, FAAN
Dean and Professor
University of Louisville, School of Nursing
Louisville, Kentucky

Kiersten Henry, DNP, ACNP-BC, CCNS, CCRN-CMC
Chief Advanced Practice Clinician
MedStar Montgomery Medical Center
Olney, Maryland

Cheryl Holsworth, MSA, RN, CBN, CMSRN
Senior Specialist for Bariatric Surgery
Sharp Memorial Hospital
San Diego, California

Robert C. Ingram, BSN, MSN, MHA, DNPc, RN, CEN
Assistant Professor
Lourdes University, College of Nursing
Sylvania, Ohio

Tonia Kennedy, MSN, EdD, RN-BC, CCRN-K
Associate Professor
Liberty University, School of Nursing
Lynchburg, Virgina

Sara Knippa, MS, RN, CCRN, PCCN, ACCNS-AG
Clinical Nurse Specialist and Educator
Cardiac ICU
University of Colorado Hospital
CHealth
Aurora, Colorado

Marianna LeCron Presley, MSN, RN, CCRN
Critical Care Nurse
Medical Intensive Care
Atrium Health Pineville
Charlotte, North Carolina

KellyAnne Lee, MSN, MBA, RN, CCRN
Healthcare Consultant
Coasta Consulting Group, LLC
Mount Pleasant, South Carolina

Tanaya C. Lindstrom, MSN, RN, CCRN, CNL
Clinical Nurse Educator
Surgical/Medical Intensive Care Units
North Florida South Georgia Veterans Health System
Gainesville, Florida

Yvette Lowery, MSN/Ed, DNP, FNP-c, CCRN, CEN, PCCN
Family Nurse Practitioner
Emergency Department
Memorial Hospital
Jacksonville, Florida

Karen A. Matos, MSN, RN, CCRN
Clinical Nurse Expert of Medical and Surgical Intensive Care Units and Telemetry
Nursing Education
Ralph H. Johnson Veterans Administration Hospital
Charleston, South Carolina

Paige McCraney, DNP, APRN
Adult Health Nurse Practitioner
Assistant Professor
University of North Georgia Department of Nursing
Dahlonega, Georgia

Denise M. McEnroe-Petitte, AS, BSN, MSN, PhD, RN
Associate Professor Nursing
Kent State University – Tuscarawas
New Philadelphia, Ohio

Katina M. Meyer, BSN, RN
Registered Nurse
Medical Intensive Care Unit
Stormont Vail Health
Topeka, Kansas

Samantha Palmer Noah, MSN, APRN, FNP-BC, AGACNP-BC
Nurse Practitioner
Flourish Health Network
Gainesville, Florida

DaiWai M. Olson, PhD, RN, CCRN, FNCS
Professor of Neurology & Neurotherapeutics
Professor of Neurosurgery
Distinguished Teaching Professor
University of Texas Southwestern Medical Center
Dallas, Texas

Sarah Peacock, DNP, APRN, ACNP-BC
Lead Advanced Provider
Department of Critical Care Medicine
Mayo Clinic
Jacksonville, Florida

Deidra Pennington, MSN, RN
Assistant Professor
Nursing
Jefferson College of Health Sciences
Roanoke, Virginia

Ruthie Robinson, PhD, RN, CNS, FAEN, CEN, NEA-BC
Director, Graduate Nursing Studies
JoAnne Gay Dishman School of Nursing
Lamar University
Beaumont, Texas

Emily Rogers, DNP, AGACNP-BC, CCRN, APRN
Nurse Practitioner, Department of Critical Care
Mayo Clinic
Jacksonville, Florida

Janet Czermak Russell, DNP, RN, APN-BC
Associate Professor of Nursing
Nursing/Biology
Essex County College
Newark, New Jersey

Peter D. Smith, BA, MSN, RN
Clinical Education Specialist
Nursing Education
Kindred Healthcare
St. Louis, Missouri

Diane Fuller Switzer, DNP, ARNP, FNP-BC, ENP-BC, ENP-C, CCRN, CEN, FAEN
Assistant Clinical Professor
Seattle University, College of Nursing
Seattle, Washington

Ashley N. Thompson, DNP, AGACNP-BC
Acute Care Nurse Practitioner, Assistant Professor
UF Health/University of Florida
Gainesville, Florida

Preface

Since the early 1970s, the American Association of Critical-Care Nurses (AACN) and its *AACN Core Curriculum* have stood at the forefront of the continuing evolution of critical care nursing to better meet the highly specialized needs of the patients and families they serve. The *AACN Core Curriculum* has now undergone eight editions, during which time it has maintained its reputation as the source of all things critical care. Among several steps we took to help prepare for this edition, AACN and I issued a reader survey and gathered together a cross-section of expert clinicians for a focus group during the organization's National Teaching Institute & Critical Care Exposition in 2019. Our goal was to gather information to ensure that this newest edition kept pace with the expanding role of nurses in the critical care profession. Participants confirmed the many ways the *AACN Core Curriculum* is used: as a clinical reference in caring for progressive and critical care patients, as a resource for CCRN certification exam preparation, for the creation of critical care courses and curricula, as a cornerstone for new nurse orientation, and in the development of competency content. Several nurses with whom we spoke stated that the *AACN Core Curriculum* was their "critical care bible," affirming that after all these years it is still an actively sought-after resource within critical care nursing practice.

As we listened to readers and collected information from multiple sources, we confirmed that the purpose of the *AACN Core Curriculum* remains, as it always has been, to articulate the knowledge base that underlies progressive and critical care nursing practice. Each edition of this work attempts to redefine that knowledge base for nurses who practice in this ever-expanding specialty area.

The eighth edition has been retitled *AACN Core Curriculum for Progressive and Critical Care Nursing*. Critical care practice and nursing have evolved over the past decade. Acutely ill patients are treated in many units of the hospital, from the Medical-Surgical departments to progressive and intermediate care units and elsewhere. Patients requiring critical care also are found outside the intensive care unit. Specialty nursing units have been created to meet these evolving health care needs; critical care nurses and patients are found in cardiac catheterization labs, emergency departments, and tele-ICUs. Sometimes they are even found at home awaiting heart transplant with inotropic medications and a left ventricular assist device. Changing the title of the text as we have done brings the resource more in line with the varied settings in which we find critically ill patients, and it signals to readers outside the traditional ICU that they are included in our base of readers.

Several similarities still exist between the seventh and eighth editions. The current edition continues to use the CCRN Examination blueprint and task statements as a starting point for determining relevant content and its apportionment throughout the book. We continue with the embellished outline format, and body systems are again used to divide the major content areas into chapters. Subsections related to physiologic anatomy, pathophysiology, and patient assessment; generalized patient care; and unique characteristics of specific disorders also have been retained.

Readers can still find the AACN Synergy Model for Patient Care woven throughout this edition. When it was developed in the late 1990s, the Synergy Model became the conceptual framework for certified practice in critical care and has since been widely incorporated across the discipline. Chapter 1 describes the model in detail, and each chapter includes in the assessment section a reminder of the model's prevalence. A key premise of the Synergy Model is that patient characteristics drive the competencies that nurses need in order to provide holistic, healing care that achieves optimal patient outcomes. A knowledge base of critical care nursing underlies clinical practice and reflects a foundational requirement for the development of these nursing competencies.

AACN's Competency Based Assessment (CBA) framework was incorporated as "leveling" guidance using the Synergy Model for Patient Care and the expanded outline format and embellishment items within the text. The terms *novice, advanced beginner, proficient,* and *expert* were used to operationalize the nurse competency and leveling of content within the *AACN Core Curriculum.*

The Novice or Advanced Beginner is encouraged to focus on the following content for foundational knowledge:

Section 1: System Wide Elements

- Anatomy and Physiology Review
- Assessment
- Patient Care
- The new "Key Concept" highlight boxes have been expanded throughout the text, and replace "Key Points" from the seventh edition

Proficient or Expert learners are encouraged to focus on the following content for expert knowledge:

Section 2: Specific Patient Health Problems

- Health Problems
- Pathophysiology, Etiology, Signs and Symptoms, Diagnostic Findings, Management of Patient Care, Complications, End Organ Diseases
- The new "Expert Tip" highlight boxes have been expanded throughout the text, and replace the "Clinical Pearls" from the seventh edition

To keep pace with the expanding role of progressive and critical care nursing practice and the evolving health care arena, the following items have been added or updated:

- Reorganization of content into four sections:
  Part I: Foundations of Progressive and Critical Care Nursing
  Part II: Critical Care of Patients with Issues Affecting Specific Body Systems
  Part III: Critical Care of Patients with Multisystem Issues
  Part IV: Critical Care of Patients with Special Needs
- Removal of all subchapters
- A new Perioperative Care chapter
- The text features improved navigation, format, and usability with a new, full-color, user-friendly interior design that uses high-contrast text colors and a larger font.
- A Crosswalk was created at the beginning of each chapter that interfaces or maps foundational nursing content within key educational and clinical documents including the following:
  - Quality and Safety in Nursing Education (QSEN) competencies
  - National Patient Safety Goals
  - American Nurses Association (ANA) Standards for Professional Nursing Practice
  - American Association of Critical-Care Nurses (AACN) Standards for Progressive and Critical Care Nursing Practice
  - American Association of Critical-Care Nurses Healthy Work Environments
  - Progressive and Critical Care Nursing Certification
- All chapters, tables, figures, boxes, and terminology are based on the most recently published AACN/ANA Scope of Practice and Standards of Care.
- QSEN content has been incorporated within chapters of the text.
- The newest sepsis guidelines content has been added to Chapter 10.

- All references complement and reinforce current AACN and critical care standards and guidelines of care.
- References and bibliographies for all chapters are now available online on the Evolve site at http://evolve.elsevier.com/AACN/corecurriculum/.
- Each chapter was carefully reviewed by AACN clinical practice specialists as well as by a nurse in current critical care practice. A clinical pharmacist also reviewed all medications for correct indication and dosages.

The contributors, reviewers, AACN clinical practice specialists, and I have worked tirelessly and made every attempt to provide the most current and relevant knowledge base of information related to progressive and critical care nursing. I welcome your comments about this edition and your suggestions for future editions of the *AACN Core Curriculum*.

Tonja M. Hartjes, DNP, APRN, CNS, CCRN, CNEcl, FAANP
Editor of the *AACN Core Curriculum for Progressive
and Critical Care Nursing*, 8th edition
tonjahartjes@gmail.com

Acknowledgments

This eighth edition of the *AACN Core Curriculum* is possible only because of the tireless dedication and professionalism of many others, whose commitment to this project made all the difference.

First, I would like to thank the devoted readers of the *AACN Core Curriculum*, who provided their time and thoughtful comments over the years regarding the use of the text and suggestions for its evolution as nursing practice has evolved. Improvements in content and design come in large part from their recommendations.

Many thanks to the contributors and reviewers whose enthusiasm, expertise, and experiences have been shared with the readers. Their continued strength and resilience during this especially important time (during the pandemic) is a testament to their commitment to nursing. Development of this resource is made possible through the sustained efforts of each contributor, whose insightful comments created an effective and useful clinical reference and CCRN review.

Sincere thanks and special recognition go to AACN's publishing staff, Michael Muscat and Katie Spiller, and the clinical practice specialists who provided endless time and dedication to me, to the contributors, to critical care nurses, and to the patients and families we serve. Special thanks to Linda Bell, Julie Miller, Mary Stahl, Cindy Cain, and Marian Altman for painstakingly reading through each chapter to offer suggestions.

I also wish to acknowledge those involved directly with the publication process. The Elsevier staff provided considerable administrative support, and their organizational skills and resources were a tremendous asset in the planning, preparation, and execution of this text: Lee Henderson, Laura Selkirk, and Manchu Mohan.

Special thanks to my friend and mentor Suzanne Burns, without whose prior contributions to critical care nursing I would not be in this position. She has served as a role model and mentored me throughout my career and the publishing process.

As always, I thank my family and friends who have been patient with my necessary absences and whose love, support, and encouragement have inspired me throughout this journey.

Contents

PART II   Critical Care of Patients with Issues Affecting Specific Body Systems

Daniel N. Storzer, DNP, ACNPC, ACNP-BC, CNRN, CCRN, CCEMT-P, FCCP, FCCM

Andrea Efre, DNP, ARNP, ANP, FNP and Bryan Boling, DNP, AG-ACNP, CCRN-CSC, CEN

Chapter 5 **Neurologic System** 354

Patricia A. Blissitt, PhD, ARNP-CNS, CCRN, CNRN, SCRN, CCNS, CCM, ACNS-BC

Chapter 6 **Renal System** 490

Bryan Boling, DNP, AG-ACNP, CCRN-CSC, CEN

Chapter 9   **Gastrointestinal System**   631

Patricia Radovich, PhD, CNS, FCCM

PART III   **Critical Care of Patients with Multisystem Issues**

Chapter 10   **Sepsis and Septic Shock**   686

Diane McLaughlin, DNP, AGACNP-BC, CCRN

CHAPTER

1

Professional Caring and Ethical Practice

Anna Dermenchyan, MSN, RN, CCRN-K, CPHQ

CROSSWALK

- **Quality and Safety in Nursing Education (QSEN):** Patient-centered care, Teamwork and collaboration, Evidence-based practice, Quality improvement, Safety, Informatics
- **National Patient Safety Goals:** Identifies patients correctly, Improve staff communication, Use medicines safely, Uses alarms safely, Prevents infection, Identify patient safety risks, Prevents mistakes in surgery
- **American Nurses Association (ANA) standards for Professional Nursing Practice:** Standard 1. Assessment, Standard 2. Diagnosis, Standard 3. Outcomes identification, Standard 4. Planning, Standard 5. Implementation, Standard 6. Evaluation, Standard 7. Ethics, Standard 8. Culturally congruent practice, Standard 9. Communication, Standard 10. Collaboration, Standard 11. Leadership, Standard 12. Education, Standard 13. Evidence-based practice and research, Standard 14. Quality of practice, Standard 15. Professional practice evaluation, Standard 16. Resource utilization, Standard 17. Environmental health
- **AACN Scope and Standards for Progressive and Critical Care Nursing Practice:** Standard 1. Quality of practice, Standard 2. Professional practice evaluation, Standard 3. Education, Standard 4. Communication, Standard 5. Ethics, Standard 6. Collaboration, Standard 7. Evidence-based practice/research/clinical inquiry, Standard 8. Resource utilization, Standard 9. Leadership, Standard 10. Environmental health
- **AACN Standards for Establishing and Sustaining Healthy Work Environments (HWE):** Skilled communication, True collaboration, Effective decision-making, Appropriate staffing, Meaningful recognition, Authentic leadership
- **PCCN content:** Professional Caring and Ethical Practice—All items
- **CCRN content:** Professional Caring and Ethical Practice—All items

AMERICAN ASSOCIATION OF CRITICAL-CARE NURSES MISSION, VISION, AND VALUES (AACN, 2020 a,b,c)

MISSION

1. Patients and their families rely on nurses at the most vulnerable times of their lives. Acute and critical care nurses rely on AACN for expert knowledge and the influence to fulfill their promise to patients and their families. AACN drives excellence because nothing less is acceptable.

VISION

1. AACN is dedicated to creating a healthcare system driven by the needs of patients and families where acute and critical care nurses make their optimal contribution.

VALUES

1. As AACN works to promote its mission and vision, it is guided by values that are rooted in, and arise from, the Association's rich history, traditions, and culture. AACN's members, volunteers, and staff will honor the following:
   a. *Ethical accountability and integrity* in relationships, organizational decisions, and stewardship of resources.
   b. *Leadership to enable individuals to make their optimal contribution* through lifelong learning, critical thinking, and inquiry.
   c. *Excellence and innovation* at every level of the organization to advance the profession.
   d. *Collaboration* to ensure quality patient- and family-focused care.

SYNERGY OF CARING

KEY RESPONSIBILITIES OF REGISTERED NURSES (AMERICAN NURSES ASSOCIATION [ANA], 2020)

1. Perform physical examinations and health histories before making critical decisions.
2. Provide health promotion, counseling, and education.
3. Administer medications and other personalized interventions.
4. Coordinate care, in collaboration with a wide array of healthcare professionals.

WHAT ACUTE AND CRITICAL CARE NURSES DO (AACN, 2019)

1. Restore, support, promote, rehabilitate, or palliate to maintain the physiologic and psychosocial stability of patients of all ages across the life span.
2. Synthesize and prioritize information to take immediate and decisive evidence-based, patient-focused action using clinical judgment and clinical inquiry.
3. Anticipate and respond with confidence, and adapt to rapidly changing patient conditions.
4. Respond to the unique needs of patients and families coping with unanticipated illness or injury and treatment, and advocate for their choices in quality-of-life and end-of-life decisions.
5. Establish and maintain a healthy work environment that is safe, respectful, healing, and caring for nurses, peers, patients, families, and the interprofessional team.
6. Demonstrate the financial contribution of nursing through appropriate resource utilization, cost effectiveness, innovation, and efficiency, resulting in optimal safety and quality outcomes.
7. Demonstrate the contribution of nursing to the quality and financial stability of the facility through stewardship of resources.
8. Promote and maintain care for self and coworkers to foster resilience.
9. Ensure the delivery of safe, compassionate, and high-quality patient care.

THE ENVIRONMENT OF PROGRESSIVE AND CRITICAL CARE NURSES (AACN, 2019)

1. Acutely and critically ill patients require complex assessment and therapies, high-intensity interventions, and continuous vigilance.

2. Progressive care nurses provide direct care or influence care for acutely ill patients who are moderately stable with an elevated risk for instability.
3. Critical care nurses provide direct care or influence care for acutely/critically ill patients who are at high risk for actual or potential life-threatening health problems, regardless of the setting for their nursing care.
4. Progressive and critical care nurses practice in settings where patients require complex assessments and interventions. These settings are not defined by the patient's location in a designated unit, but by the needs of the patient. Nurses lead and participate in collaborative interprofessional teams to create safe, respectful, healing, and caring environments in which:
   a. Patient and family values and preferences are central to the development of informed care decisions made in collaboration with and using the expertise of the interprofessional healthcare team.
   b. Ethical decision-making is supported, fostered, and promoted.
   c. Nurses are valued and committed partners on the interprofessional team in decision-making that impacts patient care, the practice environment, and organizational operations.
   d. Nurses act as advocates on behalf of patients, families, and communities.
   e. Collaboration and collegiality are embraced.
   f. Practice is based on research and best evidence.
   g. Leadership skill development is fostered at all levels.
   h. Professional and organizational leadership encourages and supports effective decision-making, lifelong learning, and professional growth.
   i. Individual talents and resources are optimized.
   j. Innovation, creativity, and clinical inquiry are recognized and valued.
   k. Diversity is recognized, supported, and respected.
   l. Skilled communication is demonstrated on all levels.
   m. A professional practice model drives the delivery of nursing care.
   n. Burnout is recognized; self-care and building resilience are supported.
   o. Nurses are recognized and recognize others for the value each brings to the work of the organization.
   p. The standards of a healthy work environment are implemented to support the health and safety of the interprofessional team.
   q. Zero tolerance is the standard for inappropriate behavior, bullying, or violent behavior.
   r. Appropriate nurse staffing ensures the matching of patient needs and nurse competencies to promote safety and quality outcomes (Barden, 2015).
5. **Patient safety**
   a. The National Academy of Medicine (NAM), formerly the Institute of Medicine (IOM), notes the occurrence of medical errors and adverse medication events increasing at an alarming rate in the United States as it relates to healthcare service delivery processes. NAM has published two landmark reports on patient safety including:
      i. To Err is Human: Building a Safer Health System (2000)
      ii. Crossing the Quality Chasm: A New Health System for the 21st Century External Link Disclaimer (2001).
   b. The Joint Commission (TJC) first established the National Patient Safety Goals in 2005. For 2020, it includes the following goals.*

---

*Visit TJC website for the most current goals: http://www.jointcommission.org

i. Improve the accuracy of patient identification by using at least two patient identifiers when providing care, treatment, and services. This will eliminate transfusion errors related to patient misidentification.

ii. Improve the effectiveness of communication among caregivers by reporting critical results of tests and diagnostic procedures on a timely basis to the right person.

iii. Improve the safety of using medications by labeling all medications, medication containers, and other solutions on and off the sterile field in perioperative and other procedural settings. In addition, reduce the likelihood of patient harm associated with the use of anticoagulant therapy. Maintain and communicate accurate patient medication information.

iv. Reduce the harm associated with clinical alarm systems by improving the safety of clinical alarm systems.

v. Reduce the risk of healthcare-associated infections by complying with either the current Centers for Disease Control and Prevention (CDC) hand hygiene guidelines or the current World Health Organization (WHO) hand hygiene guidelines. In addition, implement evidence-based practices to prevent: (a) healthcare-associated infections because of multidrug-resistant organisms in acute care hospitals, (b) central line–associated bloodstream infections (CLABSI), (c) surgical site infections (SSIs), and (d) indwelling catheter-associated urinary tract infections (CAUTI).

vi. The hospital identifies safety risks inherent in its patient population such as reduce the risk of suicide, conduct a preprocedure verification process, mark the procedure site, and perform a time-out before the procedure.

c. The Institute of Healthcare Improvement (IHI, 2020) focuses on making care continually safer by reducing harm and preventable mortality. IHI's focus on patient safety includes:

i. Galvanizing the safety agenda: Spearhead a multiorganizational initiative to create a national action plan for the prevention of harm in healthcare.

ii. Engaging leadership in change: Provide strategic guidance and innovative thinking to help leaders at all levels embrace, create, and implement tools and strategies that drive change.

iii. Fostering cultures of safety: Provide tactical tools and frameworks to assess safety culture, identify areas for improvement, and implement system-wide changes that affect culture.

iv. Building skills: Offer a range of programs to teach key safety and improvement skills at every level—from students to executives.

d. Agency for Healthcare Research and Quality (AHRQ, 2018) promotes 10 Safety Tips for Hospitals:

i. Prevent central line-associated bloodstream infections.

ii. Reengineer hospital discharges.

iii. Prevent venous thromboembolism.

iv. Educate patients about using blood thinners safely.

v. Limit shift durations for medical residents and other hospital staff if possible.

vi. Consider working with a Patient Safety Organization.

vii. Use good hospital design principles.

viii. Measure your hospital's patient safety culture.

ix. Build better teams and rapid response systems.

x. Insert chest tubes safely.

> **KEY CONCEPT**
> Patient safety is an essential component in the practice of nursing. Registered nurses protect, pro-
> mote, and optimize health and facilitate healing. It is the nurses' professional obligation to raise
> concerns regarding any practices that put patients or themselves at risk of harm. Furthermore, it is the
> responsibility of all members of the interprofessional team to ensure that patients receive safe and
> compassionate care.

THE AACN SYNERGY MODEL FOR PATIENT CARE

1. Synergistic practice and patient and family safety: The AACN Synergy
   Model for Patient Care is a conceptual framework that aligns patient needs with
   nurse competencies in achieving optimal outcomes and nurse satisfaction. The
   model's premise is that the needs of the patient and their family system drive
   the competencies required by the nurse. When this occurs, synergy is produced
   and optimal outcomes can be achieved. The synergy created by practice based on
   the Synergy Model helps the patient-family unit safely navigate the healthcare
   system.
2. The Synergy Model and ethical practice: The Synergy Model provides a
   foundation for addressing ethical concerns related to critical care nursing
   practice. The model focuses on the characteristics of patients, the competencies
   needed by the critical care nurse to meet the patient's needs based on these
   characteristics, and the outcomes that can be achieved through the synergy
   that develops when nursing competencies are driven by the patient's needs.
   AACN is committed to helping members deal with ethical issues through
   education.

AACN SYNERGY MODEL FOR PATIENT CARE (AACN, 2020a,b,c)

ORIGIN OF THE SYNERGY MODEL

1. In 1992 AACN developed a vision of a healthcare system driven by the needs of
   patients and their families in which critical care nurses can make their optimal
   contribution. AACN, in conjunction with the Certification Corporation,
   reconsidered the contributions of certification to the care of patients. Patient needs
   and outcomes must be the central focus of certification. A think tank was convened
   to conceptualize certified practice.

PURPOSE

1. Before the development of the Synergy Model, the certification process
   conceptualized nursing practice according to the dimensions of the nurse's role,
   the clinical setting, and the patient's diagnosis. The Synergy Model conceptualized
   certified practice to recognize that the needs and characteristics of patients and
   families influence and drive the characteristics or competencies of nurses. The
   synergy that develops when this occurs influences the outcomes of individual
   patients, the nurse's practice, and the organization.

OVERVIEW OF THE SYNERGY MODEL

1. Description of the Synergy Model (Fig. 1.1): The synergy that occurs when patient
   and family characteristics or needs drive the competencies that nurses need to
   achieve optimal outcomes for the patient, nurse, and organization.

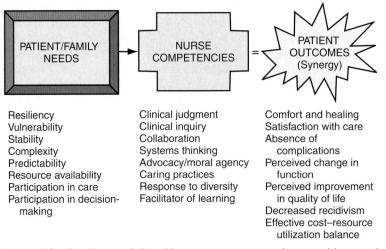

PATIENT/FAMILY NEEDS	NURSE COMPETENCIES	PATIENT OUTCOMES (Synergy)
Resiliency	Clinical judgment	Comfort and healing
Vulnerability	Clinical inquiry	Satisfaction with care
Stability	Collaboration	Absence of
Complexity	Systems thinking	complications
Predictability	Advocacy/moral agency	Perceived change in
Resource availability	Caring practices	function
Participation in care	Response to diversity	Perceived improvement
Participation in decision-making	Facilitator of learning	in quality of life
		Decreased recidivism
		Effective cost–resource utilization balance

Fig. 1.1 Patient and family characteristics drive nurse competencies to achieve optimal (synergistic) outcomes.

2. **Assumptions of the Synergy Model**
   a. All patients are biologic, psychologic, social, and spiritual entities who have similar needs and experiences at a particular developmental stage across wide ranges or continuum from health to illness. The whole patient must be considered.
   b. The dimensions of a nurse's practice as determined by the needs of a patient and family can also be described along a continuum.
   c. The patient, family, and community all contribute to providing a context for the nurse-patient relationship.
   d. Optimal outcomes can be achieved through the synergy resulting in alignment of nurse competencies with patient and family needs. For example, a peaceful death can be an acceptable outcome.
3. **Patient characteristics: The more critically ill the patient, the more likely he or she is to be highly vulnerable, unstable, and complex. Acute and critical care nurses' practice in settings where patients require complex assessment and therapies, high-intensity interventions, and high-level continuous nursing vigilance. Patient characteristics in the acutely and critically ill population can be defined along the continuum described by the Synergy Model (Table 1.1):**
   a. *Resiliency:* The capacity to return to a restorative level of functioning using compensatory coping mechanisms; the ability to bounce back quickly after an insult.
   b. *Vulnerability:* Susceptibility to actual or potential stressors that may adversely affect patient outcomes.
   c. *Stability:* The ability to maintain a steady-state equilibrium.
   d. *Complexity:* The intricate entanglement of two or more systems (e.g., body, family, therapies).
   e. *Resource availability:* The body of resources (e.g., technical, fiscal, personal, psychologic, social) that the patient, family, and community bring to the situation.
   f. *Participation in care:* Extent to which the patient and/or family engages in aspects of care.
   g. *Participation in decision-making processes:* Extent to which the patient and family engages in decision-making.
   h. *Predictability:* A summative characteristic that allows one to expect a certain trajectory of illness.

TABLE 1.1	**The Synergy Model: Patient Characteristics**
Characteristic and Description	**Continuum of Health and Illness**
INTRINSIC CHARACTERISTICS	
Resiliency The capacity to return to a restorative level of functioning using compensatory and coping mechanisms; the ability to bounce back quickly after an insult	Level 1: Minimally resilient • Unable to mount a response • Failure of compensatory/coping mechanisms • Minimal reserves • Brittle Level 3: Moderately resilient • Able to mount a moderate response • Able to initiate some degree of compensation • Moderate reserves Level 5: Highly resilient • Able to mount and maintain a response • Intact compensatory/coping mechanisms • Strong reserves • Endurance
Vulnerability Susceptibility to actual or potential stressors that may adversely affect patient outcomes	Level 1: Highly vulnerable • Susceptible • Unprotected, fragile Level 3: Moderately vulnerable • Somewhat susceptible • Somewhat protected Level 5: Minimally vulnerable • Safe; out of the woods • Protected, not fragile
Stability The ability to maintain a steady-state equilibrium.	Level 1: Minimally stable • Labile; unstable • Unresponsive to therapies • High risk of death Level 3: Moderately stable • Able to maintain steady state for limited period of time • Some responsiveness to therapies Level 5: Highly stable • Constant • Responsive to therapies • Low risk of death
Complexity The intricate entanglement of two or more systems (e.g., body, family, therapies)	Level 1: Highly complex • Intricate • Complex patient/family dynamics • Ambiguous/vague • Atypical presentation Level 3: Moderately complex • Moderately involved patient/family dynamics Level 5: Minimally complex • Straightforward • Routine patient/family dynamics • Simple/clear-cut • Typical presentation

Continued

TABLE 1.1 **The Synergy Model: Patient Characteristics —cont'd**	
Characteristic and Description	**Continuum of Health and Illness**
Predictability A characteristic that allows one to expect a certain course of events or course of illness	Level 1: Not predictable • Uncertain • Uncommon patient population or illness • Unusual or unexpected course • Does not follow critical pathway or no critical pathway developed Level 3: Moderately predictable • Wavering • Occasionally noted patient population or illness Level 5: Highly predictable • Certain • Common patient population or illness • Usual and expected course • Follows critical pathway
EXTRINSIC CHARACTERISTICS	
Resource availability Extent of resources (e.g., technical, fiscal, personal, psychologic, and social) the patient, family, and community bring to the situation	Level 1: Few resources • Necessary knowledge and skills not available • Necessary financial support not available • Minimal personal/psychologic supportive resources • Few social systems resources Level 3: Moderate resources • Limited knowledge and skills available • Limited financial support available • Limited personal/psychologic supportive resources • Limited social systems resources Level 5: Many resources • Extensive knowledge and skills available and accessible • Financial resources readily available • Strong personal/psychologic supportive resources • Strong social systems resources
Participation in care Extent to which patient and/or family engage in aspects of care	Level 1: No participation • Patient and/or family unable or unwilling to participate in care Level 3: Moderate participation • Patient and/or family need assistance in care Level 5: Full participation • Patient and/or family fully able and willing to participate in care
Participation in decision-making Extent to which patient and/or family engages in decision-making	Level 1: No participation • Patient and/or family have no capacity for decision-making; require surrogacy Level 3: Moderate participation • Patient and/or family have limited capacity; seek input/advice from others in decision-making Level 5: Full participation • Patient and/or family have capacity, and make decisions themselves

From American Association of Critical-Care Nurses (AACN), 2020. AACN synergy model for patient care. Retrieved from https://www.aacn.org/nursing-excellence/aacn-standards/synergy-model.

4. **Nurse characteristics: Nursing care is an integration of knowledge, skills, experience, and individual attitudes. The type of nurse characteristics is derived from the patient's needs and range from a competent to expert level (Table 1.2).**

   a. *Clinical judgment:* Clinical reasoning, which includes clinical decision-making, critical thinking, and a global grasp of the situation, coupled with nursing skills acquired through a process of integrating education, experiential knowledge, and evidence-based guidelines.

   b. *Advocacy/moral agency:* Working on another's behalf and representing the concerns of the patient/family and nursing staff; serving as a moral agent in identifying and helping to resolve ethical and clinical concerns within and outside the clinical setting.

TABLE 1.2 **The Synergy Model: Nurse Characteristics**	
Characteristic and Description	**Level of Expertise (Levels 1 to 5 Range From Competent to Expert)**
Clinical judgment Clinical reasoning, which includes clinical decision-making, critical thinking, and a global grasp of the situation coupled with nursing skills acquired through a process of integrating education, experiential knowledge, and evidence-based guidelines	Level 1 • Collects and interprets basic-level data • Follows algorithms, protocols, and pathways with all populations and is uncomfortable deviating from them • Matches formal knowledge and clinical events to make basic care decisions • Questions the limits of one's ability to make clinical decisions and defers the decision-making to other clinicians • Recognizes expected outcomes • Often focuses on extraneous details Level 3 • Collects and interprets complex patient data focusing on key elements of case; able to sort out extraneous detail • Follows algorithms, protocols, and pathways and is comfortable deviating from them with common or routine patient population • Recognizes patterns and trends that may predict the direction of illness • Recognizes limits and uses appropriate help • Reacts to and limits unexpected outcomes Level 5 • Synthesizes and interprets multiple, sometimes conflicting, sources of data • Makes judgments based on an immediate grasp of the "big picture," unless working with new patient populations; uses past experiences to anticipate problems (applies principles from old situations to new situations) • Helps patient and family see the "big picture" • Recognizes the limits of clinical judgment and seeks interprofessional collaboration and consultation with comfort • Recognizes and responds to the dynamic situation (following patient/family lead) • Anticipates unexpected outcomes • Acts on and directs others to act on identified clinical problems • Assists nursing staff in identifying daily goals for patients

Continued

TABLE 1.2   **The Synergy Model: Nurse Characteristics—cont'd**

Characteristic and Description	Level of Expertise (Levels 1 to 5 Range From Competent to Expert)
Advocacy/moral agency Working on another's behalf and representing the concerns of the patient/family and nursing staff; serving as a moral agent in identifying and helping to resolve ethical and clinical concerns within and outside the clinical setting	**Level 1** • Works on behalf of the patient and self Begins to self-assess personal values • Aware of ethical conflicts/issues that may surface in clinical setting • Makes ethical/moral decisions based on rules/guiding principles and on own personal values • Represents patient if consistent with own framework • Aware of patient rights • Acknowledges death as an outcome **Level 3** • Works on behalf of patient and family • Considers patient values and incorporates in care even when differing from personal values • Supports patients, families, and colleagues in ethical and clinical issues; identify internal resources • Moral decision-making can deviate from rules • Demonstrates give and take with patients/family, allowing them to speak/represent themselves when possible • Aware of and acknowledges patient and family rights • Recognizes that death may be an acceptable outcome • Facilitates patient/family comfort in the death and dying process **Level 5** • Works on behalf of patient, family, and community • Advocates from patient/family perspective, whether similar to or different from personal values • Advocates for resolution of ethical conflict and issues from patient, family, or colleague's perspective; uses and participates in internal and external resources • Recognizes rights of patient/family to drive moral decision-making • Empowers the patient and family to speak for/represent themselves • Achieves mutuality within patient/family/professional relationships
Caring practices Nursing activities that create a compassionate, supportive, and therapeutic environment for patients and staff with the aim of promoting comfort and healing and preventing unnecessary suffering. These caring behaviors include but are not limited to vigilance, engagement, and responsiveness. Caregivers include family and healthcare personnel.	**Level 1** • Focuses on basic and routine needs of the patient • Bases care on standards and protocols • Maintains a safe physical environment **Level 3** • Responds to subtle patient and family changes • Engages with the patient to provide individualized care • Uses caring and comfort practices to provide individualized care for patient/family • Optimizes patient/family environment **Level 5** • Has astute awareness and anticipates patient/family changes and needs • Fully engaged with and senses how to stand alongside the patient/family and community • Patient/family needs determine caring practices • Anticipates hazards, and promotes safety, care, and comfort throughout transitions along the healthcare continuum

TABLE 1.2   The Synergy Model: Nurse Characteristics—cont'd

Characteristic and Description	Level of Expertise (Levels 1 to 5 Range From Competent to Expert)
	• Initiates the establishment of an environment that promotes caring • Provides patient/family the skills to navigate transitions along the healthcare continuum (e.g., facilitates safe passage)
Collaboration Working with others (e.g., patients, families, healthcare providers) in a way that promotes each person's contributions toward achieving optimal and realistic patient/family goals. Collaboration involves interprofessional work with colleagues and community.	**Level 1** • Willing to be taught, coached, and/or mentored • Participates in team meetings and discussions regarding patient care and/or practice issues • Open to various team members' contributions **Level 3** • Willing to be taught/mentored • Participates in precepting and teaching • Initiates and participates in team meetings and discussions regarding patient care and/or practice issues • Recognizes and critiques interprofessional participation in care decisions **Level 5** • Seeks opportunities to role model, teach, mentor, and to be mentored • Facilitates active involvement and contributions of others in team meetings and discussions regarding patient care and/or practice issues • Involves/recruits interprofessional resources to optimize patient outcomes • Role models, teaches, and/or mentors professional leadership and accountability for nursing's role within the healthcare team and community
Systems thinking Body of knowledge and tools that allow the nurse to manage whatever environmental and system resources exist for the patient/family and staff, within or across healthcare and nonhealthcare systems.	**Level 1** • Uses previously learned strategies or standardized processes • Identifies problems but unclear of healthcare systems to resolve problems • Sees patient and family within the isolated environment of the unit • Sees self as key resource for patient/family • Applies personal experiences to identify patient/family needs **Level 3** • Develops processes/strategies based on needs and strengths of patient/family • Able to make connections within pieces or components of the healthcare system • Sees and begins to use negotiation as a tool for practice-based decisions • Recognizes and reacts to needs of patient/family as they move through healthcare systems • Recognizes how to obtain and use resources within the healthcare system **Level 5** • Develops, integrates, and applies a variety of strategies that are driven by the needs and strengths of the patient/family • Recognizes global or holistic interrelationships that exist within and across both healthcare and nonhealthcare systems • Knows when and how to negotiate and navigate through the system on behalf of patients and families

Continued

TABLE 1.2 The Synergy Model: Nurse Characteristics—cont'd

Characteristic and Description	Level of Expertise (Levels 1 to 5 Range From Competent to Expert)
	• Develops core plans based on anticipated needs of patients/families • Uses a variety of resources as necessary to optimize patient/family outcomes
Response to diversity The sensitivity to recognize, appreciate, and incorporate differences into the provision of care. Differences may include, but are not limited to, cultural, spiritual, gender, race, ethnicity, lifestyle, socioeconomic, age, and values.	Level 1 • Assesses diversity and acknowledges differences but uses standardized plans of care • Provides care based on own belief system • Practices within the culture of the healthcare environment • Recognizes barriers • Recognizes practices based upon diversity that have potential negative outcomes Level 3 • Inquiries about cultural differences and considers their effect on care • Accommodates personal and professional differences in plans of care • Helps patient/family understand the culture of the healthcare system • Recognizes barriers and seeks strategies for resolution • Identifies and uses resources that promote and support diversity Level 5 • Anticipates needs of patient/family based on identified diversities and develops plans accordingly • Acknowledges and incorporates differences • Adapts healthcare culture, to the extent possible, to meet the diverse needs and strengths of the patient/family • Anticipates and intervenes to reduce/eliminate barriers • Incorporates patient/family values with evidence-based practice for optimal outcomes
Clinical inquiry The ongoing process of questioning and evaluating practice and providing informed practice; creating changes through evidence-based practice, research utilization, and experiential knowledge.	Level 1 • Follows policies, procedures, standards, and guidelines without deviation • Uses research-based practices as directed by others • Recognizes the need for further learning to improve patient care • Recognizes obvious changing patient situation (e.g., deterioration, crisis) and seeks assistance to identify patient problems and solutions • Participates in data collection (e.g., research, quality improvement, evidence-based practice) Level 3 • Uses policies, procedures, standards, and guidelines, adapting to patient needs • Applies research findings when not in conflict with current clinical practice • Accepts advice or information to improve patient care • Recognizes subtle changes in patient condition and begins to compare and contrast possible care alternatives • Participates on team (e.g., CQI, survey, research) Level 5 • Improves, modifies, or individualizes policies, procedures, standards, and guidelines for particular patient situations or populations based on experiential or published data

TABLE 1.2 **The Synergy Model: Nurse Characteristics—cont'd**	
Characteristic and Description	**Level of Expertise (Levels 1 to 5 Range From Competent to Expert)**
	• Questions and/or evaluates current practice based on patient/family's responses, review of the literature, research, and education/learning
• Seeks to validate whether research answers clinical questions
• Embraces lifelong learning and acquires knowledge and skills needed to address questions arising in practice to improve patient care
• Evaluates outcomes of studies and implements changes (converging of clinical inquiring and clinical judgment allows for anticipation of patient needs)
Facilitator of learning

The ability to facilitate learning for patients and families, nursing staff, other members of the healthcare team, and community; includes both formal and informal facilitation of learning. | Level 1
• Follows planned educational programs using standardized educational materials
• Sees patient/family education as a separate task from delivery of care
• Provides information without seeking to assess learner's readiness or understanding
• Has basic knowledge and/or understanding of the patient/family's educational needs
• Focuses educational plan on nurse-identified patient/family needs
• Sees the patient/family as a passive recipient

Level 3
• Adapts planned educational programs to meet individual patient's needs
• Begins to recognize and integrate different ways of implementing education into delivery of care
• Assesses patient's/family's readiness to learn, develops education plan based on identified needs, and evaluates learner understanding
• Recognizes the benefits of educational plans from different healthcare providers' perspectives
• Sees the patient/family as having input into educational goals
• Incorporates patient's/family's perspective into individualized education plan

Level 5
• Creatively modifies or develops patient/family education programs
• Integrates patient/family education throughout delivery of care
• Evaluates patient/family readiness to learn and provides comprehensive individualized education evaluating behavior changes related to learning, adjusting to meet the educational goal
• Collaborates and incorporates all healthcare providers' ideas into ongoing educational plans for the patient/family
• Sees patient/family as having choices and consequences that are negotiated in relation to education |

From American Association of Critical-Care Nurses (AACN), 2020. AACN synergy model for patient care. Retrieved from https://www.aacn.org/nursing-excellence/aacn-standards/synergy-model.

    c. *Caring practices:* Nursing activities that create a compassionate, supportive, and therapeutic environment for patients and staff with the aim of promoting comfort and healing and preventing unnecessary suffering. These caring behaviors include but are not limited to vigilance, engagement, and responsiveness. Caregivers include family and healthcare personnel.

    d. *Collaboration:* Working with others (e.g., patients and families, healthcare providers) in a way that promotes each person's contributions toward achieving optimal and realistic patient and family goals. Collaboration involves interprofessional work with colleagues and community.

    e. *Systems thinking:* The body of knowledge and tools that allow the nurse to manage whatever environmental and system resources exist for the patient, family, and staff within or across healthcare and nonhealthcare systems.

    f. *Response to diversity:* The sensitivity to recognize, appreciate, and incorporate differences into the provision of care. Differences may include, but are not limited to, cultural, spiritual, gender, race, ethnicity, lifestyle, socioeconomic, age, and values.

    g. *Clinical inquiry or innovation and evaluation:* The ongoing process of questioning and evaluating practice and providing informed practice; creating changes through evidence-based practice, research utilization, and experiential knowledge (Melnyk et al., 2014).

    h. *Facilitator of learning:* The ability to facilitate learning for patients and families, nursing staff, other members of the healthcare team, and community; includes both formal and informal facilitation of learning.

5. **Outcomes of patient-nurse synergy (Fig. 1.2)**

    a. Patient-derived outcomes

       i. Behavior change: Based on the dispensing and receiving of information. Requires caregiver trust. Patients and families grow in their knowledge about health and take greater responsibility for their own health.

      ii. Functional change and quality of life: Interprofessional measures that can be used across all populations of patients but provide specific information to a population of patients when analyzed separately.

     iii. Satisfaction ratings: Subjective measures of individual health and quality of health services. Satisfaction measures query about expectations (technical care provided, trusting relationships, and education experiences) and the extent to which they are met. Often linked with functional change and quality-of-life perceptions.

     iv. Comfort ratings and perceptions: Quality-of-care outcomes based on caring practices with the aim of promoting comfort and alleviating suffering.

    b. Nurse-derived outcomes

       i. Physiologic changes: Require monitoring and managing instantaneous therapies and noting changes. The nurse expects a specific trajectory of changes when he or she "knows" the patient.

      ii. The presence or absence of preventable complications: Through vigilance and clinical judgment, the nurse creates a safe and healing environment.

     iii. Extent to which care and treatment objectives were attained: Reflects the nurse's role as an integrator of care that requires a high degree of collaboration.

    c. System-derived outcomes

       i. Recidivism: Decrease in readmission, which adds to the personal and financial burden of care.

      ii. Cost and resource utilization: Organizations usually evaluate financial cost based on an episode of care. Achieving cost-effective care requires knowing the patient and providing continuity of care. Resource utilization can affect patient

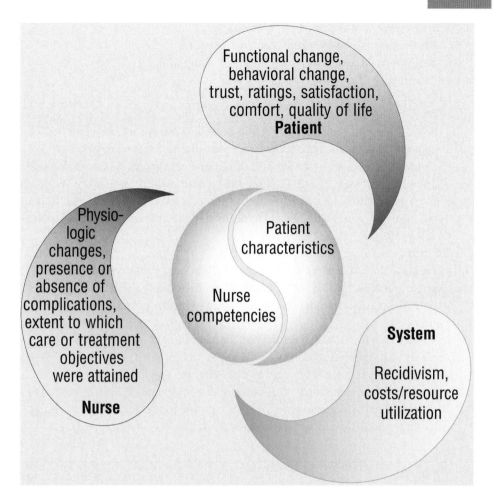

Fig. 1.2 Three levels of outcomes delineated by the AACN Synergy Model for Patient Care: Those derived from the patient, those derived from the nurse, and those derived from the healthcare system. (Reprinted from Curley, M. (1998). Patient-nurse synergy: optimizing patients' outcomes. *American Journal of Critical Care*, 7, 69. © American Association of Critical-Care Nurses. All rights reserved. Figure adapted with permission.)

outcomes when there is not enough care given by competent nurses. When nurses cannot provide care at an appropriate level to meet patient needs, they are dissatisfied and turnover is high, which results in increased costs for the organization (Ulrich et al., 2019).

APPLICATION OF THE SYNERGY MODEL

1. **The Synergy Model is the keystone of AACN certifications. It is also used as a professional practice model, a foundation for nursing school curricula and a model for professional advancement. There are many applications for the model in clinical operations, clinical practice, education, and research:***
   a. Clinical operations
      i. Leadership: Using the model for organizational infrastructure for achieving excellence in practice, improving financial outcomes, and establishing clinical advancement programs.

---

*Refer to the AACN website for up-to-date application of the Synergy Model for Patient Care: https://www.aacn.org/nursing-excellence/aacn-standards/synergy-model.

      ii. Development of continuity-of-care models.

      iii. Foundation model for family-centered care practice.

      iv. Basis for making care assignments and making nursing rounds.

  b. Clinical practice

      i. Development of clinical strategies.

      ii. Direct patient care.

      iii. AACN is developing an approach to nursing competence based on the Synergy Model. The core focus is the introduction of Synergy Nurse Competencies as an essential part of nursing competence, both at the level of entry to practice on a nursing unit and in continuing competence. The eight nurse characteristics described in the preceding section are adapted to define the knowledge and skill the nurse needs to demonstrate in practice, applicable across all.

  c. Education

      i. Basis for critical care registered nurse (CCRN) and acute/critical care clinical nurse specialist (CCNS) certification examinations since 1999.

      ii. Potential use as a foundation for education of healthcare teams.

  d. Research

      i. Validated in the AACN Certification Corporation Study of Practice.

      ii. Underwent theoretical review.

      iii. Further research needed related to consumer perspective, staffing and productivity implications for nursing, patient outcomes measurement, and development of a quantitative tool based on the model for rapidly assessing patients and determining nursing characteristics.

KEY CONCEPT

AACN Synergy Model for Patient Care accounts for the needs and characteristics of patients and families, which then drive the characteristics or competencies of nurses. Synergy results when the needs and characteristics of a patient, clinical unit, or system are matched with a nurse's competencies.

FAMILY PRESENCE: VISITATION IN THE ADULT ICU (AACN PRACTICE ALERT, 2016)

1. Evidence shows that the unrestricted presence and participation of a support person (e.g., family as defined by the patient) can improve the safety of care and enhance patient and family satisfaction. This is especially true in the intensive care unit (ICU), where the patients are usually intubated and cannot speak for themselves.

2. Family presence can improve communication, facilitate a better understanding of the patient, advance patient- and family-centered care, and enhance staff satisfaction.

3. Families and other partners are welcomed 24 hours a day according to the patient's preference.

EXPERT TIP

The use of the AACN Practice Alert can direct nurses to the evidence of Family Visitation in the Adult ICU.

HEALTHY WORK ENVIRONMENT STANDARDS (AACN, 2016)

1. AACN believes that all workplaces can be healthy if nurses and employers are resolute in their desire to address not only the physical environment but also less tangible barriers to staff and patient safety. The ingredients for success are described in the AACN Standards for Establishing and Sustaining Healthy Work Environments:
   a. Skilled communication: Nurses must be as proficient in communication skills as they are in clinical skills.
   b. True collaboration: Nurses must be relentless in pursuing and fostering true collaboration.
   c. Effective decision-making: Nurses must be valued and committed partners in making policy, directing and evaluating clinical care, and leading organizational operations.
   d. Appropriate staffing: Staffing must ensure the effective match between patient needs and nurse competencies.
   e. Meaningful recognition: Nurses must be recognized and must recognize others for the value each brings to the work of the organization.
   f. Authentic leadership: Nurse leaders must fully embrace the imperative of a healthy work environment, authentically live it, and engage others in its achievement.

> **EXPERT TIP**
> A web-based Healthy Work Environment Assessment Tool is available to collectively measure your work environment's current health. Learn more at https://www.aacn.org/nursing-excellence/healthy-work-environments.

GENERAL LEGAL CONSIDERATIONS RELEVANT TO CRITICAL CARE NURSING PRACTICE

NATIONAL GOVERNING BODIES

1. TJC accredits more than 22,000 healthcare organizations and programs in the United States. A majority of state governments recognize TJC accreditation as a condition of licensure and the receipt of Medicare and Medicaid programs (https://www.jointcommission.org).
2. National Council of State Boards of Nursing (NCSBN) is a not-for-profit membership organization comprised of the State Boards of Nursing. It collaborates with the state boards on matters of common interest and concern affecting public health, safety, and welfare including the development of nursing licensure examinations (https://www.ncsbn.org/index.htm).
3. The American Nurses Credentialing Center (ANCC) gives Magnet accreditation to hospitals that demonstrate nursing excellence (https://www.nursingworld.org/ancc/).

STATE NURSE PRACTICE ACTS (Russell, 2017)

1. Purpose: To protect the public.
2. Statutory laws: Written by the individual states.
3. Usual authorization: Board of nursing to oversee nursing (by use of regulations or administrative law).
4. Content: Define scope of practice for nurses.

SCOPE OF PRACTICE

1. **Provides guidance for acceptable nursing roles and practices, which vary from state to state.**
   a. Nurses are expected to follow the nurse practice act and not deviate from usual nursing activities.
   b. Advanced nursing practice: Expanded roles for nurses include nurse practitioner, clinical nurse specialist, certified registered nurse anesthetist, and certified nurse-midwife. These roles require education beyond the basic nurse education and usually involve a master's degree. Certain responsibilities associated with these roles are not interchangeable (ANA, 2020).
   c. Based on the Synergy Model, a scope and standards for acute care nurse practitioner practice (2017) and acute care clinical nurse specialist practice (2014) was published by AACN.

STANDARDS OF CARE

1. **A standard of care is any established measure of extent, quality, quantity, or value; an agreed-upon level of performance or a degree of excellence of care that is established.**
2. **Standards are established by usual and customary practice, institutional guidelines, association guidelines, and legal precedent.**
3. **Standards of care, standards of practice, policies, procedures, and performance criteria all establish an agreed-upon level of performance or degree of excellence.**
   a. ANA standards: The ANA has generic standards and also specialty standards (e.g., for medical-surgical nursing).
   b. AACN scope and standards for acute and critical care nursing practice.
   c. AACN scope and standards for acute care clinical nurse specialist practice.
   d. AACN scope and standards for acute care nurse practitioner practice.
4. **National facility standards: Include those published by TJC and the National Committee for Quality Assurance (NCQA).***
5. **Community and regional standards: Standards prevalent in certain areas of the country or in specific communities.**
6. **Hospital and medical center standards: Standards developed by institutions for their staff and patients.**
7. **Unit practice standards, policies, and protocols: Specific standards of care for specific groups or types of patients or specific procedures (e.g., insulin or massive blood transfusion protocols).**
8. **Precedent court cases: Standard of a "reasonable prudent nurse" (e.g., what a reasonable prudent nurse would have done in the given situation).**
9. **Other nursing and interprofessional specialty organization standards: The American Heart Association, the Society of Critical Care Medicine, and the Association of periOperative Registered Nurses.**

KEY CONCEPT

Nurses provide care in a variety of healthcare settings. All nurses have the right to practice in work environments that support and allow them to act in accordance with professional and legal standards (ANA, 2020).

---

*NCQA website contains the various standards the committee endorses and/or publishes: http://www.ncqa.org

CERTIFICATION IN A SPECIALTY AREA

1. Certification is a process by which a nongovernmental agency, using predetermined standards, validates an individual nurse's qualification and knowledge for practice in a defined functional or clinical area of nursing.
2. A common goal of specialty certification programs is to promote consumer protection and to promote high standards of practice.
3. The certified nurse may be held to a higher standard of practice in the specialty than the noncertified nurse; certification validates the nurse's knowledge in a specialty area.
4. Critical care certifications are awarded by AACN Certification Corporation, established in 1975. AACN Certification Corporation is accredited by the National Commission for Certifying Agencies, the accreditation arm of the National Organization for Competency Assurance.
   a. The AACN Certification Corporation develops and administers the CCRN, CCRN-E, CCRN-K, PCCN, ACNPC, ACNPC-AG, CCNS, ACCNS-AG, ACCNS-P, and ACCNS-N specialty examinations, and the CMC and CSC subspecialty examinations.
   b. CCRN certification: Separate certification processes for critical care nurses practicing with neonatal, pediatric, or adult populations.
   c. CCNS certification: Advanced practice certification of nurses in acute care clinical nurse specialist practice. Separate certification processes for CNSs practicing with neonatal, pediatric, or adult populations.
   d. ACNPC and ACNP-AG certification: Advanced practice certification of acute care nurse practitioners. Separate certification processes for ACNPs practicing with adult and adult-geriatric populations.
5. Certification provides patients and families with validation that the nurses caring for them have demonstrated knowledge that exceeds that which is assessed in entry-level licensure examinations (AACN Certification Corporation, 2020a,b,c).
   a. Certification has been linked to patient safety.
   b. Units with higher numbers of certified nurses reported lower frequency of falls or pressure ulcer development.
   c. Certification has also been linked to patient satisfaction, from both patients' reports and nurses' perceptions.

PROFESSIONAL LIABILITY

1. Professional negligence: An unintentional act or omission. It is the failure to do what the reasonable prudent nurse would do under similar circumstances, or an act or failure to act that leads to an injury of another. Six specific elements are necessary for professional negligence action and must be established by a person bringing a suit against a nurse (plaintiff):
   a. Duty: To protect the patient from an unreasonable risk of harm.
   b. Breach of duty: Failure by a nurse to do what a reasonable prudent nurse would do under the same or similar circumstances. The breach of duty is a failure to perform within the given standard of care. The standard defines the nurse's duty to the patient.
   c. Proximate cause: Proof that the harm caused was foreseeable and that the person injured was foreseeably a victim. This element can determine the extent of damages for which a nurse may be held liable.
   d. Injury: The harm done.
   e. Direct cause of injury: Proof that the nurse's conduct was the cause of or contributed to the injury to the patient.
   f. Damages: Proof of actual loss, damage, pain, or suffering caused by the nurse's conduct.

2. **Malpractice: Specific type of negligence that takes account of the status of the caregiver as well as the standard of care. Professional negligence is malpractice. It is differentiated from ordinary negligence (e.g., failure to clean up water from the floor).**
   a. Professional misconduct, improper discharge of professional duties, or a failure by a professional to meet the standard of care that results in harm to another person.
   b. Malpractice is the failure of a professional person to act in accordance with prevailing professional standards or a failure to foresee consequences that a professional person who has the necessary skills and education would foresee.
   c. Most common types of malpractice or negligence in critical care settings include medication errors, failure to prevent patient falls, failure to assess changes in clinical status, and failure to notify the primary provider of changes in patient status.

3. **Delegation and supervision**
   a. Definitions (National Council of State Boards of Nursing, 2020):
      i. Delegation: Transferring to a competent individual the authority to perform a selected nursing task in a selected situation. The nurse retains accountability for the delegation.
      ii. Accountability: Being responsible and answerable for actions or inactions of self or others in the context of delegation.
      iii. Authority: Deemed present when a registered nurse (RN) has been given the right to delegate based on the state nurse practice act and also has the official power from an agency to delegate.
      iv. Unlicensed assistive personnel (UAP): Any unlicensed personnel, regardless of title, to whom nursing tasks are delegated.
      v. Delegator: The person making the delegation.
      vi. Delegatee: The person receiving the delegation.
      vii. Competent: Demonstrating the knowledge and skill, through education and experience, to perform the delegated task.
   b. The five "rights" of delegation
      i. Right task: The RN ensures that the task to be delegated is appropriate to be delegated for that specific patient. Example: Delegating suctioning of a tracheostomy in a stable patient to a licensed practical nurse is appropriate. If the patient is a head injury patient who becomes bradycardic and hypotensive during suctioning, then delegation of this task for this patient may not be appropriate.
      ii. Right circumstances: The RN ensures that the setting is appropriate and that resources are available for successful completion of the delegated task.
      iii. Right person: The RN delegates the right task to the right person to be performed on the right patient.
      iv. Right direction and communication: The delegating nurse provides a clear explanation of the task and expected outcomes. The RN sets limits and expectations for performance of the task.
      v. Right supervision: The RN does appropriate monitoring and evaluation, and intervenes as needed. The RN provides feedback to the delegatee and establishes parameters for receiving feedback about the outcome of the task.
   c. Model of the delegation decision-making process: The nurse must ensure that delegation of nursing tasks is based on appropriate assessment, planning, implementation, and evaluation.
   d. Nurse executives must ensure the following:
      i. Policies and procedures concerning supervision and delegation are in place and are consistent with state nurse practice acts.

      ii. Job descriptions for UAPs do not include responsibilities for whose performance a license is required.

      iii. Adequate training and consistent orientation for UAPs are provided.

      iv. A mechanism for regular evaluation of UAPs is in place.

  e. In the complex critical care environment, many of the concepts for delegation to UAPs can also be applied to delegation of care to other professional nurses and licensed practical or vocational nurses (through assignments made by charge nurses or nurse managers).

      i. The job descriptions and scope of practice for personnel with various levels of expertise and for various roles must be clearly defined.

      ii. When assignments are made, the patient's characteristics (as defined by the Synergy Model) and required care procedures guide the decision regarding the competency level of the nurse who should provide the care.

      iii. Nurse executives and nurse managers must ensure that nurses have demonstrated and documented levels of expertise necessary to provide the care required by specific patients.

      iv. Additional training and experience are required for performance of many of the complex therapies needed by vulnerable critically ill patients.

4. Adequate staffing

  a. Staffing is a process and an outcome. The term can refer to the process by which human resources are used within a nursing care unit or to the number of staff members required to provide care. The individuals managing healthcare services have ethical responsibilities to ensure that policies and processes are in place to ensure the safety of the patients and the staff (Box 1.1).

  b. The optimal use of RN time and expertise depends on a number of variables: allocating acute and critical care beds based on patient need; ensuring availability of adequate numbers of qualified competent nursing and support staff; establishing sufficient support systems; following and adhering to legal and regulatory requirements; and evaluating services through outcome and quality measures.

  c. Patient- and family-focused care requires matching the right caregiver to each patient, identifying systems that provide the right support in delivering care, incorporating legal and regulatory considerations, and measuring the outcomes of care.

  d. ANA (2015a) recommendations for staffing policy include the following:

      i. Optimal staffing is essential for providing professional nursing value. Greater benefit can be derived from staffing models that consider the number of nurses and/or the nurse-to-patient ratios and can be adjusted to account for unit and shift level factors.

BOX 1.1   Ethical Responsibilities of Healthcare Delivery Managers

In order of priority, the following are the ethical responsibilities of those managing health service delivery systems:
1. Ensuring the safety of the services delivered.
2. Ensuring a safe environment for those receiving and those delivering the healthcare services.
3. Ensuring the responsible use, care, and distribution of the materials needed for safe delivery of services.
4. Carefully developing and implementing a budget.
5. Developing responsible institutional policies.
6. Intelligently interpreting and implementing institutional policies.
7. Knowing and adhering to all applicable laws governing practice and personnel management.

Modified from American Nurses Association, 2015b. Code of ethics for nurses with interpretive statements. Retrieved from http://www.nursingworld.org/codeofethics.

ii. Factors that influence nurse staffing needs include: patient complexity, acuity, or stability; number of admissions, discharges, and transfers; professional nursing and other staff skill level and expertise; physical space and layout of the nursing unit; and availability of or proximity to technologic support or other resources.

iii. Appropriate nurse staffing decreases medical and medication errors, patient mortality, hospital readmission, and hospital length of stay (Aiken et al., 2018).

DOCUMENTATION

1. **Mandates of regulatory agencies**
   a. Federal requirements: Related to narcotics, controlled substances, organ transplantation.
   b. National voluntary requirements: TJC requirements related to quality improvement activities.
   c. State requirements: May exist in specific situations (e.g., in relation to minors).
   d. Community (regional or local) standards: May include enhanced documentation in specific areas of practice (e.g., epidural medication).
   e. Hospital, medical center, or health maintenance organization requirements.
2. **Purposes of nursing care documentation in the patient record**
   a. To provide clear and concise communication between providers.
   b. To facilitate planning and evaluation of care, and demonstrate use of the nursing process.
   c. To show progress of patient treatment, changes in condition, and continuity of care and to record patient status, appearance, and behavior.
   d. To protect the patient; the medical record may be used in litigation.
   e. To protect healthcare professionals and institutions and reduce risk for possible litigation.
3. **Documentation requirements**
   a. General requirements regarding patient records
      i. Contain accurate and factual observations.
      ii. Include times, dates, and signatures for notations and events entered.
      iii. Reflect patient status and unusual events.
      iv. Reflect documentation of the nursing process on a continuing basis throughout the hospitalization.
      v. Note omissions of care and rationale.
      vi. Show that the provider was informed of unusual or adverse situations and record the nature of the provider's response.
      vii. Note deviations from standard hospital practice and the rationale for such deviations.
      viii. Should be legible.
      ix. Carefully document method of the patient's admission, condition on admission, discharge planning, and condition on discharge.
   b. Specific regulatory requirements mandated by regulatory agencies.
      i. Patient's name, address, date of birth, and name of any legally authorized representative.
      ii. Legal status of patient receiving mental health services.
      iii. Emergency care, if any, provided to the patient before arrival.
      iv. Findings of the patient assessment including assessment of pain status, learning needs and barriers to learning, and cultural or religious needs that may affect care.

v. Conclusions or impressions drawn from the medical history and physical examination.

vi. Diagnosis or diagnostic impression.

vii. Reasons for admission or treatment.

viii. Goals of treatment and the treatment plan; evidence of interprofessional plan of care.

ix. Evidence of known advance directives or documentation that information about advance directives was offered.

x. Evidence of informed consent when required by hospital policy.

xi. Diagnostic and therapeutic orders, if any.

xii. Records of all diagnostic and therapeutic procedures and all test results.

xiii. Records of all operative and other invasive procedures performed with acceptable disease and operative terminology that includes etiology, as appropriate.

xiv. Progress notes made by the medical staff and other authorized persons.

xv. All reassessments and any revisions of the treatment plan.

xvi. Clinical observations and reports of patient's response to care.

xvii. Evidence of patient education.

xviii. Consultation reports.

xix. Records of every medication ordered or prescribed for an inpatient.

xx. Records of every medication dispensed to an ambulatory patient or an inpatient on discharge.

xxi. Records of every dose of medication administered and any adverse medication reaction.

xxii. All relevant diagnoses established during the course of care.

xxiii. Any referrals and communications made to external or internal care providers and to community agencies.

xxiv. Conclusions at termination of hospitalization.

xxv. Discharge instructions to the patient and family.

xxvi. Clinical discharge summaries or a final progress note or transfer summary. Discharge summary contains reason for hospitalization, significant findings, procedures performed, and treatment rendered, patient's condition at discharge, and instructions to the patient and family, if any, including pain management plan.

c. An Electronic Health Record (EHR) is an electronic version of a patient's medical history maintained by the provider and the health system over time. The EHR automates access to information and has the potential to streamline the clinician's workflow (Centers for Medicare and Medicaid Services [CMS], 2012a). The EHR can improve patient care by:

i. Reducing the incidence of medical error by improving the accuracy and clarity of medical records.

ii. Making the health information available, reducing duplication of tests, reducing delays in treatment, and patients well informed to make better decisions.

d. CMS has an incentive program for hospitals to achieve meaningful use in certified EHR for the following reasons:

i. Improve quality, safety, efficiency, and reduce health disparities.

ii. Engage patients and family.

iii. Improve care coordination and population and public health.

iv. Maintain privacy and security of patient health information.

GOOD SAMARITAN LAWS

1. Various states have enacted laws to allow healthcare personnel and citizens trained in first aid to deliver needed emergency care without fear of incurring criminal and civil liability (CMS, 2012b).
2. Laws vary among states: Nurses should be familiar with the relevant state law. Look for these elements when evaluating the state's law:
   a. Who is covered under the law?
   b. Where does the coverage extend?
   c. What is covered?
3. Most laws require that care be given in good faith and that it be gratuitous.
4. There is no legal duty to render care to strangers in distress.

ETHICAL CLINICAL PRACTICE

FOUNDATION OF ETHICAL NURSING PRACTICE

1. **ANA Code of Ethics (ANA, 2015b)**
   a. The foundation of ethical practice for nursing is the ANA Code of Ethics. The ANA code is a statement of the ethical obligations and duties of every nurse, a nonnegotiable ethical standard for the profession, and an expression of the nursing profession's commitment to society.
   b. The Code, consisting of nine provisions and the accompanying interpretive statements, provides a succinct statement of the ethical values, obligations, and duties of every individual who enters the nursing profession. It also serves as the profession's nonnegotiable ethical standard and expresses nursing's own understanding of its commitment to society.

> **KEY CONCEPT**
> The primary commitment of professional registered nurses is to the patient, family, and community.

EMERGENCE OF CLINICAL ETHICS

1. **Definition of clinical ethics:** The systematic identification, analysis, and resolution of ethical issues in clinical medicine associated with the care of particular patients.
2. **Goals**
   a. Promote patient-centered decision-making that honors the rights and interests of the patient (see American Nurses Association, Code of Ethics for Nurses with Interpretive Statements at www.nursingworld.org/codeofethics).
   b. Facilitate the involvement of all clinicians (e.g., providers, nurses, social workers, and other healthcare professionals) who require assistance in this complex field.
   c. Promote organizational commitment, as well as cooperation among all involved parties to implement plans on behalf of the patient.
3. **Religion and clinical ethics**
   a. "Clinical ethics" now refers to secular bioethics.
   b. Bioethics is the application of ethics to the field of medicine and healthcare. Ethicists and bioethicists ask relevant questions more than provide sure and certain answers.
   c. Religious leaders continue to play a role in the deliberation of moral and ethical dilemmas and often provide wisdom to the secular community.
   d. Religious convictions of competent adults should be honored and respected. This can be difficult for healthcare providers when it involves decision making by parents for dependent children.

e. Spiritual values (apart from religious beliefs) may affect health. Healthcare providers should be sensitive to the spirituality of their patients.

4. **Cultural competence and clinical ethics: Cultural competence is the ability to identify the effects of a patient's culture on the health of the patient. The healthcare provider should use a framework of ethical decision-making that factors in the patient's culture while avoiding cultural stereotyping.**

5. **Organizational ethics and clinical ethics: Articulating, evaluating, and applying consistently the values of an organization that are defined internally and externally. The mission of the organization should be consistent with the expectations of the employees. The healthcare provider's ethical obligations supersede any organization's processes or requirements.**

6. **Ethics across the life span:**

   a. Before pregnancy: Carrier screening for genetic disorders; testing for human immunodeficiency virus; in vitro fertilization and related technologies; potential for human cloning; stem cell research; and surrogacy.

   b. During pregnancy: Manipulation of embryos; substance abuse during pregnancy; abortion; prenatal genetic diagnosis; implications of multiple births because of reproductive technologies.

   c. Infants: Treatment of infants born with severe impairments.

   d. Children and adolescents: Role in decision-making.

   e. Older adult: Issues related to truth telling and confidentiality have shifted for this generation; planning with patient for potential lapses in decision-making; emphasis on advance directives for this age group; end-of-life care issues.

   f. Caring for the family: Although the rights of the individual patient are still presumed to outweigh those of the family, this is being challenged in many situations and often leads to significant ethical conflicts. Conflicts center on autonomy and confidentiality. A philosophy of family-centered care has the potential to prevent such conflicts or reduce their effects on the care provided patients.

   g. In the context of family-centered care, it is essential to ensure that providers and nurses act responsibly in maintaining a patient's best interests by using knowledge of underlying ethical principles, understanding professional duties, and adopting processes for mediation and conflict resolution.

STANDARD ETHICAL THEORY

1. **Deontology**

   a. Duty-based ethics; healthcare providers have special duties of care to their patients.

   b. Associated with German philosopher Immanuel Kant.

2. **Utilitarianism**

   a. Belief that actions are morally evaluated based on the extent to which they facilitate or promote happiness or well-being; healthcare providers' actions often based on achieving a desired outcome or preoccupation with consequences of an intervention.

   b. Associated with English philosophers John Locke and John Stuart Mill.

ETHICAL PRINCIPLES (ANA, 2015b)

1. **Patient autonomy and self-determination**

   a. Principle that a competent adult patient has the right to make his or her own healthcare decisions.

   b. Autonomy refers to the potential to be self-determining; clinically supported through the informed consent process, which facilitates decision-making that is individualized based on the patient's own values.

c. *Paternalism* is the term used when healthcare providers make the decisions for the patient based on the rationale that it is in the patient's best interest. This practice denies the patient the autonomy to make his or her own decisions.

2. **Beneficence**
   a. Principle that the competent patient or appropriate surrogate is the best judge of the patient's best interests.
   b. Source of common ethical conflicts when there are disagreements between provider and patient or surrogate. Conflict may arise between the provider's perceived obligation to do good and obligation to respect the patient's expressed wishes.

3. **Nonmaleficence**
   a. Principle to "do no harm."
   b. Often considered same principle as beneficence.

4. **Justice**
   a. Principle that everyone fundamentally deserves equal respect.
   b. Point of reference for social policy related to access to healthcare.
   c. Distributive justice in health care usually involves how resources are allocated (e.g., scarcity of organs for donation, availability of ICU beds or healthcare staff, futility of care versus patient autonomy, cost-benefit ratio of treatments, and limiting of access to expensive treatments).
      i. Macroallocation decisions (e.g., public health policy).
      ii. Microallocation decisions (e.g., triage during wartime); area of distributive justice involving the clinician role.

COMMON ETHICAL DISTINCTIONS

1. **It is important to determine whether these distinctions are logically valid (e.g., capable of sorting actions into two different groups without ambiguity) and morally relevant (e.g., one of the actions identified is morally justifiable whereas the other is not).**
   a. Active versus passive means to an end (or commission versus omission).
      i. Often associated with euthanasia.
      ii. Validity questioned because the decision to omit medical interventions to bring about a certain end often involves active behaviors, such as calling a meeting.
      iii. Involves serious moral issues similar to those in the distinction between "killing" and "letting die." For instance, it can be argued that it is justifiable to actively hasten a death if the alternative is to passively stand by while a patient suffers a prolonged death.
      iv. Recommended not to use this distinction in clinical ethics assessments.
   b. Ordinary versus extraordinary means
      i. Attempts to identify interventions based on whether they are standard of practice or not.
      ii. Practice standards reflect what is being done, not necessarily what should or should not be done based on scientific principles. Should a patient be required to accept any kind of standard means of extending life even if properly grounded in science?
      iii. Not recommended as part of a clinical ethics assessment unless a patient adheres to a particular faith that prohibits a specific intervention(s).
   c. Killing versus letting die
      i. "Killing" infers a deliberate and physically active process, such as giving a lethal injection; "letting die" refers to letting the disease process take its course. No

one has a moral obligation to rescue a person if the attempt would not prolong life or the attempt would put the rescuer at risk for significant harm.

    ii. The distinction appears to be valid and morally relevant but creates significant ethical dilemmas, especially in relation to assisted suicide.

  d. Withholding versus withdrawing

    i. "Withholding" means never starting a given treatment; "withdrawing" means removing or stopping a treatment already started.

    ii. Logical validity is questionable, because there are only a few situations in which the distinction between the two actions is clear. There is no legal basis for the distinction.

    iii. No clear distinction in terms of moral relevance. Is it more justifiable not to intubate a patient than to extubate a patient when the end point is similar in both situations?

    iv. Despite the lack of logical validity and moral relevance, this distinction is commonly applied in clinical ethics.

ADVANCE CARE PLANNING

1. **Advance directive: A document in which a person gives directions in advance about medical care or designates who should make medical decisions if he or she should lose decision-making capacity.**

  a. Provides instructions that describe the kind of care a person would want or not want under particular conditions.

  b. Providers, other members of the healthcare team, and family members use these documents to ensure that a person's preferences are honored.

  c. The two most common types of advance directives are the Living Will and a Durable/Medical Power of Attorney (POA). Both documents are executed only if the person lacks decision-making capacity and is unable to make personal treatment decisions.

    i. Living Will: Document that expresses wishes about medical treatment at the end of life. It takes effect only in situations of terminal illness or permanent unconsciousness.

      (a) Generic term for an advance directive; some states do not recognize this.

      (b) Not binding for medical practitioners.

      (c) Does not protect practitioner from criminal or civil liability.

    ii. Medical or Durable POA: Allow competent adults to designate someone to make their healthcare decisions for them if they become unable to make their own decisions.

      (a) POA can also be activated in any situation in which a person is unable to make decisions—whether the circumstances are terminal or not.

    iii. A legally recognized Living Will

      (a) Must be developed by a competent adult 18 years of age or older.

      (b) Must be witnessed by two persons; some states put restrictions on who can witness.

      (c) May be revoked by physically destroying, revoking in writing, or verbally rescinding.

      (d) Remains valid until revoked.

      (e) Becomes effective only when the person becomes qualified (e.g., is terminally ill or has an irreversible condition with loss of decision-making capacity). Usually two providers must certify that procedures or treatments will not prevent death but merely prolong it.

(f) Does not apply to medications and therapies given to prevent suffering and to provide comfort.

d. Medical or provider directive: Allowed in some states; lists a variety of treatments and procedures that the patient may want depending on the patient's condition at the time he or she cannot make his or her own decisions; similar to a living will and with equal legal worth (e.g., POLST in Oregon).

e. Natural death acts: Enacted by many states to protect practitioners from civil and criminal lawsuits and to ensure that the patient's wishes are followed if the patient is not competent to make his or her own healthcare decisions.

f. Uniform Rights of the Terminally Ill Act: Adopted in 1980 and revised in 1989.
   i. Similar to natural death acts.
      (a) Narrow in scope and limited to treatment that is life prolonging in patients with a terminal or irreversible condition.
      (b) Patients who are in a persistent vegetative state are not qualified to use the provisions of this act.

g. Patient Self-Determination Act of 1990
   i. Mandates patient education about advance directives and provides assistance in executing such directives.
   ii. States that providers may not discriminate against a patient based on the presence or absence of an advance directive.

h. Medical Aid in Dying
   i. Some states have enacted legislation which authorizes medical aid in dying and allows a terminally ill adult to end his or her life in a peaceful manner. Each state's requirements vary, but all include stringent requirements, such as:
      (a) A prognosis of 6 months or less;
      (b) Reached an age of 18 years or older;
      (c) Mental capacity to make an informed decision;
      (d) A prescribed length of residency in state; and
      (e) Has requested and obtained a prescription for medical aid-in-dying medication.
   ii. Medical aid for dying legislation has specific requirements for both physicians and patients (e.g., Colorado End-of-Life Options).

2. **Do-Not-Resuscitate (DNR) and Do-Not-Intubate (DNI)**
   a. Institution-based policies that allow patients and providers to make a decision not to resuscitate and/or intubate in the event of cardiopulmonary arrest (Dzeng et al., 2015).
   b. Some states have out-of-hospital DNR laws that allow an individual to request not to be resuscitated by emergency personnel. These orders are still in effect for outpatient treatment, including emergency department care, unless revoked.
   c. Some hospitals do not recognize DNR orders during surgery. Others believe that the decision to resuscitate or not to resuscitate should be made together by the patient, the surgeon, and the anesthesiologist. Whatever decision is made should be clearly documented in the medical record before surgery.
      i. DNR: A documentation that expresses patient's wish to avoid cardiopulmonary resuscitation in the event that he or she is unresponsive and apneic, with or without pulses. The order addresses resuscitation interventions, which may include rescue breathing, chest compressions, defibrillation, and advanced cardiovascular life support interventions.
      ii. DNI: A documentation that directs caregivers not to intubate the patient and initiate mechanical ventilation in the event of acute respiratory distress or apnea.

3. **Pain management**
   a. All patients should receive pain treatment and "comfort care" regardless of their decision about life support.
   b. Comfort care includes offering pain medication, hygiene temperature control, management of nausea, and massage.
4. **Clinical Practice Guidelines for Quality Palliative Care (2018) (see Ch. 21, Palliative and End-of-Life Care):**
   a. Patient- and family-centered care that optimizes quality of life by anticipating, preventing, and treating pain and symptoms.
   b. Care is provided and services are coordinated by an interprofessional team (e.g., chaplains, nurses, providers, social workers).
   c. Services are available concurrently with or independent of curative or life-prolonging care.
   d. Palliative care should be considered for seriously and terminally ill patients who are unlikely to recover or stabilize.
   e. The registered nurse will provide adequate dosage of analgesics and sedatives as appropriate to achieve patient comfort during the dying phase and address concerns and fears using narcotics and of analgesics hastening death.
   f. Patient and family hopes for peace and dignity are supported throughout the course of illness, during the dying process, and after death (Su et al., 2018).

> **EXPERT TIP**
> Palliative and End-of-Life care is one of the toughest issues critical care nurses face every day. Sharpen your palliative care assessment skills and learn research-based protocols by taking a course online at https://www.aacn.org/clinical-resources/palliative-end-of-life.

5. **Hospice care**
   a. Team-oriented approach to expert medical care, pain management, and emotional and spiritual support expressly tailored to the patient's needs and wishes.
   b. Focus is on caring, not curing, for people facing a life-limiting illness or injury.
6. **Nonbeneficial care (formerly known as *Futile care*):**
   a. Medical futility remains ethically controversial for several reasons.
   b. Definitions of futility lack consensus and are value laden, but futile care involves interventions that sustain life for prolonged periods even when there is no hope of improvement or achieving the goals of therapy. Many questions remain unresolved and lead to ethical dilemmas and conflict.
   c. There is often serious disagreement between healthcare team members and families regarding the benefits to the patient of continued treatment.
   d. Medical futility disputes are best avoided by strategies that optimize communication between healthcare members and surrogates:
      i. Provide families with accurate, current, and frequent prognostic estimates.
      ii. Address the emotional needs of the family and try to understand the problem from the family's perspective.
      iii. Facilitate excellent palliative care through the course of the illness.

THE LAW IN CLINICAL ETHICS (Department of Health & Human Services, 2020)

1. **Informed consent for clinical care: Providers have a separate duty to provide needed facts to a patient so that the patient can make an informed healthcare decision. The right to treat a patient is based on a contractual relationship grounded in mutual consent of the parties.**

> **KEY CONCEPT**
> Informed consent is given by a patient or a patient's surrogate to a provider for treatment and/or procedure with full knowledge of the possible risks and benefits.

a. Types of consent
   i. Expressed consent: Given directly by written or verbal words.
   ii. Implied consent: Presumed in emergency situations or implied by the patient's behavior, such as presenting an arm to the practitioner to have blood drawn.
   iii. Partial or complete consent: A patient may give consent for only part of a proposed therapy. For example, consenting to a breast biopsy but not to a mastectomy should it be needed.
b. Elements of informed consent for clinical treatment
   i. Explanation of treatment or procedure.
   ii. Name and qualifications of the person to perform the procedure and those of any assistants.
   iii. Explanation of significant risks (those that may lead to serious harm, including death).
   iv. Explanation of alternative therapies to the procedure or treatment, including the risk of doing nothing at all.
   v. Explanation that the patient can refuse the treatment or procedure without having alternative care or support discontinued.
   vi. Explanation that the patient can still refuse the treatment or procedure even after it has started.
c. Standards of informed consent disclosure
   i. Medical community standard (reasonable medical practitioner standard): Disclosure of facts related to the treatment or procedure that a reasonable medical practitioner in a similar community would disclose.
   ii. Objective patient standard (prudent patient standard): Disclosure of risks and benefits based on what a prudent person in the given patient's situation would deem material.
   iii. Subject patient standard (individual patient standard): Disclosure of facts relevant to a particular patient's situation and what he or she would deem important to know to make an informed decision.
   iv. Medical disclosure laws: Requirement by some states that certain risks and consequences be printed on a consent form.
   v. Patient and provider determine together what informed consent means to them; patient must communicate his or her values and expectations of the procedure or treatment to the provider, ask questions and seek clarification of the provider-patient discussion, evaluate symptoms and report impressions of how well the treatment or procedure is working or worked, and make good-faith efforts to participate in the treatment.
d. Exceptions to informed consent
   i. Emergency situations: Consent is implied if there is no time for disclosure and informed consent.
   ii. Therapeutic privilege: Primary healthcare providers are allowed to withhold information that they feel would be detrimental to the patient's health (e.g., likely to hinder or complicate necessary treatment, cause severe psychologic harm, or cause enough anxiety to make a rational decision by the patient impossible).

iii. Patient waiver: The patient may waive full disclosure while consenting to the procedure. The healthcare provider cannot suggest this; the patient must initiate the waiver.

iv. Prior patient knowledge: If the patient has had the same procedure previously and knows the risks and benefits as explained for the first procedure, then consent can be waived.

e. Accountability for obtaining informed consent

i. The provider has full accountability for obtaining informed consent.

ii. A hospital is responsible for informed consent only if those obtaining the consent are used by the hospital or if the hospital fails to take appropriate actions when informed consent was not obtained and the hospital is aware it was not obtained.

iii. The nurse's role in obtaining informed consent varies with the situation, institution, and state law.

(a) Nurses should explain all nursing care procedures to patients and families. Such procedures rely on orally expressed consent or implied consent. If a patient refuses a procedure or care, this must be honored.

(b) Some states allow providers to delegate the obtaining of informed consent to nurses. They do so at their own risk, but the nurse must ensure that all aspects of an informed consent are disclosed. Some hospitals do not allow nurses to obtain informed consent to limit the hospital's liability.

(c) If a nurse has knowledge that an already signed consent form does not meet the criteria for informed consent or the patient revokes the consent, the nurse must notify the supervisor and/or provider.

iv. To obtain blood at the request of law enforcement personnel without consent, five conditions must be present and documented:

(a) The suspect is under arrest.

(b) The likelihood exists that the blood drawn will produce evidence for criminal prosecution.

(c) A delay in drawing blood would lead to destruction of evidence.

(d) The test is reasonable and not medically contraindicated.

(e) The test is performed in a reasonable manner.

2. **Consent forms**

a. Blanket consent: Required before admission and covers routine and customary care.

b. Specific consent forms are often mandated by states. A detailed consent form should have the following elements:

i. Signature of a patient deemed to have medical decision-making capacity, or deemed competent, or by their legally authorized representative

(a) "Competent" is a legal term which means that the patient has not been declared incompetent by a court of law and the person is able to understand the consequences of his or her actions.

(b) Medical decision-making capacity is the ability of a patient to understand the benefits and risks of, and the alternatives to, a proposed treatment or intervention (including no treatment). Capacity is the basis of informed consent. It is determined clinical by the patient's providers and requires ongoing assessment.

(1) The signature cannot be coerced.

(2) The patient cannot be impaired because of medications previously received.

ii. Name and description of procedure in lay language.

      iii. Description of risks and alternatives to treatment (including nontreatment).

      iv. Description of probable consequences of proposed procedure.

      v. Signatures of one or two witnesses as mandated by state law; the witness is attesting that the patient actually signed the form.

3. **Informed consent in human research**

   a. Since 1974, the U.S. Department of Health & Human Services has required an institutional review board to approve protocols for human research.

   b. Special precautions are in place to protect vulnerable patient populations, such as minors, mentally disabled persons, children, and prisoners.

   c. Informed consent must include the following basic elements:

      i. A description of the purpose of the research, procedures that are experimental and those that are part of regular care, and expected duration of the subject's participation.

      ii. The number of subjects to be enrolled in the study.

      iii. Description of foreseeable risks or discomforts.

      iv. Benefits, if any, to the subject versus disclosure of alternatives courses of treatment available.

      v. Description of how confidentiality of information will be maintained.

      vi. Explanation of any compensation that will be provided and explanation of medical care that will be provided if injury occurs.

      vii. Contact information for further questions about the research and the subject's rights as a research volunteer.

      viii. A clear statement that the subject understands that he or she is a volunteer and has not been coerced into participating; also a statement that the subject may withdraw consent to participate any time during the procedure without loss of benefits or penalties to which the subject is entitled.

      ix. Language that is easy to understand and includes no exculpatory wording, such as that the researcher has no liability for the patient's outcome.

      x. Notification of any additional cost that the subject may incur from participating in the research.

4. **Declaration of death**

   a. World Medical Association (WMA) Declaration on End-of Life Medical Care.

   b. Uniform Determination of Death Act (UDDA) guidelines developed by the President's Commission for the Study of Ethical Problems in Medicine and in Biomedical and Behavioral Research state that "any individual who has sustained either irreversible cessation of circulatory and respiratory functions, or irreversible cessation of all functions of the entire brain, including the brain-stem, is dead."[†] Most states have adopted these guidelines.

   c. Confusion and controversy still exist over the term *brain death* and the relation of such death to donorship for organ transplantation.

   d. Procedural guidelines for the declaration of death.

      i. Triggering of a neurologic evaluation: As soon as the responsible provider has a reasonable suspicion that an irreversible loss of all brain functions has occurred, he or she should perform the appropriate tests and procedures to determine the patient's neurologic status.

      ii. Obligation to declare a patient dead.

        (a) Cardiopulmonary criteria for determining death are recognized in all states. When the provider determines that the patient has experienced an

---

irreversible cessation of cardiopulmonary functions, he or she declares the patient dead.

(b) Consent of the surrogate, family, or concerned friends is not required. Sensitivity to family or surrogate needs is required in declaring brain death. Family members have the option to obtain a second opinion about brain death.

iii. Cessation of treatment after a declaration of death: Once the declaration of death has been made, all treatment of the patient ordinarily should cease; exceptions to this might be when efforts are made to use the body or body parts for purposes stated in the Uniform Anatomic Gift Act (education, research, advancement of medical or dental science, therapy, transplantation) or when the patient is pregnant and efforts are being made to save the life of the fetus.

iv. In cases involving organ donation, healthcare professionals who make the declaration of death:

(a) Should not be members of the organ transplantation team.

(b) Should not be a member of the patient's family.

(c) Should not have malpractice charges pending against them that are related to the case.

(d) Should not have any other special interest in declaration of the patient's death (e.g., stand to inherit anything according to patient's will).

5. **Organ donation**

a. World Medical Association Statement on Organ and Tissue Donation and Transplantation (World Medical Association, 2020).‡

b. Types of organ donors

i. Tissue donor or living organ donor: Donor may be alive (e.g., bone marrow, kidney donor) or deceased (e.g., eye donor). Organ donation by living donors poses special concerns because of the increased risk to the donors' lives.

ii. Heart-beating donor: Donor is brain dead but respiratory function is supported mechanically while cardiac function continues spontaneously.

iii. Nonheart-beating donor: Organs are procured immediately after cessation of cardiorespiratory function.

KEY CONCEPT

Organ donation can save lives. People of all ages and medical conditions can be potential donors. A national computer system and strict standards are in place to ensure ethical and fair distribution of organs. Organs are matched by blood and tissue typing, organ size, medical urgency, waiting time, and geographic location.

---

6. **Emergency Medical Treatment and Labor Act (EMTALA)**

a. A 1986 law requiring hospitals participating in Medicare to screen patients for emergency medical conditions and stabilize them or provide protected transfers for medical reasons (CMS, 2012b).

b. Failure to adhere to the law results in large fines or loss of Medicare funding.

c. Patients may sue hospitals in federal or state court for damages under EMTALA's private right of action provision.

---

‡The professional obligations of providers and hospitals related to organ donation and transplantation can be found: https://www.wma.net/policies-post/wma-statement-on-organ-and-tissue-donation/.

7. **Legal barriers to end-of-life care**
   a. The legal context of care affects interventions and outcomes.
   b. Legal myths and counteracting reality.
      i. *Myth:* Forgoing life-sustaining treatment for a patient without decision-making capacity requires evidence that this is the patient's wish.
         Reality: Only a few states require "clear and convincing evidence." Most states will allow forgoing life-sustaining treatment based on a surrogate's word that it was the patient's wish. Some states even allow termination of such treatment if no one knows the patient's wishes and it is deemed in the patient's "best interest."
      ii. *Myth:* Withholding or withdrawing artificial nutrition or hydration from terminally ill or permanently unconscious patients is illegal.
         Reality: Just like any other therapy, fluids and nutrition may be withheld if it is the patient's or surrogate's wish.
      iii. *Myth:* Risk management personnel must be consulted before life-sustaining medical treatment can be stopped.
         Reality: This may be a hospital policy, but there is no legal requirement to notify risk management personnel.
      iv. *Myth:* Advance directives must be developed using specific forms, are not transferable to other states, and govern all future decisions. Advance directives given orally are not enforceable.
         Reality: Oral statements made by the patients may be legally valid directives. The patient does not have to be competent to revoke an advance directive but does have to be competent to make one. There are no specific forms required by any law to be used to document advance directives. Most states honor directives developed in other states.
      v. *Myth:* There are no legal options for easing suffering in a terminally ill patient whose suffering is overwhelming despite palliative care.
         Reality: Terminal sedation is an option to treat otherwise intractable symptoms in patients imminently dying. The 1997 Supreme Court decision on assisted suicide leaves states free to legalize or prohibit the practice. Currently, five states (CA, OR, MT, VT, and WA) have legalized physician-assisted suicide, which gives the provider the right to prescribe oral medication to competent patients who intend to commit suicide with the medication. The patient must take his or her own medication. The provider can only prescribe the medications.

CLINICAL ETHICS ASSESSMENT

1. **Identification of ethical issues and ethical decision-making models**
   a. Distinction between ethical and nonethical problems and dilemmas: Three characteristics must be present for a problem to be deemed an ethical one:
      i. The problem cannot be resolved with just empirical data.
      ii. The problem is inherently perplexing.
      iii. The result of the decision-making will affect several areas of human concern.
   b. There are many decision-making models. Common elements include the following actions:
      i. Gather all data (including information from all the stakeholders) related to the issue.
      ii. Analyze and interpret the data: Is it an ethical issue versus a legal or policy issue? What ethical principles are involved? What ethical conflicts are present? What are the capabilities of the stakeholders involved?
      iii. Identify courses of action and analyze the benefits and burdens of each course; project the consequences of the action.

      iv. Choose a plan of action and implement the plan; provide support to the stakeholders as needed.

      v. Evaluate the consequences of the actions taken.

      vi. Evaluate the ethical decision-making process.

2. Ethical conflicts

  a. Conflicts between moral principles.

  b. Conflicts between interpretations of a patient's best interest.

  c. Conflicts between moral principles and institutional policy or the law.

KEY CONCEPT

Facilities which receive federal funding are required to have an Ethics Committee, which is an interdisciplinary team who reviews potential ethical dilemmas.

---

3. Institutional ethics committees

  a. Interprofessional team resource for patients and families, clinicians, and the institution.

    i. Assist with clarifying issues.

    ii. Assist with the development of institutional policies and procedures related to clinical ethical issues.

  b. Goals include promoting the rights of patients, fostering shared decision-making between patients and clinicians, promoting fair policies and procedures that maximize the likelihood of good patient-centered outcomes, and enhancing the ethical practice of healthcare professionals and healthcare institutions.

  c. Educate staff and the community to achieve goals.

  d. Ethics consultation: The most common situations triggering consultations by providers include the following:

    i. End-of-life care.

    ii. Patient autonomy.

    iii. Conflicts among persons involved.

  e. Composition: Should include representatives of all disciplines and of the institution administration and community-at-large members.

4. Ethics consultation: Process elements

  a. Who has access to the process (e.g., all clinicians, patients, families) should be delineated.

  b. Patients (or surrogates), if appropriate, and attending providers should be notified (providing reason for the consultation, describing the process, and inviting participation).

  c. Documentation should be in the patient record or some other permanent record.

  d. Case review or process evaluation should be done to promote accountability.

5. Core skills and knowledge required for effective ethics consultations

  a. Core skills

    i. Ethical assessment skills required to identify the nature of the ethical dilemma or conflict.

    ii. Process skills required to focus on efforts to resolve the ethical dilemma or conflict.

    iii. Interpersonal skills critical to the consultation process.

  b. Core knowledge area as it relates to ethics consultation

    i. Moral reasoning and ethical theory

    ii. Bioethical issues and concepts

    iii. Healthcare systems

    iv. Clinical knowledge

    v. Knowledge of the healthcare institution and institution policies

    vi. Beliefs and perspectives of the patient and staff populations

    vii. Relevant code of ethics, standards of professional conduct, and guidelines of accrediting organizations

    viii. Health law

NURSE'S ROLE AS PATIENT ADVOCATE AND MORAL AGENT

1. **Organizational ethics and the nurse as patient advocate: AACN takes the position that the role of the acute care nurse includes being a patient advocate. The healthcare institution is instrumental in providing an environment in which patient advocacy is expected and supported. Patient advocacy is a fundamental nursing characteristic in the Synergy Model. As a patient advocate, the critical care nurse does the following:**

    a. Respects and supports the right of the patient or the patient's designated surrogate to autonomous informed decision-making.

    b. Intervenes when the best interest of the patient is in question.

    c. Helps the patient obtain necessary care.

    d. Respects the values, beliefs, and rights of the patient.

    e. Provides education and support to help the patient or the patient's designated surrogate make decisions.

    f. Represents the patient in accordance with the patient's choices.

    g. Supports the decisions of the patient or the patient's designated surrogate or transfers care to an equally qualified critical care nurse.

    h. Intercedes for a patient who cannot speak for self in situations that require immediate action.

    i. Monitors and safeguards the quality of care the patient receives.

    j. Acts as liaison among the patient, the patient's family, and healthcare professionals.

2. **Patient rights**

    a. Patients' Bill of Rights informs patients about what they should expect during their hospital stay with regard to their rights and responsibilities (American Hospital Association, 2020).

    b. Ethics of restraints: The use of restraints in critical care has the potential to violate several ethical principles and thus should be undertaken with caution.

        i. Nonmaleficence, or preventing harm, and beneficence, or doing good. Restraints are often used to prevent harm, but unintended consequences may violate this principle. The patient's autonomy is breached, and restraints often cause significant physical harm. In many cases, use of restraint does not prevent the disruption of medical therapy.

        ii. Informed consent should be obtained from the patient and/or family before use of restraints. A discussion of alternative treatments should be included. A patient with decision-making capacity should be able to choose to forego restraint. Paternalism is involved in situations in which one overrides another's decision to prevent harm to the person or maximize the benefits of treatment. There may be justifications for such actions in the critical care environment. If the patient lacks decision-making capacity and no surrogate decision maker is available, the nurse is obligated to use restraints to prevent significant or irreversible harm.

        iii. Trust is important to the patient and family members. They trust nurses, and thus ongoing communication about restraint decisions is crucial. Family members become upset when the patient is restrained without their knowledge.

BOX 1.2   **Core Concepts of Patient- and Family-Centered Care**
1. *Dignity and Respect.* Healthcare practitioners listen to and honor patient and family perspectives and choices. Patient and family knowledge, values, beliefs, and cultural backgrounds are incorporated into the planning and delivery of care. 2. *Information Sharing.* Healthcare practitioners communicate and share complete and unbiased information with patients and families in ways that are affirming and useful. Patients and families receive timely, complete, and accurate information to effectively participate in care and decision-making. 3. *Participation.* Patients and families are encouraged and supported in participating in care and decision-making at the level they choose. 4. *Collaboration.* Patients, families, healthcare practitioners, and healthcare leaders collaborate in policy and program development, implementation and evaluation; in research; in facility design; and in professional education, as well as in the delivery of care.

Reprinted with permission from the Institute for Patient- and Family-Centered Care: www.ipfcc.org. Core Concepts of Patient- and Family-Centered Care. Retrieved from http://www.ipfcc.org/about/pfcc.html.

   c. Ethics of pain management:
     i. Patients have the right to have their reports of pain believed.
     ii. Patients have the right to have pain addressed appropriately.
     iii. Clinicians, patients, and families must be educated about pain treatment.
     iv. Pain and pain management must be made visible and emphasized in organizations.
     v. Policies on reimbursement for the services of health professionals, medications, and other palliative treatments must be designed so that they do not create barriers to symptom treatment.
     vi. Development of policies to ensure adequate treatment of symptoms should take precedence over legalization of physician-assisted suicide and euthanasia.

3. Patient- and family-centered care
   a. Patient- and family-centered care is an approach to the planning, delivery, and evaluation of health care that is grounded in mutually beneficial partnerships among healthcare providers, patients, and families.
   b. Patient- and family-centered care is a partnership approach to healthcare decision-making between the family and healthcare provider. Patient- and family-centered care is considered the standard of pediatric healthcare by many clinical practices, hospitals, and healthcare groups.
   c. Patient- and family-centered practitioners recognize the vital role that families play in ensuring the health and well-being of infants, children, adolescents, and family members of all ages.
   d. The family has a vital role in supporting the patient through a critical illness. Family and friend visits can improve patients' sense of well-being, decrease anxiety, and keep the physiologic indices within normal limits.
   e. When family members' needs are not attended to or met, significant conflict occurs.
   f. Improving family communications at the end of life can be cost effective for the family and institution.
   g. The family-centered care philosophy was developed by pediatric practitioners. Box 1.2 summarizes the core concepts of the patient- and family-centered care philosophy.

References and bibliography information are available at http://evolve.elsevier.com/AACN/corecurriculum/.

Psychosocial Aspects of Critical Care

Deborah Chapa, PhD, ACNP-BC, FAANP, ACHPN; Bimbola Fola Akintade, PhD, MBA, MHA, ACNP-BC, NEA-BC, FAANP

CROSSWALK

- **Quality and Safety in Nursing Education (QSEN):** Patient-centered care, Teamwork and collaboration, Safety
- **National Patient Safety Goals:** Indentify patients correctly, Improve staff communication, Use medicines safely, Identify patient safety risks
- **American Nurses Association (ANA) Standards for Professional Nursing Practice:** Standard 1. Assessment, Standard 2. Diagnosis, Standard 3. Outcomes identification, Standard 4. Planning, Standard 5. Implementation, Standard 6. Evaluation, Standard 7. Ethics, Standard 8. Culturally congruent practice, Standard 9. Communication, Standard 10. Collaboration, Standard 11. Leadership, Standard 12. Education, Standard 15. Professional practice evaluation, Standard 16. Resource utilization, Standard 17. Environmental health
- **AACN Scope and Standards for Progressive and Critical Care Nursing Practice:** Standard 1. Quality of practice, Standard 2. Professional practice evaluation, Standard 3. Education, Standard 4. Communication, Standard 5. Ethics, Standard 6. Collaboration, Standard 8. Resource utilization, Standard 10. Environmental health
- **AACN Standards for Establishing and Sustaining Healthy Work Environments (HWE):** Skilled communication, True collaboration, Effective decision-making, Appropriate staffing
- **PCCN content:** Behavioral and Psychosocial—Delirium, Aggression, Violence, Psychologic disorders, Substance abuse, Abuse disorders
- **CCRN content:** Neurologic—Delirium; Behavioral and Psychosocial—All

SYSTEMWIDE ELEMENTS

REVIEW OF PSYCHOSOCIAL CONCEPTS

1. **Psychosocial considerations**
   a. Critical illness is a crisis for both the patient and family members. This crisis situation can present numerous, oftentimes complex psychosocial issues and problems that require the expertise of the critical care nurse working collaboratively with the interprofessional team. The crisis of a critical illness may be superimposed on other chronic stressors (e.g., substance abuse).
   b. Patient
      i. Critically ill patients share some common, predicable psychosocial needs (e.g., the need for reassurance and support).
      ii. Specific patient psychosocial needs vary depending on patient and family characteristics and the patient's status on the health-to-illness continuum.
      iii. The more compromised the patient, the more complex the patient's needs.

  iv. Critically ill patients' psychosocial needs are based on underlying pathophysiology of the disease process, age, sex, race/ethnicity, genomics, and social determinants of health.

  v. Other contributing factors include anxiety, depression, acute stress disorder (ASD), cognitive disorders, delirium, memory gaps imposed by coma or delirium, agitation, use of psychotropic medications, sedatives, hypnotics, medication and alcohol withdrawal, and sleep deprivation.

 c. Family

  i. Definition of family: *Family* is defined by the patient or, in the case of minors or those without decision-making capacity, by their surrogates. In this context, the family may be related or unrelated to the patient. They are individuals who provide support and with whom the patient has a significant relationship (Davidson et al., 2017, p 105).

  ii. Families of critically ill patients share a variety of predictable psychosocial needs and include the following:

   (a) To obtain information

   (b) Engagement in care

   (c) Participation in decision-making

   (d) To receive support and reassurance

   (e) To be with the patient

  iii. Specific psychosocial needs of family members may vary depending on patient characteristics, family characteristics, and the patient's status on the health-to-illness continuum (e.g., cultural diversity issues).

  iv. It is a duty to serve the family. Family care is essential for long-term recovery of the patient and maintaining the health of the family.

 d. Critical care nurse

  i. Critical care nurse characteristics influence the extent to which patient and family psychosocial needs are met. Continuum of nursing characteristics (AACN Synergy Model) includes clinical judgment, advocacy and moral agency, caring practices, collaboration, systems thinking, response to diversity, clinical inquiry, and facilitation of learning.

 e. Interprofessional collaboration

  i. Members of the critical care team include the nurse, physician, psychiatrist, psychologist, advanced practice provider, palliative care practitioner, geriatrician, respiratory therapist, pharmacist, dietitian, social worker, clergy, physical therapist, occupational and speech therapist, and others as needed.

  ii. Psychosocial needs of the patient and family are met through the collaborative efforts of an interprofessional team; each member brings a unique perspective and specific expertise to the shared plan of care and patient goals.

 f. Critical care environment (interaction among elements—hence complexity)

  i. High-technology, fast-paced environment presents challenges to meeting psychosocial needs.

 g. Challenges of meeting psychosocial needs

  i. Psychosocial care includes addressing family grief, powerlessness, coping, anxiety, depression, and maintaining family integrity during crisis. This is challenged by the fact that family members are not patients and not a reimbursable service.

  ii. Value systems in critical care units inappropriately often emphasize performing nursing tasks over attending to the psychosocial needs of the patient and family.

iii. Meeting psychosocial needs demands a coordinated, interprofessional approach to care.

iv. The critical care environment and space are often a barrier to effectively meeting psychosocial needs.

v. Growing evidence supports an interrelationship between psychologic, biologic, and social (Fig. 2.1).

h. Postintensive Care Syndrome (PICS): The critical care setting may cause a cluster of health problems that can remain with the patient after discharge from the intensive care unit (ICU). These symptoms encompass new or worsening impairments in the patient's physical, cognitive, or psychologic status arising after critical illness and persisting beyond the acute hospitalization.

i. ICU-acquired weakness: At-risk patients include those on mechanical ventilation, with infections or sepsis, and an ICU stay of 1 week or more. Activities of daily living, such as bathing and dressing can be difficult, and assistance is often required at home.

ii. Cognitive or brain dysfunction: Upward of 30% to 80% of patients experience problems remembering, organizing, and staying on task after leaving the ICU. There may be some improvement in the first-year postdischarge, but some patients may never recover, which can affect their ability to balance a checkbook and other daily activities. In addition, only 50% of patients are able to return to work within 1 year, and many do not return to work or to the job they had before their illness.

iii. Other mental health disorders: Sleep disorders may be common related to noise, light, and the effect of commonly used vasoactive agents on nightmares, hallucinations, and cognition. Nightmares and other unwanted memories of their ICU stay may cause anxiety, depression, or symptoms of posttraumatic stress disorder (PTSD).

iv. There are strategies that families can use to assist the patient with this process:

(a) Talk about things known to the patient, reorient to date and time.

(b) Keep a diary or journal about the ICU stay.

(c) Read aloud to the patient.

(d) Bring in familiar items from home.

(e) Help with patient's exercises at the bedside.

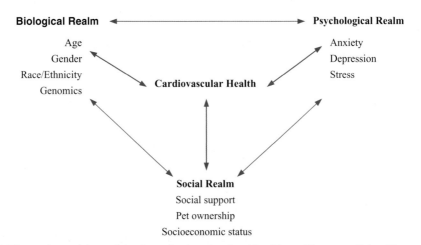

Fig. 2.1 Biopsychosocial model of cardiovascular health. (From Thomas, S.A., Chapa, D.W., Friedmann, E., et al. (2008). Depression in patients with heart failure: prevalence, pathophysiological mechanisms, and treatment. *Critical Care Nurse*, 28, 40–55.)

    (f) Educate families about what to look for as early signs, such as anxiety, depression, sleep disorders, and nightmares. Early intervention with primary care physician for psychology consult is recommended.

    (g) Medication screening by pharmacy for offending agents. Beers list for those over 65 years.

  i. PICS-F: PICS for families. Some 30% of family members are also at risk to develop this syndrome. Symptoms of anxiety, depression, and PTSD signal this syndrome. Families also exhibit sleep disorders, decreased physical functioning, social issues, such as marital and financial strain, loss of family integrity.

    i. Encourage family members to engage in self-care activities.

    ii. Encourage families to participate in the decision making and care of their loved one.

    iii. Educate family members about symptoms to look for and to discuss with their primary physician for psychology consult.

2. Common elements

  a. Life cycle

    i. Patients and family members come to critical care units at all phases of the life cycle.

    ii. Growth and development of the patient and family members influence psychosocial needs, response to critical illness, and behaviors (e.g., body image changes may present serious psychologic stressors to young adults).

  b. Needs of the patient

    i. Maslow categorized needs in terms of a hierarchy:

      (a) Physiologic requirements

      (b) Safety and security

      (c) Love and sense of belonging

      (d) Self-esteem

      (e) Self-actualization

    ii. Basic needs must be satisfied before higher-level needs can be met.

    iii. Needs change throughout the life cycle.

    iv. Critical illness may require refocusing on the achievement of basic needs.

  c. Family issues

    i. Family system theories

      (a) Derived from general system theory: A method of viewing systems composed of related parts that interact together as a whole.

      (b) Can be used by critical care nurses to understand family cultural patterns and dynamics, including communication patterns, power, economics, and interaction. May affect consenting process and surrogate decision-making. Also helps give insight into family relationships.

EXPERT TIP

There is evidence to support that family visitation for patients decreases anxiety, confusion, agitation, cardiovascular complication, length of ICU stay, and increases patient satisfaction and quality and safety. This can occur in person, virtually and by phone or writing.

---

    ii. Family systems

      (a) Groups of individuals bonded together by their interests.

      (b) Community whose members nurture and support one another.

      (c) Members have a set of rules, roles, power structure, forms of communication, and styles of problem solving that allow tasks to be accomplished effectively.

      (d) Critical illness alters rules, roles, power, and so on, in the family, which creates stress and the need for adaptation to a new environment and situation.

      (e) Influenced by cultural factors, spiritual support.

      (f) Communication, information, and emotional support are key factors for families when considering satisfaction scores.

      (g) Allowing for shared decision-making is a strategy that improves family satisfaction.

      (h) It is important to meet the individual needs of family members.

      (i) Communicating in ways that foster hope can decrease family emotional distress.

   iii. Caregiver concerns

      (a) Family caregivers are exposed to environmental stressors; may lead to role strain.

      (b) Can lead to exhaustion if not recognized and managed effectively.

      (c) Depression and health risk behaviors can occur in caregivers of critically ill patients and is recognized as caregiver burden.

d. Critical care environment

   i. Can directly affect the ability to meet a patient's needs, including the need for rest and sleep (e.g., lack of doors on patient rooms, fluorescent overbed lighting, lack of availability of sleep surface or sleep space for the family).

   ii. Staff awareness and behaviors also can have a profound effect on modifying environmental influences that affect the patient.

   iii. Unusual patterns of light and noise, together with the constant activity of a critical care unit, alter the patient's biologic rhythms and may negatively affect patient outcomes.

   iv. Environmental factors may lead to sensory overstimulation or sensory deprivation.

      (a) Noise: Sources of noise include staff conversations, alarms, and equipment. Critically ill patients have reported the sound of human voices and alarms. Adverse effects of noise (such as alarms) and associated sleep deprivation include increased adrenaline levels, diminished immune function, and decreased pain tolerance.

      (b) Lights: Ceiling lights, computers, medical equipment, and glare disturb patients.

   v. Strategies for creating a healing environment are listed in Box 2.1.

e. Stress

   i. Definition: Condition that exists in an organism when it encounters stimuli.

   ii. Critical illness is a stressful situation. Directed interventions by the nurse may lessen stress and/or the effect of stress on the patient and family. Nursing presence, respect, the anticipation of patient needs, caring attitude, competence, and allowing patients to have control when appropriate have been reported to be associated with less stressful critical care experiences.

   iii. Selye identified two types of stress:

      (a) Eustress: Condition that exists in an organism when it meets with nonthreatening stimuli.

      (b) Distress: Condition that exists in an organism when it meets with noxious stimuli.

   iv. Common psychologic stressors for critically ill patients and their families

      (a) Powerlessness (lack of control)

      (b) Sleep deprivation

      (c) Grief and loss

      (d) Sensory overload or deprivation

BOX 2.1   Strategies for Creating a Healing Environment

- Provide the patient with reassurance that the patient is being closely watched and that you are available to meet the patient's needs
- Create a personalized space for the patient, keep the patient's personal items (such as eyeglasses) within reach, and display cherished items (such as family pictures)
- Ensure privacy and dignity (e.g., close curtains and doors and talk quietly during sensitive conversations)
- Provide information about caregivers (e.g., write the names of nurses and other caregivers on a dry-erase board in the room)
- Use dimmers to adjust the brightness of lights and incandescent lighting if possible
- Adjust the curtains to block out bright lights
- Provide natural light and outside views when possible
- Aromatherapy and acupressure may decrease anxiety and aid sleep
- Decrease sensory deprivation by allowing family visitation, surrounding the patient with familiar items, providing radio or television, etc., according to the patient's desires
- Use music therapy or sound-masking therapy, which provides comforting background noise and helps manage stress, anxiety, and pain
- Adjust the alarms to be individualized for the patient
- Earplugs
- Provide structured quiet time
- Acoustic absorbers

    (e) Pain

    (f) Fear

    (g) Isolation

  v. Response to stress

    (a) Multiple stressors in the intensive care setting elicit a stress response, pain, underlying disease process, psychologic distress.

    (b) Major neural response to a stressful stimulus is activation of the sympathetic nervous system; however, multiple pathways are involved.

    (c) Relationship between psychologic stress and health: psychoneuroimmunologic research has identified a relationship between stress and immune function (e.g., an increased stress response is associated with decreased immunity).

f. Physiology of the stress/immune response

  i. Activation of the hypothalamic-pituitary-adrenal (HPA) axis

  ii. Locus caeruleus/norepinephrine-autonomic nervous system

  iii. Renin-angiotensin-aldosterone system

  iv. Activation of cytokine cascades

  v. Neurohormones involved: Corticotropin-releasing factor, cortisol, norepinephrine, epinephrine, aldosterone, angiotensin II, cytokines

  vi. Fear and helplessness activate pathways in the limbic system that lead to ASD and PTSD in patients and families.

EXPERT TIP

Activation of the stress response increases likelihood of psychologic responses, such as anxiety, depression, and PTSD which in turn will increase the response and potentially decrease healing.

ASSESSMENT

1. **Patient history**

  a. Identify preexisting psychiatric, psychologic, and social concerns

  b. Identify preillness coping mechanisms

   c. Identify sources of support (e.g., family, friends, spiritual support, pets)
   d. Identify patient proxy, Living Will, Durable Power Of Attorney, code status, physician orders for life-sustaining treatment (POLST), medical orders for life-sustaining treatment (MOLST), or advance directives
   e. Assess for medical nonadherence

> **EXPERT TIP**
> Medical nonadherence may also be related to depression or social determinants of health.

2. **Family history: Obtain on admission or as soon as possible**
   a. Healthcare proxy or family spokesperson
   b. Contact information (e.g., home and cell phone numbers, pager numbers)
   c. Diversity issues (culture, language, etc.) that affect the patient and family
   d. Coping strategies versus family caregivers
   e. Support systems (family, friends, church group, other spiritual support)
   f. Special family needs (e.g., young children, disabilities, etc.)
   g. Family concerns and goals regarding this hospitalization
   h. Family preference for presence and engagement
   i. Preferred method of meeting and communicating with the ICU team members (e.g., participation in scheduled ICU rounds, scheduled evening meetings, phone calls)
   j. Past experience with critical illness
3. **Physical examination**
   a. Cognitive assessment (e.g., ability to concentrate, level of judgment, delirium assessment)
   b. Behavioral assessment (sleep patterns, level of agitation, interaction with family and staff)
   c. Review of findings from other diagnostic studies (e.g., computed tomographic [CT] scan, electroencephalogram [EEG], etc.)
   d. Appraisal of patient characteristics: Almost all patients with a critical illness experience some psychosocial issues during the course of their illness. However, each patient and family is unique and brings a unique set of characteristics to the care situation. Examples of clinical attributes that the nurse should assess when caring for a patient with an acute respiratory disorder are the following: resiliency, vulnerability, stability, complexity, resource availability, desire for participation in care, preferred decision-making model, and predictability.
   e. Diagnostic studies
      i. Laboratory studies
      ii. EEG
      iii. Cerebral blood flow studies

> **EXPERT TIP**
> Sleep hygiene may decrease the development of agitation and delirium.

PAIN, AGITATION, DELIRIUM, IMMOBILITY AND SLEEP DISRUPTION (PADIS) (Devlin et al., 2018)

1. **Description of the problem**
   a. PADIS is a syndrome of interrelated conditions that can affect acutely ill persons. A systematic, interprofessional approach is required.
   b. Benefits of implementing the PADIS guidelines (Box 2.2)

> **BOX 2.2 Benefits for Adapting Pain, Agitation/Sedation, Delirium, Immobility, and Sleep Disruption**
>
> ↓ Duration of mechanical ventilation and associated complications
> ↓ Intensive care unit (ICU) length of stay
> ↓ Hospital length of stay
> ↓ Patient transfers to skilled nursing facilities
> ↓ ICU, hospital, and postdischarge mortality rates
> ↓ ICU, hospital, societal costs per patient
> ↓ Long-term societal burdens of ICU survivors (postintensive care syndrome)
> ↑ ICU patient throughput and bed availability
> ↓ Prevalence and duration of ICU delirium
> ↑ Long-term cognitive function and mobility
> ↓ Number of ICU patients discharged to home

From Devlin, J.W., Skrobik, Y., Needham, D.M., et al. (2018). Clinical practice guidelines for the prevention and management of pain, agitation/sedation, delirium, immobility, and sleep disruption in adult patients in the ICU. *Critical Care Medicine*, 46(9), e825–e873.

> **KEY CONCEPT**
> Untreated or inadequately treated pain can cause agitation and delirium. Assess for and treat pain first.

2. Treatment strategies
   a. Treat pain first because it can often be the cause of agitation/sedation delirium, immobility, and sleep disruption.
   b. Oral gabapentin or carbamazepine should be administered as first line for neuropathic pain.
   c. Neuraxial analgesia is only for patients with rib fractures or abdominal aortic surgery.
3. Optimize sedation management and use light level of sedation (see Ch. 19, Sedation).
   a. Not recommended for daily use
4. Delirium
   a. Identify and eliminate potential contributing factors: Approximately "50%–80% of mechanically ventilated patients and 20%–50% of patients with illness of lower severity, resulting in prolonged hospitalization, increased mortality and increased cost. Long-term effects on the patient include increased risk of mortality and long-term cognitive impairment" (Devlin et al., 2018).
   b. Recommend delirium assessment tool daily.
   c. If elimination of offending agents does not help, then first use nonpharmacologic (reorientation, access to eyeglasses and hearing aids, maintaining sleep-wake cycle, advancing mobility, light in room, attempt normal sleep-wake cycle) followed by pharmacologic (adequate analgesia, discontinuation of benzodiazepines, resume psychiatric medications, treatment of medication withdrawal syndromes, and antipsychotics if needed). Haloperidol is contraindicated.
5. **Encourage family to serve as mobility coach and provide diversionary activities to keep awake intubated patients distracted from removing the endotracheal tube. Use cognitive strengthening activities such as picture recall, memory exercises, and simple mathematical problem solving.**

SLEEP DEPRIVATION

1. **Description of problem:** Sleep deprivation in the critically ill patient involves a decrease in the amount, consistency, and/or quality of sleep that occurs in a 24-hour period. Studies have shown that, because of light, noise, and clinical care, critically ill patients suffer from sleep deprivation. Patients in the ICU do not reach the deeper stages of sleep and have been known to have 6.2 awakenings every hour. The more critically ill a patient is, the more likely the patient will have sleep deprivation. The healing from sleep is prohibited in the intensive care environment.
2. **Patient outcomes**
   a. Patient states that he or she feels rested.
   b. Patient does not demonstrate signs and symptoms of sleep deprivation, including the following:
      i. Altered mental status (e.g., confusion, delusions)
      ii. Decreased alertness
      iii. Irritability
      iv. Aggressive behavior
      v. Restlessness
      vi. Anxiety
      vii. Exhaustion
3. **Interprofessional collaboration:** Nurse, physician, advanced practice provider, pharmacist, social worker, clergy
4. **Interventions**
   a. Increase total sleep time, promote N3 and rapid eye movement (REM) sleep
   b. Cluster activities so that the patient is allowed periods of rest
   c. Prioritize activities to allow a stable patient to have periods without unnecessary, frequent assessments
   d. Decrease the noise level to promote sleep
   e. Decrease overhead lighting and provide eye masks to promote sleep
   f. Provide adequate pain relief
   g. Teach the patient and family relaxation techniques to promote rest and sleep
   h. Consult with a pharmacist to identify offending agents that alter quality of sleep or cause agitation, review Beers list for contradicted medications in the older adult
   i. Decrease use of antihistamines, benzodiazepines, and narcotics
   j. Promote nonpharmacologic sleep hygiene such as music therapy, back rub, bathing, and so on
   k. Discharge planning may include referral to a sleep specialist
   l. Individualize alarm settings to avoid nuisance alarms (e.g., irregular heart rhythm in atrial fibrillation)

> **EXPERT TIP**
> Benzodiazepines can be associated with the development of delirium, and long-term use can abolish stage IV sleep.

ASD AND PTSD

1. **Definition:** *PTSD* is a chronic and common anxiety disorder that can manifest following exposure to a traumatic life event, such as a natural disaster, military combat, physical or sexual assault, and so on. *ASD* is the initial response to stress in the first month. After 1 month, if patients still experience symptoms, then it is

classified as PTSD. The symptoms are essentially the same, although, with ASD, dissociative symptoms of numbing, decreased awareness, depersonalization, derealization, and amnesia may be present.

2. Pathophysiology: Life events that illicit fear, horror, or helplessness may lead to the development of ASD/PTSD. Disruption in at least five key systems of the brain is involved with the pathophysiology of ASD/PTSD. These systems are the HPA axis, endocannabinoid system, serotonergic (5HT) system, noradrenergic/norepinephrine, and opioid system.

3. Incidence rates
   a. ASD from motor vehicle accidents are 13% to 24%
   b. PTSD occurs in approximately 6% to 8% of the population in the United States. Patients who develop ASD may develop PTSD in 60% to 80% of cases.
   c. The rate of PTSD among women in the United States is approximately one in every nine, which is greater than in men

4. Risk factors
   a. Serious illness
   b. Traumatic life event
   c. Military exposure
   d. Sexual assault
   e. Major depression
   f. Anxiety
   g. Illicit medication use
   h. Multiple hospitalizations
   i. Comorbid medical conditions
      i. Heart disease
      ii. Diabetes
      iii. Peptic ulcer disease
      iv. Gastrointestinal problems

5. Diagnostic study findings
   a. Diagnostic procedures
      i. Self-report screening measures
      ii. Clinical interviews
   b. Diagnostic criteria: Requires experiencing symptoms from at least four clusters:
      i. Recurrent, involuntary, and intrusive memories
      ii. Traumatic nightmares
      iii. Dissociative reactions (e.g., flashbacks)
      iv. Intense or prolonged distress after exposure of traumatic reminder
      v. Marked physiologic reactivity after exposure to trauma-related stimuli (e.g., increased heart rate or shortness of breath)
      vi. The duration of symptoms lasts longer than a month (PTSD)
      vii. The disturbances cause clinically significant distress or impairment in functioning
      viii. The disturbances are not attributed to the physiologic effects of a substance or other medical condition
   c. Interprofessional collaboration: Nurse, physician, advanced practice provider, pharmacist, social worker, clergy, psychiatrist, psychologist,

6. Management of patient care
   a. Initial posttrauma period (ASD)
      i. Formal treatment may not be required.

    ii. Good social support is essential.

    iii. Accessing/minimizing/eliminating exposure to stressor may aid in the recovery process.

    iv. Patient and family may benefit from consult for psychiatrist early in the management process.

    v. Cognitive behavioral therapy (may be appropriate for patients in acute distress for the first month postincident).

    vi. Eye movement desensitization and reprocessing (this may aid in lowering emotional arousal of traumatic memories).

  b. Late posttrauma period (second-line strategy; PTSD)

    i. Communication of emotions and providing patient and family with meaningful activities to help provide purpose during crisis is important

    ii. Medications

      (a) Antidepressants (paroxetine, sertraline, and venlafaxine)

      (b) Alpha-blockers (prazosin)

      (c) Medications to avoid: Benzodiazepines (no evidence their use is beneficial, and may risk paradoxical disinhibited behaviors)

DELIRIUM (ACUTE CONFUSIONAL STATE)

1. **Definition: Characterized by acute onset and fluctuating course of inattention accompanied by either a change in cognition or a perceptual disturbance. Common psychiatric illness in critically ill patients may be a significant predictor for morbidity and mortality.**

2. **Etiology and risk factors**

  a. Incidence (rates)

    i. 70% to 83% of the critically ill experience delirium

    ii. 80% of terminally ill develop delirium near death

3. **Delirium caused by a general medical condition**

  a. Hypoxia

  b. Hypercapnia

  c. Metabolic acidosis

  d. Heart, kidney, liver failure versus hyperthyroidism or hypothyroidism

  e. Hyperparathyroidism

  f. Cerebrovascular accident, transient ischemic attack

  g. Concussion

  h. Postictal state

  i. Electrolyte imbalances (hyperkalemia, hypokalemia)

  j. Hyperglycemia or hypoglycemia

  k. Alcohol or medication withdrawal

  l. Infection

  m. Pain

4. **Substance-induced delirium (because of a medication, toxin exposure, medication abuse)**

  a. Anesthetics (emergence delirium)

  b. Analgesics

  c. Sedatives (e.g., benzodiazepines)

  d. Antiemetics

  e. Cardiac medications (e.g., antihypertensives, digoxin)

  f. Steroids

  g. Anticholinergics

h. Delirium caused by multiple causes

i. Other (not able to be specified)

5. **Signs and symptoms**

   a. Cognitive

      i. Sleep disturbances

      ii. Diminished attention span

      iii. Reduced ability to focus

      iv. Disorientation to person, place, time

      v. Confusion over daily events

      vi. Hallucinations (visual are more common)

      vii. Abnormal results on a mental status examination (e.g., Folstein Mini-Mental State Examination)

   b. Behavioral: May vary markedly from patient to patient

      i. Excessive restlessness

      ii. Sluggishness and lethargy

      iii. Inappropriate behavior

      iv. Irritability

      v. Picking or groping at bed linens, gown

      vi. Attempting to get out of bed (when unsafe)

      vii. Crying out, screaming, moaning, muttering

      viii. Personality changes

      ix. Changes in affect

   c. Physiologic

      i. Tremors and/or seizures (alcohol withdrawal)

6. **Diagnostic study findings: Dependent on the underlying problem (e.g., may have abnormal electrolyte levels, CT scan, etc.)**

7. **Collaborative diagnoses of patient needs**

   a. Assess for possible factors that could contribute to delirium

   b. Decrease the use of medications that could contribute to delirium

8. **Patient outcomes**

   a. Patient is oriented to person, time, and place

   b. Patient does not demonstrate signs or symptoms of anxiety, fear, and confusion

   c. Patient responds to simple, concrete questions

9. **Management of patient care**

   a. Anticipated patient trajectory: With treatment of the underlying cause of delirium, the problem can be managed and eliminated

      i. Treatments

         (a) Nonpharmacologic

            (1) Assess for delirium (e.g., Confusion Assessment Method [CAM]-ICU or the Intensive Care Delirium Screening Checklist [ICDSC])

            (2) Provide for adequate rest and sleep

            (3) Consider reorientation and early/progressive mobility

            (4) Review medication list with the physician and discontinue suspect medications

            (5) Monitor and manage electrolyte and acid-base disorders

            (6) Consult a psychiatrist if delirium does not resolve with standard management

            (7) The use of restraints are not recommended

            (8) Explain to family members the nature of delirium and why it occurs. Stress the temporary nature of the condition in hospitalized patients.

        (9) Give family members updates on patient management and progress (e.g., findings related to the underlying cause of the delirium)

        (10)Reassure the family that the patient is not in control or responsible for his or her behaviors

    (b) Pharmacologic: Avoid offending agents, assess for alcohol withdrawal using Clinical Institute Withdrawal Assessment for Alcohol (CIWA) and substance withdrawal using Clinical Opiate Withdrawl Scale (COWS), treat as indicated.

  b. Discharge planning

    i. May require follow-up with primary care provider.

    ii. Education to caregiver/patient about prevention (e.g., adherence to medication schedule, proper diet/electrolyte imbalance for early identification/treatment of causes of delirium).

    iii. Avoid deliriogenic medications. Pharmacy consult for medication reconciliation and to identify potentially deliriogenic agents.

10. **Interdependence: Many psychosocial issues and concerns of the critically ill patient are interdependent. For example, inadequately managed pain may lead to feelings of powerlessness, anxiety, and depression that, in turn, heighten the patient's perception of pain.**

POWERLESSNESS

1. **Description of problem**

  a. Perceived lack of control over the outcome of a specific situation. The ability of an event to engender a sense of powerlessness is influenced by the individual's self-esteem and self-concept and where the individual is in the life cycle.

  b. Critically ill patients lose their ability to control even the most basic of functions, including the ability to communicate, to breathe on their own, and to control bladder and bowel functions. Depending on the philosophy and organization of the critical care environment, they may also lose the ability to participate in decision-making about their own healthcare and future.

2. **Patient outcomes**

  a. Helplessness as an antecedent to stress disorders

  b. Patient communicates needs and wishes verbally or nonverbally

  c. Patient (and family as appropriate) participates in decision-making regarding the plan of care

  d. Signs of dysfunction are not demonstrated by the patient and family members that are associated with powerlessness, such as:

    i. Withdrawal

    ii. Aggressive behavior

    iii. Demanding behavior

    iv. Excessive repetition of the same questions

    v. Placing of unrealistic demands on the staff

    vi. Blaming of the staff for the patient's condition

  e. Patient participates in decision-making regarding daily care activities (e.g., timing of bath, sleep, visiting hours)

3. **Interprofessional collaboration: Nurse, physician, advanced practice provider, pharmacist, physical therapist, social worker, case manager, psychiatrist, psychologist**

4. **Interventions**

  a. Engage patient and family in direct care and decision-making

  b. Promote patient-nurse communication

      i. This intervention presents significant challenges, particularly if the patient is intubated or speaks a language other than English (or the predominant language at the facility).

KEY CONCEPT

Encourage active engagement in rounds. Provide patient/family with opportunity to add information during rounding process (e.g., reactions to previous treatments or medications, preferences).

---

      ii. Methods of communication should be based on patient preferences and abilities. Common communication techniques for use with intubated patients include lip reading, picture or alphabet boards, pen or pencil and paper, and computer.

      iii. Use available interpreter services for non—English-speaking patients and family members.

      iv. Encourage family engagement in the communication process.

  c. Engage the patient and family in bidirectional care planning process and decision-making

      i. Ask the patient (or healthcare proxy) what level of involvement he or she would like in the care planning process.

      ii. Encourage the patient and family members to keep a record of questions and concerns.

      iii. Provide the patient, proxy, or a family member with daily (or more frequent) updates regarding the patient's status and care plan.

  d. Encourage the patient and family members to meet with spiritual support persons if they would find this helpful.

  e. Prepare the patient for procedures. Explain what will be happening, when it will happen, and how the patient will be affected.

5. **Assure patient and family are active participants in care planning and delivery. Encourage active engagement in rounds. Provide patient/family with opportunity to add information during rounding process (e.g., reactions to previous treatments or medications, preferences).**

ANXIETY

1. **Pathophysiology: Anxiety is the apprehensive anticipation of future danger or misfortune accompanied by a feeling of dysphoria or somatic symptoms of tension. Focus of anticipated danger may be internal or external (American Psychiatric Association [APA], 2020; Devlin et al., 2018). Anxiety is stimulated in the central nervous system by neurohormones of norepinephrine, serotonin, dopamine, and gamma aminobutyric acid (GABA). In the peripheral nervous system, it is stimulated by the sympathetic nervous system.**

2. **Etiology and risk factors: Results from multiple sources in the ICU, including the following:**

  a. Unstable physiologic status (e.g., hypoxemia with shortness of breath, cardiac arrhythmias)

  b. Pain

  c. Fear of the unknown

  d. Procedures

  e. Separation from family and support system

  f. Underlying psychiatric disorder (including panic disorders, phobias, and PTSD)

  g. Lack of autonomy/control

3. **Signs and symptoms (Box 2.3)**
4. **Diagnostic study findings**
   a. When behavioral manifestations of anxiety are present, possible physiologic causes (e.g., hypoxemia and hypoglycemia) must be ruled out.
   b. Toxicology screen: To assess for possible medication-induced anxiety
   c. Mental status examination: Findings may be abnormal with severe anxiety
5. **Interprofessional collaboration: Nurse, physician, advanced practice provider, pharmacist, physical therapist, social worker, clergy, psychiatrist, psychologist, and so on**
6. **Management of patient care**

EXPERT TIP

Nonpharmacologic therapies, such as aromatherapy, pet and music therapy aid reduction of anxiety in intensive care patients.

---

   a. Goals of care: Patient does not demonstrate signs or symptoms of anxiety (e.g., no tachypnea, tachycardia, muscle tension, etc.) and can verbalize he/she does not have anxiety.
      i. Interventions
         (a) Nonpharmacologic
             (1) Reassure the patient and give explanations about the patient's condition and treatment plan
             (2) Involve family in appropriate patient care activities (massage, passive range of motion, applying lotion, assist with bathing)
             (3) Ask the patient to discuss fears and worries

---

BOX 2.3   Clinical Manifestations of Anxiety

COGNITIVE
- Apprehension
- Difficulty concentrating
- Hypervigilance
- Impaired judgment
- Self-consciousness
- Worry

BEHAVIORAL
- Easy fatigue
- Fidgeting
- Refusal of medical treatment
- Restlessness
- Sleep disturbances
- Unrealistic demands for attention

PHYSIOLOGIC
Cardiac
- Chest pain
- Dysrhythmias
- Increased blood pressure
- Palpitations
- Tachycardia

RESPIRATORY
- Choking sensation
- Shortness of breath
- Tachypnea

NEUROMUSCULAR
- Dilated pupils
- Dizziness
- Light-headedness
- Muscle and motor tension
- Tremors

GASTROINTESTINAL
- Anorexia
- Nausea
- Vomiting

GENITOURINARY
- Frequency
- Urgency

PAIN
- See Chapter 20

        (4) Assure the patient that adequate sedation and pain medication will be provided during painful procedures

        (5) Allow family members to stay with the patient as much as possible to provide support

        (6) Use music therapy

        (7) Use pet therapy if available

     (b) Pharmacology

        (1) Avoid benzodiazepines

        (2) Minimize sedatives and hypnotics

        (3) Pain medication (if indicated)

  ii. Potential complications

     (a) Teach the patient and family methods of anxiety reduction (e.g., imagery distraction, music) to prevent PTSD.

     (b) Patient and family may require post-ICU follow-up (psychiatric and/or social services) for unresolved anxiety issues.

     (c) Patient may require follow-up teaching regarding pharmacologic and nonpharmacologic interventions to treat anxiety.

DEPRESSION

1. **Definition/pathophysiology: Mood state characterized by feeling of sadness, lowered self-esteem, pessimistic thinking, and guilt. Depressive episodes and depressive disorders are psychiatric diagnoses given to patients based on specific criteria (e.g., etiology, symptoms, length of depression). Underlying pathophysiology is depletion of neurotransmitters serotonin, norepinephrine, or dopamine in the central nervous system.**

2. **Etiology and risk factors**

  a. Incidence in hospitalized patients ranges from 6% to 14%.

  b. Rates can vary between different medical illnesses. The highest rates are those with neurologic disorders.

3. **Causes of depression**

  a. Psychodynamic

    i. Illness progression

    ii. Fear and anxiety regarding the illness and the outcome of the illness

    iii. Illness-related regime

    iv. Reaction to loss and deprivation

    v. Partial or complete loss of self-esteem

  b. Cognitive: Patient's beliefs (thoughts such as "It's all my fault") may lead to depression

  c. Biochemical

    i. Neurotransmitter imbalance

    ii. Thyroid dysfunction

    iii. Hypocalcemia or hypercalcemia

    iv. Medications (e.g., antihypertensives, thiazides, spironolactone, beta-blockers, digoxin toxicity, steroids, benzodiazepines, cocaine withdrawal, alcohol)

  d. Social

    i. Lack of social support

    ii. Abandonment or isolation

  e. Other

    i. Lack of sleep

    ii. Chronic or acute unmanaged pain

4. **Signs and symptoms (Box 2.4)**
5. **Diagnostic study findings**
   a. Diagnosis based on history and clinical examination (e.g., cognitive and behavioral changes)
   b. Diagnostic test results may be abnormal if there is an underlying physiologic problem contributing to the depression (e.g., digoxin toxicity).
   c. PHQ-9 (Patient Health Questionnaire) is a validated and reliable assessment tool for adults with depression.
   d. Interprofessional collaboration: Nurse, physician, advanced practice provider, respiratory therapist, pharmacist, physical therapist, social worker, clergy, case manager
6. **Management of patient care**
   a. Anticipated patient trajectory: With counseling, ongoing support from family and friends, and when indicated, pharmacologic therapy, patients with depression can resume and maintain normal lives.
   b. Treatments
      i. Nonpharmacologic
      ii. Assist in performing a differential diagnosis: Grief reaction, mood disorder, organic brain syndrome, delirium, dementia, metabolic conditions presenting as depression (e.g., hypercapnia, metabolic acidosis, uremia)
      iii. Discuss the treatment plan and progress with the patient—engage the patient in care planning as appropriate
      iv. Discuss concerns over possible or actual depressed state
      v. Acknowledge that a depressed mood can be normal during or following a serious illness
      vi. Provide a mechanism to increase social support (family support, social services)
      vii. Attend to any suicidal ideation (Is the patient a threat to self or others?)

BOX 2.4   **Clinical Manifestations of Depression**

COGNITIVE
- Decreased ability to concentrate
- Difficulty with decision-making

BIOLOGIC
- Psychomotor agitation
- Abnormal sleep patterns
- Apparent sadness (tears, furrowed brow, downturned corners of the mouth, lack of eye contact)
- Fatigue
- Weight loss or weight gain
- Poor appetite
- Loss of libido

BEHAVIORAL
- Recurrent thoughts of death
- Loss of interest or pleasure
- Guilt
- Illness as punishment

SOCIAL
- Withdrawal
- Difficulties with relationships
- Impaired role functioning

viii. Secure a psychiatric referral as appropriate

ix. Pharmacologic: Antidepressants (e.g., tricyclics, selective serotonin reuptake inhibitors)

c. Discharge planning

i. Provide information to the patient and family about depression and available treatments.

ii. Discuss pharmacologic therapy, including mechanism of action, benefits, and side effects.

iii. Patient and family may require follow-up evaluation and teaching on pharmacologic and nonpharmacologic treatments for depression.

SUBSTANCE MISUSE, DEPENDENCE, AND WITHDRAWAL

1. **Definition**
   a. Substance misuse is the use of pharmacologic medications or alcohol for nonmedical purposes
   b. Dependence happens when a person feels the positive effects of using the substance are so strong that a loss of control occurs for the use of the substance. ICD-10 states that there must be three of the following items that exist for a period of 12 months: loss of control with respect to use, craving, withdrawal symptoms, development of tolerance with dose escalation, neglect of alternative interests, and continued use despite negative consequences.
   c. Withdrawal is the presence of a characteristic syndrome that develops after the cessation of (or reduction in) heavy and prolonged substance use.
2. **Etiology of withdrawal: Abrupt cessation of medications/alcohol use in persons with a physical dependence. Type of medications may include over the counter, prescription, and illegal medications.**
3. **Signs and symptoms of medication/opioid withdrawal: Usually occurs within 24 hours. Symptoms peak 2 to 3 days from last ingestion and may last 5 to 10 days. Withdrawal assessment tools, such as the CIWA and the Objective Opiate Withdrawal Scale (OOWS) may be used to objectively assess withdrawal over time.**
   a. Physical withdrawal
      i. Muscle pain
      ii. Abdominal cramps
      iii. Diarrhea
   b. Psychologic withdrawal
      i. Anxiety
      ii. Insomnia
      iii. Strong craving
   c. Objective
      i. Watery eyes
      ii. Frequent yawning
      iii. Acute rhinitis
      iv. Sweating
      v. Chills
      vi. Piloerection
4. **Diagnostic study findings for medication/opioid withdrawal**
   a. Electrolyte disturbances
   b. Elevated blood urea nitrogen, creatinine if dehydrated
   c. Toxicology screen

    d. Medication screens (urine, serum, saliva, sweat, hair) for multiple medication use

    e. Screening for associated infections (hepatitis B, hepatitis C, human immunodeficiency virus [HIV], tuberculosis, sexually transmitted disease)

5. **Signs and symptoms of alcohol withdrawal occurs from few hours to few days. Usually begins within 6 hours. If longer than 1 week, consider something other than alcohol withdrawal. Withdrawal syndrome includes two or more symptoms of autonomic hyperactivity (e.g., sweating, pulse >100 beats/minute, insomnia, agitation).**

    a. Mild to moderate withdrawal

    b. Agitation

    c. Anxiety

    d. Tremors

    e. Nausea and vomiting

    f. Weakness

    g. Diaphoresis

    h. Hallucinations

    i. Delirium tremens

    j. Anxiety attacks

    k. Sleeplessness

    l. Disorientation

    m. Confusion

    n. Cognitive impairment

    o. Delirium

    p. Tachycardia

    q. Fever

    r. Grand mal seizure

6. **Diagnostic study findings**

    a. Medication screens (urine, serum, saliva, sweat, hair) for multiple medication use

    b. Screening for associated infections (hepatitis B, hepatitis C, HIV, tuberculosis, sexually transmitted disease)

    c. Liver function studies: values may be elevated

    d. CIWA, revised (CIWA-Ar)

7. **Interprofessional collaboration: Nurse, physician, advanced practice provider, respiratory therapist, pharmacist, dietician, physical therapist, social worker, clergy, case manager**

8. **Management of patient care**

EXPERT TIP

Main pharmacologic treatment for alcohol withdrawal includes benzodiazepines and beta-blocker.

---

    a. Anticipated patient trajectory: With aggressive pharmacologic and nonpharmacologic management, patients undergoing acute alcohol withdrawal/medication/opioid withdrawal should recover without incident. However, in situations of critical illness, mortality may reach 50% for delirium tremens. Life-long counseling and support (e.g., Alcoholics Anonymous) is recommended for patients with an alcohol addiction. Patient does not demonstrate signs or symptoms of withdrawal (e.g., seizures, agitation, irritability) that affect patient, family, and staff safety.

b. Treatments
    i. Nonpharmacologic
        (a) Protect the patient, family, and staff from harm (e.g., use padded bed rails).
        (b) Use a nonthreatening, nonjudgmental supportive approach with the patient.
        (c) Engage the patient in short, directed conversations.
        (d) Decrease stimulation that could precipitate aggressive or violent behaviors.
    ii. Pharmacologic
        (a) Administer medications to a patient who is at risk for withdrawal or who demonstrates withdrawal behaviors
        (b) For alcohol withdrawal, benzodiazepines (give based on results of CIWA-Ar or Severity Assessment Scale) and adjunctive pharmacologic treatment (e.g., thiamine, folate, multivitamins)
        (c) For opioid withdrawal, administer opioid agonists, partial opioid agonists, alpha-2 agonists, baclofen and/or trimethobenzamide (nausea), dicyclomine (abdominal cramps), ibuprofen (pain), passionflower (emotions)
c. Discharge planning
    i. Educate patient on substance misuse/dependence/withdrawal of alcohol and opioids. Patient verbalizes understanding.
    ii. Patient referral to Alcoholics Anonymous for current and future management
    iii. Referral of family members to Al-Anon or Alateen

AGGRESSION AND VIOLENCE

1. **Definition: Aggression is forceful physical or verbal behavior that may or may not cause harm to others. Violence is the ultimate maladaptive coping response and is the acting out of aggression that results in injury to others or destruction of property.**
2. **Etiology and risk factors: Violence in the critical care setting may be triggered by the accumulation of stress in patients or family members who have feelings of desperation and lack coping skills and/or resources to resolve a situation by other means. Aggression and violence can be present with the following:**
   a. Personality disorders
   b. Organic illness
   c. Psychiatric illness
   d. Substance abuse or withdrawal
3. **Signs and symptoms**
   a. Cognitive
       i. Inability to think clearly and rationally
       ii. Paranoia
   b. Behavioral
       i. Anger, yelling, use of profanity
       ii. Agitation
       iii. Pacing (family member)
       iv. Verbal threats
       v. Striking, pushing, kicking of staff
   c. Physiologic
       i. Tachycardia
       ii. Tachypnea
       iii. Increased blood pressure
       iv. Increased muscle tension

4. **Diagnostic study findings**
   a. Mental status examination: To help rule out organic brain disease
   b. Laboratory tests: To rule out metabolic problems
   c. Medication screens: May reveal toxic medication levels, high blood alcohol levels
   d. Interprofessional collaboration: Nurse, physician, advanced practice provider, pharmacist, social worker, clergy, case manager, psychiatrist, psychologist
5. **Management of patient care**
   a. Anticipated patient trajectory: With ongoing support and counseling, patients exhibiting aggressive and/or violent behaviors have the potential to modify these behaviors and live normal lives
   b. Treatments
      i. Nonpharmacologic
         (a) Review medication list and discontinue suspect medications
         (b) Identify and remove other possible causes or stimuli that precipitate aggressive or violent behaviors (e.g., argumentative, challenging family members)
         (c) Involve social service personnel early in the patient's stay, particularly in high-risk situations (e.g., known alcohol abuse in family members)
      ii. Patient issues
         (a) Start with increased communication
         (b) Provide control as much as possible
         (c) Remove offending agents from medication administration record (MAR)
         (d) Assess triggers and communicate to others
         (e) Medication reconciliation
         (f) Patient and family member issues
         (g) Speak in a calm, soft, noncondescending manner
         (h) Allow the patient and family member to vent verbally without interruption
         (i) Focus on the particular incident at hand
         (j) Place clear limits on what will and will not be tolerated—outline the consequences of aggressive or violent behavior
         (k) Do not attempt to educate the patient and family about aggression and violence during the aggressive or violent episode
         (l) Consider a behavioral contract
         (m) Obtain psychiatric consultation as needed
         (n) Administrative discharge according to hospital policy for those who understand the consequences of their actions and continue threatening staff despite behavioral contract

> **EXPERT TIP**
> Violence may be triggered by accumulation of stress.

      iii. Pharmacologic
         (a) Anxiolytics
         (b) Neuroleptics
      iv. Discharge planning
         (a) Discuss strategies for avoiding aggression or violence in the future
         (b) Post-ICU support and psychiatric follow-up may be required
         (c) Refer the individual to anger management classes

SUICIDE

1. **Definition: A suicide attempt is the actual implementation of a self-injurious act with the express purpose of ending one's life. Often patients who have been unsuccessful in their suicide attempt are admitted to the ICU for actual or potential medical problems related to the attempt (e.g., respiratory depression, liver failure following acetaminophen overdose). A patient who has attempted suicide may be admitted to the ICU to determine whether they meet the criteria for brain death.**
   a. In 2019 The Joint Commission (TJC) identified suicide prevention as a National Patient Safety Goal "Reduce the risk for Suicide". This includes assessing individuals for suicidal ideations, links to validated screening tools, to evaluate the environment for risks to attempt suicide and safety at discharge (https://www.jointcommission.org/en/resources/patient-safety-topics/suicide-prevention/).

2. **Etiology and risk factors**
   a. Self-destructive behaviors resulting from a perceived, overwhelming threat to oneself
   b. Important differential diagnoses include unintentional medication overdose or other injury (e.g., gunshot) related to altered mental status, cognitive impairment, or physical disability (visual impairment)
   c. Elder or spousal abuse

3. **Signs and symptoms: May vary markedly depending on the type and extent of the injury present and the time that has elapsed since the injury**
   a. Cognitive and behavioral
   b. Altered level of consciousness and orientation
   c. Severe anxiety (if conscious)
   d. Severe depression (if conscious)
   e. Marked disorientation or confusion
   f. Physiologic (related to the agent used in the suicide attempt, the extent of injury and the time that has elapsed; see Ch. 14, Toxin Exposure)
   g. Medication overdose
      i. Tachycardia (amphetamines)
      ii. Bradycardia (digitalis)
      iii. Tachypnea (salicylates)
      iv. Heart block (beta-blockers and tricyclic antidepressants)
      v. Abnormal heart rhythm (selective serotonin reuptake inhibitors [SSRIs])
      vi. Bradypnea (barbiturates, opiates)
      vii. Dilated pupils (amphetamines)
      viii. Constricted pupils (opiates)
      ix. Serotonin syndrome (SSRIs)
   h. Trauma (gunshot wounds, stabbing, motor vehicle crash)
      i. Cardiovascular involvement: Hypotension, shock
      ii. Pulmonary involvement: Pneumothorax, lung contusions

4. **Diagnostic study findings**
   a. Related to the mechanism of attempted suicide
   b. Elevated liver enzyme levels: Acetaminophen overdose
   c. Abnormal CT scan: Gunshot wound to the head
   d. Abnormal arterial blood gas levels
      i. Metabolic acidosis: Salicylate, methanol overdose
      ii. Respiratory acidosis: Barbiturate, benzodiazepine, and/or opiate overdose
      iii. Respiratory alkalosis: Lower doses of salicylates

   e. Electrolyte abnormalities: Hyperkalemia with digitalis overdose

   f. Abnormal coagulation results (increased international normalized ratio and prothrombin time): Warfarin overdose

   g. Hypoglycemia: Insulin overdose

   h. Medication screens: Urine and blood

5. **Interprofessional collaboration: Nurse, physician, advanced practice provider, pharmacist, social worker, clergy, case manager, psychiatrist, psychologist**

6. **Management of patient care (see Box 2.5 for more information related to the nursing care of the suicidal patient)**

EXPERT TIP

Patients who have been suicidal in the past can live normal lives if they receive treatment, counseling, and support.

---

   a. Anticipated patient trajectory: Outcomes for patients who have attempted suicide vary significantly depending on the mechanism and extent of injury. Many suicidal patients can live normal lives if they receive treatment, counseling and support. Patient remains free from harm.

   b. Treatments (will be specific to the mechanism of injury)

     i. Stabilize the airway, breathing, and circulation.

     ii. Institute specific treatment related to toxin ingestion, wounds (e.g., gastric lavage for medication overdose when indicated). Consult the poison control center.

     iii. Assess the patient's risk for future suicide attempts.

     iv. If the patient is at continued risk for a suicide attempt, provide protection from injury (e.g., constant observation, removal of dangerous items). See TJC standards for the use of physical restraints at http://www.jointcommission.org.

     v. Once the patient's condition has stabilized, allow for opportunities to discuss the attempted suicide and the patient's feelings (e.g., hopelessness, anger, shame, sadness) in a private setting.

     vi. Obtain a mental health consultation (patient's private psychiatrist, staff psychiatrist, or advanced practice nurse).

     vii. Facilitate supervised visits from the patient/family support system (friends, clergy).

     viii. Allow family members to verbalize their feelings and concerns related to the suicide or attempted suicide.

BOX 2.5   Characteristics of Suicidal Patients

- The acute crisis period or high-lethality time is of short duration; it can be counted in hours or days. Suicidal patients are usually ambivalent about dying. At the same time that they plan suicide, they have fantasies of rescue.
- People who commit suicide may have talked about it or may not have talked about it.
- Suicidal persons usually give clues about their intentions.
- Suicidal behavior has no racial, social, religious, cultural, or economic boundaries.
- Suicide has no characteristic genetic qualities; however, its incidence is higher in families in which there have been previous suicides.
- Suicidal behavior does not necessarily mean that the person is mentally ill; in some cases, suicide is viewed as a logical last step by someone who is overwhelmed by stress.
- Most important, directly asking a person about suicidal intent will not cause suicide.

From Bolton, J. M., Gunnell, D., Turecki, G. (2015). Suicide risk assessment in patients with mental illness. *British Medical Journal*, 351(8034), h4978–5012.

c. Discharge planning
  i. Varies depending on patient factors (e.g., physical and psychologic state) and family and social support systems.
  ii. Provide information on a 24-hour suicide prevention hotline.
  iii. Provide phone numbers and websites for illness-specific support services.
  iv. TJC provides resources and recommendations for safety at discharge (https://www.jointcommission.org/en/resources/patient-safety-topics/suicide-prevention/).
d. Ethical issues: Attempted assisted suicide by the patient and family in cases of terminal disease or unbearable chronic condition (see Ch. 1, Professional Caring and Ethical Practice).

DYING PROCESS AND DEATH

1. **Description: Process of dying in the critical care setting can take many forms. Patients may die suddenly as a result of the injury or condition, after a protracted illness, after the withdrawal of life support, or as a result of brain death.**
   a. Care of patients and family members during or following the dying process is heavily influenced by the circumstances surrounding the patient's death.
   b. Kübler-Ross described five psychologic stages of the dying process:
     i. Denial or isolation
     ii. Anger, rage, envy, resentment
     iii. Bargaining
     iv. Depression
     v. Acceptance
2. **Signs and symptoms**
   a. Cardiorespiratory death: Loss of cardiac and respiratory function
   b. Brain death: Lack of brainstem function (see Ch. 5, Neurologic System)
3. **Diagnostic study findings: Most commonly used in the diagnosis of brain death. Studies include EEG, cerebral blood flow studies (see Ch. 5, Neurologic System).**
4. **Collaborative diagnoses of patient needs**
   a. Use of palliative care and end-of-life strategies will help ensure that patient goals for care are met (e.g., does not experience discomfort [pain, shortness of breath, etc.] or anxiety) during the dying process.
5. **Management of patient care (see Ch. 21 Palliative and End-of-Life Care)**
   a. Anticipated patient trajectory: A peaceful death, in the manner desired by the patient and family, is the expected outcome
     i. Treatments: Nonpharmacologic
       (a) Ensure discussions regarding goals of care and advanced care planning are honored.
       (b) Allow the patient and family members to discuss fears and concerns regarding the dying process.
       (c) Allow the patient and family members time to be alone (if desired).
       (d) Use nonpharmacologic methods of pain relief (see Ch. 20, Pain).
       (e) Determine cultural preferences related to the dying process and postmortem care.
       (f) Assist the dying person and his or her family members to validate their feelings (e.g., anger, pain).
       (g) Acknowledge the grieving that accompanies the dying process.
       (h) Help the patient and family to prepare for the dying process by describing possible symptoms and how they can be treated and that they are normal as you are watching it with them to decrease fear.

      (i) Explain the role of pain medication (to relieve pain versus to hasten dying).

      (j) Determine the patient's and family's desires for spiritual support and assist in obtaining support (e.g., notify clergy, etc.). Facilitate spiritual rituals as indicated by faith/culture.

      (k) Allow family members to be present if they choose.

  ii. Role model how to touch the patient, hold hands, wipe brow during dying process.

 iii. Help family to make meaningful connections, talk to the patient, talk about memories, resolve issues that may need resolution.

      (a) Provide family members with bedside activities to engage in during death: Life review, honoring past achievements, wiping brow, handholding.

 iv. Create memories if desired (lock of hair, handprint, electrocardiogram strip) before death.

      (a) Provide patient comfort (e.g., mouth care, positioning, suctioning).

      (b) Assist with withdrawal of life support.

      (c) Clean the patient and the room so that families do not have a last memory of blood or soiled linens.

      (d) Remove unnecessary equipment, dim lights, bring in extra chairs/tissues.

      (e) For do-not-resuscitate patients, turn off any unnecessary alarms, review treatment plan to discontinue medications and treatments that would not provide comfort during impending death. Ask families whether others need to be informed, come in to pay respects. Cue them to remember cultural obligations. "Is there anything we can do for you given your culture or faith?"

  v. Treatment: Pharmacologic

      (a) Pain medication

      (b) Sedatives

      (c) Oxygen therapy

      (d) Diuretics and other agents as needed for patient comfort

 vi. Discharge planning: Bereavement support services for the family after the patient's death

      (a) Return belongings, rings. Leave dentures in the mouth to retain shape of face in the event of open-casket funeral.

References and bibliography information are available at http://evolve.elsevier.com/AACN/corecurriculum/.

CHAPTER

3

Pulmonary System

Daniel N. Storzer, DNP, ACNPC, ACNP-BC, CNRN, CCRN, CCEMT-P, FCCP, FCCM

CROSSWALK

- **Quality and Safety in Nursing Education (QSEN):** Patient-centered care, Teamwork and collaboration, Evidence-based practice, Quality improvement, Safety, Informatics
- **National Patient Safety Goals:** Identify patients correctly, Improve staff communication, Use medicines safely, Use alarms safely, Prevent infection, Identify patient safety risks
- **American Nurses Association (ANA) standards for Professional Nursing Practice:** Standard 1. Assessment, Standard 2. Diagnosis, Standard 3. Outcomes identification, Standard 4. Planning, Standard 5. Implementation, Standard 6. Evaluation, Standard 7. Ethics, Standard 8. Culturally congruent practice, Standard 9. Communication, Standard 10. Collaboration, Standard 11. Leadership, Standard 12. Education, Standard 13. Evidence-based practice and research, Standard 14. Quality of practice, Standard 15. Professional practice evaluation, Standard 16. Resource utilization, Standard 17. Environmental health
- **AACN Scope and Standards for Progressive and Critical Care Nursing Practice:** Standard 1. Quality of practice, Standard 2. Professional practice evaluation, Standard 3. Education, Standard 4. Communication, Standard 5. Ethics, Standard 6. Collaboration, Standard 7. Evidence-based practice/research/clinical inquiry, Standard 8. Resource utilization, Standard 9. Leadership, Standard 10. Environmental health
- **AACN Standards for Establishing and Sustaining Healthy Work Environments (HWE):** Skilled communication, True collaboration, Effective decision-making, Appropriate staffing
- **PCCN content:** Respiratory—All items
- **CCRN content:** Respiratory—All items

SYSTEMWIDE ELEMENTS

ANATOMY AND PHYSIOLOGY REVIEW

1. **Respiratory circuit**
   a. The pulmonary system exists for the purpose of gas exchange. Oxygen (O_2) and carbon dioxide (CO_2) are exchanged across the pulmonary capillary membrane.
   b. Atmospheric O_2 is consumed by the body through cellular aerobic metabolism, which supplies the energy for life.
   c. CO_2, a by-product of aerobic metabolism, is eliminated primarily through lung ventilation.
   d. The respiratory circuit includes all structures and processes involved in the transfer of O_2 between atmospheric air and the individual cell, and the transfer of CO_2 between the cell and atmospheric air.
   e. Cellular respiration cannot be directly measured but is estimated by the amount of CO_2 produced ($\dot{V}CO_2$) and the amount of O_2 consumed ($\dot{V}O_2$).

    f. Exchange of O_2 and CO_2 at the alveolar-capillary level (external respiration) is the ratio of the CO_2 produced to the O_2 taken up per minute.

    g. Proper functioning of the respiratory circuit requires efficient interaction of the respiratory, circulatory, and neuromuscular systems.

    h. In addition to its primary function of O_2 and CO_2 exchange, the lung also carries out metabolic and endocrine functions as a source of hormones and a site of hormone metabolism. In addition, the lung is a target of hormonal actions by other endocrine organs (e.g., surfactant production and potentially activation of bradykinin).

2. Steps in the gas exchange process

    a. *Step 1—Ventilation:* Volume change or the process of moving air between the atmosphere and the alveoli and distributing air within the lungs to maintain appropriate concentrations of O_2 and CO_2 in the alveoli

      i. Structural components involved in ventilation

        (a) Lung

          (1) Anatomic divisions: Right lung (three lobes—upper, middle, lower); left lung (two lobes—upper, lower). Lobes are divided into bronchopulmonary segments (10 right, nine left). Bronchopulmonary segments are subdivided into secondary lobules.

          (2) Lobule: Smallest gross anatomic units of lung tissue; contain the primary functional units of the lung (terminal bronchioles, alveolar ducts and sacs, pulmonary circulation). Lymphatics surround the lobule, keep the lung free of excess fluid, and carry macrophages to remove inhaled particles from distal areas of the lung.

          (3) Bronchial artery circulation: Systemic source of circulation for the tracheobronchial tree and lung tissue down to the level of the terminal bronchiole. Alveoli receive their blood supply directly from the pulmonary circulation.

        (b) Conducting airways: Airways are a series of rapidly branching tubes of ever-diminishing diameter that eventually terminate in the alveoli. The entire area from the nose to the terminal bronchioles where gas flows, but is not exchanged, is called anatomic dead space. Amount is approximately 150 mL but varies with patient size and position.

          (1) Nose

            a) Serves as a passageway for air movement into the lungs

            b) Preconditions air by the mucosal cells and turbinate bones

              1) Warms air to within 2° to 3° F of the body's temperature; humidifies it to full saturation before it reaches the lower trachea

              2) Filters by trapping particles larger than 6 μm in diameter

          (2) Pharynx: Posterior to nasal cavities and mouth

            a) Separation of food from air is controlled by local nerve reflexes

            b) Opening of eustachian tube regulates middle ear pressure

            c) Lymphatic tissues control infection

          (3) Larynx: Complex structure consisting of incomplete rings of cartilage and numerous muscles and ligaments.

            a) Vocal cords: Speech function

              1) Contraction of muscles of the larynx causes the vocal cords to change shape

2) Vibration of the vocal cords produces sound. Speech is a joint function of the vocal cords, lips, tongue, soft palate, and respiration with control by temporal and parietal lobes of the cerebral cortex

3) Glottis: Opening between the vocal cords

b) Valve action by the epiglottis helps to prevent aspiration

c) Cough reflex: Cords close resulting in intrathoracic pressure increases to permit coughing or Valsalva maneuver

d) Cricoid cartilage

1) Only complete cartilage ring

2) Narrowest part of the child's airway

3) Inner diameter sets the limit for the size of an endotracheal tube passed through the larynx

(4) Trachea: Tubular structure consisting of 16 to 20 incomplete, or C-shaped, cartilaginous rings that stabilize the airway and prevent complete collapse with coughing

a) Begins the tracheobronchial tree

b) Warms and humidifies air

c) Mucosal cells trap foreign material

d) Cilia propel mucus upward through the airway

e) Cough reflex present especially at the point of tracheal bifurcation (carina)

f) Smooth muscle innervated by the parasympathetic branch of the autonomic nervous system

g) Carina—the point at which the trachea divides to form the mainstem bronchi

(5) Major bronchi and bronchioles

a) Right mainstem bronchus is shorter and wider than the left

(6) Terminal bronchioles

a) Smooth muscle walls (no cartilage); bronchospasm may narrow the lumen and increase airway resistance

b) Ciliated mucosal cells become flattened with progressive loss of cilia toward the alveoli

c) Sensitive to CO_2 levels: Increased levels induce bronchiolar dilation, decreased levels induce constriction

(c) Gas exchange airways: Semipermeable membrane permits the movement of gases according to pressure gradients. These airways are not major contributors to airflow resistance but do contribute to the ability of the lung to distend. The acinus (terminal respiratory unit) is composed of the respiratory bronchiole and its subdivisions (Fig. 3.1).

(1) Respiratory bronchioles and alveolar ducts

a) Terminal branching of airways

b) Distribution of inspired air

c) Smooth muscle layer diminishes

(2) Alveoli and alveolar bud

a) Most important structures in gas exchange

b) Alveolar surface area is large and depends on body size. Total surface area is about 75 to 80 m² in a normal adult. Thickness of the respiratory membrane is about 0.6 μm. The large surface area

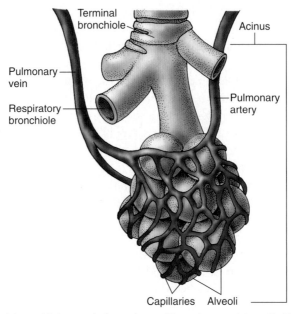

Fig. 3.1 The terminal bronchioles and the acinus. (From Ignatavicius, D. D., Workman, M. L., Blair, M., et al. [2016]. *Medical-surgical nursing: patient-centered collaborative care* 8th ed. St. Louis: Elsevier.)

distributes a large quantity of perfused blood into a very thin film to ensure near equalization of O_2 and CO_2.

   c) Alveolar cells

      1) Type I: Squamous epithelium, adapted for gas exchange, sensitive to injury by inhaled agents, structured to prevent fluid transudation into the alveoli

      2) Type II: Large secretory, highly active metabolically; origin of surfactant synthesis and type I cell genesis

      3) Alveolar macrophages: Phagocytize foreign materials

   d) Pulmonary surfactant

      1) Phospholipid monolayer at the alveolar air-liquid interface; able to vary surface tension with alveolar volume

      2) Enables surface tension to decrease as alveolar volume decreases during expiration, which prevents alveolar collapse

      3) Decreases the work of breathing, permits the alveoli to remain inflated at low distending pressures, reduces net forces causing tissue fluid accumulation

      4) Reduction in surfactant production makes lung expansion more difficult; the greater the surface tension, the greater the pressure needed to overcome it

      5) Surfactant also detoxifies inhaled gases and traps inhaled and deposited particles

   e) Alveolar-capillary membrane (alveolar epithelium, interstitial space, capillary endothelium)

      1) Bathed by interstitial fluid; lines the respiratory bronchioles, alveolar ducts, and alveolar sacs; forms the walls of the alveoli

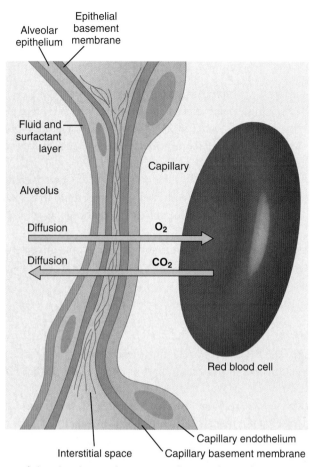

Fig. 3.2 Ultrastructure of the alveolar respiratory membrane, shown in cross section. (From Hall, J. E., Hall, M.E. [2021]. *Guyton and Hall textbook of medical physiology* 14th ed. Philadelphia: Elsevier.)

      2) About 1 μm or less thick (less than one red blood cell); permits rapid diffusion of gases; any increase in thickness, such as from inflammation or fluid accumulation, diminishes gas diffusion

    f) Gas exchange pathway (Fig. 3.2): Alveolar epithelium→alveolar basement membrane→interstitial space→capillary basement membrane→capillary endothelium→plasma→erythrocyte membrane→erythrocyte cytoplasm

ii. Alveolar ventilation ($\dot{V}_A$): That part of total ventilation taking part in gas exchange and, therefore, the only part useful to the body

  (a) Alveolar ventilation is one component of minute ventilation

    (1) Minute ventilation ($\dot{V}_E$): Amount of air exhaled in 1 minute. Equal to exhaled tidal volume (V_T) multiplied by respiratory rate (RR or f). Normal resting minute ventilation in an adult is about 6 L/min:

$$V_T \times RR = \dot{V}_E \left(500 \text{ mL} \times 12 = 6000 \text{ mL}\right)$$

Tidal volume is easily measured at the bedside by handheld devices or a mechanical ventilator. Exhaled minute ventilation is a routinely measured parameter for patients on ventilators.

(2) Minute ventilation is composed of both alveolar ventilation ($\dot{V}_A$) and physiologic dead-space ventilation ($\dot{V}D_{phys}$):

$$\dot{V}_E = \dot{V}D_{phys} + \dot{V}_A$$

where $\dot{V}$ = volume of gas per unit of time
Physiologic dead-space ventilation is that volume of gas in the airways that does not participate in gas exchange. It is composed of both anatomic dead-space ventilation ($\dot{V}D_{ana}$) and alveolar dead-space ventilation ($\dot{V}D_{phys}$).

(3) Ratio of dead space to tidal volume (V_D/V_T) measured to determine how much of each breath does not contribute to gas exchange. Normal values for spontaneously breathing patients range from 20% to 40% of V_T.

(b) Alveolar ventilation is not measured directly; it is inversely related to arterial CO_2 pressure ($PaCO_2$) in a steady state by the following formula:

$$\dot{V}_A = \frac{\dot{V}CO_2 \times 0.863}{PaCO_2}$$

where 0.863 = correction factor for differences in measurement units and conversion to standard temperature [0° C] and pressure [760 torr], dry (STPD)

(c) Because $\dot{V}CO_2$ remains the same in a steady state, measurement of the patient's $PaCO_2$ reveals the status of the alveolar ventilation.

(d) To assess ventilation, $PaCO_2$ must be measured. $PaCO_2$ is the only adequate indicator of effective matching of alveolar ventilation to metabolic demand.

(e) If $PaCO_2$ is low, alveolar ventilation is high; hyperventilation is present

(f) If $PaCO_2$ is within normal limits, alveolar ventilation is adequate

(g) If $PaCO_2$ is high, alveolar ventilation is low and hypoventilation is present

iii. Defense mechanisms of the lung

(a) Although an internal organ, the lung is unique in that it has continuous contact with particulate and gaseous materials inhaled from the external environment. In the healthy lung, defense mechanisms successfully fight against these natural materials by the following means:

(1) Structural architecture of the upper respiratory tract, which reduces deposited and inhaled materials

(2) Processing system including respiratory tract fluid alteration (e.g., increasing secretions) and phagocytic activity

(3) Mucociliary system, which removes material from the lung

(4) Humoral and cell-mediated immune responses, which may be the most important bronchopulmonary defense mechanisms

(b) Loss of normal defense mechanisms may be precipitated by disease, injury, surgery, insertion of an endotracheal tube, or smoking.

(c) Upper respiratory tract warms and humidifies inspired air, absorbs selected inhaled gases, and filters out particulate matter. Normally, no bacteria are present below the larynx.

(d) Inhaled and deposited particles reaching the alveoli are coated by surface fluids (surfactant and other lipoproteins) and are rapidly phagocytized by pulmonary alveolar macrophages.

(e) Macrophages and particles are transported in mucus by bronchial cilia, which beat toward the glottis and move materials in a mucus-fluid layer, eventually to be expectorated or swallowed. Pulmonary lymphatics also drain and transport some cells and particles from the lung.
(f) Antigens activate the humoral and cell-mediated immune systems, which add immunoglobulins (Igs) to the surface fluid of the alveoli and activate alveolar macrophages.
(g) Disruption of or injury to these defense mechanisms predisposes to acute or chronic pulmonary disease.
iv. Structural components of the thorax
(a) Sternum, spine, ribs offer protection
(b) Pleura
(1) Visceral layer next to the lungs
(2) Parietal layer next to the chest wall
(3) Pleural fluid between layers; allows smooth movement of the visceral layer over the parietal layer
(c) Adherence: Pleural space is normally a potential space (vacuum); because of a constant negative pressure (less than atmospheric pressure by 4–8 mm Hg), any change in the volume of the thoracic cage is reflected by a similar change in the volume of the lungs.
(d) Nerve supply: Parietal pleura has fibers for pain transmission, but visceral pleura does not.
v. Lung mechanics
(a) Muscles of respiration: Act of breathing is accomplished through muscular actions that alter intrapleural and pulmonary pressures and thus change intrapulmonary volumes.
(1) Muscles of inspiration: During inspiration, the chest cavity enlarges. This enlargement is an active process brought about by the contraction of the following:
a) Diaphragm: Major inspiratory muscle
1) Normal quiet breathing is accomplished almost entirely by this dome-shaped muscle, which divides the chest from the abdomen
2) Divided into the right and left hemidiaphragms
3) Downward contraction increases the superior-inferior diameter of the chest and elevates the lower ribs
4) Innervation is from the C3 to C5 level through the phrenic nerve
5) Normally accounts for 75% of tidal volume during quiet inspiration
6) Facilitates vomiting, coughing and sneezing, defecation, and childbirth

KEY CONCEPT
Injury at or above C3 to C5 level often leads to ventilator dependency.

b) External intercostal muscles
1) Increase the anterior-posterior (A-P) diameter of the thorax by elevating the ribs
2) A-P diameter is about 20% greater during inspiration than during expiration
3) Innervation is from T1 to T11

  c) Accessory muscles in the neck: Scalene and sternocleidomastoid
    1) Lift upward on the sternum and ribs and increase A-P diameter
    2) Are not used in normal, quiet ventilation
  (2) Muscles of expiration: During expiration, the chest cavity decreases in size. This is a passive act unless forced, and the driving force is derived from lung recoil. Muscles used when increased levels of ventilation are needed are the following:
    a) Abdominals: Force abdominal contents upward to elevate the diaphragm
    b) Internal intercostals: Decrease A-P diameter by contracting and pulling the ribs inward
(b) Pressures within the chest: Movement of air into the lungs requires a pressure difference between the airway opening and alveoli sufficient to overcome the resistance to airflow of the tracheobronchial tree.
  (1) Air flows into the lungs when intrapulmonary air pressure falls below atmospheric pressure.
  (2) Air flows out of the lungs when intrapulmonary air pressure exceeds atmospheric pressure.
  (3) Intrapleural pressure is normally negative with respect to atmospheric pressure as a result of the elastic recoil of the lungs, which tend to pull away from the chest wall. This "negative" pressure prevents the collapse of the lungs.
  (4) Increased effort (forced inspiration or expiration) may produce much greater changes in intrapulmonary and intrapleural pressures during inspiration and expiration.
(c) Resistances
  (1) Elastic resistance (static properties)
    a) The lung, if removed from the chest, collapses to a smaller volume because of lung elastic recoil. This tendency of the lungs to collapse is normally counteracted by the chest wall tendency to expand. Volume of air in the lungs depends on the equal and opposite balance of these forces.
    b) Compliance (C_L) is an expression of the elastic properties of the lung and is the change in volume (ΔV) accomplished by a change in pressure (ΔP):

$$C_L = \frac{\Delta V}{\Delta P}$$

      If compliance is high, the lung is more easily distended; if compliance is low, the lung is stiff and more difficult to distend
  (2) Flow resistance (dynamic properties)
    a) Airway resistance must be overcome to generate flow through the airways.
    b) Changes in airway caliber affect airway resistance. Examples are changes caused by bronchospasm or secretions, as seen in chronic obstructive pulmonary disease (COPD) or asthma.
    c) Flow through the airway depends on pressure differences between the two ends of the tube as well as resistance. Driving pressure for flow in airways is the difference between atmospheric and alveolar pressures.

     (d) Work of breathing

        (1) To minimize the work required to maintain a given level of ventilation, the body automatically changes the respiratory pattern.

        (2) Work performed must be sufficient to overcome the elastic resistance and the flow resistance.

        (3) In diseased states, the workload increases.

  vi. Control of ventilation: Although the process of breathing is a normal rhythmic activity that occurs without conscious effort, it involves an intricate controlling mechanism within the central nervous system (CNS). Basic organization of the respiratory control system is outlined in Fig. 3.3.

     (a) Respiratory generator: Located in the medulla and composed of two groups of neurons

        (1) One group initiates respiration and regulates its rate.

        (2) One group controls the "switching off" of inspiration and thus the onset of expiration.

     (b) Input from other regions of the CNS

        (1) Pons: Input is necessary for normal, coordinated breathing.

        (2) Cerebral cortex: Exerts a conscious or voluntary control over ventilation.

     (c) Chemoreceptors: Contribute to a feedback loop that adjusts respiratory center output if blood gas levels are not maintained within the normal range

        (1) Central chemoreceptors: Located near the ventrolateral surface of the medulla (but are separate from the medullary respiratory center)

          a) Respond to the pH of the extracellular fluid (ECF) surrounding the chemoreceptor and not directly to blood partial pressure of carbon dioxide ($PACO_2$)

          b) Feedback loop for CO_2 is summarized as follows: Increased arterial $PACO_2 \rightarrow$ increased brain ECF $PACO_2 \rightarrow$ decreased brain ECF pH $\rightarrow$ decreased pH at chemoreceptor $\rightarrow$ stimulation of central

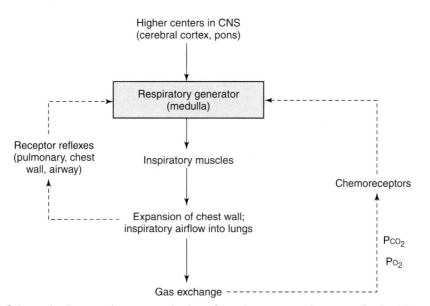

Fig. 3.3 Schematic diagram shows organization of respiratory control system. *Dashed lines* show feedback loops affecting the respiratory generator. *CNS,* Central nervous system; *PCO_2,* partial pressure of carbon dioxide; *PO_2,* partial pressure of oxygen. (From Weinberger, S. E., Cockrill, B. A., Mandel, J. [2019]. *Principles of pulmonary medicine* 7th ed. Philadelphia: Elsevier.)

chemoreceptor → stimulation of medullary respiratory center → increased ventilation → decreased arterial $PACO_2$

(2) Peripheral chemoreceptors: Located in the carotid body and aortic body

　　a) Sensitive to changes in the partial pressure of oxygen (PAO_2) with hypoxemia stimulating chemoreceptor discharge

　　b) Minor role in sensing $PACO_2$

(d) Other receptors

(1) Stretch receptors in the bronchial wall respond to changes in lung inflation

　　a) As the lung inflates, receptor discharge increases

　　b) Contribute to the start of expiration

(2) Irritant receptors in the lining of the airways respond to noxious stimuli, such as irritating dust and chemicals

(3) "J" (juxtacapillary) receptors in the alveolar interstitial space

　　a) Cause rapid shallow breathing in response to deformation from increased interstitial volume because of high pulmonary capillary pressures (such as in heart failure or inflammation)

　　b) Stimulation can also cause bradycardia, hypotension, and expiratory constriction of the glottis

(4) Receptors in the chest wall (in the intercostal muscles)

　　a) Involved in the fine tuning of ventilation

　　b) Adjust the output of the respiratory muscles for the degree of muscular work required

b. *Step 2—Diffusion:* Process by which alveolar air gases are moved across the alveolar-capillary membrane to the pulmonary capillary bed and vice versa. Diffusion occurs down a concentration gradient from a higher to a lower concentration. No active metabolic work is required for the diffusion of gases to occur.

　i. Ability of the lung to transfer gases is called the diffusing capacity of the lung (D_L). Diffusing capacity measures the amount of gas (O_2, CO_2, carbon monoxide) diffusing between the alveoli and pulmonary capillary blood per minute per mm Hg mean gas pressure difference.

　ii. CO_2 is 20 times more diffusible across the alveolar-capillary membrane than O_2. If the membrane is damaged, its decreased capacity for transporting O_2 into the blood is usually more of a problem than its decreased capacity for transporting CO_2 out of the body. Thus the diffusing capacity of the lungs for O_2 is of primary importance.

　iii. Diffusion is determined by several variables:

　　(a) Surface area available for gas exchange

　　(b) Integrity of the alveolar-capillary membrane

　　(c) Amount of hemoglobin (Hb) in the blood

　　(d) Diffusion coefficient of gas, as well as contact time

　　(e) Driving pressure: Difference between alveolar gas tensions and pulmonary capillary gas tensions. This is the force that causes gases to diffuse across membranes.

　　　(1) During the breathing of 100% O_2, the alveolar O_2 tension (PAO_2) becomes so large that the difference between PAO_2 and PvO_2 (mixed venous O_2 tension) significantly increases, proportionately increasing the driving pressure.

　　　(2) Therefore hypoxemia caused solely by diffusion defects is usually improved by breathing 100% O_2

iv.   A–a gradient (PAO_2– PaO_2) is the alveolar to arterial O_2 pressure difference (e.g., the difference in the partial pressure of O_2 in the alveolar gas spaces [PAO_2] and the pressure in the systemic arterial blood [PaO_2]). This gradient is always a positive number.

   (a) Normal gradient in young adults is less than 10 mm Hg (on atmospheric air) but increases with age and may be as high as 20 mm Hg in people over age 60 years.

   (b) A–a gradient provides an index of how efficient the lung is in equilibrating pulmonary capillary O_2 with alveolar O_2. It indicates whether gas transfer is normal.

   (c) Large A–a gradient generally indicates that the lung is the site of dysfunction (except with cardiac right-to-left shunting).

   (d) Normally, A–a gradient increases with age and increased fraction of inspired oxygen (FiO_2)

   (e) Pathologic conditions that increase the A–a gradient (difference) include the following:

      (1) Mismatching of ventilation ($\dot{V}$) to perfusion ($\dot{Q}$) ($\dot{V}/\dot{Q}$ abnormalities)

      (2) Shunting

      (3) Diffusion abnormalities

c. *Step 3—Transport of gases in the circulation*

   i. Oxyhemoglobin dissociation curve (Fig. 3.4)

   (a) Relationship between O_2 saturation (and content) and PaO_2 is expressed in an S-shaped curve that has great physiologic significance. It describes the ability of Hb to bind O_2 at normal PaO_2 levels and release it at lower PAO_2 levels.

   (b) Relationship between the content and pressure of O_2 in the blood is not linear.

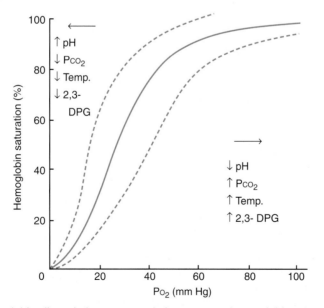

Fig. 3.4 Oxyhemoglobin dissociation curve, relating percent hemoglobin saturation and partial pressure of oxygen (*PAO₂*). Oxygen content can be determined on the basis of hemoglobin concentration and percent hemoglobin saturation. Normal curve is depicted with *solid line*. Curves shifted to right or left (and conditions leading to them) are shown with *broken lines*. *2,3-DPG*, 2,3-Diphosphoglycerate; *PACO₂*, partial pressure of carbon dioxide; *Temp*, temperature. (From Weinberger, S. E., Cockrill, B. A., Mandel, J. [2019]. *Principles of pulmonary medicine* 7ᵗʰ ed. Philadelphia: Elsevier.)

(1) Upper flat portion of the curve is the arterial association portion. Dissociation relationship in this range protects the body by enabling Hb to retain high saturation with O_2 despite large decreases (down to 60 mm Hg) in PaO_2.

(2) Lower steep portion of the curve is the venous dissociation portion. Dissociation relationship in this range protects the body by enabling the tissues to withdraw large amounts of O_2 with small decreases in PaO_2.

(c) Hb O_2 binding is sensitive to O_2 tension. The binding is reversible; the affinity of Hb for O_2 changes as PAO_2 changes.

(1) When PAO_2 is increased (as in pulmonary capillaries), O_2 binds readily with Hb.

(2) When PAO_2 is decreased (as in tissues), O_2 unloads from Hb.

(d) Increase in the rate of O_2 utilization by tissues causes an automatic increase in the rate of O_2 release from Hb.

(e) Shifts of the oxyhemoglobin curve

(1) Shifts to the right: More O_2 is unloaded for a given PAO_2, which thus increases O_2 delivery to the tissues. These shifts are caused by the following:

   a) pH decrease (acidosis), the Bohr effect

   b) $PACO_2$ increase

   c) Increase in body temperature

   d) Increased levels of 2,3-diphosphoglycerate (2,3-DPG). 2,3-DPG is an intermediate metabolite of glucose that facilitates the dissociation of O_2 from Hb at the tissues. Decreased levels of 2,3-DPG impair O_2 release to the tissues. This may occur with massive transfusions of 2,3-DPG–depleted blood and anything that decreases phosphate levels.

(2) Shifts to the left: O_2 is not dissociated from Hb until tissue and capillary O_2 are very low, which thus decreases O_2 delivery to the tissues. These shifts are caused by the following:

   a) pH increase (alkalosis), the Bohr effect

   b) $PACO_2$ decrease

   c) Decrease in body temperature

   d) Decreased levels of 2,3-DPG

   e) Carbon monoxide poisoning

ii. Ability of Hb to release O_2 to the tissues is commonly assessed by evaluating the P_{50}.

(a) P_{50} = the partial pressure of O_2 at which the Hb is 50% saturated, standardized to a pH of 7.40

(b) Normal P_{50} is about 26.6 mm Hg

iii. Each gram of normal Hb can maximally combine with 1.34 mL of O_2 when fully saturated (values of 1.36 or 1.39 are sometimes used).

iv. Amount of O_2 transported per minute in the circulation is a factor of both the arterial O_2 concentration (CaO_2) and cardiac output. This amount reflects how much O_2 is delivered to tissues per minute and is dependent on the interaction of the circulatory system (delivery of arterial blood), erythropoietic system (Hb in red blood cells), and respiratory system (gas exchange) according to the following equations:

(a) O_2 content (CaO_2 is calculated from O_2 saturation, O_2 capacity, and dissolved O_2)

    (1) O_2 capacity is the maximal amount of O_2 the blood can carry. It is expressed in milliliters of O_2 per deciliter (100 mL) of blood (mL/dL) and is calculated by multiplying Hb in grams by 1.34.

    (2) O_2 saturation is the percentage of Hb actually saturated with O_2 (SaO_2 or SvO_2) and is usually measured directly. It is equal to the O_2 content divided by the O_2 capacity multiplied by 100.

    (3) O_2 content is the actual amount of O_2 the blood is carrying (oxyhemoglobin plus dissolved O_2)

$$O_2 \text{ content} = (O_2 \text{ capacity} \times O_2 \text{ saturation}) + (0.0031 \times PaO_2)$$

(b) Systemic O_2 transport

    (1) Normal cardiac output = approximately 5 to 6 L/min (range, 4–8 L/min)

    (2) Normal arterial O_2 content = approximately 20 mL/dL

    (3) Systemic O_2 transport averages about 1000 to 1200 mL/min

v. Focusing only on the O_2 tension of the blood is unwise because an underestimation of the severity of hypoxemia may result. O_2 content and transport are more reliable parameters because they take into account the Hb concentration and cardiac output.

vi. Arterial-mixed venous differences in O_2 content ($CaO_2 - CvO_2$) is the difference between arterial O_2 content (CaO_2) and mixed venous O_2 content (CvO_2) and reflects the actual amount of O_2 extracted from the blood during its passage through the tissues.

    (a) Normal $CaO_2 - CvO_2$ is 4.5 to 6 mL/dL

    (b) Fall in CvO_2 resulting in a rise in the $CaO_2 - CvO_2$ gradient signifies decreased cardiac output and inadequate tissue perfusion if $\dot{V}O_2$ is constant.

    (c) These are average values; actual O_2 utilization is different for different tissues. The heart uses almost all the O_2 it receives.

vii. CO_2 transport: CO_2 is carried in the blood in three forms, as follows:

    (a) Physically dissolved ($PaCO_2$), which accounts for 7% to 10% of CO_2 transported in the blood

    (b) Chemically combined with Hb as carbaminohemoglobin. This reaction occurs rapidly, and reduced Hb can bind more CO_2 than oxyhemoglobin. Thus unloading of O_2 facilitates loading of CO_2 (Haldane effect) and accounts for about 30% of CO_2 transport.

    (c) As bicarbonate (HCO_3^-) through a conversion reaction:

$$CO_2 + H_2O \overset{CA}{\longleftrightarrow} H_2CO_3 \longleftrightarrow H^+ + (\text{Hb buffer}) + HCO_3^-$$

    where CA = carbonic anhydrase

    (1) Reaction accounts for 60% to 70% of CO_2 in the body

    (2) Reaction is slow in plasma and fast in red blood cell owing to the CA enzyme

    (3) When the concentration of these ions increases in red blood cells, HCO_3^- diffuses but H^+ remains

(4) To maintain electrical neutrality, chloride diffuses from the plasma (the "chloride shift")

viii. Pulmonary circulation (pulmonary artery, arterioles, capillary network, venules, and veins)

(a) Pulmonary vessels maintain a delicate balance of flow and pressure distribution that optimizes gas exchange. They are richly innervated by the sympathetic branch of the autonomic nervous system.

(b) Pulmonary circulation is a low-resistance system. Pulmonary arteries have far thinner walls than systemic arteries do, and vessels distend to allow for increases in volume from systemic circulation. Intrapulmonary blood volume increases or decreases of approximately 50% occur with changes in the relationship between intrathoracic and extrathoracic pressure.

(c) Pulmonary arteries accompany the bronchi within the lung and give rise to a rich capillary network within the alveolar walls. Pulmonary veins are not contiguous with the bronchial tree.

(d) Primary function of the pulmonary circulation is to act as a transport system.

(1) Transport of blood through the lung

a) Driving pressure for flow in the pulmonary circulation is the difference between the inflow pressure in the pulmonary artery and the outflow pressure in the left atrium.

b) In the lung, measurement of flow resistance is pulmonary vascular resistance (PVR).

$$PVR = [\text{mean pulmonary artery pressure} - \text{mean left atrial (or pulmonary artery occlusive) pressure}] \div \text{cardiac output}$$

c) About 9% of the total blood volume of the body is in the pulmonary circulation at any given time.

d) Normal pressures in the pulmonary vasculature

1) Mean pulmonary artery pressure: 10 to 15 mm Hg
2) Mean pulmonary venous pressure: 4 to 12 mm Hg
3) Mean pressure gradient: Approximately 10 mm Hg (considerably less than the systemic gradient)
4) Pressures are higher at the base of the lung than at the apex
5) Perfusion is better in the dependent areas of the lung

e) Pulmonary arterial bed constricts in response to hypoxia. Diffuse alveolar hypoxia causes generalized vasoconstriction, which results in pulmonary hypertension. Localized hypoxia causes localized vasoconstriction that does not increase pulmonary hypertension. This localized vasoconstriction directs blood away from poorly ventilated alveoli and thus improves overall gas exchange.

f) Chronic pulmonary hypertension (increased PVR) can result in right ventricular hypertrophy (cor pulmonale).

1) Transvascular transport of fluids and solutes

a) Transvascular fluid filtration in the lung (and all other organs) is described by the Starling equation. This means that fluid and solutes move because of increases or decreases in hydrostatic or osmotic filtration pressures or because of changes in the permeability of vessel walls to fluids or proteins.

   b) Pulmonary edema can result from either a net increase in hydrostatic pressure forces (favoring filtration) or a decreased resistance to filtration.

  2) Endocrine function

   a) All cardiac output passes through the lung before reaching systemic circulation. Pulmonary circulation can influence the composition of the blood supplying all organs.

   b) Several humoral substances are added, extracted, or metabolized in the lung. Examples are inactivation of vasoactive prostaglandins, conversion of angiotensin I to angiotensin II, and inactivation of bradykinin.

 d. *Step 4—Diffusion between the systemic capillary bed and body tissue cells*

  i. Pressure gradients allow for the diffusion of O_2 and CO_2 among systemic capillaries, interstitial fluid, and cells (Figs. 3.5 and 3.6).

  ii. Within the mitochondria of each individual cell, O_2 is consumed through aerobic metabolism. This process produces the energy stored in the bonds of adenosine triphosphate (ATP) and the waste products of CO_2 and water.

3. Hypoxemia: A state in which the O_2 pressure or saturation of O_2 in arterial blood, or both, is lower than normal. Hypoxemia is generally defined as PaO_2 less than 55 mm Hg or SaO_2 below 88% at sea level in an adult breathing atmospheric air. Disorders that lead to hypoxemia do so through one or more of the following processes:

 a. Low inspired O_2 tension

  i. Reduced ambient pressure (P_B) or reduced O_2 concentration of inspired air (FiO_2)

  ii. If the lungs are normal, the A–a gradient will be normal

  iii. Reduced P_B occurs at high altitudes in healthy humans and in enclosed spaces, such as mine cave-ins where fresh air is not replenished; FiO_2 remains normal

 b. Alveolar hypoventilation (increased $PaCO_2$)

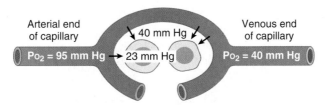

Fig. 3.5 Diffusion of oxygen from a peripheral tissue capillary to the cells. (PAO_2 in interstitial fluid = 40 mm Hg, and in tissue cells = 23 mm Hg.) *PAO_2*, Partial pressure of oxygen. (From Hall, J. E., Hall, M.E. [2021]. *Guyton and Hall textbook of medical physiology* 14th ed. Philadelphia: Elsevier.)

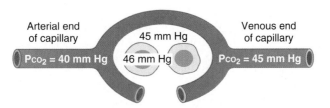

Fig. 3.6 Uptake of carbon dioxide by the blood in the tissue capillaries. ($PACO_2$ in tissue cells = 46 mm Hg, and in interstitial fluid = 45 mm Hg.) *$PACO_2$*, partial pressure of carbon dioxide. (From Hall, J. E., Hall, M.E. [2021]. *Guyton and Hall textbook of medical physiology* 14th ed. Philadelphia: Elsevier.)

    i. Decrease in alveolar ventilation from disorders of the respiratory center, peripheral nerves that supply the muscles of respiration, the respiratory muscles of the chest wall, or the lungs; medications that diminish ventilation

    ii. This causes an increase in $PaCO_2$, which results in a fall in PAO_2 according to the alveolar air equation

    iii. If the lungs are normal, the A–a gradient will be normal. Hypoxemia will improve with ventilation

c. $\dot{V}/\dot{Q}$ mismatch

    i. Most common cause of hypoxemia; A–a gradient increased.

    ii. Ideally, ventilation of each alveolus is accompanied by a comparable amount of perfusion. Fig. 3.7 presents in simplified form the possible relationships between ventilation and perfusion in the lung.

    iii. When $\dot{V}/\dot{Q}$ is decreased (<0.8), a decrease of ventilation in relation to perfusion has occurred. This is similar to a right-to-left shunt because more deoxygenated blood is returning to the left side of the heart. Low $\dot{V}/\dot{Q}$ ratios and hypoxemia occur together, because good areas of the lung cannot be overventilated to

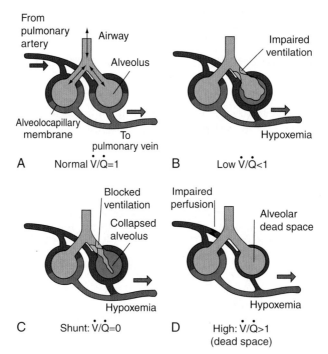

Fig. 3.7 The theoretical respiratory unit with graphic representation of the relationship between ventilation and perfusion in different clinical conditions. **A**, The ideal ventilation-perfusion ratio is $\dot{V}/\dot{Q}$ = 1. **B** and **C**, Lung diseases characterized by a loss of alveolar volume (e.g., acute respiratory distress syndrome) create V/Q ratios that are either low (0 < $\dot{V}/\dot{Q}$ < 1)—shown in **B**—or zero ($\dot{V}/\dot{Q}$ = 0 which is the definition for intrapulmonary shunt)—shown in **C**. Importantly, low $\dot{V}/\dot{Q}$ alveolar units are responsive to oxygen administration (i.e., results in an increase in partial pressure of oxygen [PaO_2]), whereas $\dot{V}/\dot{Q}$ = 0 alveolar units (intrapulmonary shunt) are not responsive to oxygen administration. **D**, High $\dot{V}/\dot{Q}$ units (dead-space ventilation) are created under any circumstances in which pulmonary perfusion is reduced while alveolar ventilation is maintained. Thus any clinical condition that decreases right ventricular output (e.g., full cardiac arrest) or increases pulmonary vascular resistance (e.g., excessive positive end-expiratory pressure) will result in increased dead-space ventilation. (From Hazinski, M. F. [2013]. *Nursing care of the critically ill child* 3rd ed. St. Louis: Elsevier.)

compensate for the underventilated areas. (Hb cannot be saturated to more than 100%.) Atelectasis, pneumonia, and pulmonary edema are clinical examples of intrapulmonary shunt.

iv. When $\dot{V}/\dot{Q}$ is increased (>0.8), a decreased perfusion relative to ventilation exists, the equivalent of dead space or wasted ventilation. Examples of cases in which this occurs are pulmonary emboli and cardiogenic shock.

v. Hypoxemia that is thought to be caused by $\dot{V}/\dot{Q}$ mismatch can be corrected by giving the patient a simple incremental FiO_2 test. For example, if the PaO_2 increases significantly in response to an FiO_2 change from 0.30 to 0.60, the primary problem is low $\dot{V}/\dot{Q}$. If the PaO_2 does not increase significantly, a right-to-left shunt exists.

d. Shunting

i. Shunting occurs when a portion of venous blood does not participate in gas exchange. An anatomic shunt may occur (a portion of right ventricular blood does not pass through the pulmonary capillaries) or a portion of pulmonary capillary blood may pass by airless alveoli.

ii. Normal physiologic shunting amounts to 2% to 5% of cardiac output.

iii. Shunting occurs in arteriovenous malformations, adult respiratory distress syndrome (ARDS), atelectasis, pneumonia, pulmonary edema, pulmonary embolus, vascular lung tumors, and intracardiac right-to-left shunts.

iv. Breathing at an increased FiO_2 level does not correct shunting because not all blood comes into contact with open alveoli, and shunted blood passes directly from pulmonary veins to arterial blood. Lack of improvement of hypoxemia with O_2 therapy is a hallmark of shunting.

v. Usually, shunting does not result in elevated $PaCO_2$, even though shunted blood is rich in CO_2. Brain chemoreceptors sense elevated $PaCO_2$ and respond by increasing ventilation.

vi. Shunting is measured by comparing mixed venous O_2 (from the pulmonary artery catheter) to arterial O_2 ($CaO_2 - CvO_2$). Amount of true shunt can be estimated by having the patient breathe 100% O_2 for 15 minutes, which eliminates the effects of abnormal $\dot{V}/\dot{Q}$ and diffusion defects. Normal shunt is 5 vol% (5 mL/dL).

e. Diffusion defects

i. Seen in patients with a thickened alveolar-capillary membrane, as in pulmonary fibrosis, which enlarges the distance between alveolar gas and the pulmonary capillaries

ii. May be overcome by diffusion because the rate of diffusion always depends on the pressure gradient.

iii. Is rarely a cause of hypoxemia by itself at rest but may contribute to hypoxemia in patients with $\dot{V}/\dot{Q}$ mismatch and/or shunting caused by a disease state or in certain patients during exercise.

4. **Acid-base physiology and blood gases**

a. Terminology

i. Acid: Donor of hydrogen ions (H^+); substance with a pH below 7.0

ii. Acidemia: Condition in which the blood pH is below 7.35

iii. Acidosis: Process (metabolic or respiratory) that causes acidemia

iv. Base: Acceptor of H^+ ions; any substance with a pH above 7.0

v. Alkalemia: Condition in which the blood pH is above 7.45

vi. Alkalosis: Process (metabolic or respiratory) that causes alkalemia

vii. pH: Negative logarithm of the H⁺ ion concentration
(a) Increase in [H⁺] = lower pH, more acidic
(b) Decrease in [H⁺] = higher pH, more alkaline
b. Buffering: Normal body mechanism that occurs rapidly in response to acid-base disturbances to prevent changes in [H⁺].
i. Bicarbonate (HCO_3^-) buffer system

$$[H^+] + HCO_3^- \leftrightarrow H_2CO_3 \leftrightarrow CO_2 + H_2O$$

This system is very important because HCO_3^- can be regulated by the kidneys and CO_2 can be regulated by the lungs.
(a) Normal 22 to 26 mEq/L
ii. Phosphate system
iii. Hb and other proteins
c. Henderson-Hasselbalch equation: Defines the relationship between pH, $PACO_2$, and bicarbonate. Arterial pH is determined by the logarithm of the ratio of bicarbonate concentration to arterial $PACO_2$. Bicarbonate is regulated primarily by the kidney and $PACO_2$ is regulated by alveolar ventilation:

$$pH = pK + \log \frac{[HCO_3^-]}{PaCO_2}$$

where pK = a constant (6.1)
i. As long as the ratio of HCO_3^- to CO_2 is about 20:1, the pH of the blood will be normal. It is this ratio, rather than the absolute values of each, that determines blood pH.
ii. pH must be maintained within a narrow range of normal because the functioning of most enzymatic systems in the body depends on the H⁺ concentration (Fig. 3.8).
d. Normal adult blood gas values (at sea level): Table 3.1.
e. Effect of altitude on blood gas values
i. PaO_2 and SaO_2 are lower at high altitudes because of a lower ambient O_2 tension
ii. Normal for 5280 feet (Denver) = PaO_2 of 65 to 75 mm Hg, SaO_2 of 94% to 95%
f. Respiratory parameter ($PaCO_2$): If the primary disturbance is in the $PaCO_2$, the patient has a respiratory disturbance.
i. $PaCO_2$ is a reflection of alveolar ventilation.
(a) Normal 35 to 45
(b) If increased, hypoventilation is present
(c) If decreased, hyperventilation is present
(d) If normal, adequate ventilation is present
(e) To assess relationships, measurements of both $PaCO_2$ and minute ventilation are needed
ii. Respiratory acidosis (elevated $PaCO_2$, caused by hypoventilation of any etiology may be acute or chronic). Treatment generally consists of improving alveolar ventilation.
(a) Obstructive lung disease, sleep apnea, and other lung diseases resulting in inadequate elimination of CO_2
(b) Traumatic brain injury or sedation from anesthesia or medications affecting respiratory drive
(c) Neuromuscular disorders: Guillain–Barré syndrome

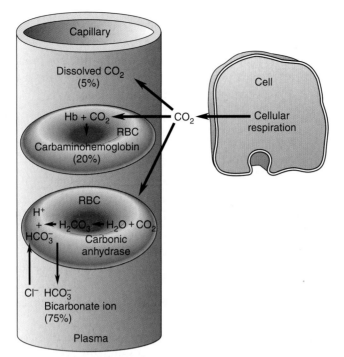

Fig. 3.8 Carbon dioxide (CO_2) is transported in three forms in the blood. Transportation of CO_2 (1) as dissolved gas, (2) as bicarbonate ion (HCO_3^-), and (3) in association with hemoglobin (*Hb*). *RBC*, Red blood cell. (From Banasik, J. L., Copstead, L. E. C. [2019]. *Pathophysiology* 6th ed. St. Louis: Elsevier.)

TABLE 3.1	**Normal Adult Blood Gas Values (at Sea Level)**	
	Arterial	**Mixed Venous**
pH	7.40 (7.35–7.45)	7.36 (7.31–7.41)
PaO_2	80–100 mm Hg	35–40 mm Hg
SaO_2	≥95%	70%–75%
$PaCO_2$	35–45 mm Hg	41–51 mm Hg
HCO_3^-	22–26 mEq/L	22–26 mEq/L
Base excess	−2 to +2	−2 to +2

HCO_3^-, Bicarbonate; $PaCO_2$, partial pressure of carbon dioxide; PaO_2, partial pressure of oxygen; SaO_2, arterial oxygen saturation.
From Kacmarek, R. M., Stoller, J. K., Heuer, A. J. (2019). *Egan's fundamentals of respiratory care* 12th ed. St. Louis: Elsevier.

(d) Pneumothorax, flail chest, or other types of chest wall trauma that interfere with breathing mechanics

(e) Incorrect mechanical ventilator settings

iii. Respiratory alkalosis (low $PaCO_2$) caused by hyperventilation of any etiology. Treatment consists of correcting the underlying cause.

(a) Nervousness and anxiety

(b) Hypoxemia, interstitial lung disease

(c) Excessive ventilation with mechanical ventilator as a response to metabolic acidosis (diabetic ketoacidosis) or from respiratory stimulant medications, such as salicylates, theophylline, catecholamines

(d) Pregnancy

(e) Pulmonary embolus, pulmonary edema

(f) Bacteremia (sepsis), liver disease, or fever

(g) CNS disturbances, such as brainstem tumors and infections

g. Nonrespiratory (renal) parameters (HCO_3^-): If the primary disturbance is in the bicarbonate level, the patient has a metabolic disturbance.

   i. Concentration influenced by metabolic processes

     (a) When HCO_3^- is elevated, metabolic alkalosis results

       (1) Loss of nonvolatile acid

       (2) Gain of HCO_3^-

     (b) When HCO_3^- is decreased, metabolic acidosis results.

       (1) H^+ is added in excess of the capacity of the kidney to excrete it

       (2) HCO_3^- is lost at a rate exceeding the capacity of the kidney to regenerate it

   ii. Causes of metabolic alkalosis (elevated HCO_3^-)

     (a) Chloride depletion (vomiting, prolonged nasogastric suctioning, diuretic therapy)

     (b) Cushing syndrome, hyperaldosteronism, potassium deficiency, renal artery stenosis, licorice ingestion

     (c) Exogenous administration of alkali (massive blood transfusions containing citrate, bicarbonate administration, ingestion of antacids)

   iii. Causes of metabolic acidosis (decreased HCO_3^-)

     (a) Increase in unmeasurable anions (acids that accumulate in certain diseases and poisonings); high anion gap

       (1) Diabetic ketoacidosis, starvation

       (2) Medications: Salicylates, ethylene glycol, methanol alcohol, paraldehyde

       (3) Lactic acidosis resulting from tissue hypoperfusion and subsequent anaerobic metabolism (shock, sepsis)

       (4) Renal failure, uremia

     (b) No increase in unmeasurable anions, normal anion gap

       (1) Diarrhea, ureterosigmoidostomy

       (2) Drainage of pancreatic fluids

       (3) Rapid intravenous (IV) infusion of nonbicarbonate-containing solutions causing a dilutional acidosis

       (4) Certain medications

       (5) Renal tubular acidosis

       (6) Hyperalimentation (causes hyperchloremic acidosis)

h. Compensation for acid-base abnormalities: Physiologic response to minimize pH changes by maintaining a normal bicarbonate to $PACO_2$ ratio

   i. pH returned to near normal by changing component that is not primarily affected.

   ii. Respiratory disturbances result in kidney compensation, which may take several days

     (a) Compensation for respiratory acidosis

       (1) Kidneys excrete more acid

       (2) Kidneys increase HCO_3^- reabsorption

       (3) Compensation is slow (days)

     (b) Compensation for respiratory alkalosis

       (1) Kidneys excrete HCO_3^-

       (2) Compensation is slow (days)

      iii. Metabolic disturbances result in pulmonary compensation, which begins rapidly but takes a variable amount of time to reach maximal levels.
- (a) Compensation for metabolic acidosis
  - (1) Hyperventilation to decrease $PaCO_2$
  - (2) Compensation is rapid (begins in 1–2 hours and reaches maximum in 12–24 hours)
- (b) Compensation for metabolic alkalosis
  - (1) Hypoventilation (limited by the degree of the rise in $PaCO_2$)
  - (2) Compensation is rapid (minutes to hours)

      iv. Body does not overcompensate. The acidity or alkalinity of the pH identifies the primary abnormality if there is only one. Abnormalities may be multiple; each is not a discrete entity. Mixed acid-base disturbances often occur.

  i. Correction of acid-base abnormalities: Caused by a physiologic or therapeutic response
      i. pH returned to normal by altering the component primarily affected; blood gas values are returned to normal
      ii. Correction for respiratory acidosis: Increased ventilation, treatment of cause
      iii. Correction for respiratory alkalosis: Decreased ventilation, treatment of cause
      iv. Correction for metabolic acidosis
- (a) Treatment of underlying cause
- (b) Administration of bicarbonate intravenously or orally (given only under specific circumstances)

      v. Correction for metabolic alkalosis
- (a) Treatment of underlying cause
- (b) Acetazolamide (carbonic anhydrase inhibitor-diuretic) used in certain situations

  j. Arterial blood gas (ABG) analysis
      i. Purpose
- (a) Shows end result of what occurs in the lung
- (b) Confirms the presence of respiratory failure and indicates acid-base status
- (c) Guides the care of patients in acute respiratory failure (ARF) and patients on mechanical ventilation

      ii. Main components: PaO_2, $PaCO_2$, pH, base excess, HCO_3^-, SaO_2, O_2 content, Hb. Both FiO_2 and body temperature must be measured for proper interpretation. It is also essential to know whether HCO_3^- and SaO_2 are directly measured or are calculated.

  k. Guidelines for interpretation of ABG levels and acid-base balance
      i. Examine pH first (Table 3.2)

TABLE 3.2	Analysis of the Acid-Base Balance of an Arterial Blood Gas	
pH	↑	Alkalemia
	↓	Acidemia
$PaCO_2$	↑	Acidemia: pH should be ↓
	↓	Alkalemia: pH should be ↑
HCO_3^-	↑	Alkalemia: pH should be ↑
	↓	Acidemia: pH should be ↓

pH and $PaCO_2$ go in opposite directions; pH and HCO_3^- go in the same direction. HCO_3^-, Bicarbonate; $PaCO_2$, arterial partial pressure of carbon dioxide.

From Kacmarek, R. M., Stoller, J. K., Heuer, A. J. (2019). *Egan's fundamentals of respiratory care* 12th ed. St. Louis: Elsevier.

(a) If pH is reduced (<7.35), the patient is acidemic.

    (1) If $PaCO_2$ is elevated, the patient has respiratory acidosis.

    (2) If HCO_3^- is reduced, the patient has metabolic acidosis.

    (3) If $PaCO_2$ is elevated and HCO_3^- is reduced, the patient has combined respiratory and metabolic acidosis.

(b) If pH is elevated (>7.45), the patient is alkalemic.

    (1) If $PaCO_2$ is decreased, the patient has respiratory alkalosis.

    (2) If HCO_3^- is elevated, the patient has metabolic alkalosis.

    (3) If $PaCO_2$ is decreased and HCO_3^- is elevated, the patient has combined metabolic and respiratory alkalosis.

(c) Expected change in pH for changes in $PaCO_2$: Commonly used rule is that the pH rises or falls 0.08 (or 0.1) in the appropriate direction for each change of 10 mm Hg in the $PaCO_2$.

(d) If the pH is normal (7.35–7.45), alkalosis or acidosis may still be present as a mixed disorder (Box 3.1).

  ii. Assess the hypoxemic state and tissue oxygenation state (Box 3.2)

(a) Arterial oxygenation is considered compromised when Hb saturation is less than 88% (PaO_2 is <55 mm Hg). If the PaO_2 is below 55 mm Hg, hypoxemia is present.

(b) If the patient is receiving supplemental O_2 therapy, PaO_2 values must be interpreted in relation to the FiO_2 delivered. One way involves examination of the two as a ratio (PaO_2/FiO_2). Normal PaO_2/FiO_2 ratio is 286 to 350, although levels as low as 200 may be clinically acceptable.

(c) Excessively high PaO_2 (>100 mm Hg) is generally not necessary and in such cases FiO_2 should be reduced.

(d) Assessment of cardiac output and O_2 transport determines tissue oxygenation. $P\overline{v}O_2$ and $S\overline{v}O_2$ may be useful guides in evaluating the adequacy of overall tissue oxygenation.

(e) Effectiveness of O_2 transport may be judged clinically by examining the patient carefully for mental status, skin color, urine output, and heart rate.

BOX 3.1   Arterial Blood Gas Analysis: Acid-Base Example

MEASUREMENTS

pH: 7.38
$PaCO_2$: 70 mm Hg
HCO_3^-: 32 mEq/L
PaO_2: 65 mm Hg
SaO_2: 92%

ANALYSIS

pH: Normal, but on acidic side
$PaCO_2$: Elevated—acidotic
HCO_3^-: Elevated—alkalotic
Primary disorder is respiratory acidosis (pH is on the acidic side and $PaCO_2$ is elevated).
Secondary disorder is metabolic alkalosis (HCO_3^- is elevated) as compensation.

INTERPRETATION

Compensated respiratory acidosis (e.g., patient with stable chronic obstructive pulmonary disease).

HCO_3^-, Bicarbonate; $PaCO_2$, arterial partial pressure of carbon dioxide; PaO_2, arterial partial pressure of oxygen; SaO_2, arterial oxygen saturation.
From Kacmarek, R. M., Stoller, J. K., Heuer, A. J. (2019). *Egan's fundamentals of respiratory care* 12th ed. St. Louis: Elsevier.

BOX 3.2   Arterial Blood Gas Analysis: Oxygenation Example

MEASUREMENTS

pH: 7.38
$PaCO_2$: 70 mm Hg
HCO_3^-: 32 mEq/L
PaO_2: 65 mm Hg
SaO_2: 92%
CaO_2: 19.0 g/dL
Hb: 18 g/dL
Hct: 54%
On 2 L/min O_2 by nasal cannula, at sea level

ANALYSIS

pH: Normal, not in lactic acidosis from hypoxia
PaO_2: Low but adequate
SaO_2: Low but adequate
CaO_2: Within normal limits
Hb: Elevated
Hct: Elevated

INTERPRETATION

Adequate oxygenation on 2 L/min O_2. Hb/Hct elevated as compensatory mechanism to increase
   O_2-carrying capacity and compensate for underlying lung disease (chronic obstructive pulmonary disease)
producing hypoxemia.

CaO_2, Arterial oxygen concentration; *Hb*, hemoglobin level; *Hct*, hematocrit; HCO_3^-, bicarbonate; $PaCO_2$, arterial partial pressure of carbon dioxide; PaO_2, arterial partial pressure of oxygen; SaO_2, arterial oxygen saturation.
From Kacmarek, R. M., Stoller, J. K., Heuer, A. J. (2019). *Egan's fundamentals of respiratory care* 12th ed. St. Louis: Elsevier.

ASSESSMENT

1. **History: Nursing history follows the sequence and length of the standard history-taking process and is modified as needed for acutely ill patients.**
    a. Patient health history: Patient's interpretation of his or her signs and symptoms and the emotional response to them play a significant role in the development or exacerbation of symptoms, especially as related to dyspnea.
        i. Common symptoms
            (a) Dyspnea: Subjective feeling of shortness of breath or breathlessness
                (1) Difficult to quantify objectively
                    a) Count the average number of words the patient is able to speak between breaths, or whether the patient can speak in full sentences.
                    b) Ask the patient to rate breathing comfort on a visual analog or dyspnea scale from 1 to 10.
                (2) Emotional problems may cause an increased awareness of respirations and complaints of inability to get enough air, despite normal blood gas values.
                (3) Dyspnea caused by increased work of breathing accompanies both obstructive and restrictive lung diseases, as well as the dysfunction of nerves, respiratory muscles, or thoracic cage.
                (4) Question the patient regarding exercise tolerance; some dyspnea with exercise is normal, but a decrease in exercise tolerance is abnormal.

      (5) Assess whether the patient's dyspnea is acute or chronic and whether it has recently increased or decreased. Determine all circumstances under which dyspnea occurs (walking, stair climbing, eating) and how long the patient has experienced dyspnea with those activities.

      (6) Assess orthopnea or dyspnea when the patient is lying flat; ask how many pillows the patient generally uses for sleep and whether for comfort or shortness of breath.

      (7) Assess for paroxysmal nocturnal dyspnea by asking whether dyspnea ever awakens the patient from sleep.

      (8) Determine whether dyspnea is accompanied by other symptoms, such as cough, wheezing, or chest pain.

      (9) In some patients, it is difficult to differentiate cardiac from pulmonary dyspnea.

    (b) Cough: Normal when it occurs as a lung defense mechanism

      (1) Determine whether cough is acute and self-limiting or chronic (lasting more than 6 weeks) and persistent.

      (2) Note any change in character and frequency.

      (3) Determine what the timing is (both daily and seasonal) and whether the cough is accompanied by sputum production, hemoptysis, wheezing, chest pain, syncope, or dyspnea.

      (4) Most common etiologic mechanisms

        a) Inhaled irritants or airway diseases (asthma, bronchitis)

        b) Aspiration or lung diseases (pneumonia, lung abscess, tumor)

        c) Left ventricular failure (pulmonary edema)

        d) Side effect of medications (some angiotensin-converting enzyme inhibitors)

    (c) Sputum production

      (1) Quantify amount by asking how many teaspoons, cups, or shot glasses of sputum are coughed up daily.

      (2) Determine aggravating and alleviating factors.

      (3) Assess the character of the sputum (color, odor, consistency).

      (4) Determine whether current sputum characteristics (quantity and quality) are changed from usual.

    (d) Hemoptysis: Expectoration of blood from the lungs or airways

      (1) Determine whether patient is prescribed antiplatelet or antithrombotic agents.

      (2) Determine whether the material coughed up is grossly bloody blood, streaked, or blood-tinged.

      (3) Try to differentiate from hematemesis. Product of hemoptysis is often frothy, alkaline, and accompanied by sputum; product of hematemesis is nonfrothy, acidic, and dark red or brown with food particles.

      (4) Determine the approximate amount of blood produced in hemoptysis using a reasonable measurement guideline, such as the number of teaspoons or shot glasses per day. Assess whether all expectorated specimens contain blood or whether this is an isolated event.

      (5) Blood may originate from the nasopharynx, airways, or lung parenchyma; blood from these sites remains red because of the contact with atmospheric O_2.

(6) Etiologic mechanisms of hemoptysis fall into three categories by location: Airways, pulmonary parenchyma, and vasculature.
   a) Airways disease: Most common; bronchitis, bronchiectasis, and bronchogenic carcinoma
   b) Parenchymal causes: Often infectious—tuberculosis (TB), *Mycobacterium avium* complex (MAC) including *M. avium* and *M. intracellulare*, lung abscess, pneumonia
   c) Cardiovascular disease: Mitral stenosis, pulmonary embolism (PE), pulmonary edema
   d) Autoimmune disorders: Granulomatosis with polyangiitis, Goodpasture syndrome
(7) Suspect neoplasm if hemoptysis occurs in a patient without prior respiratory symptoms.
   (e) Chest pain: As a reflection of the respiratory system, does not originate in the lung, because the lung is free of sensory nerve fibers
      (1) Chest wall pain: Arises from the parietal pleura, intercostal muscles, ribs, or overlying skin
         a) Well localized
         b) Often exacerbated by deep inspiration
         c) Often reproducible with palpation
      (2) Diaphragm pain: Often caused by an inflammatory process; pain often referred to the ipsilateral shoulder
      (3) Mediastinal pain: Caused by a mass or air in the mediastinum (pneumomediastinum); pain is substernal and dull
   ii. Miscellaneous symptoms of respiratory disease: Postnasal drip, sinus pain, epistaxis, hoarseness, general fatigue, weight loss, fever, sleep disturbances, night sweats, anxiety, nervousness, anorexia
   iii. Past medical history
      (a) Question the patient regarding the presence of any allergy to either medications (herbal, over the counter) or food. Obtain a description of the type and severity of the reaction.
      (b) Determine past instances of the present illness with treatment and outcome. Assess for previous episodes of TB, exposure to TB, or positive TB skin test result or history of abnormal chest x-ray. Assess for childhood lung diseases or infections, such as asthma, pneumonia, and whooping cough. Record the treatment given (if any) and the length of time the patient followed the medication regimen.
      (c) Identify past surgeries or hospitalizations: Dates, diagnosis, and complications; previous use of O_2, steroids, inhalers or nebulizers, or mechanical ventilation.
      (d) Question about previous chest radiographs: Dates, reasons, findings.
      (e) Determine whether any pulmonary function tests were performed previously and the results if known.
b. Family history
   i. Assess for similar illness or signs and symptoms in the patient's parents, siblings, and grandparents.
   ii. Determine the current state of health or cause of death for parents, siblings, and grandparents.

      iii. Find out if there is a family history of diseases, such as asthma, cystic fibrosis, bronchiectasis, and α_1-antitrypsin deficiency (emphysema).

      iv. Determine whether a family member ever had TB with consequent exposure of the patient.

  c. Social history and habits

      i. Personal status: Assess education, socioeconomic class, marital status, general life satisfaction, interests.

      ii. Health habits

        (a) Smoking

          (1) Determine whether the patient is a current or past smoker of cigarettes, cigars, or pipe.

            a) Calculate pack-year history:

$$\text{Number of packs per day} \times \text{Number of years smoked} = \text{Pack} - \text{years}$$

            b) Determine whether the patient has tried to quit and, if so, what methods were used and whether the effort was successful. If the patient is a former smoker, determine the time since the last cigarette; otherwise, determine the desire for information on smoking cessation resources and readiness to quit.

          (2) Ascertain whether the patient has smoked marijuana or another inhaled recreational drugs (e.g., crack cocaine). This includes the use of e-cigarettes and vapor cigarettes. If so, attempt to quantify the amount and frequency of drug use.

          (3) Determine whether the patient chews tobacco. If so, quantify the type chewed and the amount per day.

        (b) Drinking habits: Determine the frequency and amount consumed, and the type of alcoholic and caffeine-containing beverages.

        (c) Eating habits: Assess the quantity of meals (adequacy or excess) and determine whether any respiratory symptoms occur with eating (e.g., meal-induced dyspnea or cough).

        (d) Sexual history: Question about sexual activity tolerance.

      iii. Home conditions: Assess economic conditions, housing quality, presence of any pets and their health, presence of allergens.

        (a) Assess for the use of home hot tubs. If so, determine whether they are cleaned and maintained.

      iv. Occupational history: Assess past and present work conditions.

        (a) Determine whether the patient was exposed to heat and cold, industrial toxins, or pollutants during work or military duty.

        (b) Assess the duration of exposure and the use of protective devices.

      v. History of recent travel

      vi. Immunization status

        (a) Influenza vaccine

        (b) Pneumococcal vaccine

        (c) Hepatitis status

  d. Medication history (prescription and over-the-counter medications, herbal or home remedies)

      i. Determine current and recent medications, dosage, and the reason for prescribing.

      ii. Assess whether the patient is using any inhaled medications.

(a) Identify the device used: Metered-dose inhaler (MDI), nebulizer, or other delivery device.

(b) Assess the frequency of use (i.e., on an as-needed basis or on a regular schedule).

(c) If possible, have the patient demonstrate the technique for inhaling medication. Many patients use an incorrect technique when inhaling their medications, which results in reduced deposition of the medication in the lung and reduced efficacy. Patients should exhale completely, inhale the medication slowly and deeply, and then hold the breath for 10 seconds if possible.

(d) Preferred delivery methods: Powder delivery devices (nonaerosol), MDI with spacer, nebulizer, MDI with open mouth, MDI with closed mouth (least amount of medication delivered).

2. **Physical examination**
   a. Physical examination data
      i. Inspection
         (a) Ensure that the patient is disrobed to the waist and, if possible, seated. Be sure proper steps for maintaining privacy and modesty are taken.
            (1) Warm room and good lighting should be available
            (2) Nurse must have a thorough knowledge of anatomic landmarks and lines (Fig. 3.9)
               a) Manubrium, body, and xiphoid process of the sternum, right and left sternal borders
               b) Angle of Louis, point of maximal impulse, suprasternal notch
               c) Interspaces, ribs, costal margins, costal angle, and spinous processes
               d) Pulmonary lobes and areas of contact with the chest wall (Fig. 3.10)
               e) Lines: Midclavicular, midsternal, anterior-axillary, midaxillary, posterior-axillary, vertebral, and midscapular
         (b) Observe general condition and musculoskeletal development
            (1) State of nutrition, debilitation, evidence of chronic disease
            (2) Pectus carinatum: Sternum protrudes instead of being lower than the adjacent hemithoraces
            (3) Pectus excavatum: Sternum is abnormally depressed between the anterior hemithoraces
            (4) Kyphosis: Exaggerated A-P curvature of the spine
            (5) Scoliosis: Lateral curvature of the spine causing widened intercostal spaces on the convex side and crowding of the ribs on the concave side; when accompanied by kyphosis, it is called kyphoscoliosis. If severe, it can result in restrictive lung disease.
         (c) Observe the A-P diameter of the thorax; normal A-P diameter is approximately one-third the transverse diameter. In patients with obstructive lung disease, the A-P diameter may be as great as or greater than the transverse diameter ("barrel chest").
         (d) Observe the general slope of the ribs.
            (1) Ribs are normally at a 45-degree angle in relation to the spine.
            (2) In patients with emphysema, the ribs may be nearly horizontal.
         (e) Observe for asymmetry
            (1) One side may be larger because of tension pneumothorax or pleural effusion.
            (2) One side may be smaller because of atelectasis or unilateral fibrosis.
            (3) If asymmetry is present, the abnormal side will move less than the normal side.

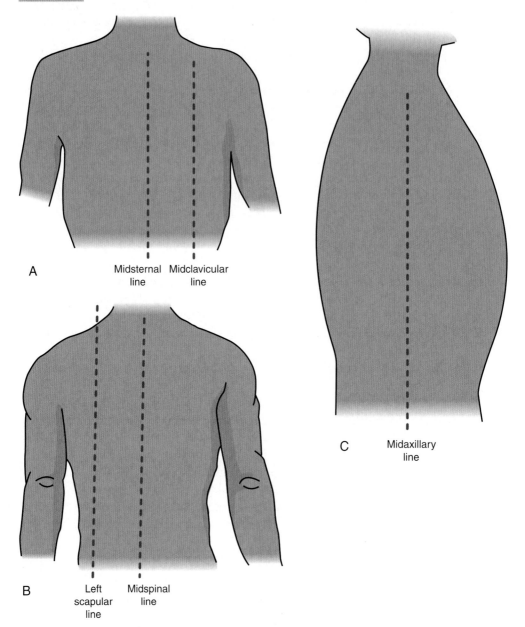

Fig. 3.9 Landmarks of the chest. **A**, Anterior chest wall. **B**, Posterior chest wall. **C**, Lateral chest wall. (Courtesy American Association of Critical-Care Nurses, Aliso Viejo, CA.)

(f) Look for retraction or bulging of the interspaces.
  (1) Retraction of the interspaces, which can be observed during inspiration, indicates more negative intrapleural pressure because of obstruction of the inflow of air or increased work of breathing.
  (2) Bulging of the interspaces may result from a large pleural effusion or pneumothorax, often seen during a forced expiration in patients with asthma or emphysema.
(g) Observe the pattern of ventilation
  (1) Assess the level of dyspnea and the work of breathing.
    a) Position in which the patient can breathe most comfortably. Patients with COPD often assume a forward-leaning position, resting the arms on the knees or a bedside table.

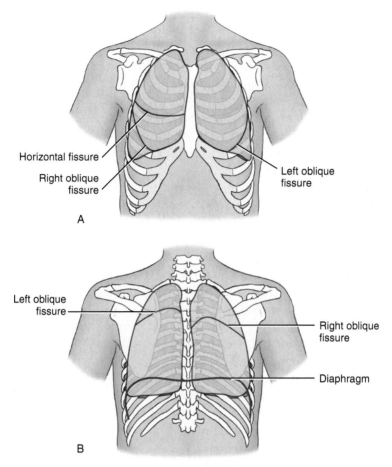

Fig. 3.10 Topographic position of lung fissures on anterior chest (**A**) and posterior chest (**B**). (From Heuer, A. J., Scanlan, C. L. [2018]. *Wilkins' clinical assessment in respiratory care* 8th ed. St. Louis: Elsevier.)

      b) Use of accessory muscles of breathing
      c) Use of pursed-lip breathing
      d) Flaring of the nares during inspiration, a common sign of air hunger, especially in ventilated patients
      e) Paradoxical movement of the diaphragm
  (2) Assess for inspiratory stridor; low-pitched or crowing inspiratory sounds that occur when the trachea or major bronchi are obstructed for one of the following reasons:
      a) Tumor (intrinsic or extrinsic), foreign body
      b) Severe laryngotracheitis, laryngeal edema postextubation, or crushing injury
      c) Goiter, scar, or granulation tissue
  (3) Observe for expiratory stridor; low-pitched crowing sound heard on expiration. Causes include foreign body or intrathoracic, tracheal, or mainstem tumor.
  (4) Observe for unusual movements with breathing; on inspiration, the chest and abdomen should expand or rise together. Paradoxical breathing occurs with respiratory muscle fatigue: on inspiration, the chest rises and the abdomen is drawn in because the fatigued

diaphragm does not descend on inspiration as it should. Instead, the diaphragm is drawn upward by the negative intrathoracic pressure during inspiration.

(5) Observe and assess the ventilatory pattern
   a) Normal, quiet respirations
   b) Bradypnea: Abnormally slow rate of ventilation
   c) Tachypnea: Rapid rate of ventilation
   d) Hyperpnea: Increase in the depth and, perhaps, in the rate of ventilation. Overall result is increased tidal volume and minute ventilation
   e) Apnea: Complete or intermittent cessation of ventilation
   f) Biot's breathing: Two to three short breaths alternating with long, irregular periods of apnea
   g) Cheyne-Stokes respiration: Periods of increasing ventilation, followed by progressively more shallow ventilations until apnea occurs; pattern typically repeats itself. Sometimes occurs in normal persons when asleep, and usually indicates CNS disease, heart failure, or sleep apnea.
   h) Kussmaul respiration: Deep and labored breathing pattern often associated with severe metabolic acidosis. Commonly seen in diabetic ketoacidosis (DKA).
(6) Splinting of respirations: Act of resisting full inspiration in one or both lungs as a result of pain
(7) Flail chest: Inward movement of a portion of the chest on inspiration, usually associated with trauma to the chest; from fracture of the rib cage in two or more sections

(h) Other observations
   (1) General state of restlessness, pain, altered mental status, fright, or acute distress. Earliest signs of hypoxemia often include a change in mental status and restlessness.
   (2) If O_2 is being administered, record the amount (flow in liters per minute), type of device (liquid, compressed gas), and method of delivery (nasal cannula, high flow nasal cannula, oxygen reservoir nasal cannula [Oxymizer] or mask).
   (3) Inspect the extremities
      a) Clubbing of the fingers is a late sign of a chronic pulmonary or cardiac disease.
      b) Cigarette stains on the fingers suggest a current smoking habit.
      c) Lower-extremity edema indicates possible right-sided heart failure from chronic pulmonary disease and hypoxemia-induced pulmonary hypertension.
   (4) Observe for cyanosis
      a) Fundamental mechanism of cyanosis is an increase in the amount of reduced (deoxygenated) Hb in the vessels of the skin caused by one of the following:
         1) Decrease in the O_2 saturation of the capillary blood
         2) Increase in the amount of venous blood in the skin as a result of the dilation of venules and capillaries
      b) Visible cyanosis requires the presence of at least 5 g of reduced Hb per deciliter of blood

1) This is an absolute, not a relative, value. It is not the percentage of deoxygenated Hb that causes cyanosis, but the amount of deoxygenated hemoglobin without regard to the amount of oxyhemoglobin. Presence or absence of cyanosis may be an unreliable clinical sign.

2) In anemia, cyanosis may be difficult to detect because the absolute amount of Hb is too low. Conversely, patients with polycythemia may be cyanotic at higher levels of arterial O_2 saturation than those with normal Hb levels.

  c) Discoloration suggestive of cyanosis may occur in patients with abnormal blood or skin pigments (methemoglobinemia, sulfhemoglobin, argyria).

  d) Factors influencing cyanosis include the rate of blood flow, perfusion, skin thickness and color, the amount of Hb, cardiac output, and the perception of the examiner.

  e) Central versus peripheral cyanosis

1) Central cyanosis implies arterial O_2 desaturation or an abnormal Hb derivative. Both mucous membranes and skin are affected.

2) Peripheral cyanosis without central cyanosis may result from the slowing of perfusion to the tissues (cold exposure, shock, decreased cardiac output). O_2 saturation may be normal.

  f) In carbon monoxide poisoning, O_2 saturation may be dangerously low without obvious cyanosis because carboxyhemoglobin causes the skin to turn a cherry red.

(i) Assess for neck vein distention, neck masses, and enlarged nodes.

(j) Examine the neck, eyelids, and hands for any edema; if present, consider superior vena cava syndrome.

(k) As patients age, the following physical changes may be noted: Flattening of the ribs and diaphragm, decreased chest expansion, use of accessory muscles, marked bony prominences, loss of subcutaneous tissue, pronounced dorsal curve of the thoracic spine, increased A-P diameter relative to lateral diameter, dyspnea on exertion, dry mucous membranes, decreased ability to clear mucus, and hyperresonance from increased distension of the lung.

ii. Palpation

(a) Palpate the thoracic muscles and skeleton, feeling for any of the following: Pulsations, tenderness, bulges, or depressions in the chest wall. In addition, the presence of tactile fremitus is assessed.

(b) Expansion of the chest wall

(1) Examiner's hands should be placed over the lower lateral aspect of the chest, with the thumbs along the costal margin anteriorly or meeting posteriorly in the midline.

(2) Movement of the hands is noted on inspiration and expiration. Asymmetry of movement is always abnormal. Reduced chest wall movement is often seen in patients with barrel chest and emphysema.

(c) Position and mobility of the trachea

(1) Deviations of the trachea toward the defect are seen in atelectasis, pleural effusion, unilateral pulmonary fibrosis, pneumonectomy, hemidiaphragm paralysis, and the inspiratory phase of flail chest.

  (2) Deviation of the trachea to the side opposite the lesion is seen with neck tumors, thyroid enlargement, tension pneumothorax, pleural effusion, mediastinal mass, and the expiratory phase of flail chest.

(d) Point of maximal impulse: Deviates with mediastinal shift.

(e) Palpation of ribs and chest for tenderness, pain, or air in subcutaneous tissue (crepitus).

(f) Vocal fremitus, palpable vibration of the chest wall, produced by phonation

  (1) Patient should be instructed to say the word "ninety-nine" loud enough so that the fremitus can be felt with uniform intensity. Some soft-spoken women may need to falsely lower their voice so that the fremitus can be felt. Examiner should place the hands on the patient's chest wall.

  (2) Diminished fremitus is seen in any condition that interferes with the transference of vibrations through the chest.

   a) Pleural effusion or thickening, pleural tumors

   b) Pneumothorax with lung collapse or emphysema

   c) Obstruction of the bronchus

  (3) Increased fremitus results from any condition that increases the transmission of vibrations through the chest, such as the following:

   a) Pneumonia, consolidation

   b) Atelectasis (with open bronchus)

   c) Pulmonary infarction or pulmonary fibrosis

   d) Secretions with a patent airway

(g) Pleural friction fremitus or rub

  (1) Occurs when inflamed pleural surfaces rub together during ventilation, producing a "grating" sensation that coincides with the respiratory excursion

  (2) May be palpable during both phases of ventilation but sometimes is felt only during inspiration

(h) Rhonchal fremitus (rhonchi)

  (1) Produced by the passage of air through thick exudate, secretions, or an area of stenosis in the trachea or major bronchi

  (2) Unlike friction fremitus, rhonchal fremitus can be relieved by coughing, suctioning, or clearing the secretions from the tracheobronchial tree.

(i) Subcutaneous emphysema: Indicates a leak of air under the skin because of a communication with the airway, mediastinum, or pneumothorax

  (1) Crepitus may be palpated over the area, and on auscultation, may be mistaken for crackles (rales)

EXPERT TIP

Air tends to rise, so examination of the neck and supraclavicular areas are best to locate crepitus.

---

 iii. Percussion

  (a) Nature of the sound produced depends on the density of the structures immediately under the area percussed. Sound vibrations produced by percussion probably do not penetrate more than about 4 to 5 cm below the surface; therefore solid masses deep in the chest cannot be outlined with percussion. In addition, because a lesion must be several centimeters in diameter to be detectable by percussion, only large abnormalities can be located.

(b) Procedure: Accomplished by striking the dorsal distal third finger of one hand, held against the thorax, with the distal tip of the flexed third finger of the other hand

   (1) Striking finger must strike only the stationary finger instantaneously and then be immediately withdrawn.

   (2) All movement is executed at the wrist.

   (3) Examiner must be sensitive to the sounds that are received from the chest wall.

   (4) One side of the chest is compared with the other side.

   (5) Percussion of the posterior chest: Patient flexes the head forward and rests the forearms on the thighs to move the scapulae laterally.

   (6) Percussion begins at the apices and continues downward to the bases, alternating side to side.

(c) Percussion sounds over the lung

   (1) Resonance: Sound heard normally over the lungs

   (2) Hyperresonance: Sound heard over the lungs in normal children, in the apices of the lungs relative to the base in an upright adult, and throughout the lung fields in adults with emphysema or pneumothorax.

      a) Lower in pitch than normal resonance

      b) Relatively intense and easy to hear

      c) Indicates increased air (less dense)

   (3) Tympany: Produced by air in an enclosed chamber; does not occur in the normal chest except below the dome of the left hemidiaphragm, where it is produced by air in the underlying stomach or bowel.

      a) Relatively musical sound

      b) Usually higher-pitched than normal resonance; the higher the tension within the viscus, the higher the pitch

   (4) Dullness: Sound that is heard with lung consolidation, atelectasis, masses, pleural effusion, or hemothorax.

      a) Short, not sustained

      b) Soft, not loud; similar to a dull thud

      c) Indicates that fluid or solid material is in the underlying thorax

      d) Normally heard over the liver and heart

(d) Percussion for diaphragmatic excursion: Range of motion of the diaphragm may be estimated with percussion.

   (1) Instruct the patient to take a deep breath and hold it.

   (2) Determine the lower level of resonance-to-dullness change (the level of the diaphragm) by percussing downward until a definite change is heard in the percussion note.

   (3) After instructing the patient to exhale and hold the breath, repeat the procedure.

   (4) Distance between the levels at which the tone change occurs is the diaphragmatic excursion.

      a) Normal diaphragmatic excursion is about 3 to 4 cm; partial descent of the diaphragm may be caused by weakness or paralysis of the diaphragm or hemidiaphragm. Suspect nerve injury in postoperative patients with these signs following thoracic or spinal surgery.

b) Diaphragm is normally higher on the right than the left.
c) Diaphragm is elevated in conditions that increase intraabdominal pressure (pregnancy, ascites) and conditions that decrease thoracic volume (atelectasis).
d) Diaphragm is fixed and lower than normal in emphysema.
e) It is difficult to differentiate between an elevated diaphragm and a thoracic disease that causes dullness to percussion (e.g., pleural effusion).

iv. Auscultation
   (a) Basic points
      (1) Diaphragm of the stethoscope is more sensitive to higher-pitched tones and is thus best for hearing most lung sounds.
      (2) Place the stethoscope firmly on the chest to exclude extraneous sounds and eliminate sounds that result from light contact with the skin or air. Confusing sounds may be produced by moving the stethoscope on the skin or hair, breathing on the tubing, sliding the fingers on the tubing or chest piece, or listening through clothing.
      (3) Patient should be asked to breathe through the mouth a little more deeply than usual. This minimizes turbulent flow sounds produced in the nose and throat.
      (4) Examiner should always compare one lung to the other by moving the stethoscope back and forth across the chest starting at the top of the thorax and moving downward.
      (5) Listening to the anterior chest will cover the upper and middle lobes; listening to the back covers the lower lobes (see Fig. 3.10).
   (b) Normal breath sounds vary according to the site of auscultation
      (1) Vesicular (always normal)
         a) Soft sounds heard over the anterior, lateral, and posterior chest
         b) Heard primarily during inspiration
      (2) Bronchial (may be normal or abnormal, depending on the location of the sounds)
         a) Heard normally over the trachea
         b) High-pitched, harsh sound with long and loud expirations
         c) When heard over the lung fields, the sound is abnormal and suggests consolidation
      (3) Bronchovesicular (normal or abnormal, depending on the location)
         a) Heard over large bronchi (near the sternum, between the scapulae, over the right upper lobe apex)
         b) Abnormal when heard over the lung fields; signifies consolidation
   (c) Abnormalities of breath sounds
      (1) Absent or diminished sounds caused by decreased airflow (airway obstruction, COPD, muscle weakness, splinting) or increased insulation blocking the transmission of sounds to the stethoscope (obesity, pleural disease or fluid, pneumothorax).
      (2) Bronchial sounds heard over the lung fields suggest consolidation or increased density of lung tissue (e.g., atelectasis, pulmonary infarction, pneumonia, large tumors with no airway obstruction).
   (d) Adventitious sounds: Abnormal sounds that are superimposed on underlying breath sounds.
      (1) Evaluate whether position and coughing affect the sounds

(2) Terminology

    a) Crackles (rales): Signify the opening of collapsed alveoli and small airways

        1) Described as fine or coarse

        2) Heard as small pops or crackles; the sound of fine crackles can be mimicked by rubbing together a few pieces of hair near one's ear. Sound of coarse crackles can be mimicked by pulling open Velcro material

        3) Fine crackles occurring late in inspiration imply conditions that cause restrictive ventilatory defect

        4) Fine crackles heard early in inspiration are often atelectasis, caused by small airway closure

        5) Coarse early inspiratory crackles are associated with bronchitis or pneumonia

    b) Wheeze: Indicates an obstruction to airflow or air passing through narrowed airways

        1) Continuous high-pitched sound with musical quality

        2) Commonly heard during expiration but may be heard during inspiration

        3) Causes: Asthma, bronchitis, foreign body, tumor, pulmonary edema, pulmonary emboli, poorly mobilized secretions

    c) Rhonchi: Result from the passage of air through secretions in the large airways

        1) Low-pitched, continuous sounds

        2) May have a snoring quality when very large airways are involved ("sonorous" wheezes)

        3) Tend to improve or disappear after coughing

    d) Pleural friction rub: Indicates inflammation and loss of pleural fluid

        1) Grating, harsh sound in inspiration and expiration; disappears with breath-holding. Sound can be mimicked by cupping a hand over one's ear and rubbing the fingers of the other hand over the cupped hand.

        2) Heard with pleural infections, infarction, pulmonary emboli, fractured ribs. Located in the area of most intense chest wall pain.

(e) Voice sounds: Spoken words are modified by disease in a manner similar to breath sounds, which results in the increased or decreased conduction of sound.

    (1) Increased conduction occurs when normal lung tissue is replaced with denser, more solid tissue; it is associated with bronchial breath sounds.

        a) Bronchophony: Spoken word (e.g., ninety-nine) is heard distinctly but normal sound is muffled

        b) Egophony: E sound changes to A; sound has the quality of sheep bleating

        c) Whispered pectoriloquy: Whispered sounds are heard with clarity, as if the patient were speaking into the diaphragm of the stethoscope, but normal sound is muffled

    (2) Decreased conduction of sound occurs in the presence of obstructed bronchi, pneumothorax, or large collections of fluid or tissue between the lung and the chest wall

        a) Decreased ability to hear voice sounds

        b) Accompanied by decreased fremitus

b. Monitoring data
  i. Pulse oximetry
    (a) Noninvasive estimate of arterial O_2 saturation (SpO_2) using an infrared light source placed at the finger or other acceptable extremity, forehead, or earlobe
    (b) Uses two principles for measurement
      (1) Spectrophotometry measures the infrared light absorption of Hb (to distinguish saturated from reduced Hb)
      (2) Photoplethysmography uses light to measure the arterial pressure waveforms generated by the pulse (pulse rate and strength) in the capillaries of the tissue at the measurement site
    (c) Pulse oximeters are generally accurate in the SpO_2 range of 70% to 100% but are inaccurate in states of low blood flow (decreased perfusion because of hypovolemia, hypotension, or vasoconstriction).
    (d) SpO_2 accuracy is adversely affected by the following:
      (1) Motion of the extremity (false pulse rate and waveform artifact)
      (2) Light dilution (interferes with the probe's ability to detect the correct light wavelength)
      (3) Abnormal Hb (device cannot distinguish between oxyhemoglobin and carboxyhemoglobin and thus overestimates saturation); methemoglobin may interfere with light absorption
      (4) Some fingernail polish colors (e.g., metallic, dark colors, such as black) interfere with light absorption
      (5) Anemia (Hb level <5 g/dL may result in insufficient signal to process readings)
    (e) Useful for identifying the trend of changes in PaO_2 or when weaning from mechanical ventilation or monitoring the use of analgesia or sedative medications.
    (f) Extreme caution must be exercised not to over-rely on a normal SpO_2 level to indicate normal oxygenation in all cases. Numerous clinical situations (e.g., COPD) may cause erroneous readings. If in doubt, get an ABG.
  ii. SvO_2 monitoring
    (a) Mixed venous oxygen saturation (SvO_2) is monitored in the pulmonary artery at the distal end of a flow-directed thermodilution pulmonary artery catheter.
    (b) Catheter holds an optical module that contains a light-emitting source, a photodetector, and a microprocessor to analyze reflected light.
    (c) Reflectance spectrophotometry is used to differentiate oxygenated blood from deoxygenated blood through light wavelengths in the red and infrared spectra.
    (d) Continuous SvO_2 monitoring allows for assessment of global oxygenation. It can detect cardiopulmonary instability and changes before changes in other hemodynamic parameters (Table 3.3). Some specific indications include the following:
      (1) High-risk cardiovascular surgery, end-stage heart failure, acute myocardial infarction
      (2) Acute hypoxemic respiratory failure (e.g., ARDS, pulmonary embolus)
      (3) Severe burns, multisystem organ failure
      (4) Neurosurgery
      (5) High-risk obstetrics

TABLE 3.3	Factors Associated With Fluctuations in Mixed Venous Oxygen Saturation (SvO$_2$)
Changes	**Causative Factors**
CHANGES THAT DECREASE SvO$_2$	
Decrease in cardiac output	Hypovolemia or cardiac tamponade Shock Myocardial infarction Arrhythmias Increases in positive end-expiratory pressure (PEEP)
Decrease in oxygen saturation	Pulmonary edema Adult respiratory distress syndrome Decrease in inspired oxygen
Decrease in hemoglobin level	Anemia Hemorrhage Dysfunctional hemoglobin
Increase in oxygen consumption	Pain Anxiety or fear Agitation or restlessness Hyperthermia or burns Tachycardia Shivering Activity (positioning, suctioning)
CHANGES THAT INCREASE SvO$_2$	
Decrease in oxygen consumption	Use of analgesics and anesthetics Neuromuscular blockade or use of paralytics Use of β-antagonists Hypothermia Hypothyroidism Sepsis (dysoxia, shunting) Cyanide poisoning Sleep or rest
Increase in oxygen saturation	Increase in fraction of inspired oxygen or hyperoxia Intracardiac shunt or arteriovenous fistula Severe mitral valve regurgitation Distal migration of a pulmonary artery catheter
Increase in cardiac output	Optimal preload Use of positive inotropic agents Use of mechanical-assist devices

From Kacmarek, R. M., Stoller, J. K., Heuer, A. J. (2019). *Egan's fundamentals of respiratory care* 12th ed. St. Louis: Elsevier.

(e) SvO$_2$ reflects the delicate balance between O$_2$ delivery and O$_2$ utilization. Identifying the trend in measurements allows for real-time assessment and intervention. Because of this, the measure can be used for the following:
  (1) Evaluate the adequacy of tissue oxygenation.
  (2) Detect adverse changes in O$_2$ delivery and O$_2$ consumption or impaired tissue oxygenation.
  (3) Evaluate the effectiveness of interventions to improve the balance between O$_2$ delivery and consumption including administration of fluids or medications and the use of mechanical assistance (e.g., intraaortic balloon pump [IABP], positive end-expiratory pressure [PEEP]).
  (4) Evaluate the effects of routine medical and nursing procedures on tissue oxygenation (Figs. 3.11 and 3.12).
  (5) Diagnose intracardiac shunting, cardiac tamponade.

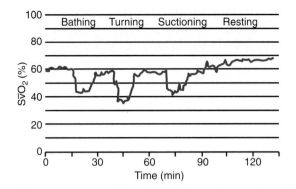

Fig. 3.11 Effects of routine nursing procedures (bathing, turning, and endotracheal suctioning) on mixed venous oxygen saturation ($S\bar{v}O_2$). (From Jesurum J: $S\bar{v}O_2$ monitoring. In Chulay, M., Gawlinski, A., editors. (1998). *Hemodynamic monitoring protocols for practice*. Aliso Viejo, CA: American Association of Critical-Care Nurses. Used with permission.)

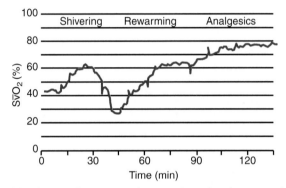

Fig. 3.12 Effects of shivering, active rewarming, and analgesics on mixed venous oxygen saturations ($S\bar{v}O_2$) after cardiac surgery. (From Jesurum J: $S\bar{v}O_2$ monitoring. In Chulay, M., Gawlinski, A., editors. (1998). *Hemodynamic monitoring protocols for practice*. Aliso Viejo, CA: American Association of Critical-Care Nurses. Used with permission.)

        (6) Assist in the differential diagnosis of pathologic conditions.
     (f) Normal SvO_2 value is 70%.
        (1) Values lower than 60% may indicate either inadequate delivery of O_2 or increased O_2 consumption (e.g., decreased Hb level, decreased SaO_2, decreased cardiac output, an increase in tissue metabolic demands).
        (2) Values higher than 80% may indicate either increased O_2 delivery or decreased O_2 demand (e.g., increased cardiac output, decreased metabolic demand, reduced ability of the cells to use oxygen).
     (g) Accuracy of SvO_2 monitoring may be affected by the following:
        (1) Blood pH and hematocrit level
        (2) Blood flow characteristics and blood temperature (including the flow of IV fluid past the catheter tip)
        (3) Motion artifacts because of catheter "whip" against the vessel wall
   iii. End-tidal CO_2 monitoring
     (a) Noninvasive sampling and measurement of exhaled CO_2 tension at the patient-ventilator interface.

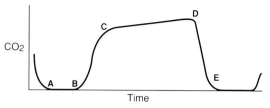

Fig. 3.13 Normal capnogram. **AB**, Beginning exhalation, dead space; **BC**, initial alveolar empty-ing; **CD**, end-alveolar emptying; **D**, end-tidal carbon dioxide (CO_2); **E**, inspiration (CO_2-free gas). (From Odom-Forren. [2018]. *Drain's perianesthesia nursing* 7th ed. St. Louis: Elsevier.)

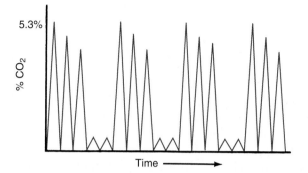

Fig. 3.14 Representative capnogram demonstrating Cheyne-Stokes breathing. (From Cairo, J. M. [2020]. CO_2, carbon dioxide. *Pilbeam's mechanical ventilation* 7th ed. St. Louis: Elsevier.)

  (b) Devices (capnographs) typically use infrared analysis of respired gas using different light wavelengths to measure the absorption of CO_2 molecules.

    (1) Requires either a simple transducer or a tubing connection to the ventilator circuitry, which is then tied into a standard hemodynamic pressure monitoring module or, by ventilator electronic interface, directly into a physiologic monitoring system.

    (2) Displayed airway pressure tracings can be helpful in identification of patient-ventilator dyssynchrony, assessment of the inspiratory work of breathing, and detection of auto-PEEP.

  (c) Graphic display of exhaled CO_2 generated during the ventilatory cycle (Fig. 3.13).

  (d) Provides both numerical and graphic display of CO_2 waveform on a breath-by-breath basis or at a slower speed for identification of trends (Fig. 3.14)

    (1) Normal speed shows the phases of CO_2 elimination

    (2) Slow speed shows trends over minutes to hours

  (e) $PaCO_2$ to postapneic end-tidal carbon dioxide pressure ($PetCO_2$) gradient is 1 to 4 mm Hg (normal $\dot{V}/\dot{Q}$ matching is assumed in the lungs); in critically ill patients, the gradient may exceed 20 mm Hg.

  (f) Application is limited for reliably predicting changes in alveolar ventilation except in patients with normal pulmonary perfusion and $\dot{V}/\dot{Q}$ ratios.

  (g) Measurement of $PetCO_2$ depends on adequate blood flow to the lungs to eliminate CO_2.

  (h) Gradual narrowing of the gradient over time represents improved ventilation-perfusion matching, decreased CO_2 production, or decreased pulmonary perfusion.

(i) Increased gradient may indicate hypoventilation, increased production of CO_2 (e.g., in fever, seizures), or absorption of CO_2 from an outside source. Rapid rise in the gradient may indicate malignant hyperthermia.

(j) Sudden drop to a low level indicates incomplete sampling, possibly because of a system leak or partial air obstruction; a zero value indicates a disconnect in the system.

(k) Pulse oximetry assesses oxygenation only; $PetCO_2$ measurement for monitoring ventilation in patients undergoing deep sedation or undergoing resuscitation efforts and may be useful to detect changes over time in other patients, even those not on ventilators. End-tidal carbon dioxide pressure ($ETCO_2$) also used to confirm a tracheal intubation after the procedure.

iv. Blood gas analysis
   (a) Acid-base balance (pH, $PaCO_2$, HCO_3^-)
   (b) Oxygenation status (PaO_2, SaO_2, CaO_2)

v. Respiratory (ventilator) waveform analysis (Fig. 3.15)
   (a) Provides real-time information to assess changes in lung mechanics over time. Less useful in high-frequency or oscillation ventilation modes.
   (b) Visual representation of respiratory waveforms is available with most ventilators.
      (1) Volume mode: Volume is preset, pressure varies with patient compliance and resistance
      (2) Pressure mode: Pressure is preset, volume varies
   (c) Pressure-time waveforms
      (1) Used to assess the following:
         a) Ventilator mode
         b) Patient-ventilator synchrony
         c) Inspiratory attempts in heavily sedated or paralyzed patients
         d) End expiration for hemodynamic monitoring
      (2) Positive pressure or upward stroke is the ventilator breath.
      (3) Negative deflection is from the patient's spontaneous breathing (or attempts).

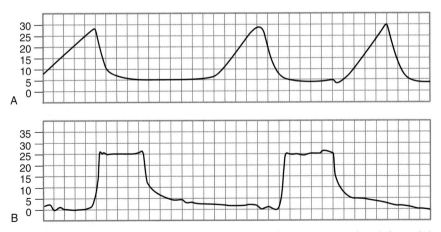

Fig. 3.15 Pressure-time waveforms. **A**, Pressure-time waveform indicating breakthrough breathing (*arrow*) on a patient receiving neuromuscular blockade. **B**, Pressure-time waveform of pressure support ventilation. All breaths have square pressure configuration. (From Good, V., Kirkwood, P. [2018]. *Advanced critical care nursing* 2nd ed. St. Louis: Elsevier.)

(4) Volume breath waveform starts at zero or the preset PEEP, builds gradually, looks like a shark fin (Fig. 3.15A).

(5) Pressure waveform shows a constant pressure, a characteristic "square wave" (Fig. 3.15B).

(6) Modes of ventilation can be identified through the waveform signature (Fig. 3.16).

(7) Patient-ventilator synchrony

    a) Normal ratio of inspiration to expiration is 1:2 or 1:3

    b) Flow rate can be adjusted faster or slower to match the patient's need

    c) Inadequate flow rate is identified by a "scooped-out" appearance on the inspiratory waveform

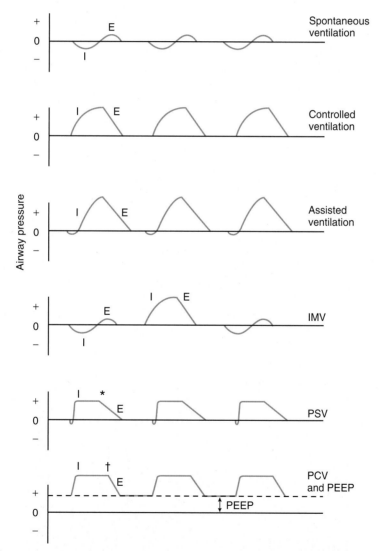

Fig. 3.16 Airway pressure during spontaneous ventilation and during mechanical ventilation with several different ventilatory patterns. *E*, Expiration; *I*, Inspiration; *IMV*, intermittent mandatory ventilation; *PCV*, pressure-controlled ventilation; *PEEP*, positive end-expiratory pressure; *PSV*, pressure support ventilation. *Inspiratory positive-pressure support ceases when the patient's flow rate falls below a threshold level. †The relative timing of inspiration and expiration is controlled by physician-determined ventilator settings. (From Weinberger, S. E., Cockrill, B. A., Mandel, J. [2019]. *Principles of pulmonary medicine* 7ᵗʰ ed. Philadelphia: Elsevier.)

(8) Auto-PEEP occurs when expiration is not long enough to empty the lungs. If auto-PEEP is present, the baseline pressure will rise when an end-expiratory hold maneuver is performed.

(d) Flow-time waveforms (Fig. 3.17)

    (1) Used to assess auto-PEEP and patient response to therapy

    (2) Volume breath: Flow of gas is constant throughout the breath; referred to as a square-flow waveform.

    (3) Pressure breath: Flow is higher at the beginning and slower at the end; referred to as a decelerating flow pattern.

    (4) Spontaneous breaths: Decelerating but more rounded.

    (5) Auto-PEEP is identified when the expiratory waveform does not reach baseline.

    (6) Bronchospasm reduces expiratory flow. If therapy is effective, expiratory flow will be faster and reach baseline more quickly.

(e) Pressure-volume and flow-volume loops

    (1) Pressure-volume loops: Pressure and volume are plotted on different axes; result looks like a loop (Fig. 3.18)

        a) Spontaneous breaths show negative movement (to left of graph) on inspiration, positive movement (to right) on expiration

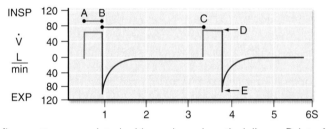

Fig. 3.17 Square flow pattern associated with a volume breath delivery. Points A-B and C-D represent inspiration. The expiratory limb of the waveform is below the baseline. The peak expiratory flow is indicated by E. Units are liters per minute. *EXP, INSP* (From Good, V., Kirkwood, P. [2018]. *Advanced critical care nursing* 2nd ed. St. Louis: Elsevier.)

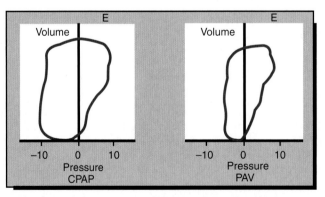

Fig. 3.18 Pressure-volume loop changes comparing continuous positive airway pressure (*CPAP*) with proportional assist ventilation (*PAV*) and showing inspiration (I) and expiration (E). PAV reduces the work of breathing (WOB). Inspiratory WOB is the area within the loop to the left of the vertical axis. Expiratory WOB is the area within the loop to the right of the vertical axis. (From Cairo, J. M., Philbeam, S.P. [2010]. *Mosby's respiratory care equipment* 8th ed. St. Louis: Elsevier.)

      b) Ventilator breaths (volume and pressure) have loops that go counterclockwise on the right (positive) side of the graph; the lower portion shows inspiration; the higher portion shows expiration

      c) Monitor resistance and compliance over time

         1) Increased compliance shifts the slope to the right and down

         2) Increased resistance produces a bow-shaped inspiratory curve

   (2) Flow-volume loops plot flow and volume on different axes. Expiratory portion of the loop helps assess the effectiveness of bronchodilator therapy.

      a) Allows continuous monitoring of waveforms integrated with hemodynamic monitoring

      b) Useful as a backup to monitor system disconnects

      c) Zeroing should occur with initial setup and any disconnection

      d) Damping of the waveform occurs with fluid in the tubing or leaks; check for disconnects and leaks, clear the tubing by flushing with an air-filled syringe

3. Appraisal of patient characteristics: Patients with acute, life-threatening pulmonary problems may present in critical care units with an array of clinical findings that represent the highest priority of patient needs. Their clinical course may resolve quickly, slowly, or not at all. Examples of clinical attributes that the nurse should assess when caring for a patient with an acute respiratory disorder are the following: resiliency, vulnerability, stability, complexity, resource availability, participation in care and decision-making, and predictability.

DIAGNOSTIC STUDIES

  a. Laboratory

    i. Sputum examination

     (a) Obtain a specimen through voluntary coughing and expectoration, induction of sputum by inhalation of an aerosol, nasotracheal or endotracheal suctioning, transtracheal aspiration, or bronchoscopy.

     (b) Assess characteristics: Compare to the patient's normal state

       (1) Color and consistency: Green—*Pseudomonas* infection; yellow—bacterial infection; rust colored—pneumococcal infection

       (2) Volume: More than 25 mL/day is excessive

       (3) Odor: Should be odorless

         a) Foul smell may indicate an anaerobic process

         b) Musty odor may indicate *Pseudomonas* infection

       (4) Microscopic examination

         a) Cytologic study for malignant cells

         b) Smear for examination for bacteria or fungi

         c) Sputum cultures to diagnose infection and assess medication resistance

         d) Stains on cultures for mycobacteria (acid-fast bacilli), *Pneumocystis jiroveci*, *Legionella pneumophila*

    ii. Pleural fluid examination

     (a) Diagnostic thoracentesis is performed to obtain a specimen.

     (b) Determine if the fluid is a transudate or an exudate based on the protein and lactate dehydrogenase (LDH) levels in the pleural fluid compared with the blood

     (c) Examine specimen for cell counts, protein and LDH levels, glucose level, amylase level, and pH; Gram staining for bacteria is performed; cytologic analysis for malignant cells and microorganisms is conducted

        (d) Biopsy of parietal pleura may be performed
- iii. Skin tests
  - (a) Type I hypersensitivity (mediated by IgE): To pollens, molds, grass
  - (b) Type II hypersensitivity (mediated by T lymphocytes): Purified protein derivative testing for TB
  - (c) Fungal diseases
  - (d) As controls to assess anergy: Mumps, *Candida* infection
- iv. Serologic tests determine the causative pathogen in bacterial, viral, mycotic, and parasitic diseases
  - (a) Quantiferon Gold test commonly used to test for TB in addition to skin testing

b. Radiologic
- i. Chest radiograph precedes all other studies
  - (a) Posteroanterior and lateral views most common
  - (b) Portable anteroposterior views are obtained in progressive and critical care settings when the patient cannot be moved. These radiographs are generally of lesser quality than an erect posteroanterior film for the following reasons:
    - (1) Difficulty in positioning the patient
    - (2) Short film distance from the chest; variable distances in serial films
    - (3) Less powerful x-ray generator; interference from attached tubes, lines, equipment
  - (c) Lateral decubitus views are used if fluid levels need to be identified (as with pleural effusions and abscesses).
  - (d) Oblique views may be used to localize lesions and infiltrates.
  - (e) Lordotic views are used to evaluate the apical portion of the lung and the middle lobe or lingula and can help determine whether a lesion is anterior or posterior.
  - (f) Expiratory films are used for visualizing pneumothorax or air trapping.
- ii. Computed tomography (CT) scan
  - (a) To scan axial cross sections of the body
  - (b) Particularly useful in detecting subtle differences in tissue density. Gives better definition of small or questionable lesions; particularly useful for determining whether a lesion has calcification. Also used to in the detection of pulmonary embolus.
  - (c) High-resolution CT (HRCT) for three-dimensional images of the lung to detect a pattern of emphysema, progression of fibrosis
- iii. CT pulmonary angiogram: Visualizes the pulmonary arterial tree through the injection of radiopaque dye
  - (a) Risk of acute kidney injury or allergic reaction from the radiopaque dye
- iv. Ventilation-perfusion lung scanning
  - (a) Involves injection or inhalation of radioisotopes; performed to obtain information on pulmonary blood flow and ventilation
  - (b) Can detect pulmonary emboli and assess regional lung function preoperatively
  - (c) Less specific in patients with underlying pulmonary disease
- v. Ultrasonography
  - (a) Useful in evaluating pleural disease
  - (b) Can detect small amounts of pleural fluid and loculations within the pleural space
  - (c) Can distinguish fluid from pleural thickening

   (d) Can localize the diaphragm and detect disease immediately below it, such as a subphrenic abscess
   (e) Not useful for defining structures or lesions within the pulmonary parenchyma (the ultrasonic beam penetrates air poorly)
   (f) Used to monitor during special procedures—catheter or chest tube insertion, bronchoscopy, thoracentesis
 vi. Fluoroscopy
   (a) Shows the movement of pulmonary structures and the diaphragm. Used to determine diaphragm function.
   (b) Exposure of the patient to radiation is greater during fluoroscopy than during a standard radiographic examination.
 vii. Pulmonary angiography: Visualizes the pulmonary arterial tree through the injection of radiopaque dye.
   (a) Useful to investigate thromboembolic disease of the lung, congenital circulatory abnormalities, masses.
   (b) Some risks; dangerous to perform in pulmonary hypertension; O_2 desaturation has occurred in some patients with the injection of contrast medium. Hemodynamic parameters should be measured before the procedure.
 c. Pulmonary function tests: Box 3.3 and Fig. 3.19.
 d. Bronchoscopy: Insertion of a fiberoptic scope into the airways for direct visualization and possible obtaining of specimens.
   i. Indicated for diagnosis of lung malignancy, evaluation of hemoptysis, removal of foreign body or secretions, and sampling of lung tissue via washings, brushings, or biopsy.
   ii. After the procedure, the patient must be observed for respiratory depression (because of sedatives), decreased ventilation, and hypoxemia.
   iii. Supplemental O_2 is administered during the procedure.
   iv. If transbronchial biopsy is performed, hemoptysis or pneumothorax is a possible complication.

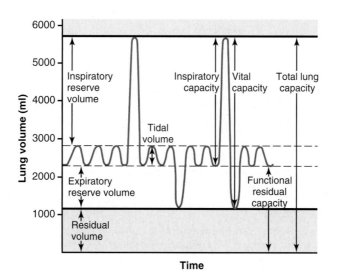

Fig. 3.19 A diagram showing respiratory excursions during normal breathing and during maximal inspiration and maximal expiration. (From Hall, J. E., Hall, M.E. [2021]. *Guyton and Hall textbook of medical physiology* 14th ed. Philadelphia: Elsevier.)

BOX 3.3 Pulmonary Function Tests

PURPOSE

- Classify pulmonary function as normal or exhibiting a restrictive or obstructive defect.
- Describe disease early and in physiologic terms.
- Follow the patient in quantitative terms for future comparisons.
- Assist in evaluation of the risk of surgery.

LUNG VOLUMES AND CAPACITIES

- Measured with the patient in the upright position; values obtained are compared with predicted values
- Volumes: There are four discrete and nonoverlapping lung volumes:
    1. Tidal volume (V_T): Volume of gas inspired and expired during each respiratory cycle
    2. Inspiratory reserve volume (IRV): Maximal volume of gas that can be inspired after a tidal breath is taken
    3. Expiratory reserve volume (ERV): Maximal volume of gas that can be expired from the end-expiratory position
    4. Residual volume (RV): Volume of gas remaining in the lungs at end of a maximal expiration
- Capacities: There are four capacities, each of which includes two or more of the primary volumes:
    1. Total lung capacity (TLC): Volume of gas contained in the lung at the end of a maximal inspiration

$$TLC = V_T + IRV + ERV + RV$$

    2. Vital capacity (VC): Maximal volume of gas that can be expelled from the lungs following a maximal inspiration

$$VC = V_T + IRV + ERV$$

    3. Inspiratory capacity (IC): Maximal volume of gas that can be inspired from the resting expiratory level

$$IC = V_T + IRV$$

    4. Functional residual capacity (FRC): Volume of gas remaining in the lungs at resting end expiration

$$FRC = ERV + RV$$

VENTILATORY MECHANICS

- Provide information about dynamic lung function. Subjects perform forced breathing maneuvers.
- Forced expiratory spirograms
  FVC: Forced vital capacity; reduced in restrictive disease or in obstructive disease if there is air trapping
  FEV_t: Forced expiratory volume in t (seconds); usually measured at 0.5, 1, and 3 seconds. Reduced in obstructive disease. Most useful measurements are FEV_1 and FEV_6.
  $FEV_1/VC\%$: Forced expiratory volume at 1 second as a percentage of vital capacity. Evaluates obstruction to flow. FEV_1/VC: Normally >75% in adults.
  FEF: Forced expiratory flows ($FEF_{25\%-75\%}$, $FEF_{75\%-85\%}$). These tests assess flows over a range of lung volumes.
  Values for timed flow studies are decreased out of proportion to vital capacity in obstructive disease
- Flow-volume loop studies: Volume and flow during inspiration and expiration are graphically plotted. Obstructive disease produces abnormal flow-volume loops; restrictive disease produces normal-appearing but smaller flow-volume loops.
- Maximum voluntary ventilation (MVV)
    - Volume of air ventilated with maximal effort over a short period of time
    - May be used to predict the patient's ability to undergo procedures that require ventilatory reserve (e.g., surgery, extubation)

LUNG COMPLIANCE STUDIES

- Assess the distensibility of the lungs; lung compliance (C_L) is the reciprocal of elastance
- Expressed as the increase in volume (V) per increase in transpulmonary pressure (P)

$$C_L = \frac{\Delta V}{\Delta P}$$

BOX 3.3   **Pulmonary Function Tests—cont'd**

- Static compliance (C_{st}) is measured in the absence of airflow.
  - In the patient on a ventilator, it is measured by dividing VT by the plateau pressure (minus positive end-expiratory pressure [PEEP]) and is called the *effective static compliance*.
  - Normal values are around 100 mL/cm H_2O.
- Dynamic compliance (C_{dyn}) is measured under conditions of flow
  - In patients on a ventilator, it is measured by dividing V_T by the peak inspiratory pressure (minus PEEP) and is called the *effective dynamic compliance*.
  - Normal range is between 40 and 50 mL/cm H_2O.
- Compliance is decreased in conditions that make the lungs or thorax stiffer or reduce expansibility. Such conditions include atelectasis, pneumonia, pulmonary edema, fibrotic changes, pleural effusion, pneumothorax, kyphoscoliosis, obesity, abdominal distention, flail chest, and splinting because of pain.
- Increases in compliance occur with age or emphysema.
- Compliance curves (serial changes in volume plotted against changes in pressure) are useful in monitoring patients on volume ventilators. Determinations of the best pressure-volume combinations for the patient may be made. Comparisons of static and dynamic pressure-volume curves help determine which component (airway, lung, or chest wall) is contributing to changes in compliance.

GAS TRANSFER AND EXCHANGE STUDIES

- Blood gas and acid-base analysis
  - Fundamental to the diagnosis and management of pulmonary problems
  - See Physiologic Anatomy
- Diffusing capacity (D_L)
  - Measures the amount of functioning alveolar-capillary surface area available for gas exchange
  - Values decrease with ventilation-perfusion mismatching and membrane problems and with decreases in pulmonary capillary blood volume.

GUIDELINES FOR INTERPRETATION OF PULMONARY FUNCTION TEST RESULTS

- Values are compared with predicted values for age, height, and gender.
- Restrictive pulmonary impairment generally results in decreased volumes and capacities.
- Decreased static lung compliance suggests parenchymal disease.
- Obstructive defect generally results in decreased values on tests of dynamic ventilatory function. This change may be reversible with the use of bronchodilators.
- Chronic obstructive pulmonary disease with long-term air trapping and destruction of parenchyma results in increased FRC, RV, and TLC.
- Patient preparation and cooperation are necessary to obtain reliable and valid data for most pulmonary function tests.

From Hyatt, R. E., Scanlan, P. D., Nakamura, M. (2014). *Interpretation of pulmonary function tests* 4th ed. Philadelphia: Lippincott Williams & Wilkins.

---

    e. Lung biopsy
       i. Needle biopsy can diagnose malignancy or infection; pneumothorax may be a complication. Approach may be percutaneous or bronchoscopic.
      ii. Open lung biopsy requires a thoracotomy or thoracoscopic examination but has better diagnostic yields.
    f. Mediastinoscopy is performed for the diagnostic exploration of the mediastinum and to obtain biopsy specimens.

PATIENT CARE

1. Inability to establish or maintain a patent airway.
    a. Description of problem: Blocked airway caused by physiologic or mechanical obstruction and the inability of the patient to clear or maintain the airway. Clinical findings vary with the degree of obstruction and include abnormal breath sounds, altered respiratory rate or depth, cough, cyanosis (late), and dyspnea.

b. Goals of care
   i. Airway patency is maintained
   ii. Breath sounds are clear with no adventitious sounds
   iii. Secretions are easily expectorated or suctioned
c. Interprofessional collaboration: Nurse, physician, advanced practice provider, respiratory therapist.
d. Interventions
   i. Assist the patient to deep breathe
      (a) Position to maximize inspiratory muscle length and to maximize ventilation (Semi-Fowler's to high Fowler's position, depending on patient comfort).
      (b) Ask the patient to take slow, deep breaths; assess volume (e.g., functional residual capacity [FRC] to total lung capacity [TLC]); ask the patient to hold the breath several seconds.
      (c) Provide the patient with cues or devices to motivate independent deep-breathing exercises (e.g., incentive spirometer).
   ii. Position the patient to facilitate coughing
      (a) Help the patient assume a comfortable cough position (high Fowler's), with knees bent and a lightweight pillow over the abdomen to augment the expiratory pressures and minimize discomfort.
      (b) Teach the patient alternate cough techniques (controlled cough, the forced expiratory technique known as "huff cough" or quad-assist cough). For controlled cough, the patient takes a slow maximal inspiration, holds the breath for several seconds, and follows with two or three coughs. Huff cough consists of one or two forced exhalations (huffs) from middle to low lung volumes with the glottis open.
      (c) Guaifenesin (an expectorant) may help liquefy secretions
   iii. Provide an artificial airway and ventilation if indicated.
      (a) Oropharyngeal airway
         (1) Purpose: Maintains the airway by holding the tongue anteriorly in an unconscious patient
         (2) Technique: Correct size measures from the corner of the patient's mouth to the angle of the jaw following the natural curve of the airway. Rotate the airway 180 degrees before insertion. As the tip of the airway reaches the hard palate, rotate the airway again by 180 degrees, aligning it as before in the pharynx.
         (3) Contraindications: Do not use in a conscious patient because it may stimulate the gag reflex and cause vomiting.
         (4) Complications: Vomiting and aspiration with an intact gag reflex; malpositioning because of improper length; worsening of obstruction by pushing the tongue back further into the pharynx because of incorrect placement
      (b) Nasopharyngeal airway
         (1) Purpose: Useful when an oral airway cannot be used; more readily tolerated than the oropharyngeal airway
         (2) Technique: Generously lubricate the tip of the airway with water soluble lubricant. Gently guide the tip posteriorly and toward the ear, along the nasal passage until the flange rests on the nostril opening.
         (3) Contraindications: Patients on anticoagulant therapy, prone to epistaxis, facial trauma, suspected basilar skull or cribriform plate fracture

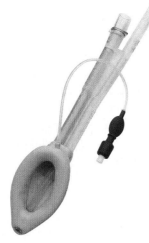

Fig. 3.20 Laryngeal mask airway. (From Hagberg, C. A. [2018]. *Hagberg and Benumof's airway management* 4th ed. Philadelphia: Elsevier.)

       (4) Complications: Nosebleed, nasal mucosa irritation
       (5) Adequate lubrication before insertion and humidification is essential to ensure the patency of a narrow lumen
       (6) Airway is intended for short-term use only

KEY CONCEPT
Do not use a nasopharyngeal airway in the trauma patient if there is a risk of skull fracture.

    (c) Cricothyrotomy: Restricted to extreme emergencies when other methods fail or are unavailable. Incision must be made through the cricothyroid membrane.
    (d) Laryngeal mask airway (Figs. 3.20 and 3.21)
       (1) For use by experienced, trained providers only—usually an anesthesiologist or certified registered nurse anesthetist (CRNA)
       (2) Can be used with spontaneous respirations or mechanical ventilation
       (3) Laryngeal mask airway sits tightly over the larynx
       (4) Disadvantages: Suctioning is difficult, may not prevent aspiration, the patient may dislodge it if agitated
    (e) Laryngeal tube can be inserted blindly through the oropharynx into the hypopharynx to create an airway for ventilation. Can be used as an alternative airway device for medical personnel who are not experienced in tracheal intubation.
    (f) Endotracheal intubation: Box 3.4 and Fig. 3.22.
    (g) Tracheostomy
       (1) Purpose and indications
          a) To facilitate removal of secretions from the tracheobronchial tree
          b) To decrease dead-space ventilation
          c) To bypass an upper airway obstruction or provide an alternate airway
          d) To aid in patient comfort when assisted or controlled ventilation is needed for an extended period of time

(2) Principles of care

    a) Stoma is kept clean and dry

    b) Frequency of inner cannula tube exchanges with disposable tubes and of routine cleaning of inner cannulas with reusable inner cannulas follows hospital or institutional guidelines.

       1) Be prepared for complications during any cleaning procedure

       2) Keep the following equipment at the bedside:

          a) Self-inflating manual resuscitation bag and mask

          b) Suction equipment (include catheters, O_2 flow meter, tubing)

          c) Intubation materials

          d) Tracheal tube and stoma cleaning supplies

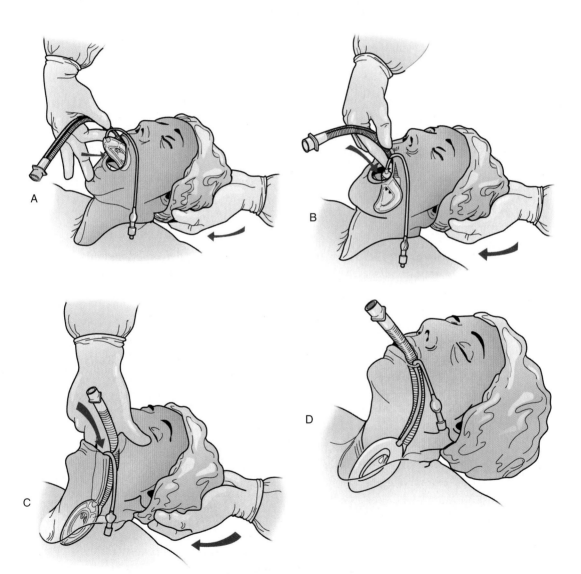

Fig. 3.21 Placement of laryngeal mask airway (LMA). **A**, The LMA is held like a pencil and inserted into the open mouth with only the slightest neck extension. **B**, The LMA is directed posteriorly and down to the oropharynx. **C**, The LMA is advanced with the opposite hand and guided into the posterior pharynx. **D**, The final location of the LMA after correct placement. (From Cairo, J. M. [2018]. *Mosby's respiratory care equipment* 10th ed. St. Louis: Elsevier.)

BOX 3.4   Endotracheal Intubation and Extubation

KEY PRINCIPLES FOR INTUBATION

- Thorough training and retraining in this procedure are absolute necessities for competency.
- Preoxygenate with 100% O_2 for 3 to 5 minutes if possible.
- Check for correct placement of the tube after insertion.
  1. Feel air movement through the tube opening.
  2. Assess for bilateral chest excursion during inspiration and expiration.
  3. Auscultate over epigastrium and lung bases and apices for bilateral breath sounds.
  4. Attach a disposable end-tidal CO_2 detector-monitor or esophageal balloon to confirm lung versus esophagus placement.
  5. Obtain a chest radiograph (gold standard); tip of the tube should be about 2 to 3 cm above the carina.
  6. Provide manual ventilation using a self-inflating resuscitation bag connected to a 100% O_2 source set at 10 to 15 L/min.

Nasotracheal Intubation

- Sometimes used when the oral route is not available
- Risk of paranasal sinusitis, as well as bleeding is increased
- Should not be used if the patient has a bleeding abnormality or on anticoagulant therapy

Nursing Care Considerations for the Intubated Patient

- Provide frequent mouth care including dental care (every 2–4 hours).
- Suction the mouth and pharynx every four hours.
- Check the placement of the tube immediately after insertion, each shift and after tube position adjustments.
- Carefully secure the tube to prevent movement and to decrease tracheal damage.
- Provide adequate humidity regardless of whether nasal or oral intubation is used.
- Assess the oral mucosa each shift and move oral tubes from side to side when necessary. Note and document the centimeter marking on the tube at the teeth or gum line as a reference point (21 cm for women and 23 cm for men is common).
- Be aware that infection may result from contaminated equipment or nonsterile procedures. Suction equipment and tubing should be changed at least every 24 hours.
- Suction as required according to the patient's need, not at a routine interval. Use a sterile technique.
  1. Use either a single-use or closed-suction catheter system, depending on hospital policy.
  2. Provide presuctioning and postsuctioning oxygenation (with each pass of the suction catheter) with three to five deep inflations of 100% O_2 for 30 seconds using either the manual two-handed technique or the manual demand breath by ventilator.
  3. Keep the duration of suctioning brief (no more than 1 second) to minimize the amount of O_2-containing air that is evacuated from the lungs; apply suction only when withdrawing the catheter.
  4. Monitor the electrocardiogram for arrhythmias during and after suctioning; observe for changes in O_2 saturation by pulse oximetry if available.
  5. Observe and document the amount and type of secretions.

Tracheal Tube Cuffs

- Cuff design characteristics
  - Low sealing pressure; intracuff pressure should not exceed the capillary filling pressure of the trachea ($\leq$25 cm H_2O or $\leq$20 mm Hg) to avoid tracheal mucosal injury.
  - Cuff pressure is distributed over a large contact area.
- Large volumes of air are accepted with minor increases in balloon tension.
  - Provides sufficient pressure to maintain an adequate seal during inspiration and expiration (necessary to allow positive pressure ventilation and the use of positive end-expiratory pressure [PEEP]). Also may help prevent pulmonary aspiration of large food particles but does not protect against aspiration of liquids, such as water and enteral formula feedings.
  - Does not distort tracheal wall
- Low-pressure, high-volume cuffs generally meet the desired characteristics and have replaced low-residual-volume, high-pressure cuffs.
- Principles of cuff inflation and deflation
  - Inflation of low-pressure cuffs: Most cuffs are sufficiently inflated with less than 10 mL of air.
  - Need for increasing amounts of air to obtain a seal may be caused by tracheal dilation or to a leak in the cuff or pilot balloon valve; the condition should be corrected
  - Routine deflation is not necessary. Periodic deflation may be useful so that the patient can breathe around the tube to facilitate speech (often difficult to accomplish when the patient is receiving mechanical ventilation).

Continued

BOX 3.4   Endotracheal Intubation and Extubation—cont'd

KEY PRINCIPLES FOR EXTUBATION

- Extubation will depend on whether or not the underlying patient condition that led to the need for intubation has improved or reversed to the extent that the artificial airway is no longer necessary. Generally accepted criteria for extubation include the following:
  - Hemodynamic stability
  - Patient is able to protect airway
  - Patient is able to clear secretions

Assess Readiness for Extubation

- Ventilatory parameters or measurements (such as presence of cuff leak, maximum inspiratory pressure and negative inspiratory force, spontaneous tidal volume, minute ventilation, rapid shallow breathing index, and vital capacity within acceptable limits)

Postextubation monitoring

1. Reassess oxygenation and ventilation status within 30 minutes after extubation or sooner as indicated.
2. Observe for laryngospasm. Auscultate the trachea with a stethoscope for stridor and breathing difficulties. Treatment may consist of racemic epinephrine inhalation, administration of steroids to reduce laryngeal edema, and possibly reintubation.
3. Postextubation stridor may occur immediately or take several hours to develop.
4. Monitor the patient's tolerance of extubation by clinical observation, auscultation of breath sounds, measurement of arterial blood gas levels, observation for stridor, and ventilatory measurements.
   - Racemic epinephrine administered via small volume nebulizer; intent is to reduce subglottic edema by inhalation of a potent vasoconstrictor

Hoarseness

- Common following either short-term or long-term endotracheal intubation
- Usually disappears during the first week

Aspiration

- Aspiration of food, saliva, or gastric contents if the swallowing mechanism is impaired
- Presence of the tube over extended periods results in a loss of the usual protective reflexes of the larynx
- Monitor the patient carefully during feedings; watch for excessive coughing; start with clear liquids after tube removal

Difficulty Removing Tracheostomy Tube

- More frequently seen in infants but occurs in adults as well
- Related to the narrow lumen of the trachea, which is further reduced by swelling

LATE POSTEXTUBATION COMPLICATIONS

Fibrotic Stenosis of the Trachea

- Caused by prolonged use of any tube with a rigid inflatable cuff
- Follows earlier ulceration and necrosis of the site
- Lesions may become advanced before the appearance of clinical evidence (dyspnea, stridor); a tracheoesophageal fistula may form
- Prevented by the use of low-pressure cuffs and proper monitoring of cuff pressures

Stenosis of the Larynx

- Caused by the discrepancy between the anatomy of the larynx and the size and shape of the tube
- Treatment
- Dilation or surgical intervention
- Permanent tracheostomy

3) Have an extra tracheostomy tube of the same size and type at the bedside; keep a tube obturator at the bedside in case the tube must be reinserted emergently.

4) Be prepared to intubate or otherwise support ventilation.

c) Uncuffed tubes are commonly used in children and adults with laryngectomies and are sometimes used during decannulation or weaning (progressive downsizing of tube).

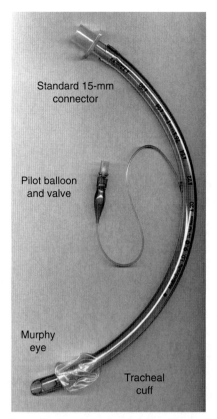

Standard 15-mm connector

Pilot balloon and valve

Murphy eye

Tracheal cuff

Fig. 3.22 The components of a cuffed endotracheal tube. (From Cairo, J. M. [2018]. *Mosby's respiratory care equipment* 10ᵗʰ ed. St. Louis: Elsevier.)

      d) Cuffed tubes are used when the patient is receiving mechanical ventilation (Fig. 3.23). Tube may have an air-filled or self-inflating foam cuff, depending on the brand.

      e) Suctioning is always a sterile procedure except at home, where a clean technique may be used.

  (3) Weaning from the tracheostomy tube

      a) Criteria (see discussion of extubation criteria in Box 3.4)

      b) Patient must demonstrate physiologic and psychologic independence from an artificial airway. Techniques include the use of the following:

        1) Cuff deflation periods with the tube opening capped to allow breathing through the upper airway

        2) Tracheostomy button

        3) Fenestrated tube with the cuff inflated or deflated with the external tube opening capped or occluded to permit airflow to be directed to the upper airway

        4) Progressive downsizing of the tube from the original size to a smaller one

      c) Patient is monitored carefully to see how weaning is tolerated; blood gas studies as needed and clinical observations are used.

      d) Complete sealing of the tracheotomy incision may occur within 72 hours of extubation. Patients cannot produce adequate coughing pressure until this is accomplished.

  iv. Prevent complications of airway intubation: Box 3.5.

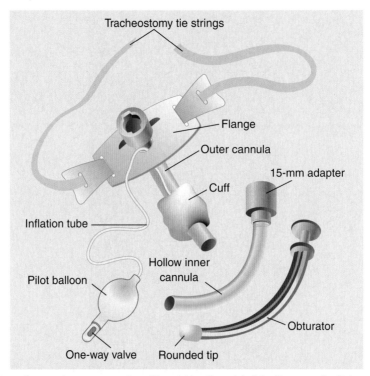

Fig. 3.23 Parts of a tracheostomy tube. (From Harding, M. M., Kwong, J., Roberts, D., et al. [2020]. *Lewis's medical-surgical nursing: assessment and management of clinical problems* 11th ed. St. Louis: Elsevier.)

BOX 3.5 Prevention of Complications of Airway Intubation

PHYSIOLOGIC ALTERATIONS CAUSED BY AIRWAY DIVERSION

- Supplemental humidification of inspired gases is required to help thin secretions and prevent irritation of delicate pulmonary membranes.
- Endotracheal tubes prevent effective coughing and removal of secretions because of eliminating the glottis from the air route preventing the development of increased intrathoracic pressures, which makes effective coughing difficult.
- Accumulated oral secretions and bacteria provide a good medium for bacterial growth and may precipitate ventilator-associated pneumonia.
- Bypassing the larynx produces aphonia

COMPLICATIONS DURING PLACEMENT OF THE AIRWAY

Endotracheal Tube

- Mucous membrane disruption and tooth damage or dislodgment
- Right mainstem bronchial intubation; tube must be repositioned immediately
  - Decreased or absent breath sounds on the left side
  - Decreased arterial partial pressure of oxygen (PaO_2) or arterial O_2 saturation by pulse oximetry (SpO_2)
  - Arrhythmias, including pulseless electrical activity
  - Shift of the trachea to the left (late)
- With the nasotracheal route, one may see the following:
  - Nosebleed
  - Submucosal dissection
  - Introduction of a polyp or plug from the nose into the lungs, which results in infection or obstruction
  - Sinusitis

BOX 3.5   Prevention of Complications of Airway Intubation—cont'd

Tracheostomy and Cricothyrotomy

Percutaneous tracheostomy is now commonly performed at the bedside.
- Mediastinal emphysema
- Hemorrhage
- Pneumothorax
- Cardiac arrest
- Damage to adjacent structures in the neck

COMPLICATIONS OCCURRING WHILE THE TUBE IS IN PLACE

Obstruction Because of
- Plugging with secretions. This is entirely preventable by systemic hydration and proper use of humidification and suctioning.
- Herniation of the cuff over the end of the tube
- Kinking of the tube
- Cuff overinflation

Displacement or Dislodgement

Displacement or dislodgement out of the trachea (endotracheal or tracheostomy tube) and inadvertent movement into a false passage or pretracheal space (tracheostomy tube)
- Especially hazardous during the first 3 to 5 days of tracheostomy. Avoid by using a tube of the proper length and fixing it securely to the patient. Although securing the tube is important, care of the stoma and surrounding skin to prevent skin breakdown or pressure sores from the tube neck plate is also important.
- Dislodgement out of the trachea into tissue causes mediastinal emphysema, subcutaneous emphysema, and pneumothorax. Diagnosis is determined by observation of reduced or absent airflow movement from the tube opening, deterioration in blood gas values and/or vital signs, observations of neck and local tissue swelling with crepitations by palpation, poor chest excursion and respiratory distress, and inability to pass a suction catheter properly through the tube.
- Low tube placement into one bronchus or at the level of the carina results in obstruction or atelectasis of the nonventilated lung. Check the placement of the endotracheal tube by auscultation, followed by radiographic examination or use of a fiberoptic scope.
  - Displacement into one bronchus: Signs and symptoms are as follows:
    - Decreased or delayed motion on one side of the chest
    - Unilateral diminished breath sounds
    - Excessive coughing
    - Localized expiratory wheeze
  - Placement at the level of the carina: Signs and symptoms are as follows:
    - Excessive coughing
    - Localized expiratory wheeze
    - Difficulty in introducing the suction catheter
    - Bilateral diminished breath sounds

Other Complications
- Poor oral hygiene; mouth care is absolutely essential.
- Local infection of tracheostomy wound, tracheal tissue, or lungs; tracheostomy should be treated as a surgical wound and specimens for culture should be obtained if active infection is suspected.
- Massive hemorrhage resulting from erosion of the tracheostomy tube into the innominate vessels; may be fatal. Occurs most often with low placement of the tube, excessive rubbing of the tube within the trachea, or pulling torsion on the tube; watch for pulsations moving the tube with the heartbeat.
- Disconnection between the tracheal tube and ventilator
  - Most likely to occur when the patient is being turned.
  - All ventilators must have adequate alarms.
  - Frequent checking of all connections should be routine.
- Leaks caused by broken or malfunctioning cuff balloon or pilot valve
  - Diagnosis is confirmed by the ability of a previously aphonic patient to talk, detection of air movement at the nose and mouth, pressure changes on the ventilator, and decreased exhaled volumes as measured with a hand-held portable respirometer or ventilator spirometer.
  - Tube must be removed and replaced. Always check the cuff for leaks before inserting; note the cuff pressure and amount of air required to fill the cuff and compare with later values.
- Tracheal ischemia, necrosis, dilation

Continued

Pulmonary System

3

BOX 3.5	**Prevention of Complications of Airway Intubation—cont'd**

- Because of the oval shape of the trachea and the round shape of the tube, there is a tendency for erosion in the anterior and posterior trachea.
- Diagnosis is indicated by the necessity to use larger and larger amounts of air to inflate the balloon to maintain the seal.
- May progress to tracheoesophageal fistula; this is indicated if food is aspirated through the trachea or air is in the stomach or if the results of a methylene blue dye test are positive.

From Kacmarek, R. M., Stoller, J. K., Heuer, A. J. (2019). *Egan's fundamentals of respiratory care* 12th ed.. St. Louis: Elsevier.

2. **Impaired respiratory mechanics**
   a. Description of problem: Patient is unable to maintain adequate oxygen supply because of structural impediments (e.g., airway constriction, closure, or obstruction by secretions; a flattened diaphragm; respiratory muscle fatigue; loss of structural integrity of the thoracic cage). Clinical findings may include dyspnea, tachypnea, fremitus, abnormal ABG values, cyanosis (late finding), cough, nasal flaring, use of accessory muscles of respiration, assumption of a three-point position or the use of pursed-lip breathing, prolonged expiratory phase, increased A-P chest diameter, and altered chest excursion.
   b. Goals of care
      i. Respiratory rate, tidal volume, and maximal inspiratory pressure are within normal limits for the patient
      ii. Dyspnea at rest is minimal; exertional dyspnea is decreased
      iii. Patient takes bronchodilator medications as prescribed.
      iv. Patient is able to pace the activities of daily living (ADLs) with ventilatory function.
   c. Interprofessional collaboration: Nurse, physician, advanced practice provider, respiratory therapist, speech therapist, physical or occupational therapist
   d. Interventions
      i. Teach pursed-lip breathing, abdominal stabilization, and directed or controlled coughing techniques to minimize the energy expenditure of respiratory muscles. Pursed-lip breathing forces the patient to breathe slowly and establishes a back pressure in the airway, which helps to stabilize the airway and diminish dyspnea, especially after exertion.
      ii. Evaluate the status of the inspiratory muscles and, if appropriate, initiate inspiratory muscle training.
         (a) Inspiratory muscle training may improve the conscious control of the respiratory muscles and decrease the anxiety associated with increased respiratory effort.
         (b) Improved respiratory muscle strength may improve exercise tolerance and decrease dyspnea.
         (c) Monitor O_2 saturation via pulse oximetry as a measure of tolerance during training.
      iii. Teach the patient medication names, doses, method of administration, schedule, and appropriate behavior should an adverse effect occur. Instruct in the consequences of improper use of medications.
         (a) β-agonists and anticholinergics are bronchodilators commonly prescribed to decrease airflow resistance and the work of breathing. Methylxanthines

are less commonly prescribed but may also be used for COPD
exacerbations.

(b) Patient should be able to demonstrate the proper technique for MDI self-
administration. Spacer may be attached to the MDI to optimize medication
delivery. If technique is poor or the patient is unable to use an MDI, assess
the need for an alternative delivery device such as a small-volume nebulizer.

iv. Teach the patient to modify ADLs within ventilatory limits.

(a) Encourage periodic hyperinflation of the lungs with a series of slow, deep
breaths.

(b) Hyperinflation therapy helps to prevent atelectasis and reduced lung
compliance by expanding the alveoli, which are partially closed, and by
mobilizing airway secretions.

v. Monitor the rate and pattern of respiration, breath sounds, use of accessory
muscles of respiration, and sensation of dyspnea. Clinical manifestations of
respiratory muscle fatigue include the following:

(a) Shallow, rapid breathing in early stages

(b) Use of accessory muscles and a paradoxical breathing pattern

(c) Active use of expiratory muscles, magnified sense of dyspnea

3. **Impaired alveolar ventilation**

a. Description of problem: Inability to maintain spontaneous ventilation.
Clinical findings include an ineffective breathing pattern, dyspnea, tachypnea
or apnea, accessory muscle use, abnormal ABG levels, excess work of
breathing.

b. Goals of care

i. Respiratory rate and breathing pattern are normal for the patient

ii. ABG levels are within acceptable limits for the patient

iii. Dyspnea is decreased with no air trapping at the end of expiration

iv. No evidence of ventilator-related complications is apparent

c. Interprofessional collaboration: Nurse, physician, advanced practice provider,
respiratory therapist, pharmacist

d. Interventions

i. Promote normal rest and sleep patterns. Plan activities to allow rest periods.
Rest allows energy reserves to be replenished. Sleep deprivation blunts the
patient's respiratory drive.

ii. Provide an appropriate level of mechanical ventilatory support as warranted
(Box 3.6).

iii. Prevent the development of complications associated with the use of positive
pressure ventilation (Box 3.7).

(a) The Awakening and Breathing Coordination, Delirium monitoring/
management and Early exercise/mobility (ABCDEF) bundle
(ICUdelirium.org)

(b) Clinical Guidelines Prevention and Management of Pain, Agitation/
Sedation, Delirium, Immobility, and Sleep Disruption in Adult
Patients in the ICU (PADIS) https://www.sccm.org/ICULiberation/
Guidelines

KEY CONCEPT

Bundles of care use three to five identified best practices in a structured way at the point of care.
These interventions when used together are proven to improve patient outcomes.

BOX 3.6 Levels of Ventilatory Support

OBJECTIVES OF MECHANICAL VENTILATION

Physiologic Objectives
- To support or otherwise manipulate pulmonary gas exchange
  - Alveolar ventilation (e.g., arterial partial pressure of carbon dioxide and pH)
  - Arterial oxygenation (e.g., partial pressure of oxygen, arterial oxygen saturation, and oxygen content)
- To increase lung volume
  - End-inspiratory lung inflation
  - Functional residual capacity
- To reduce or otherwise manipulate the work of breathing

Clinical Objectives
- To reverse hypoxemia
- To reverse acute respiratory acidosis
- To relieve respiratory distress
- To prevent or reverse atelectasis
- To reverse ventilatory muscle fatigue
- To permit sedation and/or neuromuscular blockade
- To decrease systemic or myocardial oxygen consumption
- To reduce intracranial pressure
- To stabilize the chest wall

POSITIVE PRESSURE VENTILATORS

- Most common type of ventilatory support used in critical care. Apply positive pressure to the airways during the clinician-selected pattern of ventilation.
- Response of the breath delivery system to patient efforts
  - Triggering: Initiation of gas delivery. Significant ventilatory loads can be imposed by insensitive or unresponsive ventilator triggering systems. Oversensitive valves can result in spontaneous ventilator cycling independent of patient effort.
  - Gas delivery: Flow from the ventilator is governed (or limited) by a set flow (flow limited) or set pressure (pressure limited) on most machines.
  - Cycling: Gas delivery can be terminated at a preset volume, time, or flow.
- Response of patient efforts to ventilator settings
  - Alteration of the activity of mechanoreceptors in the airways, lungs, and chest wall
  - Alteration of arterial blood gas (ABG) values
  - Elicitation of respiratory sensations in conscious or semiconscious patients
  - Result is a change in rate (ventilatory demand), depth, and timing of respiratory efforts (synchrony between patient and ventilator) through neural reflexes, chemical (chemoreceptors), and behavioral responses

STANDARD MODES OF MECHANICAL VENTILATION

Modes of mechanical ventilation are classified according to initiation of the inspiratory cycle:
- *Spontaneous respiration:* With most ventilators, the patient can breathe spontaneously through the ventilator circuit when the ventilator rate is set at zero. Positive airway pressure can be applied when the patient is breathing through the circuit.
- *Assist control (A/C):* Every breath is supported by the ventilator. Backup control ventilatory rate is set, but the patient may choose any rate above the set rate. Most ventilators deliver A/C ventilation using volume-cycled or volume-targeted breaths. Pressure-limited or pressure-targeted A/C is available on certain ventilators.
- *Intermittent mandatory ventilation (IMV):* Mode of ventilation and weaning that combines a preset number of ventilator-delivered mandatory breaths of predetermined tidal volume with the capability for intermittent patient-generated spontaneous breaths. In a subtype of this mode, called *synchronized intermittent mandatory ventilation* (SIMV), a demand valve is incorporated into the IMV system that senses the start of a patient breath. The demand valve opens, and the mandatory breath is delivered in synchrony with the patient's effort.
- *Pressure control ventilation:* Applies a constant pressure for a preset time. The application of constant pressure throughout inspiration results in a square pressure-overtime waveform during inspiration and a decelerating inspiratory flow waveform as the pressure gradient falls between the ventilator (pressure remains constant) and the patient (pressure rises as the lung fills). Flow in this breath format is variable and this leads to variable tidal volumes. Flow depends on the resistance of the lung, the compliance of the lung, and patient effort. With this type of breath, changes in airway resistance or lung/chest-wall compliance will alter tidal volume (e.g., worsening of airway resistance or lung compliance results in a decrease in tidal volume).
  1. Used in acute respiratory distress syndrome (ARDS) to reduce barotrauma.

BOX 3.6 Levels of Ventilatory Support—cont'd

- *Volume control ventilation:* Ensures the delivery of a preset tidal volume (unless the peak pressure limit is exceeded). On most ventilators, the setting of peak inspiratory flow rate and the choice of inspiratory flow waveform determine the length of inspiration. Some ventilators change the peak inspiratory flow rate to maintain constant inspiratory time on switching between a constant flow and decelerating flow waveforms. With volume control breaths, worsening airway resistance or lung/chest-wall compliance results in increases in peak inspiratory pressure with continued delivery of the set tidal volume (unless the peak pressure limit is exceeded).
- *Pressure support ventilation (PSV):* Pressure-targeted, flow-cycled mode of ventilation in which each breath must be triggered by the patient. Application of positive pressure to the airway is set by the clinician. This augmentation to inspiratory effort starts at the initiation of inhalation and typically ends when a minimum inspiratory flow rate is reached. There are two applications for this mode:
  1. Used in conjunction with SIMV to improve patient tolerance and decrease the work of spontaneous breaths, especially from demand-flow systems and endotracheal tubes with a narrow inner diameter
  2. Used as a stand-alone ventilatory mode for patients under consideration for weaning or during the stabilization period
- *Continuous positive airway pressure (CPAP):* Designed to elevate end-expiratory pressure to above atmospheric pressure to increase lung volume and oxygenation. All breaths are spontaneous, and therefore an intact respiratory drive is required. Can be used in intubated as well as nonintubated patients via a face or nasal mask. Depending on machine type, CPAP is delivered via a continuous flow or demand valve system.
- *Bilevel positive airway pressure (BiPAP):* This noninvasive ventilatory assist device uses a spontaneous breathing mode with the baseline pressure elevated above zero. Unlike CPAP, BiPAP allows separate regulation of inspiratory and expiratory pressures. Application of BiPAP is essentially a combination of PSV with CPAP. The differences between inspiratory and expiratory positive airway pressures (IPAP and EPAP, respectively) contribute to the total ventilation. Enhances the capabilities of home CPAP for obstructive sleep apnea to provide nocturnal support in a variety of restrictive and obstructive disorders. Affords a noninvasive means of augmenting alveolar ventilation in hypercapnic respiratory failure.

ALTERNATE MODES OF MECHANICAL VENTILATION

Some ventilatory support strategies are aimed at limiting or reducing lung inflation volumes and/or pressures to avoid ventilator-associated lung injury

- *Pressure Regulated Volume Control (PRVC):* This is a mode of ventilation in which the ventilator attempts to achieve set tidal volume at lowest possible airway pressure.
- *Airway pressure release ventilation (APRV):* This is an inverse ratio, pressure-controlled, intermittent mandatory ventilation with unrestricted spontaneous breathing. There are both mandatory breaths, as well as spontaneous breaths. It has advantages over conventional ventilation, including alveolar recruitment, improved oxygenation, preservation of spontaneous breathing, improved hemodynamics and potential lung-protective benefits. APRV is used mainly for the difficult to oxygenate patients with acute lung injury and acute respiratory distress syndrome.
- *High-frequency ventilation:* Provides a faster respiratory rate (60–3000 breaths/min) and lower tidal volume (1–3 mL/kg) than other ventilator systems, to reduce barotrauma/volutrauma and cardiac depression. Three types of mechanical system are capable of delivering high-frequency ventilation:
  - High-frequency positive pressure ventilation (HFPPV): Time-cycled, volume-limited ventilation that delivers a preset tidal volume 60 to 100 times per minute.
  - High-frequency jet ventilation (HFJV): Delivers jets of high-pressure gas through a small catheter in the trachea or an endotracheal tube at frequencies of 60 to 600 breaths/min.
  - High-frequency oscillation (HFO): Moves a volume of gas to and fro in the airway, through laminar flow at rates of 600 to 3000 cycles/min (50 Hz) throughout the lungs.
- *Inverse-ratio ventilation (IRV):* Ventilatory support strategy that uses a prolonged inspiratory to expiratory ratio (I/E) greater than or equal to 1:1. Breath delivery is either pressure controlled (PC-IRV) or volume controlled (VC-IRV).
  - Major function of prolonged inspiratory time is to allow for recruitment of alveolar units with long time constants.
  - Increase in mean airway pressure is key to the beneficial effects related to oxygenation, as well as to potential adverse hemodynamic effects (decreased cardiac output).
  - Because of the abnormal I/E ratio, patient desynchrony with the ventilator is common, and sedation and/or paralysis is usually required.
  - Development of auto-positive end-expiratory pressure (auto-PEEP) is common and should be routinely monitored; during PC-IRV, tidal volume varies according to respiratory mechanics.

Continued

BOX 3.6 Levels of Ventilatory Support —cont'd

GUIDELINES FOR VENTILATOR ADJUSTMENT DURING MECHANICAL VENTILATION

All ventilator controls and settings are adjusted according to the patient's underlying disease process and the results of ABG analysis.

- *Minute ventilation:* Usually 6 to 10 L/min but may be much higher, depending on patient needs
- *Tidal volume:* Governed by estimated tidal volume; normally varies from 5 to 8 mL/kg ideal body weight to prevent lung overinflation and potential stretch injury to the lung tissue. Lower tidal volumes are used in ARDS. Intentional use of lower tidal volumes may cause an increase in arterial CO_2 levels and is therefore referred to as *permissive hypercapnia*. Low tidal volume has been shown to lower mortality in some settings.
- *Respiratory rate:* Varies from 8 to 12 breaths/min for most clinically stable patients; rates above 20 breaths/min are sometimes necessary
- *Flow rate:* Adjusted so that inspiratory volume delivery can be completed in a time frame that allows adequate time for exhalation. Inspiratory flow rate range of about 40 to 100 L/min is most commonly used. Slow flow rates are preferred for optimal air distribution in normal lungs; faster flow rates are beneficial in patients with obstructive lung disease. Altering the flow rate may reduce the work of breathing, improve patient-ventilator synchrony, and increase the comfort of patients who are restless while undergoing mechanical ventilation.
- *I/E ratio:* Normal ratio is 1:2 to 1:3
- *Inspiratory flow of gas from the ventilator:* Depending on the model, can be delivered using one of several flow patterns, such as decelerating, square wave, or sine wave
- *Oxygen concentration:* Initially, the fraction of inspired oxygen (FiO_2) is deliberately set at a high value (often 1.0) to ensure adequate oxygenation. An ABG sample is obtained, and the FiO_2 is adjusted according to the patient's arterial partial pressure of oxygen (PaO_2) and SpO_2. Inspired partial pressure of O_2 is adjusted so that PaO_2 is acceptable for the patient's condition. This is usually a PaO_2 higher than 55 mm Hg or SpO_2 of 88% or higher. Excessively high levels for prolonged periods can cause oxygen toxicity. The lowest FiO_2 that achieves an acceptable PaO_2 and SaO_2 should be used.
- *PEEP:* Used as appropriate to reduce the FiO_2 to safe levels
- *Humidification:* Continuous humidification is mandatory, with inspired air warmed to near body temperature. Standard humidifiers using a water feed system must be monitored closely for water condensation in the tubing and emptied routinely. Heat and moisture exchanges (HME) are sometimes used.
- *Sensitivity:* Established parameters are followed for sensitivity settings (when the patient can trigger the machine for "assistance"); sensitivity is adjusted so that minimal patient effort is required, usually −0.50 to −1.5 cm H_2O; certain ventilators allow for a flow-triggering mechanism and should be set to their maximum sensitivity (1–3 L/min)
- *Pressure limit alarms:* Should be set at approximately 10 to 15 cm H_2O above the patient's normal peak inflation pressure (PIP) or airway pressure. Goal is to keep PIP below 35 to 40 cm H_2O if possible. Peak inspiratory plateau is equal to or less than 35 cm H_2O. Certain ventilators provide a low-airway-pressure alarm feature. Check that all other alarms are operational and on at all times.

ASSESSMENT OF THE EFFECTIVENESS OF MECHANICAL VENTILATION

- Some general measures include the following:
  - All patients on life support equipment should be monitored and clinically observed routinely according to institutional policy.
  - Physical assessment should be performed each shift.
  - Ventilator system and its current settings should be assessed.
  - Manual self-inflating resuscitation bag should be open and ready for use.
  - Suction equipment should be in working order and ready for use.
  - When medications are to be given, orders must be written clearly and precisely (e.g., a bronchodilator can be administered as scheduled or continuously by aerosol or via the ventilator circuit by metered-dose inhaler).
  - Many patients have an arterial line, cardiac monitor, intravenous line, pulse oximetry and/or $EtCO_2$ monitoring if they are on continuous ventilatory support.
- General monitoring for patients on continuous ventilatory support
  - Hemodynamic monitoring
  - Cardiac output assessment, monitoring, heart sounds, pulses, pulse pressures, electrocardiogram as needed or as part of standard intensive care unit routine
  - Vital capacity, negative inspiratory pressure, minute ventilation, maximum voluntary ventilation
  - Biochemical, hematologic, electrolyte studies, and chest radiographs
  - Measurement of intake and output, body weight
  - Respiratory pattern assessment, breath sounds, symmetry in chest movement, vital signs
  - Inspection of dressings and drainages, tubes, and suction apparatus
  - Assessment of neurologic state, level of consciousness, pain, level of anxiety
  - Evaluation of response to treatments and medications

BOX 3.6   Levels of Ventilatory Support —cont'd

VENTILATORY MONITORING OF ANY PATIENT ON CONTINUOUS VENTILATION

- Ventilation checks performed routinely
  - When blood gas samples are drawn
  - When changes are made in ventilator settings
  - Hourly or more frequently for any patient in unstable condition
  - Routinely throughout each shift
- Components of the ventilator to be recorded in the medical record
  - Blood gas values
    Record source (arterial, mixed venous) with ventilator settings and measurements so that decisions about changes may be made.
    It often is valuable to document the patient's position at the time of the blood gas drawing because position changes (side lying, upright, supine) influence ventilation-perfusion relationships and, hence, blood gas analysis results.
  - Ventilator settings to be read from the machine ventilator mode (e.g., SIMV or A/C).
    Tidal volume, machine preset rate, pressure support level (if used), preset minute volume, inspiratory flow rate or time and preset I/E ratio (depending on mode and ventilator)
    Temperature of the humidification device, temperature of the inspired gas
    Oxygen concentration
    Peak inflation airway pressure limit
    PEEP level set
    Alarms on
  - Ventilator measurements to be taken
    PIP, plateau, and/or mean airway pressures if requested, and PEEP level (measurement of auto-PEEP may be required for some patients)
    FiO_2, alveolar to arterial gradient or PaO_2/FiO_2 ratio, shunt fractions (if ordered)
    Minute ventilation (exhaled), respiratory rate (both patient and machine), tidal volume (exhaled)
    Effective compliance, static and dynamic; compliance curves (depending on institutional policy)
    I/E ratio (displayed), dead space/tidal volume ratio (if requested)
  - Respiratory monitoring techniques during mechanical ventilation
    Pulse oximetry: noninvasive estimate of arterial oxygen saturation (SpO_2). See discussion in Monitoring Data under Patient Assessment.
    End-tidal CO_2 ($PetCO_2$) monitoring: noninvasive sampling and measurement of exhaled CO_2 tension at the patient-ventilator interface. See discussion in Monitoring Data under Patient Assessment.

From Kacmarek, R. M., Stoller, J. K., Heuer, A. J. (2019). *Egan's fundamentals of respiratory care* 12th ed. St. Louis: Elsevier.

BOX 3.7   Complications Associated With Positive Pressure Ventilation

CARDIAC EFFECTS

Decreased Cardiac Output

- Caused by decreased venous return to the heart and reduced transmural pressures (intracardiac minus intrapleural pressures). In addition, there are increases in PVR and juxtacardiac pressure from the surrounding distended lungs.
- Pulse changes, decreased urine output and blood pressure
- Treatment
  - Positioning with the head flat and legs elevated (modified Trendelenburg's position)
  - Administration of fluids to increase preload
  - Adjustment of volumes delivered by ventilator
  - Careful positive end-expiratory pressure (PEEP) titration; avoidance of auto-PEEP

Possible Dysrhythmias

- Causes: Hypoxemia and pH abnormalities
- Patients in unstable condition on ventilators should have cardiac monitoring

PULMONARY EFFECTS AND OTHER VENTILATOR ASSOCIATED EVENTS

Barotrauma and/or Volutrauma (Pneumothorax, Pneumomediastinum, Subcutaneous Emphysema)

- Occurs when a high pressure gradient between the alveolus and adjacent vascular sheet causes the overdistended alveolus to rupture. Gas is forced into the interstitial tissue of the underlying perivascular sheet. The gas

Continued

BOX 3.7 Complications Associated With Positive Pressure Ventilation—cont'd

may dissect centrally along the pulmonary vessels to the mediastinum and into the fascial planes of the neck and upper torso; high inflation volumes, or volutrauma, has also been described as an important risk factor.
- Positive pressure ventilation, especially with PEEP, subjects patients to the risk of pneumothorax, particularly if high pressures and volumes are used.
- Barotrauma can occur with mainstem intubation, in patients with acute respiratory distress syndrome (ARDS) or chronic obstructive pulmonary disease (COPD), and in other patients with acute lung injury.
- Diagnosis
  - Increases in airway peak pressure
  - Decreased breath sounds and chest movement on the affected side
  - Changes in vital signs, restlessness, possible cyanosis
  - Chest radiographic changes

Atelectasis
- Collapse of lung parenchyma from the occlusion of air passage, with reabsorption of gas distal to the occlusion
- Causes
  - Obstruction (e.g., secretions, endobronchial mass, bronchiectasis)
  - Possible lack of periodic deep inflations in patients ventilated with small tidal volumes
- Diagnosis
  - Diminished breath sounds or bronchial breath sounds, rales or crackles
  - Chest radiographic evidence
  - Alveolar to arterial (A–a) gradient increases, ratio of arterial partial pressure of oxygen (PaO_2) to fraction of inspired oxygen (FiO_2) decreases, and compliance decreases
- Prevention
  - Use of lower tidal volumes
  - Humidification, vigorous tracheal suctioning based on need
  - Chest physical therapy, repositioning

TRACHEAL DAMAGE, TRACHEOESOPHAGEAL FISTULA, VESSEL RUPTURE
- Cause: Excessive tube cuff pressures because of overinflation or reduced tracheal blood flow causing ischemia
- Prevention
  - Careful monitoring of intracuff pressures or volumes
  - Avoidance of frequent manipulation and pulling of endotracheal tube

Oxygen Toxicity
- Pathology: Impaired surfactant activity, progressive capillary congestion, fibrosis, edema and thickening of interstitial space
- Cause: Prolonged administration of high oxygen concentrations (FiO_2 of >0.50)
- Prevention: Careful monitoring of blood gas levels. Goal is to use the lowest FiO_2 that achieves adequate oxygenation (PaO_2 over 55 mm Hg and arterial oxygen saturation [SaO_2] over 88%).

Inability to Liberate (Wean) From Ventilator
- Can occur in any patient, particularly those with COPD, cystic fibrosis, debilitation, malnutrition, and musculoskeletal disorders
- Mechanical ventilation eases the work of breathing for these patients, which makes the transition to breathing off the ventilator (e.g., weaning) difficult

Hypercapnia–Respiratory Acidosis
- Inadequate ventilation leads to acute retention of carbon dioxide and decreased pH.
- Patients can tolerate increased arterial partial pressure of carbon dioxide ($PaCO_2$) and decreased pH under certain circumstances.
- Corrected by improving alveolar ventilation and treating the underlying cause.

Hypocapnia-Respiratory Alkalosis
- Because of hyperventilation, which causes increased elimination of carbon dioxide and increased pH
- If carbon dioxide is decreased too rapidly, shock or seizures may result, particularly in children. Maintain ventilation to produce a normal pH, not necessarily a normal partial pressure of carbon dioxide ($PaCO_2$).
- Treatment
  - Decrease the respiratory rate
  - Decrease the tidal volume if inappropriately high
  - Add mechanical dead space

BOX 3.7   Complications Associated With Positive Pressure Ventilation —cont'd

FLUID IMBALANCE

- Fluid retention: Because of overhydration by airway humidification and decreased urinary output because of possible antidiuretic hormone effects. Symptoms include the following:
  - Increased A–a gradient, decreased PaO_2/FiO_2 ratio
  - Decreased vital capacity and compliance
  - Weight gain, intake greater than output
  - Increased dead space/tidal volume ratio
  - Hemodilution (decreased hematocrit and decreased sodium values)
  - Increased bronchial secretions
- Dehydration related to decreased enteral or parenteral intake in relation to urinary and/or gastrointestinal output, and overdiuresis. In addition, insensible losses average 300 to 500 mL/day and increase with fever. See Chapter 6, Renal System clinical findings.
- Signs and parameters to be monitored
  - Daily weight changes (often more accurate than intake and output measurement)
  - Skin turgor, moistness of the oral mucosa
  - Hemoglobin and hematocrit values
  - Character of pulmonary secretions
  - Airway humidification

INFECTION AND VENTILATOR-ASSOCIATED PNEUMONIA

- Patients at risk: Debilitated, aged, immobile, early postoperative, or immunocompromised individuals
- Intubation bypasses normal upper airway defenses and makes oral care more difficult.
- Ventilatory equipment and therapy, particularly aerosols, may be the carrier.
- Suctioning technique may not be sterile.
- There may be cross-contamination between patients and staff or autocontamination.
- Pulmonary patients may have indwelling catheters of various types.
- Nonsterile solutions may be left out in open containers.
- Patients may be improperly positioned so that aspiration is possible, or the endotracheal tube cuff may not be inflated to minimal occlusive volume.
- Preventive measures (VAP Bundle)
  - See ICU Liberation Guidelines (ABCDEF, PADIS) from the Society of Critical Care Medicine at https://www.sccm.org/ICULiberation/Guidelines
  - Daily sedation interruption and spontaneous breathing trial
  - Early, Progressive Mobility
  - Use of intermittent rather than continuous sedation
  - Peptic ulcer prophylaxis
  - Aseptic airway and tracheostomy technique
  - Subglottic suction to prevent pooling of secretions above endotracheal tube cuff
  - Sterile suction technique using an open-suction or closed-suction catheter system
  - Elevation of the head of the bed to 30 to 45 degrees continuously or as patient condition warrants
  - Rigorous hand washing, which is mandatory and critical, as well as the use of personal protective equipment as necessary
  - Meticulous oral care with chlorhexidine to assist in prevention, including toothbrushing to remove dental bacteria, which should be performed regularly
  - Bronchial hygiene, chest physical therapy as indicated
  - Isolation techniques as needed
  - Routine cultures of specimens from patients and machines
  - Avoidance of routine tracheal instillation of normal saline for lavage
  - Early recognition and response to clinical and laboratory signs of infection
  - Change of ventilator tubing, including humidifier reservoirs, according to institutional policy; verify the length of time that the ventilator circuit is left in place before changing
  - Emptying and changing of reservoir water per institutional policy; empty water in tubing into a waste receptacle every 1 to 2 hours and as needed

GASTROINTESTINAL EFFECTS

Complications

- Stress ulcer and bleeding
- Adynamic ileus
- Gastric dilatation from loss of adequate nerve supply; fluid shifts may lead to shock

Continued

BOX 3.7 **Complications Associated With Positive Pressure Ventilation—cont'd**

Prevention and Treatment
- Routine auscultation of bowel sounds
- Antacids, histamine antagonists
- Hemoccult or gastroccult and pH stomach aspirate testing; stool check for blood

DYSYNCHRONY

Causes
- Incorrect ventilator setup for the patient's needs (e.g., inspiratory flow rate less than needed)
- Acute change in patient status
- Obstructed airway, pneumothorax
- Ventilator malfunction
- Acute anxiety
- Acute pain

Management
- Perform a rapid bedside check of the patient and ventilator.
- Disconnect the patient from the ventilator and provide manual ventilation with 100% oxygen via a self-inflating bag.
- Check vital signs, chest expansion, and bedside monitoring equipment.
- Suction the airway and check the patency of the endotracheal or tracheostomy tube.
- Obtain arterial blood gas values.
- Sedate the patient if indicated and order for acute anxiety, and give analgesics if pain is present; observe for hypoventilation and be prepared to adjust the ventilator setting to meet the patient's needs.

PRINCIPLES FOR MATCHING VENTILATION TO PATIENT NEEDS
- Do not assume that the patient will adjust to the ventilator; the reverse is desirable.
- Vary the cycle frequency, tidal volume, triggering sensitivity, and inspiratory flow rate until the correct combination is achieved.
- Provide calm reassurance and moderate sedation as indicated.

From Kacmarek, R. M., Stoller, J. K., Heuer, A. J. (2019). *Egan's fundamentals of respiratory care* 12th ed. St. Louis: Elsevier.

    (c) Assess, prevent, and manage pain

    (d) Both spontaneous awakening trials and spontaneous breathing trials (to reduce respiratory muscle weakness and shorten ventilator days)

    (e) Choice of analgesia and sedation

KEY CONCEPT

Use intermittent analgesia and sedation rather than continuous.

    (f) Delirium: Assess, prevent, and manage

    (g) Early mobility and exercise

EXPERT TIP

Early mobility helps prevent weakness and deconditioning associated with prolonged bed rest.

    (h) Family engagement and empowerment

  iv. Provide optimal methods for weaning (also called liberating) patients from continuous mechanical ventilation. Use of nurse or respiratory therapy driven weaning protocols can significantly reduce ventilator days and critical care length of stay. These evidenced-based guidelines incorporate aspects of the ABCDEF bundle of care.

(a) Indications for weaning or liberation (term usually reserved for the gradual withdrawal of ventilatory support, although it includes the overall process of discontinuing ventilator support):

    (1) Underlying disease process is resolved; original signs and symptoms for ventilatory support are no longer present.

    (2) Patient's strength, vigor, and nutritional status are adequate.

    (3) Patient does not require more than 5 cm H_2O of PEEP or an FiO_2 greater than 0.5 to maintain an acceptable PaO_2 (usually at least 55 mm Hg).

    (4) Patient has stable, acceptable hemodynamic parameters and Hb level.

    (5) Patient has stable and acceptable values for ABGs, V_T, vital capacity, respiratory rate, minute ventilation, maximum inspiratory and expiratory pressures.

    (6) Level of consciousness is acceptable.

    (7) Patient is psychologically prepared, emotionally ready, and cooperative.

    (8) Predictors of successful weaning and criteria for liberation trial:

        a) Resting minute volume of less than 10 L and ability to double this value during a maximum voluntary ventilation effort

        b) Maximum inspiratory pressure more negative than –20 cm H_2O

        c) Spontaneous V_T greater than 5 mL/kg (or 10–15 L/min)

        d) Spontaneous respiratory frequency (f) equal to or less than 30 breaths/min

        e) Vital capacity above 10 mL/kg body weight

        f) PaO_2/FiO_2 ratio higher than 200

        g) f/V_T ratio less than 60 to 105 (rapid shallow breathing index)

(b) Principles of liberation (See ICU Liberation Guidelines [ABCDEF, PADIS] from the Society of Critical Care Medicine at https://www.sccm.org/ICULiberation/Guidelines)

    (1) Explain the procedure. Place the patient in an upright position for better lung expansion. Obtain baseline measurements of vital signs.

    (2) Obtain ventilatory measurements or weaning parameters. Measure minute ventilation, rate, V_T, maximum inspiratory pressure, V_c, and maximum voluntary ventilation.

    (3) Techniques of discontinuing ventilator support (intermittent mandatory ventilation, pressure-supported ventilation, continuous positive airway pressure [CPAP]: Box 3.8.

    (4) Mechanisms contributing to failure to wean include insufficient ventilatory drive, hypoxemia, high ventilatory requirement, respiratory muscle weakness, low compliance, and excessive work of breathing. The longer it takes to resolve the problem that precipitated the need for ventilatory support, the more difficult it may be to wean.

(c) Treatment of the difficult-to-wean patient

    (1) Monitor the color, consistency, and volume of sputum. Change in sputum characteristics may indicate infection, which may increase the work of breathing.

BOX 3.8   Techniques for Discontinuing Ventilator Support

INTERMITTENT MANDATORY VENTILATION

In intermittent mandatory ventilation (IMV), the amount of support provided by the ventilator is gradually reduced and the amount of respiratory work done by the patient is progressively increased.

- Transition period may be several hours to several days, depending on the length of time ventilatory support was required as well as institutional policy.
- Pace of decreasing the IMV rate is determined by clinical assessment and ABG analysis.
- Pressure support ventilation (PSV) is often used with IMV in lower amounts (5–10 cm H_2O); the IMV rate is reduced while the PSV level is held constant.

PRESSURE SUPPORT VENTILATION

Stand-alone mode of PSV is also used as a means of gradually reducing the level of ventilator support.

- PSV level is initially titrated to a spontaneous tidal volume of 10 to 12 mL/kg and then reduced in increments of 3 to 6 cm H_2O based on clinical assessment and ABG analysis.
- PSV is titrated down until a low level of support is reached (5–10 cm H_2O).

CONTINUOUS POSITIVE AIRWAY PRESSURE

With continuous positive airway pressure (CPAP) ventilatory support, the patient breathes spontaneously (with no mechanical assistance) against a threshold resistance, with pressure above atmospheric levels maintained at the airway throughout breathing.

- CPAP level is initially set at 3 to 5 cm H_2O
- May be helpful for patients with dynamic hyperinflation and auto-positive end-expiratory pressure
- When weaning trials are completed, the patient is usually extubated from CPAP at 3 to 5 cm H_2O

In theory, CPAP prevents or limits the deterioration in oxygenation that often occurs when patients switch from mechanical ventilation to spontaneous breathing. Some data refute this notion.

See ICU Liberation Guidelines (ABCDEF, PADIS) from the Society of Critical Care Medicine at https://www.sccm.org/ICULiberation/Guidelines

---

  (2) Physical therapy and rehabilitation efforts are very important (with both physical and psychological advantages).

  (3) Monitor the rate and depth of respiration, breath sounds, use of accessory muscles of respiration, and dyspnea.

  (4) Monitor the patient for clinical signs of respiratory muscle fatigue, including shallow, rapid breathing (early); increased $PaCO_2$, decreased respiratory rate (late).

  (5) Monitor the ratio of inspiratory time (T_i) to total duration of respiration (T_{tot}); an increase in the T_i/T_{tot} ratio indicates decreased respiratory muscle endurance.

  (6) Observe for abnormal chest wall motion as an indication of respiratory muscle dysfunction.

    a) Paradoxical motion of the chest wall is characterized by expansion of the rib cage and inward motion of the abdomen during inspiration.

    b) Asynchronous chest wall motion is characterized by disorganized and uncoordinated respiratory motion.

  (7) Administer appropriate medication therapy for maintenance of ventilation (Box 3.9).

4. **Impaired respiratory gas exchange**

  a. Description of problem: Inability to maintain adequate respiratory gas exchange. Clinical findings include confusion, anxiety, somnolence, restlessness, irritability, inability to mobilize secretions, hypercapnia, hypoxemia, hypoxia, dyspnea, cyanosis, tachycardia, and dysrhythmias.

BOX 3.9   Medication Therapy for Maintenance of Ventilation

NARCOTICS

- Morphine sulfate, dilaudid, and fentanyl dosed to effect (intermittent administration is preferred over continuous infusions)
- If used, administer intermittently to manage discomfort, rather than continuously, and before any sedation.
- Act as a respiratory depressant; good euphoric agents and excellent analgesics
- Sensation of dyspnea is reduced
- Large dosages may cause increased venous capacitance
- Medication tolerance may develop with prolonged use

NARCOTIC ANTAGONISTS

- Used in cases of narcotic overdose to reverse the effects of narcotics
- They are not stimulants but compete with narcotic molecules for cellular receptors in medication-depressed neurons

BENZODIAZEPINES

- These agents may contribute to the occurrence of delirium and are not recommended.
- Lorazepam and midazolam are the most commonly used agents in the critical care setting.
- These medications cause a central nervous system (CNS) depressant effect, which can lead to alveolar hypoventilation and respiratory acidosis, particularly in geriatric patients and in those with liver disease.
- Severe respiratory depression and apnea can result if they are used with other CNS depressant medications.
- As with any sedative agent, the routine use of a validated sedation scale for monitoring and assessing the degree of sedation is important.
- Recommended to use intermittently rather than continuously.
- Daily sedation holiday (see Ch. 19, Sedation).

ANESTHETIC AGENTS

- Propofol and dexmedetomidine are used as sedative agents in the intensive care unit setting. It is unrelated to any of the currently used barbiturate, opioid, and benzodiazepine agents.
- Respiratory and hemodynamic monitoring are essential during continuous infusion.

PARALYTIC AGENTS

- Provide pharmacologic intervention at the myoneural junction, which results in muscle paralysis.
- If the patient is conscious, sedation is mandatory.

Nondepolarizing Muscle Relaxants

- Administered intravenously (IV)
- Compete with acetylcholine at the receptor site
- Vecuronium and rocuronium are the most common agents used in the critical care setting
- Loading doses given (different for each medication), followed by maintenance doses, with careful monitoring
- Use of peripheral nerve stimulator for determining train-of-four at least every 2 hours; the goal is one or two out of four twitches
  - Use of end-tidal carbon dioxide monitoring for visual detection of respiratory efforts; in-line airway pressure graphic monitoring may also be helpful
  - Skeletal muscle weakness and disuse atrophy occur when these agents are administered for prolonged periods; full recovery of muscles may take from weeks to months
  - Neuromuscular blockade and sedation should be stopped at least once daily to assess the patient's underlying level of sedation and also to reevaluate the need for continued paralysis or sedation

Depolarizing Muscle Relaxant (Succinylcholine)

- Attaches to the muscle cell wall and causes depolarization
- Used primarily for inducing short-duration muscle relaxation in anesthesia and endotracheal intubation
- Bolus dose is typically 1.0 to 1.5 mg/kg IV; onset of action is approximately 45 to 60 seconds; duration of action after a single dose is approximately 2 to 10 minutes

BRONCHODILATORS

β-Agonists

- Stimulate β-receptors in the bronchial smooth muscle, which results in bronchial smooth muscle relaxation; the most potent bronchodilators currently available

Continued

BOX 3.9 Medication Therapy for Maintenance of Ventilation —cont'd

- Epinephrine: Stimulates β_1- and β_2-receptors; given by inhalation or parenterally, with rapid action either way; duration of action is 0.5 to 2 hours
- Albuterol: Mostly β_2 selective; given in inhaled and oral forms; duration of action is 4 to 6 hours inhaled and 5 to 8 hours in oral form

Anticholinergic Bronchodilators
- Block cholinergic constricting influences on bronchial muscle
- Work predominantly on the large airways
- Atropine and ipratropium: Given in inhaled form
- Tiotropium (Spiriva): 24-hour duration of action, given by powder inhalation

Antiallergy Medications
- Block immunoglobulin E-dependent mast cell release of mediators of bronchoconstriction, such as histamine and leukotrienes
- Montelukast: Given orally in the evening to counteract hormonal variation in bronchoconstriction

Corticosteroids
- Augment the effects of β-agonist bronchodilators and are antiinflammatory; often started at high dosage, then tapered off
- Dosage should be kept low to minimize adrenocortical and pituitary suppression and side effects
- Prednisone: Oral dose often given once daily, in the early morning to minimize systemic side effects
- Methylprednisolone given IV
- Inhaled steroids: Given after inhaled β-agonists
  - Provide beneficial pulmonary steroid effects with minimal systemic absorption
  - When steroids are taken by inhalation, the patient must use a spacer device and rinse the mouth with water after each use to prevent fungal infection (candidiasis) of the oropharynx or larynx.

---

b. Goals of care
   i. Hypoxemia resolves or improves.
   ii. Eucapnia is present or the patient's usual compensated $PaCO_2$ and pH levels are observed.
   iii. Patient performs ADLs and modifies self-care activity with or without supplemental O_2.
   iv. Patient indicates that he or she is able to breathe comfortably.
c. Interprofessional collaboration: Nurse, physician, advanced practice provider, respiratory therapist, dietitian, physical or occupational therapist
d. Interventions
   i. Assess oxygenation status
      (a) Hypoxia-hypoxemia relationships
         (1) Hypoxia: Decrease in oxygenation at the tissue level (a clinical diagnosis); must be corrected; in some cases, O_2 therapy alone may not correct tissue hypoxia.
         (2) Hypoxemia: Decrease in arterial blood O_2 tension (a laboratory diagnosis). A normal PaO_2 alone does not guarantee adequate tissue oxygenation.
         (3) Organs most susceptible to lack of O_2: Brain, adrenal glands, heart, kidneys, liver, and retina of the eye.
         (4) Factors governing effective oxygenation
            a) Sufficient O_2 supply in inspired air
            b) Sufficient ventilation to enable gas exchange between atmospheric air in the alveoli and dissolved gases in the pulmonary capillaries
            c) Ready diffusion of gases across the alveolar-capillary membrane

    d) Adequate circulation of blood from the lungs to tissues; adequate volume of blood and Hb level. Falling cardiac output leads to a compensatory rise in O_2 extraction at the tissue level.

    e) O_2 brought to tissues must be readily released from the Hb molecule and be readily diffused into and taken up by various tissues

(b) Assessment of hypoxemia-hypoxia

  (1) Clinical signs and symptoms: see Description of Problem; may also include apprehension, headache, angina, impaired judgment, hypotension, abnormal respirations, hypoventilation, yawning

  (2) ABG analysis, including oxyhemoglobin saturation, and content; Hb level; arteriovenous O_2 content differences (if pulmonary artery catheter is in place)

  (3) Noninvasive O_2 monitoring

    a) Pulse oximetry (SpO_2): see Patient Assessment

ii. Provide O_2 therapy

  (a) Principles of O_2 therapy

    (1) Remember the airway; no O_2 treatment is of any use without a patent and adequate airway.

    (2) O_2 is a medication and should be administered in a prescribed dose (the FiO_2 is the dose).

    (3) Response to O_2 administration should be interpreted in terms of its effect on tissue oxygenation rather than only its effect on ABG values.

    (4) Disease pathology is the major determinant of the effectiveness of O_2 therapy.

    (5) Delivered concentration of gas from any appliance is subject to the condition of the equipment, the application technique, and the cooperation and pattern of ventilation of the patient.

    (6) Low-flow O_2 systems do not provide the total inspired gas (the patient breathes some atmospheric air) and therefore are adequate only if tidal volume is adequate, respiratory rate is not excessive, and ventilator pattern is stable. Variable O_2 concentrations (21%–90%) are provided, but FiO_2 varies greatly with changes in tidal volume and pattern of ventilation.

    (7) High-flow O_2 systems provide the total inspired gas (the patient breathes only gas supplied by the apparatus) and are adequate only if flow rates exceed the inspiratory flow rate and minute ventilation. Both high and low O_2 concentrations (24%–100%) may be delivered.

  (b) Rationale for the use of low-flow O_2 systems in patients with COPD and chronic CO_2 retention

    (1) Central chemoreceptors become desensitized to chronically high blood CO_2 levels, so CO_2 no longer serves as a respiratory stimulus; the only remaining stimulus to increase ventilation is hypoxemia. As a result, high concentrations of O_2 depress the ventilatory drive, which leads to $\dot{V}/\dot{Q}$ mismatching, the Haldane effect, depressed minute ventilation, and increased $PaCO_2$.

    (2) Nursing implications

      a) Administer only enough O_2 to keep PaO_2 at adequate levels for the patient (typically 55–60 mm Hg)

      b) Safety lies in the use of controlled low flow rates, monitoring of ABG levels, and careful observation.

      c) Hazards of O_2 therapy

(3) O_2-induced hypoventilation
   a) Prevent by the use of low flow rates and O_2 concentrations (FiO_2 of 0.24–0.30)
   b) Patient is at greatest risk when the $PaCO_2$ is chronically elevated above normal
   c) Use O_2 therapy with caution in patients with chronic CO_2 retention; priority is to correct hypoxemia; if $PaCO_2$ increases and pH decreases, may need to intubate or use bilevel positive airway pressure (BiPAP)
(4) Absorption atelectasis: Because of the elimination of nitrogen (nitrogen washout) and the effect of O_2 on pulmonary surfactant
(5) Retinopathy of prematurity in neonates
(6) O_2 toxicity: Rarely seen in adults
   a) Because of lung exposure to a high concentration (exact level is controversial; usually considered to be FiO_2 >0.50–0.70) over an extended time (longer than 48–72 hours)
   b) May be mild or fatal
   c) Early signs and symptoms
      1) Retrosternal retractions, dyspnea, coughing
      2) Restlessness, paresthesias in the extremities
      3) Nausea, vomiting, anorexia
      4) Fatigue, lethargy, malaise
   d) Late signs and symptoms include progressive respiratory difficulty to asphyxia, cyanosis
   e) Pathologic process
      1) Local toxicity to the capillary endothelium leads to interstitial edema, which thickens the alveolar-capillary membrane. Type I alveolar cells are destroyed by an exudative response. In the end stages, hyaline membranes form in the alveolar region, followed by fibrosis and pulmonary hypertension.
      2) Biochemical changes are most likely owing to the overproduction of oxygen free radicals, which produce oxidation reactions that inhibit enzyme functions and/or kill cells. High PAO_2 values can also release additional free radicals from neutrophils and platelets, which instigate the capillary endothelial damage described.
   f) Both the concentration and duration of O_2 administration are critical (50% O_2 or higher over several days is potentially dangerous). Even low-flow O_2 (1–2 L/min) has been shown to produce cellular changes over time.
   g) Clinical changes in O_2 toxicity: Decreased compliance and vital capacity, increased A–a gradient, reduced PaO_2/FiO_2 ratio
(7) Prevention of complications caused by O_2 therapy
   a) O_2 is a potent medication that should be used only when indicated and according to preestablished goals of therapy.
   b) If high concentrations are necessary, the duration of administration should be kept to a minimum and the concentration reduced as soon as possible.
   c) Objective: Maintain PaO_2 of at least 55 to 60 mm Hg to produce an acceptable SaO_2 of 88% to 90% without causing lung injury or inducing CO_2 retention.

     d) Reassessment of ABG levels is mandatory during the initial titration of O_2 therapy and when pulse oximetry values are questionable.

     e) Patients should never be exposed to dangerous levels of hypoxemia for fear of development of O_2 toxicity. Hypoxia is far more common than O_2 toxicity and must be corrected. One hundred percent oxygen should never be withheld in an emergency.

  (c) Methods of O_2 delivery (low-flow and high-flow systems): Box 3.10.

iii. Administer PEEP: Oxygenation adjunct treatment modality

  (a) Pressure above the atmospheric level is maintained at the airway opening at the end of expiration to prevent alveolar collapse.

  (b) At the end of quiet expiration, lung volume is increased; therefore FRC is increased. Increase in FRC depends on both the amount of PEEP used and the functional state of the lungs. Alveolar volume is increased; recruitment of alveoli occurs.

  (c) Major goal of PEEP is enhanced O_2 transport by improvement in PaO_2 and SaO_2. PEEP reduces the shunt effect of collapsed alveoli and may increase PaO_2 dramatically. Another important goal of PEEP is to avoid increasing FiO_2, which could lead to O_2 toxicity.

  (d) Clinical use of PEEP

    (1) ARDS and the presence of diffuse pulmonary infiltrates, characterized by closure of the airways or the collapse of alveoli at end expiration, which results in refractory hypoxemia and increased FiO_2 requirements.

    (2) ARF that has caused a persistent hypoxemia with an FiO_2 of 0.5 or greater.

    (3) Cardiogenic pulmonary edema

    (4) Avoidance of pulmonary O_2 toxicity from high FiO_2 values

  (e) PEEP is tailored to the patient's need. Determination of the optimal level requires accurate assessment of cardiopulmonary function, including measurement of peak and plateau airway pressures, blood pressure, and cardiac output when available. PEEP levels above 12 to 15 cm H_2O are generally considered high.

  (f) Side effects of PEEP

    (1) Exacerbation of the same hemodynamic consequences that occur with positive pressure breathing (see Box 3.7). Patients with poor cardiovascular dynamics are at most risk. Adequate intravascular volume is essential.

    (2) Barotrauma: Rupture of lung tissue at high PEEP levels, especially in patients with acute lung injury. Associated with high peak and plateau inflation pressures and high mean airway pressures.

  (g) Monitoring guidelines

    (1) It is essential to monitor the parameters that indicate the status of cardiac output and tissue perfusion (see Ch. 4, Cardiovascular System).

    (2) If a significant drop in cardiac output occurs, PEEP may need to be reduced, or vasoactive medication support for blood pressure may be indicated. Hypovolemia, if present, must be corrected when this is a contributing factor to decreased cardiac output. Short-term inotropic therapy may sometimes be used to correct decreased cardiac output in a normovolemic patient with known or suspected ventricular dysfunction.

BOX 3.10 **Methods of Oxygen Delivery**

MASKS

General Points
- Useful if O_2 is needed quickly and for short periods
- Concentrations of 24% to 100% O_2 are delivered, depending on the device

Disadvantages
- Uncomfortable and hot
- Irritation of the skin caused by tight fit
- Difficult to control the fraction of inspired O_2 (FiO_2) precisely, except when the Venturi mask is used
- Must be removed when the patient eats, so O_2 delivery is lost

Possible Complications
- Patients who are prone to vomit may experience aspiration
- May cause CO_2 retention and hypoventilation if the flow is too low and exhalation ports are obstructed

Types of Mask
- Simple
  - 35% to 60% O_2 at flows of 6 to 10 L/min
  - FiO_2 varies considerably with changes in tidal volume, ventilatory pattern, and inspiratory flow rate and with a tight or loose fit of the mask
- Partial rebreathing
  - Delivers 35% to 60% O_2 or higher at flows of 6 to 10 L/min
  - Portion of exhaled breath enters the reservoir bag to be rebreathed with incoming 100% O_2 in the next breath
  - Flows must be adjusted so that the reservoir bag does not completely collapse during inspiration; otherwise, CO_2 retention may occur
- Nonrebreathing
  - Delivers 90% or more O_2 concentration, provided there are no leaks in the system; a one-way valve between the reservoir bag and mask prevents rebreathing from the 100% O_2 gas source
  - Ideal method of delivering a high O_2 gas concentration for the short term
  - Reservoir bag must not collapse during inspiration
- Air entrainment (Venturi mask)
  - Adjustments allow for the delivery of precise O_2 concentrations of 24% to 50%
  - Total airflow must be adequate for the ventilatory needs of the patient
  - Best suited to patients who must have a consistent FiO_2

NASAL CANNULA
- Low O_2 concentrations are delivered (<40%), but level depends on the patient's tidal volume
- FiO_2 can be estimated as a 4% increase in FiO_2 for each liter of O_2 flow; generally not run at flow rates beyond 5 or 6 L/min
- Humidifier not necessary unless flow rates exceed 4 L/min

HIGH FLOW NASAL CANNULA
- Can provide high O_2 concentrations at a high flow rate (e.g., 100% FiO_2 at 50 liters of flow)

Advantages
- Easy to apply
- Light
- Economical
- Disposable
- Patient mobility allowed

Disadvantages
- Easily dislodged
- High flow rates uncomfortable (dryness and bleeding)
- Possible skin breakdown around the ears caused by tubing, nasal dryness, and breakdown of mucous membranes from the prongs

OXYMIZER

Combines the concepts of low flow and reservoir delivery systems. Reservoir cannula stores about 20 mL of O_2 during exhalation. Pendant reservoir delivery system is situated over the anterior chest wall.

BOX 3.10 Methods of Oxygen Delivery —cont'd

Advantages
- Decreased flow needed for a given FiO_2
- Reduced O_2 costs
- Allows longer periods away from a stationary O_2 source

Disadvantages
- Patients may object to the appearance of a reservoir cannula
- FiO_2 variability still exists
- Amount of O_2 savings varies greatly, depending on individual patient needs

HYPERBARIC OXYGEN THERAPY
- O_2 is administered at pressures greater than 1 atmosphere
  - Administered in a single patient chamber
  - Monitoring systems and ventilators can be adapted to allow treatment of critically ill patients
- Indications: Primary treatment for decompression of divers, air or gas embolism, carbon monoxide and/or cyanide poisoning, acute traumatic ischemia (compartment syndrome, crush injury), clostridial gangrene, necrotizing soft tissue infection, ischemic skin grafts or flaps, enhanced healing of problem wounds, refractory osteomyelitis
- Complications: Barotrauma, tympanic membrane rupture, pneumothorax, air embolism, O_2 toxicity, fire risk, reversible visual changes, claustrophobia, sudden decompression, radiation necrosis, central nervous system (CNS) toxic reaction (rare)

OTHER MEDICAL GAS THERAPIES
- Helium therapy: Used as an adjunct in managing large airway obstruction and status asthmaticus. Because of helium's low density, the driving pressure to move gas in and out of the larger airways is decreased, and therefore the work of breathing is reduced.
  - Administered in prepared gas cylinders delivering a mixture with a helium/O_2 ratio of either 80%:20% or 70%:30%.
  - Because of the high diffusibility of helium, the gas is generally administered via a nonrebreathing mask; it can be used with mechanical ventilation.
  - In a nonintubated patient, speech may be distorted during helium administration.
- Nitric oxide therapy: Used in the treatment of diseases characterized by pulmonary hypertension and hypoxia. Not approved by the U.S. Food and Drug Administration for these applications, except as an investigational medication. In very low concentrations (2–20 parts per million) mixed with O_2, nitric oxide selectively dilates pulmonary blood vessels, reduces intrapulmonary shunt, and improves arterial oxygenation.
  - Commonly administered via ventilator with a special analyzer for precise and stable nitric oxide dose titration; can be given to a nonintubated patient through a tight-fitting face mask.
  - Toxic effects are possible with inhaled nitric oxide, including production of nitrous dioxide, methemoglobinemia, production of peroxynitrite, platelet inhibition, increased left ventricular filling pressure, rebound hypoxemia, and pulmonary hypertension.

From Kacmarek, R. M., Stoller, J. K., Heuer, A. J. (2019). *Egan's fundamentals of respiratory care* 12th ed. St. Louis: Elsevier.

    (3) PEEP is lost if the patient is disconnected from the ventilator for suctioning. For this reason, closed-suction catheter systems are often used for mechanically ventilated patients to maintain PEEP levels during suctioning. If a precipitous drop in SpO_2 occurs during suctioning, preoxygenation before the procedure becomes critical.

  iv. Administer CPAP (see Box 3.6).

    (a) Similar to PEEP but used in spontaneously breathing patients via a nasal mask. May also be used in ventilator-dependent patients to improve PaO_2 and saturation levels.

    (b) Used during weaning from mechanical ventilation and for obstructive sleep apnea.

  v. Encourage the patient to take deep breaths.

  vi. Position the patient to facilitate $\dot{V}/\dot{Q}$ matching ("good side down").

  vii. Provide rest periods between activities to minimize O_2 demands.

    viii. Alleviate or minimize anxiety, which may increase O_2 demands.

    ix. Monitor the patient's response to any activity. If deterioration occurs, assist the patient with care including helping with turning and transfer, and passive range-of-motion exercises.

    x. Teach the patient and significant others techniques of self-care that will minimize O_2 consumption.

    xi. Maintain body temperature at a normal level; avoid patient shivering.

SPECIFIC PATIENT HEALTH PROBLEMS

ACUTE RESPIRATORY FAILURE (ARF)

1. **Pathophysiology**
   a. Respiratory system cannot carry out its two major functions: (1) delivery of an adequate amount of O_2 into the arterial blood and (2) removal of a corresponding amount of CO_2 from mixed venous blood. As an "acute" disorder, the onset must be relatively sudden; however, the onset can occur over days, as may be seen in patients with preexisting lung disease, or within minutes to hours, as may be seen in patients with no preexisting lung disease.
   b. The abnormalities in ABG levels may be in PAO_2 (hypoxemic respiratory failure), in $PACO_2$ (hypercapnic respiratory failure), or both. Critical value for the diagnosis based on arterial hypoxemia is PaO_2 lower than 55 mm Hg or SaO_2 lower than 88%; lower values can cause a marked decrease in oxyhemoglobin saturation and, therefore a considerable drop in O_2 content. Corresponding critical value for the diagnosis of acute hypercapnic respiratory failure is $PaCO_2$ above 50 mm Hg (with an accompanying acidemia, or pH of <7.30).
   c. Four major pathophysiologic mechanisms cause ARF—hypoventilation, ventilation-perfusion mismatching, shunt, and diffusion impairment. Two major processes involved are the following:
      i. Increase in extravascular lung water
         (a) Characterized by severe hypoxemia with normal to low $PaCO_2$
         (b) Occurs in patients with cardiogenic or noncardiogenic pulmonary edema and other parenchymal infiltrates
      ii. Impaired ventilation
         (a) Characterized by elevated $PaCO_2$ and decreased PaO_2
         (b) Occurs with intrapulmonary disorders (airway disease) or extrapulmonary problems (neuromuscular or chest wall diseases, alterations in respiratory drive). Other causes include low inspired oxygen tension (PiO_2) because of high altitude or inhalation of toxic gases and low mixed-venous oxygenation secondary to anemia, hypoxemia, inadequate cardiac output, or increased O_2 consumption.

2. **Etiology and risk factors**
   a. Increase in extravascular lung water (ARDS, pulmonary edema, aspiration, pneumonia, atelectasis)
   b. Impaired ventilation
      i. Intrapulmonary problems (see causes listed under Impaired Respiratory Mechanics and Impaired Alveolar Ventilation)
      ii. Extrapulmonary problems: Pleural effusion, kyphoscoliosis, multiple rib fractures, thoracic surgery, peritonitis; neuromuscular defects, such as polio, Guillain-Barré syndrome, multiple sclerosis, myasthenia gravis, brain or spinal injuries; medication effects (narcotics, barbiturates, tranquilizers, anesthetic agents); cerebral infarction

   c. Patient history
      i. Past medical history: Chronic airway obstruction, restrictive defects, neuromuscular defects, or respiratory center damage; history of conditions that impair gas exchange and diffusion
      ii. Family history: Any significant pulmonary disease in parents, grandparents, or siblings. One form of emphysema caused by a deficiency of the enzyme α_1-antitrypsin is an inherited disorder.
      iii. Social history: Current or past smoking; calculate the pack-year history for smokers (number of packs smoked per day times the number of years smoked)
      iv. Medication history: Prescribed and over-the-counter medications, their dosages, and last time taken. Assess for evidence of nonadherence in taking prescribed medications (e.g., missed doses or overdoses).

KEY CONCEPT

Patients who are diagnosed with COPD in their 40s should be evaluated for α_1-antitrypsin deficiency. Smoking cessation is the most important treatment.

---

3. **Signs and symptoms**
   a. Patient's chief complaint
      i. Most often dyspnea or increased work of breathing
      ii. Other symptoms include the following:
         (a) Increased pulmonary secretions
         (b) Manifestations of hypoxemia
         (c) Manifestations of hypercapnia with acidemia: Headache, confusion, inability to concentrate, irritability, somnolence, dizziness
   b. Nursing examination of patient
      i. Inspection
         (a) General observations
            (1) Posture, skin color, cyanosis, tissue perfusion, lung expansion
            (2) Signs of right-sided heart failure, such as pitting edema of the lower extremities, jugular venous distention
            (3) Signs of hypercapnia with acidemia: Muscle twitching, asterixis, miosis, papilledema, engorged fundal veins, diaphoresis
         (b) Thoracic abnormalities, such as increased A-P diameter (barrel chest), intercostal retractions, bulging interspaces on expiration (obstruction to air outflow), pectus carinatum or excavatum, spinal deformities
         (c) Pattern of ventilation
            (1) Use of accessory muscles of respiration
            (2) Abnormal rate, depth, or rhythm of breathing
            (3) Inspiration to expiration ratio (normal ratio is 1:2 or 1:3)
            (4) Inspiratory and/or expiratory stridor indicative of upper airway airflow obstruction
      ii. Palpation
         (a) Skin temperature and texture
         (b) Vocal fremitus
      iii. Percussion
         (a) Dullness over dense lung tissue (consolidation or fulminant pulmonary edema)
         (b) Hyperresonance with air trapping (COPD) or pneumothorax

iv. Auscultation
  (a) Decreased breath sounds with less air movement or less dense lung tissue (COPD)
  (b) Bronchial and bronchovesicular breath sounds over areas of consolidation, atelectasis, pulmonary edema
  (c) Adventitious sounds: Crackles or rales, rhonchi or wheezes, pleural friction rub with pleuritis

4. **Diagnostic study findings**
  a. Laboratory: ABG analysis
    i. Respiratory failure is defined by ABG measurements as hypoxemic (decreased PaO_2) and/or hypercapnic (increased $PaCO_2$ and decreased PaO_2).
    ii. Criteria: PaO_2 below 55 mm Hg, $PaCO_2$ above 50 mm Hg, or both
      (a) Acute: Acidosis, normal or mildly increasing blood buffer (HCO_3^-) levels
      (b) Chronic: Relatively normal pH, elevated blood buffer levels
    iii. Shunt studies: Demonstrate intrapulmonary shunt greater than 15%
  b. Radiologic: Findings depend on the primary disease

5. **Goals of care**
  a. Impaired respiratory gas transport: FiO_2 is sufficient for the patient's O_2 supply needs; respiratory rate, tidal volume, ABG levels are within normal limits for the patient
  b. Impaired alveolar ventilation
    i. Respiratory rate and breathing pattern are normal for the patient.
    ii. Patient has a minimal sensation of dyspnea with no auto-PEEP.
    iii. No ventilator-associated infections or other complications are present.
  c. Impaired respiratory gas exchange
    i. Hypoxemia resolves or improves.
    ii. Eucapnia or the usual compensated $PaCO_2$ and pH levels are observed.
    iii. Mental status is normal and the patient is breathing comfortably.
    iv. Patient performs techniques that maximize $\dot{V}/\dot{Q}$ matching

6. **Interprofessional collaboration: Nurse, physician, advanced practice provider, respiratory therapist, dietitian, pharmacist, social worker**

7. **Management of patient care**
  a. Anticipated patient trajectory
    i. Positioning: Keep the head of the bed elevated at least 30 degrees to maximize ventilation and prevent aspiration; turn as warranted to maximize $\dot{V}/\dot{Q}$ matching, consider physical therapy and early mobility.
    ii. Skin care: Progressive mobility should be used to mobilize secretions and maintain skin integrity.
    iii. Pain management: Provide nonpharmacologic pain relieving interventions, or administer pain medication to relieve the discomfort of tubes and treatment.
    iv. Nutrition: Obtain dietitian consult and collaboration; provide adequate nutrition to maintain cellular function and healing with the increased work of breathing.
    v. Transport: Same level of care and all precautions as on the unit need to be maintained if the patient requires transport within or outside the facility.
    vi. Discharge planning: Initiate early with the patient and family, especially if the patient will require continued care at home; evaluate the need for support and rehabilitation on discharge; anticipate home care equipment needs; provide a social services consult to arrange for the transition to home care, if warranted.

      vii. Pharmacology: Antibiotics, provide nonpharmacologic pain relieving interventions, sedatives, or analgesics as warranted. Instruct the patient and family in medications, inhalers, spirometry to be used at home.

     viii. Psychosocial issues: Psychosocial effect is affected by the circumstances of the patient's admission (abrupt because of trauma vs. slow deterioration at a skilled care facility), prior hospitalizations in acute care units, the effects on family dynamics and household income, and many other variables. Degree, nature, and extent of support must be tailored to patient and family needs and incorporate as wide an array of healthcare services as warranted.

      ix. Treatments
- (a) Noninvasive
  - (1) O$_2$ delivery systems
  - (2) Bilevel positive airway pressure
  - (3) Average volume assured pressure support (AVAPS): Effective in patients with acute exacerbation of COPD with hypercapnic encephalopathy, neuromuscular disease and obesity hypoventilation.
- (b) Invasive
  - (1) Intubation and mechanical ventilation

      x. Ethical issues: Issues related to the use and withdrawal of artificial means of ventilation represent a common source of ethical decision-making requirements involving the patient (with or without an advance directive in place), family members, members of the health care team, and possibly others, such as a hospital ethics committee (see Ch. 1 coverage of these issues).

  b. Potential complications
- i. Hospital-associated infections (HAIs)
  - (a) Mechanism: Patient vulnerable because of position changes and possible need for enteral feedings, probable use of a urinary catheter, foreign airway object, recumbent position, and the need for cleansing and removal of oropharyngeal secretions.
  - (b) Management: see Positioning, Skin Care, and Infection Control
- ii. Complications related to the therapies used for ventilatory support (e.g., O$_2$ toxicity barotrauma, volutrauma, tracheal damage, gastric ulcers, inability to wean from the ventilator)
  - (a) Causes: see Box 3.7.
  - (b) Management: see Box 3.7.
  - (c) Prevention of ventilator-associated pneumonia (VAP): see Box 3.7.

CHEST TRAUMA
(See Ch. 11, Multisystem Trauma)

ACUTE RESPIRATORY DISTRESS SYNDROME (ARDS)
1. **Pathophysiology**
   a. ARDS refers to a group of manifestations of an evolving severe diffuse lung injury. Some patients survive and recover completely, although may have some residual impairment, however slight. Others, notably those with sepsis (particularly of abdominal origin), have a high mortality because their ARDS evolves into a chronic form.
   b. Acute phase of ARDS is characterized by damaged integrity of the blood-gas barrier. There is extensive damage to type I alveolar epithelial cells with increased endothelial permeability. Interstitial edema is found along with the leakage of protein-containing fluid into the alveoli. This alveolar fluid contains erythrocytes and leukocytes in addition to amorphous material comprising strands of fibrin.

There is also impaired production and function of surfactant. Resultant physiologic abnormalities are as follows:

    i. Shunting of blood through atelectatic or fluid-filled lung units causes a widening of the A–a difference in PAO_2; the resultant hypoxemia is resistant to high FiO_2 but is often responsive to PEEP.

    ii. Physiologic dead space is increased, frequently exceeding 60% of each breath; consequently, very large minute ventilation may be required to maintain acceptable levels of arterial $PACO_2$.

    iii. Compliance of certain portions of lung parenchyma is reduced. Increased stiffness of the lungs is associated with decreased FRC and a requirement for high peak inspiratory pressures during mechanical ventilation. Other lung areas have relatively normal specific compliance and thus are not so much stiff as they are small.

    iv. Resistance to blood flow through the lungs is increased by narrowing or obstruction of pulmonary vessels. As a result, peak airway pressure (PAP) is often increased while pulmonary artery occlusive pressure (PAOP) remains normal or low. Chest radiographs reveal diffuse bilateral infiltrates suggesting noncardiogenic pulmonary edema.

  c. Chronic phase of ARDS is characterized by thickening of the endothelium, epithelium, and interstitial space. Type I cells are destroyed and replaced by type II cells (neutrophils), which proliferate but do not differentiate into type I cells as normal. Interstitial space is greatly expanded by edema fluid, fibers, and a variety of proliferating cells. Fibrosis commences after the first week. Within the alveoli, the protein-rich exudate may organize to produce the characteristic "hyaline membrane," which effectively destroys the structure of the alveoli.

  d. Resultant physiologic abnormalities are the following:

    i. Increased vascular resistance

    ii. Hypoxemia caused by $\dot{V}/\dot{Q}$ mismatch or possible diffusion defect

    iii. Decreased tissue compliance

2. **Etiology and risk factors**

  a. Direct injury: Pulmonary contusion, gastric aspiration, near-drowning, inhalation of toxic gases and vapors, some infections, fat embolus, amniotic fluid embolus, radiation, bleomycin

  b. Indirect injury: Septicemia, shock or prolonged hypotension, nonthoracic trauma, cardiopulmonary bypass, drug overdose, head injury, pancreatitis, diabetic coma, multiple blood transfusions

3. **Signs and symptoms**

  a. Patient's chief complaint is severe dyspnea.

  b. Increased work of breathing manifested by tachypnea, hyperpnea, nasal flaring, intercostal retractions, use of accessory muscles

  c. Production of frothy, pink sputum, dullness to percussion, bronchovesicular breath sounds over most lung fields, and diffuse crackles over all lung fields if substantial pulmonary edema is present

  d. Diminished lung expansion

  e. Diminished level of consciousness if hypoxemia is severe

4. **Diagnostic study findings: To exclude other causes of pulmonary edema**

  a. Brain natriuretic peptide level below 100 pg/mL favors ARDS

KEY CONCEPT

Need to rule out congestive heart failure (CHF), which can look very similar to ARDS on chest imaging.

b. ABG analysis
   i. Hypoxemia is the hallmark of ARDS and is caused by intrapulmonary shunting. Hypoxemia is refractory to O_2 therapy (e.g., PaO_2 is below 55 mm Hg or SaO_2 is below 90% with FiO_2 above 0.5).
   ii. Respiratory alkalosis occurs in the early phases of ARDS because of hyperventilation.
   iii. Hypercapnia not usually seen initially; it is an ominous sign if present.
   iv. Shunt studies demonstrate large right-to-left shunt (usually >20% of cardiac output) measured during 100% O_2 breathing.
   v. Increased A–a gradient.
   vi. Reduced PaO_2/FiO_2 ratio
       (a) Mild: 200 to 300—27% mortality
       (b) Moderate: 100 to 200—32% mortality
       (c) Severe: <100—45% mortality
c. Radiologic: Chest radiograph demonstrates diffuse bilateral interstitial and alveolar infiltrates without cardiomegaly or pulmonary vascular redistribution in the acute phase; a fine or coarse reticular pattern evolves in the chronic phase.

5. **Goals of care**
   a. Hypoxemia resolves or improves with or without O_2 supplementation or mechanical ventilation
   b. Respiratory rate, depth, and breathing pattern are normal for the patient
   c. Arterial pH, $PACO_2$, and PAO_2 normalize to acceptable values
   d. Patient has minimal or no sensation of dyspnea
   e. There is no clinical evidence of any complications related to equipment or therapies.

6. **Interprofessional collaboration: Nurse, physician, advanced practice provider, respiratory therapist, dietitian, pharmacist.**

7. **Management of patient care**
   a. Most patients require intubation and mechanical ventilation.
       i. Low tidal volumes and high levels of PEEP
           (a) National Institutes of Health (NIH), National Heart, Lung, and Blood Institute (NHLBI) ARDS Network at http://www.ardsnet.org
       ii. Extracorporeal membrane oxygenation
       iii. Consider prone positioning
   b. Potential complications
       i. Fluid overload
           (a) Management: Monitor input and output closely; observe for signs of fluid overload; use the lowest intravascular volume compatible with adequate tissue perfusion.
       ii. Barotrauma/volutrauma because of physical stress of positive pressure ventilation on acutely damaged alveolar membranes
           (a) Pneumothorax less common with low tidal volume ventilation which reduces plateau airway pressures.

VAPING

1. **Inhaling of an aerosol that is created by heating a liquid or wax containing various substances. Several devices are available including battery-operated electronic cigarettes and vape pens.**
   a. Nicotine
   b. Cannabinoids, such as tetrahydrocannabinol, cannabidiol
   c. Flavoring and additives, such as glycerol, propylene glycol

    i. E-cigarette or vaping has led to vaping-associated pulmonary injury. Initially described in 2019, this has resulted in an acute or subacute respiratory illness that can be severe and life-threatening. The pathogenesis is not well known. Vitamin E acetate has been linked, but the mechanism of toxicity is not known. Treatment is mainly supportive care although some patients have gone on to lung transplantation.

TRANSFUSION-RELATED LUNG INJURY

1. Pathophysiology
   a. Transfusion-related acute lung injury can occur with the transfusion of any blood or blood product; however, it is most frequently associated with plasma-rich products, such as whole blood, platelets, and fresh frozen plasma.
   b. Transfusion-related acute lung injury is marked by acute respiratory distress that develops within minutes to hours after a blood transfusion.
   c. The alveoli fill with protein and fluid as a result of pulmonary endothelial and alveolar damage.
   d. Suggested mechanisms include donor leukocyte antibodies that react against recipient white cells, recipient antibody to donor plasma, and/or a two hit model where some associated process, such as sepsis or systemic inflammation causes endothelial activation which is then further activated by transfusion therapy mediated lipid or other mediator.
   e. Most common major transfusion reaction
   f. Causes one-third of transfusion-related deaths
   g. Occurs in approximately every 1/500 to 1/5000 units of products transfused
   h. Occurs during or less than 6 hours after transfusion
   i. Most often plasma containing products, but can occur with any blood product
2. Signs and symptoms
   a. Symptoms may be mild to severe and may include dyspnea, hypoxemia, tachypnea, fever, and cyanosis.
   b. The patient also develops large amounts of frothy, pink secretions.
   c. When performing lung auscultation, crackles and decreased breath sounds are noted bilaterally. These signs and symptoms occur without any indication of circulatory overload in patients who do not have a preexisting lung injury.
3. Treatment
   a. Treatment for transfusion-related acute lung injury is primarily supportive and the syndrome is often self-limiting. However, patients who experience this transfusion reaction usually require mechanical ventilation. Vasopressors may also need to be used.
   b. Use of steroids. Not routinely recommended.
   c. Lasix (Furosemide) is NOT appropriate. Diuretics are best avoided to prevent lowering the intravascular pressures, which could worsen the patient's hypotension.
   d. Symptoms may subside within 96 hours.
4. Prevention
   a. Limit FFP/platelets from females

PULMONARY EMBOLISM

1. Pathophysiology
   a. PE, an obstruction of the pulmonary artery by an embolus, affects lung tissue, the pulmonary circulation, and the function of the right and left sides of the heart.

Degree of compromise correlates with the extent of embolic vascular occlusion and the degree of preexisting cardiopulmonary disease.

b. Most emboli (>90%) arise from deep venous thromboses (DVTs) in the iliofemoral system. Because of increased use of central venous catheters, upper extremity DVT is rising in incidence. It represents about 5% of PE sources. Other sites include the right side of the heart and the pelvic area. Nonthrombotic emboli, such as fat, air, and amniotic fluid, also occur but are relatively uncommon.

c. Distribution of emboli is related to the size of emboli and blood flow. Very large emboli have an effect in a large artery; however, the thrombus may break up and block several smaller vessels. Lower lobes are frequently involved because they have greater blood flow.

d. Pulmonary infarction (death of the embolized tissue) occurs infrequently. More often, there is distal hemorrhage and atelectasis, but alveolar structures remain viable. Infarction is more likely if the embolus completely blocks a large artery or if there is preexisting lung disease. Infarction results in alveolar filling with extravasated red blood cells and inflammatory cells and causes opacity on a radiograph. Occasionally, the infarct becomes infected, which leads to an abscess.

e. Effects of acute pulmonary artery obstruction
   i. Altered gas exchange because of right-to-left shunting and $\dot{V}/\dot{Q}$ inequalities. Possible etiologic mechanisms for these alterations include the following:
      (a) Overperfusion of the uninvolved lung, which lowers $\dot{V}/\dot{Q}$ ratios
      (b) Eventual reperfusion of atelectatic areas distal to the embolic obstruction
      (c) Development of postembolic pulmonary edema
   ii. Degree of hemodynamic compromise correlates with the degree of vascular occlusion in patients with no underlying heart or lung disease
      (a) Initial hemodynamic consequence is acute reduction in the pulmonary vascular cross-sectional area with a subsequent increase in the resistance to blood flow through the lungs.
      (b) If cardiac output remains constant or increases, pulmonary arterial pressure must rise.
   iii. If cardiac or pulmonary disease exists and has already impaired the pulmonary vascular reserve capacity, a small degree of vascular occlusion will result in greater pulmonary artery hypertension and more serious right ventricular dysfunction.

2. **Etiology and risk factors**
   a. Factors favoring venous thrombosis (Virchow's triad) include the following:
      i. Blood stasis
         (a) Surgery or anesthesia, prolonged immobilization
         (b) Heart failure, acute myocardial infarction
         (c) Shock (bacteremic or nonbacteremic)
      ii. Blood coagulation alterations
         (a) Diabetes mellitus, polycythemia vera, dysproteinemia
         (b) Estrogen administration
         (c) Pregnancy
         (d) Recent childbirth
         (e) Malignancy

KEY CONCEPT
Need to consider evaluation for inherited blood clotting disorders (e.g., factor V Leiden, etc.)

      iii. Vessel wall abnormalities

        (a) Trauma (especially fractures of the spine, pelvis, or legs with fat emboli)

        (b) Venous disease of a lower extremity

   b. Previous pulmonary embolus

KEY CONCEPT
Recurrent DVT/PE makes lifelong anticoagulation mandatory.

---

   c. Central line removal or disconnection (air embolus)

   d. Recent pelvic or lower abdominal surgery (fat embolus)

   e. Burns

   f. Obesity

   g. Amniotic fluid embolus

3. **Signs and symptoms**

   a. Patient's chief complaint varies considerably, depending on the severity and type of embolism. Sudden onset of chest pain (usually pleuritic), cough, and hemoptysis (only 13% of PEs, which suggests pulmonary infarction) are commonly reported.

   b. Massive PE (>50% vascular occlusion): Mental clouding, anxiety, feeling of impending doom and apprehension.

   c. Other symptoms may be vague and nonspecific and may mimic myocardial infarction or CHF.

      i. Dyspnea, tachypnea, increased work of breathing

      ii. Tachycardia, diffuse chest discomfort, reduced blood pressure

      iii. Anxiety, restlessness, apprehension, agitation, syncope

      iv. Asymmetric chest expansion because of pleuritic pain

      v. Petechiae over the thorax and upper extremities (fat emboli commonly seen in the axilla)

      vi. Diaphoresis, cold and clammy skin, and cyanosis

      vii. Increased fremitus with a large hemorrhagic pulmonary infarct; pleural friction fremitus may be palpated in patients with pleural inflammation distal to an infarct.

      viii. Resonance heard throughout the lung fields except dullness to percussion over the area of infarction

      ix. Pleural friction rub; inspiratory crackles (rales) may be heard; increased intensity of the pulmonic second sound (P_2); fixed splitting of the second heart sound (S_2) is an ominous finding caused by marked right ventricular overload. A murmur over the affected lung field, augmented by inspiration, and is generated by flow through a partially obstructed pulmonary artery. Murmur may be absent initially and then develop as an embolus resolves.

4. **Diagnostic study findings**

   a. Laboratory: ABG levels may indicate respiratory alkalosis (caused by hyperventilation) and hypoxemia; A–a gradient is increased; in a small percentage (6%) of patients, the A–a gradient may be normal.

      i. D-dimer, which may be nonspecific, but if normal makes the diagnosis of PE less likely

      ii. Cardiac enzymes may be elevated with right heart strain. Frequently leads to misdiagnosis of CHF.

    b. Radiologic
- i. Chest radiograph: Nonspecific, frequently normal. Pleural effusion occurs in 30% to 50% of cases but is small; atelectasis and elevated hemidiaphragm on the affected side may be seen. Useful to detect other things causing similar symptoms.
- ii. Lower-extremity Doppler ultrasonography: Negative findings on serial ultrasonographic scans reduce the likelihood of PE.
- iii. Pulmonary angiography: Most definitive test (gold standard) for PE; should be considered when results of noninvasive tests are equivocal or contradictory or as an initial diagnostic test if the patient is hemodynamically unstable.
- iv. CT-angio or CT-PA very sensitive and done more often than pulmonary angiography.

    c. Electrocardiogram (ECG): In massive PE may reveal "P pulmonale," right-axis deviation, or incomplete or new right bundle branch block. ECG often demonstrates sinus tachycardia or, less frequently, atrial fibrillation or flutter. In addition, an S wave in lead 1, Q waves in lead III, ST elevation or T wave inversion in lead III may be seen.

    d. Radionuclide testing: Lung ventilation-perfusion scan not definitive but suggestive of PE; less risky than angiography; performed for clinically stable patients with suspected PE.

5. **Goals of care**
   - a. Pulmonary artery blood flow is restored
   - b. Hemodynamic parameters return to normal
   - c. Recurrence or worsening of embolization and thrombosis is prevented
   - d. Chest pain is relieved

6. **Interprofessional collaboration: Nurse, physician, advanced practice provider, respiratory therapist, pharmacist, dietitian**

7. **Management of patient care**
   - a. Anticipated patient trajectory
     - i. Positioning: Keep the head of the bed elevated at 30 to 45 degrees to enhance ventilation and prevent aspiration. Instruct the patient to avoid crossing the legs or sitting with the feet dependent for long periods. Vary position and do range-of-motion manipulations to enhance peripheral blood flow.
     - ii. Skin care: Inspect skin integrity regularly, especially on the lower legs. Promptly report the patient's development of pain, swelling, tenderness, rubor, and localized warmth in a lower extremity (suggestive of phlebitis, possible thrombosis).
     - iii. Pain management: Administer analgesics for relief of chest pain (can be severe).
     - iv. Discharge planning: Provide patient education and follow-up related to the prevention of phlebitis and DVT, facilitation of venous return, and safe use of anticoagulants.
     - v. Pharmacology: Administer anticoagulants as ordered; monitor for signs of bleeding; administer thrombolytic therapy, and pain medication as ordered.
     - vi. Treatments
       - (a) O_2 administration, as needed
       - (b) Early mobility with turning and ambulation, promotion of coughing and deep breathing
       - (c) Use of elastic stockings, pneumatic compression stockings (if not contraindicated with systemic anticoagulation), leg elevation
       - (d) Adequate fluid intake to avoid dehydration and increased blood viscosity

    (e) Thrombolytic therapy: Can be given systemically (less invasive) or catheter-directed (more invasive). This can be considered for patients with severe hypoxemia or shock or subacute PE.

    (f) Anticoagulant therapy, heparin or low-molecular-weight heparin, warfarin

    (g) Placement of filter device in inferior vena cava (limited indications and reserved for those patients who cannot be anticoagulated).

    (h) Surgical embolectomy, rarely performed now

    (i) Direct oral anticoagulants: Xarelto (rivaroxaban), Eliquis (apixaban), Savaysa (edoxaban), and Pradaxa (dabigatran) are all approved for treatment of DVT/PE

  b. Potential complications

    i. Bleeding

      (a) Mechanism: Risk of anticoagulation therapy

      (b) Management: Judicious, closely monitored use of anticoagulants

CHRONIC OBSTRUCTIVE PULMONARY DISEASE (COPD)

1. Pathophysiology

  a. COPD is an inclusive and nonspecific term referring to a condition in which patients have chronic cough and expectoration and various degrees of dyspnea either at rest or with exertion, with a significant and progressive reduction in expiratory airflow as measured by the forced expiratory volume in 1 second (FEV_1). This airflow abnormality does not show major reversibility in response to pharmacologic agents.

  b. Affects more than 5% of the population and is associated with high morbidity and mortality.

  c. Fourth-ranked cause of death in the United States, killing more than 120,000 people each year.

  d. COPD is usually divided into two subtypes: Chronic bronchitis and emphysema.

    i. Chronic bronchitis: Clinical diagnosis defined as the presence of chronic cough with sputum production on a daily basis for a minimum of 3 months a year for not less than 2 successive years. Many patients exhibit chronic hypoxemia with resultant episodes of cor pulmonale. They may also have reduced responsiveness of the respiratory center to hypoxemic stimuli, a trait that is probably inherited. Some of the pathophysiologic findings of chronic bronchitis are the following:

      (a) Increase in the size of the tracheobronchial mucous glands and goblet cell hyperplasia, which results in increased sputum production

      (b) Epithelial mucous cell metaplasia, which results in a decreased number of cilia. Hypersecretion of mucus and impaired cilia lead to a chronic productive cough.

      (c) Increase in bronchial wall thickness with progressive obstruction to airflow (chronic obstructive bronchitis)

      (d) Exacerbations are usually because of infection, with the following clinical picture:

        (1) Increased amount of sputum and retained secretions

        (2) Increased $\dot{V}/\dot{Q}$ abnormalities, which increase hypoxemia, CO_2 retention, and acidemia

        (3) Hypoxemia and acidemia increase pulmonary vessel constriction, raising PAP and ultimately leading to right-sided heart failure (cor pulmonale).

ii. Emphysema: Anatomic alteration of the lung characterized by an abnormal enlargement of the air spaces distal to the terminal, nonrespiratory bronchioles, accompanied by destructive changes in the alveolar walls. Emphysema patients often exhibit increased dyspnea and breathing effort owing to an inherent increased responsiveness to hypoxemia. Resultant clinical picture is typically that of a well-oxygenated and dyspneic patient. Pulmonary abnormalities seen in emphysema are the following:

   (a) Gas exchange surface of the respiratory bronchioles, alveolar ducts, and alveoli is reduced.

   (b) Air trapping is increased because of the loss of elastic recoil in airway support structures (causes increased A-P diameter).

   (c) Air sacs are replaced by bullae and capillary area is proportionately diminished.

   (d) $\dot{V}/\dot{Q}$ inequality occurs and FRC is increased.

   (e) Increased work of breathing results in greater resting O_2 consumption.

iii. Asthma/COPD overlap

   (a) Many individuals have inflammatory features of both asthma and chronic bronchitis/emphysema.

   (b) Characterized by persistent airflow limitation with several features usually associated with asthma and several features associated with COPD

   (c) A subgroup of patient with eosinophilia may experience lung function improvement with antiinterleukin-5 receptor monoclonal antibodies that deplete blood and sputum eosinophils.

2. **Etiology and risk factors (chronic bronchitis and emphysema)**

   a. Various forms of tobacco inhalation which include cigarette smoking—the most important factor and the major toxic stimulus, cigars and vaping

   b. Environmental pollution, occupational exposure

   c. Predisposition because of genetic makeup, especially α_1-antitrypsin deficiency. Should be considered in nonsmokers or young patients with emphysema. Current guidelines recommend testing every COPD patient for this genetic finding.

3. **Signs and symptoms: These diseases may present as pure entities, but it is common for patients to have a combination of the symptoms of the two.**

   a. Chronic bronchitis

      i. Chief complaint is usually chronic cough and sputum production.

      ii. Wheezing

      iii. Observe for signs of right-sided heart failure: Peripheral edema, distended neck veins, skin color that is dusky or cyanotic. Patients with chronic bronchitis show little sign of respiratory distress or dyspnea at rest.

      iv. Chest expansion may be normal; vocal fremitus may be normal or increased because of copious bronchial secretions.

      v. Resonance may be heard on percussion if there are no areas of secretion retention or consolidation.

      vi. Dullness to percussion is heard in areas of increased lung density (consolidation).

      vii. Coarse crackles and/or expiratory wheezes are commonly heard.

   b. Emphysema

      i. Chief complaint is dyspnea on exertion (early symptom) and eventually dyspnea at rest.

      ii. Skin color is often pink because the patient is well oxygenated

      iii. Weight loss, inability to perform ADLs

    iv. Barrel chest; note posture (tripod) and work of breathing both at rest and during exercise; use of accessory muscles of respiration is common.

    v. Pursed-lip breathing

    vi. Reduced chest excursion because of hyperinflated lungs and flattened diaphragm from chronic air trapping

    vii. Reduced vocal fremitus because of less dense, more hyperinflated lungs

    viii. Hyperresonance throughout all lung fields

    ix. Distant, quiet breath sounds because of reduced air movement and air trapping; wheezes heard on occasion

4. Diagnostic study findings

  a. Chronic bronchitis

    i. Laboratory

      (a) ABG analysis: Hypoxemia and often hypercapnia with compensated respiratory acidosis

      (b) Other laboratory findings: Polycythemia on complete blood count (CBC) in some patients

    ii. Pulmonary function: Reduction in the ratio of FEV_1 to FVC and all other measures of expiratory airflow; some reversibility following bronchodilator therapy in selected patients

  b. Emphysema

    i. Laboratory: ABG analysis—may be normal or abnormal, depending on the type and severity of $\dot{V}/\dot{Q}$ abnormalities. Hypoxemia, if present, may be mild with normal $PaCO_2$

    ii. Radiologic: Chest radiographs often show low, flattened diaphragms. In severe emphysema, lung fields may be hyperlucent and show hyperinflation, with diminished vascular markings and bullae. Disease is most prominent in the upper lung zones except in α_1-antitrypsin deficiency, in which a basilar predominance may be seen. Chest radiographs are of value during acute exacerbation to exclude complications, such as pneumonia and pneumothorax.

    iii. Pulmonary function: Increased FRC, residual volume, and TLC. Reduced FEV_1 with the ratio of FEV_1 to FVC of less than 75% (>80% is normal) and reduction in other expiratory airflow measures, which is typically nonreversible following administration of bronchodilators. Increased lung compliance and decrease in static recoil. Decreased diffusion capacity indicating a reduction in alveolar capillary gas exchange area.

5. Goals of care

  a. Both disorders

    i. The entirety of the tracheobronchial tree remains patent and free of secretions

    ii. Oxygenation improves

    iii. Alveolar ventilation improves

    iv. Work of breathing is minimized; ABG levels, vital signs, and tidal volume are within normal limits for the patient.

  b. Chronic bronchitis

    i. Constricted airways are dilated

    ii. Patient is able to effectively clear secretions

    iii. There are minimal to no signs and symptoms of right-sided heart failure

    iv. Patient reports taking bronchodilator medications as prescribed

c. Emphysema
   i. Breathing pattern is normal for the patient
   ii. Sensation of dyspnea is decreased
   iii. There is no air trapping at the end of expiration (auto-PEEP)
6. **Interprofessional collaboration: Nurse, physician, advanced practice provider, respiratory therapist, dietitian, pharmacist, physical and occupational therapist.**

EXPERT TIP

Physical therapists and occupational therapists can be very helpful with pulmonary rehabilitation and development of routines that maximize the pulmonary function that they have remaining.

---

7. **Management of patient care**
   a. Anticipated patient trajectory
      i. Positioning: Keep the head of the bed elevated 30 to 45 degrees unless medically contraindicated to improve ventilation and prevent aspiration. Allow the patient to assume a position of comfort for breathing to diminish dyspnea. Patients with emphysema may need an overbed table for best positioning.
      ii. Skin care: Many of these patients have little adipose tissue owing to the increased work of breathing. Skin integrity may be compromised by consistent use of corticosteroids over the course of the disease. Others may exhibit peripheral edema related to right-sided heart failure. In either case, skin integrity warrants frequent monitoring and active care so that pressure injury or other breaks do not lead to infection.
      iii. Nutrition: Labored ventilation and the increased work of breathing associated with these disorders often precipitate the need for dietitian consultation to ensure that sufficient protein and calorie intake are paired with judicious fluid intake.
      iv. Infection control: These patients are especially vulnerable to HAIs.
      v. Transport: If transport is necessary, ensure that optimal levels of patient care, patient monitoring, O_2 supply, humidification, and positioning are maintained throughout transport.
      vi. Discharge planning: Discuss the need for smoking cessation; instruct in the proper use of an inhaler, effective coughing techniques, follow-up care at home. Consultation with social services to address the medical and social services support as needed. Outpatient pulmonary rehabilitation if eligible.
      vii. Pharmacology: Bronchodilators, steroids, and antibiotics as needed; sedatives and pain medication sufficient to enable therapies to be performed and to keep the patient comfortable. For patients with documented α_1-antitrypsin deficiency receiving α_1-proteinase inhibitor (Prolastin), provide medication monitoring instruction.
      viii. Psychosocial issues: Determine patient and family needs for support, because COPD can have a major effect on family roles, dynamics, and income. Identify issues important to the patient and family and communicate these to the social services member of the team.
      ix. Treatments
         (a) Carefully administer O_2 using the lowest FiO_2 that produces adequate oxygenation; observe for CO_2 retention.
         (b) Observe for signs of fluid overload; monitor intake and output closely.

     (c) Monitor ABG levels; notify the physician immediately if PaO_2 drops below the patient's known baseline or target level (usually PaO_2 of 55 mm Hg or higher) or if $PaCO_2$ rises significantly beyond the established baseline value. In a patient with chronic CO_2 retention, monitoring $PaCO_2$ is less important than observing pH changes.

     (d) Advocate for the administration of influenza and pneumococcal vaccine.

  x. Ethical issues: Determine whether an advance directive is in place, and determination of code status upon admission, as intubation may be a terminal event.

KEY CONCEPT

Palliative care counseling can be very helpful to support the patient, determine goals of care, symptom management and stress from the illness

---

  b. Potential complications
    i. Hospital-associated infections
    ii. Inability to wean or liberate from the ventilator
    iii. Deconditioning secondary to steroid use or lack of muscle work
    iv. Cor pulmonale
     (a) Mechanism: Right-sided heart failure develops secondary to increased resistance to blood flow and increased pressures in the right side of the heart, the pulmonary artery, and the venous circuit owing to COPD.
     (b) Management: Symptomatic management of problems, such as fluid balance, peripheral edema, cough

ASTHMA AND STATUS ASTHMATICUS

1. Pathophysiology
  a. Asthma: Chronic disease of variable severity characterized by airway hyperreactivity that produces airway narrowing of a reversible nature
    i. Increased responsiveness of the airways to various stimuli
    ii. Widespread narrowing of the airway with changes in severity; airway closure may occur
    iii. Cellular infiltration and mucosal edema
    iv. Airway hyperreactivity, with smooth muscle contraction and excessive mucus production and diminished secretion clearance
    v. $\dot{V}/\dot{Q}$ abnormalities
    vi. Increased work of breathing and airway resistance
    vii. Hyperinflation of the lung, with an increase in residual volume
    viii. Host defect of altered immunologic state
    ix. Some patients develop airway remodeling, then respond as in COPD
  b. Status asthmaticus: Severe asthma attack that is refractory to bronchodilator therapy, including β-adrenergic agents
    i. Severely reduced spirometric values for peak expiratory flow rate (PEFR), FVC, and FEV_1.
    ii. Hypoxemia is present with a widened A–a O_2 tension gradient or reduced PaO_2/FiO_2 ratio.
    iii. Airway narrowing because of the following:
     (a) Bronchial smooth muscle spasm (minor component)

(b) Inflammation of bronchial walls, which leads to increased mucosal permeability and basement membrane thickening

(c) Mucus plugging from airways because of increased production and reduced clearance of secretions. Mucus plugging, mucosal edema, and secretions account for the apparent resistance to bronchodilator therapy in patients in status asthmaticus.

2. **Etiology and risk factors**
   a. Respiratory infection
   b. Allergic reaction to inhaled antigen (pollen, grass, perfume, smoke)
   c. Poor bronchodilator use and management
   d. Idiosyncratic reaction to aspirin or other nonsteroidal antiinflammatory medications
   e. Emotional stress, exercise
   f. Occupational or environmental exposure (air pollution)
   g. Use of nonselective β-blocking agents (propranolol, timolol maleate)
   h. Mechanical stimulation (coughing, laughing, and cold air inhalation)
   i. Sinusitis, reflux esophagitis
   j. Genetic predisposition
   k. Elevated IgE levels

3. **Signs and symptoms**
   a. Chief complaints are usually dyspnea, wheezing, cough, and chest tightness; severity ranges from intermittent, mild symptoms to severe respiratory symptoms despite intensive therapy.
   b. Physical exhaustion, inability to sleep or rest, anxiety
   c. Difficulty speaking in sentences, minimal chest excursion with inspiration
   d. Production of thick, tenacious sputum
   e. Increased work of breathing evidenced by the following:
      i. Posture—habitus often leaning forward, with head lowered
      ii. Respiratory distress, tachypnea, hyperpnea at rest, expiratory stridor
      iii. Use of pursed-lip breathing with prolonged expiration
      iv. Nasal flaring, bulging of interspaces on expiration, diaphoresis
   f. Signs of dehydration
   g. Vocal fremitus may be decreased (decreased density with lung hyperinflation); rhonchal fremitus with copious secretions
   h. Hyperresonance throughout the lung fields, low diaphragm, and limited diaphragmatic excursion on percussion
   i. Expiratory wheezes or rhonchi (as air and secretions move through narrowed airways). Severe wheezing may be audible without a stethoscope.
   j. Decreased breath sounds throughout constitute an ominous sign. Asthmatic patient is then not moving enough air and will likely need to be intubated.

EXPERT TIP
Patients will often know and tell you when they need to be intubated.

---

4. **Diagnostic study findings**
   a. Laboratory
      i. Evidence of infection (e.g., positive sputum culture results), elevated white blood cell (WBC) count
      ii. ABG analysis

(a) May initially show low normal or decreased $PaCO_2$, increased pH, and decreased PaO_2 (<55 mm Hg)

(b) In severe asthmatic attacks, progression to a "normal" or increased $PaCO_2$ level may be a sign of impending respiratory failure.

b. Radiologic: Chest radiograph may be normal or hyperlucent. Used to confirm or rule out a diagnosis of pneumonia, atelectasis, pneumothorax, or other condition that mimics asthma.

c. Pulmonary function: Reduced FEV_1 and PEFRs. Serial measurements of these parameters indicating the response to bronchodilators are essential to establish the severity of the obstruction and assess the adequacy of the response to therapy. In patients requiring hospitalization, PEFR may be less than 60 L/min initially or may not improve to more than 50% of the predicted value after 1 hour of treatment. FEV_1 may be less than 30% of the predicted value or may not improve to at least 40% of the predicted value after 1 hour of aggressive therapy.

d. Fraction of exhaled nitric oxide (FENO)

5. **Goals of care**

a. Diameter and patency of the airways are improved

b. Airway secretions and coughing are reduced

c. Dyspnea and the work of breathing are reduced

d. Oxygenation and ABG values are optimized

6. **Interprofessional collaboration: Nurse, physician, advanced practice provider, respiratory therapist, dietitian, pharmacist.**

7. **Management of patient care**

a. Anticipated patient trajectory

   i. Positioning: Keep the head of the bed elevated 30 to 45 degrees to maximize ventilation, enhance coughing effectiveness, and prevent aspiration. Assist the patient to his or her own position of comfort.

   ii. Discharge planning: Teach correct inhaler technique, teach peak flow and symptom monitoring, and instruct the patient and family on avoidance of allergens and situations that trigger episodes and on the importance of taking medications properly.

   iii. Pharmacology: Administer long-acting beta agonist and inhaled corticosteroids and monitor effects (salmeterol is contraindicated during an acute asthma attack because of its delayed onset of action; albuterol or some other bronchodilator with a rapid onset of action should be used); administer steroids and antibiotics as needed. Leukotriene receptor antagonists are added if symptoms persist despite high-dose inhaled corticosteroids and long-acting beta-agonist therapy. Severe and persistent asthma with concurrent allergen sensitization and an elevated IgE level warrants consideration of omalizumab therapy.

   iv. Psychosocial issues: Asthmatic attacks are stressful and frightening to the patient and family; the intensive care unit (ICU) environment may only add further anxiety. Need to work with the family as a unit because the ramifications of asthma may extend to the physical home environment and interpersonal dynamics, and ability to work and function in customary roles.

   v. Treatments:

(a) Administer BiPAP, CPAP, heliox (helium and oxygen mixture).

(b) Intubation and mechanical ventilation become necessary.

(c) Administer fluids and humidification to keep airway secretions thin and easily expectorated.

(d) Perform close objective monitoring of ABG values, acid-base status, and ventilatory parameters (especially FEV_1 or peak flow rates if spirometry is not available).

(e) If beta-blocker therapy is required, ensure patient is on a selective agent rather than nonselective.

> **KEY CONCEPT**
> It is important to know if a patient has been intubated in the past.

b. Potential complications: see Chronic Obstructive Pulmonary Disease.

PNEUMONIA

1. **Pathophysiology**
   a. Inflammatory process of the alveolar spaces caused by infection.
   b. Possible pathogenic mechanisms for the development of pneumonia include the following:
      i. Aspiration: Anaerobic bacteria and oral flora
      ii. Inhalation
      iii. Inoculation
      iv. Direct spread from contiguous sites
      v. Hematogenous spread
      vi. Colonization in chronic lung disease (e.g., COPD, cystic fibrosis)
   c. Acquisition of infection depends on the nature of the infecting organism, the immediate environment, and the defense status of the host.
   d. Important constituents of the pulmonary defense system
      i. Upper airway defenses: Adversely affected by nasotracheal intubation, endotracheal intubation, suction catheters, nasogastric tubes
         (a) Nasopharyngeal filtration
         (b) Mucosal adherence
         (c) Bacterial interference
         (d) Saliva
         (e) Secretory IgA
      ii. Lower airway defenses: May be impaired or inactivated by old age; underlying diseases, such as diabetes, chronic bronchitis, malnutrition; and medication or O_2 therapy
         (a) Cough reflex
         (b) Mucociliary clearance
         (c) Humoral factors
         (d) Cellular factors

2. **Etiology and risk factors**
   a. Normal host infected with usual organisms
      i. *Streptococcus pneumoniae* (pneumococcus): Most common cause of community acquired bacterial pneumonia worldwide, declining because of immunization and reduction in smoking.
      ii. *Mycoplasma pneumoniae:* Spread by droplet nuclei; may occur in epidemics. Can shear off cilia.
      iii. *Haemophilus influenzae:* With encapsulated type B organisms, is more likely to cause bacteremia; nontypable *H. influenzae* is seen more in the older adult population and in those with cystic fibrosis and COPD disease.

iv. Viruses: Relatively uncommon cause of pneumonia in adults; influenza A virus is the most common cause. Pneumonia caused by cytomegalovirus (CMV), respiratory syncytial virus, and herpes simplex virus are often seen in immunocompromised patients.

v. *Chlamydia pneumoniae*: Causes a spectrum of illnesses from mild upper respiratory symptoms to pneumonia and produces a ciliostatic factor.

vi. Fungi: Inhalation of *Histoplasma capsulatum* results in acute severe pulmonary histoplasmosis. Similar reactions occur in patients infected with *Blastomyces dermatitidis, Cryptococcus, Coccidioides immitis, Aspergillus fumigatus*, and *Candida albicans*. Geographic location is important in identifying certain organisms.

EXPERT TIP

Candida in the respiratory system is generally only a pathogen in the immunocompromised or transplant population.

---

b. Normal host infected with unusual organisms
   i. *Legionella pneumophila* infections may be sporadic or occur in localized outbreaks in institutions.
   ii. *Bacillus anthracis* infects humans who have been in contact with anthrax-infected animals.
   iii. *Yersinia pestis* causes plague; transmitted from wild animals and their fleas, or via the respiratory route.
   iv. *Francisella tularensis* causes pleuropulmonary tularemia, endemic in certain parts of the United States; transmitted by ticks or, possibly, by inhalation from infected animals.
   v. Group A *Streptococcus* and *Meningococcus* bacteria reside in the upper respiratory tract; pneumonia occurs in individuals housed in groups, such as in military service. *Streptococcus pyogenes* causes pneumonia typically after outbreaks of viral infections.
   vi. *Mycobacterium tuberculosis* infection or atypical TB can produce life-threatening pulmonary complications in hosts whose only risk factor is age.

c. Abnormal host infected with usual organisms: Compromised states can result from the presence of chronic underlying disease, poor nutrition, trauma, or surgery, or subsequent to immunosuppression
   i. Pneumococcal pneumonia is more severe in this population.
   ii. Gram-negative bacilli, such as *Escherichia coli, Pseudomonas aeruginosa, Serratia, Proteus vulgaris, Acinetobacter* and *Klebsiella pneumoniae*, and *Moraxella catarrhalis*, can be the causative organisms.
   iii. Anaerobic bacteria, such as Bacteroides, cause severe pulmonary infections in the abnormal host.
   iv. *Staphylococcus aureus* pneumonia is seen in diabetic patients, in patients with a recent history of influenza (postinfluenza pneumonia), and institutionalized or hospitalized patients.
   v. *K. pneumoniae* causes a virulent, necrotizing pneumonia often seen in alcoholic or debilitated patients; abscess formation is common.

d. Abnormal host infected with unusual organisms
   i. Enterococcal pneumonia is associated with the use of third-generation cephalosporins.

    ii. Group B *S. pneumoniae* pneumonia is often seen in older patients with underlying diseases.

    iii. Hospital-acquired *L. pneumophila* pneumonia occurs in renal transplant patients and those who are debilitated and immunocompromised.

    iv. *Legionella micdadei*, the Pittsburgh pneumonia agent, may infect renal transplant patients during corticosteroid therapy.

    v. Fungi, including *A. fumigatus* and *Aspergillus flavum*, produce pneumonia mostly in patients who have received high doses of steroids and broad-spectrum antibiotics.

    vi. *Nocardia asteroides* pneumonia is seen in renal transplant patients and patients with hematologic malignancies.

    vii. *Pneumocystis jirovecii* infections, with typical and atypical mycobacteria, and CMV infections are seen in patients with acquired immunodeficiency syndrome.

  e. Multidrug-resistant organisms, vancomycin-resistant enterococci, and methicillin-resistant *S. aureus* are becoming more prevalent in the community, so that patients may enter facilities with the infection or colonization rather than acquire it in the hospital.

  f. Pneumonias can be categorized by their mode of origin as follows:

    i. Community-acquired pneumonia (CAP) occurs in a nonhospitalized patient who has not had healthcare contact. There are more than 100 microbes that can cause community-acquired pneumonia. Influenza remains the predominant viral cause of CAP in adults.

    ii. Hospital-acquired pneumonia (HAP) occurs 48 hours or more after hospital admission and does not appear to be incubating at the time of admission.

    iii. VAP develops more than 48 to 72 hours after endotracheal intubation.

3. Signs and symptoms

  a. Chief complaint varies depending on the organism. Some common presentations include the following:

    i. Pneumococcal pneumonia: Abrupt shaking chills or rigor, fever, dyspnea, pleuritic pain, and cough productive of rusty sputum

    ii. Mycoplasma: Fever, myalgias, headache, minimally productive cough, and nonpleuritic chest pain

    iii. *H. influenzae*: Fever, chills, and cough with purulent sputum

    iv. Klebsiella: Sudden onset, blood-tinged sputum, and tachypnea

  b. Clinical features: Hypoxemia, increased work of breathing, impaired alveolar ventilation, impaired respiratory gas exchange

    i. Asymmetric chest expansion with dullness or flatness to percussion over affected areas

    ii. Breath sounds may be decreased; fine inspiratory crackles or bronchial breath sounds over areas of consolidation (lobar pneumonia)

    iii. Bronchophony; whispered pectoriloquy and egophony may also be heard with consolidation

4. Diagnostic study findings

  a. Laboratory

    i. Sputum examination

      (a) Color and consistency vary with the pathogen.

      (b) Initial Gram staining and microscopic examination

        (1) Good sputum specimen contains few (<5) squamous epithelial cells picked up in transit through the upper respiratory tract. When

sputum cannot be expectorated, a specimen may be obtained by other means, such as suctioning, transtracheal aspiration, or fiberoptic bronchoscopy.

(2) Examination of expectorated sputum specimens has relatively poor sensitivity and specificity.

(3) Staining demonstrates polymorphonuclear leukocytes (PMNs) and bacterial agents; large numbers of PMNs are seen in most bacterial pneumonias; fewer PMNs and more mononuclear inflammatory cells are seen in mycoplasmal and viral pneumonias.

(4) Sputum cultures are done with initial Gram staining and microscopic examination; however, some bacteria are relatively difficult to grow, so the initial Gram stain result is just as important in making the etiologic diagnosis.

  ii. Blood cultures

(a) Obtaining a blood sample is very important in the evaluation because of the high specificity of a positive culture result, especially in hospitalized patients with pneumococcal pneumonia.

(b) Blood and sputum cultures are obtained before antibiotic administration.

(c) Patients with documented bacteremic pneumonia have a worse prognosis than those with nonbacteremic pneumonia.

  iii. Leukocyte counts

(a) Often elevated in lobar pneumonia; may be normal with atypical pneumonia

(b) Normal or reduced in the older adult, in immunocompromised patients, in patients with overwhelming infections, and in those with viral infection

  iv. ABG analysis: May indicate hypoxemia and hypocapnia in lobar pneumonia

  b. Radiologic: Chest radiographic findings vary with involvement

    i. Segmental or lobar consolidation, infiltrates, air bronchograms

    ii. Particularly helpful in detecting parapneumonic effusions, abscesses, and cavities

  c. Thoracentesis: May be indicated when significant pleural effusion is present

5. Goals of care

  a. Pulmonary infection is halted and reversed.

  b. Oxygenation and ventilation are improved.

  c. Removal of airway secretions is facilitated.

  d. Vital signs, ABG values, and respiratory dynamics are restored to within normal limits for the patient.

  e. Dyspnea at rest and with exertion are minimized.

6. Interprofessional collaboration: Nurse, physician, advanced practice provider, respiratory therapist, pharmacist.

7. Management of patient care

  a. Anticipated patient trajectory:

    i. Positioning: Change position to mobilize secretions; avoid the supine position, consider physical therapy and early mobility.

    ii. Skin care: Turn frequently to drain lungs and maintain skin integrity.

    iii. Pain management: Pleuritic chest pain control may be achieved by antiinflammatory agents, analgesics, or intercostal nerve blocks; may consider nonpharmocologic interventions, and pain medications need to relieve the discomfort of tubes and treatment and prevent interference with turning, coughing, deep breathing, incentive spirometry, ambulation.

    iv. Nutrition: Enlist assistance from a dietitian to ensure that nutritional intake is adequate to restore strength, facilitate ventilator weaning, and support healing and recovery; if possible, use the enteral route to reduce infection risk.

    v. Infection control: Regular, thorough oral care with brushing (vs. swabbing) and cleansing appears to reduce morbidity and mortality from pneumonia. Use strict infection control procedures; avoid unnecessary invasive procedures or limit their duration of use.

    vi. Pharmacology: Administer antibiotics within 8 hours of admission, preferably within 4 hours, and monitor response; administer sedatives and pain medication as needed.

      (a) Duration of therapy should be based upon the clinical response. A short duration of therapy (e.g., 7 days) is sufficient for most patients with uncomplicated HAP or VAP who have had a good clinical response.

      (b) Chest radiograph findings usually clear more slowly than clinical improvement.

  b. Potential complications

    i. Superimposed HAI(s)

    ii. Difficulty weaning or liberating from mechanical ventilation

VENTILATOR-ASSOCIATED PNEUMONIA AND EVENT

1. **Pathophysiology**
   a. VAP develops 48 hours or longer after mechanical ventilation is provided by means of an endotracheal tube or tracheostomy.
   b. Results from the invasion of the lower respiratory tract and lung parenchyma by organisms.
   c. Microaspiration occurs when patients have asymptomatic aspiration of small volumes of oropharyngeal secretions or gastric fluid into their lungs.
   d. Intubation compromises the integrity of the oropharynx and trachea and allows oral and gastric secretions to enter the lower airways.
2. **Etiology and risk factors**
   a. Complication, in as many as 28% of patients who receive mechanical ventilation
   b. Increases with the duration of mechanical ventilation with estimated risk of 3% per day
   c. Mortality rate for VAP is 27% to 76%
   d. Higher risk in trauma patients
   e. Late onset usually associated with antibiotic-resistant organisms
3. **Signs and symptoms**
   a. Fever
   b. Purulent secretions
4. **Diagnostic study findings**
   a. Noninvasive study findings
      i. Leukocytosis
      ii. Chest x-ray: Infiltrates consistent with pulmonary infection
      iii. Chest CT: Infiltrates consistent with pulmonary infection
   b. Invasive study findings
      i. Bronchoscopy may show purulent secretions.
5. **When the combination of radiologic infiltrates and two clinical criteria are met, the sensitivity of diagnosing VAP is 69% and the specificity is 75%.**
6. **Interprofessional collaboration: Nurse, physician, advanced practice provider, respiratory therapist, infectious disease specialist.**

7. **Management of patient care**
   a. VAP bundle components
   b. Prevention: Head of bed elevation at least 30 degrees
   c. Use of subglottic suction
   d. Cuff pressures should be maintained at greater than 20 cm of water to prevent aspiration around the endotracheal tube
   e. Frequent changes of the ventilator circuit have not been shown to reduce the risk of VAP and are not recommended
   f. Frequent oral care and use of chlorhexidine
8. **Interventions**
   a. Antibiotics
   b. May require mechanical ventilation to support gas exchange
9. **Potential complications**
   a. Increased oxygen demand
   b. Development of ARDS
   c. Difficulty weaning or liberating from mechanical ventilation
   d. Exposure to antibiotics (e.g., c-diff)
   e. Increased length of ICU and hospital stay

KEY CONCEPT
Prevention with the utilization of the VAP bundle is the most important.

DROWNING

1. **Pathophysiology**
   a. Drowning is defined as primary respiratory impairment from submersion in a liquid. Drowning is the third leading cause of unintentional injury, accounting for 7% of all injury-related deaths worldwide.
   b. Electrolyte change: There is a tendency toward hemoconcentration in saltwater drowning and toward hemodilution in fresh water drowning. Aspiration of more than 11 mL/kg of body weight must occur before blood volume changes occur and more than 22 mL/kg before electrolyte changes take place.
   c. Pulmonary effects: The water aspirated may contain mud, sand, algae, chemicals, and/or vomitus.
      i. In freshwater aspiration, water rapidly enters the circulation; in saltwater aspiration, the hypertonic sea water draws fluid from the circulation into the lungs. However, near-drowning victims of saltwater and freshwater immersion have the same initial pathophysiologic aberrations: Major insults include hypoxemia and tissue hypoxia, hypoxic brain injury with cerebral edema, hypercapnia, and acidemia. Hypothermia, pneumonia, and (rarely) disseminated intravascular coagulation (DIC), acute kidney injury, and hemolysis may also occur.
      ii. Organic and inorganic contents of the aspirated fluid, regardless of the type of water, produce an inflammatory reaction in the alveolar-capillary membrane that leads to an outpouring of plasma-rich exudate into the alveolus, displacement of air, and deposition of proteinaceous material.
      iii. There is destruction of surfactant by aspirated water and proteinaceous exudate, which results in large areas of atelectasis.
      iv. Regional hypoxia promotes hypoxic vasoconstriction, which raises pulmonary intravascular pressures, promotes further interstitial fluid flux, and frequently gives rise to pulmonary edema.

v. In some patients, hyaline membranes develop on the walls of injured bronchioles, alveolar ducts, and alveoli. This results in reduced compliance and increased ratio of dead space to tidal volume, increased respiratory work, and $\dot{V}/\dot{Q}$ mismatch.

2. **Etiology and risk factors**
   a. Freshwater or saltwater immersion because of young age and inability to swim
   b. Prior alcohol or drug ingestion
   c. Head and neck trauma and loss of consciousness associated with epilepsy, diabetes, syncope, or dysrhythmias
   d. Barotrauma associated with scuba diving; CO_2 narcosis ("the bends")

3. **Signs and symptoms**
   a. Patient's chief complaint: Respiratory distress, coughing
   b. Unconsciousness, neurologic deficits if cerebral anoxia has occurred
   c. Tachypnea and intercostal retractions in the conscious patient (must generate greater negative inspiratory forces to inflate fluid-filled, less compliant lungs)
   d. Apnea in the unconscious patient; may also see cyanosis, other signs of hypoxemia, anoxia
   e. Hypothermia or fever
   f. Diminished chest expansion owing to low lung compliance; dullness to percussion over most lung zones (possible diffuse pulmonary edema); possible diffuse crackles on inspiration

4. **Diagnostic study findings**
   a. Laboratory
      i. Minimal electrolyte and Hb changes
      ii. ABG levels: Hypoxemia and metabolic acidosis
      iii. Leukocytosis
      iv. Coagulation studies: Coagulation disorders including DIC, have been reported in near-drowning victims.
   b. Radiologic: Initial chest imaging may be normal or show infiltrates or pulmonary edema.
   c. ECG: May show dysrhythmias, nonspecific changes. Few victims die of ventricular fibrillation. Acidemia, CO_2 retention, and hypoxemia result in marked irregular bradycardia, which precedes asystole and cardiac arrest.

5. **Goals of care**
   a. Effective ventilation and perfusion are restored (cardiopulmonary resuscitation [CPR], Advanced Cardiac Life Support at the scene)
   b. Patient is rewarmed to normothermia if hypothermic.
   c. Gastric contents are evacuated.
   d. ABG levels, oxygenation, electrolyte levels, and fluid balance values are normalized.
   e. Early complications are minimized, and late complications are prevented.
   f. There is no good evidence to support the routine use of steroids or prophylactic antibiotics.

6. **Interprofessional collaboration: Nurse, physician, advanced practice provider, respiratory therapist, pharmacist.**

7. **Management of patient care**
   a. Anticipated patient trajectory
      i. Positioning: Keep the patient's head and neck in the neutral position and avoid hyperextension of the cervical spine until spinal cord and head trauma injuries have been ruled out.

    ii. Skin care: If the patient was submerged in cold water, use core rewarming to gradually return body temperature to the normal range. Monitor and maintain skin integrity via hypothermia-hyperthermia devices.

    iii. Pharmacology: Patient may require vasopressors for blood pressure support, sodium bicarbonate for metabolic acidosis, β-agonists for bronchospasm, diuretics for fluid balance.

    iv. Psychosocial issues: If incident was not accidental or was secondary to alcohol/drug abuse, the circumstances of the near-drowning episode may warrant follow-up and counseling. Patient prognosis will affect the need for family support and home care issues.

  b. Potential complications

    i. Hypothermia

    ii. Fluid and electrolyte imbalances

    iii. Seizures

    iv. ARDS

    v. Aspiration pneumonia

    vi. Pulmonary edema

    vii. Sepsis

PULMONARY PROBLEMS IN SURGICAL/THORACIC SURGERY PATIENTS

1. **Pathophysiology**

  a. Surgery represents a stress to the respiratory system. Pulmonary problems are the major cause of morbidity after surgery.

  b. Changes in pulmonary function occur normally during the immediately postoperative period. These changes are most evident following abdominal or thoracic surgery.

    i. Reduction in FVC is consistent with a restrictive defect; it is significant but usually temporary.

    ii. Reduction in lung volumes, especially FRC, also occurs, caused in part by pain and the supine position.

    iii. Reduced lung compliance is present, resulting in reduced tidal volume and increased respiratory frequency.

  c. Microatelectasis is the most common cause of hypoxemia; the increased respiratory frequency leads to respiratory alkalosis.

  d. Bacterial invasion of the lower airways and reduced clearance postoperatively predispose to respiratory infection.

  e. Aspiration of gastric and oropharyngeal contents occurs postoperatively in patients who have a disturbance in consciousness.

  f. Arterial hypoxemia caused by $\dot{V}/\dot{Q}$ mismatching is common in the postoperative period in normal patients and is exaggerated in patients with COPD.

2. **Etiology and risk factors**

  a. History of COPD or cigarette smoking is the most important risk factor. Preoperative hypercapnia is a serious risk factor

  b. Obesity results in decreased vital capacity.

  c. Very young and older adult persons are at increased risk.

  d. People with underlying chronic diseases are at greater risk.

  e. Prolonged anesthesia time increases risk.

  f. Thoracic and abdominal surgery are especially hazardous to patients at risk. Maximal inspirations are voluntarily limited because of pain, which thereby increases the risk of atelectasis.

3. **Signs and symptoms**
   a. Patient's chief complaint varies with the type of surgery but is often incisional pain.
   b. Cough with or without sputum production and fear of or reluctance to cough, deep breathe, and move about after surgery
   c. Tachypnea, shallow respirations because of splinting with incisional pain may progress to signs of respiratory distress, increased work of breathing, dyspnea.
   d. If atelectasis progresses to pneumonia, clinical signs include those related to fever and infection.
4. **Diagnostic study findings**
   a. Preoperative medical evaluation includes chest radiography, ECG, sputum examination, and pulmonary function tests.
      i. FEV_1, FVC, and PEFR values are used to predict the development of postoperative pulmonary complications.
      ii. Split pulmonary function studies estimate the amount of pulmonary function that will remain postoperatively after lung resection.
      iii. Other diagnostic tests may be ordered preoperatively, depending on preexisting pulmonary or cardiac disease. These include CT scan of the chest and $\dot{V}/\dot{Q}$ scan.
   b. For patients with abnormal pulmonary function study results, ABG analysis is performed preoperatively. Presence of hypoxemia or CO_2 retention at baseline indicates that postoperative ABG levels should be followed closely.
   c. Cardiac stress test, possible cardiac catheterization. If the stress test results are positive, elective surgery should be postponed until the cause is corrected.
5. **Goal of care: Prevent or minimize postoperative pulmonary complications**
6. **Interprofessional collaboration: Nurse, physician, advanced practice provider, anesthesiologist, respiratory therapist**
7. **Management of patient care**
   a. Anticipated patient trajectory:
      i. Treatments
         (a) Provide preoperative training in effective techniques for turning, deep breathing, coughing, ambulation, activity exercises, and active and passive range-of-motion exercises; suggest oral hygiene care.
         (b) Encourage cessation of smoking at least 48 hours before surgery. Cessation before elective surgery should be as long as possible.
         (c) Familiarize the patient with respiratory therapy equipment and techniques, such as incentive spirometry, chest physiotherapy, and the postoperative exercise program.
         (d) Provide early ambulation and leg exercises, chest physiotherapy, and postural drainage.
         (e) Guide the patient to perform intensive deep breathing exercises and support chest and abdominal incisions during coughing.
   b. Potential complications
      i. Acute pneumonia
      ii. Acute respiratory failure
      iii. Difficulty weaning from ventilator

AIR LEAK SYNDROMES

1. **Pathophysiology: High transpulmonary pressures are applied to the lungs which causes the alveoli to overdistend and rupture. Air then leaks into the interstitium.**
   a. Gas may remain local or spread
   b. Pneumothorax: Can be life-threatening if under tension
      i. Primary spontaneous: Occurs without a precipitating event. Smoking is a risk factor. Certain disease states, such as Marfan syndrome, can be a risk factor.
      ii. Secondary spontaneous: Occurs as a complication of underlying lung disease, such as COPD. Rupture of subpleural blebs.
      iii. Traumatic
      iv. Iatrogenic: Occurs with procedures such as central line insertion, lung biopsies, thoracentesis.
   c. Pneumomediastinum
      i. Spontaneous occurrence is rare
      ii. Result of trauma
      iii. Mechanical ventilation
      iv. Thoracic surgery
2. **Etiology and risk factors**
   a. Mechanical ventilation with high pressures
   b. Trauma
   c. Bullous lung disease
   d. ARDS
3. **Signs and symptoms**
   a. Restriction from trapped gas
   b. Atelectasis
   c. Inflammatory response at the site of rupture
   d. Hypoxemia
   e. Dyspnea
   f. Subcutaneous emphysema
   g. Neck and/or chest pain
   h. Cough
   i. Voice change
   j. Hemodynamic instability
4. **Diagnostic study findings**
   a. Noninvasive study findings
      i. Chest x-ray: Lucency
      ii. Chest CT: Lung collapse, blebs with bullous disease
5. **Interprofessional collaboration: Nurse, physician, advanced practice provider, respiratory therapist.**
6. **Management of patient care**
7. **Goals of care**
   a. Supportive care
   b. Oxygenation
   c. Bronchial hygiene
   d. Prevent complications
8. **Interventions**
   a. Emergent needle decompression
   b. Chest tube insertion: Small tubes, such as pigtail catheters or large bore if blood or fluid present

c. May require mechanical ventilation to support gas exchange

d. Observation may be appropriate for a small pneumothorax in patients who are hemodynamically stable.

e. Supplemental oxygen should be administered to facilitate resorption of the pleural air.

f. Video-assisted thoracoscopic surgery for persistent air leak or failure of the lung to fully expand

g. Chemical pleurodesis

h. Thoracotomy if unable to perform thoracoscopy

9. **Potential complications**

a. Infection

b. Bleeding

c. Nerve damage

d. Diaphragmatic paralysis

e. Subcutaneous emphysema

10. **Recognition and management**

a. Assess lung sounds

b. Assess for crepitus by palpating the skin

c. Hemodynamic monitoring

d. Anticipate chest tube insertion

11. **Additional nursing considerations**

a. Manage pain

ACUTE PULMONARY INHALATION INJURIES
(See Ch. 12, Burns)

NEOPLASTIC LUNG DISEASE

1. **Pathophysiology: Almost all lung cancers fall within one of four histologic categories: Squamous cell carcinoma, small cell carcinoma, adenocarcinoma, and large cell carcinoma. In addition, malignant mesothelioma is discussed. In the United States, lung cancer occurs in about 225,000 patients and causes over 160,000 deaths annually.**

a. Squamous cell carcinoma: Constitutes approximately 20% of all bronchogenic carcinomas. These tumors originate in the epithelial layer of the bronchial wall. Series of progressive histologic abnormalities results from chronic or repetitive cigarette smoke-induced injury.

i. Initially, there is metaplasia of the normal bronchial columnar epithelial cells, which are replaced by squamous epithelial cells.

ii. Squamous cells become more atypical until a well-localized carcinoma (carcinoma in situ) develops.

iii. These cells tend to be located in relatively large or proximal airways, most commonly at the subsegmental, segmental, or lobar level. With the growth of tumor into the bronchial lumen, the airway may become obstructed and the lung distal to the obstruction frequently becomes atelectatic and may develop a postobstructive pneumonia.

iv. At times, a cavity develops within the tumor mass; cavitation is more common with squamous cell carcinoma than other bronchogenic carcinomas.

v. Metastasis beyond the airway usually involves the following:

(a) Direct extension to the pulmonary parenchyma or to other neighboring structures

(b) Invasion of the lymphatics with spread to local lymph nodes in the hilum or mediastinum

vi. Squamous cell tumors tend to remain within the thorax and cause problems by intrathoracic complications rather than by distant metastasis.

b. Small cell carcinoma: Comprises about 13% of all lung cancers and consists of several subtypes. These tumors generally originate within the bronchial wall, most commonly at a proximal level.

i. Oat cell carcinoma, the most common subtype, shows a submucosal growth pattern, but the tumor quickly invades the lymphatics and submucosal blood vessels. Hilar and mediastinal nodes are involved early in the course of the disease and these involved nodes are frequently the most prominent aspect of the radiographic presentation.

ii. Metastasis to distant sites is a common early complication; common sites are the brain, liver, bone (and bone marrow), and adrenal glands.

iii. Propensity for early metastasis gives small cell carcinoma the worst prognosis among the major categories of bronchogenic carcinoma.

c. Adenocarcinoma: Accounts for about 38% of all lung tumors, with the majority occurring in the periphery of the lung

i. Characteristic tendency to form glands and to produce mucus.

ii. Usually presents as a peripheral lung nodule or mass. Occasionally, tumors can arise within a relatively large bronchus and therefore may present with complications of localized bronchial obstruction.

iii. May spread locally to adjacent regions of the lung, to the pleura, or to the hilar or mediastinal lymph nodes; may metastasize to distant sites—liver, bone, CNS, and adrenal glands. In contrast to small cell carcinoma, it is more likely to be localized at the time of presentation.

iv. Overall prognosis is intermediate between that of squamous cell and that of small cell carcinoma.

d. Large cell carcinoma: Accounts for about 5% of all lung cancers. Carcinomas are defined by the characteristics that they lack (e.g., the specific features that would otherwise classify them as one of the other three cell types). It is difficult to pinpoint the cells of origin from which these tumors arise.

i. Behavior is similar to that of adenocarcinoma.

ii. Found in the periphery of the lungs, although it tends to be somewhat larger than adenocarcinoma.

iii. Tumor spread and prognosis are the same as for adenocarcinoma.

e. Other nonsmall cell carcinomas, which cannot be further classified, account for about 18% and other lung cancers account for about 6% of all lung cancers.

f. Malignant mesothelioma

i. Involves the pleura rather than the airways or pulmonary parenchyma

ii. Eventually traps the lung and spreads to mediastinal structures

iii. No clearly effective form of therapy is available, and fewer than 10% of patients survive 3 years

2. **Etiology and risk factors**

a. Smoking is the single most important risk factor for the development of carcinoma of the lung. Each of the four major categories of carcinoma is associated with cigarette smoking; however, the statistical association between smoking and the individual cell types is greatest for squamous cell and small cell carcinomas, which are seen almost exclusively in smokers. Even though smoking increases the risk for adenocarcinoma and large cell carcinoma, these cell types are also observed in nonsmokers. In addition, smoking does not appear to be a risk factor for bronchial carcinoids or malignant mesothelioma.

b. Occupational factors

    i. Asbestos, a fibrous silicate used for its fire resistant and thermal insulatory qualities, is the most widely studied of the environmental and occupationally related carcinogens. Carcinoma of the lung is the most likely malignancy to complicate asbestos exposure, although other tumors, especially mesothelioma, are strongly associated with prior asbestos exposure. Risk for development of lung cancer is particularly high in a smoker exposed to asbestos, in which case the two risk factors have a multiplicative effect. There is a long time lag (>20 years) after exposure before the tumor becomes apparent.

    ii. Other occupational exposures implicated in the development of lung cancer also have a long latent period of at least 2 decades between exposure and presentation of the tumor. Examples include exposure to arsenic, ionizing radiation (uranium, gamma radiation, x-rays), haloethers (chemical industry), polycyclic aromatic hydrocarbons (mineral oils, soots, coal tar, and foundry work), synthetic mineral fibers (rock wool or slag wool), diesel exhaust, and crystalline silica.

c. Radon decay products: Radon gas is a decay product of naturally occurring uranium in the earth that may cause bronchogenic carcinoma or contribute to cancer risk only when inhaled into the respiratory system, where it interacts with pulmonary epithelial or other cells.

d. Common nonmodifiable risk factors: Gender, race, inherited predisposition.

3. **Signs and symptoms**

a. Patient's chief complaints: Cough (50%–75% of patients) and hemoptysis (20%–40% of patients) are the most common presenting symptoms in patients with lung cancer. Other symptoms vary, depending on the region of tumor involvement.

b. Dyspnea secondary to an obstructed bronchus or large pleural effusion

c. Chest pain from pleural involvement

d. Dysphagia from tumor involvement of the adjacent esophagus

e. Hoarseness from vocal cord paralysis

f. Edema of the face and upper extremities from superior vena cava obstruction

g. Nonspecific symptoms: Anorexia, weight loss, wasting, dyspnea, diminished chest expansion, bronchial breath sounds over a large tumor or postobstructive pneumonia, dullness over a large tumor near the chest wall or a pleural mass, signs of pleural effusion

4. **Diagnostic study findings**

a. Laboratory: Cytologic examination of sputum, washings, or brushings or of material aspirated from the tumor with a small-gauge needle

b. Radiologic

    i. Chest radiograph: May reveal a nodule or mass in the lung, involvement of the hilar or mediastinal nodes, or pleural involvement.

    ii. CT, magnetic resonance imaging (MRI), and positron emission tomography (PET): Help define the location, extent, and spread of tumor

c. Bronchoscopy: Allows direct examination of the airways intrabronchially and sampling for cytologic evaluation. Forceps biopsy specimens used for both histologic and cytologic analysis; bronchial washings used extensively in the diagnosis of bronchogenic carcinoma. Cytologic analysis of bronchial brushings is an effective diagnostic procedure, especially when used in combination with forceps biopsy.

  d. Electromagnetic navigation bronchoscopy. Lung tumors near the center of the chest can be biopsied during bronchoscopy, but bronchoscopes have trouble reaching the outer part of the lungs. The abnormal area is identified, and a computer helps guide a bronchoscope to the area of biopsy. The bronchoscope has special attachments that allow it to reach further than a regular bronchoscope. This takes extra equipment and training and is not widely available.

  e. The development of endobronchial ultrasound (EBUS) with bronchoscopy has revolutionized investigation of mediastinal lymphadenopathy by facilitating minimally invasive sampling of lymph nodes at the site of disease.

  f. Transbronchial needle aspiration can be useful in the diagnosis of a tumor presenting as a submucosal lesion or as a mass that compresses the bronchial lumen externally. Patients with necrotic lesions or lesions from which significant bleeding is anticipated are candidates for this technique.

  g. Mediastinoscopy: For staging of lung cancer if CT is not diagnostic of lymph node involvement

  h. Staging of lung cancer is based on the following:
  i. Size, location, and local complications, such as direct extensions to adjacent structures or obstruction of the airway lumen
  ii. Mediastinal lymph node involvement
  iii. Distant metastasis

5. **Goals of care**
  a. Patent airway is established and maintained.
  b. Ventilation and respiratory gas exchange are maximized to the extent possible.
  c. Every effort is made to ensure that the patient is pain free.
  d. Hospital-acquired and surgery-related complications are prevented.

6. **Interprofessional collaboration: Nurse, physician, advanced practice provider, respiratory therapist, pharmacist, oncology nurse navigator, oncologist, radiation oncologist, social worker.**

7. **Management of patient care**
  a. Anticipated patient trajectory: Follows the course for specific clinical problems related to the nature, extent, and location of the tumor and the surgery and other treatments used
  i. Pain management: Some forms of lung cancer can be exquisitely painful, so special attention to this aspect of care is warranted. See content related to pain in Chapter 20, Pain.
  ii. Nutrition: Dietitian consultation at the time of cancer diagnosis is encouraged because patients may encounter significant weight loss and wasting with various aspects of care, such as chemotherapy and/or radiation therapy.
  iii. Infection control: Of major concern, especially when the patient may be imminently in need of undergoing chemotherapy and/or radiation therapy, which will further weaken the immune system.
  iv. Discharge planning: Nature and extent of postdischarge needs must be evaluated, including outpatient follow-up care, chemotherapy or radiation therapy, home care supplies, equipment and care needs, and the nature of health care required in relation to the ancillary staff resources. If appropriate, provide referral to hospice care services.
  v. Pharmacology: Chemotherapy may prolong survival; antibiotics are administered as needed and the results monitored; pain medication needs to ensure patient comfort. Immunotherapy for the treatment of advanced-stage lung cancer is rapidly evolving and extending survival. Tailored treatment based

on mutation testing and immune inhibition has implications for treatment at the time of the initial evaluation and diagnosis.

    vi. Psychosocial issues: Patient and/or family may require considerable support in dealing with this diagnosis, its treatment both in the hospital and in the community and home, its potential outcomes, and its prognosis. Pastoral care may be supportive and comforting if the patient and/or family desires this. Other means of support include working with social services or the American Cancer Society in arranging for another patient with a similar diagnosis who has successfully coped with this situation to visit the patient to provide encouragement and sharing of experiences.

    vii. Treatments: Planning for chemotherapy or radiation therapy may be completed while the patient is in the high-acuity setting.

    viii. Ethical issues: Determine whether an advance directive is in place if the patient situation warrants it.

  b. Potential complications
    i. Hospital-acquired infection
    ii. Vary with the nature, extent, location, and staging of the neoplasm, as well as the patient's response to treatment

PULMONARY FIBROSIS

1. **Pathophysiology: Idiopathic pulmonary fibrosis, also called cryptogenic fibrosing alveolitis is a specific form of chronic, progressive, fibrosing interstitial pneumonia of unknown cause. Associated with histiopathologic and/or radiologic pattern of usual interstitial pneumonia. More fibrotic than inflammatory.**
2. **Etiology and risk factors: Occurs in adults (majority are >55 years old). Limited to lungs. Mean rate of decline is approximately 150 to 200 mL/year.**
3. **Signs and symptoms: Dyspnea, exercise intolerance**
4. **Diagnostic study findings**
  a. Noninvasive study findings
    i. Chest x-ray: Reticular markings
    ii. Chest CT: High resolution. Typical findings include subpleural, bibasilar predominance of reticular markings and honeycombing.
  b. Invasive study findings
    i. Lung biopsy: Video-assisted thoracoscopic or open
5. **Interprofessional collaboration: Nurse, physician, advanced practice provider, respiratory therapist, pharmacist, palliative medicine/palliative care**
6. **Management of patient care**
  a. Goals of care
  b. Interventions: No U.S. Food and Drug Administration–approved therapy has been shown to be efficacious
    i. Supportive care (supplemental oxygen)
    ii. Participation in clinical trials
    iii. Selected medications (e.g., pirfenidone, nintedanib, phosphodiesterase inhibitors)
    iv. Referral for lung transplant
    v. Identify and treat comorbidities
    vi. Palliative care
7. **Potential complications**
  a. Impaired oxygenation
  b. Spontaneous pneumothorax

OBSTRUCTIVE SLEEP APNEA

1. **Pathophysiology**
   a. Apnea is defined as cessation of airflow for more than 10 seconds. Sleep apnea is defined as repeated episodes of upper airway obstruction associated with obstructive apnea and hypopnea during sleep together with daytime sleepiness or altered cardiopulmonary function. Epidemiologic studies estimate that the condition affects about 26% of adults between the ages of 30 to 70 years.
   b. Upper airway dysfunction and the specific sites of narrowing or closure are influenced by the underlying neuromuscular tone, upper airway muscle synchrony, and the stage of sleep.
      i. These events are most prominent during rapid eye movement sleep secondary to hypotonia of the upper airway muscles characteristic of this stage of sleep.
      ii. Definitive event in obstructive sleep apnea is the posterior movement of the tongue and palate into apposition with the posterior pharyngeal wall, which results in occlusion of the nasopharynx and oropharynx.
      iii. Following the obstruction and resultant apnea, progressive asphyxia develops until there is a brief arousal from sleep, restoration of upper airway patency, and resumption of airflow. Patient quickly returns to sleep, only to experience the sequence of events over and over again.
      iv. Patients with sleep apnea are at increased risk for diurnal hypertension, pulmonary hypertension, nocturnal dysrhythmias, right and left ventricular failure, myocardial infarction, atrial fibrillation, and stroke.
      v. Hypoxemia, hypercapnia, polycythemia, and cor pulmonale may complicate the late stages of the disease.
2. **Etiology and risk factors**
   a. Obesity: Increased upper body obesity, as reflected by neck circumference (neck size 17 inches and larger in males, 16 inches and larger in females)
   b. Nasal obstruction such as severe septal deviation or nasopharyngeal infection or blockage
   c. Adenoidal or tonsillar hypertrophy (seen in children)
   d. Micrognathia, retrognathia, or macroglossia
   e. Vocal cord paralysis
   f. Genetically determined craniofacial features or abnormalities of ventilatory control (CNS) may be the reason that sleep apnea is common in some families
3. **Signs and symptoms**
   a. Patient's chief complaint: Excessive daytime sleepiness
      i. Epworth Sleepiness Scale questionnaire
      ii. STOP-BANG assessment: http://www.stopbang.ca
   b. Fatigue as well as related personality changes and cognitive difficulties (patient may come to the hospital following an accident caused by daytime sleepiness)
   c. Chronic loud snoring
   d. Morning headaches
   e. Loss of libido
4. **Diagnostic study findings**
   a. Laboratory: ABG analysis is not diagnostic of sleep apnea but is performed as part of a diagnostic workup to determine baseline ventilation and oxygenation.
   b. Polysomnography (sleep study) for sleep staging, airflow and ventilatory effort, arterial O_2 saturation, ECG, body position, and periodic limb movement evaluation.

   c. Home evaluation and testing
      i. Pulse oximetry, portable (home) monitoring of cardiopulmonary channels such as airflow, ventilatory effort, and heart rate.
   d. Pulmonary function studies may be done to exclude or confirm concomitant intrinsic lung disease, such as obstructive or restrictive lung disease.
5. **Goals of care: Apneic episodes during sleep are prevented.**
6. **Interprofessional collaboration: Nurse, physician, advanced practice provider, respiratory therapist, sleep center staff.**
7. **Management of patient care: If the patient is obese, see Bariatric Patients in Chapter 15 for all aspects of care.**
   a. Anticipated patient trajectory
      i. Positioning: Keep the head of the bed elevated 30 to 45 degrees; avoid the supine position; maintain a neutral position for head and neck alignment; avoid neck flexion.
      ii. Nutrition: Obtain a dietary consult to initiate a weight reduction program if obesity is a contributing factor.
      iii. Transport: Maintain body alignment, especially of the head and upper torso, to keep the airway patent at all times.
      iv. Discharge planning: Educate the patient regarding the proper use and care of oral or dental devices or CPAP equipment. Side effects of the use of oral or dental devices include excessive salivation and temporomandibular joint discomfort.
      v. Pharmacology: Instruct the patient to avoid alcoholic beverages, narcotics, and sedatives before sleep.
      vi. Psychosocial issues: Daytime demeanor and social interactions may improve considerably after the disorder is effectively treated.
      vii. Treatments
         (a) O_2 delivery via a CPAP or BiPAP device as ordered
            (1) Instruct on the proper use and maintenance of equipment.
            (2) Teach care of the skin surrounding the nose area where the mask is applied.
            (3) Assess for intolerance to nasal CPAP machine noise and airway pressure.
         (b) Postoperative monitoring and instruction following surgical treatment or correction for sleep apnea if indicated
            (1) Preoperative and postoperative teaching for patients requiring tracheostomy; if the neck is thick, the decannulation process may be difficult.
            (2) Repeat the sleep study or nocturnal oximetry following tracheostomy tube placement because the patient may still hypoventilate secondary to central sleep apnea or intrinsic lung disease.
            (3) Provide tracheostomy tube and stoma care instruction to the patient and family.

END-STAGE PULMONARY CONDITIONS: LUNG TRANSPLANTATION

1. **Pathophysiology: Specific pathophysiologic mechanisms responsible for end-stage pulmonary disease depend on the underlying etiologic factors.**
   a. Transplantation of one or both lungs as a treatment for end-stage pulmonary failure has become a commonly accepted practice. The total number of lung transplantations performed in the United Stated was 2487 (in the 2017 report) and that number continues to increase annually.
   b. Primary underlying diagnoses for patients with end-stage lung disease
      i. Emphysema: 40% of the total

    ii. Pulmonary fibrosis: 22%

    iii. Cystic fibrosis: 16%

    iv. α_1-antitrypsin deficiency: 6%

    v. Pulmonary hypertension: 4%

    vi. Other disorders (bronchiectasis, eosinophilic granuloma, lymphangioleiomyomatosis, obliterative bronchiolitis, sarcoidosis): 12%

  c. United Network for Organ Sharing (UNOS) reports that nearly 4000 people in the United States await lung transplantation and about 500 die waiting. Median wait time in the United States is slightly more than 3 years.

  d. Survival rates following lung transplantation are 69% at 1 year and 51% at 3 years. Survival rates are highest for those with pulmonary fibrosis or pulmonary hypertension and lowest for those with emphysema.

2. **Etiology and risk factors: Pulmonary transplantation is appropriate for patients with irreversible, progressively disabling, end-stage pulmonary disease whose life expectancy is to be less than 18 months despite the use of appropriate medical or alternative surgical therapies. These include patients with the following disorders:**

  a. Emphysema and α_1-antitrypsin deficiency (which together account for 46% of all cases)

    i. Patients with COPD and an FEV_1 lower than 20% to 25% of the predicted value, hypercarbia ($PaCO_2$ of >50 mm Hg), or mean pulmonary artery pressure without O_2 of more than 30 mm Hg have a 2-year survival rate of less than 70%.

    ii. Usually, patients who receive a transplant have an FEV_1 of less than 20% of the predicted value.

  b. Cystic fibrosis

    i. Patients with cystic fibrosis who have an FEV_1 of less than 30% of that predicted, a PaO_2 of less than 55 mm Hg, or a $PaCO_2$ of more than 50 mm Hg have a 2-year survival rate of approximately 70%.

    ii. Women and younger patients with cystic fibrosis have lower survival rates than men or the older adult, and is a consideration for transplantation earlier.

  c. Pulmonary hypertension (primary and secondary): Patients with a mean pulmonary artery pressure of more than 45 mm Hg

  d. Idiopathic pulmonary fibrosis or interstitial lung disease

    i. Such patients tend to have the highest mortality while awaiting transplantation.

    ii. These patients often have an FEV_1 and FVC of less than 50% of the predicted values.

3. **Signs and symptoms**

  a. Patient's chief complaint: Varies, depending on the type of underlying respiratory disorder and the degree of disability. At the initial screening or clinic visit virtually all patients have some degree of dyspnea and shortness of breath, either at rest or on minimal exertion.

  b. Physical findings vary widely, depending on the underlying pulmonary condition and the degree to which pulmonary function is impaired.

  c. Traditional selection criteria for lung transplant recipients used until recently are the following:

    i. Age of 65 years or younger for a single lung transplant; age of 60 years or younger for a bilateral lung transplant

    ii. No other underlying significant systemic disease such as renal or hepatic insufficiency or neoplastic disease

     iii. Demonstrated past and current adherence with medical regimens

     iv. No evidence of serious psychiatric illness, such as functional psychosis or organic brain disease, major depression, or severe characterologic disturbances with a history of self-destructive acts (alcohol, drug abuse)

     v. No immune markers or contraindication to immunosuppression

     vi. Abstinence from tobacco use for longer than 6 months

     vii. No extrapulmonary site of infection

     viii. Ambulatory with rehabilitation potential with O$_2$ as required

     ix. Without significant coronary artery disease

     x. Longer time on the wait list

  d. "Transplant benefit": Revised lung allocation system instituted by the Organ Procurement and Transplantation Network and UNOS to provide an evidence-based, individualized, clinical data-driven system for allocating lungs for transplantation.

     i. Replaces the system heavily based on the length of time on that waiting list with an approach that balances the waiting list urgency and the likely duration of benefit from transplantation.

     ii. Intention is that candidates who are most urgently in need of a transplant and who are expected to receive the greatest survival benefit from the transplant will receive priority for available lungs.

     iii. Patient's health data are entered online into the UNOS database system, called UNet, to generate a lung allocation score (LAS), which ranges from 0 to 100. If data change, new or revised data can be entered online by healthcare staff. Time on the waiting list is used only to select among candidates with equal LASs. Candidate with the highest LAS gets priority.

     iv. Some of the criteria used in determining the LAS include the following:

      (a) Need for continuous mechanical ventilation

      (b) Presence of type 1 or 2 diabetes mellitus

      (c) Need for O$_2$ at rest

      (d) Cardiac catheterization data (pulmonary artery systolic pressure, mean PAP, PAOP), FVC

      (e) Pulmonary diagnoses

      (f) Age

      (g) Body mass index

      (h) New York American Heart Association class

     v. Verify the patient's commitment to transplant candidacy.

      (a) Discussion among the patient, family, and transplant team about the transplantation process and provision of the opportunity to explore options, ask questions, and voice concerns

      (b) Decision by the patient as to whether or not to proceed with the formal evaluation

      (c) Formal evaluation performed on either an inpatient or outpatient basis, depending on the degree of pulmonary impairment

4. Diagnostic study findings

  a. Laboratory

     i. Infectious disease testing: Purified protein derivative or TB Quantiferon Gold test, mumps, Candida testing

     ii. Serologic studies: CMV titer, varicella-zoster titer, herpes simplex titer, Epstein–Barr titer

     iii. Human immunodeficiency virus antigen-antibody levels, hepatitis screen, blood type and cross-match

      iv. Serum electrolyte levels, CBC with differential, prothrombin time, partial thromboplastin time, platelet count, creatinine clearance, liver function tests, levels of nutritional markers (albumin, total protein), urinalysis

      v. Thyroid and endocrine function tests

      vi. ABG levels

  b. Radiologic

      i. Chest radiograph, posteroanterior and lateral

      ii. High-resolution or spiral CT of the chest (considered the gold standard)

      iii. Quantitative $\dot{V}/\dot{Q}$ scan

  c. Pulmonary function

      i. Spirometry (includes prebronchodilator and postbronchodilator studies if obstruction is present)

      ii. Lung volumes using nitrogen washout and plethysmography

      iii. Diffusion capacity of carbon monoxide

  d. Cardiovascular studies: ECG, echocardiogram with pulse Doppler imaging, cardiac catheterization studies

5. **Goals of care**

  a. Alveolar ventilation and tissue oxygenation are optimized.

  b. Hemodynamic stability, acid-base balance, electrolyte levels, and fluid balance are maintained.

  c. Family is prepared for and supported during the preoperative, postoperative, and discharge events related to lung transplantation.

  d. Patient is able to manage postdischarge care and follow-up.

6. **Interprofessional collaboration: Nurse, physician, advanced practice provider, respiratory therapist, pulmonary rehabilitation team, physical therapist, occupational therapist, and infection control specialist, all members of the lung transplantation team—pulmonologist, thoracic surgeon, anesthesiologist, pharmacist, dietitian, psychiatric social worker, organ procurement coordinator.**

7. **Management of patient care**

  a. Anticipated patient trajectory:

      i. Positioning: Keep the head of the bed elevated at least 30 to 45 degrees to enhance ventilation, prevent aspiration, and promote drainage from the thoracic pleural space.

      ii. Pain management: Pain medication to relieve the discomfort of surgical wounds, tubes, and dressings and to prevent treatment interference.

        (a) Provide adequate thoracotomy pain control according to patient needs via IV or epidural pain management, patient-controlled analgesics, or oral analgesics.

        (b) Consider pain control needs before exercise and chest physiotherapy sessions.

        (c) Use pain control to enhance sleep and rest. Early postoperative phase often results in fragmented sleep, confusion, and irritability.

      iii. Nutrition: Comprehensive nutritional plan via dietary consult

        (a) Administer enteral feedings when the gastrointestinal system is functional and the patient is unable to take food by mouth; advance the diet as tolerated.

        (b) Administer total parenteral nutrition only when the gastrointestinal tract is not available or nonfunctional.

        (c) Avoid excessive carbohydrates to limit CO_2 production and respiratory workload.

(d) Avoid excessive fluids, particularly in patients with renal insufficiency.

iv. Infection control

(a) Of utmost importance, especially when immunosuppressive therapy will be used and when the patient is already malnourished

(b) Maintain sterile technique when caring for arterial or venous access devices or any invasive line.

v. Discharge planning

(a) Initiate patient and family education early in the preoperative phase (see details under Psychosocial Issues later.)

(b) Early postoperative period: Encourage patient participation in inpatient rehabilitation

(1) Range-of-motion exercises (12–24 hours postoperatively)

(2) Progressive resistance exercises within the first 2 to 3 days after transplantation if cardiovascular stability is established

(3) Ambulation for short distances; if mechanical ventilation is required, the patient may ambulate short distances using a manual resuscitation bag for assisted ventilations.

(c) After the patient leaves the ICU: Ambulation progresses as rapidly as tolerated.

(1) Special walker to hold O_2 tanks and IV pole or pumps, a urinary drainage bag, chest tubes, portable suction, and pulse oximeter

(2) Weaning from O_2 therapy

(3) Return of the patient to the treadmill for endurance training

(d) Conduct comprehensive education as part of the discharge planning process. Teach the patient the benefits of participating in an outpatient rehabilitation program following discharge.

(1) Endurance program progresses to home exercise

(2) Progression of musculoskeletal program: Improved functional ability to perform ADLs. Instruct on the need for the patient to continue ongoing medical follow-up with a private doctor and the transplant center.

a) Periodic pulmonary function, O_2 assessment

b) Signs and symptoms to report

c) Maintenance of logs of laboratory and spirometry records, medication dosages

d) Medication regimen: see Pharmacology

vi. Pharmacology: Antibiotics as needed, immunosuppression and pain medication

(a) Reduce pulmonary artery pressures with epoprostenol administered via continuous ambulatory medication delivery (CADD) pump, sildenafil, or nitrates.

(b) Teach self-administration of medication, as with MDIs.

(c) Teach the role of immunosuppression therapy in survival.

(d) Teach medication dose scheduling, monitoring for side effects, and the importance of early reporting of adverse reactions to the physician or nurse.

vii. Psychosocial issues: Provide psychosocial support throughout the hospital stay via active involvement of the patient and family in all aspects of the process.

(a) Prepare the patient and support person or family for the preoperative evaluation and waiting period: Relocation to a transplant center for lung transplantation.

(1) Living arrangements

(2) Support group

(3) Consent forms signed with the surgeon

(4) Medical follow-up and ongoing care while transplantation is awaited
(b) Conduct preoperative education of the patient and support person or family concerning the rationale for the preoperative tests, responsibilities of the patient while awaiting transplantation, operative procedure, and expected postoperative course, including activity and medication regimen.
   (1) Familiarize with the organization or program coordinating organ availability (e.g., placement on a national computerized waiting list; donor availability, selection, and preparation; donor-recipient matching [ABO compatibility, size]; lung allocation process and priorities).
   (2) Use of pagers or cellular phones for coordination of transplantation
       a) Gather information regarding the available donor
       b) Notify the retrieval team and the patient
   (3) Role of the transplant nurse coordinator and when to call.
   (4) Operative procedures and pretransplantation and posttransplantation care including anticipated hospital surgical and anesthetic preparation, surgical technique, time in the operating room, ICU stay.
   (5) Pretransplantation rehabilitation program for conditioning
       a) Goals and expected outcomes
       b) Exercise prescription of O_2 therapy
       c) Supervision and monitoring (e.g., SpO_2 measurement)
   (6) Daily self-assessment by the patient to detect early changes in medical and pulmonary condition
       a) Progression of endurance training
       b) Periodic reevaluation of exercise tolerance
       c) Postoperative planning
           1) Discuss anticipated feelings and issues related to the patient's return to independence and to the transition to a less active role on the part of the support person(s) or family.
           2) Encourage the patient's self-care activities, such as making appointments and scheduling laboratory work.
           3) Offer early involvement of the hospital or transplant chaplain or pastoral services.
   viii. Ethical issues: Discussions at the time of candidacy and selection need to include planning by the patient and family for decisions regarding ethical issues that may arise at any point in the transplantation process. Advance directive, healthcare power of attorney, and other necessary documents need to be on file and readily available.
b. Potential complications
   i. Intrathoracic hemorrhage
       (a) Major intrathoracic surgery involving major vascular supply to the cardiopulmonary system
       (b) Management
           (1) Monitor for intrathoracic and/or intraabdominal bleeding postoperatively.
           (2) Assess pleural and mediastinal chest tubes, verify that the suction level is as ordered, note the color and consistency of drainage, calculate the volume and rate of drainage output.
           (3) Assess the abdomen for distention and tenderness, and volume and consistency of nasogastric drainage.

(4) Monitor chest radiographic changes.

(5) Monitor and maintain the stability of hemodynamic parameters.

    a) Obtain hemodynamic profiles as ordered or routinely if the pulmonary artery catheter is in place

    b) Titrate vasoactive medications as necessary

(6) Transfuse as ordered using CMV-negative blood products; autotransfusion setups must be routinely available to allow quick response to blood loss.

  ii. Fluid overload

    (a) Mechanism: May have preexisting pulmonary infiltrates related to underlying pulmonary disorder, right-sided heart failure owing to pulmonary hypertension and vascular resistance.

    (b) Management

      (1) Monitor intake and output and fluid status with particular attention to avoiding volume overload

        a) Measure urine output; maintain at over 30 mL/h.

        b) Monitor serum blood urea nitrogen and serum creatinine levels.

        c) Monitor urine and serum electrolyte levels.

      (2) Administer diuretics as indicated

  iii. Infection

    (a) Mechanism: Numerous sources, including aspiration, incisional contamination, poor wound healing, surgery, transplant

    (b) Management

      (1) Optimize pulmonary care in the early postoperative phase

        a) Provide frequent and thorough oral care that includes brushing, cleansing, and removal of secretions; verify that the cuff of the endotracheal tube is sealed properly so oral secretions cannot pass.

        b) Provide pulmonary hygiene, positioning, chest physical therapy, inhaled bronchodilator treatment as ordered, suctioning based on need.

        c) Monitor trends in peak and mean inspiratory pressures, exhaled V_T, breathing effort, synchrony with ventilator.

      (2) Wean or liberate from mechanical ventilation as soon as possible.

  iv. Rejection of transplanted lung

    (a) Mechanism: Transplanted lung(s) represent foreign body that immune system normally rejects

    (b) Management

      (1) Monitor for rejection and infection of transplanted lung

        a) Administer immunosuppressive agents

        b) Monitor donor and recipient bronchoscopy culture results

        c) Administer antimicrobial therapy

        d) Maintain proper isolation procedures

      (2) Assess pulmonary function via arterial to alveolar ratio, A–a gradient, ABG levels, end-tidal CO_2 level, pulse oximetry; hypoxemia may indicate fluid volume overload, lung infection, or lung rejection.

References and bibliography information are available at http://evolve.elsevier.com/AACN/corecurriculum/.

Cardiovascular System

Andrea Efre, DNP, ARNP, ANP, FNP and Bryan Boling, DNP, AG-ACNP, CCRN-CSC, CEN

CROSSWALK

- **Quality and Safety in Nursing Education (QSEN):** Patient-Centered Care, Teamwork and Collaboration, Evidence-based practice (EBP), Quality Improvement (QI), Safety
- **National Patient Safety Goals:** Identify patients correctly, Improve staff communication, Use medicines safely, Use alarms safely, Prevent infection, Identify patient safety risks
- **American Nurses Association (ANA) standards for Professional Nursing Practice:** *Standard 1. Assessment, Standard 2. Diagnosis, Standard 3. Outcomes identification, Standard 4. Planning, Standard 5. Implementation, Standard 6. Evaluation, Standard 7. Ethics, Standard 10. Collaboration, Standard 12. Education, Standard 13. Evidence-based practice and research, Standard 14. Quality of practice, Standard 15. Professional practice evaluation, Standard 16. Resource utilization*
- **AACN Standards for Progressive and Critical Care Nursing Practice:** *Standard 1.* Quality of practice, *Standard 2.* Professional practice evaluation, *Standard 3.* Education, *Standard 4.* Communication, *Standard 5.* Ethics, *Standard 6.* Collaboration, *Standard 7.* Evidence-based practice/research/clinical inquiry, *Standard 8.* Resource utilization, *Standard 9.* Leadership
- **AACN Standards for Establishing and Sustaining Healthy Work Environments (HWE):** Skilled communication, True collaboration, Effective decision-making, Appropriate staffing
- **PCCN content:** Cardiovascular—all items
- **CCRN content:** Cardiovascular—all items

SYSTEMWIDE ELEMENTS

ANATOMY AND PHYSIOLOGY REVIEW

1. **Heart (Figs. 4.1 and 4.2)**
   a. The heart lies in the middle mediastinum, slightly left of the midline. It is a muscular organ that pumps blood through the circulatory and pulmonary systems.
   b. Its long axis is oriented from the right shoulder blade to the left upper quadrant of the abdomen.
   c. The base (top wide area) of the heart (atria and great vessels) is located diagonally at the second intercostal space, right and left sternal borders.
   d. The apex, or tip, of the heart (junction of the ventricles and ventricular septum) is usually located at the fifth intercostal space on the left midclavicular line.
2. **Cardiac wall structure**
   a. Pericardium: Fibrous sac surrounding the heart and containing small amounts (15–50 mL) of pericardial fluid. This lubricated space protects the heart from friction, allowing it to easily change volume and size during contractions. The pericardium also keeps heart muscle anchored within the mediastinum.

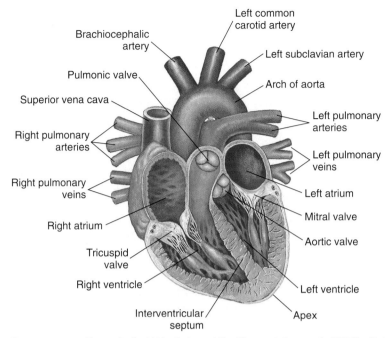

Fig. 4.1 Cardiac anatomy. (From Ball, J.W., Dains, J.E., Flynn, J.A., et al. (2019). *Seidel's guide to physical examination*, 9th ed. St. Louis: Elsevier.)

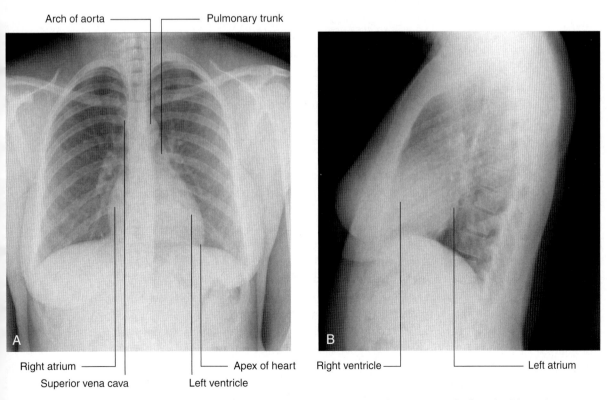

Fig. 4.2 Chest radiographs. **A,** Standard posteroanterior view of the chest. **B,** Standard lateral view of the heart. (From Drake, R.L., Vogl, A.W., Mitchell, A.W.M. (2020). *Gray's anatomy for students*, 4th ed. Philadelphia: Churchill Livingstone.)

    b. Epicardium: Outer surface of the heart (includes epicardial coronary arteries, autonomic nerves, adipose tissue, lymphatics)

    c. Myocardium: Muscular, contractile portion of the heart. Muscle fibers wrap around the heart in multiple, interlacing layers.

    d. Endocardium: Inner surface of the heart

    e. Papillary muscles: Myocardial structures extending into the ventricular chambers and attaching to the chordae tendineae

    f. Chordae tendineae: Strong tendinous attachments from the papillary muscles to the tricuspid and mitral valves; prevent prolapse of the valves into the atria during systole

3. **Chambers of the heart**

    a. Atria: Thin-walled, low-pressure chambers

       i. Right and left atria act as reservoirs of blood for their respective ventricles

      ii. Right atrium (RA), located above and to the right of the right ventricle, receives systemic venous blood via the superior vena cava and inferior vena cava, and venous blood from the heart via the coronary sinus

      iii. Left atrium (LA), superior and posterior to the other chambers, receives oxygenated blood returning to the heart from the lungs via the pulmonary veins

      iv. When the mitral and tricuspid valves open, there is rapid filling of blood passively from atria into ventricles (about 80%–85% of total filling)

      v. At the end of diastole, atrial contraction (also referred to as atrial kick) forcefully adds 15% to 20% more to the ventricular volume

    b. Ventricles: Major muscular chambers, responsible for pumping action of the heart

       i. Right ventricle (RV) is anterior under the sternum

         (a) Thin-walled, low-pressure system

         (b) Contracts and propels deoxygenated blood into the pulmonary circulation via the pulmonary artery (the only artery in the body that carries deoxygenated blood)

      ii. Left ventricle (LV) is the strongest part of the heart as a pump: Conical (ellipsoid) structure behind and to the left of the RV

         (a) Thick-walled, high-pressure system

         (b) Squeezes and ejects blood into the systemic circulation via the aorta during ventricular systole

      iii. Interventricular septum is functionally more a part of the LV than of the RV. It forms the anterior wall of the LV. Its curved shape protrudes into the RV cavity.

4. **Cardiac valves**

    a. Atrioventricular (AV) valves

       i. Location and structure: Situated between the atria and the ventricles (tricuspid valve on the right, mitral valve on the left)

         (a) Tricuspid valve is composed of three leaflets: The large anterior leaflet and the two smaller posterior and septal leaflets

         (b) Mitral valve is composed of two leaflets: The long, narrow posterior (mural) leaflet (like a toilet seat) and an oval anterior (aortic) leaflet (like a toilet lid)

      ii. Function: These are one-way valves that permit unidirectional blood flow from the atria to the ventricles during ventricular diastole and prevent retrograde flow during ventricular systole

         (a) With ventricular diastole, the ventricles relax and the valve leaflets open

      (b) With ventricular systole, the valve leaflets close completely

      (c) First heart sound (S_1) is produced as the mitral (M_1) and tricuspid (T_1) valves close. M_1 is the initial and major component of S_1.

  b. Semilunar valves

    i. Location and structure

      (a) Pulmonary valve is situated between the RV and the pulmonary artery. It consists of three semilunar cusps that attach to the wall of the pulmonary trunk.

      (b) Aortic valve is situated between the LV and aorta. It consists of three slightly thicker valve cusps, the bases of which attach to a valve annulus (fibrous ring).

    ii. Function: Permit unidirectional blood flow from the outflow tract during ventricular systole and prevent retrograde blood flow during ventricular diastole

      (a) With ventricular systole, the valves open when the respective ventricle contracts and pressure is greater in the ventricle than in the artery.

      (b) After ventricular systole, pressure in the artery exceeds pressure in the ventricles. This and retrograde blood flow cause the valve to close.

      (c) Second heart sound (S_2) is produced when the aortic (A_2) and pulmonic (P_2) valves close. A_2 is normally the initial and major component of S_2.

5. Coronary vasculature (Fig. 4.3)

  a. Arteries

    i. Two main arteries branch off at the base of the aorta, supplying blood to the heart

    ii. Right coronary artery (RCA)

      (a) Originates behind the right coronary cusp of the aortic valve

      (b) Supplies

        (1) RA and RV

        (2) Sinoatrial (SA) node and AV node

        (3) Inferior-posterior wall of the LV (in 90% of hearts)

        (4) Inferior-posterior third of the interventricular septum

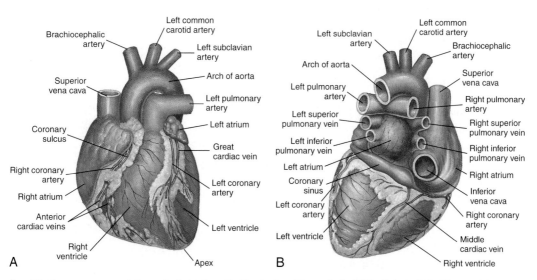

Fig. 4.3 Coronary vasculature. **A,** Anterior. **B,** Posterior. (From Ball, J.W., Dains, J.E., Flynn, J.A., et al. (2019). *Seidel's guide to physical examination*, 9th ed. St. Louis: Elsevier.)

(c) Main branches
  (1) SA node in 55% of hearts
  (2) RV branch
  (3) AV node in 90% of hearts
  (4) Posterior descending artery (supplying the inferior-posterior wall of the LV in 85% of hearts)

iii. Left coronary artery (LCA)
  (a) Left main coronary artery (LMCA): Branches into the left anterior descending (LAD) and circumflex arteries
  (b) LAD artery
    (1) Supplies the anterior two-thirds of the interventricular septum and the anterior wall of the LV
    (2) Branches include diagonals (two to six other diagonals may be present), septal perforators (three to five other perforators may be present)
  (c) Left circumflex (LCX) artery also branches from the LMCA
    (1) LCX artery supplies
      a) SA node in 45% of hearts
      b) AV node in 10% of hearts
      c) Inferior-posterior LV in 10% of hearts
      d) Lateral posterior surface of the LV via the obtuse marginal branches (OMBs)
      e) Posterior descending artery arises from the LCX artery in 15% of hearts (see description under RCA)
    (2) Branches of the LCX include the OMBs (may be one to three), which supply the lateral wall of the LV and occasionally, the posterior lateral muscular branch

iv. Coronary collaterals: Potential vascular connections between the RCA and LCA exist
  (a) They may open, if stenosis of one of the coronary arteries occurs, to supply blood from the other artery
  (b) They cannot augment flow to meet acute requirements for increased flow

b. Cardiac veins
  i. Return deoxygenated blood to the RA, mostly through the coronary sinus
  ii. Follow paths similar to those of the arteries; have no valves

c. Coronary blood flow
  i. Coronary vascular reserve: Coronary circulation has the ability to increase flow to meet added needs up to approximately 6 times normal
  ii. Coronary blood flow is about 70 to 90 mL/min
  iii. The heart uses most of the oxygen available in the coronary circulation; little oxygen reserve exists
  iv. Most of coronary blood flow is in diastole, because in systole, coronary artery blood flow usually decreases because of ventricular compression and contraction
  v. Coronary blood flow is reduced by
    (a) Hypotension
    (b) Tachycardia: Decreased LV diastolic filling times
    (c) Mechanical obstruction (coronary stenosis or spasm)

6. Neurologic control of the heart
  a. Autonomic nervous system: Influences contractility, depolarization-repolarization, and rate of conductivity

    i. Sympathetic stimulation: Norepinephrine release is the main impetus of stimulation to the heart; its two effects include the following:

      (a) α-adrenergic: Causing peripheral arteriolar vasoconstriction

      (b) β-adrenergic

        (1) Increases SA node discharge, increasing heart rate (positive chronotropy)

        (2) Increases the force of myocardial contraction (positive inotropy)

        (3) Accelerates AV conduction time

    ii. Parasympathetic stimulation: Occurs via the 10th cranial (vagus) nerve. Acetylcholine release is the main parasympathetic impetus to cardiac effects.

      (a) Decreases the rate of SA node discharge, slowing heart rate (negative chronotropy)

      (b) Slows conduction through AV tissue

    iii. Ventricles have mainly sympathetic innervation and only sparse vagal innervation

    iv. Parasympathetic influences normally predominate in the conducting system (SA node, AV node)

  b. Chemoreceptors: Afferent receptors located in the carotid and aortic bodies. Sensitive to changes in partial pressure of oxygen, partial pressure of carbon dioxide, and pH, causing changes in heart rate and respiratory rate via stimulation of vasomotor center in the medulla.

  c. Baroreceptors: Stretch receptors in the heart and blood vessels that respond to pressure and volume changes

7. **Cardiac muscle microanatomy and contractile properties**

  a. Cardiac muscle fibers (myocardial) have contractile properties allowing them to shorten and to develop force. The fibers are arranged in a lattice-style pattern, and when one fiber is stimulated, all become stimulated (known as syncytium). The cardiac myocyte is composed of bundles of myofibrils that contain myofilaments. The myofibrils (termed sarcomeres) are the contractile unit of the myocardial cell, and changes in their length affect the force of the heart's contraction. Sarcomeres are composed of:

    i. Contractile proteins: Myosin and actin (their interactions help to produce contraction, fiber shortening)

    ii. Regulatory proteins: Tropomyosin and troponin (they inhibit myosin-actin interactions)

    iii. Troponin C binds $Ca2+$; troponin I (TnI), binds to actin and inhibits myosin-actin interactions; and troponin T (TnT), binds to tropomyosin

  b. Intercalated discs interlock cardiac muscle fibers together at the ends and provide quick transmission of electrical impulse

  c. Myocardial working cells: Enable chemical energy to be transformed into mechanical actions (contraction and relaxation)

  d. The excitation and contraction process is how an action potential triggers the myocardial cell to contract (action potential is detailed later in the Electrophysiology section).

    i. During excitation (depolarization), calcium enters the working cell interior across sarcolemma

    ii. Calcium binds with troponin, and myosin-actin inhibition is lost

    iii. Actin and myosin may now interact, using adenosine triphosphate for energy

    iv. Sarcomeres shorten, which results in muscle fiber shortening and subsequent cardiac muscle contraction

    v. Calcium is then pumped out of cell, allowing fiber to relax again until process repeats

8. **Anatomy of the cardiac conduction system (Fig. 4.4)**
   a. SA node
      i. Normal pacemaker of the heart, possessing the fastest inherent rate of automaticity (~70 beats/min)
      ii. Located in the right superior wall of the RA at the junction of the superior vena cava and the RA
   b. Internodal atrial conduction
      i. Impulse is conducted from the SA node through the RA and LA musculature to the AV node
      ii. Although the atria do not have specialized high-speed conduction tracts comparable to the ventricular bundles and fascicles, there are preferred conduction pathways (e.g., Bachmann's bundle, which conducts impulses from the SA node to the LA)
   c. AV node
      i. Delays the impulse from the atria before it goes to the ventricles. This allows time for both ventricles to fill before ventricular systole.
      ii. Inherent rate of automaticity is approximately 40 beats/min
      iii. Located in the right interatrial septum, above the tricuspid valve's septal leaflet
   d. Bundle of His: Arises from the AV node and conducts the impulse to the bundle branch system. The bundle of His is close to the annulus of the tricuspid valve.
   e. Bundle branch system: Pathways that arise from the bundle of His and branch at the top of the interventricular septum
      i. Right bundle branch is the smaller, direct continuation of the bundle of His. It transmits the impulse down the right side of the interventricular septum to the RV myocardium.
      ii. Left bundle branch is the larger branch from the bundle of His. It transmits the impulse to the septum and the LV. The left bundle branch divides into three parts:
         (a) Left anterior fascicle: Transmits the impulse to the anterior and superior endocardial surfaces of the LV
         (b) Left posterior fascicle: Transmits the impulse over the posterior-inferior endocardial surface of the LV
         (c) Septal bundle

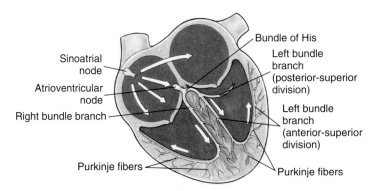

Fig. 4.4 Anatomy of the cardiac conduction system. (From Ball, J.W., Dains, J.E., Flynn, J.A., et al. (2019). *Seidel's guide to physical examination*, 9th ed. St. Louis: Elsevier; Canobbio, M.M. (1990). *Cardiovascular disorders*, St. Louis: Elsevier.)

   f. Purkinje system

      i. Arises from the distal portion of the bundle branches, forming networks on the ventricle's endocardial surface

     ii. Transmits the impulse into the subendocardial and myocardial layers of both ventricles

    iii. Provides for depolarization of the myocardium (from endocardium to epicardium)

    iv. Ventricles have their own inherent rate of automaticity of approximately 20 to 30 beats/min

9. **Electrophysiology**

   a. Electrophysiologic properties of cardiac muscle cells

      i. Excitability: Ability to depolarize and form an action potential when sufficiently stimulated

     ii. Automaticity: Ability to generate an impulse without an outside stimulus

    iii. Conductivity: Ability to conduct an electrical impulse to neighboring cells, spreading the impulse throughout the heart to achieve total depolarization

    iv. Refractoriness: Temporary inability of the depolarized cell to become excited and generate another action potential

   b. Resting membrane potential (RMP): Electrical charge of cardiac muscle cell at rest. Cell ions consist primarily of sodium, potassium, and calcium.

      i. Sodium ion concentration is greater *outside* the cell

     ii. Potassium ion concentration is greater *inside* the cell

    iii. Calcium ion concentration is greater *outside* the cell

   c. Depolarization: Change in the electrical charge of a stimulated cell from negative to positive by the flow of ions across the cell membrane. Sodium moves into the cell, potassium moves out.

   d. Repolarization: Recovery or recharging of a cell's normal polarity. Sodium moves back out of the cell, potassium moves into the cell. The cell recovers its negative charge.

   e. Threshold potential: The electric voltage level at which cardiac cells become activated and produce an action potential, which leads to muscular contraction

   f. Stimulation of myocardial cells

      i. Stimulus may be chemical, electrical, or mechanical

     ii. When the cell is stimulated, the electrical charge inside the cell becomes less negative, and depolarization occurs

    iii. When the threshold potential is reached, changes occur in the membrane

    iv. SA and AV nodes achieve threshold potential first

     v. Cell membrane permeability is altered, and specialized channels in the membrane open, which allows the entry of sodium and calcium ions into the cell

   g. Action potential: As cardiac cells reverse polarity, the electrical impulse generated during that event creates an energy stimulus that travels across the cell membrane—a high-speed, short-lived, self-reproducing current (heart only). This is represented on an action potential curve.

      i. Phase 0—Depolarization: A quick upstroke (several milliseconds) representing the initial phase of excitation

     ii. Phase 1—Initial phase of repolarization

    iii. Phase 2—Plateau phase of repolarization: Slow inward current of calcium (and sodium, to a lesser extent); potassium diffuses out of the cells

    iv. Phase 3—Last phase of repolarization: Outward current of potassium increases, and the slow, inward current of sodium and calcium decreases. Cells rapidly repolarize, returning to normal RMP.

    v. Phase 4—Membrane at RMP

h. Cardiac pacemaker cells (SA and AV nodes) action potential

    i. Pacer cells, having increased automaticity, spontaneously depolarize in phase 4 without a stimulus. Other cells of the heart, having repolarized, require another stimulus to become depolarized.

        (a) Rate of automaticity may be altered by increasing or decreasing the slope of phase 4

        (b) Increasing the slope speeds heart rate; decreasing the slope slows heart rate

    ii. Spontaneous depolarization of pacer cells is caused by a steady influx of sodium and efflux of potassium

    iii. SA node has the fastest rate of depolarization

i. Refractoriness of heart muscle

    i. Absolute refractory period (effective refractory period): Another stimulus to the cell will not produce another action potential (phases 0, 1, and 2 and part of phase 3 of the action potential curve)

    ii. Relative refractory period: Only a very strong stimulus can initiate an action potential and cause depolarization (latter part of phase 3)

    iii. Supernormal period: Weak stimulus (one that would not normally elicit an action potential) can evoke an action potential and cause depolarization (at the end of phase 3)

10. **Events in the cardiac cycle (Fig. 4.5)**

a. Ventricular systole: Contraction and emptying of the ventricles

    i. First phase of ventricular contraction (systole) is called isovolumetric contraction. Pressure increases, but no blood is ejected until LV pressure exceeds aortic pressure (and opens the aortic valve).

    ii. As pressure rises in the ventricles, the AV valves close, associated with the first heart sound (S_1, composed of mitral [M_1] and tricuspid [T_1] components)

    iii. The "c" wave of the atrial pressure curve is produced when the AV valves are pushed backward toward the atria as ventricular pressure builds

    iv. When LV pressure exceeds the pressure in the aorta, the aortic valve opens (comparable events in the RV occur with the pulmonic valve)

    v. Blood is rapidly ejected into the aorta (systolic ejection)

    vi. LV pressures decrease, falling below the pressure in the aorta, ventricular ejection stops, and the aortic valve closes. (Comparable events occur in the pulmonary artery, closing the pulmonic valve.)

    vii. Closing of the aortic and pulmonic valves is associated with the second heart sound (S_2, composed of aortic [A_2] and pulmonic [P_2] components)

    viii. Aortic valve closure is represented by the dicrotic notch in the aortic pressure waveform

    ix. Repolarization of the ventricles occurs at this time and produces the T wave on the electrocardiogram (ECG)

    x. After the aortic valve closes, pressure in the LV falls rapidly (isovolumetric relaxation phase); no blood enters the ventricle

    xi. The atrial "v" wave is produced by rapid filling of the atria during ventricular systole, against closed AV valves. This marks the end of systole.

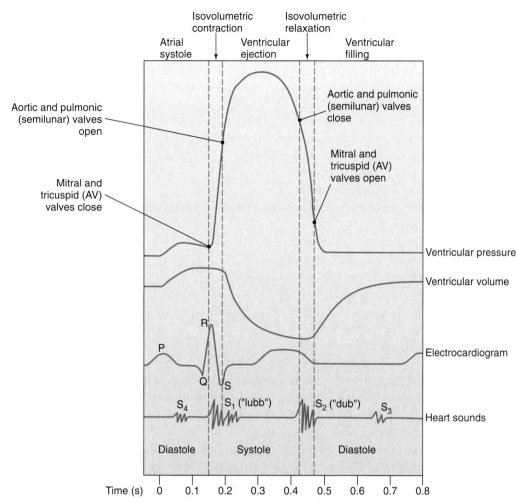

Fig. 4.5 Events of the cardiac cycle. *AV,* Atrioventricular. (From Ignatavicius, D.D., Workman, M.L., Rebar, C.R., et al. (2021). *Medical-surgical nursing: concepts for interprofessional collaborative care*, 10th ed. St. Louis: Elsevier.)

   b. Ventricular diastole: Filling phase of the ventricles
     i. When pressure is lower in the ventricles than in the atria, the AV valves reopen, which initiates the early rapid filling phase of the ventricles during diastole. This marks the start of diastole.
     ii. Pressure in the atria is higher than diastolic pressure in the ventricles, so blood flows from the atria into the ventricles
     iii. "a" wave: Atrial pressure rises with atrial contraction
     iv. P wave (electrocardiogram [ECG]): In late diastole, represents atrial depolarization (an electrical event)
11. Variables affecting LV function and cardiac output (CO)
   a. CO: Amount of blood ejected by the LV in 1 minute
     i. CO is the product of stroke volume (SV) and heart rate (HR): $CO = SV \times HR$
     ii. SV is the amount of blood ejected by the LV with each contraction or the difference between left ventricular end-diastolic volume (LVEDV) and left ventricular end-systolic volume (LVESV): $SV = LVEDV - LVESV$; (60–130 mL)
     iii. Normal resting CO = 4 to 8 L/min
     iv. CO is determined by preload, afterload, contractility, and heart rate

b. Preload: The degree to which muscle fibers are lengthened (stretched) before contraction
   i. In the intact heart, preload is secondary to the volume (size) of the chamber. This is determined by the amount of blood filling the chamber.
   ii. Increases in preload increase the CO as described by the *Frank-Starling law* of the heart
   iii. Muscle fibers can reach a point of stretch beyond which contraction is no longer enhanced, and further increases in preload do not yield any further increase in CO
   iv. Increased preload occurs with
      (a) Increased circulating volume
      (b) Venous constriction (decreases venous pooling and increases venous return to heart)
      (c) Medications: Vasoconstrictors
   v. Decreased preload occurs with
      (a) Hypovolemia
      (b) Mitral stenosis
      (c) Medications: Vasodilators (e.g., nitrates), diuretics
      (d) Cardiac tamponade
      (e) Constrictive pericarditis
c. Afterload: Initial resistance that must be overcome by the ventricles to develop force and contract, opening the semilunar valves and propelling blood into the systemic and pulmonary circulatory systems (systolic contraction)
   i. Factors affecting afterload include arterial resistance (wall stress and thickness), aortic impedance, and blood viscosity
   ii. Systemic vascular resistance (SVR) is used as a rough estimate of afterload
   iii. To calculate SVR: Mean arterial pressure (MAP) minus central venous pressure (CVP); this number is divided by CO; the resulting value then is multiplied by 80 and converted into dynes/s/cm^{-5} (1 dyne is the force that gives a mass of 1 g an acceleration of 1 cm/s^2):

$$SVR = \frac{MAP - CVP}{CO} \times 80$$

   iv. Normal SVR = 900 to 1400 dynes/s/cm^{-5}
   v. Excessive afterload: Increases LV stroke work, decreases SV, increases myocardial oxygen demands, and may result in LV failure
   vi. Increased afterload is seen in
      (a) Aortic stenosis
      (b) Peripheral arteriolar vasoconstriction
      (c) Hypertension
      (d) Pulmonary hypertension
      (e) Polycythemia
      (f) Vasoconstriction
      (g) Vasoconstrictor medications (e.g., epinephrine and norepinephrine)
      (h) Hypovolemia
      (i) Hypothermia
   vii. Decreased afterload is seen in
      (a) Hyperthermia
      (b) Sepsis

      (c) Use of arterial vasodilators (e.g., nitrates)

      (d) Hypotension

  d. Contractility (inotropic state): Heart's contractile strength

    i. There is no way to measure contractility directly. Contractile state can be assessed indirectly through its effects on CO or with noninvasive imaging.

    ii. Factors increasing the contractile state of the myocardium include

      (a) Use of positive inotropic medications (e.g., digitalis, milrinone, epinephrine, dobutamine)

      (b) Increased heart rate (Bowditch's phenomenon)

      (c) Sympathetic stimulation (via β_1 receptors)

    iii. Factors decreasing the contractile state of the myocardium include

      (a) Negative inotropic medications (e.g., type 1 A antiarrhythmics, β-blockers, calcium channel blockers, barbiturates)

      (b) Hypoxia

      (c) Hypercapnia

      (d) Myocardial ischemia or infarction

      (e) Metabolic acidosis

  e. Heart rate

    i. Influenced by many factors, including

      (a) Blood volume status

      (b) Sympathetic and parasympathetic tone

      (c) Medications

      (d) Temperature

      (e) Respiration

      (f) Arrhythmias

      (g) Peripheral vascular tone

      (h) Emotions

      (i) Metabolic status (increases with hyperthyroidism)

    ii. Determinant of myocardial oxygen supply and demand

      (a) Increased heart rates increase myocardial oxygen consumption

      (b) Fast heart rates (>150 beats/min) decrease diastolic coronary blood flow (shorter diastole)

  f. Cardiac index (CI)

    i. CI is CO corrected for differences in body size (CO of 4 L/min may be adequate for a 100-lb person but inadequate for a 200-lb person)

    ii. Based on body surface area (BSA) as estimated from a height and weight nomogram: CI = CO/BSA

    iii. Normal CI is 2.5 to 4.0 L/min/m²

  g. Ejection fraction (EF)

    i. Percentage of blood in the ventricle ejected with every beat

      (a) Normal LVEF = 50% to 75%

      (b) Not clinically significant until less than 50%

    ii. Good reflection of LV performance

  h. Ventricular function curve: Shows how to relate the contributions of preload, afterload, and contractility (but *not* heart rate) to ventricular function

12. Systemic vasculature

  a. Major functions: Provides tissues with blood, nutrients, and hormones and removes metabolic wastes

  b. Resistance to flow: Depends on diameter of vessels (especially arterioles), viscosity of blood, and elastic recoil in vessel walls

c. Circulating blood volume: There is approximately 5 L of total circulating blood volume in the adult body

d. Major components of the vascular system
   i. Arteries
      (a) Strong, compliant, elastic-walled vessels that branch off the aorta, carry blood away from the heart, and distribute it to capillary beds throughout the body
      (b) A high-pressure circuit
      (c) Able to stretch during systole and recoil during diastole because of elastic fibers in the arterial wall
   ii. Arterioles
      (a) Control SVR and thus arterial pressure
      (b) Have strong smooth muscle walls innervated by the autonomic nervous system
      (c) Autonomic nervous system
         (1) Adrenergic (stimulatory) system: Releases two neurotransmitters: epinephrine and norepinephrine. Epinephrine stimulates β-receptors (increases heart rate, increases contractility, dilates arterioles). Norepinephrine stimulates α-receptors (vasoconstriction).
         (2) Cholinergic (inhibitory) system: Releases acetylcholine (decreases heart rate; releases nitric oxide, causing vasodilatation)
      (d) Lead directly into capillaries, supply tissue beds
   iii. Capillary system
      (a) Tissue bed exchange of oxygen and carbon dioxide and solutes between blood and tissues; site of fluid volume transfer between plasma and interstitium
      (b) Gas exchange caused by diffusion. Diffusion of a substance is from an area of high concentration to an area of low concentration until equilibrium is established.
      (c) Fluid homeostasis
         (1) Increased capillary hydrostatic pressure moves fluid from the vessel into the interstitium
         (2) Greater capillary osmotic pressure moves fluid from the interstitium into the vessels
         (3) Plasma protein concentration in the capillaries provides the osmotic gradient
         (4) Retains fluid in the intravascular space
         (5) Prevents edema formation in the interstitium
         (6) Albumin accounts for 75% of total plasma osmotic pressure; fibrinogen accounts for a small amount
         (7) Serum albumin level is a good indicator of a patient's colloid osmotic pressure
      (d) Capillaries lack smooth muscle
   iv. Venous system
      (a) Stores about 65% of total blood volume
      (b) Receives blood from capillaries
      (c) Conducts blood back to the heart within a low-pressure system
      (d) No muscle layer: Veins are compressed by the contraction of surrounding skeletal muscle
      (e) Valves in the veins prevent reverse blood flow
      (f) Venous pressure in the lower extremities is normally 20 mm Hg or less

13. **Control of peripheral blood flow**
    a. Autoregulation: Ability of the tissues to control their own blood flow (vasodilatation, vasoconstriction)
       i. Coronary blood flow remains fairly constant over a wide range of blood pressures (BPs)
       ii. As coronary perfusion pressure drops below 50 mm Hg, autoregulatory ability becomes impaired
    b. Autonomic regulation of vessels
       i. Vasoconstriction occurs when norepinephrine is released by stimulation of the sympathetic nervous system (adrenergic effect)
       ii. Vasodilatation occurs when acetylcholine is released by stimulation of the parasympathetic nervous system (cholinergic effect) or by inhibition of vasoconstriction
    c. Stretch receptors: Baroreceptors (pressoreceptors) keep MAP constant
       i. Receptor sites in the arteries (aortic arch, carotid sinus, pulmonary arteries, and atria)
       ii. Action with increased BP
           (a) Respond to stretching of arterial walls
           (b) Impulse transmitted from the aortic arch via the vagus nerve to the medulla
           (c) Parasympathetic nervous system stimulated; sympathetic nervous system inhibited
           (d) Result: Decreased heart rate and contractility, dilation of peripheral vessels, decreased SVR, decreased BP
       iii. Action with decreased BP
           (a) Sympathetic nervous system stimulated, parasympathetic nervous system inhibited
           (b) Result: Increased heart rate and contractility, arterial and venous constriction (which preserves blood flow to the brain and heart), and increased BP
14. **Arterial pressure**
    a. Neurohumoral regulation
       i. Renin-angiotensin-aldosterone system also helps control arterial pressure (see Ch. 6, Renal System)
       ii. Renin is a protease secreted by the kidneys; converts angiotensinogen to angiotensin I
       iii. Renin release from the kidneys is affected as follows:
           (a) Decreased BP (e.g., hemorrhage, dehydration, diuretics, sodium depletion) → increases in renin secretion
           (b) Rise in sympathetic output (β stimulation) → increases in renin secretion
           (c) Fall in sodium concentration → increases in renin secretion (decreased volume)
           (d) Increased BP → decreases in renin secretion
       iv. Angiotensin I is converted to angiotensin II. (These effects are blocked by angiotensin-converting enzyme [ACE] inhibitors.)
       v. Angiotensin II, the most potent vasoconstrictor known, is produced when increased renin secretion stimulates its formation
           (a) Effects of angiotensin II include the following:
               (1) Arteriolar constriction, which increases systolic and diastolic pressures

        (2) Stimulation of the adrenal cortex to secrete aldosterone, which causes sodium and water retention

        (3) Increase in extracellular fluid volume, which shuts off the stimulus that initiated renin secretion so that BP is maintained at the normal level

    (b) Effects of angiotensin II are blocked at its receptors by angiotensin II receptor blockers (ARBs)

  b. Pulse pressure: Difference between systolic and diastolic pressures

    i. Function of SV and arterial capacitance

    ii. Normal pulse pressure: 30 to 40 mm Hg

    iii. Changes in SV (with exercise, shock, heart failure [HF]) are reflected in similar changes in pulse pressure

  c. MAP: Average arterial pressure during the cardiac cycle; dependent on mean arterial blood volume and elasticity of the arterial wall

    i. $\text{MAP} = \dfrac{(\text{diastolic pressure} \times 2) + \text{systolic pressure}}{3}$

    ii. Example: BP of 120/60 mm Hg

$$\text{MAP} = \frac{[(60 \times 2) + 120]}{3}$$

$$\text{MAP} = \frac{(120 + 120)}{3}$$

$$\text{MAP} = \frac{240}{3} = 80$$

ASSESSMENT

1. **History**

  a. Chief complaint: Patient's explanation for seeking medical assistance

  b. History of present illness: The events and symptoms that have occurred before cardiac complaint.

EXPERT TIP

When collecting subjective data, it is useful to use a mnemonic, such as OLDCART. This is especially helpful in evaluating chest pain.

*O*nset
*L*ocation
*D*uration
*C*haracter
*A*ggravating and *A*lleviating factors, and *A*ssociated symptoms
*R*adiation
*T*reatment and *T*iming

---

    i. Other signs and symptoms

      (a) New onset of fatigue: With or without activity

      (b) Edema: Location, degree, duration

      (c) Syncope or presyncope

      (d) Diaphoresis

      (e) Dyspnea: Orthopnea, paroxysmal nocturnal dyspnea, dyspnea on exertion (determine how much exercise it takes to induce symptoms, e.g., number of blocks, flights of stairs, etc.)

    (f) Palpitations: Nature, length, associated symptoms

    (g) Cough or hemoptysis

    (h) Claudication: How many feet can you walk?

    (i) Recent weight gain or loss

    (j) Recent changes in sleep patterns or difficulty sleeping or sleep apnea

    (k) Change or limitations in activities of daily living

c. Medical history: Identify all previous illnesses, injuries, and surgical procedures

  i. Patient's assessment of general health for last several years

  ii. Coronary risk factors: Age, sex, race, hypertension, dyslipidemia, smoking, family history of cardiac disease, diabetes, metabolic syndrome, obesity, lack of physical activity, history of drugs or alcohol, or connective tissue disease

  iii. Last medical examination, hospitalizations, prior relevant cardiac tests (e.g., echocardiography, catheterization)

  iv. Heart history: Coronary artery disease (CAD), angina, myocardial infarctions (MIs), hypertension, valvular disease, arrhythmias, trauma, peripheral vascular disease, congenital heart defects, heart murmurs, rheumatic fever, cerebrovascular accident (CVA), and transient ischemic attacks

d. Medications: Identify all prescribed or over-the-counter medications. Determine why and how often the patient is taking medication(s), dosages, any side effects, compliance issues. Include medications that they may take that are prescribed to others.

e. Allergies: Medications, foods (e.g., shellfish), environmental substances, latex, or iodine (potential reaction to contrast medium used during cardiac catheterization procedures)

f. Family history: Identify

  i. State of health or cause of death; age at death of immediate family members

  ii. Hereditary, familial diseases pertaining to cardiovascular system

    (a) Diabetes mellitus, hypertension, cardiovascular disease, sudden death or syncope, lipid disorders, stroke, or collagen vascular disease

g. Social history: Identify

  i. Present and past work experiences and occupational exposures

  ii. Level of activity, exercise, type and quantify amount per week

  iii. Smoking/tobacco use (present or past, pack per year history), quantify amount and method used (smoke, chew, vape). Note if using electronic cigarettes and any additives used—such as flavoring or marijuana.

  iv. Address alcohol use (amount, how often and type). Note: Alcohol overuse and hepatic insufficiency may lead to HF.

  v. Recreational drug use (past or present) and quantify type, amount, and how often

Note: Ask about cannabis (marijuana) products. These may be taken as a medical adjunct or recreational depending on state laws and may be used orally, topically, smoked, or vaped. Identify the cannabinoid being used, as the cannabinoid that appears to increase cardiac risk is tetrahydrocannabinol (THC), but there is no current indication that cannabidiol (CBD) has cardiac concerns.

Note: Cocaine has many cardiac implications, as do amphetamines, methamphetamine, and synthetically produced chemical drugs (e.g., spice, K2, and bath salts)

  vi. Nutrition: Foods eaten, meals per day, who prepares meals (quantify fast food per week)

  vii. Support system: Relationship with significant others

  viii. Cultural issues and language barriers

      ix. Daily living patterns (particularly in children and the older adult)

      x. Safety concerns (e.g., dangerous hobbies, unsafe behaviors)

2. Physical examination

  a. General overall appearance

     i. Physical appearance (e.g., disheveled, signs of distress, anxiety, or tearful)

     ii. Nonverbal signs of pain (e.g., facial grimace with movement)

  b. Vital signs

     i. Pulses: Palpate bilaterally

      (a) Check rate, rhythm, and quality

      (b) Describe pulses, using scale of 0 to 3

        (1) 0 = absent pulses

        (2) Doppler only

        (3) 1 + = palpable but thready, easily obliterated

        (4) 2 + = normal, not easily obliterated

        (5) 3 + = bounding, easily palpable, cannot obliterate

      (c) Sites for palpation of arteries

        (1) Carotid

        (2) Upper extremities: Brachial, radial

        (3) Lower extremities: Femoral, popliteal, dorsalis pedis, and posterior tibialis

      (d) Describe pulse characteristics

        (1) Normal pulse character

        (2) Pulsus alternans: Pulse waves alternate, every other beat is weaker; caused by impaired myocardium; noted in severe LV failure

        (3) Water hammer (Corrigan's pulse)

          a) Abrupt, rapid upstroke followed by rapid downstroke

          b) Palpated in patients with aortic insufficiency or patent ductus arteriosus (PDA)

     ii. Blood pressure (BP)

      (a) Sphygmomanometer or electronic BP device

        (1) Width of cuff important

          a) Ideal width is 40% of the circumference of the arm

          b) For obese patients, use appropriate cuff size or a thigh cuff

        (2) Positioning of cuff: No less than 2.5 cm from the antecubital fossa

        (3) Falsely low measurement: Cuff too large for arm, arm above heart level, inability to accurately hear first Korotkoff sound

        (4) Falsely high measurement: Cuff too small for arm, loose cuff not centered over brachial artery, arm below heart level

      (b) Take BP in both arms. More than a 10- to 15-mm Hg difference in systolic pressures may indicate diminished arterial flow on the side with the lower reading (obstruction, dissection)

      (c) Orthostatic BP drop: Assess at-risk patients

        (1) Check BP supine, sitting, standing

        (2) Fall of more than 20 mm Hg of systolic pressure and/or increase of HR of more than 15 beats per minute within 3 minutes of standing, signifies orthostatic hypotension

        (3) Caused by vasodilating medications, volume depletion

      (d) Pulsus paradoxus: Exaggeration of the normal physiologic response to inspiration (BP lower on inspiration than on expiration)

        (1) Examine with the patient breathing normally

(2) Inflate sphygmomanometer until no Korotkoff sounds are heard; slowly deflate cuff until Korotkoff sounds first heard on expiration; note pressure reading

(3) Continue to deflate cuff until sounds heard during both expiration and inspiration; note reading

(4) Subtract second reading from first to determine pulsus paradoxus

(5) Normally, on inspiration, the difference between inspiration and expiration is less than 11 mm Hg. With pulsus paradoxus, fall in BP on inspiration is 11 mm Hg or greater.

(6) May be seen in:

    a) Cardiac tamponade

    b) Constrictive pericarditis

    c) Emphysema, asthma

    d) Hemorrhagic shock

    iii. Respiratory rate, rhythm, regularity

    iv. Temperature

    v. Oxygen saturation

c. Skin inspection

    i. Skin color (e.g., pallor, cyanosis), temperature, and turgor

    ii. Petechiae, angiomas, or scars

    iii. Mucous membrane moisture, color, and ulcerations

d. Neck examination

    i. Neck veins give important clues regarding fluid status

    (a) Jugular veins reflect RA and RV filling pressures

    (b) Internal jugular veins are harder to visualize than external jugular veins, but they more accurately reflect pressure and volume changes in the RA (CVP)

    (c) Check for jugular vein distention (JVD) and pulsation

      (1) Elevate the head of the bed until jugular waves can be seen

      (2) Shine a bright light tangentially to illuminate vessels, if not obvious

    (d) Determine jugular venous pressure

      (1) The sternal angle (angle of Louis) is roughly 5 cm above the atrium (when the patient is upright or lying down)

      (2) Measure the distance in centimeters from the sternal angle to the top of the distended neck vein

      (3) The value obtained plus the 5 cm provides a rough estimate of CVP

    ii. Check for hepatojugular reflux

    (a) Place the patient at a 45-degree angle

    (b) Compress the upper right abdomen for 30 to 45 seconds (causes additional venous return from liver to heart)

    (c) If hepatojugular reflux is present, the jugular pulses become more pronounced, and the level of filling of neck veins will rise (signifies inability of the right side of the heart to deal with the added volume)

    iii. Carotid artery: Auscultate the left and right arteries with both the diaphragm of the stethoscope (for high pitched) and bell of the stethoscope (for low pitched) to assess for carotid bruit(s). If bruit is present, do not palpate.

    iv. Thyroid: Inspect for visible enlargement of the thyroid (goiter)

e. Chest examination

    i. Inspect chest wall and skin, noting any injury/trauma, ecchymosis, discolorations, rash, or previous surgical scars

      ii. Consider shape and contour of the chest, asymmetry or irregularity

      iii. Inspect inspiratory and expiratory effort

  f. Pulmonary examination (see Ch. 3, Pulmonary System)

  g. Cardiac examination

      i. Palpate the chest over valves and cardiac apex. Heaves, lifts, or thrills may be felt with valve dysfunction or ventricular aneurysm. Thrills are palpable vibrations (analogous to the sensation felt on the throat of a purring cat) and signify turbulence or murmur loud enough to feel (aortic stenosis, mitral stenosis, PDA, ventricular septal defect [VSD]). Locations include:

        (a) Aortic: Second intercostal space (ICS) at the right sternal border (RSB)

        (b) Pulmonic: Second ICS at LSB

        (c) Tricuspid: Fourth ICS at LSB

        (d) Mitral: Fifth ICS at left midclavicular line (MCL)

        (e) Cardiac apex: Fifth to sixth ICS, left MCL

      ii. Palpate the point of maximum impulse (PMI), also known as the apical pulse site, approximately 2 to 3 cm in diameter and located over the left ventricle. For many patients, this is fifth to sixth ICS, left MCL. It may be assessed seated, leaning forward, or in a left lateral decubitus position. It is not usually palpable in the supine or semirecumbent position. The ventricular tapping is palpated over the left ventricle and indicates size and location of the heart. Displaced PMI may be related to:

        (a) LV dilatation or LV volume overload, aortic insufficiency, mitral regurgitation, dilated cardiomyopathy (DCM)

          (1) A forceful, *sustained* apical impulse may indicate LV hypertrophy

          (2) Nonsustained but forceful apical impulses are created by high-output states (e.g., fever, anemia, anxiety, hyperthyroidism)

      iii. Left peri-sternal lift: The heel of the hand rests slightly left of the sternum with the fingers lifted slightly off the chest. A heave or a lift suggests RV dilatation.

      iv. Auscultation of the heart

        (a) Listen for normal and abnormal heart sounds with both the diaphragm and the bell (Table 4.1).

EXPERT TIP

When using the bell of the stethoscope, press lightly; otherwise, the underlying skin functions as a diaphragm and low-pitched sounds will not be heard.

---

        (1) Main auscultation areas on the chest (Fig. 4.6)

          a) Aortic area (second ICS, RSB)

          b) Pulmonic area (second ICS, LSB)

          c) Tricuspid area (fourth ICS, LSB)

          d) Mitral (fifth ICS, MCL)—Depending on the female anatomy, the fifth ICS may lie beneath breast tissue that must be moved; recommend above the breast in seated position or leaning forward, and below the breast supine and left lateral

---

EXPERT TIP

To ensure diagnostic sounds are heard, listen for heart sounds with the diaphragm and the bell of the stethoscope in three positions: Sitting upright (with or without leaning forward), supine, and left lateral decubitus.

TABLE 4.1 Abnormal Heart Sounds

Abnormal Heart Sound	Cause/Circumstance	Seen In	Characteristics
Fixed splitting of S_2		Atrial septal defect	Does not change with expiration (no respiratory variation)
Persistent (wide) splitting of S_2	Occurs with any increase in right ventricular (RV) volume or pressure, prolonged RV ejection and delayed pulmonary valve closure, or delay in RV systole (right bundle branch block)	Right bundle branch block Pulmonary hypertension of any cause Pulmonary stenosis Ventricular septal defect	Second heart sound is split on expiration and more widely split on inspiration
Paradoxical splitting (reversed splitting) of S_2 (e.g., P_2 earlier than A_2)	Occurs when left ventricular (LV) ejection time is prolonged, resulting in delayed aortic closure; therefore pulmonic valve closes first	Left bundle branch block Severe aortic stenosis Patent ductus arteriosus	Split widens on expiration and narrows on inspiration (P_2 precedes A_2)
Third heart sound (S_3): Ventricular gallop	Occurs during rapid phase of ventricular filling in early diastole; caused by resistance to ventricular filling, resulting from increased volume load or decreased ventricular compliance	Can normally be heard in children and young adults, and in women during the last trimester of pregnancy (physiologic S_3) Abnormal when heard in older age groups or in association with disease states (left-sided heart failure, ischemia, right-sided heart failure, fluid overload) Heard transiently in patients with ischemia	Sound is low pitched (heard best with bell) When originating in LV, heard best at the apex with patient in left lateral decubitus position When originating in RV, heard best along fourth intercostal space, left sternal border, in inspiration Sound directly follows S_2, and sounds like cadence of "see" in "Tennessee"
Atrial gallop (presystolic or S_4)	Occurs during atrial contraction, just before S_1 during late phase of ventricular filling Occurs when there is volume overload of either ventricle or decreased ventricular compliance	Often a normal finding in adults Heard also in patients with myocardial ischemia or infarction, systemic and pulmonic hypertension, ventricular failure	Left-sided S_4 is usually heard best at the apex (does not change with respirations) Right-sided S_4 (less common) is usually louder on inspiration, over left lower sternal border Sound is immediately before S_1, and sounds like cadence of "a" in "appendix" or "Ken in Kentucky"
Summation gallop	Simultaneous occurrence of atrial (S_4) and ventricular (S_3) gallop	Heard with tachycardias (which cause shortening of diastole) and heart failure	Additional galloping sounds heard: the S_4 just before S_1 and the S_3 just after S_2

Modified from Bickley, L.S., Szilagyi, P.G. (2016). *Bates' guide to physical examination and history taking*, 11th ed. Philadelphia: Lippincott William & Wilkins; Fang, J.C., O'Gara, P.T. (2019). The history and physical examination: an evidence-based approach. In D.P. Zipes, P. Libby, R.O. Bonow, et al., editors, *Braunwald's heart disease: a textbook of cardiovascular medicine*, 11th ed. (pp 83-101). Philadelphia: Elsevier.

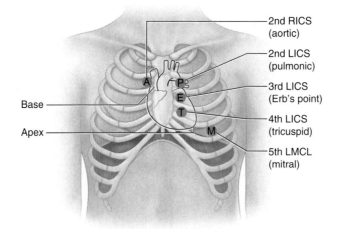

Fig. 4.6 Auscultation areas of the heart. *LICS*, Left intercostal space; *LMCL*, left midclavicular line; *RICS*, right intercostal space. (From Silvestri, L.A., Silvestri, A.E. (2020). *Saunders comprehensive review for the NCLEX-RN© examination*, 8ᵗʰ ed. St. Louis: Elsevier.)

(2) Origin of heart sounds: Opening and closing of valves (see Fig. 4.5) and rapid acceleration or deceleration of blood produce either low- or high-pitched sounds

(3) Normal heart sounds

    a) First heart sound (S_1): Produced by mitral and tricuspid valve closure, and best heard at the apex

---

EXPERT TIP

The diaphragm picks up high-pitched sounds and is used for S_1, S_2, and many murmurs. The bell is for low-pitched sounds and is used for S_3, S_4, and the low rumble of mitral stenosis (best heard in left lateral position over the mitral area of the apex).

---

        1) Marks the onset of ventricular systole

        2) LV depolarizes and contracts before the RV

        3) Component parts of S_1 may be split (mitral component [M_1] before tricuspid component [T_1]), but this is not commonly audible

        4) Coincides with carotid artery pulse wave

    b) Second heart sound (S_2): Produced by aortic and pulmonic valve closure and best heard at the base of the heart.

        1) Listen at the pulmonic area

        2) Both component parts of S_2 may be heard: Aortic component [A_2] before pulmonary component [P_2]. Normal P_2 is heard only at pulmonic area.

    c) Physiologic (normal) split of S_2 (A_2P_2) (see Table 4.1)

        1) P_2 is delayed on inspiration when the RV is slower to contract than the LV

        2) Delay because of increased volume loading of the RV in inspiration caused by increased venous return to the heart

3) RV ejection of blood is prolonged and delays pulmonic valve closure, prolonging the time from aortic closure (A_2) to pulmonic closure (P_2). A resulting split occurs between A_2 and P_2 during inspiration.

4) A_2 precedes P_2 and is generally louder

5) Split of S_2 is generally heard over the pulmonic area

6) Best heard in quiet respiration when the patient is sitting or standing

d) Third heart sound (S_3) is a low-pitched sound heard after S_2 (in systole). It is a low-pitched sound and best heard at the apex using the bell of the stethoscope. It is an early sign of fluid overload. It may be a normal finding in a child or pregnant female. The S_3 is sometimes referred to as a ventricular gallop.

e) Fourth heart sound (S_4) is a low-pitched sound heard before S_1 (at end diastole) and is best heard with the bell of the stethoscope over the apex. It is pathologic and related to a noncompliant ventricle. It is sometimes referred to as an atrial gallop and can be a sign of diastolic HF.

(4) Extracardiac sounds

a) Ejection click: Sharp, high-pitched sound just after S_1; caused by tensioning of the great vessels as they distend in early systole

b) Pericardial friction rub

1) Likened to the sound of leather rubbing or new snow crunching

2) Usually heard with the diaphragm in full expiration (are loudest when the patient is leaning forward)

3) Often have three components (ventricular systole, ventricular filling, and atrial systole)

c) Opening snap: Sound produced by a stenotic mitral valve snapping into the open position

d) Prosthetic valve: Crisp, sometimes metallic clicking, with both opening and closure heard

(5) Murmurs

a) Sounds produced by turbulent blood flow (Box 4.1)

b) Determine whether the murmur is systolic (occurring with or just after S_1) or diastolic (with or after S_2), then determine location to assist in defining the cause

c) Abnormal murmurs (hemodynamically significant) (Table 4.2)

h. Extremities examination

i. Edema: May indicate right-sided HF, venous stasis, venous insufficiency

ii. Color, temperature changes: May indicate arterial insufficiency (especially if asymmetrically cool)

iii. Skin condition: Petechiae, jaundice

iv. Hair loss: May indicate arterial disease

v. Ulcerations: May indicate stasis, ischemia

vi. Peripheral pulses: See Vital Signs

vii. Motor and sensory function: Numbness, foot drop (in advanced peripheral ischemia)

viii. Clubbing of nail beds: May indicate chronic pulmonary disease or HF

ix. Varicosities

x. Gangrene

BOX 4.1 Evaluating Murmurs

DETERMINE WHETHER MURMUR IS SYSTOLIC OR DIASTOLIC

1. Concentrate first on systole (S_1 to S_2)
   - Listen at all areas, starting with the base (the aortic and pulmonic areas) and moving down to the apex (the tricuspid and mitral areas)
2. Listen to all areas in diastole (S_2 to S_1)
3. Listen to all areas with the diaphragm and the bell
   - If possible, listen in three positions: seated, supine, and left lateral position

DETERMINE CHARACTERISTICS OF THE SOUND TO INCLUDE

- Site of maximal intensity
- Radiation of sound (murmurs radiate in the direction of blood flow)
- Timing, duration, and location
- Effect of respirations on murmur, whether increased or decreased with either inspiration or expiration
- Effect of patient position on the murmur's intensity

DESCRIBE PATTERNS, INTENSITY, AND QUALITY OF MURMURS

1. Patterns
   - *Crescendo:* Builds up in intensity
   - *Decrescendo:* Decreases in intensity
   - *Crescendo-decrescendo:* Peaks and then decreases in intensity
2. Intensity: Based on a grade of I to VI; recorded with grade over VI to show scale used
   - *I/VI:* Barely audible; the clinician can hear only after listening a while
   - *II/VI:* Easily audible
   - *III/VI:* Loud; not associated with a thrill
   - *IV/VI:* Loud and may be associated with a thrill
   - *V/VI:* Very loud; can be heard with the stethoscope partly off the chest (tilted); associated with a thrill
   - *VI/VI:* Very loud; can be heard with the stethoscope off the chest; associated with a thrill
3. Quality: May be described as blowing, musical, rough, harsh, honking, vibratory, cooing
4. Pitch: High pitched, low pitched

CHARACTERISTICS OF SPECIFIC HEART SOUNDS

- *Ejection murmurs:* Usually rough, extending into or through systole (e.g., aortic stenosis or sclerosis)
- *Regurgitant murmurs:* Are usually a more pure, uniform sound (e.g., mitral regurgitation)
- *Pansystolic (holosystolic) murmurs:* Heard from S1 through S2

COMMENTS ON FUNCTIONAL, INNOCENT MURMURS

- Hemodynamically insignificant, physiologic; usually ejection murmurs associated with either increased flow or volume
- Not associated with cardiovascular disease
- Common in children and pregnant women
- Heard in hyperthyroidism, anemia
- Diastolic murmurs are never functional or innocent

SOUNDS WITH BOTH SYSTOLIC AND DIASTOLIC COMPONENTS

- *Venous Hum:* Continuous murmur without interval; usually caused by turbulent blood flow through jugular veins and common in children.
  - Best heard above the medial third of the right clavicle, and described as a humming or roaring.
- *Pericardial Friction Rub:* May have three short components representing ventricular systole (S_1 to S_2), then ventricular diastole (early S_2 to S_1), with a pause and a third sound heard in atrial systole just before S_1.
  - Best heard at the 3rd intercostal (ICS) just left of the sternum and described as scratchy
- *Patent Ductus Arteriosus:* Continuous murmur loudest in late systole
  - Best heard at the left 2nd ICS and described as harsh and machine-like.

TABLE 4.2 Abnormal Heart Murmurs: Main Characteristics

Abnormal Murmur	Location Where Heard Best	Characteristics	Comments
SYSTOLIC MURMURS			
Mitral insufficiency or regurgitation	Loudest at apex Radiates to left axilla	Blowing quality, high pitched	Pansystolic—extends through A_2 May be rough and heard at base (mitral valve prolapse)
Tricuspid insufficiency or regurgitation	Loudest at lower left sternal border Radiates to right sternal border, liver	Blowing quality, low pitched Variable in intensity (may increase with inspiration)	Pansystolic
Aortic stenosis	Maximal intensity at base of heart, usually at second intercostal space, right sternal border Radiates to neck and apex	Harsh in quality, medium or high-pitched May be crescendo-decrescendo murmur Intensity varies; no relation to severity of murmur	Systolic ejection murmur Extends to S_2 Thrill may be found at second intercostal space, right sternal border
Hypertrophic (obstructive) cardiomyopathy	Maximal intensity at second to fourth intercostal spaces, right sternal border May radiate to apex	Crescendo-decrescendo Decreases during expiration and squatting Increases with Valsalva maneuver	Ejection murmur Thrill may be found at lower left sternal border
Pulmonic stenosis	Maximal loudness at second intercostal space, left sternal border Louder when patient is supine and during inspiration	Harsh Usually grade III to IV intensity Persistent split of S_2, including expiration; the more severe the stenosis, the more pronounced the split	Pulmonary systolic ejection sound (click) Thrill may be felt at second intercostal space, left sternal border Right ventricular (RV) S_4 possible
Interventricular septal defect	Maximal loudness along lower sternal border Radiates widely	Harsh	Pansystolic or early systolic Thrill often present over left sternal border
Patent ductus arteriosus	Maximal intensity at second intercostal space, left sternal border	Machinery-like murmur	Continuous systolic and diastolic murmur Occasional thrill at second intercostal space, left sternal border

Continued

TABLE 4.2 Abnormal Heart Murmurs: Main Characteristics—cont'd

Abnormal Murmur	Location Where Heard Best	Characteristics	Comments
DIASTOLIC MURMURS			
Mitral stenosis	Maximal intensity at point of maximal intensity (PMI) May be heard only when patient lying on left side at the PMI with bell of stethoscope	Very low pitched Fading rumble Presystolic, crescendo if patient in normal sinus rhythm Intensity not affected by inspiration	Early diastolic and presystolic rumble (if in sinus rhythm) May be associated with an opening snap and accentuated S_1
Tricuspid stenosis	Maximal intensity at fourth intercostal space, left sternal border	Rumbling Low pitched Intensity should increase on inspiration, unless right ventricle has failed	Early diastolic May have an opening snap
Aortic insufficiency or regurgitation	Maximal intensity at third to fourth intercostal space, left sternal border, and at apex Radiates to apex Heard best when patient is sitting up and leaning forward, during exhalation	Blowing quality High pitched Decrescendo Intensity varies with severity	Pandiastolic (unless acute, when it is short, early diastolic murmur)
Pulmonary insufficiency or regurgitation	Maximal loudness along second left intercostal space, left sternal border Radiates along left sternal border	Blowing quality High pitched Decrescendo	Sometimes increases with inspiration

Modified from Bickley, L.S., Szilagyi, P.G. (2013). *Bates' guide to physical examination and history taking*, 11th ed. Philadelphia: Lippincott William & Wilkins; Fang, J.C., O'Gara, P.T. (2019). The history and physical examination: an evidence-based approach. In D.P. Zipes, P. Libby, R.O. Bonow, et al., editors, *Braunwald's heart disease: a textbook of cardiovascular medicine*, 11th ed. (pp 83-101). Philadelphia: Elsevier.

3. **Monitoring data (Fig. 4.7)**
   a. See Table 4.3 for types of bedside monitoring and Table 4.4 for hemodynamic pressures
   b. Complications of bedside invasive hemodynamic monitoring
      i. Arrhythmias, hemorrhage, thrombi, emboli (air, blood), infection, pneumothorax, pulmonary infarction (balloon left inflated), cardiac perforation, vascular occlusion or spasm
4. **Appraisal of patient characteristics: Patients with acute, life-threatening cardiovascular problems come to critical care units with a wide range of biochemical, metabolic, and psychosocial clinical characteristics. During their stay, their clinical status may significantly improve or deteriorate, slowly or abruptly change, involve one or all life-sustaining functions, and be readily or nearly impossible to monitor with precision. Some attributes of patients with acute cardiac disorders that the nurse needs to assess are the following: Resiliency, vulnerability, stability, complexity, resource availability, participation in care and decision making, and predictability.**

DIAGNOSTIC STUDIES

1. **12-lead ECG**
   a. The 12-lead ECG gives a visual impression of the electrical conduction and cardiac abnormalities. It records the electrical activity of the heart and identifies:
      i. Arrhythmias and conduction defects
      ii. Ischemia or infarction
      iii. Electrolyte abnormalities

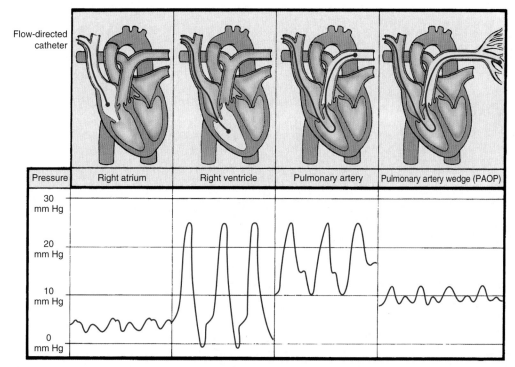

Fig. 4.7 Bedside hemodynamic monitoring via flow-directed, balloon-tipped catheter capable of thermodilution cardiac output determination. *PAOP,* Pulmonary artery occlusion pressure. (From Urden, L.D., Stacy, K.M., Lough, M.E. (2022). *Critical care nursing: diagnosis and management,* 9th ed. St. Louis: Elsevier.)

TABLE 4.3   Common Types of Bedside Monitoring

Type of Monitoring	Uses	Measurements	Comments
Direct arterial BP monitoring: Catheter inserted into artery and attached to pressure transducer that converts and amplifies arterial pressure to electrical waveform for continuous readings	Monitor BP trends (e.g., during cardiac surgery, in critically ill patients, with IABP, potent vasopressors or vasodilators) For ventilated patients, frequent ABG testing, monitoring for acid-base imbalances Radial artery most commonly used	Reference (air fluid interface) stopcock closest to pressure transducer at heart level (phlebostatic axis; see Bedside Hemodynamic Monitoring later in table); radial line should be at same level	Allen's test: Check adequacy of ulnar circulation before radial catheter insertion 1. Have patient clench fist tightly 2. Occlude both radial and ulnar arteries 3. Have patient open hand; observe for pallor 4. Release pressure over ulnar artery; color should return within 2 to 3 seconds if artery patent 5. If no capillary filling in 3 seconds, test result is negative
CVP monitoring: Use of a single or multilumen catheter positioned in superior vena cava (inferior vena cava for femoral lines) attached to pressure transducer	Continuous monitoring of blood volume, RV function, CVP Fluid, blood, and medication administration Vein sites: Internal or external jugular, femoral, subclavian	Normal CVP varies from patient to patient Monitor trends in CVP Normal CVP: 2 to 6 mm Hg	Decreased CVP: Hypovolemia, venodilation, negative-pressure ventilators, RV assist devices, central venous obstruction (masses), decreased venous return Increased CVP: Increased blood volume, right-sided heart failure, cardiac tamponade, positive pressure breathing, straining
Bedside hemodynamic monitoring via continuous monitoring via flow-directed, balloon-tipped catheter capable of thermodilution cardiac output determination (PA catheter); see Fig. 3.7 Various catheters are available with capabilities of continuous CO monitoring, transvenous pacing, and mixed venous oxygen saturation measurements, and with additional fluid and medication administration ports	Assess and manage hemodynamics via continuous monitoring: fluid balance, intracardiac pressures, CO, CI, SVR, SvO$_2$, ScvO$_2$ Evaluate trends; report significant changes Monitoring RA and PAOP is preferable to assess RV and LV function PA mean: used primarily for hemodynamic calculations of pulmonary vascular resistance	RA pressure is measured through proximal port of catheter; reflects RVEDP RV pressures are seen when floating catheter into position during insertion; RV waveform is distinct with sharp upstroke after the QRS and downstroke, no dicrotic notch PAP and PAOP measured through distal port (see Fig. 3.7 and Table 4.4) PA systolic pressure represents pressure produced by RV	Phlebostatic axis: Obtain pressure reading with patient in comfortable position (0–60 degrees), as long as transducer is at same phlebostatic level as marked axis (intersection of following two lines): 1. Draw a line from fourth intercostal space at sternum toward edge of chest and down to side 2. Draw second line on side of chest, halfway between anterior and posterior portions of chest (midaxillary), running head to foot 3. Mark intersection of lines on side of chest; place transducer at level horizontal to that mark
		PA diastolic pressure generally reflects LVEDP and is used as measure of LV function and diastolic filling pressures; usually 2 to 4 mm Hg higher than mean PAOP or mean LA pressure PAOP is a reflection of LA pressure and is used to assess LVEDP filling pressure = "a" wave; balloon of catheter is inflated, wedges in small branch of PA (see Fig. 3.7); PAOP should be 2 to 4 mm Hg less than PA diastolic pressure	Catheter must not be left in RV (ventricular tachycardia occurs) PA diastolic pressure: Correlates well with mean PAOP in the normal heart, during myocardial infarction, and in LV failure; often used instead of PAOP if obtaining accurate wedge is impossible CO can also be measured manually via proximal port by means of thermodilution (an average of three rapid injections of 10 mL D5W or NS is used to calculate CO, CI, SVR by computer)

ABG, Arterial blood gas; *BP,* blood pressure; *CI,* cardiac index; *CO,* cardiac output; *CVP,* central venous pressure; *D5W,* dextrose 5% in water; *IABP,* intraaortic balloon pump; *LA,* left atrial; *LV,* left ventricular; *LVEDP,* left ventricular end-diastolic pressure; *NS,* normal saline; *PA,* pulmonary artery; *PAP,* pulmonary artery pressure; *PAOP,* pulmonary artery occlusive pressure; *RA,* right atrial; *RV,* right ventricular; *RVEDP,* right ventricular end-diastolic pressure; *SvO$_2$,* venous oxygen saturation; *ScvO$_2$,* central venous oxygen saturation; *SVR,* systemic vascular resistance.

From Schroeder P, Barbeito A, Bar-Yosef S, Mark JB (2015). Cardiovascular monitoring. In R.D. Miller, editor: *Miller's anesthesia,* 8th ed. Philadelphia, Elsevier.

TABLE 4.4 Hemodynamic Pressures: Normal Values and Possible Causes of Abnormal Values

Measurements	Normal Values	Possible Causes for Increase	Possible Causes for Decrease
Right atrial pressure (RAP)/central venous pressure (CVP)	2–6 mm Hg	Pulmonary hypertension Pulmonary embolism Constrictive pericarditis Cardiac tamponade Right heart failure Pulmonic stenosis Chronic obstructive pulmonary disease (COPD) Obstructive sleep apnea (OSA) Right ventricular (RV) infarction	Hypovolemia (e.g., diuretics, blood loss, burns, vomiting) Vasodilatation (e.g., nitrates, morphine, hypersensitivity reactions)
RV pressures	Systolic: 15–30 mm Hg Diastolic: 2–6 mm Hg	Pulmonary hypertension (e.g., left-sided heart failure, ventricular septal defect, left ventricular [LV] ischemia, infarct, mitral regurgitation or stenosis, cardiomyopathy) Pulmonary disease (e.g., pulmonary embolism, hypoxemia, COPD) OSA Eisenmenger syndrome: Pulmonary hypertension associated with right-to-left shunt, cyanosis	Same as previous
Pulmonary artery (PA) pressures	Systolic: 20–30 mm Hg Diastolic: 5–10 mm Hg Mean: 10–20 mm Hg	Atrial or ventricular septal defects (increased pulmonary blood flow because of left-to-right shunt) Pulmonary hypertension Hypertension Pulmonary emboli COPD LV failure Mitral stenosis or regurgitation Volume overload Ischemia	

Continued

TABLE 4.4 Hemodynamic Pressures: Normal Values and Possible Causes of Abnormal Values—cont'd			
Measurements	Normal Values	Possible Causes for Increase	Possible Causes for Decrease
Pulmonary artery occlusive pressure (PAOP)	4–12 mm Hg	Fluid overload LV failure Ischemia Mitral stenosis or regurgitation Constrictive pericarditis	Hypovolemia Venodilating medications
Systemic vascular resistance (SVR)	900–1400 dynes/s/cm^{-6}	Hypovolemia Hypothermia Vasoconstriction	Vasodilating medications Shock: Septic, neurogenic, or anaphylactic
Pulmonary vascular resistance (PVR)	50–250 dynes/s/cm^{-5}	Pulmonary embolism, large Pulmonary hypertension Hypoxemia	Pulmonary vasodilating medications
Cardiac output (CO)	4–8 L/min	Sepsis Intra- and extracardiac shunts	Decreased preload Increased afterload Decreased contractility Arrhythmias
Cardiac index (CI)	2.5–4.0 L/min/m^2	Sepsis	Same as for CO Respiratory failure Right-to-left heart shunts
Stroke volume variation (SVV)	<10%–15% (on mechanical ventilation)	Fluid volume deficit	N/A
Mixed venous oxygen saturation (SvO$_2$) Central venous oxygen saturation (ScvO$_2$)	60%–80% (Scvo$_2$ runs approx. 5% to 10% higher than Svo$_2$)	Sepsis Left-to right intracardiac shunt Thyrotoxicosis Anesthesia Same as previous SvO$_2$	Hypoxemia Anemia, bleeding Fever Heart failure Arrhythmias Respiratory failure Right to left heart shunts Same as previous SvO$_2$

From Schroeder, B., Barbeito, A., Ben-Yosef, S., Mark, J.B. (2015). Cardiovascular monitoring. In R.D. Miller, editor: *Miller's anesthesia*, 8th ed. Philadelphia: Elsevier; Edwards Lifesciences, Stroke volume variation: Can we use fluid to improve hemodynamics? Retrieved from http://ht.edwards.com/resourcegallery/products/minivasive/pdfs/stroke_volume_variationpdf.pdf; Reyer E. (2013). The hemodynamic and physiologic relevance of continuous central venous oxygenation monitoring: It's not just for sepsis. Retrieved from http://www.icumed.com/media/402627/M1-1430%20Reyer%20%20-%20SCVO2%20Oximetry%20White%20Paper%20Rev.01-Web.pdf.

    iv. Medication or illicit drug effects and toxicities
     v. Hypertrophy of the ventricles and enlargement of the atria
    vi. Anatomic orientation of the heart
   b. Each tracing on the graph paper corresponds to electrical components within the
      heart (Fig. 4.8). Evaluate for arrhythmias, conduction delays or abnormalities of
      rhythm, rate, or complexes. Report changes to provider.
       i. The horizontal axis records time, with the normal speed of paper: 25 mm/s
          (a) Each small box is 1 mm = 0.04 second
          (b) Each large box is 5 mm = 0.20 second
          (c) Time intervals for complexes are recorded in seconds
              (1) P wave represents atrial depolarization as the impulse is initiated in the
                   SA node
              (2) PR interval represents the time taken for the impulse to travel from
                   atria to ventricles via the AV node (normal is 0.12–0.20 second).
              (3) The QRS complex represents ventricular depolarization (normal length
                   is 0.8–0.12 second)
      ii. The vertical axis records amplitude and voltage with a usual calibration standard
           of 10 mm = 1 mV
          (a) Each small box (1 mm) = 0.1 mV
          (b) Each large box (5 mm) = 0.5 mV
          (c) Height or elevation of complexes or ST segment are recorded in millimeters
              (1) ST elevation indicates acute myocardial injury (possibly MI)
              (2) ST depression and T-wave inversions indicate myocardial ischemia

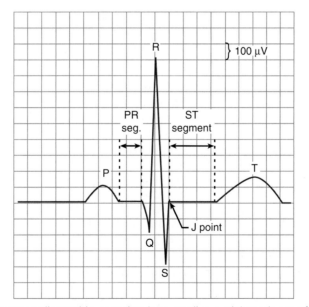

Fig. 4.8 Normal electrocardiographic complex (one cardiac cycle) made up of P, Q, R, S, and T waves. Also shown are the PR segment, ST segment, and J point, which marks the end of the QRS complex and the beginning of the ST segment. ST segment deviation is measured by the number of millimeters or microvolts (1 mm = 1 μV) the ST segment is deviated (i.e., elevated or depressed) from the PR segment and typically is measured at one of three locations: (1) the J point, (2) J point + 60 ms past the J point, or (3) J point + 80 ms past the J point. (From Moser, D.K., Riegel, B. (2007). *Cardiac nursing: a companion to Braunwald's heart disease*, Philadelphia, Elsevier.)

(3) Q waves indicate prior injury (prior MI) leading to nonconductive tissue

(4) Height and shape of complexes is useful in detection of atrial and ventricular hypertrophy

---

KEY CONCEPT

ST elevation is a medical emergency requiring immediate intervention. Follow Advanced Cardiac Life Support (ACLS) guidelines and call the provider.

---

  c. ECG waves: Representation, measurement, abnormalities—See Table 4.5 and Fig. 4.8
    i. Deflections: Waves of the ECG recording are either above or below the isoelectric line.
      (a) Positive deflections occur when the heart's depolarization wave moves toward the positive electrode of the recording lead.
      (b) Negative deflections occur when the heart's depolarization wave moves away from the positive electrode of the recording lead.
      (c) Biphasic deflections occur when the heart's depolarization wave is moving both toward and away from the positive electrode. If the wave of depolarization is perpendicular to the positive electrode, waves may be small or absent.
  d. A 12-lead ECG uses four limb leads and six chest leads to visualize the heart from multiple angles (Table 4.6 and Fig. 4.9).
    i. Limb leads: Two electrodes of opposing polarity (positive and negative) are used to record electrical activity. These bipolar electrodes are placed on each of the patient's arms and/or legs.
    ii. Augmented limb leads: Electrical activity is recorded between one positive electrode (unipolar) and the electrical sum of other two standard limb electrodes. The wave's amplitude is augmented (enhanced voltage) for ease of visualization.
    iii. Precordial (chest) V leads: Record electrical activity between one positive electrode (unipolar) and the electrical sum of the three standard limb electrodes.
      (a) As the chest leads are positioned from V_1 to V_6, the ECG will reflect R waves progressively getting taller, known as normal R-wave progression (note: R in V_5 is a little taller than V_6).
      (b) The chest leads may also be placed on the right chest wall to create a right-sided ECG that is useful when evaluating right ventricular infarcts. An individual chest lead may also be used: V_4R (analogous to V_4, only on right side).
  e. ST changes and acute findings on the 12-lead ECG: Monitor for ST elevation or depression, T wave changes, arrhythmias, or new findings not noted on previous ECG.

KEY CONCEPT

ST elevation is indicative of an MI. The location of the elevation on the ECG identifies the area of the MI (Table 4.7). The ST elevation is significant if it measures 1 mm or more in a limb lead (I-AVF) or 2 mm or more in a chest lead (V1–V6).

TABLE 4.5 Electrocardiogram Waves and Intervals: Description, Characteristics, and Abnormalities

ECG	Description	Characteristics	Causes for Abnormalities
P wave	Represents atrial depolarization Right atrium (RA) begins depolarization earlier than the left atrium (LA)	Normal duration: <0.10 second Normal amplitude: ≤2.5 mm P waves >2.5 mm in amplitude in any lead are abnormal "2.5×2.5 rule" (handy rule of thumb): P wave should not be wider than 2.5 mm (LA enlargement) or taller than 2.5 mm (RA enlargement)	Atrial enlargement: Increased P amplitude or width RA enlargement: • Tall, peaked P waves in lead II, III, and aVF • May show tall or biphasic P waves in V_1 (>2.5 mm in amplitude) LA enlargement: • Wide, notched P waves in limb leads and V_4 to V_6 and/or P waves with broad negative deflection in lead V_1 (>1 mm); • P >2.5 mm in width
PR interval	Represents time required for conduction through atrioventricular (AV) node PR segment represents normal delay of impulse in AV node	Normal interval: 0.12–0.20 second Measure from beginning of P wave to beginning of QRS complex PR segment is normally isoelectric	Prolonged delay (PR interval >0.20 second) indicates diseased AV node, ischemia, medication effects, or increased vagal tone, WPW with delta wave (resulting in a shortened PR, as can beats that originate from the AV junction). Depressed PR segments occur with pericarditis
QRS complex	Represents ventricular depolarization Atrial repolarization occurs during this time period but is obscured by QRS	Normal duration: 0.06 to 0.10 second; borderline at 0.11 second Measured from onset of Q wave (or R wave if no Q wave is present) to end of QRS	Abnormal if ≥0.12 second; indicative of intraventricular conduction delay; seen in patients with bundle branch blocks (≥0.12), Wolff-Parkinson-White (WPW) syndrome, and hyperkalemia (sine wave)
Q wave	Present if the first deflection of the QRS is negative	Small physiologic Q waves are usually seen in leads I, aVL, V_5, and V_6, as well as in inferior leads II, III, and aVF	Q waves are pathologic when >0.04 second wide (>0.03 second in inferior leads II, III, and aVF) and >25% of R wave amplitude Q waves in leads III, aVR, and V_1 are normal Pathologic Q waves result from myocardial infarction
R wave	First positive deflection occurring in the QRS complex		Prominent R waves may be seen with ventricular hypertrophy and in young adults, persons with thin chests, and patients with WPW syndrome

Continued

TABLE 4.5 **Electrocardiogram Waves and Intervals: Description, Characteristics, and Abnormalities—cont'd**

ECG	Description	Characteristics	Causes for Abnormalities
S wave	Negative deflection that follows an R wave		
ST segment	Represents initial ventricular repolarization	Measure immediately after QRS complex to beginning of T wave; normally isoelectric	Elevated ST segment is caused by pericarditis, injury, acute infarctions, myocarditis, LV aneurysms, and normal variation (early repolarization) Depressed ST segment may indicate subendocardial injury or ischemia, electrolyte disturbances, medication effect, or early repolarization, or it may be nonspecific
T wave	Represents ventricular repolarization		Inverted T waves may be associated with infarctions, ischemia, injury, or hypertrophy Tall, peaked T waves may be caused by hyperkalemia or acute injury or may be a normal variant
QT interval	Represents complete duration of ventricular depolarization and repolarization	Corrected QT interval (QTc) takes heart rate into account and provides a normal range corrected for heart rate	Causes of prolonged QTc: Ischemia, electrolyte imbalances (hypocalcemia), hypertrophy, congenital prolongation and numerous medications (e.g., antiarrhythmic, antipsychotic, antidepressant, and antihistamine medications—see https://crediblemeds.org). Prolonged QTc is associated with an increased incidence of polymorphic ventricular tachycardia (torsades de pointes) and, potentially, sudden death Causes of shortened QTc: Acute ischemia, hypercalcemia, and medications (digitalis)
	QT interval varies with heart rate, sex, and age	In general, QTc of ≥0.44 second in males and ≥0.45 second in females is considered abnormal. QT is measured from the beginning of the Q wave to the end of the T wave, then QTc is calculated. Most commonly used formula is Bazett: QTc = QT/√RR-interval (Note: many hemodynamic monitors will automatically calculate the QTc and display it alongside the QT)	

Modified from Mirvis, D.M., Goldberger, A.L. (2019). Electrocardiography. In D.P. Zipes, P. Libby, R.O. Bonow, et al., editors. *Braunwald's heart disease: a textbook of cardiovascular medicine*, 11th ed. Philadelphia: Elsevier; Bickley, L.S., Szilagyi, P.G. (2013). *Bates' guide to physical examination and history taking*, 11th ed. Philadelphia: Lippincott William & Wilkins; Fang, J.C., O'Gara, P.T. (2019). The history and physical examination: an evidence-based approach. In D.P. Zipes, P. Libby, R.O. Bonow, et al., editors, *Braunwald's heart disease: a textbook of cardiovascular medicine*, 11th ed. Philadelphia: Elsevier.

4

	TABLE 4.6	**Location of Electrodes and Lead Connections for the Standard 12-Lead Electrocardiogram and Additional Leads**	
Lead Type	**Positive Input**		**Negative Input**
STANDARD LIMB LEADS[a]			
I	Left arm		Right arm
II	Left leg		Right arm
III	Left leg		Left arm
AUGMENTED LIMB LEADS			
aVR	Right arm		Left arm plus left leg
aVL	Left arm		Right arm plus left leg
aVF	Left leg		Left arm plus right arm
PRECORDIAL LEADS			
V_1	Right sternal margin, 4th ICS		Wilson central terminal
V_2	Left sternal margin, 4th ICS		Wilson central terminal
V_3	Midway between V_2 and V_4		Wilson central terminal
V_4	Left midclavicular line, 5th ICS		Wilson central terminal
V_5	Left anterior axillary line at the same horizontal plane as for the V_4 electrode[b]		Wilson central terminal
V_6	Left midaxillary line at the same horizontal plane as for the V_4 electrode		Wilson central terminal
POSTERIOR CHEST LEADS			
V_7	Posterior axillary line at the same horizontal plane as for the V_4 electrode		Wilson central terminal
V_8	Posterior scapular line at the same horizontal plane as for the V_4 electrode		Wilson central terminal
V_9	Left border of spine at the same horizontal plane as for the V_4 electrode		Wilson central terminal
RIGHT-SIDED CHEST LEADS			
V_3R to V_6R	The right-sided precordial leads are placed in mirror image of the precordial leads on the right side of the chest. Evaluate for right ventricular infarct.		Wilson central terminal

[a]Limb electrodes should be placed near the wrists and ankles or, at a minimum, distal to the shoulders and hips.
[b]If the anterior axillary line is difficult to delineate, the electrode may be placed midway between the V_4 and V_6 electrode positions.
ICS, Intercostal space.
Modified from Mirvis, D.M., Goldberger, A.L. (2015). Electrocardiography. In D.L. Mann, D.P. Zipes, P. Libby, et al., editors. *Braunwald's heart disease: a textbook of cardiovascular medicine,* 10th ed. (p. 116). Philadelphia: Elsevier.

f. Additional telemetry monitoring techniques for more views with less leads: To see chest lead views that usually are only visible on a 12-lead ECG recording, the electrode position may be modified/repositioned.
    i. Modified chest lead first position (MCL_1, or Marriott's chest lead): Using a three-lead telemetry monitor, place red or positive electrode in the fourth ICS, right sternal border in the usual V_1 position of pectoral chest leads. Typically, the PQRST complexes are negative. Typically, this position is used to differentiate ventricular arrhythmias.
    ii. Modified chest lead sixth position (MCL_6) is placing the red or positive electrode in the V_6 position of the fifth ICS midaxillary line.
    iii. Five-lead telemetry systems: Modify the position of the brown chest lead.

Note: See Box 4.2 for ECG and rhythm assessment checklist and Table 4.8 for descriptions of cardiac arrhythmias and conduction defects (see AACN's Practice Alert: Accurate Dysrhythmia Monitoring in Adults and Ensuring Accurate ST-Segment Monitoring at https://www.aacn.org/clinical-resources/practice-alerts/dysrhythmia-monitoring).

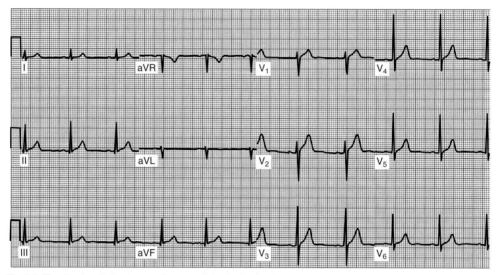

Fig. 4.9 Twelve-lead electrocardiogram (sinus rhythm).

TABLE 4.7	12-Lead Electrocardiogram Contiguous Lead Identifying Area of Infarct, Vasculature, and Possible Complications		
Area of Infarct	**Electrocardiogram Leads**	**Associated Coronary Artery**	**Potential Complications**
Inferior wall	II, III, aVF	Right coronary, possibly left circumflex	May affect SA node and AV node function (atrial arrhythmias) or valve dysfunction
Septal wall	V_1-V_2	Left anterior descending	Ventricular arrhythmias and LV failure
Anterior wall	V_2-V_4	Left anterior descending	Ventricular arrhythmias and LV failure
Lateral wall, high	I, aVL	Left circumflex	
Lateral wall, low	V_5-V_6	Left anterior descending	Ventricular arrhythmias and LV failure
Posterior	V_7-V_9[a]	Posterior descending, right coronary, or left circumflex	AV nodal conduction disturbance
Right ventricle[b]	V_4R[b]	Right coronary	AV nodal disturbance, valve dysfunction, hypotension

[a]Leads are placed on the left posterior chest wall at the fifth intercostal space, beginning at the left posterior axillary line.
[b]Leads are placed on the right chest wall fifth intercostal midclavicular line: if positive follow with a full right-sided chest lead position to evaluate right ventricular infarct, which is most likely to be combined with an acute inferior myocardial infarction.
AV, Atrioventricular; *ECG,* electrocardiogram; *LV,* left ventricular; *SA,* sinoatrial.

From Mirvis, D.M., Goldberger, A.L. (2019). Electrocardiography. In D.P. Zipes, P. Libby, R.O. Bonow, et al., editors. *Braunwald's heart disease: a textbook of cardiovascular medicine,* 11th ed. Philadelphia: Elsevier; Fang, J.C., O'Gara, P.T. (2019). The history and physical examination: an evidence-based approach. In D.P. Zipes, P. Libby, R.O. Bonow, et al., editors, *Braunwald's heart disease: a textbook of cardiovascular medicine,* 11th ed. Philadelphia: Elsevier.

BOX 4.2   **Interpretation of 12-Lead Electrocardiogram**

ANALYZE ELECTROCARDIOGRAM RHYTHMS SYSTEMATICALLY

- *Rhythm:* Regular, irregular, pattern if irregular
- *Rate:* Atrial (P waves) and ventricular (QRS).
    - For example, bradycardia <60 beats per minute, tachycardia >100 beats per minute, supraventricular tachycardia >150 beats per minute
- *P wave:* Identification, configuration or morphology, and relation to QRS (before, after)
- *PR interval:* Measurement
- *QRS complex:* Measurement, configuration, width and height
- *ST segment:* Elevation, depression or isoelectric
- *T wave:* Size, shape, direction (inversion)
- *Q-Wave:* Pathologic Q waves grouped in locations suggest previous infarct
- *Identify Rhythm:* For example normal sinus rhythm. Identify arrhythmias and origin

---

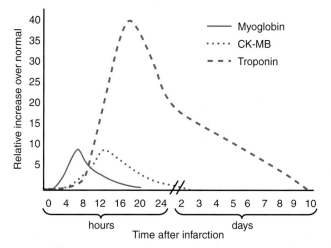

Fig. 4.10 Time course of the appearance of serum levels of creatine kinase MB isoenzyme *(CK-MB)*, myoglobin, and troponin in a patient with an ST-segment elevation myocardial infarction. (From Henry, J.B. (2001). *Clinical diagnosis and management by laboratory methods*, Philadelphia: Elsevier.)

2. Laboratory

a. Cardiac troponin T and troponin I are two of the three troponin proteins released from the myocardium during cardiomyocyte necrosis. Elevated values of either troponin suggest MI, or myocarditis, but there may be chronic elevations in patients with HF and renal failure (usually troponin T is more affected by renal failure).

   i. A value more than 0.1 ng/L is rare in a healthy individual, and therefore levels above 0.1 ng/L are monitored for elevation over time.

   ii. Levels increase 2 to 6 hours following MI, which is usually the time of symptom onset, peak at 18 to 24 hours, and fall slowly over 7 to 14 days (Fig. 4.10).

   iii. Most facilities measure troponin I, which is available in bedside point of care.

b. Creatine kinase (CK) is an enzyme found in the heart, brain, and skeletal tissues. CK-MB isoenzyme is found primarily in cardiac muscle. It elevates 4 to 6 hours after acute MI, peaks at 18 to 24 hours, and then returns to normal in 2 to 3 days.

c. Myoglobin is a heme protein found in muscle. May assist in the diagnosis of muscle injury but is not cardiac specific. Level rises 2 to 3 hours after injury, peaks 8 to 12 hours after infarct, and then rapidly returns to normal in 18 to 24 hours. It can be elevated with cardiopulmonary resuscitation (CPR), falls, and injections.

TABLE 4.8 **Cardiac Arrhythmias and Conduction Defects**

Rhythm	Mechanism	Characteristics	Comments
SINUS RHYTHMS			
Sinus rhythm	Originates in sinoatrial (SA) node	Rate: 60–100 beats/min Rhythm: Regular P wave: • Normal and upright in leads II, III, aVF • Precede each QRS • Identical size and shape in any given lead PR interval: 0.12–0.20 second 	Optimal cardiac rhythm Sinus arrhythmia: if rhythm varies (PP or RR interval varies >0.16 second) usually related to respirations (RR intervals decrease with inspiration) Causes: Vagal responses (children, young adults), SA node disease (in older adult)
Sinus bradycardia		Rate: <50 beats/min PQRST: Complexes and intervals are normal 	Causes: May be normal during sleep and in athletes and young hearts; seen in hypothermia, increased intracranial pressure, decreased sympathetic tone, increased parasympathetic tone, Valsalva maneuver, carotid massage, vomiting, medications, hypothyroidism
Sinus tachycardia		Rate: 100–200 beats/min Rhythm: Regular PQRST: Complexes and intervals normal	Causes: Secondary to anxiety, exercise, pain, hyperthyroidism, shock, anemia, fever, hypoxia, hypercapnia, heat exposure, medications, heart failure (early sign)

TABLE 4.8 Cardiac Arrhythmias and Conduction Defects—cont'd

Rhythm	Mechanism	Characteristics	Comments
Sinus arrest or sinus pause	SA node fails, no impulse initiated, atrial standstill	PQRST complex: Not seen	Causes of sinus blocks and pauses: increased vagal stimulation (e.g., by suctioning), myocardial infarction (MI), myocarditis, medication effects (e.g., from digitalis)
ATRIAL RHYTHMS			
Premature atrial contraction (PAC)	Early atrial impulse, interrupting the inherent regular rhythm	Normal QRS complex if ventricular repolarization was complete Abnormal QRS complex if conducted aberrantly (ventricle partially repolarized)	Causes: stimulants (caffeine, tobacco, alcohol), hypoxia, medications, digitalis toxicity, atrial enlargement

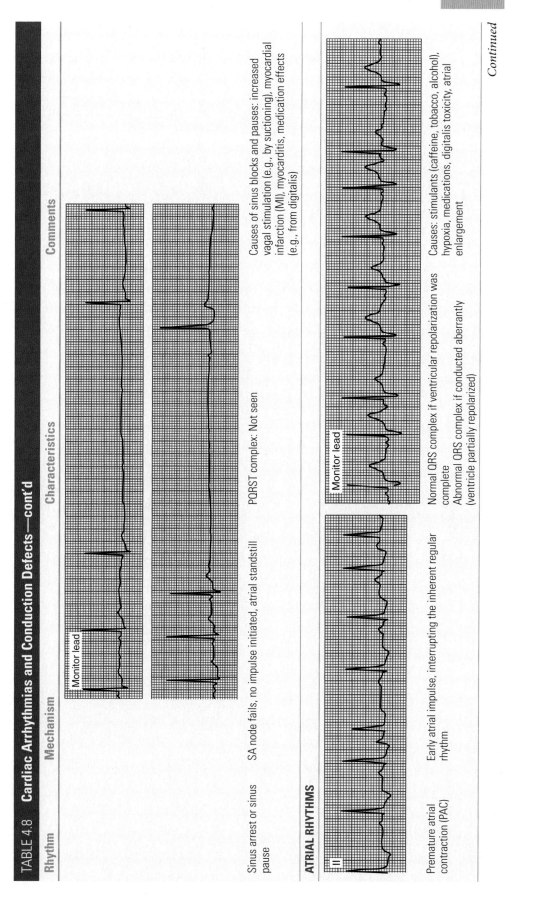

Continued

TABLE 4.8   Cardiac Arrhythmias and Conduction Defects—cont'd

Rhythm	Mechanism	Characteristics	Comments
		No QRS complex if beat arrived too early during the ventricle's absolute refractory period (e.g., nonconducted PAC) Usually no compensatory pause, but may have a partial pause	
Atrial flutter	Origin: reentry	 Atrial rates: 200–350 beats/min Ventricular rates, along with rhythm, may be constant at 2:1, 3:1, 4:1 or may vary; if there is a variable atrioventricular (AV) conduction block Flutter waves may appear as wide, sawtooth waves representing rapid atrial depolarization, persist through QRS complexes, and are best seen in leads II, III, and aVF	According to the "rule of 150," a supraventricular tachycardia (SVT) at a rate of 150 beats/min is usually atrial flutter with a 2:1 block
Atrial fibrillation	Chaotic, random, and rapid atrial activity Atrial impulses are randomly conducted through the AV junction	 Atrial rates: 350–650 beats/min Irregular fibrillatory waves of varying amplitude; best seen in V_1 P wave: Not seen Ventricular rhythm is irregular QRS complex: Often looks normal, but aberrantly conducted beats are often seen when a long RR interval is followed by a short RR interval, before ventricle is fully repolarized	Risk of atrial thrombi with atrial fibrillation If ventricular rhythm becomes regular ("regularization of atrial fibrillation"), digitalis toxicity should be suspected

TABLE 4.8 Cardiac Arrhythmias and Conduction Defects—cont'd

Rhythm	Mechanism	Characteristics	Comments
JUNCTIONAL RHYTHMS			
AV junctional beats	Originate in AV junction, spreading both antegrade and retrograde	If conduction to atria and ventricles is simultaneous, P wave is buried in QRS complex (not visible) and QRS usually normal 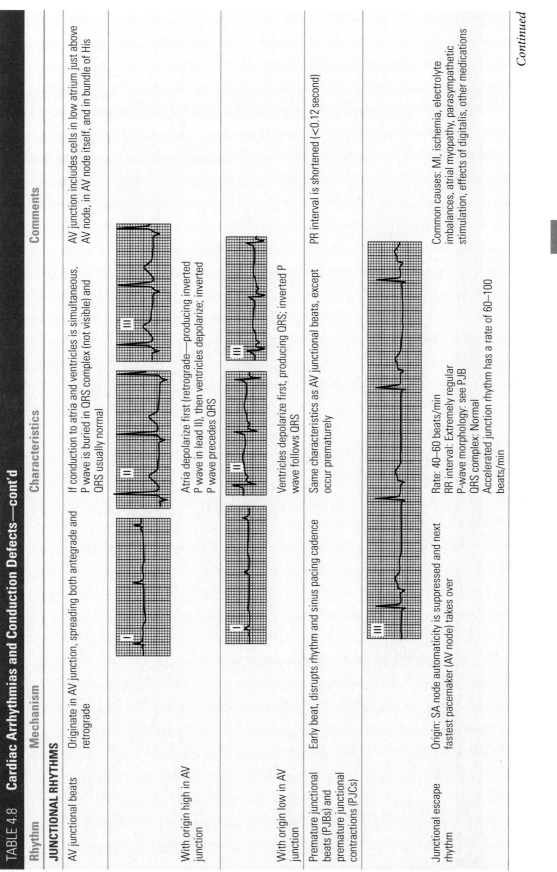	AV junction includes cells in low atrium just above AV node, in AV node itself, and in bundle of His
With origin high in AV junction		Atria depolarize first (retrograde—producing inverted P wave in lead II), then ventricles depolarize; inverted P wave precedes QRS	
With origin low in AV junction		Ventricles depolarize first, producing QRS; inverted P wave follows QRS	PR interval is shortened (<0.12 second)
Premature junctional beats (PJBs) and premature junctional contractions (PJCs)	Early beat, disrupts rhythm and sinus pacing cadence	Same characteristics as AV junctional beats, except occur prematurely	
Junctional escape rhythm	Origin: SA node automaticity is suppressed and next fastest pacemaker (AV node) takes over	Rate: 40–60 beats/min RR interval: Extremely regular P-wave morphology: see PJB QRS complex: Normal Accelerated junction rhythm has a rate of 60–100 beats/min	Common causes: MI, ischemia, electrolyte imbalances, atrial myopathy, parasympathetic stimulation, effects of digitalis, other medications

Continued

4 Cardiovascular System

TABLE 4.8 **Cardiac Arrhythmias and Conduction Defects—cont'd**

Rhythm	Mechanism	Characteristics	Comments
AV junctional tachycardia	An usurping rhythm	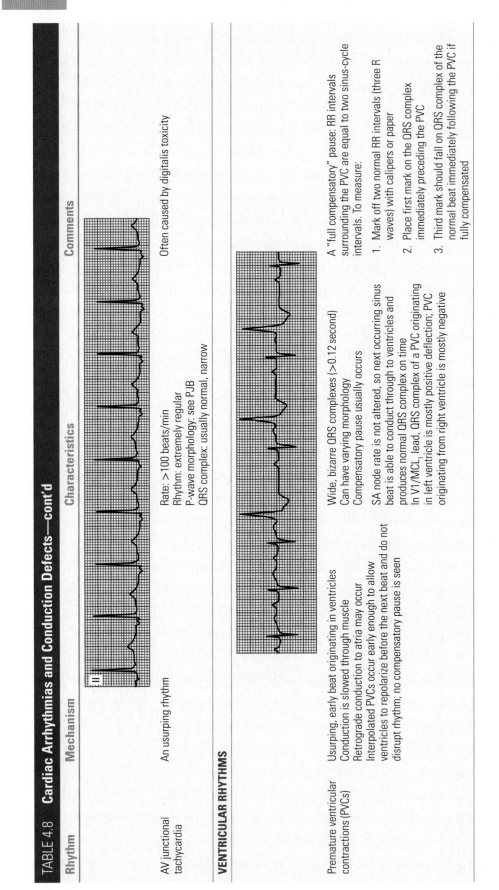 Rate: >100 beats/min Rhythm: extremely regular P-wave morphology: see PJB QRS complex: usually normal, narrow	Often caused by digitalis toxicity
VENTRICULAR RHYTHMS			
Premature ventricular contractions (PVCs)	Usurping, early beat originating in ventricles Conduction is slowed through muscle Retrograde conduction to atria may occur Interpolated PVCs occur early enough to allow ventricles to repolarize before the next beat and do not disrupt rhythm; no compensatory pause is seen	Wide, bizarre QRS complexes (>0.12 second) Can have varying morphology Compensatory pause usually occurs SA node rate is not altered, so next occurring sinus beat is able to conduct through to ventricles and produces normal QRS complex on time In V1/MCL₁ lead, QRS complex of a PVC originating in left ventricle is mostly positive deflection; PVC originating from right ventricle is mostly negative	A "full compensatory" pause: RR intervals surrounding the PVC are equal to two sinus-cycle intervals. To measure: 1. Mark off two normal RR intervals (three R waves) with calipers or paper 2. Place first mark on the QRS complex immediately preceding the PVC 3. Third mark should fall on QRS complex of the normal beat immediately following the PVC if fully compensated

TABLE 4.8   Cardiac Arrhythmias and Conduction Defects—cont'd

Rhythm	Mechanism	Characteristics	Comments
Ventricular escape rhythm	Impulses from higher centers (SA or AV node) either are not generated or are blocked; ventricles initiate "escape" rhythm based on inherent automaticity of the ventricular tissue	Rate: 20–40 beats/min (usually 20–30 beats/min), rarely <20 beats/min Rhythm: usually very regular QRS complex: wide, bizarre No P wave association with QRS complex	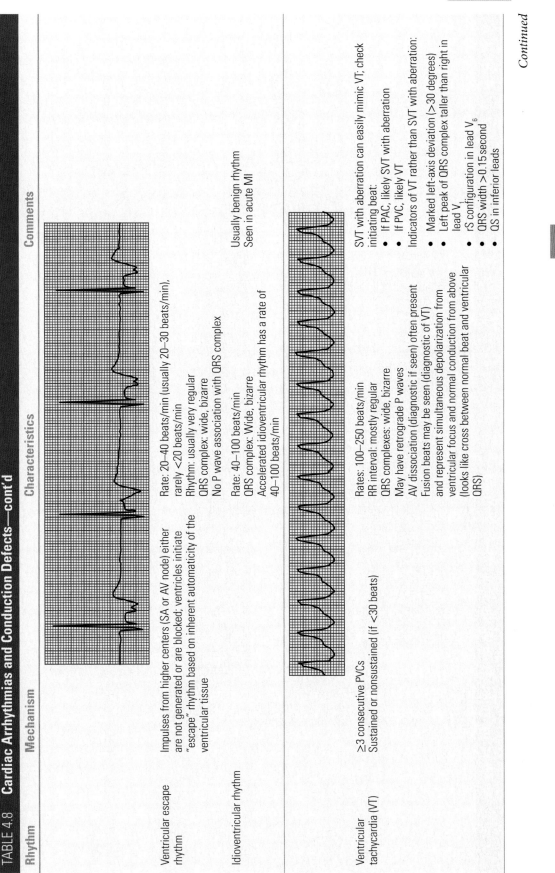
Idioventricular rhythm		Rate: 40–100 beats/min QRS complex: Wide, bizarre Accelerated idioventricular rhythm has a rate of 40–100 beats/min	Usually benign rhythm Seen in acute MI
Ventricular tachycardia (VT)	≥3 consecutive PVCs Sustained or nonsustained (if <30 beats)	Rates: 100–250 beats/min RR interval: mostly regular QRS complexes: wide, bizarre May have retrograde P waves AV dissociation (diagnostic if seen) often present Fusion beats may be seen (diagnostic of VT) and represent simultaneous depolarization from ventricular focus and normal conduction from above (looks like cross between normal beat and ventricular QRS)	SVT with aberration can easily mimic VT; check initiating beat: • If PAC, likely SVT with aberration • If PVC, likely VT Indicators of VT rather than SVT with aberration: • Marked left-axis deviation (>30 degrees) • Left peak of QRS complex taller than right in lead V_1 • rS configuration in lead V_6 • QRS width >0.15 second • QS in inferior leads

Continued

4   Cardiovascular System

TABLE 4.8 **Cardiac Arrhythmias and Conduction Defects—cont'd**

Rhythm	Mechanism	Characteristics	Comments
Torsades de pointes (twisting of points)	Polymorphic VT	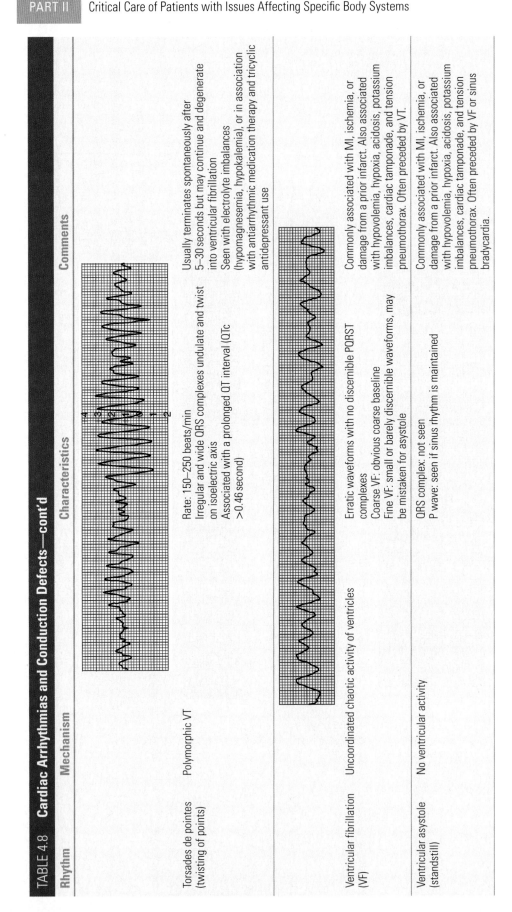Rate: 150–250 beats/min Irregular and wide QRS complexes undulate and twist on isoelectric axis Associated with a prolonged QT interval (QTc >0.46 second)	Usually terminates spontaneously after 5–30 seconds but may continue and degenerate into ventricular fibrillation Seen with electrolyte imbalances (hypomagnesemia, hypokalemia), or in association with antiarrhythmic medication therapy and tricyclic antidepressant use
Ventricular fibrillation (VF)	Uncoordinated chaotic activity of ventricles	Erratic waveforms with no discernible PQRST complexes Coarse VF: obvious coarse baseline Fine VF: small or barely discernible waveforms, may be mistaken for asystole	Commonly associated with MI, ischemia, or damage from a prior infarct. Also associated with hypovolemia, hypoxia, acidosis, potassium imbalances, cardiac tamponade, and tension pneumothorax. Often preceded by VT.
Ventricular asystole (standstill)	No ventricular activity	QRS complex: not seen P wave: seen if sinus rhythm is maintained	Commonly associated with MI, ischemia, or damage from a prior infarct. Also associated with hypovolemia, hypoxia, acidosis, potassium imbalances, cardiac tamponade, and tension pneumothorax. Often preceded by VF or sinus bradycardia.

TABLE 4.8   Cardiac Arrhythmias and Conduction Defects—cont'd

Rhythm	Mechanism	Characteristics	Comments
AV CONDUCTION DEFECTS			
First-degree AV block	Impulse is delayed at AV junction	PR interval: is consistent each beat and is >0.20 second Every sinus beat is conducted to the ventricles, producing normal QRS complex for every P wave	Most commonly associated with ischemic damage or following cardiac surgery. May also be associated with degenerative diseases, infections, rheumatic disease, neuromuscular disorders, metabolic causes, or drug/toxin effects
Second-degree AV block	Impulses are not all conducted through AV node		
Second-degree AV block type I or Wenckebach	Progressive delay in conduction through AV node until a QRS complex is dropped	PR interval: gradually increases until impulse fails to conduct through AV junctional tissue; produces dropped QRS at varying or constant intervals PR interval: shortest after each dropped beat PP interval: constant if in sinus rhythm (untrue, if sinus arrhythmia) RR interval: progressively shortens P waves and QRS: normal	Related to infarction, medication effect, or vagal effect

Continued

TABLE 4.8   Cardiac Arrhythmias and Conduction Defects—cont'd

Rhythm	Mechanism	Characteristics	Comments
Second-degree AV block type II	SA node discharges regularly Produces constant PP interval One or more atrial impulses fails to conduct to ventricles (no QRS complex seen)	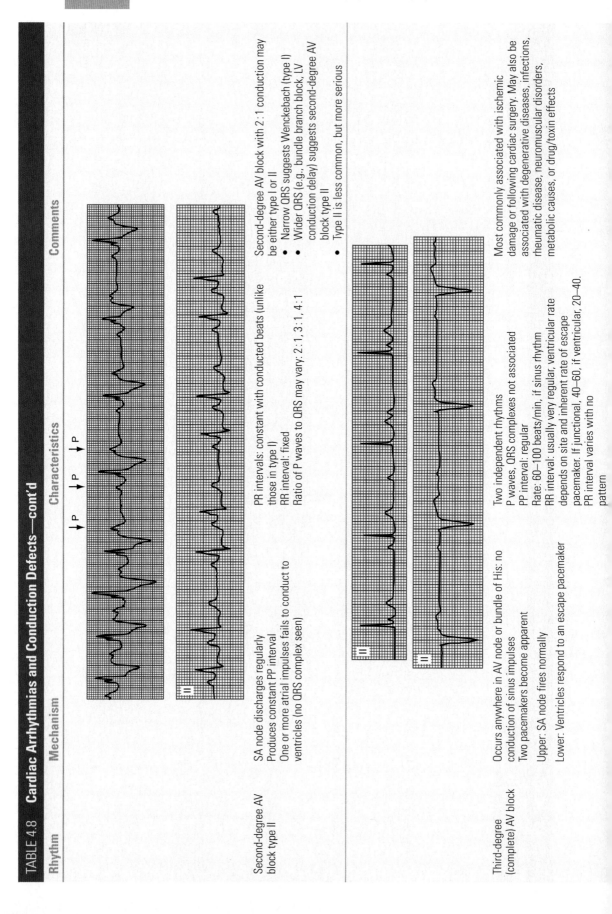 PR intervals: constant with conducted beats (unlike those in type I) RR interval: fixed Ratio of P waves to QRS may vary: 2:1, 3:1, 4:1	Second-degree AV block with 2:1 conduction may be either type I or II • Narrow QRS suggests Wenckebach (type I) • Wider QRS (e.g., bundle branch block, LV conduction delay) suggests second-degree AV block type II • Type II is less common, but more serious
Third-degree (complete) AV block	Occurs anywhere in AV node or bundle of His: no conduction of sinus impulses Two pacemakers become apparent Upper: SA node fires normally Lower: Ventricles respond to an escape pacemaker	Two independent rhythms P waves, QRS complexes not associated PP interval: regular Rate: 60–100 beats/min, if sinus rhythm RR interval: usually very regular, ventricular rate depends on site and inherent rate of escape pacemaker. If junctional, 40–60, if ventricular, 20–40. PR interval varies with no pattern	Most commonly associated with ischemic damage or following cardiac surgery. May also be associated with degenerative diseases, infections, rheumatic disease, neuromuscular disorders, metabolic causes, or drug/toxin effects

TABLE 4.8   Cardiac Arrhythmias and Conduction Defects

Rhythm	Mechanism	Characteristics	Comments
ECG CHANGES WITH ELECTROLYTE IMBALANCES			
Potassium Imbalances			

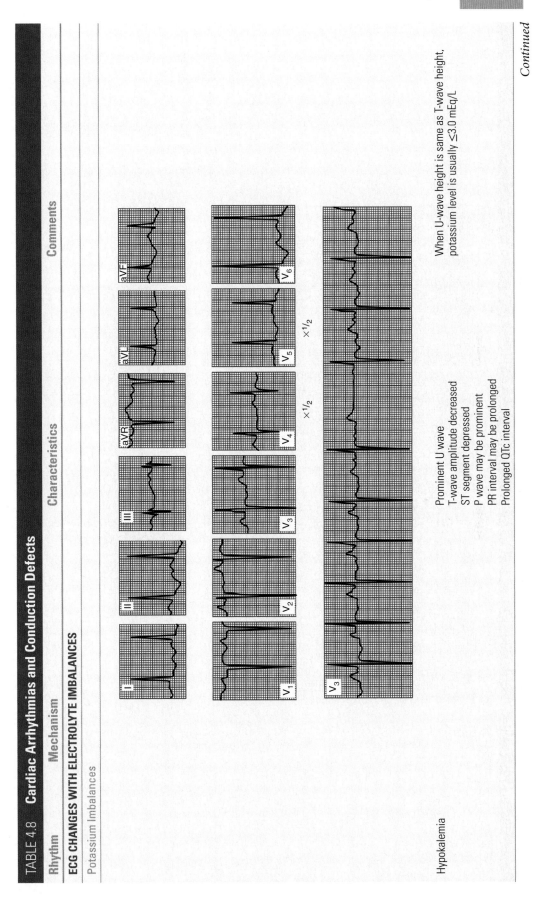

Hypokalemia

Prominent U wave
T-wave amplitude decreased
ST segment depressed
P wave may be prominent
PR interval may be prolonged
Prolonged QTc interval

When U-wave height is same as T-wave height, potassium level is usually ≤3.0 mEq/L

Continued

TABLE 4.8 **Cardiac Arrhythmias and Conduction Defects—cont'd**

Rhythm	Mechanism	Characteristics	Comments
Hyperkalemia		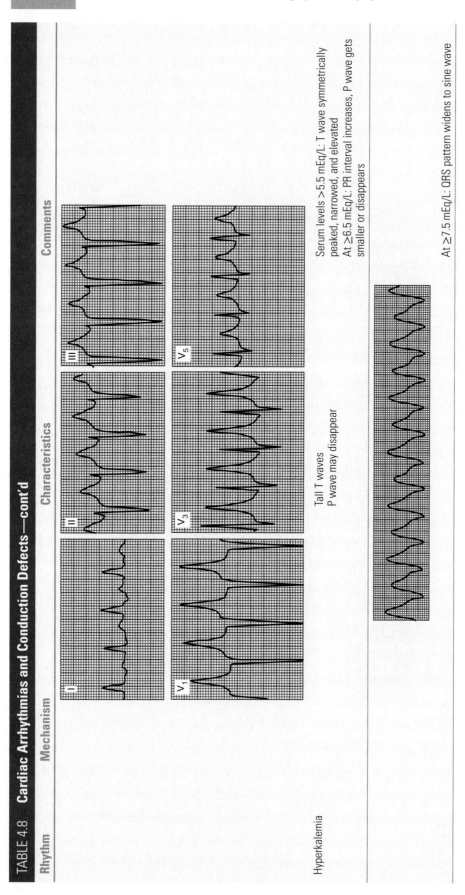 Tall T waves P wave may disappear	Serum levels >5.5 mEq/L: T wave symmetrically peaked, narrowed, and elevated At ≥6.5 mEq/L: PR interval increases, P wave gets smaller or disappears At ≥7.5 mEq/L: QRS pattern widens to sine wave

TABLE 4.8   Cardiac Arrhythmias and Conduction Defects—cont'd

Rhythm	Mechanism	Characteristics	Comments

CALCIUM IMBALANCES

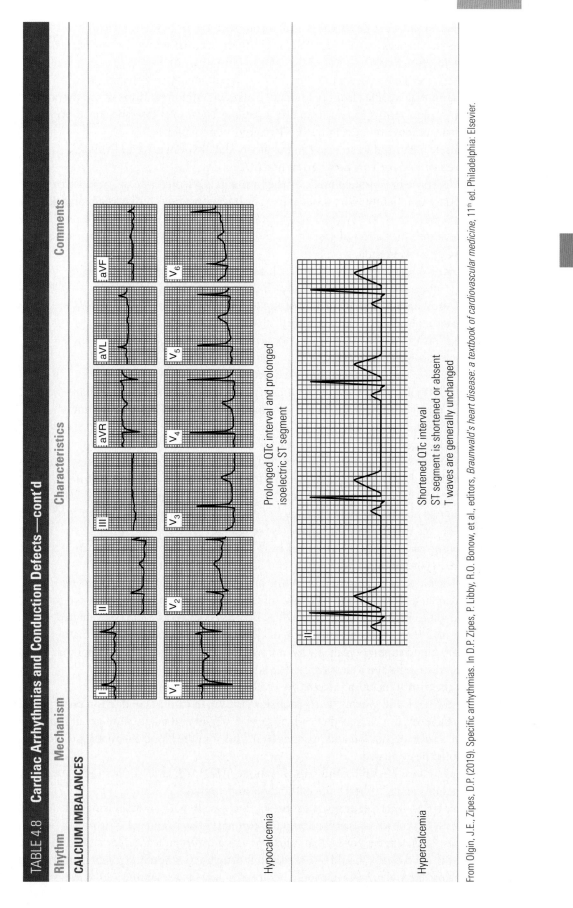

Hypocalcemia

Prolonged QTc interval and prolonged isoelectric ST segment

Hypercalcemia

Shortened QTc interval
ST segment is shortened or absent
T waves are generally unchanged

From Olgin, J.E., Zipes, D.P. (2019). Specific arrhythmias. In D.P. Zipes, P. Libby, R.O. Bonow, et al., editors, *Braunwald's heart disease: a textbook of cardiovascular medicine*, 11th ed. Philadelphia: Elsevier.

d. Brain natriuretic peptide (BNP) is a substance secreted from the ventricles in response to changes in pressure. Released with myocardial stretch and correlates with LV dysfunction.

    i. Used to evaluate HF (both LV and RV) and pulmonary emboli and to differentiate cardiac from pulmonary causes of pulmonary distress and dyspnea

    ii. Falsely low results can occur in obese patients because of clearance in adipose tissue (adipose tissue removes BNP from the circulation)

    iii. Falsely high results can occur in the older adult, hypertensive individuals, females, and patients being given nesiritide

e. C-reactive protein is protein made by the liver and is released into the bloodstream in response to inflammation, tissue injury, or infection, and is tested as a biomarker of inflammation.

    i. Elevations may also indicate an acute infection, inflammatory disease processes, and possible uremia

f. Clotting profile (prothrombin time [PT], activated partial thromboplastin time [aPTT], international normalized ratio [INR], and activated clotting time [ACT])

    i. PT is a vitamin K–dependent clotting test, often used with INR and used to detect a bleeding or clotting disorder.

    ii. aPTT is a measure of time taken for a clot to form. Used as a measure in monitoring heparin levels.

    iii. INR: Used for measuring the effectiveness of anticoagulant therapy

        (a) INR of 2.0 to 3.0 is therapeutic for atrial fibrillation and nonvalvular thromboembolic diseases (pulmonary embolism [PE] and deep venous thrombosis [DVTs])

        (b) INR of 2.5 to 3.5 is therapeutic for mechanical valves

g. ACT: Bedside test to measure the time required for blood coagulation. Prolongation may indicate deficiency in coagulation factors or GPIIb/IIIa inhibitor treatment.

h. D-dimer is a fibrin degradation product, a small protein fragment, released with endogenous fibrinolysis in the presence of an acute clot. Used in the diagnosis of DVT, PE, and disseminated intravascular coagulation (DIC).

Note: Clotting profile may be abnormal in the presence of hepatic dysfunction, lupus, hypothermia, hypovolemia, hypervolemia, and affected by medications.

    i. Complete blood cell count (CBC): White blood count (WBC), hemoglobin (Hb) level, hematocrit (HCT), and platelets. Infection, anemias, and hypoxia related to abnormalities in the CBC may affect the cardiac system and should be evaluated and treated. Platelets are an indication of clotting ability and affect clot formation in coronary blood supply, which is why antiplatelet medications are used in coronary disease treatments and following cardiac stent placement.

    j. Blood chemistry: Including electrolyte levels, blood urea nitrogen (BUN) level, creatinine level, and glucose level. Potassium is used in cardiac conduction and abnormal levels can cause lethal arrhythmias. Calcium and magnesium are useful tests in cardiac evaluation and may not be included in the blood chemistry profile but should be evaluated.

    k. Thyroid studies: Thyroid stimulating hormone (TSH), T3, and T4. Thyroid dysfunction can affect heart rate and induce arrhythmias.

    l. Toxicology: Many street drugs affect the cardiac system with cocaine being one of the most well-known causes of chest pain, coronary spasm, and MI. The presence of cocaine, amphetamines, or methamphetamine is a contraindication for a treadmill stress test. All patients should be asked about drug use (without judgment or threat). A urine or serum drug screen should be done in patients presenting with chest pain.

m. Digoxin levels should be evaluated

n. Fasting serum lipid profile: Total cholesterol, high-density lipoprotein (HDL), low-density lipoprotein (LDL); Triglycerides

Note: Guidelines place atherosclerotic risk above treating to a goal number. They recommend statin therapy should be used based on risk or LDL greater than 190 or triglycerides over 500 mg/dL.

o. Homocysteine level: To identify folic acid-responsive hyperlipidemia. Normal level is 5 to 15 μmol/L. Elevated levels considered an independent risk factor for CAD.

3. **Radiography**

a. Chest radiograph is used to visualize
   i. Cardiac size and position
   ii. Abnormalities of the heart, great vessels, lungs, pleura, and ribs
   iii. Pulmonary vasculature
   iv. Position of catheters, lines, and pacemaker leads

4. **Echocardiogram**

a. Provides information on the chamber size and function, and the valvular morphology and function, including:
   i. LV systolic function: EF
   ii. LV wall motion (shows areas of hypokinesis, akinesis, dyskinesis), wall thickness, cavity size
   iii. LV diastolic function
   iv. Chamber size
   v. Regurgitation
   vi. Prosthetic valve function
   vii. Stenotic valves
   viii. Congenital defects and shunts
   ix. Intracardiac masses, including tumors, thrombi, and vegetation
   x. Pericardial disease
   xi. Pericardial effusion
   xii. Cardiac tamponade

b. Types of echocardiogram
   i. M mode: Used to measure intracardiac dimensions; measures chamber size and wall thickness
   ii. Two-dimensional echocardiography provides real-time imagery of the heart and its structures using a two-dimensional ultrasonic beam
   iii. Doppler echocardiography is used to demonstrate the velocity and direction of blood flow through the heart and great vessels
   iv. Color flow imaging: Doppler signals are processed to depict real-time velocities superimposed on a two-dimensional echocardiogram. Red represents flow toward the transducer; blue represents flow away from the transducer. Lighter shades mean higher velocity. Used to evaluate shunts, regurgitation, stenosis.
   v. Contrast echocardiography
   vi. Bubble echo (agitated saline): Used to detect congenital or acquired shunts, patent foramen ovale
   vii. Enhancing agents: Contrast media used to enhance the LV endocardial border and help identify myocardial infarct or ischemia
   viii. Transesophageal echocardiography (TEE): Transducer is placed in the esophagus
      (a) Capable of exquisite definition of cardiac structure and function because of the proximity of the transducer to the heart

(b) Used in the operating room when the adequacy of valvular repair is to be evaluated and when more detail is needed (in cases of prosthetic valves or suspected patent foramen ovale, LA thrombus, or aortic dissection; in patients with poor acoustic penetration of the ultrasonic signal from the chest, such as patients with chronic obstructive pulmonary disease or a heavy build)

  ix. Stress echocardiography: Images obtained before, during, and after exercise or pharmacologic stress (states of increased myocardial oxygen demand). Stress tests are discussed in the next paragraph.

    (a) Methods used include treadmill (most common) and pharmacologic stressing (dobutamine, dipyridamole, adenosine)

    (b) Ischemia results in a region of hypokinesis (decreased wall motion)

    (c) Evaluates extent and location of CAD and ischemic mitral regurgitation

  x. Intravascular ultrasonography (IVUS): A small ultrasonic transducer attached to a catheter tip is threaded into the coronary artery over a guidewire. It provides high-resolution images of the inside of the artery. Invaluable in the catheterization laboratory for interventional procedures. Assesses the following:

    (a) Size of the lumen, degree of stenosis

    (b) Structure of the arterial wall

    (c) Proper coronary stent placement

5. **Exercise electrocardiography (exercise stress testing)**

  a. 12-lead ECG is monitored during exercise, and the level of difficulty of the exercise activity is gradually increased at regular intervals. The exercise may be a bicycle, but more commonly uses a treadmill using a Bruce Protocol (speed and incline are increased every 3 minutes). A predetermined target heart rate is established as a goal and the exercise capacity is reported in terms of estimated metabolic equivalents (METs) of tasks. When target heart rate is reached and sustained for 1 minute, the treadmill is slowed to a stop, the recovery stage begins, and monitoring continues.

  b. The 12-lead ECG is monitored continuously throughout all stages, for changes (such as ST elevation, ST depression, T wave changes) or arrhythmias (such as ventricular ectopy) that may indicate ischemia or cardiac concerns.

  c. BP is also measured during each interval and into recovery, as are any symptoms.

  d. Indications for exercise testing

    i. To identify suspected CAD

    ii. To rule out ischemia

    iii. To perform a functional assessment in patients known to have CAD (such as patients who have had an MI or angioplasty, or are undergoing coronary bypass surgery) to assess risk, severity, and prognosis

    iv. To evaluate the effectiveness of revascularization or medical therapy for CAD

    v. To evaluate arrhythmias, especially exercise-induced ventricular tachycardia (VT)

    vi. To evaluate patients with rate-responsive pacemakers

    vii. To measure the exercise capacity: Reported in terms of estimated METs

    viii. To screen persons entering physical fitness programs or high-risk professions (e.g., airline pilots) for CAD

  e. Contraindications to exercise testing

    i. Acute MI

    ii. Unstable (preinfarction) angina (on effort)

    iii. Uncompensated HF

    iv. Severe aortic stenosis or moderate stenotic valvular heart disease

    v. Uncontrolled hypertension or severe atrial hypertension

    vi. Severe illness, such as fulminant infection, asthma, renal failure, acute aortic dissection, acute pulmonary embolus, or pulmonary infarction

    vii. Acute pericarditis or myocarditis

    viii. Electrolyte imbalance

    ix. Tachyarrhythmias, bradyarrhythmias, high-degree AV block, or arrhythmias that cause hemodynamic compromise

    x. Positive cocaine finding on drug screen

6. **Myocardial imaging: Radioisotope is injected into a peripheral vein and its cardiac uptake can be imaged to enhance the accuracy of an exercise stress test or provide an alternative to exercise by using pharmacologic agents. Myocardial perfusion imaging is more sensitive and specific (80%–85%) than exercise ECG-stress testing alone (70%).**

    a. Nuclear imaging/myocardial scintigraphy: Usually a radiotracer (Tc-99 sestamibi, Myoview, or thallous chloride 201) is injected into a peripheral IV during the test to identify ischemia, infarct, and myocardial viability. Two images are taken, one at baseline when the heart is at rest and one with activity or pharmacologic stimulation to rate or blood flow. The images are compared to see if the uptake of isotope is the same at rest and with stimulation. Decreased isotope uptake indicates decreased myocardial perfusion; ischemic sites show normal uptake at rest and decreased uptake on exercise. Infarcted sites show no uptake at all.

    b. Exercise or pharmacologic agents are used with the nuclear images

        i. Exercise stress test (sometimes referred to as a thallium stress test) involves walking on a treadmill (or exercise bicycle) using Bruce Protocol (as previously discussed). Once target is reached the second isotope is added and activity continued for 60 seconds.

        ii. Pharmacologic nuclear stress tests involve pharmacologic agents used to simulate the effects of exercise (potentially to induce ischemia) in patients who are unable to exercise.

           (a) Regadenoson (Lexiscan) activates A2A adenosine receptors producing coronary vasodilation and increased blood flow. If the flow is inhibited by atherosclerosis, the isotope uptake will be limited in the nuclear image.

           (b) Dipyridamole (Persantine) inhibits platelet adenosine uptake and dilates coronary arteries.

           (c) Adenosine (Adenoscan) activates A1 and A2 adenosine receptors producing coronary vasodilation and increases blood flow.

           (d) Dobutamine (Dobutrex) stimulates beta-1 adrenergic receptors and increases cardiac stimulation and heart rate.

Note: In a similar way to the exercise nuclear stress test, the second isotope is given at a specific point in the pharmacologic stress test (timing is based on the medication and goal of the test).

    c. Multiple-gated acquisition (MUGA) scan is an additional type of nuclear image

        i. Used to measure the EF of the LV

        ii. Very accurate unless the patient has an irregular rhythm because multiple images cannot be gated (superimposed) on ECG

7. **Electrophysiologic studies (EPS)**

    a. Series of programmed electrical stimuli are applied within the heart to the endothelium through electrodes in the cardiac chambers under fluoroscopic guidance. Used to induce cardiac arrhythmias. The purpose is to reproduce

arrhythmias in a controlled environment to assess the best mode of therapy for their control (e.g., medications, pacemaker, ablation).
   b. Selection criteria may include:
      i. Patients with ventricular or supraventricular tachyarrhythmias
      ii. Patients at high risk for sudden cardiac death
      iii. Patients with unexplained recurrent syncopal episodes with suspected cardiac cause
      iv. Patients who have survived a cardiac arrest without identified cause
      v. Candidates for an implantable defibrillator
      vi. Candidates for ablation therapy
8. **Cardiac computed tomography (CT): May use a multidetector computed tomography (MDCT) or an electron-beam computed tomography (EBCT). Because of the high speed of the scanner, it is used to produce high-quality pictures of the heart in motion and detect calcium in the coronary arteries.**
   a. Provides two-dimensional image of cardiovascular structures
   b. Visualizes coronary calcium, silent atherosclerosis
      i. Amount of calcium can be predictive of multivessel CAD
      ii. Not sufficiently specific
9. **Coronary computed tomography angiography (CCTA): A heart imaging test that helps determine whether plaque buildup has narrowed a patient's coronary arteries**
   a. IV contrast is used
10. **Magnetic resonance imaging (MRI): Safe diagnostic technique involving no ionizing radiation. Used with contrast to produce a magnetic resonance angiogram (MRA).**
   a. Provides a three-dimensional view of cardiovascular structure
   b. Creates a computer-assisted image; measures tissue proton density
   c. MRI may be used to determine or identify
      i. Anatomy of the heart
      ii. Congenital heart defects
      iii. Masses in the myocardium or pericardium
      iv. Ventricular aneurysm
      v. Aortic dissection
      vi. Arterial disease (MRA)
      vii. Tissue changes, such as sarcoidosis, myocarditis
   d. Safe alternative to radiography for children and pregnant women
   e. As a magnetic device, MRI machine:
      i. Devices (pacemakers and automated implantable cardioverter defibrillator) implanted since 2000 should be MRI safe. Labeled "MRI Conditional", but it is still recommended to interrogate devices after an MRI is completed.
      ii. MRIs should not be used for patients with prosthetic metallic devices (valves, prosthetic joints), as the magnet may displace or damage such devices. Caution following arterial stents (coronary or peripheral) as the magnetic force may displace the stent, especially if newly inserted.
   f. Infarct-avid imaging (myocardial infarct indicators)
      i. Technetium Tc 99 m pyrophosphate is injected into a peripheral vein.
      ii. Infarcted areas of the heart show increased levels of radioactivity as "hot spots." These appear within 4 hours of infarction, may not peak until 12 to 24 hours later, and remain positive for 2 to 7 days.
      iii. Limited usefulness in acute MI; useful when ECG changes are not definitive or when enzyme levels have already returned to normal

11. **Cardiac catheterization and angiography: Radiopaque contrast medium is injected into the coronary arteries for visualization of the coronary arteries by x-ray digital imaging; recordings are made on digital media. Still photographs may be produced for patient records. The cardiac images may be used as a diagnostic tool and interventions, such as angioplasty or stenting, are treatments that may be initiated immediately. (For more information on cardiac catheterization, please see STEMI and Box 4.3.)**
   a. Patients selected include
      i. Asymptomatic patients with
         (a) Evidence of significant ischemia or severe LV dysfunction on noninvasive testing
         (b) Positive stress test results but asymptomatic
         (c) Valvular heart disease
      ii. Symptomatic patients with
         (a) Angina—unstable or stable
         (b) Atypical chest pain
         (c) Recent MI
         (d) Valvular disease
         (e) Congenital heart defects
         (f) Aortic disease
         (g) LV failure
         (h) Survival after a sudden cardiac death event

BOX 4.3	**Key Concepts in Nursing Care After Percutaneous Coronary Intervention Procedures**

GENERAL NURSING CARE
1. Observe for complications.
2. For a femoral procedure, maintain the patient on bed rest for 2 to 6 hours with progressive elevation of head of bed (initially <30 degrees). Time of restrictions depends on procedure, medications, and method of postprocedure closure. Closure may include manual pressure (e.g., 15–20 minutes directly to femoral site), mechanical closure device (e.g., FemoStop), collagen closure plugs (e.g., Angio-Seal), or percutaneous suture devices (e.g., Perclose).
3. For the transradial procedure, the patient is able to ambulate and eat immediately after procedure. A transradial compression device (e.g., TR band) is applied by interventionist before sheath removal at the end of the procedure and the air pressure is removed by RN at bedside.
4. Affected limb should be kept straight and immobile. For radial approach, IV access or blood pressure monitoring should be avoided on the affected arm for at least 24 hours if possible.
5. Patient may be positioned in reverse Trendelenburg's position to facilitate eating and comfort, and repositioned on side by log rolling, if procedure site is not bleeding.
6. Take electrocardiogram upon return from procedure and if chest discomfort is present.
7. Ensure that blood work is done for serial measurement of cardiac markers.
8. Monitor vital signs closely, including telemetry for ST segments and arrhythmias.
9. Monitor pulses, warmth, sensation of affected limb; assess for bleeding and hematoma at procedural site.
10. If there is bleeding or hematoma, hold direct pressure until bleeding has stopped.
11. Mark hematoma and closely watch for signs of increased size. Inflatable femoral or arterial compression system may be applied to maintain hemostasis. Unstable hematoma and especially those with lower back and abdominal pain may require ultrasound to rule out retroperitoneal bleed.
12. Finger foods are easier for patient while head-of-bed elevation is restricted. (Transradial access will require patient to do no lifting or movement of affected wrist.)
13. Assess need for medication for back, wrist, and groin discomfort.
14. Maintain IV fluids as ordered and encourage drinking of fluids (to facilitate excretion of catheterization dye by kidneys).
15. Ensure adequate output. Urinary catheter may be necessary for patients who cannot void (within 2–4 hours), for patients who are unable to void in bed at required position, or for patients who are at high risk for bleeding.

Continued

BOX 4.3 **Key Concepts in Nursing Care After Percutaneous Coronary Intervention Procedures—cont'd**

16. Patient may be on anticoagulant or antiplatelet medications after percutaneous coronary intervention and require coagulation levels. With most antiplatelet IV medications, CBC done 8 hours postprocedure and following AM; however, follow the protocol in your facility. Perform other monitoring to detect bleeding problems (check urine, vomit, stools; watch for nosebleeds; monitor neurologic status). Heparin should be stopped 1 to 4 hours before sheath removal.
17. Check activated coagulation time if sheath is to come out (if <150 seconds, sheath may be removed if patient is stable and without ischemic pain).
18. Various closure devices are used, each with its own postcatheter protocol.

POSTPROCEDURE NURSING CARE DURING SHEATH REMOVAL

Check with your facility procedures regarding competency training required before attempting a procedure.

1. Explain removal process to patient.
2. Medicate patient before removal to diminish discomfort. Medications include morphine or other fast-acting analgesics along with local anesthesia to site.
3. Have normal saline bolus and atropine (0.5 mg IV) readily available at bedside for vasovagal reactions (hypotension, bradycardia, diaphoresis, nausea).
4. Gather all other equipment for removal: suture removal kit; syringes; gloves, goggles, and gown; dressings; Doppler device, compression devices, if used.
5. Aspirating 5 to 10 mL of blood from each sheath (both venous and arterial lines) ensures that there are no clots on the tip of the sheath to embolize on withdrawal and that any heparin is removed from the patient's system.
6. Locate arterial pulse. Apply manual, direct pressure just above puncture site (and over arterial pulse) for a minimum of 20 minutes after sheath removal until hemostasis is complete. Pulling the arterial sheath first and then the venous sheath after hemostasis avoids potential risk of arteriovenous fistula.
7. If using a compression device, follow protocols for safe use during and after sheath removal.

POSTPROCEDURE NURSING CARE AFTER SHEATH REMOVAL

1. After sheath removal check vital signs every 15 minutes 4 times, every 30 minutes 4 times, and then every hour.
2. Continue to monitor and document pulses and assess for bleeding or hematoma; promptly treat with direct pressure until hemostasis is complete. Notify physician if bleeding recurs.
3. Maintain bed rest for 2 to 6 hours after sheath removal per protocol for closure method and procedure site (e.g., radial, femoral). Elevate head of bed progressively (initially less than 30 degrees) with affected limb immobilized.
4. Continue to medicate for discomfort from bed rest.
5. Auscultate for systolic bruit at site of sheath insertion at least every 8 hours: positive bruit along with localized pain and pulsatile mass suggests possible pseudoaneurysm; notify physician immediately. Surgery or ultrasonographically guided compression is necessary for closure. Patients at high risk for pseudoaneurysm include the following:
   - Obese patients (difficult to apply direct pressure)
   - Patients in whom sheath size larger than No. 8 French was used (larger injury to artery)
   - Patients receiving postprocedure anticoagulants (hemostasis problem)
   - Older adult patients (artery wall changes with age)
   - Females (fat distribution, smaller arteries, potential for multiple punctures during catheterization procedure)

DISCHARGE AFTER PERCUTANEOUS CORONARY INTERVENTION

1. Teach discharge activities, symptoms to report (e.g., masses, bleeding, increased localized pain and bruising at the site of insertion, tingling or numbness, extremity weakness, shortness of breath, chest discomfort), medications, diet, risk factors, and actions to take:
   a. Call provider and apply pressure for bleeding or swelling at catheter site.
   b. Limit activities for 2 days. Do not lift more than 10 lb. Limit movement of wrist for 48 hours (i.e., no golf, tennis, lifting).
   c. Do not drive for 1 day.
   d. Medication compliance (e.g., antiplatelet therapy).
   e. Schedule follow-up with cardiologist and PCP.
2. Give the patient a stent information packet and an identification stent card and ensure that questions regarding care are answered.
3. Provide clear instructions regarding all medications (types, rationales, dosages, side effects) to the patient and significant others.

CBC, Complete blood count; *IV*, intravenous; *PCP*, primary care provide; *RN*, registered nurse.

   b. Technique
      i. Right-sided heart catheterization performed via the femoral or brachial vein, with the catheter advanced into the RA and then past the tricuspid valve through the RV into the pulmonary artery to record pressures, perform angiography, determine CO and resistances, and define anatomy
      ii. Left-sided heart catheterization performed in a retrograde manner via the femoral, brachial, or radial artery (or transseptal approach through the RA and intra-atrial septum); catheter is advanced into the LV to determine pressure. Transradial percutaneous transluminal coronary intervention (PCI) is associated with lower vascular and bleeding complication rates and less complications at the access site than with transfemoral access (Bajaj et al., 2019).
   c. Left ventriculography
      i. Technique: Radiopaque contrast medium is injected into the LV cavity
      ii. Purposes
         (a) Evaluate ventricular wall motion and chamber size
            (1) Identify akinetic areas and wall motion abnormalities
            (2) Detect hypokinetic areas: Weaker than normal contractions in systole
            (3) Detect dyskinetic areas: Areas bulge outward during systole instead of contracting
         (b) Assess function, determining
            (1) End-diastolic volume
            (2) End-systolic volume
            (3) Stroke volume
            (4) EF
         (c) Detect ventricular aneurysms
         (d) Evaluate mitral, aortic valves
         (e) Demonstrate ventricular-level left-to-right intracardiac shunts (VSD)
   d. Aortography
      i. Technique: Contrast injected into aortic root or descending aorta
      ii. To assess: Aortic valve insufficiency, aneurysms or dissections of ascending aorta, coarctation of the aorta, diseases of the aorta, presence of saphenous vein grafts, presence of PDA
   e. Coronary arteriography
      i. Radiopaque contrast material injected into the ostia of the LCA and RCA, allowing multiple views and recordings of coronary arterial circulation
         (a) To assess the extent of significant CAD by identifying the presence and severity of lesions
         (b) To guide therapeutic options in ischemic heart disease
         (c) To assess possible coronary arterial spasm
         (d) To administer intracoronary thrombolytics and medications
         (e) To perform transcatheter interventional procedures: PCI, coronary stent placement, atherectomy, and percutaneous transluminal coronary angioplasty (PTCA)
   f. Complications of diagnostic cardiac catheterization
      i. Death
      ii. MI
      iii. Neurologic events (stroke)
      iv. Acute renal failure or oliguria caused by contrast medium and inadequate hydration
      v. Transient cardiac arrhythmias, bradycardia, conduction disturbances

      vi. Hemorrhage or hematoma at insertion site

     vii. Allergic reactions to contrast medium

    viii. Arterial perforation, thrombosis, embolus, and dissection

     ix. Hypovolemia (because of diuresis from contrast medium and nothing-by-mouth [NPO] status)

  g. Additional procedures that may be done during cardiac catheterization include:

      i. Rotoblation of a blocked artery

     ii. Cardiac implant closure devices (such as closure of some congenital heart defect)

    iii. Treatment of some heart valves defects (such as a MitraClip for mitral valve regurgitation)

     iv. Permanent and temporary pacemaker implantations

PATIENT CARE

1. **Acute chest pain (refer to Assessment Section)**

  a. Assess the subjective and objective data (as discussed in previous section)

  b. Interprofessional collaboration: Nurse, physician, advanced practice provider, pharmacist, occupational and physical therapists, dietitian, social worker

  c. Interventions

      i. Ask the patient to notify the nurse immediately at the onset of chest discomfort or other associated symptoms of distress. Stress the importance of early recognition and treatment of chest discomfort.

     ii. Administer oxygen per unit protocol

    iii. Check vital signs, monitor ECG

     iv. Do a 12-lead ECG immediately

      v. Ensure that the patient has a patent IV line

     vi. Administer and titrate medications to alleviate angina (see Specific Patient Health Problems)

    vii. Notify the provider

    viii. Collaborate with the provider on medication needs (types, dosages, frequency, and route) and titrations and adjustments of medications, depending on the patient response

     ix. Monitor the patient's pain

       (a) Assess quality, duration, intensity, frequency of the pain

       (b) Assess the effectiveness of medications

       (c) Look for trends and medication interactions and identify other possible comfort measures

      x. Provide other comfort interventions as appropriate

     xi. Alert the provider if pain continues so that further actions can be determined. Cardiac pain means the myocardium is in jeopardy, and immediate interventions are needed.

  d. Monitoring and management of patient care

      i. Chest pain or possible acute coronary syndrome (ACS) without objective evidence of myocardial ischemia (nonischemic initial ECG and normal cardiac troponin) may be observed in a chest pain unit or telemetry unit with serial ECGs and cardiac troponin at 3- to 6-hour intervals (see specific health problems section for ACS). Continuous ST segment monitoring should be used (see AACN's Practice Alert: Ensuring Accurate ST-Segment Monitoring at https://www.aacn.org/clinical-resources/practice-alerts/st-segment-monitoring).

ii. Chest pain or possible ACS with normal serial ECGs and cardiac troponins should have a treadmill ECG, stress myocardial perfusion imaging, or stress echocardiography, before discharge or within 72 hours after discharge

iii. For patients with chest pain or possible ACS and a normal ECG, normal cardiac troponins, and no history of CAD, it is reasonable to initially to use a coronary CT angiography to assess coronary artery anatomy or rest myocardial perfusion imaging with technetium

2. **Decreased CO**

   a. Description of problem: Decreased CO can be caused by either mechanical or electrical cardiac dysfunction.

   b. Goals of care

      i. Work of the heart is decreased by decreasing myocardial oxygen demands

      ii. Myocardial oxygen supply is increased (minimizing ischemia, size of infarct)

      iii. Hemodynamics are normal: CO is adequate

      iv. Heart rate is controlled, and arrhythmias are eliminated

      v. Patient is free of chest pain

      vi. Patient has normal urinary output

   c. Interprofessional collaboration: Nurse, physician, advanced practice providers, pharmacist, physical therapist.

   d. Interventions

      i. Monitor and frequently assess for signs and symptoms of decreased CO. Findings can include the following:

         (a) Changes in the patient's hemodynamics: Blood pressure, heart rate, CO

         (b) ECG changes or arrhythmias

         (c) Chest pain

         (d) Weakness, fatigue, dizziness

         (e) Shortness of breath, dyspnea, crackles

         (f) Cold and clammy skin, cyanosis, pallor

         (g) Decreased peripheral pulses

         (h) Decreased or absent urinary output (oliguria, anuria)

         (i) Diminished mentation or loss of consciousness

         (j) Jugular vein distention

3. **Activity intolerance**

   a. Description of problem: Because of cardiac dysfunction, the patient may exhibit the following clinical findings, reflecting a decreased tolerance for the activities of daily living:

      i. Fatigue, weakness

      ii. Dyspnea with progressively less exertion

      iii. Leg cramps

      iv. Discomfort in chest, neck, jaw, shoulder, arm

      v. Increased heart rate and/or BP

      vi. Arrhythmias

      vii. ST-segment and T-wave changes signifying ischemia

   b. Goals of care

      i. Cause is identified and treated

      ii. Patient engages in progressive ambulation

      iii. No complications of bed rest are present (skin intact, breath sounds clear, no signs of deep venous thromboembolism)

      iv. Patient is educated regarding the need for lifestyle modifications, diet, exercise, and weight control (as needed)

    c. Interprofessional collaboration: Nurse, advanced practice providers, physicians (specialists include cardiologist), physical and occupational therapists; cardiac rehabilitation nurse for activity plans in hospital and after discharge; social worker to assist with home equipment acquisition, home visits, nursing home placement (temporary or permanent); dietitian

    d. Interventions

      i. Assess and document the patient's response to progressive ambulation, including monitoring of heart rate and rhythm, respiration, and BP

      ii. Assist the patient with initial increases in ambulation

      iii. Administer pain medication, as needed, before planned ambulation (if the patient is pain free, progression in ambulation will be more successful)

      iv. Plan rest periods between various treatments, visits, and ambulation

      v. Teach the patient how to progress safely: Instruct in correct positioning and efficient use of body for each step

        (a) Active range-of-motion exercises

        (b) Dangling

        (c) Transfers from bed to chair or bedside commode

        (d) Ambulation in room and hallway

      vi. Ensure that the patient is instructed with regard to the availability and use of special equipment to assist in ambulation (walkers, canes, wheelchairs), if needed

      vii. If the patient becomes unstable (ischemic pain, vital signs beyond set limits, arrhythmias), help the patient back to bed and immediately evaluate the need for oxygen, medications (e.g., nitrates, antiarrhythmics), ECG, notification of the physician, emergency equipment

      viii. Arrange consultations with other health professionals, as appropriate

      ix. Encourage the patient and family to openly express feelings and ask questions regarding the ability to ambulate and lifestyle resumption and changes

4. **Inadequate knowledge of cardiac diagnosis, medications, or treatment**

    a. Description of problem

      i. Patient and/or family verbalizations indicate a lack of knowledge or inappropriate or incorrect information

      ii. Patient does not adhere with the recommended regimen, which resulted in incorrect or inappropriate care at home

      iii. Patient is easily agitated, hostile, worried, suspicious (because of misinformation, misunderstanding, or misinterpretation)

      iv. Patient and/or family is unable to plan realistic goals or home care

    b. Goals of care

      i. Patient (and family) verbalizes an understanding of the diagnosis, medications, treatment, and follow-up care

      ii. Patient demonstrates proper home care techniques

    c. Interprofessional collaboration: See Acute Chest Pain

    d. Interventions

      i. Identify learning needs

      ii. Assess readiness to learn (the patient is alert, pain free, not sleep deprived; information is not given immediately after sedatives are administered)

      iii. Determine the best methods for the patient to learn (group, one-to-one, videos)

      iv. Reinforce learning with the use of printed materials related to the disease, discharge instructions, procedures, and medications

v. Instruction sheets should be available in languages other than English

vi. Arrange for an interpreter if the patient does not understand English

vii. Document teaching and the patient's response

viii. Arrange appropriate consults: Cardiac rehabilitation; dietary, occupational, and physical therapy; home health; social work

ix. Schedule practice and return demonstrations of psychomotor skills

SPECIFIC PATIENT HEALTH PROBLEMS

ACUTE CORONARY SYNDROME

a. ACS is a term that refers to a spectrum of conditions including:
   i. Acute MI or STEMI
   ii. Q wave MI and non-Q Wave MI
   iii. Non-ST elevation MI (NSTEMI)
   iv. Unstable angina (UA)
   v. Non-ST elevation acute coronary syndromes (NSTE-ACS)

At presentation, patients with UA and NSTEMI can be indistinguishable and are therefore considered the same in the American Heart Association/American College of Cardiology (AHA/ACC) 2014 practice guidelines.

b. The leading symptom of ACS is chest pain.

c. A 12-lead ECG should be performed and interpreted within 10 minutes of symptom onset. Based on the ECG interpretation, the diagnosis is differentiated as either:

1. **MI or STEMI = ST-elevation is present on 12-lead ECG**
   a. MI may also have a new left bundle-branch block
   b. A true posterior MI is an exception and is an MI with no ST elevation

2. **NSTE-ACS = the absence of persistent ST-elevation and can be further subdivided based on cardiac biomarkers of necrosis (e.g., cardiac troponin)**

EXPERT TIP

Approximately 70% of patients presenting with an ACS have unstable angina or NSTEMI.

---

a. NSTEMI = elevated troponin

b. UA = no elevation of troponin or other biomarkers

ACUTE MYOCARDIAL INFARCTION—ST-SEGMENT ELEVATION MYOCARDIAL INFARCTION

KEY CONCEPT

The location of the STEMI is determined by identifying ST elevation patterns on the 12-lead ECG (see Table 4.7).

---

1. **Pathophysiology (see also Coronary Artery Disease)**
   a. Blood flow may be obstructed acutely by a thrombus in the coronary artery
   b. Site and amount of necrosis depend on the location of the arterial occlusion, on collateral circulation, and on the previous occurrence of any infarctions or disease
   c. Extent of necrosis
      i. Transmural: Full-thickness (endocardium to epicardium) STEMI
      ii. Nontransmural: Non-Q wave (subendocardial)

2. Etiology and risk factors

a. Approximately 30% of patients with STEMI are women, and 23% of U.S. patients with STEMI have diabetes mellitus.

b. Pathology of an MI is defined as myocardial cell death because of prolonged ischemia.

c. The most common reason is related to unstable atherosclerotic plaque that results in coronary occlusion. Some other causes may include:

   i. Coronary artery spasm

   ii. Severe anemia (decreased oxygen supply)

   iii. Severe aortic stenosis

   iv. Other causes include hyperthyroidism, emboli (endocarditis, atrial fibrillation), trauma, dissection, drugs (cocaine)

d. Additional precipitating factors include acute hypotension, ventricular tachyarrhythmia

e. Risk factors: Major risk factors include smoking, hypertension, dyslipidemia, physical inactivity, obesity, diabetes mellitus, and recreational drugs, such as cocaine (also see Coronary Artery Disease)

3. Signs and symptoms

a. Patient history continues to be the most important factor in differentiating the MI diagnosis.

b. Chest pain is a significant symptom, but approximately one-third of patients with MI experience symptoms other than chest pain.

> **EXPERT TIP**
> The chest pain associated with an MI may be differentiated from angina if the pain lasts longer than 20 minutes and is unrelieved with rest or nitrates.

c. Pain may radiate to neck, jaw, arms, and back. These areas may be the only locations of discomfort.

d. Other findings vary with the size and extent of the infarction, the patient's status, and the history of previous MI. They may include:

   i. Pallor, diaphoretic, cool, clammy skin

   ii. Weakness, light-headedness

   iii. Vagal effects, such as bradycardia, nausea, and vomiting

   iv. Dyspnea (most common presentation in the older adult)

   v. Palpitations and arrhythmias, irregular, pulse (slow, fast, and/or thready)

   vi. Low, normal, or high BP

   vii. Anxiety, apprehension, nervousness, and a new history of sleep disturbance

4. Diagnostic study findings

a. ECG: Most important diagnostic tool; changes on ECG correlate with the location of the necrosis or injury (see Table 4.7)

   i. ST elevation (>1 mm in limb leads or >2 mm in chest leads)

   ii. Abnormal Q wave

     (a) More than 0.04 second in duration (0.03 second for inferior MI)

     (b) Appears within hours of transmural MI

     (c) Other causes of Q waves

       (1) Normal Q waves: small Q wave in leads I, aVL, V_5, V_6, aVR

       (2) Normal Q wave in lead III: Less than 0.03 second, decreased with inspiration

       (3) Left bundle branch block (LBBB)

       (4) Myocarditis, cardiomyopathy

> **EXPERT TIP**
> Caution in LBBB. New LBBB should be regarded as a sign of acute MI and treated as such until proven otherwise. In addition, the presence of ST and T wave changes related to preexisting LBBB can confuse interpretation.

    iii. Serial ECGs are essential, along with those done during ischemic pain

  b. Serial cardiac isoenzymes

    i. Troponin levels (cardiac troponin T or I) are more than 0.1 ng/mL in NSTEMI within 2 to 6 hours of symptom onset and myocardial injury (false elevations may occur in renal insufficiency). The 99th percentile cutoff point at 0.01 ng/mL is well established for troponin T, but varies slightly based on assay used for troponin I.

    ii. CK-MB isoenzyme levels elevated within 6 hours. May be dissipated if 24 hours since the onset of symptoms. CK-MB levels have dramatic elevation with reperfusion therapy and decrease quickly.

    iii. Myoglobin

    iv. Leukocytosis (large MI) because of stress and tissue necrosis; peaks 2 to 4 days after the infarction

  c. Echocardiography: Assesses LV function, wall motion abnormalities, and complications, such as VSD, thrombi, aneurysms, mitral regurgitation, and pericardial effusions, but this should not hold up cardiac catheterization or PCI

  d. Coronary catheterization: This is both diagnostic and a treatment when the catheterization is used for coronary intervention (see treatments for more detail and Figs. 4.11 and 4.12).

5. **Interprofessional collaboration: Nurse, physicians (cardiologist and possibly cardiac surgeon), advanced practice providers, physical and occupational therapists, social worker, cardiac rehabilitation team, dietitian, pharmacist, and respiratory therapy and/or perfusionist may be involved.**

6. **Management of patient care (Fig. 4.13)**

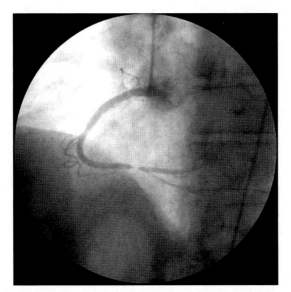

Fig. 4.11 Stenosis of the right coronary artery before percutaneous coronary intervention. (Courtesy Dr. Steve Ramee, Ochsner Clinic Foundation.)

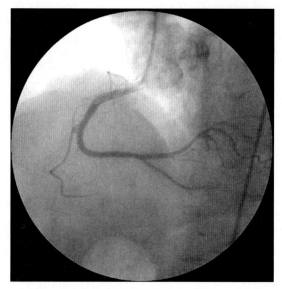

Fig. 4.12 Right coronary artery revascularization after percutaneous coronary intervention with a coronary stent procedure. (Courtesy Dr. Steve Ramee, Ochsner Clinic Foundation.)

KEY CONCEPT

The priority is revascularization: Minimize time to PCI therapy or thrombolytic to increase survival and preservation of myocardial function. PCI should occur within 90 minutes or less. If patient transfer to a PCI-capable hospital is needed, the goal is 120 minutes or less.

---

   a. Place the patient on a monitor. Monitor at least two leads (e.g., lead II and a V lead), watching closely for ST segment changes (elevations, depressions, or return to baseline). Monitor for arrhythmias, because VF is common in the early hours of MI.

   b. Oxygen: 2 to 4 L/min to keep oxygen saturation above 90%. Hypoxemia is caused by ventilation-perfusion mismatch and LV failure.

   c. Primary PCI is the recommended method of reperfusion, with a goal of 90 minutes from symptom onset (see Box 4.3 for PCI care).

   d. Patients with STEMI at non–PCI-capable hospitals should be administered fibrinolytic therapy (in the absence of contraindications, see Box 4.4 when the anticipated PCI-capable hospital exceeds 120 minutes).

   e. Ensure that the patient has at least two good IV sites for administration of medications, volume support, and reperfusion therapy.

   f. Pain management: Relieve discomfort with analgesics

     i. Relief of pain decreases elevated sympathetic response and myocardial workload (lowering heart rate and BP) and counters the arrhythmic effect of circulating catecholamines

     ii. Morphine sulfate: 2 to 4 mg IV every 5 minutes to relieve pain

       (a) Decrease dosages in the older adult and in patients with respiratory disease

       (b) Respiratory depression with morphine sulfate usually peaks 7 minutes after IV injection and is dose related (not usually a problem in patients with MI)

       (c) Orthostatic hypotension can result from volume depletion: Provide volume support

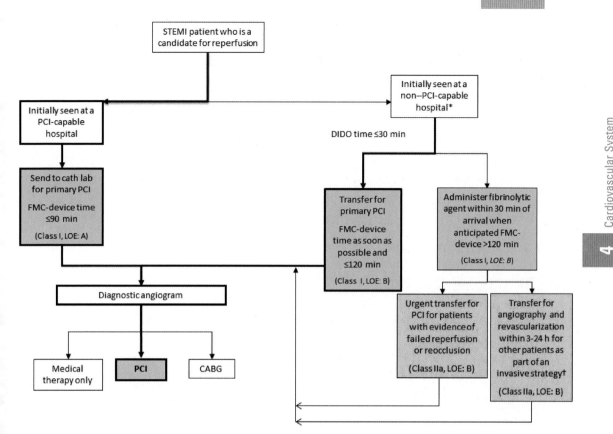

Fig. 4.13 Reperfusion therapy for patients with STEMI. The *bold arrows* and *boxes* are the preferred strategies. Performance of PCI is dictated by an anatomically appropriate culprit stenosis. *Patients with cardiogenic shock or severe heart failure initially seen at a non–PCI-capable hospital should be transferred for cardiac catheterization and revascularization as soon as possible, irrespective of time delay from MI onset (Class I, LOE: B). †Angiography and revascularization should not be performed within the first 2 to 3 hours after administration of fibrinolytic therapy. *CABG*, Coronary artery bypass graft; *DIDO*, door-in–door-out; *FMC*, first medical contact; *LOE*, Level of evidence; *MI*, myocardial infarction; *PCI*, percutaneous coronary intervention; *STEMI*, ST-elevation myocardial infarction. (From O'Gara, P.T., Kushner, F.G., Ascheim, D.D., et al. (2013). 2013 ACCF/AHA Guideline for the Management of ST-Elevation Myocardial Infarction: A Report of the American College of Cardiology Foundation/American Heart Association Task Force on Practice Guidelines. *Journal of the American College of Cardiology*, 61(4), e78-e140.)

      (d) Naloxone, 0.4 mg IV (repeated up to 3 times at 3-minute intervals), may be given to counteract narcotic-induced depressed respirations and hypotension

    iii. Remind the patient to notify the nurse immediately if discomfort reoccurs

  g. Pharmacology

EXPERT TIP

Use caution if street drugs are suspected in causing cardiac event, especially stimulators, such as cocaine, methamphetamine, or synthetic drugs. If so, use caution with beta-blockers, as there is a risk of unopposed alpha-agonist response. Goal is PCI, and thrombolytics are contraindicated in cases of severe hypertension, aortic dissection, seizures, or intracerebral hemorrhage.

BOX 4.4	**Contraindications and Cautions for the Use of Fibrinolysis in ST-Segment Elevation Myocardial Infarction[a]**

ABSOLUTE CONTRAINDICATIONS

- Any previous intracranial hemorrhage
- Known structural cerebral vascular lesion (e.g., arteriovenous malformation)
- Known malignant intracranial neoplasm (primary or metastatic)
- Ischemic stroke within 3 months except acute ischemic stroke within 4.5 hours
- Suspected aortic dissection
- Active bleeding or bleeding diathesis (excluding menses)
- Significant closed-head or facial trauma within 3 months
- Intracranial or intraspinal surgery within 2 months
- Severe uncontrolled hypertension (unresponsive to emergency therapy)
- For streptokinase, previous treatment within the previous 6 months

RELATIVE CONTRAINDICATIONS

- History of chronic, severe, poorly controlled hypertension
- Significant hypertension at initial evaluation (SBP >180 mm Hg or DBP >110 mm Hg)[b]
- History of previous ischemic stroke >3 months
- Dementia
- Known intracranial pathology not covered in Absolute Contraindications, Traumatic or prolonged (>10 minutes) cardiopulmonary resuscitation
- Major surgery (≤3 weeks)
- Recent internal bleeding (within 2–4 weeks)
- Noncompressible vascular punctures
- Pregnancy
- Active peptic ulcer
- Oral anticoagulant therapy

[a]Viewed as advisory for clinical decision making and may not be all-inclusive or definitive.
[b]Could be an absolute contraindication in low-risk patients with MI.
DBP, Diastolic blood pressure; *SBP*, systolic blood pressure.
From O'Gara, P.T., Kushner, F.G., Ascheim, D.D., et al. (2013). 2013 ACCF/AHA guideline for the management of ST-elevation myocardial infarction: a report of the American College of Cardiology Foundation/American Heart Association Task Force on Practice Guidelines. *Journal of American College of Cardiology*, 61, e78.

    i. The goal for all treatments is early primary PCI, and availability and timing of this procedure dictates pharmacology intervention. For adjunctive antithrombotic and antiplatelet therapy to support reperfusion with primary PCI (Table 4.9). If PCI is not available and antithrombotic therapy is used (Table 4.10).

    ii. Antiemetics (e.g., droperidol) may be needed because of the high degree of acute vagal tone with MI and the emetic side effects of opiate analgesia.

    iii. Anxiolytics may be used if the patient is agitated, delirious, or very anxious, or experiences sleep deprivation.

    iv. Nitroglycerin (NTG): Rapid-acting nitrate

        (a) Actions

            (1) Dilates veins and arteries

            (2) Decreases venous return by systemic pooling of blood: Decreases preload

            (3) Reduces myocardial oxygen demand and consumption

            (4) Relieves coronary artery spasm

        (b) Dosages

            (1) Sublingually 0.4 mg every 5 minutes; up to three doses

            (2) IV drip started at 5 to 10 mcg/min. Titrate until pain is relieved or adverse side effects occur (hypotension).

TABLE 4.9 Select Pharmacologic Antiplatelet and Anticoagulant Therapies

Medication/Medication Class	Actions	Administration and Dosing	Comments
ANTIPLATELET AGENTS			
Aspirin	Antiplatelet and antiinflammatory properties	Initial dosing of 162 to 325 mg, nonenteric coated, taken as soon as possible after symptom onset in patients with acute coronary syndrome (ACS) Daily doses of 75 to 162 mg for long-term treatment after percutaneous coronary intervention (PCI)	• Reduced toxicity (e.g., bleeding, gastrointestinal [GI] distress) at lower doses
Adenosine diphosphate (ADP) antagonists (e.g., clopidogrel, cangrelor, prasugrel, ticagrelor, ticlopidine)	Inhibition of $P2Y_{12}$ receptor activation leading to inhibition of platelet aggregation	Clopidogrel • Loading dose of 300-600 mg, followed by 75 mg once daily • Daily dose of 75 mg is given for up to 1 yr (or longer for those not experiencing a bleeding complication) after PCI	• If patient needs coronary artery bypass graft, clopidogrel ideally should be withheld for 5 to 10 days before surgery to minimize bleeding complications • Option for patients intolerant to aspirin (allergy, GI disturbances, bleeding disorders)
		Cangrelor • For use as an adjunct to PCI: 30 mcg/kg IV bolus administered prior to PCI followed immediately by 4 mcg/kg/min continuous IV infusion continued at least 2 hours or for the duration of PCI, whichever is longer	• An oral $P2Y_{12}$ inhibitor should be administered in follow-up to maintain platelet inhibition
		Prasugrel • ***Adults <75 years old ≥60 kg:*** 60 mg oral loading dose, then 10 mg once daily • ***Adults <75 years old <60 kg:*** 60 mg oral loading dose, then 5 mg once daily	• Use in patients 75 years and older is generally not recommended • Optimal duration of therapy is not known • Recommended patients also take 75-325 mg/day of aspirin
		Ticagrelor • For patients with ACS (including those undergoing PCI), 180 mg loading dose plus 325 mg aspirin, then starting 12 hours after the loading dose, 90 mg twice daily plus 75-100 mg aspirin daily for 1 year • After 1 year, 60 mg twice daily plus aspirin recommended	• Avoid maintenance aspirin doses above 100 mg/day due to reduced efficacy of ticagrelor
		Ticlopidine • Requires several days of therapy before reaching maximum effectiveness • Daily dose of 250 mg bid	• AHA/ACC preferentially recommend use of clopidogrel over ticlopidine for treatment of ACS due to a better safety profile and shorter onset of action • Routine blood monitoring (platelet and white blood cell counts) required when taking medication to identify neutropenia (occurs in 2% of patients), thrombotic thrombocytopenic purpura (occurs in 0.03%, more fatal)

TABLE 4.9 Select Pharmacologic Antiplatelet and Anticoagulant Therapies—cont'd

Medication/Medication Class	Actions	Administration and Dosing	Comments
Glycoprotein IIb/IIIa inhibitors: (e.g., eptifibatide, tirofiban, abciximab)	Prevent binding of von Willebrand factor and fibrinogen, combating platelet aggregation Significantly reduce death or myocardial infarction in short term Used with aspirin and heparin for patients who undergo early PCI, or are at high risk for intervention	Administered IV only for set time periods and at set dosages (before, during, and after PCI) Present dosing regimens: Eptifibatide: 180 mcg/kg bolus, then 2 mcg/kg/min for 72 to 96 hr Tirofiban: 25 mcg/kg IV within 5 minutes followed by 0.15 mcg/kg/minute for up to 18 hours. Abciximab: 0.25 mcg/kg bolus, then 0.125 mcg/kg/min (max 10 mcg/min) for 12 to 24 hr	Oral glycoprotein IIb-IIIa receptor inhibitors have not proven effective or safe to date
ANTICOAGULANT AGENTS			
Unfractionated heparin (UFH)		For UFH, a weight-based dose is given, 60 to 70 units/kg intravenous (IV) bolus (maximum 5000 units) • Initially 12 to 15 units/kg/hr (maximum 1000 units/hr) to reach activated partial thromboplastin time (aPTT) goal of 1.5 to 2 times control	Close blood monitoring required routinely (every 6 hr until therapeutic level reached and with dosage changes) to ensure tight aPTT goal maintenance control Given in conjunction with aspirin (unless contraindicated) Monitor for heparin-induced thrombocytopenia
Low-molecular-weight heparins (LMWH) (e.g., enoxaparin, dalteparin)		Enoxaparin • Administered 1 mg/kg subcutaneously every 12 hr Dalteparin • 120 units/kg subcutaneously every 12 hr	• Advantages: Avoidance of need for close blood monitoring, less likely to induce thrombocytopenia • Disadvantages: More frequent minor bleeding events are seen with its use

Data from O'Gara P.T., Kushner F.G., Ascheim D.D., et al. (2013) ACCF/AHA guideline for the management of ST-elevation myocardial infarction: a report of the American College of Cardiology Foundation/American Heart Association Task Force on Practice Guidelines. *Journal of the American College of Cardiology*, 61(4), e78–e140; Amsterdam E.A., Wenger N.K., Brindis R.G., et al. (2014). AHA/ACC guideline for the management of patients with non–ST-elevation acute coronary syndromes: a report of the American College of Cardiology/ American Heart Association Task Force on Practice Guidelines *Journal of the American College of Cardiology*, 64:e139–e228; Kumbhani DJ, Cannon CP, Beavers CJ, et al. (2020). ACC Expert Consensus Decision Pathway for Anticoagulant and Antiplatelet Therapy in Patients with Atrial Fibrillation or Venus Thromboembolism Undergoing Percutaneous Coronary Intervention or With Atherosclerotic Cardiovascular Disease. *Journal of the American College of Cardiology*, 77(6), 629-658, 2021

Clinical Pharmacology powered by ClinicalKey. www.clinicalkey.com.

TABLE 4.10 Thrombolytic Agents

Thrombotic Agent	Dose	Comments

Tenecteplase (TNK-tPA) (TNKase)	• Half-life is 90–130 minutes
	• Weight-based single IV bolus:
	  • 30 mg for weight <60 kg
	  • 35 mg for 60–69 kg
	  • 40 mg for 70–79 kg
	  • 45 mg for 80–89 kg
	  • 50 mg for >90 kg (max)
		• Single dose
		• Binds to fibrin and converts tissue plasminogen to plasmin, promoting fibrinolysis
		• The most fibrin specific of the thrombolytic agents

Reteplase (rPA)	Half-life: 13–16 minutes • Dosage: 10 million unit bolus; repeat in 30 minutes	• Two IV doses • Fibrin specific but less strong than TNK-tPA
Alteplase (tPA)	• Initial plasma Half-life: <5 minutes • 90-minute weight-based infusion Dosage: For weight >67 kg: • 15-mg bolus • Follow with 50 mg infusion over 30 minutes • Then 35 mg over 60 minutes For weight ≤67 kg: • 15-mg bolus • Follow with 0.75-mg/kg infusion over 30 minutes (not >50 mg) • Then 0.5 mg/kg over 60 minutes (not >35 mg) • Maximum dose = 100 mg	• tPA: tissue-type plasminogen activator • Fibrin specific but less strong than thromboplastin time of 50–75 seconds • Aspirin also given • Contraindicated with gentamicin allergy (medication used in preparation of t-PA)TNK-tPA • Complex dosing schedule • Concurrent heparin required to avoid reocclusion (goal is partial thromboplastin time of 50–75 sec)

Note: When thrombolytics are given for ST-segment elevation myocardial infarction (STEMI), the patient should receive anticoagulant therapy for a minimum of 48 hours, and preferably for the duration of the index hospitalization up to 8 days or until revascularization if performed. These could be unfractionated heparin (UFH), Enoxaparin or Fondaparinux. (Please see ACC/AHA guidelines for management of STEMI).

Note: IV fibrinolytic treatment not recommended in patients with NSTE-ACS (Amsterdam et al., 2014).

From O'Gara, P.T., Kushner, F.G., Ascheim, D.D., et al. (2013). 2013 ACCF/AHA guideline for the management of ST-elevation myocardial infarction: a report of the American College of Cardiology Foundation/American Heart Association Task Force on Practice Guidelines. *Journal of the American College of Cardiology*, 61(4), e78–e140; Amsterdam, E.A., Wenger, N.K., Brindis, R.G., et al. (2014). AHA/ACC guideline for the management of patients with non–ST-elevation acute coronary syndromes: a report of the American College of Cardiology/American Heart Association Task Force on Practice Guidelines. *Journal of the American College of Cardiology*, 64:e139–e228.

EXPERT TIP

Ask the patient if they have taken phosphodiesterase-5 inhibitors (PDE-5), such as sildenafil (Viagra) within 24 hours. The combined vasodilatory effects may cause severe hypotension.

a) Do not stop IV NTG abruptly. Wean gradually; observe for returning symptoms. Once dosage is 10 mcg/min, stop NTG after 15 minutes.

b) Side effects include hypotension, headache, sweating, nausea, tachycardia, and bradycardia.

c) Patients often develop tolerance of NTG's hemodynamic effects after 12 to 24 hours of administration. Infusion rate may need to be adjusted with continued use. If an NTG patch is used, it may be discontinued for 8 to 12 hours each day (usually at nighttime).

v. β-blockers: Reduce myocardial ischemia and increase hospital survival rates. Usually IV β-blockers (e.g., metoprolol) are given initially to ensure rapid lowering of heart rate, BP.

     vi. ACE inhibitors: For patients with anterior MI, pulmonary congestion, LV EF of less than 40% (unless systolic BP [SBP] is <100 mm Hg). Contraindicated in renal failure.

     vii. ARBs: For patients intolerant of ACE inhibitors

     viii. Stool softeners

     ix. Statins: Lipid-lowering therapy: Used to lower overall risk of atherosclerotic cardiovascular disease rather than a specific goal number. In addition, lifestyle modifications are vital to managing lipid control.

  h. Positioning

     i. Maintain bed rest for the first 12 hours; then use of a chair or bedside commode in the first 24 hours (follow facility protocol/provider orders)

     ii. Increase ambulation in room as tolerated during the first 48 hours

  i. Nutrition

     i. Keep the patient on NPO status until the PCI procedure is completed or until discomfort or pain is gone, then give clear liquids and progress the diet

     ii. Feed a low-fat, low-sodium diet

     iii. Earlier "coronary precautions" have now been abandoned (e.g., restriction of hot and cold fluids, avoidance of caffeine; regular caffeine drinkers develop tolerance and can experience withdrawal symptoms of increased heart rate or headaches; several cups of coffee have no ill effects)

  j. Discharge planning

     i. Teaching issues include the rationales for and descriptions of therapy, methods for treating discomfort or pain at home

     ii. Stress smoking cessation after MI. Patient may need nicotine replacement if he or she is a heavy smoker or has withdrawal symptoms.

     iii. Discharge planning following PCI (see Box 4.3)

  k. Psychosocial issues: Aggressive risk factor modification and lifestyle changes are necessary. Barriers and challenges to these goals need to be identified. Reduction of emotional stressors may improve long-term prognosis.

     i. Denial or depression are emotions many patients exhibit, both before admission and during hospitalization

     ii. Flexible visiting hours can assist in relieving anxiety and other stress that can create a situation promoting pain occurrence (depending on the patient's status, need for rest, procedures, and family dynamics)

7. **Treatment requiring intervention or surgery**

  a. Cardiac catheterization and primary PCI: Catheterization to evaluate severity of coronary artery occlusions and attempt to improve or restore coronary blood flow with angioplasty and/or stenting to open the occluded artery and limit myocardial necrosis

     i. PTCA

       (a) Balloon catheter is placed across stenosis and inflated to enlarge the lumen diameter by mechanically compressing and splitting plaque

     ii. Coronary stent placement

       (a) Devices are placed intraluminally to achieve maximal lumen size and maintain the patency of the vessel's lumen. Many PCI procedures include some form of stenting with PTCA.

       (b) Stents are made from various metals

       (c) Drug-eluting stents (DES): Made of synthetic materials with the ability to deliver medications that significantly decrease intimal hyperplasia and in-stent restenosis

iii. Key concepts for nursing care after PCI procedure and for discharge (see Box 4.3)
iv. Potential complications of PCIs
    (a) Vascular site complications
    (b) Recurrent pain: Restenosis
        (1) Mechanism of restenosis: Postprocedure, thrombosis is the cause of early reocclusion. Factors associated with increased risk of restenosis include multivessel CAD, proximal LAD stenosis, diabetes, and final lumen diameter of less than 100%.
        (2) Management: Follow interventions for acute chest pain (see earlier Acute Chest Pain under Patient Care and later Acute Coronary Syndrome section). PCI or CABG may be indicated.
    (c) Iodine contrast reaction
        (1) Mechanism: Allergic reaction (itching, rash, laryngospasm, swelling, or anaphylaxis)
        (2) Management: Treat with diphenhydramine (Benadryl) 25 to 50 mg PO/IM/IV, epinephrine 0.5 to 1 mL (1:1000 IV), IV steroids
    (d) Acute coronary occlusion
        (1) Mechanism: Results from dissection
        (2) Management: Emergency CABG
    (e) Myocardial ischemia or injury (including STEMI or NSTEMI)
v. Thrombolysis (see Table 4.10 and Box 4.4): IV thrombolytics are used if primary PCI is not available and are used as soon as possible (in the emergency department, EMS, critical care unit)
vi. Intraaortic balloon pump (IABP) or other devices may be necessary for severe hypotension or cardiogenic shock, especially in patients with low CO and ongoing ischemia (see Mechanical Circulatory Support). IABP is used during MI for the following:
    (a) Acute mitral regurgitation
    (b) Refractory ventricular arrhythmias
    (c) Post-MI angina
    (d) As a bridge to revascularization
b. CABG: Surgical revascularization of the myocardium with bypass grafting
  i. Venous graft
    (a) Saphenous vein from leg used to create a conduit. One end of the graft is sewn onto the aorta and the other end is sewn onto the affected coronary artery distal to the obstruction.
    (b) Failure rates are higher than with arterial grafts; as high as 25% within the first year
    (c) Failure rate after 1 year increases at a rate of 2% to 5% per year
  ii. Arterial graft
    (a) Left internal mammary artery (LIMA) is most common site; radial artery and right internal mammary artery (RIMA) are often used as secondary sources for additional grafts or if LIMA is a poor conduit
    (b) In IMA grafts, proximal artery remains attached to the subclavian artery from which it arises and the distal end is dissected from the anterior chest wall and sewn onto the coronary artery distal to the obstruction.
    (c) The 10-year patency rate is around 98%.

    (d) In case of radial artery grafts, preoperative evaluation of ulnar artery flow is essential to ensure that perfusion to the hand will be adequate following removal of the radial artery

    (e) Radial artery grafts at increased risk for spasm; patients may be placed on long acting nitrates or calcium channel blockers for up to 1 year

  iii. Complications during surgery: Complications may occur during the surgery or postoperatively. These may include MI, cardiac arrest, stroke, renal failure, death, reoperation, or new mechanical support.

  iv. Immediate postoperative complications

EXPERT TIP

Because of the effects of cardiopulmonary bypass on the heart and vasculature, hemodynamic instability and myocardial stunning are common in the first 24 hours after CABG. Close monitoring and prompt interventions are required to avoid life-threatening complications.

    (a) Low CO, hypotension: Because of inadequate volume replacement, fluid shifts (third spacing), hemorrhage; can decrease systemic perfusion, affecting the kidneys, brain, and heart

    (b) Hemorrhage

    (c) Hypertension (increased afterload decreases CO)

    (d) Cardiac tamponade: Suspect if decreased CO and hypotension are present with increased CVP (unless hypovolemic), narrowed pulse pressure, distended jugular veins, pulsus paradoxus, distant heart sounds

    (e) Arrhythmias: Caused by electrolyte imbalances, hypoxemia, medication toxicity, hypothermia, anesthesia, pulmonary artery catheters, and intraoperative damage to the electrical conduction pathways. Atrial fibrillation is common (15%–40% of patients undergoing CABG; 37%–50% of patients undergoing isolated valve surgeries; as high as 60% of patients undergoing combined CABG and valve procedures).

    (f) Respiratory failure: Associated with hypoxemia, alveolar hypoventilation

    (g) Prerenal azotemia: Caused by decreased CO, hypovolemia

    (h) Electrolyte imbalances: Hypokalemia, hypocalcemia, hypomagnesemia (common)

    (i) Graft closure: Can be prevented by antiplatelet aggregation therapy with risk factor modification

  v. Early extubation (usually within 6 hours) should be anticipated once the patient meets weaning criteria

  vi. Agents commonly used after CABG

    (a) Volume support (e.g., volume expander, and/or whole and packed red blood cells): To increase the preload, elevate CVP, increase SBP if it falls below predetermined parameters, and increase the HCT

    (b) Medications for acute management: See Heart Failure

    (c) Antiarrhythmic agents often administered prophylactically to decrease the incidence of atrial fibrillation

  c. Ventricular assist device (VAD): See Heart Failure

8. Potential complications of MI

  a. Postinfarction pain (persistent, recurrent)

    i. Mechanism: Common causes are ischemia, reinfarction, pericarditis (Dressler syndrome). Pericarditis does not occur in the first 24 hours.

    ii. Management

       (a) When pain is present, obtain an ECG and compare with previous ECGs

       (b) Pain recurring after MI suggests ongoing ischemia and should be treated promptly

  b. Cardiogenic shock

    i. Mechanism: Seen in the first 48 hours, especially with large anterior MI, because of ischemia or with severe mitral regurgitation

    ii. Management: See Heart Failure and Shock

  c. Arrhythmias: Atrial fibrillation, VT, VF, bradyarrhythmias

    i. Mechanism: See Cardiac Rhythm Disorders

    ii. Management

       (a) Monitor the patient's ECG and watch for hypotension and bradycardia

       (b) Watch for reperfusion arrhythmias. In the initial period after coronary blood flow is restored, ventricular arrhythmias frequently occur.

       (c) AV sequential pacing may be required for increasing CO (blocks are common)

       (d) Instruct the patient to avoid Valsalva maneuvers: Cause dramatic changes in heart rate and BP (ventricular filling) and can cause arrhythmias (especially in patients <45 years of age)

  d. Other complications

    i. Reocclusion: Symptoms include ST-segment changes, chest discomfort, arrhythmias, hypotension

    ii. LV thrombus: More likely with a CK rise of more than 3200 IU/L. Treatment includes anticoagulation for 3 to 6 months and with akinesis or dyskinesis of the anterior wall and/or apex.

    iii. VSDs: Surgical repair is needed immediately if the patient is hemodynamically unstable or if CO is low (IABP, inotropic medications, vasodilators, surgical or catheter-based closure)

    iv. LV aneurysm: Surgical repair is often combined with CABG, valve repair

    v. Severe acute mitral regurgitation: IABP, inotropic medications, catheterization, surgery

    vi. Rupture of LV free wall, ventricular septal rupture, or papillary muscle rupture. All of which would cause the patient significant symptoms including chest pain, shortness of breath, hypotension, and cardiogenic shock. Treatment includes volume support, IABP, vasoactive medications, surgery. Majority of patients with free wall rupture do not survive.

EXPERT TIP

You must always stabilize the patient and rule out MI first, then consider imposter rhythms that may cause ST elevation (e.g., pericarditis, early repolarization, electrolyte imbalance, or LBBB).

NON—ST ELEVATION MYOCARDIAL INFARCTION (SEE ACUTE CORONARY SYNDROME (NSTEMI- ACUTE CORONARY SYNDROME AND UNSTABLE ANGINA))
Unstable Angina

KEY CONCEPT

NSTEMI and UA have a similar pathophysiology and clinical presentation. In NSTEMI, the ischemia is severe enough to cause myocardial damage leading to elevations in the levels of cardiac biomarkers (troponins), and in UA, they are not elevated.

---

1. **Pathophysiology: See STEMI and Coronary Artery Disease. NSTEMI and UA are often a result of abrupt, nonexertional plaque rupture, thrombosis, vasoconstriction, or arterial occlusion, often with subsequent reperfusion.**
   a. Coronary occlusion (plaque rupture, platelet-mediated thrombosis, vasoconstriction, or arterial occlusion)
   b. Subtotal or intermittent coronary occlusion
   c. Coronary spasm (Prinzmetal angina) can temporarily occlude coronary artery flow
   d. Restenosis after PCI can create an obstruction to blood flow without spasm or thrombus
   e. Severity and number of obstructions, availability of collateral circulation, and amount of thrombus all factor into the clinical presentation
2. **Etiology and risk factors**
   a. In the United States, NSTE-ACS is a term used to group NSTEMI and UA. It is estimated that more than 80,000 persons will experience an ACS in the United States each year, and approximately 70% of these will have NSTE-ACS.
   b. Precipitating factor: Atherosclerotic plaque
   c. Risk factors: The common risk factors of CAD
   d. Identifiers of patients at high risk
      i. Prolonged pain (particularly at rest)
      ii. Arrhythmias: Bradycardias, tachycardias
      iii. Hypotension
      iv. Transient ST changes during pain
      v. New mitral regurgitation murmur, S_3, crackles
      vi. New BBB
3. **Signs and symptoms**
   a. Subjective and objective findings: May be similar to that of MI and more severe than stable angina:
      i. Symptoms occur at rest
      ii. Symptoms usually last longer than 20 minutes
   b. Physical findings
      i. Patient may appear to be anxious and nervous
      ii. Minimal movement
      iii. Visible signs of pain, possible clutching chest or facial grimacing
      iv. Tachycardia (increased sympathetic tone)
      v. Transient mitral regurgitation—new murmur
      vi. Transient rales—new symptom
      vii. Transient S_3 or S_4
      viii. Hypotension
      ix. Edema to extremities: May indicate HF
4. **Diagnostic study findings**
   a. Determination is made by:
      i. The absence of persistent ST elevation is suggestive of NSTEMI (except in patients with true posterior MI).
      ii. NSTEMI-ACS can be further subdivided on the basis of cardiac biomarkers (such as cardiac troponin).
      iii. Cardiac biomarkers are elevated = NSTEMI (see STEMI for diagnosis and treatment)
      iv. Cardiac biomarkers are not elevated = UA
   b. Laboratory

     i. Troponins or CK-MB isoenzymes are not elevated in UA. Elevations in troponin levels are strong prognostic indicators of mortality risk, should be obtained beyond 6 hours after symptom onset.

     ii. CBC: Check for cause of anemia (decreased oxygen supply)

     iii. Creatinine, BUN levels: Assess renal function (for dye administration, heparinization)

     iv. C-reactive protein (CRP; inflammatory marker) and BNP (indicates ventricular dilatation, pressure overload) are markers used to evaluate risk for future events

  c. ECG: May or may not show evidence of myocardial injury or ischemia (see ST-Segment Elevation Myocardial Infarction)

> **EXPERT TIP**
> If the initial ECG is not diagnostic but the patient remains symptomatic and there is a high clinical suspicion for ACS, serial ECGs should be performed to detect ischemic changes.

     i. Transient ST changes with pain: Occurrence of ST changes with symptoms and at rest are highly suggestive of ischemia and probably severe CAD

     ii. ST depression

     iii. Inverted T-wave changes

     iv. New BBB

     v. Sustained VT

  d. Echocardiography: May or may not show transient abnormal wall motion, valve dysfunction, hypertrophy. Identifies LV dysfunction.

  e. Pharmacologic (e.g., dobutamine, adenosine, thallium) stress echocardiography: Demonstrates ischemia, stress-induced wall motion abnormalities, ventricular dysfunction, ischemic mitral regurgitation

  f. Myocardial scintigraphy (thallium, Tc 99 m sestamibi) with pharmacologic stress (adenosine, dipyridamole) may demonstrate ischemia, infarction, and LV dysfunction

  g. Coronary catheterization with potential for PCI

5. Interprofessional collaboration: See STEMI

6. Management of patient care

  a. Anticipated patient trajectory: Therapy with effective antiplatelet agents and prompt angiography have resulted in significant gains in infarct prevention and myocardial preservation

  b. Goals of care

     i. Ischemia, MI, and death are prevented by

       (a) Decreasing myocardial oxygen demand

       (b) Improving myocardial oxygen supply

     ii. Disease process is modified

       (a) Antiplatelet and antithrombin therapy

       (b) Lifestyle modifications (smoking cessation; diet; weight, BP, and glucose control)

  c. Treatment

     i. Pharmacology: Pain and ischemia management

       (a) NTG: Rapid-acting nitrate sublingual, IV infusions (see STEMI for route, dosages, and considerations)

       (b) Morphine sulfate: Analgesic, anxiolytic, venodilation

         (1) Used when NTG is ineffective for pain relief or symptoms of pulmonary edema are present

         (2) Doses of 1 to 5 mg IV

(c) β-blockers (e.g., atenolol, metoprolol)
   (1) Action
       a) Decrease angina
       b) Decrease heart rate and contractility
       c) Decrease myocardial oxygen demand
       d) Increase diastolic filling time
       e) Increase exercise tolerance
   (2) IV administration initially is used for continued chest pain
   (3) Contraindications: Bronchial asthma, heart failure (unless caused by ischemia), AV blocks, hypotension
   (4) Side effects: Hypoglycemia, arrhythmias (including conduction blocks), central nervous system effects (decreased energy, decreased libido, nightmares, confusion), gastrointestinal effects (diarrhea, nausea, constipation)
   (5) Sudden withdrawal of the medication can have rebound effects (including angina, hypertension, MI). Gradual withdrawal or adjustment should be made, unless an emergency (e.g., bradycardia) mandates immediate discontinuation.
(d) Calcium channel antagonists: Nondihydropyridines (e.g., verapamil or diltiazem)
   (1) Actions
       a) Negative inotropic; negative chronotropic effects on SA and AV conductive tissue
       b) Increase angina threshold, reduce ischemia, increase exercise tolerance, decrease afterload
       c) Vasodilators help improve myocardial blood supply
   (2) Use cautiously in combination with β-blockers because of possible adverse effect on heart rate and LV function suppression
   (3) Contraindications: Aortic valve disease, severe anemia, AV blocks, Wolff-Parkinson-White (WPW) syndrome (verapamil)
(e) ACE inhibitors: Used if hypertension continues in a patient receiving NTG, β-blockers, especially when caused by LV dysfunction or HF symptoms
ii. Antiplatelet and antithrombotic combination therapy (see Table 4.9)
   (a) Aspirin: Blocks only one pathway to platelet aggregation
   (b) Glycoprotein IIb/IIIa (GPIIb/IIIa) receptor blockers
       (1) Block the final common pathway of platelet aggregation
       (2) Therefore may be ideal in treating ACS
iii. Positioning: See STEMI
iv. Nutrition: Low-fat, low-sodium diet
v. Discharge planning: See STEMI
vi. Psychosocial issues: See STEMI
vii. Other interventions: See STEMI
   (a) PCI: Early invasive strategy is recommended for patients with the following:
       (1) Angina or ischemia recurring at rest or with minimal activity with aggressive medical therapy
       (2) Angina or ischemia recurring with symptoms of HF (S_3, pulmonary edema, increased crackles, new or worse mitral regurgitation)
       (3) EF of less than 40%
       (4) Hemodynamic instability, hypotension with angina at rest
       (5) PCI within 6 months previously

(6) Prior CABG

(7) Sustained VT

(b) IABP: See Heart Failure

(c) VAD: See Heart Failure

(d) CABG: See STEMI

CHRONIC STABLE ANGINA PECTORIS

1. **Pathophysiology**
   a. Myocardial oxygen demand outstrips oxygen supply
   b. Progressive coronary atherosclerosis increasingly limits coronary blood flow and myocardial perfusion
2. **Etiology and risk factors**
   a. Precipitating factors
      i. Increased myocardial oxygen demand because of
         (a) Increased heart rate resulting from exertion, tachyarrhythmia, anemia, fever, anxiety, pain, thyrotoxicosis, medications, digestion, hyperadrenergic states
         (b) Increased contractility resulting from exercise, tachycardia, anxiety, medications, hyperadrenergic states
         (c) Increased afterload resulting from hypertension, aortic stenosis, medications (pressors)
         (d) Increased preload resulting from volume overload, medications
      ii. Decreased oxygen supply because of
         (a) CAD (fixed narrowing of coronary arteries)
         (b) Coronary artery spasm (cocaine abuse, cold air, medications [ergots])
         (c) Circulatory diversion (digestion, coronary artery steal)
         (d) Anemia
         (e) Hypoxemia
         (f) Hypovolemia
         (g) Shock
         (h) HF
   b. Risk factors: The common risk factors of CAD
3. **Signs and symptoms**
   a. Subjective findings: Angina discomfort is any exertional, rest-relieved symptom and may be described as burning, squeezing, aching, heaviness, pressure sensation, smothering, indigestion-like, or a band across the chest. It may occur anywhere between the ears and the umbilicus.
      i. Etiologic or precipitating factors: Elicit pertinent information from the patient
      ii. Characterize the patient's symptoms
         (a) Duration of discomfort: Chest pain from ACS generally lasts more than 20 minutes
         (b) Location and radiation of discomfort: Can include the chest, neck, jaws, arms, back, epigastrium
         (c) Patient is asked to quantify the discomfort by using a scale from 1 (the least) to 10 (the worst pain ever experienced by the patient)
         (d) Associated symptoms may include nausea, diaphoresis, palpitations, shortness of breath, syncope, and presyncope
         (e) Effect of exertion and rest: The timing of the discomfort is crucial. Was it with activity, at rest, postprandial? With what kind of activity? How often does it recur? What starts it? What relieves it?

(f) Effect of nitrates (if the patient has CAD, nitrates should decrease or abolish the discomfort in 1 to 2 minutes, not 15 to 20 minutes, but may also be effective in relieving pain caused by gastroesophageal reflux disease)

b. Objective findings:

  i. Patient may show signs of anxiety, but should not be in acute distress

  ii. Patient may have signs of pain (clutching chest, arm or facial grimacing) lasting less than 20 minutes

  iii. Breath sounds should be normal with no signs of respiratory distress

  iv. Heart sounds should be normal S_1 and S_2; if there is an S_3 present, this may be a sign of fluid overload or HF (which may also be noted in extremity edema)

c. Determine the type or form of angina discomfort

  i. UA: New-onset angina or angina that has changed in frequency, severity, or duration or occurs with less exertion or at rest. Duration of pain is usually more than 20 minutes (see Acute Coronary Syndromes).

  ii. Chronic, stable angina: Angina that has not increased in frequency or severity over time. Caused primarily by obstructive, fixed atheromatous coronary lesions.

  iii. Prinzmetal (variant) angina: Resting angina caused by coronary artery spasm, associated with transient ST-segment elevation

d. Determine class of angina: Canadian classification

  i. Canadian class I: Angina produced by strenuous exertion

  ii. Canadian class II: Angina produced by walking more than two level blocks

  iii. Canadian class III: Angina produced by walking less than two level blocks

  iv. Canadian class IV: Angina at rest

e. Other important aspects of the history include the following:

  i. Presence of risk factors for CAD

  ii. Cardiac review of systems

  iii. Medication history (including use of illicit drugs)

  iv. History of tests, interventions; CABG, PTCA

  v. Allergies to shellfish, iodine (contrast dye)

  vi. If the patient underwent intervention (PCI, CABG), try to elicit the patient's anginal history before the intervention

4. **Diagnostic study findings: No acute ECG changes and no elevation of cardiac enzymes**

5. **Interprofessional collaboration: See STEMI**

6. **Management of patient care**

a. Anticipated patient trajectory: Prognosis varies widely depending on LV function, the severity of CAD, and associated risk factors. Prompt diagnosis and treatment enables elimination of symptoms and improved longevity.

b. Goals of care

  i. Ischemia, MI, and death are prevented by

    (a) Decreasing myocardial oxygen demand (β-blockers, calcium channel blockers, nitrates)

    (b) Improving myocardial oxygen supply (nitrates)

  ii. Disease process is modified

    (a) Antiplatelet and antithrombin therapy

    (b) Lifestyle modifications (e.g., smoking cessation, diet, BP control, diabetes control, lipid management, and physical activity)

c. Treatments

  i. Discharge planning

(a) Risk factor modification teaching
   (1) Smoking cessation to reduce reoccurrence of cardiac events
   (2) Weight control
   (3) Exercise: Daily routine important
   (4) BP: Less than 130/85 mm Hg
   (5) Diabetes: Tight glucose control
   (6) Lipid control

d. Other interventions
   i. PCIs may be used in the treatment of a chronic stable angina patient to identify coronary narrowing and attempt to increase the luminal diameter of coronary arteries that have been stenosed by CAD and to increase coronary blood flow using PTCA, coronary stent placement, and atherectomy (see Figs. 4.11 and 4.12)
      (a) PTCA: Balloon catheter is placed across stenosis and inflated to enlarge the lumen diameter by mechanically compressing and splitting plaque
      (b) Coronary stent placement: Primary stenting to restore coronary blood flow and normal luminal diameter. Devices are placed intraluminally to achieve maximal lumen size and maintain the patency of the vessel's lumen. Many PCI procedures include some form of stenting with PTCA.
         (1) Bare metal stents are made from various metals
         (2) Drug-eluting stents are made of synthetic materials with the ability to deliver medications to almost eliminate the restenosis of stents
      (c) Coronary atherectomy: Removal of atheromatous material from the artery (debulking). Procedure is less popular because of improved stenting procedures.
         (1) Directional coronary atherectomy: Plaque is cut by a catheter with a rotating cutter and trapped in its chamber for removal
         (2) Transluminal extraction atherectomy: Slower rotating cutter is used with vacuum suction to withdraw atheromatous debris
         (3) Rotational atherectomy: High-speed, rotating burr grinds atheromatous material into microdebris in the bloodstream
      (d) Brachytherapy: Intracoronary radiation procedure to treat and prevent in-stent restenosis (usually used for a chronic stable patient rather than STEMI)
      (e) Key concepts for nursing care after PCI procedure (see Box 4.3)
      (f) See STEMI for PCI complications and discharge teaching

CORONARY ARTERY DISEASE
1. Pathophysiology

KEY CONCEPT

CAD is a progressive disorder in which the coronary arteries become occluded as a result of atherosclerosis. It is the most common type of heart disease and occurs over decades of time, which often makes it undetected until a blockage occurs and causes symptoms.

---

a. Injury (because of plaque formation, toxins, infections, or mechanical causes) occurs to the endothelial cells in the intima of the coronary arteries, altering cell structure
b. Platelets adhere and aggregate at the site of injury, and macrophages migrate to the area as a result of injury. Smooth muscle cells and macrophage foam cells enter the

intimal layer. These accumulations promote the development over time of a fatty fibrous plaque, and migration of LDL into the subintimal space results in lipid core.

c. This plaque is a pearly white accumulation in the intimal lining, consisting mostly of smooth muscle cells but also collagen-producing fibroblasts and macrophages. These deposits protrude into the lumen, obstructing blood flow.

d. Progressive narrowing of the vessel occurs. This process tends to occur at vessel bifurcations and at the proximal end of the artery.

e. The fatty fibrous plaque can rupture and form either a mural thrombus or an occlusive thrombus

   i. A mural thrombus can partially or totally obstruct the artery. The disrupted plaque and mural thrombus can develop into a more fibrotic, stenotic lesion, which changes the plaque's geometry.

   ii. An acute, labile, occlusive thrombus can totally obstruct the artery and create clinical complications (MI, UA, sudden cardiac death)

   iii. The ruptured plaque, caused by endothelial injury and exposure to blood flow, activates platelet and fibrin formation, enhancing thrombus formation

f. Coronary blood flow may be further diminished by vasoconstriction (resulting from the release of vasoactive agents [thromboxane A_2, angiotensin II], impaired vasodilatation, and platelet activation)

g. Atherosclerotic process causes

   i. Decreases in blood flow and oxygen supply to the myocardium

   ii. An imbalance between myocardial oxygen supply and demand, which results in myocardial ischemia

2. **Etiology and risk factors**

KEY CONCEPT

The risk factors for CAD are the same risk factors seen with the coronary diseases (e.g., hypertension).

---

a. Heredity: Familial component for premature heart disease; MI or sudden cardiac death in father, mother, or siblings

b. Age: About 85% of people who die of heart disease are over the age of 65 years. CAD is more prevalent among middle-aged and older persons (males >45 years of age; females >55 years of age). However, approximately 50% of U.S. children 12 to 19 years of age have five or more risk factors.

c. Sex: Men tend to manifest CAD 10 to 15 years earlier than women.

   i. Men: Before age 55 years, prevalence is 3 to 4 times higher among men than among women (before menopause), and initial cardiac event for men is more often MI than angina.

   ii. Women: After age 55 years, prevalence rates slowly equalize for both sexes; at age 75 years, rates are close to equal, and CAD causes more deaths in women than in men.

d. Race/ethnicity: Black Americans have the highest risk of heart disease, which may be related to increased rates of hypertension, diabetes, and obesity.

e. Smoking

   i. Enhances atherogenic progression; decreases HDL cholesterol level; influences thrombus formation, plaque instability, arrhythmias.

   ii. Dose and duration dependent: Risk of death from CAD is 2 to 6 times higher among smokers than among nonsmokers.

f. Hyperlipidemia: More than 100 million U.S. adults aged 20 years or older have total cholesterol levels of 200 mg/dL or more; almost 31 million have levels of 240 mg/dL or higher. High levels of triglycerides, LDL, and very-low-density lipoproteins are associated with an increased risk of CAD. The 2019 ACC/AHA guidelines place a greater emphasis on lifestyle modification as part of the management of atherosclerotic risk reduction. Individuals with LDL-C of 190 mg/dL (or higher) or triglycerides 500 mg/dL (or higher) should be evaluated for secondary causes of hyperlipidemia.

   i. Total cholesterol 200 mg/dL or higher
   ii. Triglycerides: Higher than 200 mg/dL
   iii. LDL-C: Higher than 190 mg/dL
   iv. HDL: Lower than 40 mg/dL (HDL level >60 mg/dL is a negative risk factor)

   Note: Guidelines focus more on atherosclerotic cardiovascular disease (ASCVD) risk than maintaining specific blood levels when addressing statin therapy.

g. Hypertension
   i. Contributes to direct vascular injury, along with the effects of increased wall stress and oxygen demands
   ii. Over 30% of American adults ages 20 years or over have hypertension, and Black American adults have among the highest prevalence of hypertension internationally.
   iii. SBP higher than 140 mm Hg and/or diastolic pressure higher than 90 mm Hg (dependent on age and history)

h. Diabetes mellitus: Patients with diabetes mellitus are twice as likely to develop CAD as persons without diabetes

i. Obesity: Positively associated with an increased rate of CAD; also contributes to the development of hypertension and diabetes
   i. Fat distribution plays a role (abdominal or central obesity carries a higher risk)
   ii. Metabolic syndrome: Recognized syndrome (also referred to as insulin resistance syndrome) associated with higher risk and identified by the presence of three or more of the following:
      (a) Abdominal obesity: Waist circumference greater than 40 inches in men and greater than 35 inches in women
      (b) Triglyceride level higher than 150 mg/dL
      (c) HDL level lower than 40 mg/dL in men and 50 mg/dL in women
      (d) BP higher than 130/85 mm Hg
      (e) Glucose level (fasting) higher than 110 mg/dL

j. Physical inactivity: Studies show a positive relationship between inactivity and CAD, mainly resulting from its aggravation of other risk factors

k. LV hypertrophy: Heart's response to chronic pressure overloads; associated with increased risk for cardiovascular events

l. Thrombogenic risk factors: Deficiencies in serum coagulation inhibitors (antithrombin III, protein C, and protein S), elevated plasma fibrinogen level, enhanced platelet aggregation

m. Hepatic: Cardiovascular risk is increased in alcoholic liver disease, nonalcoholic fatty liver disease, nonalcoholic steatohepatitis, chronic hepatitis C virus infection, all conditions featuring steatosis

n. Depression: Associations have been made between depression and adverse coronary outcomes, ACS, and CAD

3. **Signs and symptoms**
   a. CAD may be asymptomatic and may be diagnosed because of abnormal findings on tests (stress testing, echocardiography)
4. **Diagnostic study findings: No acute ECG changes and no elevation of cardiac enzymes**
5. **Interprofessional collaboration: See STEMI**
6. **Management of patient care**
   a. Anticipated patient trajectory: Primary prevention is the key to decreasing the morbidity and mortality of CAD.
   b. Goals of care
      i. Modifiable risk factors are under control and/or improved. Risk factor modification is incorporated into the patient's lifestyle and patient verbalizes an understanding of how to manage or modify the risk factors that contribute to CAD.
      ii. Patient and family have educational resources to assist in modifying lifestyle (e.g., smoking cessation program, medication information sheets, follow-up plan) to assist in implementing new health practices
      iii. Goals of the treatment program are met
   c. Treatments
      i. Nutrition
         (a) Nutritional status, dietary habits should be assessed.
         (b) Education should be provided on the rationale for compliance with a cholesterol-controlled diet if lipid levels are above the goals and provide patient and family information on low-fat, low-cholesterol foods.
         (c) Referrals should be given to hospital and community resources for follow-up and reinforcement.
         (d) Diet should include the use of monounsaturated and polyunsaturated fats (olive, sunflower, and corn oils; soft oleomargarine) and avoidance of *transfatty* acids, which should be less than 7% of total calories. Other dietary additions can include fish and ω-3 fatty acids, fiber, and flaxseed.
         (e) Goals for weight should be discussed. Weight and height should be measured. Body mass index (BMI) should be determined.

$$BMI = \frac{\text{weight in pounds}}{(\text{height in inches})^2} \times 703$$

         (1) Desirable waist circumference: Less than 41 inches in males and less than 36 inches in females
         (2) BMI: Desired = 18 to 24.9 kg/m² (25–30 kg/m² indicates overweight; >30 indicates obesity)
      ii. Pharmacology
         (a) Antiplatelet agents (such as aspirin [acetylsalicylic acid], 81 mg/day) may be included in the patient's health regimen, if not contraindicated.
         (b) Lipid-lowering agents will often be necessary; the patient should be aware of their uses and side effects and follow-up requirements.
         (c) Antihypertensive agents may be necessary (diuretics, ACE inhibitors, ARB, or β-blockers).
      iii. Psychosocial issues
         (a) An adequate support system to assist in changing to heart-healthy behaviors and lifestyle is important.

(b) Complementary and alternative medical methods to assist with stress reduction, include massage therapy, yoga, regular exercise, postural therapy, and acupuncture

iv. Other treatments

(a) Provide the patient with information regarding the risk factors for CAD

(b) Encourage the patient and significant others to quit smoking; provide information and help regarding risks, methods for stopping, and nicotine replacement.

(c) Provide information on lipid-lowering diets that have 30% or less fat, with less than 7% saturated fat.

(d) Lipid management: Guidelines make no recommendations for specific lipid targets, but instead they identify four groups of primary- and secondary-prevention patients who should be treated with statins:

(1) Individuals with clinical atherosclerotic cardiovascular disease

(2) Individuals with LDL-cholesterol levels over 190 mg/dL, such as those with familial hypercholesterolemia

(3) Individuals with diabetes aged 40 to 75 years old with LDL-cholesterol levels between 70 and 189 mg/dL and without evidence of atherosclerotic cardiovascular disease

(4) Individuals without evidence of cardiovascular disease or diabetes but who have LDL-cholesterol levels between 70 and 189 mg/dL and a 10-year risk of atherosclerotic cardiovascular disease greater than 7.5%

(5) Individuals who do not fit into any of the four groups, consider family history of premature atherosclerotic cardiovascular disease in a first-degree relative, high-sensitivity CRP over 2 mg/L, the presence of calcification on a coronary artery calcium (CAC) scan, and an ankle-brachial index (ABI) under 0.9.

(6) If the patient is hypertensive

a) BP goal: 140/90 mm Hg or lower

b) Modifications include weight control, routine exercise, moderate alcohol consumption, and sodium restriction

(e) Weight control should be discussed with the patient and a plan for weight loss developed (especially for patients who are more than 120% of their ideal weight for height). Hypertensive patients and/or patients with elevated glucose or triglyceride levels should receive information on achieving ideal body weight.

(f) Encourage exercise and physical activity (after risks are assessed, often after exercise testing in patients over 40 years of age)

(1) Goal of 30 minutes, 3 to 4 times weekly (minimum); preferably 30 to 60 minutes of moderate exercise, including walking, cycling, jogging, swimming

(2) Other opportunities for increased physical activity should be explored

(g) Increased emphasis continues to be placed on education regarding women and cardiovascular disease, aggressive medical management for women, along with the inclusion of more female patients in clinical trials

d. Potential complications: See the following sections for possible sequelae of CAD

HEART FAILURE

1. **HF is a clinical presentation of impaired cardiac function in which one or both ventricles are unable to maintain an output adequate to meet the metabolic**

demands of the body. HF can occur on either the right or the left side of the heart and is caused by systolic dysfunction (poor contraction), diastolic dysfunction (impaired filling), increased afterload (increased resistance), or alterations in heart rate (too fast, too slow).

KEY CONCEPT

HF is common in critically ill patients and may result from chronic (e.g., hypertension) or acute disease (e.g., AMI). Treatment usually involves optimizing volume status (e.g., preload and afterload) and/or increasing contractility of the heart via pharmacologic (e.g., inotropes) or mechanical (e.g., IABP) means.

---

2. **Pathophysiology**
   a. Left-sided heart failure with reduced ejection fraction (HFrEF)
      i. Impaired forward output caused by decreased LV contractility (e.g., CAD, cardiomyopathies) in which the EF is reduced to below normal
      ii. To compensate, the LV dilates and the heart rate increases in an attempt to maintain a normal output. This increase in the SV and heart rate may return the CO toward normal despite a poor EF.
      iii. LV filling pressures rise because of increased preload or decreased LV compliance (producing LV diastolic dysfunction)
      iv. LA and pulmonary venous pressures rise, producing pulmonary congestion and edema
         (a) When pulmonary capillary oncotic pressure (30 mm Hg) is exceeded, fluid leaks into the pulmonary interstitial space, creating pulmonary edema
         (b) Decreased oxygenation of the blood occurs as oxygen exchange is impeded by the presence of fluid
      v. Right-sided heart pressure increases as a result of increased pressure in the pulmonary system
      vi. Right-sided HF may then occur because of the pulmonary hypertension, resulting in peripheral and organ edema
   b. Left-sided heart failure with preserved ejection fraction (HFpEF)
      i. A noncompliant, stiff LV (because of hypertrophy, ischemia, infiltration, scarring) has less ability to relax, which interferes with adequate filling and results in rising diastolic (filling) pressures
      ii. As a consequence, LA, pulmonary venous, and pulmonary capillary pressures increase
      iii. Pulmonary artery and right-sided heart pressures rise if the condition is untreated
      iv. Up to 30% to 50% of patients with HF have normal LV systolic function
   c. Right-sided HFpEF
      i. The right side of the heart is unable to pump blood forward adequately, which results in a drop in CO
      ii. Causes include pulmonary hypertension (most common), as well as RV MI
      iii. RV dilatation and elevation of filling pressure develop, which results in peripheral edema
   d. Right-sided HFpEF: Can occur with RV hypertrophy and cardiomyopathies; analogous to left-sided heart diastolic dysfunction, except the consequence is peripheral edema rather than pulmonary edema, associated with elevated right-sided heart-filling pressures (increased jugular venous pressures)

e. Four stages of HF progression:
  i. Stage A: High risk of HF, no cardiac structural disorders
  ii. Stage B: Structural defect or disorder of the heart, no symptoms of HF
  iii. Stage C: Structural defect or disorder of the heart, present or past symptoms of HF
  iv. Stage D: End-stage cardiac disease; the patient needs continuous therapy (inotropic medications, mechanical supports, transplantation, hospice care)
3. **Etiology and risk factors: See Table 4.11 for factors related to left- and right-sided HF**
4. **Signs and symptoms: Patients generally have asymptomatic HF for an uncertain time before the recognition of symptoms. Decrease in activity tolerance and/or fluid retention are generally the first complaints identified.**

EXPERT TIP

The signs and symptoms of left HF are predominantly pulmonary (e.g., rales, shortness of breath), whereas signs and symptoms of right HF tend to be systemic (e.g., peripheral edema).

TABLE 4.11   Etiology or Precipitating Factors in Heart Failure

LEFT-SIDED HEART FAILURE		Right-Sided Heart Failure	Both Sides
Systolic	**Diastolic**		
Ischemic heart disease Myocardial infarction	Coronary artery disease Myocardial ischemia	Left-sided heart failure Atherosclerotic heart disease	Patient nonadherence regarding
Myocardial stunning, hibernation	Left ventricular hypertrophy		• Medications
Coronary artery disease	Cardiomyopathy: hypertrophic, restrictive, dilated	Acute right ventricular myocardial infarction	• Dietary restrictions
Idiopathic dilated cardiomyopathy		Pulmonary embolism	• Alcohol use Medications
Myocardial contusion	Increased circulating volume	Fluid overload, excess sodium intake	• Negative inotropic agents
Aortic insufficiency	Cardiac tamponade	Myocardial contusion Cardiomyopathy	• Causing sodium retention
Arrhythmias: Ventricular tachycardia, atrial fibrillation		Valvular heart disease	
Postpump syndrome	Constrictive pericarditis Left ventricular hypertrophy	Atrial or ventricular septal defect	
Myocarditis	Mitral stenosis or insufficiency	Pulmonary outflow stenosis	
Infectious: Viral, bacterial, fungal	Aortic stenosis or insufficiency	Chronic obstructive pulmonary disease	
Acute rheumatic fever	Age (decreased compliance of heart muscle)	Pulmonary hypertension (cor pulmonale)	
Drug abuse: Heroin, alcohol, cocaine	Diabetes mellitus	Sleep apnea	
Nutrition deficits: Protein, thiamine	Intracardiac shunts		
Electrolyte disorders: Decrease in calcium, sodium, potassium, phosphate			
Diabetes, thyroid disease			
Medications suppressing contractility (negative inotropic)			

From Mann, D.L., Felkner, G.M. (2016). *Heart failure: a companion to Braunwald's heart disease*, ed 3. Philadelphia: Elsevier.

a. History: See Table 4.12 for clinical findings in left- and right-sided HF
b. Physical examination of patient
   i. See Table 4.12
   ii. Functional therapeutic classification of patients with HF
       (a) I: Symptoms occur with strong exertion
       (b) II: Symptoms occur with normal exertion
       (c) III: Symptoms occur with minimal exertion
       (d) IV: Symptoms occur at rest

5. **Diagnostic study findings**
   a. Laboratory
      i. BNP level: Elevations reflect myocyte stretch and increased ventricular pressures; prognostic indicator
      ii. CRP level: May be elevated
      iii. HCT, Hb level: Assess for anemia
      iv. Electrolyte levels: Imbalances because of diuresis
      v. Thyroid stimulating hormone level: Hypothyroidism, hyperthyroidism
      vi. Renal function tests: BUN, creatinine levels
      vii. Liver function tests (right-sided failure)
      viii. Cardiac troponin, enzyme levels (if potential acute MI)
      ix. Human immunodeficiency virus (HIV) testing: If the patient is at high risk for this cause

TABLE 4.12 **Clinical Findings in Heart Failure**		
LEFT-SIDED HEART FAILURE		
Systolic	**Diastolic**	**Right-Sided Heart Failure**
Anxiety	Exercise intolerance	Increased fatigue
Sudden light-headedness	Orthopnea	Hepatomegaly
Fatigue, weakness, lethargy	Dyspnea, dyspnea on exertion, paroxysmal nocturnal dyspnea	Splenomegaly
Orthopnea	Cough with frothy white or pink sputum (in pulmonary edema)	Dependent pitting edema
Dyspnea, dyspnea on exertion, paroxysmal nocturnal dyspnea	Tachypnea (on exertion)	Ascites
Tachypnea (on exertion)	Basilar crackles, rhonchi, wheezes	Cachexia
Cheyne-Stokes respirations (if severe)	Pulmonary edema	Abdominal pain (from congested liver)
Diaphoresis	Symptoms of right-sided heart failure	Anorexia, nausea, emesis
Palpitations	Hypoxia, respiratory acidosis	Weight gain
Sacral edema, pitting of extremities	Elevated pulmonary artery diastolic pressure, pulmonary artery occlusive pressure	Low blood pressure
Basilar rales, rhonchi, crackles, wheezes	S_3, S_4 heart sounds	Oliguria, nocturia (increased renal perfusion, blood volume when lying in bed)
Cool, moist, cyanotic skin	Holosystolic murmur (if tricuspid, mitral regurgitation)	Venous distention
Hypoxia, respiratory acidosis		Hepatojugular reflux
Elevated pulmonary artery diastolic pressure, pulmonary artery occlusive pressure		Fatigue, weakness
		Kussmaul's sign (if constriction)
Nocturia		Murmur of tricuspid insufficiency
		S_3, S_4 heart sounds (right-sided)
Mental confusion		Elevated central venous pressure and right atrial and right ventricular pressures
Decreased pulse pressure		
Pulsus alternans		
Lateral displacement of point of maximal impulse		
S_3, S_4 heart sounds		
Murmur of mitral insufficiency		

From Mann, D.L., Felkner, G.M. (2016). *Heart failure: a companion to Braunwald's heart disease*, ed 3. Philadelphia: Elsevier.

b. Radiologic: Results often normal, abnormalities may include:
 i. Pulmonary vasculature: Edema, congestion
 ii. Cardiac silhouette: May show cardiac chamber enlargement
 iii. Pleural effusion (left-sided failure)
 iv. Valve calcifications
c. ECG
 i. Nonspecific changes
 ii. Arrhythmias, ischemic disease, conduction abnormalities, medication and electrolyte effects
d. Echocardiogram: To assess:
 i. Chamber size, wall thickness
 ii. Systolic and diastolic function
 iii. Thrombus formation
 iv. Valvular function
 v. Pericardial disease
e. Radionuclide imaging
 i. Assessment of chamber function and volume
 ii. Myocardial perfusion imaging for ischemia, infarction
f. CT and MRI: To assess structural abnormalities, tumors, vascular anomalies, pericardial disease
g. Cardiac catheterization with arteriography: To assess:
 i. Coronary anatomy (two-thirds of patients have CAD as a contributing cause)
 ii. Pressures in right and left chambers
  (a) High filling pressures represent diastolic dysfunction
  (b) Diuretic and IV NTG use can create a false-negative result by artificially normalizing the filling pressures
 iii. Ventricular contractility
 iv. Valvular function, cardiac defects

6. **Interprofessional collaboration: See STEMI, also heart failure specialist (physician or advanced practice provider), electrophysiologist, psychologist, home care, palliative care team, financial aid counselor.**

7. **Management of patient care**
a. Anticipated patient trajectory: A common clinical cardiology problem with a poor prognosis. Quality of life and longevity can be improved dramatically with available medications and therapy.
b. Goals of care
 i. Symptom relief
 ii. Hemodynamics are stabilized rapidly (using diuretics, vasodilators, inotropic agents)
 iii. Excess fluid is removed and edema is corrected
 iv. Complications from arrhythmias are prevented
c. Treatments
 i. Positioning
  (a) Sitting patient up and/or use of extra pillows may increase ease of breathing. Avoid dependent feet to help mobilize edema.
  (b) Prevent complications of DVT by range-of-motion exercises, use of thromboembolic disease hose, pneumatic antiembolic stockings
 ii. Skin care: If the patient is on prolonged bed rest, institute measures to prevent the hazards of immobility
 iii. Pain management: Administer medications to alleviate discomfort, as ordered

   iv. Nutrition

     (a) Monitor intake and output closely

     (b) Closely observe restrictions on fluid (1000–1500 mL/day) and sodium

     (c) Weigh patient daily

   v. Discharge planning: Before discharge, the patient and/or significant others should be able to do the following:

     (a) Explain HF and its prognosis

     (b) List symptoms that indicate a worsening of the condition, whether from HF or from medication side effects. Patient should know when to call for medical advice to prevent rehospitalizations and complications.

     (c) Describe each current medication: Name, purpose, dosage, frequency, side effects, and benefits of compliance

     (d) Identify the lifestyle changes necessary to prevent recurrence

       (1) Diet and weight control

         a) Sodium restriction (diet, medications)

         b) Fluid restrictions, as ordered

         c) Foods rich in potassium (important for patients taking loop diuretics)

         d) Daily weight monitoring

       (2) Cessation of high-risk activities: Smoking, alcohol, and/or drug use

       (3) Routine exercise: Increases exercise tolerance, decreases symptoms

     (e) Identify the rationale for the control of BP, lipid levels, diabetes

     (f) Demonstrate how to take the pulse; recognize the need to have BP taken routinely

     (g) Verbalize the importance of follow-up care and provide written instructions

   vi. Pharmacology

     (a) See Table 4.13 for medications commonly used in the treatment of HF

     (b) Avoid medications that decrease myocardial contractility (except β-blockers)

       (1) Antiarrhythmic medications (except amiodarone)

       (2) Calcium channel blocking agents (except for amlodipine, felodipine)

       (3) Nonsteroidal antiinflammatory drugs (NSAIDs): Cause sodium retention, renal insufficiency

       (4) Chemotherapeutic medications (e.g., daunorubicin, doxorubicin)

   vii. Psychosocial issues

     (a) Patient will likely need help at home (help arrange home services).

     (b) Noncompliance with the prescribed diet, weight, fluid intake, and medications can be devastating with this disorder. Patient and significant others need education, support, and close follow-up.

     (c) Coping with a long-standing, progressive disease becomes a strain on both patient and caregivers. Assess for signs of depression.

     (d) High costs of medications, hospitalizations, interventions create additional strains.

   viii. Other interventions

     (a) Biventricular pacing: Cardiac resynchronization therapy (CRT) has been shown to increase LV systolic function by synchronizing ventricular contraction so that the LV walls contract at the same time, which results in increased CO and improved remodeling. Pacemaker education (procedure, rationales, incision care, follow-up) is needed.

TABLE 4.13   Medications Commonly Used to Treat Heart Failure in the Critical Care Setting

Medication/Medication Class	Actions	Administration and Dosing	Comments
POSITIVE INOTROPIC AGENTS			
Milrinone	Phosphodiesterase ¾ inhibitor ↑Myocardial contractility without increasing HRRelaxes vascular (arterial and venous) smooth muscle, producing peripheral vasodilatation (↓ afterload and preload)	Dosage: 50 mcg/kg undiluted is administered over 10 to 60 min (loading dose), followed by a 0.125- to 0.75-mcg/kg/min infusion	Untoward effects include tachycardia, arrhythmias, hypotension
Dobutamine (Dobutrex)	↑Myocardial contractility ↑Stroke volume and CO ↓SVR No beneficial renal effects	Dosage: Infused at an IV rate of 2.5 to 15 mcg/kg/min Contraindications: Hypertrophic cardiomyopathy, severe AS	Monitor for tachyarrhythmias, (ventricular ectopy) Can ↓ BP in low dosages (usually associated with volume depletion, excessive diuresis, IV nitroglycerin); check for volume depletion before administering medication
VASOPRESSORS			
Dopamine (Intropin)	Used to support BP	Dosages of 2 to 10 mcg/kg/min (β-adrenergic effects) ↑ BP, cerebral and renal perfusion Dosages of >10 mcg/kg/min (α-adrenergic effects) cause peripheral vasoconstriction. ↑ SVR, ↑ afterload and BP (possible ↓ CO)	May cause tachycardia Check skin color, temperature, capillary refill; α-adrenergic stimulation causes peripheral venoconstriction. Infuse in central or large vein. Extravasation causes tissue necrosis and sloughing. If this occurs: Stop infusion and immediately inject phentolamine (Regitine), 5 to 10 mg diluted in 10 to 15 mL of saline solution, around site to lessen deleterious effects of infiltrated dopamine.
Phenylephrine (Neo-Synephrine)	Effectively increases BP by arteriolar constriction ↓ HR, ↑ SV	Dosage: 0.1 to 0.5 mg IV slowly (diluted 1 mg in 10 mL normal saline) Infusion: 0.2 to 5.0 mcg/kg/min (use lowest therapeutic dose) Onset: Immediate Duration: 15 to 20 min	
Other vasoactive medications, including vasopressin (antidiuretic hormone), norepinephrine (Levophed)			Monitor hemodynamic parameters closely, especially when using vasoactive medications (monitor arterial and hemodynamic pressures often with noninvasive BP monitoring, arterial lines, and pulmonary artery catheter)
AFTERLOAD REDUCTION			
Sodium nitroprusside (Nipride)	↓ Afterload via arterial dilation, also causing ↓ preload and BP and ↑ CO ↓ SVR and PAOP Contraindications: Severe AS, coarctation of aorta	Action: Immediate and very brief; effect ends 1 to 2 min after infusion stopped Initial dosage: Start at 0.1 mcg/kg/min; rate of infusion is titrated by BP, hemodynamics	Extravasation should be treated with phentolamine (see earlier under dopamine) to avoid necrosis at IV site Watch for cyanide toxicity with methemoglobinemia

TABLE 4.13 Medications Commonly Used to Treat Heart Failure in the Critical Care Setting—cont'd

Medication/Medication Class	Actions	Administration and Dosing	Comments
ACE inhibitor (e.g., captopril, enalapril)	Used for afterload and preload reduction and neurohormonal modulation ↑ Heart function and exercise capacity ↓ Mortality risk Contraindicated in shock, hyperkalemia (K⁺>5.5 mEq/L)	Angiotensin II receptor blockers may be used in patients who are unable to tolerate ACE inhibitors, usually due to cough	Monitor for • Symptomatic hypotension • ↑ K⁺ (increases retention) • ↑ Creatinine (decreased renal function)
Sacubitril/Valsartan (Entresto)	Neprilysin inhibitor/ARB ↓ degredation of natriuretic peptides leading to vasodilation, natriuresis, diuresis, and inhibition of fibrosis	***ACE inhibitor naïve or taking low-dose ACE inhibitor:*** Start at 24 mg sacubitril/26 mg valsartan twice daily; double dose every 2 to 4 weeks as tolerated to target maintenance dose of 97 mg sacubitril/103 mg valsartan twice daily ***Patients taking high-dose ACE inhibitor:*** Start at 49 mg sacubitril/51 mg valsartan twice daily; double dose every 2-4 weeks as tolerated to target maintenance dose of 97 mg sacubitril/103 mg valsartan twice daily	• Has been shown to be superior to enalapril in clinical trials • Benefit is most evident in patients with low LVEF • Monitor kidney function and for hypotension and angioedema
PRELOAD REDUCTION			
IV nitroglycerin	Improves left ventricular function by lowering preload via vasodilatation, to relieve discomfort		
Diuretics (e.g., torsemide, furosemide, bumetanide)	↓ Intravascular and extravascular fluid volume, and subsequently ↓ preload		Evaluate for patient response: ↑ Urinary output, ↓ edema, improved lung sounds and breathing; ↓ central venous pressure and PAOP Monitor for complications: • Electrolyte imbalances (↓ Na⁺, ↓ K⁺, ↓ Mg⁺⁺) • Impaired renal function (↑ creatinine) • Hypovolemia • Other symptoms: Fatigue, nausea, vomiting, headache, dry mouth, muscle cramps, wooziness

TABLE 4.13 Medications Commonly Used to Treat Heart Failure in the Critical Care Setting—cont'd

Medication/Medication Class	Actions	Administration and Dosing	Comments
β-blockers (e.g., carvedilol, bisoprolol, metoprolol succinate)	• Beneficial in decreasing symptoms of heart failure, increasing patient well-being, neurohormone modulation • Carvedilol combines β-blockade with vasodilatation properties		Watch for fluid retention, fatigue, hypotension, increased symptoms
Digoxin (Lanoxin)	Beneficial in decreasing symptoms, improving exercise tolerance, especially in combination therapy Also used for rate control of atrial fibrillation, atrial flutter		Dosing is based on CrCl in the acute care setting
Spironolactone (Aldactone)	Antagonist to aldosterone ↓ Mortality, hospitalization	Dosages: 12.5 to 25 mg/day	Watch K+ retention Caution in patients with kidney disease and low eGFR
Anticoagulation (warfarin)	Used for atrial fibrillation, thromboembolism risk		
Morphine sulfate	↓ Preload ↓ Venous return to heart (↑ capacitance) ↓ Pain, anxiety ↓ Myocardial oxygen consumption	3 to 5 mg IV	

ACE, Angiotensin-converting enzyme; *AS,* aortic stenosis; *BP,* blood pressure; *CO,* cardiac output; *HR,* heart rate; *IV,* intravenous; *PAOP,* pulmonary artery occlusive pressure; *SV,* stroke volume; *SVR,* systemic vascular resistance.

From Mann D.L., Felkner G.M. (2016) *Heart failure: a companion to Braunwald's heart disease,* 3rd ed, Philadelphia, Elsevier.

Hollenberg SM. Stevenson LW, Ahmad T, et al.: 2019 ACC Expert Consensus Decision Pathway on Risk Assessment, Management, and Clinical Trajectory of Patients Hospitalized with Heart Failure. *Journal of the American College of Cardiology.* 74(5), 1966-2011, 2019

Maddox TM, Januzzi JL Jr, Allen LA, et al.: 2021 Update to the 2017 ACC Expert Consensus Decision Pathway for Optimization of Heart Failure Treatment: Answers to 10 Pivotal Issues About Heart Failure With Reduced Ejection Fraction. *Journal of the American College of Cardiology.* 77(6), 772-810, 2021

Clinical Pharmacology powered by ClinicalKey. www.clinicalkey.com.

2019 ACC Expert Consensus Decision Pathway on Risk Assessment, Management, and Clinical Trajectory of Patients Hospitalized With Heart Failure: A Report of the American College of Cardiology Solution Set Oversight Committee.

2017 ACC/AHA/HFSA Focused Update of the 2013 ACCF/AHA Guideline for the Management of Heart Failure: A Report of the American College of Cardiology/American Heart Association Task Force on Clinical Practice Guidelines and the Heart Failure Society of America.

2013 ACCF/AHA Guideline for the Management of Heart Failure: A Report of the American College of Cardiology Foundation/American Heart Association Task Force on Practice Guidelines

(b) ICD: Approximately 50% of mortality in HF is caused by dysrhythmia. ICDs have been shown to prolong life span in patients who meet criteria.

(c) IABP placement: See Mechanical Circulatory Support

(d) VAD: See Mechanical Circulatory Support

(e) Extracorporeal membrane oxygenation (ECMO): See Mechanical Circulatory Support

(f) Surgery

(1) Revascularization for ischemic HF

(2) Valvular repair or replacement

(3) Transplantation

d. Potential complication: Death

PERICARDIAL DISEASE

> **KEY CONCEPT**
> Pericardial disease includes pericarditis, pericardial effusion, cardiac tamponade, and constrictive pericarditis.

1. **Pathophysiology**
   a. Pericarditis
      i. Inflammation of the pericardium with a wide variety of causes
      ii. May be acute or chronic
      iii. Acute pericarditis most commonly of viral or idiopathic origin
         (a) Produces acute illness characterized by fever, chest pain (characteristically relieved by sitting up or leaning forward), pericardial friction rub, global ST elevation, little to no pericardial effusion
         (b) Is usually self-limited and responds to NSAIDs
         (c) May be recurrent with relapses
   b. Pericardial effusion
      i. Abnormal amount of pericardial fluid can result when pericardial fluid is produced too rapidly to be reabsorbed.
      ii. If pericardial fluid accumulates slowly, the pericardium stretches with little increase in intrapericardial pressure. Cardiac filling and function are not disturbed. If effusion accumulates rapidly, intrapericardial pressure rises and tamponade may result.
      iii. Huge effusions (several liters) may develop slowly without tamponade (especially in uremic pericarditis).
      iv. Same causes as for pericarditis
   c. Cardiac tamponade
      i. Common causes are few: Aortic dissection, MI with myocardial rupture, trauma (catheter or pacemaker perforation, contusion during CPR), or laceration during pericardiocentesis (postoperative bleeding), bleeding at cardiac surgical sites
      ii. Results when pericardial fluid accumulates too rapidly to allow the pericardium to stretch. Can occur with small amounts of fluid or blood (~150 mL) in the pericardial space.
      iii. Intrapericardial pressure rises dramatically
      iv. Increased intrapericardial pressure exceeds the filling pressures of the right side (pretamponade) and then of both sides, impairing ventricular filling and output

     v. CVP and jugular venous pressures rise (may not be seen in marked hypovolemia)

    vi. Muffled heart sounds may be present

   vii. Pulsus paradoxus develops

  viii. CO falls dramatically

    ix. Compensatory tachycardia develops

    x. Hypotension and death result in minutes

  d. Constrictive pericarditis

    i. Results from chronic scarring and thickening of the pericardium after pericarditis of any cause

    ii. Most common causes are posttraumatic, postpericardiotomy, and postradiation factors; neoplasm; and tuberculosis

   iii. Epicardium becomes thickened with tough and rigid fibrous tissue that calcifies

   iv. This interferes with filling (especially of the right side of the heart) in mid to late diastole, which results in decreased CO and increased jugular venous filling pressures

    v. Syndrome of right-sided HF with decreased output develops

   vi. Pulmonary edema is not seen

   vii. Death is the usual outcome, unless life-saving but high-risk (10%–25% mortality) pericardiectomy is performed

2. Etiology and risk factors for pericarditis

  a. Idiopathic, acute, or nonspecific (most common)

  b. Infection

    i. Viral: Echovirus and coxsackievirus B (the two most common causes of acute pericarditis); adenovirus, enterovirus, and influenza, mumps, measles, smallpox, and chickenpox viruses

    ii. Bacterial: Pneumococci, staphylococci, *Mycobacterium tuberculosis*, streptococci, *Pseudomonas* species

   iii. Fungal: *Histoplasma, Aspergillus, Candida*

   iv. Rickettsial, spirochetal (Lyme disease, because of *Borrelia burgdorferi*)

    v. HIV infection and acquired immunodeficiency syndrome: Becoming a prevalent cause worldwide

  c. Neoplasms (especially metastatic tumors from the lung and breast; melanomas; lymphomas)

  d. Connective tissue diseases: Systemic lupus erythematosus, rheumatoid arthritis, polyarteritis nodosa, and scleroderma

  e. Radiation therapy to the thorax: Treatments for Hodgkin disease, breast or lung cancer

  f. Acute MI: Early inflammatory process (24–72 hours after) or delayed immunologic response (Dressler syndrome). Dressler syndrome (occurring weeks or months after MI) has decreased in incidence because of advanced MI therapy (use of thrombolytics).

  g. Postcardiotomy or postthoracotomy syndrome (occurs 2–10 days after surgery). Pericardial effusions are common. In heart transplant patients, effusions are associated with a higher incidence of acute rejection.

  h. Chest trauma, penetrating (stabbing, rib fractures) or nonpenetrating, including surgical procedures, such as pacemaker insertion

  i. Dissecting aortic aneurysm

  j. Systemic disease: Uremia, myxedema, sarcoidosis, severe hypothyroidism (pericardial effusions)

   k. Immunologic or hypersensitivity reactions: Medication reactions (e.g., to hydralazine, procainamide, penicillin, phenytoin, isoniazid)

3. Signs and symptoms
  a. Subjective and objective findings
    i. Sharp or stabbing precordial pain, increased with inspiration, lying down, swallowing or belching, or turning of thorax; may be relieved by sitting up and/or leaning forward. Pain may also be dull (hard to distinguish from MI pain).
    ii. Associated trapezius ridge pain (specific for pericarditis)
    iii. Nonspecific influenza-like complaints, such as low-grade fever, joint discomfort, fatigue, weight loss, night sweats
    iv. Weakness, exercise intolerance
    v. History of any of the etiologic findings
    vi. Recent history of taking immunosuppressive medications (e.g., corticosteroids)
    vii. Weight loss
  b. Pulsus paradoxus: In cardiac tamponade, pulsus paradoxus is the result of the influence of respiration on the beat-to-beat filling of the LV by flow from the pulmonary veins
    i. During inspiration, there is less pulmonary venous return to the left side of the heart; this is exaggerated by impaired filling caused by high intrapericardial pressure
    ii. Result is decreased left-sided heart output and decreased BP during inspiration
    iii. Pulsus paradoxus is an inspiratory decrease in BP of 11 mm Hg or greater
    iv. May not be seen in states in which LV filling is not solely dependent on pulmonary venous return (aortic insufficiency, VSD)
  c. Pericardial friction rub (audible in ~85% of patients with acute pericarditis)
    i. Has up to three components per cardiac cycle. High pitched is described as rasping, scratchy, grating, or squeaky sounds. May be very transient. Absence of a rub does not rule out pericarditis.
    ii. Heard best with the stethoscope diaphragm pressed firmly at the left lower sternal border
    iii. Most frequently heard at end expiration with the patient sitting upright and leaning forward
    iv. Having the patient hold the breath will help differentiate from pleural friction rub
  d. Other physical findings: Depending on the severity, any or all of the following symptoms may be observed:
    i. Dyspnea with or without pain, orthopnea
    ii. Cough, hemoptysis
    iii. Tachycardia
    iv. Fever
    v. Anxiety, confusion, restlessness
    vi. Pallor
    vii. Anorexia
    viii. Jugular venous distention
    ix. Kussmaul's sign (rise in CVP on inspiration): Seen in patients with constrictive pericarditis
    x. Flushing, sweating
    xi. Peripheral edema, abdominal swelling, or discomfort (constrictive pericarditis)
    xii. Increased cardiac dullness in large effusions
    xiii. Hepatojugular reflux

xiv. Heart sounds are often normal except muffled and distant sounding with effusion

xv. Pericardial "knock" in constriction (an early diastolic sound, uncommon)

4. **Diagnostic study findings**

a. Laboratory

  i. Troponin: Elevated levels mark myocardial injury and may be seen in pericarditis or MI

  ii. Moderate leukocytosis, increased sedimentation rate in acute or chronic pericarditis

  iii. CRP: Elevated levels

  iv. Blood cultures: To identify causative organisms and their sensitivity to antibiotics

  v. Antinuclear antibody test: Results positive in connective tissue diseases

  vi. BUN level: Renal status evaluation

  vii. Purified protein derivative testing: Tuberculosis

  viii. Pericardiocentesis, especially pericardial biopsy and drainage, may be helpful diagnostically

b. ECG

  i. In acute pericarditis

    (a) Diffuse ST-segment elevation in most leads or leads that are not grouped specifically in a myocardial region (see Table 4.7)

    (b) PR segment may be depressed

    (c) ST segment reverts to normal and T wave inverts after several days or upon resolution of the symptoms

  ii. Arrhythmias: Bradycardias, tachycardia (sinus or atrial arrhythmias, atrial fibrillation)

c. Radiologic: Normal or shows cardiac enlargement resulting from pericardial effusion

d. Echocardiography: To identify and quantify pericardial effusions, wall motion abnormalities, RA and RV diastolic collapse (pretamponade)

  i. Results usually normal in acute pericarditis unless effusions present

  ii. In tamponade: Identifies pericardial effusions, LA compression, and respiratory variation in LV inflow of more than 25% (tamponade)

  iii. Restriction in ventricular filling (constriction)

e. MRI, CT: To detect thickening of the pericardium, calcifications

f. Right-sided heart catheterization: Used to:

  i. Evaluate and monitor hemodynamics

  ii. Evaluate the severity of constriction

  iii. Assess the need for pericardiotomy

  iv. Assist in the differential diagnosis of constriction and restrictive cardiomyopathy

  v. Identify increased RV and LV filling pressures with equalization (constriction)

5. **Interprofessional collaboration: Nurse, physicians (cardiologist, infectious disease and possibly cardiac surgeon), advanced practice provider, physical and occupational therapists, social worker, cardiac rehabilitation team, dietitian, pharmacist.**

6. **Management of patient care**

a. Anticipated patient trajectory: Cardiac tamponade is a life-threatening condition, and the patient will die if emergent pericardiocentesis is not performed. Constrictive pericarditis is lethal and requires pericardiectomy. Pericarditis is generally self-limited.

b. Goals of care
   i. Treatment is directed toward the underlying disease.
   ii. Patient is comfortable, pain free, and without symptoms.
   iii. Hemodynamics, vital signs, and ECG are within normal limits.
   iv. Patient is free from complications (HF, tamponade).
   v. Laboratory values and clinical findings return to normal, and blood culture results are negative.
c. Treatments
   i. Positioning: Position the patient for comfort; sitting up and leaning forward will help increase comfort.
   ii. Pain management
      (a) Frequently ask the patient about pain and discomfort; if present, assess characteristics.
      (b) Give medications to relieve pain caused by the inflammatory process (acetaminophen, aspirin, antiinflammatory agents). Pain is often gone or diminished significantly in 24 to 48 hours but may last weeks. Corticosteroids are given for recurring, severe pain.
      (c) Reassure the patient regarding the nonischemic cause of the pain.
   iii. Pharmacology
      (a) Antimicrobial agents: If culture or serologic evidence of a susceptible etiologic agent is present
      (b) NSAIDs: For pericarditis, pleural effusions
      (c) Corticosteroids: If unresponsive to NSAIDs after 48 hours. Used cautiously for a short term and tapered quickly. They can contribute to recurrences because of viral proliferation.
      (d) Colchicine: May help in pain management and prevent recurrences
      (e) Anticoagulants: Withheld with pericardial effusions to lower the risk of tamponade. Heparin can be used, if necessary, because of its shorter half-life and reversibility.
      (f) Volume support (IV fluids) and/or inotropic agents (e.g., dobutamine): Used as a temporizing agent to improve CO during tamponade
   iv. Other interventions
      (a) Nursing care for cardiac tamponade
         (1) If tamponade occurs notify the provider immediately
         (2) Administer oxygen as ordered
         (3) Prepare the patient for pericardiocentesis
         (4) Emergency pericardiocentesis is life-saving. Removal of 50 to 100 mL of fluid can bring major hemodynamic improvement.
         (5) If a pericardial catheter is present, aspirate pericardial fluid per orders
         (6) Give fluids to increase preload
         (7) Discontinue agents that decrease preload (diuretics, nitrates, morphine)
      (b) Pericardiocentesis: For persistent effusions, tamponade, purulent pericarditis
         (1) Echocardiographic guidance of the procedure improves safety
         (2) Sclerosing agents may be infiltrated intrapericardially for chronic effusions
      (c) Pericardiotomy procedures for effusions and diagnostic biopsy, subxiphoid pericardiotomy, pericardial window surgery
      (d) Pericardiectomy: Treatment for constrictive pericarditis. Higher-risk surgery (10%–25% mortality) in severe or chronic disease.

d. Potential complications
  i. Cardiac tamponade: Complication of pericarditis (see Treatments earlier)
  ii. Recurrent pericarditis
    (a) Mechanism
      (1) Probable autoimmune response, may reoccur numerous times over years
      (2) Can be related to tapering or stopping of antiinflammatory agents
    (b) Management
      (1) Corticosteroids often needed to stop painful symptoms. Steroid dependency and adverse side effects are major concerns. Nonsteroidal agents (e.g., colchicine, azathioprine) can be used to help avoid reoccurrence.
      (2) Pericardiectomy is considered when medical therapy is unsuccessful

MYOCARDITIS

> **KEY CONCEPT**
> Myocarditis is an inflammation of the myocardium caused by microorganisms, medications, or chemicals. Can be acute or chronic (subacute) and focal or diffuse. There may be complete recovery or it can lead to severe cardiovascular compromise and death from DCM.

1. **Pathophysiology**
  a. Myocardial damage occurs because of infection or injury
  b. Interstitial infiltrates develop. Immune responses to inflammation ensue, and myocardial fibers become injured, hypertrophy, and begin to die.
  c. Necrosis of the myofibers may be global or spotty
  d. Vascular responses to inflammation include vasculitis and spasm, which contribute to myocardial fibrosis and necrosis
  e. Pericardial involvement often occurs at the same time
  f. Contractility and CO decrease
  g. LV function may be sufficiently impaired to cause fulminant myocarditis and HF
  h. Myocardial injury can continue after active infection as a result of persistent immune and autoimmune responses
2. **Etiology and risk factors**
  a. Causes can include viral, bacterial, rickettsial, parasitic, or mycotic organisms. There are also noninfectious causes, which include autoimmune disorders, medications, and cardiac toxins.
  b. In Europe and North America, viral infection (in particular, infection with coxsackievirus B) is the most common cause of myocarditis
  c. Viral
    i. Most common types include coxsackievirus A and B, adenovirus, and echovirus
    ii. Others include influenza virus, cytomegalovirus, HIV, hepatitis B virus, and mumps and rubella viruses
  d. Bacterial
    i. Infection with *Salmonella typhi, Coxiella burnetii*
    ii. Diphtheria: Most common cause of death
    iii. Tuberculosis
    iv. Streptococci, meningococci, clostridia, staphylococci
  e. Rickettsial

   f. Fungal: Aspergillosis

   g. Protozoal: Chagas disease *(Trypanosoma cruzi)*, seen in patients traveling to or living in Central and South America; malaria

   h. Autoimmune disorders: Systemic lupus erythematosus, Wegener granulomatosis

   i. Cardiac toxins (e.g., cocaine, catecholamines)

   j. Medications: Doxorubicin, amitriptyline

3. Signs and symptoms: Viral myocarditis is a diagnosis of exclusion. The responsible virus is very difficult to identify.

EXPERT TIP

Myocarditis may present similarly to MI; however, myocarditis is a diagnosis of exclusion. If a patient presents with chest pain, shortness of breath, nausea, and vomiting, the nurse should assume that the cause is an MI until proven otherwise.

---

   a. Clinical manifestations of viral myocarditis

      i. Patient may have complaints of a "common cold," fever, chills, sore throat, abdominal pain, nausea, vomiting, diarrhea, arthralgia, and myalgia up to 6 weeks before overt symptoms of HF appear.

      ii. Chest pain (two-thirds of patients) with no evidence of pericarditis or ischemia. Pain may be pleuritic, precordial, or associated with sweating, nausea, or vomiting. Chest pain can imitate ischemic pain.

      iii. Dyspnea: Dyspnea at rest, exertional dyspnea, paroxysmal nocturnal dyspnea, orthopnea

      iv. Palpitations

      v. Fatigue, weakness

   b. Physical findings

      i. Tachycardia

      ii. Symptoms of HF (rapid, fulminant)

      iii. Increased jugular venous pressure

      iv. Enlarged lymph nodes: Seen with sarcoidosis

      v. Pruritic rash (maculopapular): Medication reaction

      vi. Pulsus alternans (extreme HF)

      vii. Narrow pulse pressure

      viii. Hypotension

      ix. S_1 diminished (decreased contractility)

      x. S_3 gallop: Common

      xi. Murmurs: Mitral or tricuspid regurgitation (if ventricular dilatation is present)

      xii. Pericardial friction rub: Uncommon

4. Diagnostic study findings

   a. Laboratory

      i. Cultures (blood, throat, urine, stool specimens): To rule out bacterial and fungal causes

      ii. Cardiac enzyme levels

      iii. CBC: Slight to moderate leukocytosis

      iv. Erythrocyte sedimentation rate: Elevated

      v. Titers for *Rickettsia*, virus, fungus

      vi. Skin test for tuberculosis

b. Radiologic: Findings may be normal or
   i. Pulmonary congestion
   ii. Cardiomegaly
c. ECG
   i. Sinus tachycardia
   ii. ST segment can be elevated, T waves inverted; nonspecific ST- and T-wave changes
   iii. QTc interval is prolonged
   iv. ST returns to baseline in several days
   v. T-wave changes may last weeks or months (with severe myocarditis)
   vi. Arrhythmias are seen in one-third of patients
        (a) VT, supraventricular tachycardia (SVT), premature ventricular contractions
        (b) Atrial fibrillation
        (c) AV blocks
d. Echocardiography: Used to rule out other causes of HF and evaluate LV function
   i. Diffuse hypocontractility
   ii. Pericardial effusions
   iii. Valvular dysfunction
   iv. Chamber enlargement
   v. Ventricular thrombi
e. Cardiac MRI: Improvements in cardiac MRI technology have reduced the need for invasive biopsy.
f. Endocardial biopsy: Although myocarditis is a nonspecific histologic diagnosis, routine biopsy has no proven utility because of the high level of insensitivity and numerous false-negative results (up to 55% when only five specimens are obtained).
g. Right-sided heart catheterization: To evaluate CO, CI, SVR, pulmonary vascular resistance (PVR) for LV function
h. Coronary angiography: To exclude other causes of HF; CAD, valvular disease, congenital disorders
i. EPS: If history of sudden death, VF, and/or VT

5. **Interprofessional collaboration: See Pericarditis section**
6. **Management of patient care**
   a. Anticipated patient trajectory: Usually a mild disease; bed rest is important, along with management of symptoms. Patient is often in a stepdown unit, unless symptoms of HF, heart block, or other complications arise.
   b. Goals of care
      i. CO, hemodynamics, and vital signs are within normal limits
      ii. Patient has no arrhythmias
      iii. Patient has no signs or symptoms of HF
      iv. Plan is developed for progressive activities and exercise
      v. Patient shows a progressive (slow) increase in activity tolerance
   c. Treatments
      i. Positioning
         (a) Maintain bed rest at first (the patient needs activities restricted); exception would be use of a bedside commode, if tolerated
         (b) Allow patient to slowly ambulate with assistance
         (c) Monitor heart, respiratory rates, BP, and oxygen saturation with activity
      ii. Pain management: Relieve chest pain promptly
      iii. Nutrition: Low-sodium diet, fluid restriction, if signs of HF are present

  iv. Discharge planning
- (a) Instruct the patient about the need for a progressive increase in ambulation over the next 2 months
- (b) Teach the patient which symptoms to look for and report regarding activity tolerance. Patient should be able to monitor his or her pulse.
- (c) Facilitate and assist with the development of an activity and exercise program for the patient, both in the hospital and at home

  v. Pharmacology
- (a) Oxygen: Ensure adequate oxygenation; check pulse oximetry results, maintain oxygen saturations at over 92%. Hypoxia is common with myocarditis.
- (b) Diuretics
- (c) Afterload reduction agents (ACE inhibitors, ARBs): For cardiac failure
- (d) IV pressors and inotropic agents: If hemodynamic support is needed
- (e) Antiarrhythmics: As needed; monitor closely for arrhythmias—high risk for sudden death
- (f) Antiviral therapy (pleconaril): Used for enteroviruses
- (g) β-blockers: To decrease heart rate, arrhythmias
- (h) Immunosuppressive therapy: Has not proved beneficial for preservation of LV function or survival (except in a small number of patients)
- (i) NSAIDs: Ineffective; may facilitate disease process, increase mortality

  vi. Other interventions: Focused on managing symptoms
- (a) Treat causative agent if known
- (b) Temporary transvenous pacemaker for AV blocks
- (c) Temporary left ventricular assist devices (LVADs) may be required: IABP, LVAD to assist in CO and as a bridge to transplantation
- (d) Heart transplantation

d. Potential complications

  i. Arrhythmias
- (a) Mechanism: Myocardial injury, infection
- (b) Management
  - (1) SVTs: Cardioversion; unstable patients need direct current cardioversion whereas patients who are maintaining hemodynamic stability can be chemically cardioverted
  - (2) Heart blocks: Temporary transvenous pacemaker (transient condition usually not requiring permanent pacemaker)

  ii. DCM, HF
- (a) Mechanism: Can develop slowly over time
- (b) Management: Patient with myocarditis routinely followed to evaluate LV function

INFECTIVE ENDOCARDITIS

1. **Pathophysiology**
   a. Acute or chronic infection of the heart's endocardial surface, including valves, chordae tendineae, septum, and mural endothelium
   b. Infecting organisms may be present in the bloodstream (may be a very transient invasion).
   c. Valves and endothelial surface of the heart can be predisposed to injury. Infecting organisms have an affinity for traumatized areas and preexisting defects, such as with valvular disease, prosthetic valves, septal defects, or local trauma (from indwelling catheters).

> **EXPERT TIP**
> IE is a common reason for cardiac valve replacement surgery, particularly in younger patients.

   d. When traumatic injury from abnormal hemodynamic or endothelial stress has occurred, deposits of platelets and fibrin form microscopic thrombotic lesions

   e. Affected areas are then amenable to colonization by microorganisms. Bacteria and organisms from other infections in the body (skin, genitourinary tract, lungs, mouth) attach to the valves and to these thrombotic lesions.

   f. As the microorganisms colonize, they cause the deposition of platelets, leukocytes, erythrocytes, and fibrin, forming vegetations. Eventually, valvular tissue is destroyed by the infection, and the valve leaflets may become incompetent, ulcerate, rupture, abscess (ring or annular), or perforate.

   g. Valves on the left side of the heart are more often affected (85% of cases). Mitral valve is most commonly affected. Right-sided ineffective endocarditis (IE) is predominantly caused by IV drug use and generally involves the tricuspid and pulmonic valves.

   h. The bacteria and other microorganisms from the vegetations are circulated systemically, which causes bacteremia.

   i. Antibody formation increases the levels of immune complexes in the blood, which causes hypersensitivity reactions (allergic vasculitis) in peripheral parts of the body involving the arterioles, vessel walls, and cutaneous tissue.

   j. Embolization of infective material may occur throughout the body (left-sided vegetation causes systemic emboli; tricuspid valve vegetation causes pulmonary emboli).

2. **Etiology and risk factors**

   a. Median age of affected patients has increased to 50 years because of the decrease in rheumatic heart disease, increase in longevity, and emergence of nosocomial causes.

   b. Disease frequency is 2.5 times greater in men than in women.

   c. A wide variety of microorganisms cause endocarditis. Common organisms include the following:

      i. *Streptococcus* types (50%–60%)

        (a) *Streptococcus viridans:* Had been the most prevalent causative organism in subacute cases (now involved in only approximately one-third of cases)

        (b) Group B, D, or G streptococci

        (c) *Enterococci:* Often a nosocomial cause; resistant to medical therapy

      ii. *Staphylococcus* types (15%–40%)

        (a) *Staphylococcus aureus:* Most prevalent causative organism in acute and nosocomial cases (e.g., methicillin-resistant strains)

        (b) Coagulase-negative species: Often the cause of prosthetic valve endocarditis

      iii. Gram-negative rods (HACEK organisms [*Haemophilus* species, *Actinobacillus actinomycetemcomitans, Cardiobacterium hominis, Eikenella corrodens, Kingella kingae*])

      iv. Enterobacteriaceae: *Pseudomonas aeruginosa*

      v. Fungi: *Candida albicans, Aspergillus fumigatus*

      vi. Viruses: Coxsackievirus, adenovirus

   d. Surgery or procedures predisposing to IE bacteremia risk

      i. Dental procedures (extractions, surgery, cleaning) that cause mucosal or gingival bleeding: Cause 20% of cases of bacteremia

> **EXPERT TIP**
> In patients with poor dentition and dental abscesses, extraction of all teeth is common before open-heart surgery to prevent reoccurrence.

      ii. Tonsillectomy, adenoidectomy
      iii. Bowel surgeries, esophageal procedures
      iv. Genitourinary surgery, biopsies
   e. Other therapies and procedures predisposing patients to IE bacteremia risk
      i. Invasive tests and monitoring (pulmonary artery catheters)
      ii. Prolonged IV therapy (hyperalimentation)
      iii. Immunosuppressive therapy
      iv. Hemodialysis
   f. Medical conditions that predispose to IE
      i. Prosthetic valve
      ii. Rheumatic valvular disease: Previously most common predisposing condition; now rare in the United States
      iii. Previous IE episode
      iv. Congenital heart defect (e.g., PDA, coarctation of the aorta, VSD): About 14% of cases
      v. Degenerative valve disease: About 9% of cases
      vi. Mitral valve prolapse
      vii. Hypertrophic, obstructive cardiomyopathy
      viii. Abscesses on skin
      ix. Inflammatory gastrointestinal disease, gastrointestinal tumors
   g. Other factors: Intravenous drug abuse, unidentified causes of IE bacteremia (30%–40% of IE cases)

3. Signs and symptoms
   a. Subjective findings: Patient may complain of nonspecific, vague symptoms
      i. Fever (prolonged, unknown source, sudden onset)
      ii. Chills, night sweats
      iii. Fatigue, malaise
      iv. Neurologic dysfunctions: Headache, vision loss, stroke, confusion
      v. Nausea, vomiting, anorexia, weight loss
      vi. Arthralgias, myalgias
      vii. Back pain (cause unknown)
      viii. Dyspnea
   b. Physical findings: Depend on the presence of a systemic versus a local infection, the presence of systemic emboli, immune responses, and the duration of infection
      i. Fever: Higher than 100.4° F (38° C)
      ii. Signs and symptoms of HF
      iii. Petechiae (caused by emboli or allergic vasculitis): Seen in 20% to 40% of patients on the conjunctivae, neck, chest, abdomen, and mucosa of the mouth (usually a sign of a long-standing infection)
      iv. Osler's nodes (resulting from immunologically mediated vasculitis): Small, very tender, reddened, raised nodules on fingers and toe pads
      v. Roth's spots (resulting from emboli or allergic vasculitis): Round or oval white spots on the retina
      vi. Purpuric pustular skin lesions (caused by emboli)

vii. Janeway lesions (caused by septic emboli or allergic vasculitis): Large, nontender nodules on the palms of the hands, toes, and soles of the feet

viii. Splinter hemorrhages of the nails (resulting from emboli or allergic vasculitis)

ix. Conduction disturbances seen on ECG

x. Central nervous system disturbances (e.g., hemiplegia, confusion, headache, seizures, transient ischemic attacks, aphasia, ataxia, changes in the level of consciousness, psychiatric symptoms) if embolization to the brain has occurred

xi. Hematuria, oliguria, flank pain, hypertension, if the kidney is infarcted or abscessed from emboli. Glomerulonephritis frequently caused by allergic or immunologic reactions; kidney involvement is common.

xii. Tachypnea, dyspnea, hemoptysis, sudden pain in the chest or shoulder, cyanosis, and restlessness if the lung is infarcted

xiii. Abdominal pain (caused by mesenteric emboli)

xiv. Decreased or no pulses in cold limbs (emboli)

xv. Splenomegaly or pain caused by splenic infarction

xvi. If HF present, possible hepatojugular reflux, jugular venous distension, or peripheral edema

xvii. New murmurs of valvular insufficiency. Murmurs may also develop later, with therapy, and may change character.

xviii. Decreased or absent breath sounds or adventitious breath sounds if the lungs are infarcted

4. **Diagnostic study findings**
   a. Laboratory data
      i. Positive blood culture results (minimum of two separate sample sets initially, drawn 12 hours apart). Negative blood culture results do not necessarily rule out IE.
      ii. Other associated findings
         (a) Elevated sedimentation rate and CRP level (immune response)
         (b) Anemia (common in subacute endocarditis)
         (c) Leukocytosis, thrombocytopenia (associated with splenomegaly)
         (d) Proteinuria, microscopic hematuria, pyuria
         (e) Rheumatoid factor levels may be elevated, as may circulating immune complex levels
         (f) Hyperglobulinemia (common)
         (g) Abnormal laboratory values associated with affected organs (kidneys, lungs, heart)
   b. ECG
      i. Signs of ischemia or infarction if coronary artery emboli have occurred
      ii. New AV blocks, BBB
   c. Chest radiograph: Occasional pleural effusion; multiple, patchy pulmonary infiltrates
   d. Transthoracic echocardiography: Presence of vegetations on any of the valves; assesses degree of valvular dysfunction and complications (e.g., ruptured chordae tendineae, perforated valve cusps)
   e. TEE: Better sensitivity for vegetations, recommended for prosthetic valves
      i. Excellent views of prosthetic valves, mitral valve, aortic valve, ring abscesses
      ii. Evaluation of ventricular function
      iii. Assessment of the severity of mitral regurgitation
      iv. Negative TEE results does not exclude IE

    f. Catheterization: Preoperative evaluation, if valve replacement planned. Assesses the following:

      i. Valve dysfunction

      ii. Aneurysms, intracardiac shunts

      iii. Underlying CAD

    g. MRI or CT of head: With neurologic symptoms, to evaluate for infarction, abscess, or bleeding

5. **Interprofessional collaboration: See Pericarditis; plus home health nurse (IV therapy), dentist.**

6. **Management of patient care**

    a. Anticipated patient trajectory: Prompt diagnosis is difficult but important for successful treatment. Prognosis is good with effective antibiotic therapy; however, mortality remains approximately 20%. Older adult patients with symptoms of HF, renal insufficiency, or systemic embolization have a worse prognosis.

    b. Goals of care

      i. Patient is afebrile

      ii. Patient has negative blood culture results

      iii. Patient is well hydrated, as evidenced by normal skin turgor, balanced intake and output, and moist mucosa

    c. Treatments

      i. Skin care: Monitor for problems in skin integrity resulting from fever and sweating. Ensure that the patient is turning or turned often while on bed rest.

      ii. Nutrition

        (a) Assess the patient for signs of dehydration

        (b) Monitor caloric and fluid intake and output; weigh patient daily

      iii. Infection control

        (a) Monitor vital signs, especially temperature. Persistent or recurring fevers can indicate failure of or hypersensitivity to antimicrobial therapy, nosocomial infections, emboli, abscesses, thrombophlebitis, or medication reaction.

        (b) Assist in reduction of fever (e.g., administer antimicrobials, antipyretics, and cooling measures, as ordered; encourage fluid intake, if no evidence of HF)

        (c) Draw several blood culture samples initially and if temperature spikes (proper technique for drawing blood samples for culture is vital because of the difficulty in choosing antibiotics to adequately treat microorganisms)

        (d) Ensure that proper preventative measures are taken against nosocomial causes: Provide meticulous monitoring and care of indwelling catheters (change dressings and tubing; limit the duration of site use)

      iv. Discharge planning

        (a) Preventative teaching includes the following:

          (1) Discussion of the use of prophylactic antibiotics (for predisposing procedures, e.g., dental, bowel, bladder surgery). Provision of written material on high-risk procedures and recommended IE prophylaxis.

          (2) Stress good oral hygiene to decrease the frequency of bacteremia

            a) Stress the importance of close monitoring (physician appointments, laboratory work) during therapy and for several months afterward. Patient needs to be aware of the symptoms (e.g., fever, rash) to report promptly. Relapses generally occur within 2 months after therapy has been completed.

b) If the patient is to go home with continued outpatient IV antimicrobial therapy, then a demonstrated knowledge of medications, indwelling catheter care, and home health services is necessary.

  v. Pharmacology

    (a) Antimicrobial-antibiotic therapy

      (1) Initiate as soon as possible after initial blood culture results (to halt continued valvular damage and abscess formation). Patient will likely receive prolonged intravenous antibiotic therapy.

      (2) Check antimicrobial peak and trough serum levels to monitor therapeutic effects and prevent toxicity

      (3) Assess for musculoskeletal involvement (arthralgias, back pain, and myalgia are common symptoms). Antibiotic therapy usually helps decrease symptoms.

      (4) Fever usually stops after 3 days of therapy. If fever persists longer than 14 days, secondary infection or antibiotic resistance should be suspected.

      (5) If the patient is responding and stable, home outpatient IV therapy may be considered to finish the course of medication therapy

    (b) Anticoagulants: Do not prevent IE emboli and may increase bleeding risks

  vi. Other interventions

    (a) Prolonged IV administration of appropriate antimicrobials

    (b) Valve replacement surgery indicated (30%–50% of cases) if the patient has significant damage to the valves (prosthetic valves), ring or annular abscesses, HF, or refractory bacteremia

      (1) With aortic valve IE, valve replacement is imperative

      (2) In mitral or tricuspid valve IE, repair of valve is possible

d. Potential complications

  i. HF

    (a) Mechanism: Main cause of death from IE. Occurs when aortic and/or mitral valve becomes incompetent or regurgitant, or chordae tendineae rupture. May be progressive or acute (more often caused with aortic regurgitation).

    (b) Management

      (1) Assess the patient for signs and symptoms of HF

      (2) Monitor for new murmurs during hospitalization. Murmurs may change or appear during the course of the illness.

      (3) Valve replacement surgery: Immediate surgery is generally required

  ii. Embolization

    (a) Mechanism: Occurs from vegetations on the valves. May be the presenting symptom; can happen at any time and numerous events may occur. Seen in 20% to 50% of cases of IE. Often affects the central nervous system and the lower extremities, kidney, spleen, and bone.

    (b) Management

      (1) Assess the patient for signs and symptoms of systemic embolization

      (2) Monitor level of consciousness: Check for signs of cerebral emboli (e.g., headache, numbness, weakness, tingling, paralysis, ataxia, sudden blindness, or sudden hemiplegia)

      (3) Check for petechiae on neck, upper trunk, eyes, and lower extremities

      (4) Observe the extremities for painful nodes, swelling, erythema, decreased or absent pulses, coolness, decreased capillary refill

(5) Assess the patient for signs and symptoms of MI; monitor the ECG

(6) Arrange for guaiac test of stools, tests for blood in urine and nasogastric aspirations

(7) If pulmonary, myocardial, or cerebral embolism occurs, administer oxygen therapy, position the patient for comfort and ease of breathing, and give pain medications as ordered

(8) Ultrasonography, CT, and/or MRI used in diagnosis

(9) This type of embolization is not treated with anticoagulants unless the patient has a previous indication for their use (such as a prosthetic valve). Anticoagulants have not proved to be beneficial in therapy and may result in the complication of intracranial hemorrhage.

(10) Treatment is aimed at the infection and antimicrobials are given

(11) Surgery for valve replacement is considered if embolization occurs more than once, if infection is uncontrolled, or if there is persistent HF

   iii. Abscess

     (a) Mechanism: Occurs from contaminants, bacteremia

       (1) Cardiac valve ring abscess: Occurs with prosthetic valve endocarditis. Infection at the suture site of the valve can cause valve incompetency and dehiscence.

       (2) Extracardiac abscess: Often involves the spleen

     (b) Management: Splenectomy is the main therapy if the spleen is involved

   iv. Neurologic complications

     (a) Mechanism: Because of emboli and subsequent cerebral infarction, hemorrhage, cerebral abscesses, mycotic aneurysms (late complication). Neurologic complications are seen in 30% to 40% of IE patients and are associated with a high (40%) mortality rate.

     (b) Management: Watch for the development of headaches, seizures (see Ch. 5, Neurologic System)

   v. Renal insufficiency

     (a) Mechanism: Caused by immune-response glomerulonephritis, renal embolic infarcts. Azotemia develops.

     (b) Management: Usually improves with antimicrobial therapy

   vi. Conduction defects

     (a) Mechanism: Because of infectious process at the aortic valve; affects the AV node or bundle of His and includes all AV blocks, BBB

     (b) Management: Surgical intervention generally required

CARDIOMYOPATHY

> **KEY CONCEPT**
> Cardiomyopathy is a chronic or acute disorder of the heart muscle. Treatment may involve pharmacotherapy to reduce afterload and/or improve the contractility. Surgery and/or pacemaker/implantable cardiac defibrillator (ICD) placement may also be appropriate.

1. **Pathophysiology**
   a. DCM (most common type in the United States): Disorder is 2.5 times more common in males
      i. Myocardial fibers degenerate and fibrotic changes occur.

    ii. Severe dilatation of the heart occurs; includes atrial and ventricular dilatation, which creates global enlargement.

    iii. Systolic and diastolic dysfunction occurs and contractility decreases, which results in decreased SV, decreased EF, low CO, and compensatory increase in heart rate.

    iv. Mitral annular dilatation is secondary to LV dilatation and results in mitral insufficiency.

    v. HF develops, is often refractory to treatment, and is accompanied by malignant ventricular arrhythmias (often the cause of death).

b. Hypertrophic cardiomyopathy (HCM)

    i. Increased mass and thickening of the heart muscle, which results in diastolic dysfunction

    ii. Myocytes become abnormal, lose their geometric parallel arrangement, and become fibrotic.

    iii. Ventricles become rigid and stiff, restricting filling. Filling volumes decrease, and thus SV decreases.

    iv. LV chamber becomes very small (hypertrophy occurs inwardly at the expense of the LV chamber)

    v. LA becomes dilated

    vi. Contractility may be normal or increased

    vii. Obstructive form of HCM can occur: Often associated with an LV outflow tract dynamic obstruction that may be caused by concentric hypertrophy or localized hypertrophy. This obstructive form is referred to as *hypertrophic obstructive cardiomyopathy* (HOCM).

    viii. These processes may continue for years with no obvious problems and delayed onset of symptoms, or they may end with sudden cardiac death as a first sign of the disease process, because of malignant ventricular arrhythmias (VF, VT)

    ix. Men and women equally affected

c. Restrictive cardiomyopathy (least common)

    i. Restricted filling of ventricles

    ii. Usually caused by an infiltrative process, most often amyloidosis in adults

    iii. Heart loses its compliance, grows stiff, and cannot distend well in diastole or contract well in systole

    iv. Left ventricular end diastolic pressure (LVEDP) increases; contractility decreases, which results in low CO, HF, and death

2. Etiology and risk factors

a. DCM

    i. Idiopathic

    ii. Familial: 25% to 30% of cases

    iii. Infection (autoimmune reaction): Bacterial, parasitic, fungal, protozoal

    iv. Metabolic disorders: Chronic hypophosphatemia, thiamine deficiency, protein deficiency

    v. Toxins: Alcohol, lead, arsenic, uremic substances

    vi. Connective tissue disorders: Lupus erythematosus, rheumatoid disease, polyarteritis, scleroderma

    vii. Viral myocarditis

    viii. Medications: Amitriptyline, doxorubicin, cocaine

    ix. Ischemia

    x. Pregnancy (third trimester) or the postpartum period (common in multiparous women who are older than 30 years or have a history of preeclampsia)

      xi. Neuromuscular disorders: Muscular dystrophy, myotonic dystrophy

      xii. Infiltrative disorders: Sarcoidosis, amyloidosis

      xiii. Beriberi

  b. HCM

      i. Strong familial component (60%–70% of cases)

      ii. Idiopathic

      iii. Neuromuscular disorders: Friedreich ataxia

      iv. Metabolic: Hypoparathyroidism

      v. Hypertension

  c. Restrictive cardiomyopathy

      i. Idiopathic

      ii. Infiltrative: Amyloidosis, sarcoidosis, hemochromatosis, neoplasms

      iii. Endomyocardial fibroelastosis in children

      iv. Glycogen and mucopolysaccharide deposition

      v. Radiation

3. **Signs and symptoms: See Table 4.14 for physical findings associated with DCM, HCM, and restrictive cardiomyopathy. HCM may present at any age, may remain asymptomatic.**

  a. Ascertain the patient's chief complaint and the history of the present illness

  b. Patient may complain of angina, syncope, palpitations, exertional dyspnea, orthopnea, fatigue

  c. Determine whether there is a familial component (family history of cardiomyopathy or sudden death in young adults)

  d. Rule out other disease processes, such as hypertension, ischemic heart disease, amyloidosis, and preeclampsia

  e. Identify potential etiologic factors, such as recent infections, history of alcohol use, current use of medications, use of cocaine, pregnancy, and any endocrine disorders

4. **Diagnostic study findings**

  a. Laboratory

      i. Arterial blood gas (ABG) levels: Check for hypoxemia

      ii. Electrolyte levels: Decreased potassium and/or magnesium levels

      iii. Cardiac enzyme levels: Infarct

      iv. Renal function: BUN, creatinine levels

  b. Radiologic

      i. Heart normal or enlarged

      ii. Pulmonary congestion

  c. ECG

      i. Arrhythmias or conduction defects (e.g., sinus tachycardia, atrial fibrillation, ventricular ectopy, BBBs)

      ii. Atrial fibrillation: High incidence (70%–80%)

      iii. Evidence of both LA and LV enlargement: Increased QRS voltage

      iv. Abnormal Q waves

      v. VT

      vi. Prolonged QTc interval

  d. Transthoracic echocardiography

      i. LV systolic function: EF of 15% to 30% in DCM

      ii. Valvular dysfunction

      iii. LV hypertrophy (in HCM)

      iv. Marked asymmetric septal hypertrophy (in HCM, HOCM) and LV outflow tract pressure gradient (in HOCM)

      v. LA enlargement

TABLE 4.14 Physical Findings Associated With Dilated, Hypertrophic, and Restrictive Cardiomyopathy

Cardiomyopathy	Patient Complaint	Inspection	Palpation	Percussion	Auscultation
Dilated	Dyspnea on exertion, orthopnea, fatigue, palpitations	Clinical manifestations of HF, dysrhythmias on monitor, conduction defects	Narrow pulse pressure, pulsus alternans, cool skin, JVD, PMI laterally displaced, left ventricular heave, peripheral edema, hepatomegaly	Cardiac enlargement, dullness in bases of lungs	Irregular heartbeat, third and fourth heart sounds, mitral and tricuspid insufficiency, pulmonary rales
Hypertrophic	Dyspnea on exertion, orthopnea, PND, angina, syncope, palpitations	Dyspnea, orthopnea	Forceful and laterally displaced apical impulse, systolic thrill (in HOCM)		Fourth heart sound, a third heart sound may be heard, split-second heart sound, systolic ejection murmur
Restrictive	Fatigue, weakness, dyspnea on exertion, anorexia, poor exercise tolerance	Dysrhythmias, distended neck veins, Kussmaul's sign	Edema, ascites, HJR, right upper quadrant pain	Cardiac enlargement, pulmonary congestion	Third and fourth heart sounds, mitral and tricuspid insufficiency

HF, Heart failure; *HJR,* hepatojugular reflux; *JVD,* jugular venous distention; *PMI,* point of maximal impulse; *PND,* paroxysmal nocturnal dyspnea.

From Falk, R.H., Hershberger, R.E. (2015). The dilated, restrictive, and infiltrative cardiomyopathies. In D.L. Mann, D.P. Zipes, P. Libby, R.O. Bonow, E. Braunwald, editors: *Braunwald's heart disease: a textbook of cardiovascular medicine,* 10th ed. (pp 1551–1573). Philadelphia, Elsevier.

Cardiovascular System

4

    e. Radionuclide tests: May reveal increased ventricular volumes, decreased EF in DCM, increased uptake in patients with amyloidosis, defects in cardiac wall in patients with neoplasms or sarcoidosis

    f. TEE: To evaluate anatomy and rule out thrombosis

    g. Right-sided heart catheterization:

       i. Pulmonary artery occlusion pressure (PAOP) and pulmonary artery pressure (PAP) elevated, CO decreased

       ii. RV end-diastolic pressure and CVP rise in right-sided HF or with DCM

    h. Left-sided heart catheterization, angiogram, arteriogram

    i. Rule out CAD

       i. Mitral regurgitation

       ii. LV outflow tract gradient in HOCM

       iii. EPS and Holter study: To identify VF and VT and to guide therapy

    j. Endomyocardial biopsy: Used to identify the cause of restrictive cardiomyopathy

5. Interprofessional collaboration: See Heart Failure section

6. Management of patient care

    a. Anticipated patient trajectory: In most patients, cardiomyopathy may be stabilized or actually improved with medical management. A few patients will succumb to progressive HF unless transplantation is possible.

    b. Goals of care

       i. Symptoms of HF are relieved

       ii. Cause (especially if toxin) is determined and removed or treated

       iii. Sinus rhythm is maintained, if possible. Atrial fibrillation or other arrhythmias are treated promptly.

       iv. High risk of sudden death is reduced

    c. Treatments

       i. Positioning: Use preventive measures, especially for patients at high risk

         (a) Assist with passive and active exercises while the patient is confined to bed

         (b) Apply antiembolism stockings

         (c) Encourage ambulation as tolerated

         (d) Position the patient so that angulation at the groin and knees is avoided. Elevate the patient's legs when the patient is out of bed. Patient should be instructed not to cross the legs or ankles. Avoid using the knee joint on a Gatch bed.

         (e) Instruct the patient to avoid activities that may cause straining or increase the obstruction, such as strenuous exercise, Valsalva maneuvers, and sitting or standing suddenly

       ii. Pain management: Administer supportive measures as the situation dictates (e.g., oxygen therapy, pain medications, sedatives, emotional support)

       iii. Nutrition: Sodium-restricted diet, weight control

       iv. Infection control: IE prophylactic therapy

       v. Discharge planning: Patient education regarding the following:

         (a) Activities that aggravate symptoms

         (b) Benefits of weight reduction, sodium restriction, smoking and/or alcohol use cessation, exercise

         (c) BP control

         (d) Follow-up evaluations

         (e) Screening of family members (physical examination, laboratory tests, ECG, echocardiography) starting at age 12 years

       vi. Pharmacology

    (a) ACE inhibitors or ARBs: Used to decrease afterload and remodeling, improve LV EF

    (b) β-blockers (e.g., carvedilol, metoprolol, atenolol)

        (1) Function by slowing or reversing the progression of LV dysfunction (because of hyperadrenergic tone)

        (2) Increase LV EF

        (3) Decrease heart rate, increase ventricular filling time

        (4) Decrease hospitalization for HF

    (c) Antiarrhythmic agents (atrial fibrillation, VT)

    (d) Anticoagulants: For atrial fibrillation (monitor INR, aPTT; observe for bleeding)

    (e) Antibiotics: If the patient is at risk for IE, instruct the patient to notify the dentist before any dental or surgical procedures (e.g., gastrointestinal or genitourinary procedures) for prophylactic antibiotics

    (f) Treatment specific to DCM

        (1) Inotropic agents to improve myocardial contractility and decrease HF

        (2) Diuretics to relieve pulmonary congestion; monitor volume status

        (3) Afterload- and preload-reducing agents, such as ACE inhibitors, ARBs and angiotensin receptor-neprilysin inhibitor (ARNi) to decrease myocardial workload, improve CO, and decrease pulmonary venous pressure

        (4) Spironolactone: Helpful in decreasing mortality in HF

    (g) Treatment specific to HOCM

        (1) Goal is to administer medications to reduce outflow tract obstruction to relieve syncope, angina, dyspnea, and arrhythmias, and prevent sudden cardiac death. β-blockers, calcium channel blockers, or a type IA antiarrhythmic are used.

        (2) Avoid agents that decrease preload (nitrates, diuretics, or morphine). Hypovolemia can be very detrimental because the LV is very preload dependent for adequate CO.

        (3) Avoid administering isoproterenol, dopamine, or digitalis preparations because they increase contractility and hence worsen the obstruction

    (h) Treatment specific to restrictive cardiomyopathy: Avoid digoxin in patients with cardiac amyloidosis, because it concentrates in the amyloid fibrils and can result in digitalis toxicity

  vii. Psychosocial issues

    (a) Help the patient identify stressors and teach methods of stress reduction

    (b) Counseling may be needed for the patient and family members if alcohol or cocaine use is present and is suspected as a cause

  viii. Other interventions

    (a) Closely monitor vital signs, ECG, intake and output, hemodynamics, laboratory values

    (b) For HOCM patients

        (1) Surgical septal myectomy: Septal muscle creating obstruction is surgically excised. Hypertrophied muscle does not regenerate. Many patients can return to their normal lifestyles.

        (2) Septal ablation (alternative to surgery): Alcohol is injected, via a percutaneous transluminal catheter, into the small coronary artery supplying the obstructive area; muscle is destroyed and shrinks, which lessens the obstruction. Potential complications include heart blocks, arrhythmias, VSD, and MI.

(c) Biventricular synchronized pacemaker used to help improve CO in DCM and HOCM
   (1) Patients with an LV EF of less than 35%, QRS of more than 0.12 mm. Used in older patients.
   (2) Can decrease obstruction. Increases activity tolerance and quality of life, used as a bridge.
   (3) Prepare the patient for this procedure. Be knowledgeable about the pacemaker procedure, equipment, protocols.
(d) Automatic implantable cardioverter defibrillator (AICD)
   (1) Patients who have experienced sudden cardiac death should receive an AICD
   (2) Patients who have two or more risk factors for sudden cardiac death (family history of sudden cardiac death, syncope not attributable to another cause, nonsustained VT, LV wall thickness ≥30 mm, failure to increase SBP by at least 20 mm Hg from rest to peak exercise or fall of >20 mm Hg during exercise) should be strongly considered for AICD placement
(e) Patients with end-stage disease may be candidates for cardiac transplantation (see End-Stage Heart Disease)

d. Potential complications
   i. HF, LV failure (see Heart Failure)
   ii. Dysrhythmias, particularly atrial and ventricular, on ECG: Atrial fibrillation, ventricular arrhythmias (see Cardiac Rhythm Disorders). Arrhythmias attributed to HCM are a common cause of sudden cardiac death in young adults.
      (a) With atrial fibrillation: Rate and rhythm control; unstable patients should receive direct current cardioversion while hemodynamically stable patients can be converted with medication (e.g., amiodarone)
      (b) Patients at high risk for sudden cardiac death evaluated for AICD
      (c) Bradycardias, AV conduction defects may require permanent pacemakers
   iii. IE: See Infective Endocarditis section
   iv. Embolism
      (a) Mechanism: Stasis of blood can cause DVT, PE
         (1) Patients at risk are the older adult and immobile patients on bed rest; patients who are in HF or atrial fibrillation, or who have a dilated myocardium
         (2) Yearly risk of systemic embolization and stroke with HOCM and atrial fibrillation is 20%
      (b) Management: Long-term anticoagulation, use of supportive stockings, performance of range-of-motion exercises

CARDIAC RHYTHM DISORDERS

1. **Life-threatening cardiac rhythms are divided into arrhythmias that are either too slow, too fast, or unable to generate an adequate pulse. For emergency management of these conditions, be sure to consult the most current ACLS guidelines.**

Symptomatic Bradycardia

1. **Bradycardias, conduction defects, and slow escape rhythms**
2. **Pathophysiology**
   a. Dysfunction of the SA node: Result of ischemia, infarction, disease, degeneration, defects, or medication effects (SA exit blocks, severe sinus bradycardia, sinus pause, sinus arrest, sick sinus syndrome)

b. Dysfunction of the AV node: Result of ischemia, infarction, disease, defects, degeneration, or medication effects; leads to AV conduction defects—second-degree, types I and II, third-degree (complete) heart block; surgical injury or interventional effects, such as transcatheter aortic valve replacement (TAVR)

    i. AV nodal tissue slows or fails to propagate electrical impulses to the ventricles

    ii. Slower pacemaker cells in lower sites (junctional, bundle of His, ventricular) escape and take over as the cardiac pacemaker in third-degree blocks

    iii. In acute anterior MI, complete heart block develops in 6% to 10% of patients

    iv. In inferior MI, ischemia or infarction of the AV node may create a temporary conduction defect, which usually resolves in less than a week

c. Hypersensitivity of the carotid sinus: Exaggerated response to vagal stimulation causes slowing of the heart rate and conductivity and lowering of the BP

3. **Etiology and risk factors**

a. Parasympathetic or vagal stimulation: Valsalva maneuver, nausea, vomiting, suctioning

b. Aging: Structural degeneration of the conductive system

c. MI, ischemic heart disease

d. Medications: Calcium channel blockers; cardiac glycosides; β-blockers

e. Infectious process: Endocarditis, myocarditis, typhoid fever, rheumatic fever, Chagas disease

f. Metabolic disorders: Myxedema, hypothermia, hypercalcemia

g. Aortic stenosis

h. Tumors

i. Trauma

j. Postcardiac surgery or interventional procedures

k. Connective tissue disease (sarcoidosis, amyloidosis, systemic lupus erythematous, thyroid disease)

l. Dive reflex (immersion in cold water)

4. **Signs and symptoms**

a. Syncope or presyncope

b. Wooziness, light-headedness

c. Fatigue, weakness

d. Shortness of breath

e. Angina

f. Pauses in pulse longer than 3 seconds

g. Heart rates lower than 40 beats/min

h. Hypotension

i. Signs of HF, cardiogenic shock

j. Dyspnea

k. Exercise intolerance

l. Decreased CO, CI

5. **Diagnostic study findings**

a. ECG: See Table 4.8 for arrhythmia features

    i. Correlation of symptoms with documented ECG is main diagnostic tool

    ii. Pauses more than 3 seconds in duration

    iii. Third-degree heart block with inferior MI: Usually narrow QRS complex accompanies bradycardia (higher escape pacemaker)

    iv. Third-degree heart block with anterior MI: Wide QRS complex may be observed (lower escape pacemaker)

b. Holter monitoring: To identify arrhythmias not documented elsewhere and correlate with symptoms
c. EPS: To test SA and AV node function, confirm need for permanent pacemaker
d. Labs: Laboratory work required for investigation of arrhythmias includes:
   i. CBC
   ii. Serum electrolytes including calcium and magnesium
   iii. BUN, creatinine, and glucose
   iv. TSH (for hypothyroid)
   v. Medication levels if appropriate (e.g., digoxin)
   vi. Toxicology, especially cocaine and amphetamines
   vii. Cardiac biomarkers (R/O MI or coronary ischemia as cause of arrhythmia)

6. **Interprofessional collaboration: See STEMI; also Electrophysiologist**
7. **Management of patient care: Arrhythmia management usually follows ACC/AHA guidelines and ACLS**
  a. Anticipated patient trajectory: Marked bradycardia results in diminished CO, poor tissue perfusion, hypotension, and potentially loss of consciousness and death
  b. Goals of care
    i. Hemodynamics are improved via improved heart rate
    ii. Symptoms from bradycardia are decreased or absent
  c. Treatments
    i. Infection control: Proper wound care and site observation (for drainage, redness, tenderness) is necessary to decrease the potential for infection from pacemakers. Monitor temperature, laboratory results (white blood cell count).
    ii. Discharge planning: Patient education regarding the following:
      (a) Rationales, procedure, activity precautions, and wound care for pacer placement
      (b) Daily pulse checks at home (permanent pacemaker)
      (c) Symptoms to report: Wooziness, fainting, prolonged weakness, fatigue, palpitations, chest pain, difficulty breathing, fever, redness, drainage or swelling at surgical site, prolonged hiccups, electrical shocks
      (d) Follow-up care: To assess pacemaker function, adjust pacemaker parameters
      (e) Identification bracelet (medical alert)
      (f) Home (telephonic) pacemaker monitoring
    iii. Pharmacology: According to AHA's ACLS guidelines
      (a) If the patient is symptomatic, administer atropine, 0.5 to 1.0 mg IV
        (1) Given every 3 to 5 minutes IV; total IV dosage of up to 3 mg
        (2) Effective for marked sinus bradycardia, second-degree, and some third-degree blocks
        (3) Dose of less than 0.5 mg IV can cause paradoxical bradycardia
      (b) Other potential medications include dopamine, epinephrine, isoproterenol
      (c) Isoproterenol is used for heart transplant patients; because of vagal denervation, these patients will not respond to atropine
    iv. Other interventions
      (a) If the patient is in stable condition or asymptomatic: Monitor closely, notify the physician, determine possible causes, have medications and transcutaneous pacemaker equipment readily available (especially if the patient is in third-degree block or second-degree AV block type II)
      (b) Ensure adequate oxygenation: Oxygen saturations of 92% or higher
      (c) Check the patency of IV lines

(d) Pacemakers: If the patient is unable to maintain adequate CO, use of a temporary or permanent pacemaker is indicated
  (1) Purpose: To provide an extrinsic electrical impulse so that depolarization and subsequent contraction occur
  (2) Modes of pacing (Fig. 4.14)
    a) Fixed rate (asynchronous): Impulses are delivered at a predetermined rate, irrespective of any intrinsic electrical activity
    b) Demand (synchronous): Impulses are delivered at a predetermined rate only if the patient's own heart rate is less than the pacemaker's set rate
    c) Dual chamber: Pacemakers that can sense electrical activity in and pace either or both chambers to provide the normal sequence of atrial and ventricular contraction (AV sequential pacing) are the most common
    d) Rate responsive: Pacemakers increase the heart rate to meet the demands of increased activity
  (3) Components of all pacemakers
    a) Battery
      1) In temporary pacers, battery longevity depends on use and capabilities. Batteries should be checked routinely and changed per unit standards.
      2) Permanent pacemaker batteries last 7 to 10 years (varies with the degree of the patient's pacemaker dependency)
    b) Lead system: Transmission of electrical impulse as follows:

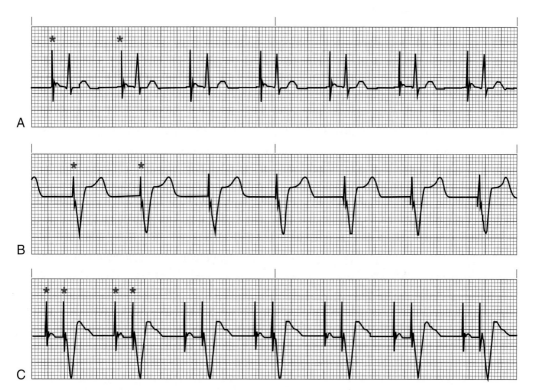

Fig. 4.14 Pacing examples. A, Atrial pacing. **B,** Ventricular pacing. **C,** Dual-chamber pacing. The *asterisk* indicates the pacemaker impulse. (From Urden, L.D., Stacy, K.M., Lough, M.E. (2022). *Critical care nursing: diagnosis and management,* 9th ed. St. Louis: Elsevier.)

1) Unipolar electrode systems: One pole is the pacing lead tip and the other pole is the pacemaker generator; produce large pacing spikes, easily seen on monitors and ECGs
2) Bipolar electrode systems (most common): Both negative and positive electrode poles are at the distal end of the pacing lead; produce small pacing spikes, often not seen on monitors and ECGs
   c) Pulse generator; pacemaker's control box
(4) Capture threshold level: Minimum pacemaker output setting required to pace the heart 100%
   a) Factors increasing the threshold: Hyperkalemia, hypoxia, medications (β-blockers, type I antiarrhythmics)
   b) Factors decreasing the threshold: Increased catecholamine levels, digitalis toxicity, corticosteroids
(e) Transcutaneous pacemaker: Emergency therapy used until a transvenous pacer can be inserted. Many have monitoring, defibrillation, and pacing capabilities.
   (1) One large anterior pacing electrode is ideally placed over the heart, and the other is placed directly posterior on the back. Other models have sternal-apex electrodes.
   (2) Pacemaker electrodes are attached to an output cable attached to a pacing unit. Pacing unit is generally part of a portable defibrillator unit.
   (3) Pacing rate and output are then set. Rate initially is set at 80 beats/min. Output is gradually increased until a pacer spike with a depolarization (pacer-generated QRS) is seen. Confirm ventricular contraction by palpating a pulse associated with the paced complex.
(f) Transvenous pacemaker: Pacing catheter is placed via the percutaneous route to the RA, RV, or biventricular for pacing. The proximal end of the catheter is attached to a pacing generator.
   (1) Initial rate usually set at 60 to 80 beats per minute
   (2) Output is set to an intermediate level (~5 mA) and decreased until capture is lost (usually at <2 mA)
   (3) Pacing output is then set to 2 to 3 times the level required for capture
(g) Epicardial transthoracic pacing: Electrode wires are attached to the epicardium (RA, RV, or both). Used during cardiac surgery in anticipation of conduction defects or arrhythmias. Proximal ends exit through the chest wall for attachment to the pulse generator.

EXPERT TIP

In the operating room, the pacemaker may be set in an asynchronous mode (e.g., DOO) to avoid interference from the electrocautery and to pace the heart as it comes off cardiopulmonary bypass. Upon arrival to the intensive care unit (ICU), pacing is typically changed to a synchronous mode (e.g., VVI, AAI, DDI) in accordance with the provider's order.

---

   (1) Electrode wires need to be insulated when not in use
   (2) May have one or two RA and one or two RV wires and a ground wire
(h) Permanent pacemaker: Leads placed in contact with the endocardium. Generator is implanted in a subcutaneous, subclavicular, or abdominal pocket. Capabilities can include sequential pacing of the RA,

RV, or both; programmability and rate responsiveness to allow for heart rate increases during exercise.

    (i) Key concepts for nursing care of patients with pacemakers (Box 4.5)

  d. Potential complications

    i. Monitor for complications of pacemaker insertion

      (a) Pneumothorax

      (b) Myocardial perforation: Can lead to hypotension, tamponade

      (c) Hematoma

      (d) Arrhythmias (premature ventricular contractions)

      (e) Infections (systemic or local)

      (f) Hiccups, muscle twitches (from stimulation of the diaphragm, abdomen)

    ii. Monitor for pacemaker malfunctions (Box 4.6 and Figs. 4.15 and 4.16)

Symptomatic Tachycardia

1. **Rhythms in this section include SVTs or VTs that cause symptoms necessitating immediate conversion or control**
2. **Pathophysiology**
  a. With increased heart rate at rest, diastolic filling period shortens and CO falls because of decreased ventricular filling

---

BOX 4.5 Key Concepts in the Nursing Care of Patients With Pacemakers

TRANSCUTANEOUS PACEMAKERS

- Patient will need sedation and analgesia because of increased output requirements (50–200 mV) for transcutaneous route
- Cardiopulmonary resuscitation may be performed safely over pacing electrodes, if needed
- Frequent inspection of skin is needed to prevent potential burns if pacing is prolonged

TRANSVENOUS PACEMAKERS

1. Ensure that chest radiograph is obtained to rule out pneumothorax if pacemaker is placed via subclavian or internal jugular approach.
2. Monitor closely for appropriate sensing and pacing.
3. Take appropriate action in case of sudden loss of capture.
    - Can signify that pacing electrode has migrated out of position or perforated right ventricle
    - Increase output to attempt recapture and notify physician
    - Do not attempt to reposition pacing electrode
    - Be prepared to use atropine, dopamine, or transcutaneous pacing
4. Ensure electrical safety when using temporary pacemaker.
    - Ensure that all equipment is grounded and in good working order
    - Wear gloves when handling electrodes
    - Place pulse generator in plastic bag or glove to protect from bodily fluids, other liquids
    - Position pulse generator in safe location (e.g., intravenous drip pole, holder strap when ambulating) to avoid dropping it or patient's rolling over on it in bed

EPICARDIAL TRANSTHORACIC PACEMAKER

- In addition to points related to transvenous pacemakers, electrode wires need to be insulated when not in use

PERMANENT PACEMAKER

1. Keep defibrillator paddles 1 to 2 inches away from permanent pacemaker site on chest.
2. Ensure pacer is interrogated after defibrillation or code is over.
3. Have magnet (doughnut) available: Used over pacer to program to asynchronous mode if pacemaker-mediated tachycardia is suspected or if electrocautery is to be used.

From Swerdlow, C.D., Wang, P., Zipes, D.P. (2015). Pacemakers and implantable cardioverter-defibrillators. In D.L. Mann, D.P. Zipes, P. Libby, R.O. Bonow, E. Braunwald, editors: *Braunwald's heart disease: a textbook of cardiovascular medicine*, 10th ed. (pp 721–747). Philadelphia, Elsevier.

BOX 4.6 Complications Associated With Pacemaker Functioning

FAILURE TO PACE

No pacer spike seen at appropriate times
Caused by:
- Battery failure
- Lead dislodgement
- Wire fracture
- Disconnection of wire or cable
- Generator failure
- Oversensing: No impulse generated because some other activity (often muscular) has been sensed and misinterpreted as a QRS complex

FAILURE TO CAPTURE

Pacer-generated QRS not seen
Caused by:
- Lead dislodgement or malposition
- Battery failure
- Pacing at voltage below capture threshold
- Faulty connections
- Lead fracture
- Ventricular perforation

FAILURE TO SENSE

Pacemaker may compete with patient's own intrinsic rhythm
Caused by:
- Sensitivity setting that is too high
- Battery failure
- Malposition of catheter lead
- Lead fracture
- Pulse generator failure
- Lead insulation break

From Swerdlow, C.D., Wang, P., Zipes, D.P. (2015). Pacemakers and implantable cardioverter-defibrillators. In D.L. Mann, D.P. Zipes, P. Libby, R.O. Bonow, E. Braunwald, editors: *Braunwald's heart disease: a textbook of cardiovascular medicine*, 10th ed. (pp 721–747). Philadelphia, Elsevier.

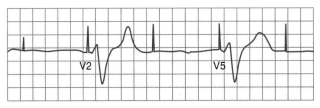

Fig. 4.15 An example of intermittent failure to capture is shown. Pacing spikes can be seen marching steadily through the tracing, but every other beat fails to elicit ventricular depolarization. This can occur because of elevated pacing thresholds, a low programmed pacemaker output, a depleted pulse generator battery, lead abnormality, or a prolonged refractory period. (From Antman, E.M. (2007). *Cardiovascular therapeutics: a companion to Braunwald's heart disease*, 3rd ed. Philadelphia: Elsevier.)

    b. Eventually, BP drops
    c. Pulmonary venous pressures increase, causing shortness of breath and dyspnea as the result of pulmonary congestion
    d. Heart rate at which CO declines is variable and depends on the patient's substrate cardiac function

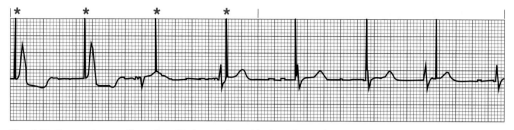

Fig. 4.16 Pacemaker malfunction: Undersensing. Notice that after the first two paced beats, a series of intrinsic beats occurs; the pacemaker unit fails to sense these intrinsic QRS complexes. These spikes do not capture the ventricle because they occur during the refractory period of the cardiac cycle. The *asterisk* indicates the pacemaker impulse. (From Urden, L.D., Stacy, K.M., Lough, M.E. (2022). *Critical care nursing: diagnosis and management*, 9th ed. St. Louis: Elsevier.)

e. Myocardial oxygen demands increase and myocardial oxygen supply decreases because of diminished coronary perfusion at rapid heart rates; subendocardial ischemia can result

f. Loss of atrial systole (kick) decreases the ventricular diastolic filling volume; SV and CO fall 10% to 15% in rhythms without a normal atrial-ventricular sequence of contraction

g. Decreased output can result in end organ dysfunction (e.g., syncope, presyncope, oliguria, ischemia)

3. **Etiology and risk factors**

  a. SVTs

    i. Acute MI

    ii. Ischemia

    iii. Reentry (most common cause of paroxysmal SVT)

    iv. Valvular heart disease

    v. Use of stimulants: Alcohol, coffee, tobacco

    vi. Congenital heart disease

    vii. Pulmonary disease

    viii. Medication toxicity: Digitalis, antidepressants

    ix. Accessory pathways (e.g., WPW syndrome)

    x. Cardiomyopathies

  b. VT: Sustained (>30 seconds)

    i. Acute MI

    ii. Ischemia

    iii. Hyperthyroidism

    iv. Tetralogy of Fallot

    v. Medications: Digitalis, antiarrhythmic agents

    vi. Electrolyte imbalances: Low potassium, magnesium

    vii. Hypoxia

    viii. LV aneurysms

    ix. Congenital or acquired long QT syndromes

    x. Valvular heart disease

4. **Signs and symptoms**

  a. Dyspnea

  b. Palpitations

  c. Shortness of breath

  d. Angina

    e. Wooziness, syncope

    f. Weakness, exercise intolerance

    g. Anxiety

    h. Mentation changes

    i. Heart rate exceeding 100 beats per minute

    j. Jugular venous distention

    k. Polyuria, oliguria

    l. Hypotension

    m. Unconsciousness

    n. Rapid, thready pulse or pulse deficit

5. **Diagnostic study findings**

    a. Laboratory: To ascertain

        i. Imbalances of electrolytes, include magnesium

        ii. ABG levels: Hypoxia, acidosis

        iii. CBC: To rule out hemorrhage, infection

    b. ECG

        i. See ECG features for VT (see Table 4.8)

        ii. See ECG features for SVTs (see Table 4.8)

    c. EPS, after the patient's condition is stabilized

6. **Interprofessional collaboration: see STEMI; also electrophysiologist, anticoagulation clinic or nurse**

7. **Management of patient care**

    a. Anticipated patient trajectory: Marked tachycardia results in diminished CO, poor tissue perfusion, hypotension, and potentially loss of consciousness and death

    b. Goals of care

        i. Rapid rhythm is terminated or rate is controlled to maintain adequate CO and tissue perfusion

        ii. Patient has relief of symptoms related to the rapid rhythm

    c. Treatments

        i. Pharmacology: According to AHA's ACLS guidelines

           (a) Stable narrow QRS supraventricular rhythms

               (1) Vagal maneuvers (bearing down, forceful coughing) often terminate AV nodal reentry tachycardia. These are more successful when performed as soon after onset as possible. Patient should be instructed as to a safe procedure for home use.

               (2) Adenosine may be administered, 6 mg IV, injected rapidly, followed by a dose of 12 mg 1 to 2 minutes later if rhythm continues

---

EXPERT TIP

Because of the short half-life of adenosine, it must be administered and flushed rapidly, through a peripheral IV.

---

                  a) Adenosine often terminates AV nodal reentry and sinus nodal reentrant tachycardia

                  b) Not used for atrial fibrillation or flutter

              (3) Atrial fibrillation: Most frequently seen supraventricular tachyarrhythmia

                  a) Main goals are to lower ventricular response rate, decrease symptoms, and convert to sinus rhythm if and when possible

b) If the duration of atrial fibrillation is longer than 48 hours (or if unknown), anticoagulation is necessary to decrease the risk of atrial thrombi and CVA. Warfarin (to an INR of 2–3) or direct oral anticoagulation (DOAC) agents should be used for a least 3 weeks before and 4 weeks after elective synchronized direct current (DC) cardioversion. DOACs are recommended over warfarin unless there are contraindications or in patients with moderate-severe mitral stenosis or a mechanical heart valve. IV heparin is initiated and continued until the treatment plan is determined.

c) If the duration is less than 48 hours, diltiazem, digoxin, or β-blockers are used for rate control

d) If the duration is less than 48 hours, amiodarone may be used to convert the rhythm before elective synchronized DC cardioversion

e) If the duration is longer than 48 hours, antiarrhythmic medications (amiodarone, procainamide) are not used because they could convert the rhythm and place the patient at risk for a thrombotic event before adequate anticoagulation

f) Rate control of chronic atrial fibrillation has better long-term outcomes than attempts to maintain sinus rhythm with antiarrhythmics

(4) Atrial flutter: Rate control with β-blockers. Calcium channel blockers and digoxin are given before synchronized DC cardioversion or radiofrequency ablation.

(5) Automatic atrial tachycardia (produced by enhanced automaticity in atrial tissue): β-blockers, propafenone (amiodarone, if poor LV function)

(b) Stable wide QRS arrhythmias

(1) VT

a) Amiodarone, 150 mg IV over 10 minutes, followed by 1 mg/min infusion for 6 hours, then maintenance infusion of 0.5 mg/min for 18 hours

1) Medication of choice with known LV dysfunction in both supraventricular and ventricular arrhythmias

2) Adverse effects: Hypotension, QT interval prolongation

b) Lidocaine, 0.5 to 0.75 mg/kg IV push, is given every 5 to 10 minutes to a total of 3 mg/kg if desired; maintenance infusion is 1 to 4 mg/min IV

c) Procainamide, if LV function is known to be good (EF <40%)

1) 20 to 30 mg/min IV, injected slowly

2) Maximum dose: 17 mg/kg

3) End points for therapy: Arrhythmia termination; hypotension; widening of QRS by more than 50%

4) If procainamide is successful at terminating VT, infusion is started at 1 to 4 mg/min

d) Treatment includes correcting the underlying cause. Choice of antiarrhythmic agent, when the patient is in stable condition, is guided by EPS or some other documented test of efficacy (e.g., serial Holter monitoring).

e) Adenosine is no longer recommended to be used with wide QRS tachycardias as a diagnostic tool

    (2) Torsades de pointes (a polymorphic form of VT)

        a) Often seen as a proarrhythmic arrhythmia as a result of antiarrhythmic medication therapy

        b) Responds to measures that shorten the QT interval (isoproterenol, phenytoin, magnesium, overdrive pacing)

        c) If the patient is unstable, synchronized cardioversion is performed immediately per ACLS guidelines for VT

    (3) AVRT—antidromic (WPW): Wide complex; procainamide used

ii. Other interventions

    (a) Evaluate stability by rapid assessment of vital signs, level of consciousness, related symptoms

    (b) Ensure adequate airway, breathing, circulation

    (c) Administer oxygen as needed to provide for oxygen saturations exceeding 92%

    (d) Synchronized DC cardioversion: If the patient is symptomatic and unstable, prepare for immediate synchronized cardioversion

        (1) Synchronized DC cardioversion is delivery (to the patient) of a selected amount of electrical energy synchronized with the R wave of the patient's intrinsic rhythm

        (2) Explain the entire procedure to the patient and significant others, including the risks

        (3) Obtain a consent form, if conditions are not deteriorating too rapidly

        (4) Sedative and anesthetic medications are given to the patient before the procedure, if the patient is conscious (an anesthesiologist is often used for elective procedures)

        (5) Attach the defibrillator monitor leads to the patient; these leads can be piggybacked to many bedside monitors for quick ECG access

        (6) Make sure the monitor is synchronized to the patient's rhythm: The "Sync" button should be on, and spikes indicating the recognition of R waves should be seen on the monitor. If spikes are not seen, check the gain on the machine, try another lead, and/or adjust the electrodes.

        (7) Code cart and suction equipment should be at bedside. Knowledge of the safe use of the defibrillator is vital.

        (8) If the patient goes into VF, deliver immediate defibrillation; turn off the "Sync" button, if necessary (most machines default to defibrillation mode after a cardioversion attempt). Remember to turn the "Sync" button back on each time, if repeated cardioversion is necessary.

    (e) Radiofrequency or cryoablation ablation: Patient may need to be prepared for catheter ablation of accessory pathways

        (1) The procedure is done in the EPS laboratory, a catheter is used to selectively damage myocardial tissue

        (2) Ablation stops the conduction of electrical impulses and disrupts the reentry circuit

        (3) Uses

           a) Accessory pathways: WPW syndrome

           b) Symptomatic SVT

           c) Junctional tachycardia: Caused by enhanced automaticity; seen in infants and children after surgery for congenital heart defects and in digitalis toxicity

      d)   Atrial flutter (treatment of choice)

      e)   VT with bundle branch reentry, refractory VT

      f)   Atrial fibrillation

   (4) Complications of ablation

      a)   Bleeding at the catheter site

      b)   DVT

      c)   Cardiac tamponade

      d)   Myocardial perforation

      e)   Infection

      f)   Ischemia

      g)   Stroke

      h)   Complete AV block

      i)   PE

      j)   Pneumothorax

   (5) Patient education issues

      a)   Procedure description, rationale

      b)   Procedure length (2–4 hours average, up to 10 hours)

      c)   Possible need for a permanent pacemaker

      d)   Recurrence rate for tachyarrhythmias: 8% to 12%

      e)   Monitor the patient and site (see Box 4.3)

(f) Atrial or transesophageal pacing (antitachycardia) may also be considered for termination of persistent stable tachycardias (atrial fibrillation, atrial tachycardia)

(g) Surgical endocardial or epicardial techniques for ablation of pathways are used in cases in which radiofrequency catheter ablation is not possible and the patient's symptoms are hindering quality of life. The surgical maze procedure is very successful in abolishing atrial fibrillation.

(h) AICD

   (1) Device is implanted into the patient with sensing leads and defibrillator coil electrodes attached to the endocardium and to a pulse generator. This is done by transvenous approach or a thoracotomy.

   (2) Capabilities include the following:

      a)   Bradycardia pacing

      b)   Overdrive pacing

      c)   Cardioversion: At 25 J

      d)   Defibrillation

      e)   ECG measurement with storage and event logs

      f)   Dual chamber pacemaker

   (3) Indications: Recurrent VT, VF; sudden cardiac death; or decreased LV EF of less than 35%

   (4) Important issues to understand and teach to the patient and significant others:

      a)   If the AICD discharges, it is not dangerous to the staff or family

      b)   Incidence of spontaneous (appropriate or inappropriate) discharge is 75% the first year

      c)   Concurrent use of antiarrhythmic agents is still necessary to decrease the frequency of events

      d)   Interrogator units can analyze the history of shocks, battery life, and heart rhythm at the time of shock

Absent or Ineffective Pulse

1. **All cases of absent or ineffective pulse are life-threatening and necessitate immediate intervention, usually CPR**
2. **Pathophysiology**
   a. No CO and, subsequently, no tissue perfusion
   b. Respirations cease. Patient is clinically dead.
   c. Rapid cell death. Brain cells start to die after 4 to 6 minutes of circulatory collapse. After 10 minutes, some degree of brain death is inevitable.
   d. VF: Inability to generate an organized impulse for muscular contraction
   e. Asystole: No electrical activity initiated
   f. Pulseless electrical activity (PEA): Electrical activity and conduction occur, with the absence of a palpable pulse and BP. Rhythms seen are any rhythm except VF or VT.
      i. Caused by lack of ventricular filling volume (hypovolemia, fluid losses, saddle emboli, tamponade)
      ii. Caused by the myocardium's inability to contract effectively: Lack of oxygen, acidotic states, electrolyte disturbances (elevated or decreased potassium levels), physical impairment to contraction (tension pneumothorax, tamponade, pericardial effusion), muscular dysfunction from necrosis (MI), thrombosis, hypothermia, medication overdose
3. **Etiology and risk factors**
   a. Causes of VF or pulseless VT
      i. MI
      ii. Ischemia
      iii. Myocardial disease: Cardiomyopathies, myocarditis
      iv. Anoxia: Smoke inhalation, drowning, respiratory failure, airway obstruction
   b. Causes of asystole
      i. Hypokalemia
      ii. Hyperkalemia
      iii. Hypothermia
      iv. Acidosis
   c. Causes of PEA
      i. Hypovolemia: Most common cause
      ii. Hypoxia
      iii. Tension pneumothorax
      iv. Acidosis
      v. Acute MI
      vi. PE
      vii. Hyper-/hypokalemia
      viii. Tamponade
      ix. Medication overdose: Calcium channel blockers, digitalis, tricyclic antidepressants, β-blockers
      x. Hypothermia
4. **Signs and symptoms**
   a. History
      i. History taking is often deferred or performed in conjunction with emergency, life-preserving measures
      ii. Determine whether the patient has a history of any of the aforementioned causes

b. Physical examination
   i. No pulse
   ii. Unconsciousness or rapidly deteriorating level of consciousness
   iii. No respiration

5. **Diagnostic study findings**
   a. ABG levels: Measured after immediate actions taken, to check oxygenation, acidosis
   b. Electrolyte levels
   c. ECG or monitor
      i. In PEA, there is organized electrical activity but no significant CO
      ii. VF (coarse versus fine)
      iii. Pulseless VT (very rapid)
   d. No invasive studies are performed until the patient's condition is stabilized

6. **Interprofessional collaboration: Nurse, physician (cardiologist, electrophysiologist, and anesthesiologist), advanced practice providers, respiratory therapist, chaplain**

7. **Management of patient care**
   a. Anticipated patient trajectory: Patient "clinically dead." Preservation of life and avoidance of brain death require prompt action.
   b. Goals of care
      i. Life is preserved
      ii. CO and tissue perfusion are restored rapidly without brain death
   c. Treatments
      i. Positioning: Lay patient flat, with a board under the back for support during CPR
      ii. Pharmacology: According to AHA's ACLS guidelines
         (a) Emergency medications for VF and pulseless VT
            (1) 100% oxygen
            (2) Epinephrine, 1 mg IV push, every 3 to 5 minutes during arrest; start after initial defibrillation
            (3) After epinephrine administration, and repeated defibrillation attempts, antiarrhythmic medications are considered
               a) Amiodarone: Dose is 300 mg IV, diluted in 20 to 30 mL dextrose 5% in water, infused rapidly; dose of 150 mg IV given for recurrent VF
               b) Lidocaine: 1 to 1.5 mg/kg IV (up to 3 mg/kg total) may be considered as an alternative to amiodarone and magnesium, 1 to 2 g IV (if polymorphic arrhythmia, hypomagnesemia; routine use of magnesium is no longer recommended in monomorphic VF/VT)
         (b) Medications for asystole and PEA
            (1) Emergency medications given in boluses
            (2) Epinephrine, 1 mg IV push, every 3 to 5 minutes during arrest
            (3) Sodium bicarbonate, 1 mEq/kg, may be used to correct severe, systemic acidosis, hyperkalemia, or in the case of tricyclic antidepressants overdose
            (4) If hypokalemia: Potassium and magnesium are given
            (5) If hyperkalemia: Sodium bicarbonate, glucose and insulin, calcium, albuterol may be given
            (6) Thrombolytic agents may be given for massive PE
         (c) IV infusions are not hung during immediate arrest; they can be hung only after the patient's heart rate and rhythm have been restored

iii. Psychosocial issues: Family needs support during this time. Chaplain, social worker, nursing supervisor, and charge nurse can assist with comforting and communicating with significant others. Consider family presence during resuscitation.

iv. Other interventions
   (a) Immediately call cardiac arrest code team
   (b) Assess airway, breathing, and circulation (ABC); perform CPR
   (c) Ensure that crash cart and emergency equipment are at bedside
   (d) Defibrillate as soon as equipment is available, without delay *if the patient is in VF, or pulseless VT*; if patient is in asystole, verify in multiple leads to ensure that it is not fine VF
      (1) Biphasic defibrillators are preferred to monophasic
      (2) Use 120 to 200 J (biphasic; 360 J monophasic) per ACLS guidelines
      (3) Single shocks followed by immediate resumption of CPR is preferred to series of stacked shock of escalating energy dosage
      (4) Be familiar with the safe use of the defibrillator. Always treat it as if it is a weapon and visually ensure that everyone at the bedside is clear from the bed before defibrillating (each time).
      (5) If the monitor shows a flat line, check the power (cables connected?), check the gain (too low?), check the other leads (activity may be seen in a different axis)
   (e) Ensure that CPR is resumed promptly after defibrillation or any assessments
   (f) Automatic external defibrillator (AED) may be the only defibrillator available in some areas of the hospital
      (1) Fully or semiautomatic models
      (2) Cables attach to two adhesive conductive pads
      (3) Machine records rhythm, analyzes data, states command to "Clear," and delivers electrical shocks
      (4) CPR must be stopped for the machine to analyze the rhythm (takes 15–20 seconds)
      (5) Most problems result from operator difficulties (learn to use the equipment properly)
   (g) Transcutaneous pacemakers for asystole: If considered, should be used early in arrest (<5 minutes after onset) for the best chance of success. May be temporizing, to help the heart pace while the causes are identified and treated.
   (h) Induced hypothermia may be used to improve neurologic outcome after sudden cardiac death survival (see Ch. 13, Hypothermia)
   (i) AICD often used if the patient survives arrest
   (j) Promptly assess and treat for the common causes of PEA
      (1) Administer immediate volume replacement. Can lift legs for immediate autoinfusion.
      (2) Listen for breath sounds; check for pneumothorax
      (3) Ensure proper oxygenation
      (4) Hyperventilate the patient: Respiratory acidosis usually occurs in arrest as a result of inadequate ventilation
      (5) Check ABG results for acidosis
      (6) Assist the physician with pericardiocentesis for tamponade, needle decompression of pneumothorax
      (7) Draw blood for measurement of electrolyte levels, medication screens

v. Ethical issues
- (a) Healthcare professionals should be aware of the patient's wishes regarding CPR before emergencies occur. Advance directives should be identified at admission and "Do not attempt resuscitation" orders initiated and communicated to all appropriate staff. Patient and family need to understand that outpatient directives must be reinstituted as a medical order when the patient is hospitalized to be valid.
- (b) Duration of resuscitative efforts depends on many factors (e.g., age, medical condition)

MITRAL REGURGITATION

> **KEY CONCEPT**
> In mitral regurgitation (MR), blood is partially regurgitated back into the LA during ventricular systole because of an incompetent mitral valve. This may happen acutely or develop as a chronic condition. Treatment is most commonly surgical repair or replacement of the mitral valve.

1. **Pathophysiology**
   a. With the failure of the mitral valve to close completely during ventricular contraction, some fraction of the LV output is ejected backward into the LA
   b. Pressures in the LA and pulmonary veins rise (dramatically if the onset is acute), and pulmonary congestion and/or edema results in dyspnea
   c. Reduced forward output results in chronic fatigue (or hypotension if acute)
   d. The pathophysiology and clinical course vary dramatically, depending on whether the onset is acute or chronic
   e. Acute onset
      i. LA diastolic pressures, along with pulmonary pressures, dramatically increase
      ii. LA has no time to compensate and initially remains small and noncompliant (which creates high pressures)
      iii. Forward output falls dramatically, and cardiogenic shock develops
      iv. Pulmonary congestion may develop as a result of high pressures within the pulmonary vascular bed, and pulmonary edema rapidly ensues
   f. Chronic process
      i. LA has time (often years) to enlarge and develop compliance to keep pressures at near-normal levels
      ii. PAPs remain relatively normal
      iii. Eventually the degree of mitral regurgitation may exceed the capacity of the LA to compensate, and pulmonary congestion and dyspnea may develop
      iv. LV compensates for chronic volume overload by dilating in an attempt to maintain normal forward output, while emptying a large volume of its output backward into the LA
      v. LV can dilate to the extent that it is unable to recover, even after surgical correction of mitral regurgitation
      vi. Pulmonary venous pressures rise, with resulting increases in PAOP and secondary pulmonary hypertension
      vii. Atrial fibrillation is often seen and occurs secondary to LA enlargement
      viii. RV will also progressively hypertrophy, and right-sided HF may follow

2. **Etiology and risk factors**
   a. Acute causes
      i. Acute rupture of the chordae tendineae as a result of endocarditis or chronic strain on the mitral valve apparatus by mitral valve prolapse, rheumatic heart disease
      ii. Papillary muscle dysfunction or rupture secondary to acute MI
      iii. Trauma
   b. Chronic causes
      i. Rheumatic heart disease
      ii. Congenital malformations of the mitral valve, chordae tendineae, or mitral annuli
      iii. Mitral valve prolapse
      iv. LV dilatation from other causes
      v. Connective tissue disease (e.g., Marfan syndrome)
      vi. IE
      vii. Calcified mitral annulus

3. **Signs and symptoms**
   a. Subjective findings: Patient complains of:
      i. Shortness of breath
      ii. Orthopnea
      iii. Paroxysmal nocturnal dyspnea
      iv. Weakness or becoming easily fatigued
      v. Palpitations
      vi. Symptoms of RV failure
   b. Objective findings: History of past rheumatic fever, streptococcal infection, endocarditis, ischemia, trauma, mitral valve prolapse
   c. Physical findings
      i. If the patient is in HF, the following may be seen:
         (a) Tachypnea
         (b) Anxiety
         (c) Diaphoresis
         (d) Cyanosis
         (e) Confusion
         (f) Edema
         (g) Jugular venous distention (right-sided HF)
         (h) Signs of pulmonary edema (frothy, pink sputum)
      ii. Other findings include the following:
         (a) Apical impulse (PMI) is laterally displaced, diffuse, and hyperdynamic (in chronic mitral regurgitation)
         (b) Apical systolic thrill may be felt
         (c) Pulse may be irregular if in atrial fibrillation
         (d) Hepatomegaly (late sign)
      iii. Auscultation
         (a) High-pitched, blowing holosystolic murmur
            (1) Heard best at apex with radiation to axilla
            (2) Begins at S_1 and extends through S_2 (aortic closure)
         (b) Rales if pulmonary congestion or edema present
         (c) S_2 may be widely split or accentuated (P_2) as a result of early closure of the aortic valve, because LV ejection time is shortened; pulmonic closure delayed because of right-sided heart pressure overload
         (d) Possible RV lift secondary to RV pressure overload

4. **Diagnostic study findings**
   a. Radiologic
      i. LA and LV enlargement in chronic mitral regurgitation
      ii. LA does not enlarge with acute onset
      iii. Calcification of mitral valve
      iv. Pulmonary edema
   b. ECG: Atrial fibrillation
   c. Echocardiography: Helps determine the cause, LV function and dimensions, indications for surgery
      i. Degree of insufficiency
      ii. LA and LV enlargement in chronic mitral insufficiency
      iii. Mitral valve prolapse, mitral annular calcification, flail leaflet, vegetations, rheumatic heart disease
      iv. Abnormal regional wall motion if papillary muscle dysfunction is the cause
   d. TEE: Used in guiding mitral valve reconstructive surgery; superior to transthoracic echocardiography in visualizing the mitral valve leaflets
   e. Cardiac catheterization
      i. Documents the severity of mitral regurgitation
      ii. Screens for CAD
      iii. Documents PAOP and right-sided heart pressures
5. **Interprofessional collaboration: See ACS**
6. **Management of patient care**
   a. Anticipated patient trajectory: Severe mitral regurgitation must be corrected, or progressive left-sided HF and early death occur
   b. Goals of care
      i. Patient is hemodynamically stable and in sinus rhythm
      ii. Symptoms of reduced CO are identified and treated promptly
      iii. Patient receives appropriate teaching regarding surgical interventions, medications, and discharge care
   c. Treatments
      i. Discharge planning
         (a) Instructions include the usual postoperative instructions for any heart surgery
         (b) If the valve is replaced, the importance of endocarditis prophylaxis and chronic anticoagulation is stressed (if the patient does not comply with the follow-up medication regimen, stroke and possibly death are highly likely)
      ii. Pharmacology
         (a) Treat atrial fibrillation: Slow the ventricular response, increase exercise capacity with β-blockers, calcium channel blockers
         (b) Antibiotics: For prophylaxis of recurrent rheumatic heart disease, prophylaxis for IE during dental procedures
         (c) Acute mitral regurgitation may respond to administration of vasodilators to decrease afterload (e.g., nitroprusside) or as a prelude to valve surgery
         (d) Diuretics, nitrates: To lower pulmonary congestion; use carefully, may lower CO
         (e) Anticoagulants: Prevent embolization if atrial fibrillation is present. If warfarin is used, goal is an INR of 2 to 3. DOAC agents are also reasonable choices.
      iii. Other interventions
         (a) IABP may be a life-saving procedure in severe cases

      (b) Transcatheter mitral valve replacement

      (c) If the valve is to be surgically reconstructed (surgical mitral valvuloplasty) or replaced, the patient and family must be counseled with regard to the surgery

         (1) Explain the disease process, preoperative routines, surgical procedure (including the replacement valve to be used), and expectations during the immediate postoperative period

         (2) Mitral valve replacement provides greater durability in comparison to repair

         (3) Chronic anticoagulant use is not necessary with reconstruction if the patient is in sinus rhythm

         (4) Postoperative general care for valve repair is similar to postoperative care for most cardiac surgical operations

  d. Potential complications

    i. Systemic emboli with atrial fibrillation requiring anticoagulation

    ii. IE: IE prophylaxis needed (see Infective Endocarditis)

MITRAL STENOSIS

> **KEY CONCEPT**
>
> Mitral stenosis is a progressive narrowing of the mitral orifice that impedes the flow of blood from the LA to the LV during ventricular diastole. Although medical therapy is available for palliation, in most cases, interventional treatment, such as surgical valve replacement or repair is needed.

1. **Pathophysiology**
   a. Progressive fibrosis, scarring, and thickening of the valve leaflets, usually from rheumatic valvular disease
   b. Extensive fusion of the leaflets and chordae tendineae develops
   c. Area of a normal adult's mitral valve orifice is 4 to 6 cm². In mild mitral stenosis, it is 2 cm² (symptoms may be experienced only with exercise, atrial fibrillation). In severe mitral stenosis, it is 1 cm², with symptoms apparent even at rest.
   d. Elevation of LA pressures results from the obstruction to the flow from the LA to the LV. As the valve continues to narrow, the LA slowly dilates and hypertrophies.
   e. Intractable atrial fibrillation usually results
   f. As atrial pressures elevate, pulmonary capillary hydrostatic pressure rises above the plasma oncotic pressure, and fluid escapes into the pulmonary interstitium and alveoli
   g. As the valve orifice narrows to smaller than 1 cm², pulmonary hypertension occurs and RV pressures increase, with eventual hypertrophy and dilatation. RV failure frequently follows.
   h. Stenotic obstruction impedes forward blood flow and alone is often enough to decrease SV and CO. Loss of atrial kick resulting from atrial fibrillation or tachycardia compound the problem, decreasing LV filling time and further decreasing CO.
   i. Atrial thrombi form in the LA appendage, and systemic or cerebral emboli may ensue

2. **Etiology and risk factors: Incidence has decreased in the United States**
   a. Rheumatic heart disease (most common cause)
   b. Congenital mitral valve disease (uncommon)

    c. Tumors of the LA (atrial myxoma)

    d. Risk factor: Pregnant women with mitral stenosis often develop cardiac decompensation in the third trimester

3. Signs and symptoms

    a. History

        i. Gradual decline in physical activity over the years

        ii. Palpitations (frequent complaint): Possibly from frequent premature atrial contractions, paroxysmal atrial fibrillation

        iii. Shortness of breath, dyspnea on exertion

        iv. Paroxysmal nocturnal dyspnea

        v. Cough (bronchial irritability), hoarseness

        vi. Orthopnea

        vii. Fatigue

        viii. Hemoptysis (ruptured bronchial vessels)

        ix. Symptoms of right-sided HF (occur later)

        x. Dysphagia (enlarged atrium displaces the esophagus)

        xi. History of systemic emboli, rheumatic heart disease

    b. Objective findings: Signs and symptoms of right-sided HF occur as late signs (see Heart Failure)

    c. Physical examination: Findings depend on the degree of HF present

        i. Inspection

          (a) Any of the signs of HF

          (b) Jugular venous distention

        ii. Palpation

          (a) May feel the RV lift if pulmonary hypertension is present; an LV "tap" may be present

          (b) Diastolic thrill may be present at the apex (with the patient in the left lateral recumbent position)

        iii. Auscultation

          (a) Pronounced S_1

          (b) Low-pitched apical diastolic murmur (best heard at the apex, radiates to the left sternal border)

          (c) Associated murmur of tricuspid insufficiency may be present if RV failure exists. Listen at the left lower parasternal area.

          (d) Pulmonary component, S_2, later and louder if pulmonary hypertension exists

          (e) Mitral opening snap present just after pulmonic component of S_2

4. Diagnostic study findings

    a. Radiologic: Chest radiograph reveals the following:

        i. LA and RV hypertrophy

        ii. Interstitial edema, pulmonary vascular redistribution to the upper lobes of the lungs (caused by high PAOP)

    b. ECG

        i. If in sinus rhythm, broad P waves: Notched in lead I, biphasic in V_1

        ii. Atrial fibrillation

        iii. RV hypertrophy pattern (with pulmonary hypertension)

    c. Transthoracic echocardiography with Doppler

        i. Reveals thickened, tethered, and doming (stuck together) anterior and posterior mitral valve leaflets

        ii. Calculates mitral valve area

      iii. Shows enlarged LA

      iv. Shows enlarged RV

      v. Assess the degree of pulmonary hypertension and mitral regurgitation, and the function of the other valves

   d. TEE: For identification of an LA appendage thrombus (seen in 20% of cases of atrial fibrillation)

   e. Cardiac catheterization: Used if the echocardiographic results are confusing or questionable given the patient presentation

      i. To assess pulmonary hypertension and CO; to measure PAOP-LV diastolic pressure gradient and calculate mitral valve area

      ii. Coronary arteriography: Used to assess the function of the other valves and rule out CAD

5. Interprofessional collaboration: See ACS, Anticoagulation clinic

6. Management of patient care

   a. Anticipated patient trajectory: Patient with mitral stenosis will gradually develop limiting symptoms and HF, with the likelihood of stroke and early death

   b. Goals of care

      i. Hemodynamics improve

      ii. Complications (including atrial fibrillation, recurrent infections, atrial thrombus) are treated and/or prevented

   c. Treatment

      i. Nutrition: Restricted sodium intake

      ii. Infection control: IE prophylactic therapy

      iii. Discharge planning: Patient education regarding the following:

         (a) Activity limitations

         (b) Medications

         (c) Anticoagulation and follow-up requirements

      iv. Pharmacology

         (a) Diuretics, nitrates: To lower pulmonary congestion; use carefully, may lower CO

         (b) β-blockers, calcium channel blockers: To treat atrial fibrillation, slow ventricular response, and increase exercise capacity

         (c) β-blocking agents may increase exercise tolerance by slowing the heart rate and lengthening the diastolic filling period. Use carefully in patients with impaired LV function.

         (d) Anticoagulants: Prevent embolization. Warfarin is the recommended agent. Mitral stenosis goal is an INR of 2 to 3. Prosthetic mitral valve goal is 2.5 to 3.5.

         (e) Antibiotics: Prophylaxis for recurrent rheumatic heart disease; prophylaxis for IE during dental procedures

      v. Other interventions

         (a) Medical management is palliative; mechanical correction is eventually required to improve CO and decrease atrial and pulmonary pressures

         (b) Current treatment options include surgical mitral valve replacement, open surgical commissurotomy, percutaneous balloon mitral valvuloplasty

         (c) If patient is unstable, synchronized DC cardioversion, or when stable, chemical cardioversion, if atrial fibrillation is present

   d. Potential complications

i. Systemic emboli or PEs from atrial thrombus
   (a) Mechanism: High risk for thrombus formation during atrial fibrillation or HF (see Ch. 3, Pulmonary System)
ii. Other complications include HF, infection

AORTIC REGURGITATION

> ### KEY CONCEPT
> In aortic regurgitation (AR), an incompetent aortic valve causes the backward flow of blood from the aorta to the LV during ventricular diastole. Although medical management may be used in milder cases, the most common treatment is surgical repair or replacement of the valve.

1. **Pathophysiology**
   a. Aortic valve can become incompetent as a result of destruction of the cusps (endocarditis), degeneration of the cusps, unhinging of the valvular apparatus (dissection), rheumatic disease, connective tissue disease, congenital heart disease, trauma, or degenerative change
   b. Acute onset
      i. Increased regurgitation into the LV produces volume overload, *markedly* increasing the LVEDP
      ii. CO falls and hypotension develops
      iii. There is a drop in the aortic diastolic pressure that diminishes the coronary blood flow
      iv. The compensatory increase in heart rate adds to the already elevated myocardial oxygen demand
      v. Patient comes for treatment with pulmonary edema, cardiogenic shock. Ischemia and sudden cardiac death may occur.
   c. Chronic process
      i. LV compensates by dilating to increase its SV to maintain an adequate forward output. This gradually increases myocardial oxygen demands.
      ii. LVEDP increases. The LV myocardial fibers stretch and hypertrophy. Preload and EF, at this point, remain relatively normal.
      iii. As the disease progresses, the LV fails and decompensates; SV and EF decrease. LV systolic and diastolic pressures increase.
      iv. Wide pulse pressure develops as a result of low aortic diastolic pressures
      v. Decreased blood flow to the coronary arteries during diastole results in myocardial ischemia
2. **Etiology and risk factors**
   a. Acute causes
      i. IE (most common cause of acute AR): Can also be a chronic cause
      ii. Aortic dissection
      iii. Blunt trauma, causing valve rupture (e.g., motor vehicle collision)
      iv. Prosthetic valve dysfunction
   b. Chronic causes
      i. Idiopathic calcification of the valve
      ii. Congenital malformations (bicuspid aortic valve)
      iii. Hypertension
      iv. Rheumatic disease

     v. Aortic aneurysms (e.g., Marfan syndrome)

     vi. Diseases of the aortic valve and root

     vii. Systemic lupus erythematosus

     viii. Medications: Appetite suppressants

     ix. Syphilis (rare)

3. **Signs and symptoms: Can be well tolerated. Symptoms often do not become evident to the patient until the disease is fairly well advanced.**

  a. Subjective findings

     i. Dyspnea (most common symptom): Caused by an increased LVEDP

     ii. Angina pectoris

     iii. Paroxysmal nocturnal dyspnea

     iv. Orthopnea

     v. Presyncope and syncope

  b. Physical examination: Many of physical findings are absent in acute AR. Widening pulse pressure of chronic disease creates these findings. Acute disease has a narrow pulse pressure.

     i. Inspection

       (a) Signs and symptoms of left-sided HF

       (b) Distinct carotid artery pulsations

       (c) Flushed appearance

     ii. Palpation

       (a) Diffuse apical impulse, displaced laterally and downward (in chronic forms); the apical impulse does not change with acute onset

       (b) Water-hammer pulse: Bounding, abrupt rise and fall in the carotid arteries and other peripheral pulses

     iii. Auscultation

       (a) High-pitched, blowing, decrescendo diastolic murmur

         (1) Loudest at lower left sternal border, third to fourth intercostal space

         (2) Starts immediately after S_2

         (3) Short (early diastole) with acute aortic insufficiency

         (4) Long (through diastole) if chronic

         (5) If hard to hear, have the patient sit up and lean forward. Assure the bell is in full contact with the skin.

       (b) S_3 common

       (c) S_4 heard in more severe disease (abnormal LV compliance)

       (d) Rales at the bases, if the onset is acute

4. **Diagnostic study findings**

  a. Radiologic: Chest radiograph reveals the following:

     i. LV enlargement (normal with acute aortic insufficiency)

     ii. Wide mediastinum (if caused by aortic dissection)

     iii. Possible aortic valve calcification

     iv. Possible interstitial pulmonary edema

  b. ECG: Often normal in mild to moderate AR

     i. LV hypertrophy: Increased amplitude of QRS

     ii. As disease progresses, ST segment and T wave depression

     iii. Sinus tachycardia (acutely)

  c. Echocardiography: Very important tool, particularly in the diagnosis of acute cases

     i. Identifies cause and severity of AR

     ii. Shows LV cavity dilatation with chronic cases

     iii. Reveals vegetation

d. MRI or CT scan: To exclude aortic dissection

e. Radionuclide imaging: Used to evaluate the severity of AR and LV function

f. TEE: To assess the ascending and descending thoracic aorta for aneurysms, dissection, and the cause and severity of aortic insufficiency

g. Cardiac catheterization

    i. Evaluates hemodynamics

       (a) CO assessment

       (b) Increased PAOP

       (c) Increased right-sided heart pressures (late)

    ii. Quantifies the degree of insufficiency

    iii. Assesses LV function and EF, reveals other abnormalities

    iv. Reveals coronary anatomy

    v. Evaluates for aortic dissection

5. **Interprofessional collaboration: See ACS; also electrophysiologist, infectious disease specialist**

6. **Management of patient care**

a. Anticipated patient trajectory: When severe, AR will ultimately result in irreversible HF and early death if not recognized and corrected with aortic valve replacement before LV dysfunction

b. Goals of care

    i. Stable hemodynamics are maintained

    ii. Afterload is reduced

    iii. Pulmonary congestion, if evident, is decreased

c. Treatments

    i. Positioning: Head of bed elevated, if signs of HF are present

    ii. Infection control: Prophylaxis for IE risk

    iii. Discharge planning

       (a) Teach the patient about the need for adherence to the medication regimen and follow-up evaluations

       (b) Prophylactic antibiotics will be used to prevent IE. Patient should understand what types of procedures require antibiotic prophylaxis.

    iv. Pharmacology

       (a) Inotropic agents (dopamine, dobutamine) to increase CO in acute AR (before surgery)

       (b) ACE inhibitors: To decrease LV remodeling and hypertrophy, reduce afterload (if necessary)

       (c) Diuretics, nitrates: With symptoms of HF, to decrease pulmonary congestion

       (d) Antibiotics: IE prophylaxis

       (e) β-blockers: Avoided in acute AR; used very cautiously because the patient often needs sinus tachycardia to support output

    v. Other interventions

       (a) Cardiac surgery

          (1) If the patient is symptomatic or asymptomatic with LV dysfunction or significant dilatation, valve replacement is the main treatment for the incompetent valve

          (2) AR caused by IE: Does not require a delay in surgery, if the patient is symptomatic

       (b) Bedside hemodynamic monitoring: To assess and monitor CO and responses to medication

       (c) EPS study: If VT is present, AICD implantation because of the high risk of sudden cardiac death

(d) Atrial pacing: May be needed to increase the heart rate, decrease regurgitation

(e) IABP contraindicated

EXPERT TIP

Because IABP therapy forces blood back toward the aortic annulus in an attempt to improve coronary artery perfusion, in the case of an incompetent aortic valve, blood will be driven back into the LV, leading to LV failure.

---

d. Potential complications
   i. IE: Most significant complication to prevent
   ii. Arrhythmias: Ventricular, heart blocks, electromechanical dissociation
   iii. HF, cardiogenic shock, death

AORTIC STENOSIS

KEY CONCEPT

Treatment is surgical repair or replacement of the valve. TAVR is now appropriate for low- and high-risk patients.

---

1. **Pathophysiology**
   a. Ejection from the LV during systole is impaired because of an obstructive narrowing. Stenosis may be supravalvular, subvalvular, or valvular (most common).
   b. Supravalvular obstructions are rare and are usually congenital.
   c. Subvalvular obstructions are associated with HCM.
   d. Valve becomes thickened and calcified, with a progressive fusing of the cusps. LV afterload gradually increases. Aortic insufficiency often develops (Fig. 4.17).
   e. Systolic pressure gradient develops between the LV and the aorta.
   f. To maintain SV and adequate CO, the LV hypertrophies in a concentric manner.
   g. LV becomes stiff and noncompliant; the LVEDP increases.
   h. LA pressures increase, which increases the pulmonary vascular pressures. Pulmonary congestion develops and eventually increases the pressures in the right chambers.

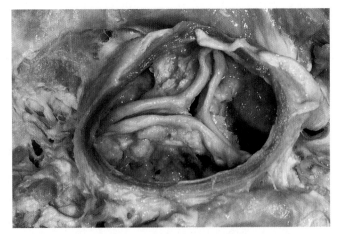

Fig. 4.17 Gross pathology of degenerative aortic stenosis. (From Crawford, M.H., DiMarco, J.P., Paulus, W.J. (eds) (2010). *Cardiology*, 3rd ed. Philadelphia: Mosby.)

i. Because the left side of the heart has to pump against increased afterload, myocardial oxygen demand is greatly increased.

j. LV hypertrophy and increased LVEDP cause a decrease in subendocardial coronary perfusion, and ischemia can result in angina and arrhythmias.

k. Because forward CO cannot be augmented to meet requirements, exertional syncope may result.

2. **Etiology and risk factors**

   a. Most common cause: Calcific or degenerative process (progressive disease in patients >65 years)

   b. IE

   c. Congenital heart defects: Bicuspid valve (symptoms usually seen in patients in their 50s and 60s); associated with other defects, especially coarctation of the aorta. Most common cause in younger adults.

   d. Rheumatic valvular heart disease (the commissure fuses, leaflets thicken and fibrose; symptoms often seen in patients in their 30s and 40s), associated with mitral valve disease

   e. Prevalence of aortic stenosis increases with age

3. **Signs and symptoms**

   a. Dyspnea on exertion (pulmonary congestion)

   b. Syncope on exertion (transient arrhythmias, decreased cardiac and cerebral perfusion) or presyncope

   c. Angina (caused by LV hypertrophy, increased myocardial demands, lowered coronary blood flow)

   d. Symptoms of LV failure

   e. Palpitations

   f. Fatigue or weakness

   g. History of a gradual decrease in physical activity to avoid dyspnea

   h. Inspection

      i. Anxiety

      ii. Labored respiration, tachypnea

      iii. Jugular veins: Presence of an "a" wave (if right-sided HF is present and the patient is in sinus rhythm)

   i. Palpation

      i. Forceful, sustained apical impulse

      ii. Systolic thrill felt rarely in the second or third right intercostal space

      iii. Pulsus parvus and tardus (small carotid upstroke and delayed peak) is variably present

   j. Auscultation

      i. Harsh, loud systolic ejection murmur, crescendo-decrescendo, loudest at the second right intercostal space, radiating up to the base of the neck and at apex

      ii. Paradoxical split S_2

      iii. S_3 (in severe LV dysfunction)

      iv. S_4 (with LV hypertrophy)

      v. Rales (LV failure)

4. **Diagnostic study findings**

   a. Radiologic: Studies may be normal in significant stenosis

      i. Cardiac enlargement in late stages

      ii. Pulmonary vascular congestion

      iii. Calcified aortic valve

      iv. Dilated ascending aorta

b. ECG: Normal in 20% to 30% of patients
   i. LV hypertrophy and strain pattern (increased QRS voltage, ST changes)
   ii. Conduction defects, such as LBBB, occasional heart block
   iii. Left axis deviation
   iv. Atrial fibrillation in late stages
c. Echocardiography: For diagnosis, follow-up
   i. Presence and severity of aortic stenosis
   ii. LV hypertrophy (concentric), impaired LV diastolic function
   iii. LA enlargement
   iv. Other valvular disease
d. Exercise treadmill study: Unsafe unless aortic stenosis is mild
e. Cardiac catheterization: Used to assess the following:
   i. CAD: 50% of patients have coexisting CAD
   ii. Hemodynamics
      (a) Increased LV systolic pressure and LVEDP
      (b) Pressure gradient between the LV and the aorta is usually more than 50 mm Hg
      (c) Calculation of the aortic valve area

5. **Interprofessional collaboration: See ACS; also infectious disease specialist, electrophysiologist, stroke team**

6. **Management of patient care**
   a. Anticipated patient trajectory: Aortic stenosis threatens the patient with limiting angina, HF, and death, and can be surgically corrected at any age
   b. Goals of care
      i. Patient is free of the signs and symptoms of complications (e.g., HF, arrhythmias, emboli)
      ii. Patient demonstrates a knowledge of the disease progress, medications, and therapies to allow active participation in decision making regarding surgical interventions
   c. Treatments
      i. Nutrition: Diet should be low in sodium
      ii. Infection control: IE prophylaxis
      iii. Discharge planning
         (a) Teach the patient about the symptoms to report promptly and disease progression: The patient is at increased risk for sudden cardiac death.
         (b) Activity restrictions: Moderate aortic stenosis—avoid competition sports. Severe aortic stenosis—low-level activity only.
      iv. Pharmacology: Medical management is palliative. Treatment is based on symptom presentation.
         (a) Antibiotics: To prevent IE
         (b) Antihypertensives: To control hypertension
         (c) Antiarrhythmics: To prevent and control rhythm disturbances (e.g., digoxin, amiodarone for atrial fibrillation)
         (d) If signs of HF, pulmonary congestion are present: Digoxin, diuretics, ACE inhibitors. Watch preload. These medications can lower CO, because the LV is very dependent on preload.
         (e) Vasodilators: Should be avoided; can cause profound hypotension
         (f) Anticoagulation: In patients with atrial fibrillation and a CHA_2DS_2-VASc score of 2 or more, anticoagulation is recommended. DOAC agents are reasonable choices.

     v. Psychosocial issues: Patient's goals and wishes are important because of the high risk of mortality. Activity limitations have a major impact on home life, finances, and morale.

    vi. Treatments

       (a) Surgery is the only effective therapy for critical aortic stenosis

         (1) Valve replacement with stented bioprosthetic mechanical valves or pulmonic autograft (Ross procedure)

         (2) Lifelong anticoagulant therapy is necessary when prosthetic mechanical valves are used

         (3) TAVR is an option for patients with high or intermediate surgical risk

       (b) Aortic percutaneous balloon valvuloplasty and debridement are not an alternative to surgery

         (1) Used as a bridge to surgery in patients with pulmonary edema or cardiogenic shock, to improve hemodynamics

         (2) Used for patients who are not surgical candidates to improve symptoms

         (3) Does not improve survival

         (4) Benefits last only a few months

  d. Potential complications

     i. Sudden cardiac death

       (a) Mechanism: High incidence after the patient becomes symptomatic, often resulting from ventricular arrhythmias

       (b) Management: AICD may be required

    ii. Other complications (see also applicable sections)

       (a) LV failure (diastolic dysfunction)

       (b) Conduction defects: Heart blocks (especially in degenerative disease)

       (c) IE (more common in younger patients)

       (d) Emboli: Stroke, vision problems

ATRIAL SEPTAL DEFECT

> **KEY CONCEPT**
>
> An atrial septal defect (ASD) can result in shortened life span and morbidity as a result of dyspnea and right-sided HF. Paradoxical emboli (right-to-left circulation) can result after the right side of the heart fails. Treatment is surgical correction of the defect.

1. **Pathophysiology**

  a. A defect in the interatrial septum that allows free communication between the right and left sides of the heart at the atrial level. Common types of ASD include the following:

     i. Secundum defect (fossa ovalis): Located in the middle of the septum in the area of the foramen ovale. This is the most common type (70%).

    ii. Primum defect (often associated with endocardial cushion defects): Located at the lower end of the septum, superior to the interventricular septum (20%)

    iii. Sinus venosus defect: Located high in the septum at the junction of the RA and superior vena cava. Frequently associated with partial anomalous pulmonary venous return of the right upper lobe vein to the superior vena cava. Least common type (5%–10%).

    iv. Patent foramen ovale: Open congenital defect found in up to 27% of adults. A flap of tissue on the left side of the septum normally closes this opening shortly after birth. If the flap does not grow to the surrounding tissue, high right atrial pressures can open the flap. Large patent foramina ovales and/or defects with right-to-left shunting are associated with cryptogenic strokes (focal neurologic deficits because of focal ischemia).

b. As a result of the defects, flow is from the normally higher-pressure LA to the RA, which creates a left-to-right shunt.

c. Right-side heart and pulmonary artery flow increase because these structures handle both the normal systemic venous return from the body and the left-to-right shunt flow through the ASD.

d. This results in volume overload of the right chambers.

e. RA, RV, and pulmonary artery dilate

f. Systolic murmur of an ASD results from increased flow across the normal pulmonic valve (flow murmur). Diastolic rumble can occur from increased flow across the tricuspid valve.

g. Spontaneous closure rarely occurs after 2 years of age.

h. Pulmonary hypertension and pulmonary vascular disease may develop over time (seen in 15%–20% of adults with this defect). In extreme cases, the shunt may reverse, becoming right to left and irreversible (Eisenmenger syndrome).

i. RV dilatation, hypertrophy, and failure can result.

j. Atrial fibrillation is often seen.

k. Mitral valve anomalies (with cleft leaflets) often occur in endocardial cushion defects (associated with ostium primum defects), resulting in mitral insufficiency.

2. **Etiology and risk factors**

a. Occurs twice as often among females

b. Exact cause unknown; may be caused by:

  i. Genetic factors

  ii. Maternal and fetal infection during the first trimester of pregnancy (e.g., rubella)

  iii. Effects of medications or medications

  iv. Dietary deficiencies during fetal development

3. **Signs and symptoms: Symptoms often develop in the fourth to sixth decades of life. Presentations vary, depending on the direction of the shunt. When the shunt reverses to right to left, signs and symptoms of severe HF with cyanosis will be present.**

a. Patient may complain of:

  i. Mild fatigue

  ii. Exertional dyspnea

  iii. Palpitations

b. Appearance is generally normal

c. Symptoms of HF may be seen in older patients

d. Cyanosis, clubbing of the fingers and toes (with right-to-left shunts)

e. Palpation: Systolic, hyperdynamic lift along the left sternal border, caused by enlarged RV

f. Auscultation

  i. Systolic ejection murmur: Heard best in the second left intercostal space; caused by increased flow across the pulmonic valve

  ii. Fixed, widely split S_2

  iii. Early, low-pitched diastolic murmur may be heard best at the lower left sternal border or xiphoid area; caused by increased blood flow across the tricuspid valve if shunt flow is large

4. **Diagnostic study findings**

a. Radiologic: Chest radiograph may be normal or may reveal the following:

  i. Mild to moderate enlargement of the RA, RV, pulmonary artery

  ii. Increased pulmonary vascular markings

b. ECG
  i. Atrial fibrillation and/or atrial flutter
  ii. PR prolongation
  iii. Incomplete RBBB
  iv. Left axis deviation in ostium primum defects
c. Echocardiography
  i. RV enlargement
  ii. Actual defect is occasionally seen with two-dimensional echocardiography, color-flow Doppler studies
  iii. IV injection of contrast medium demonstrates the shunt by the early appearance of contrast medium in the left heart chambers
d. TEE: Used to evaluate the mitral valve
e. Cardiac catheterization: Used predominantly to evaluate CAD, hemodynamics, associated heart disease. Can be used for quantifying shunt.
  i. Characteristic finding is an increase (step-up) in oxygen concentration in the RA
  ii. Increased PAPs may be documented

5. Interprofessional collaboration: See ACS; also cardiologist

6. Management of patient care
a. Anticipated patient trajectory: ASD can rob people of 2 decades of life and should be corrected as soon as recognized
b. Goals of care
  i. Prompt aggressive treatment of HF symptoms is provided
  ii. Elective repair of the defect is accomplished as soon as possible
c. Treatments
  i. Pharmacology
    (a) Antibiotics to prevent endocarditis
    (b) Medical management of HF
  ii. Other interventions
    (a) Surgical repair is the standard treatment for a significant ASD
      (1) Prepare the patient and family (parents, if the patient is a child) for the possibility of surgical repair, including providing an explanation of the disease process, preoperative routines, the surgical procedure, and expectations for the postoperative period.
      (2) Using a median sternotomy or right thoracotomy, the surgeon closes the defect with a pericardial or Dacron patch or suture.
      (3) Early defect repair is recommended to prevent pulmonary hypertension, HF, and early death.
      (4) Repair may be deferred in children but should be performed before they enter school (2–5 years of age).
      (5) In older children and young adults, the repair should be performed before pulmonary hypertension develops; pathophysiologic changes may be irreversible if the defect is not repaired.
      (6) Postoperative care for ASD repairs is similar to postoperative care for most cardiac operations; stress the importance of preventing potential complications (atrial fibrillation, embolization).
    (b) Transcatheter closure of an ASD and patent foramen ovale is used in suitable patients
    (c) Heart-lung transplantation: Becomes the only available option if the disease has progressed to include irreversible pulmonary hypertension and pulmonary vascular disease

d. Potential complications
    i. Transient heart block
        (a) Mechanism: Most common complication after closure of a septum primum defect because of edema or injury to the AV node
        (b) Management: Temporary pacing may be required. Occasionally, heart block is permanent.
    ii. Other complications include
        (a) Arrhythmias: Watch for atrial fibrillation, flutter, AV blocks (more frequent in older patients). SVTs may continue after surgery.
        (b) HF (left side and right side), pulmonary hypertension
        (c) PE or thrombosis, stroke
        (d) Brain abscess

VENTRICULAR SEPTAL DEFECT

> **KEY CONCEPT**
> Ventricular septal defects (VSDs) may close on their own in infants; however, surgical repair is needed in those that do not.

1. **Pathophysiology**
    a. An abnormal opening between the ventricles occurring in the membranous or muscular portion of the ventricular septum. Constitutes 25% of all congenital heart defects. Common types of this defect include the following:
        i. Perimembranous defects
            (a) Occur in approximately 80% of patients with a VSD
            (b) Located at the base of the septum under the aortic valve
            (c) Aortic insufficiency can result if the valve cusp is poorly supported
        ii. Muscular defects
            (a) Occur in 5% to 20%
            (b) Occasionally, multiple defects
    b. Small defects
        i. Some 75% close spontaneously before the affected individuals are 20 years of age (50% by age 4 years)
        ii. In general, create no hemodynamic disturbance or pulmonary hypertension in adults; low risk of IE
        iii. Small left-to-right shunt with high pressure gradient between the LV and RV causes a high-velocity jet and a loud (usually grade IV/VI) murmur
    c. Large defects
        i. Left-to-right shunting through the defect as a result of the higher LV pressures
        ii. Increased RV pressures and PAP occur
        iii. Increased pulmonary blood flow results in increased pulmonary venous return to the LA. LA pressures, along with the LVEDP, increase. The left heart chambers are volume overloaded, which leads to dilatation, failure, and pulmonary edema.
        iv. Over time, the pulmonary hypertension can become irreversible, often exceeding systemic pressures. The shunt then reverses, becoming right to left, with resulting cyanosis (Eisenmenger syndrome).

2. **Etiology and risk factors**
   a. Precise cause of the congenital defect is unknown
   b. Is frequently associated with other defects, such as coarctation of the aorta and PDA
   c. Factors contributing to congenital defects
      i. Genetic abnormalities
      ii. Chromosomal abnormalities (e.g., Down syndrome)
      iii. Maternal and fetal infections during the first trimester of pregnancy (e.g., rubella)
      iv. Effects of medications and medications (e.g., cocaine use) during fetal development
      v. Dietary deficiencies during fetal development
      vi. Effects of maternal smoking and/or alcohol intake during pregnancy
      vii. High altitudes
   d. Acute MI: VSD is a serious but infrequent complication of MI and rapidly leads to HF, shock, and death
3. **Signs and symptoms: Effects of large defects often become evident at 3 to 12 weeks of age. Symptoms depend on defect size and the patient's age.**
   a. Subjective findings
      i. Small defects: Patients are usually asymptomatic
      ii. Large defects
         (a) Fatigue, exercise intolerance
         (b) Exertional dyspnea
         (c) Angina-like symptoms (caused by pulmonary hypertension)
         (d) Eisenmenger syndrome
   b. Objective findings
      i. Frequently normal growth and development
      ii. Possible difficulty in feeding
      iii. May have a history of slow weight gain, small size
      iv. History of endocarditis
      v. History of frequent respiratory infections, often with bronchopneumonia
      vi. History of heart murmurs from birth
      vii. Family history of heart defects
      viii. Maternal exposure to infectious process or poor nutrition, medications, and medications in the first trimester
   c. Physical examination of the patient: Signs vary, depending on shunt direction and size. Right-to-left shunts produce signs and symptoms of severe HF and cyanosis.
      i. Inspection
         (a) Restlessness, irritability
         (b) Frail appearance, thinness, paleness, waxen complexion
         (c) Tachypnea, air hunger, grunting respirations
         (d) Excessive sweating
         (e) Hemoptysis
         (f) Symptoms of HF, cyanosis
         (g) Prominent sternum: From large RV while growing
      ii. Palpation
         (a) Systolic thrill over lower LSB, fourth intercostal space
         (b) PMI may be displaced laterally in larger defects
         (c) Lift may be felt over the left sternal border
         (d) Peripheral pulses: Rapid, thready

      iii. Auscultation

         (a) Harsh, loud, high-pitched holosystolic murmur (even with a small VSD)

           (1) Loudest at the left sternum, third to fifth intercostal space

           (2) The louder the murmur, the smaller the defect

           (3) Nonradiating murmur

         (b) Loud S_2, split but not fixed (may be single in Eisenmenger syndrome)

         (c) Mitral diastolic rumble at the apex (from increased flow through the mitral valve) indicates a large defect

         (d) Aortic insufficiency murmurs (associated with membranous defects) may be heard

         (e) Patient with Eisenmenger syndrome may not have a murmur (with equalization of right- and left-sided heart pressures)

         (f) Rales with failure

4. Diagnostic study findings

    a. Radiologic (findings may be normal for small VSDs)

      i. LA and LV enlargement

      ii. RA and RV enlargement in the presence of pulmonary artery hypertension

      iii. Increased pulmonary vascular markings

      iv. Pulmonary artery dilatation

    b. ECG

      i. Small defects produce a normal ECG

      ii. Large defects

         (a) LA enlargement and LV hypertrophy

         (b) RV hypertrophy

    c. Echocardiography

      i. Distinguishes shunt flow, increased pulmonary flow, aortic insufficiency; checks prosthetic patches (postoperatively), aneurysms (after closure complication)

      ii. Reveals chamber enlargement

      iii. Demonstrates shunting by the use of echocardiographic contrast material and color-flow Doppler studies

    d. TEE: Identifies residual shunt flow (intraoperatively)

    e. Cardiac catheterization: Can confirm and quantify shunt; assesses hemodynamics; documents the degree of pulmonary hypertension and associated disease (pulmonary stenosis, AR, CAD)

5. Interprofessional collaboration: See ACS; also dentist

6. Management of patient care

    a. Anticipated patient trajectory: Most VSDs close within the first 2 years of life, but the remainder put patients at risk of endocarditis, limitations because of dyspnea, HF, and early death if not corrected

    b. Goals of care

      i. Patient's response to the VSD is evaluated to identify the need for interventions

      ii. If symptoms or complications occur, they are promptly identified and treated

      iii. Patient is taught about infection risks, follow-up care

    c. Treatments

      i. Nutrition: Diet high in calories to assist with infant growth; nasogastric tube may be required

      ii. Infection control: IE prophylaxis

      iii. Discharge planning

         (a) Teach the patient the importance of good dental hygiene

(b) Instruct regarding the need for antibiotic prophylaxis to prevent IE (if a small, residual VSD)

   iv. Pharmacology

     (a) Antibiotics: For IE prophylaxis

     (b) Diuretics (e.g., furosemide, hydrochlorothiazide): To treat pulmonary edema, lower intravascular volumes. Electrolytes and renal function need monitoring.

     (c) Afterload reduction

   v. Treatments: Depend on defect size

     (a) Asymptomatic patients who have no pathologic changes do not require surgery. Small defects may close spontaneously over time.

     (b) Plasma exchange transfusions (if HCT >65%) for severe polycythemia

     (c) Catheter closure of VSDs done with occlusive devices especially for muscular VSDs

     (d) Patients require surgery when

       (1) Patient is symptomatic with HF

       (2) Patient is asymptomatic with a ratio of pulmonary to systemic blood flow in the shunt of 1.5 : 1 or higher

       (3) Patient shows failure to thrive (at 6 months, the prospect of spontaneous closure has diminished considerably)

       (4) Patient experiences repeated, severe respiratory infections or recurrent endocarditis

  d. Potential complications (see specific sections in chapter)

   i. HF (causes 11% of deaths from VSD)

   ii. IE: 4% to 10% risk

   iii. Arrhythmias, sudden cardiac death: Frequently seen with Eisenmenger syndrome

PATENT DUCTUS ARTERIOSUS

1. Pathophysiology

  a. A persistent patency of the fetal circulation between the aorta and the pulmonary artery that failed to close after birth, seen in 2% of adults

  b. During fetal circulation: Blood from the pulmonary artery flows through the ductus into the descending aorta to bypass collapsed lungs. Ductus functionally closes within 24 to 48 hours after birth but may remain open up to 8 weeks.

  c. Ductus closure: Contraction of smooth muscles in the ductus wall results from increased arterial oxygen tension. If the smooth muscles do not contract, the ductus remains open (e.g., hypoxia at birth). Prostaglandin inhibitors can stimulate closure.

  d. If the ductus has not closed spontaneously by 3 months of age, it probably will not

  e. Because the aorta has higher pressures, blood flows back through the patent ductus into the lower-pressure pulmonary artery in a *left-to-right* shunt, and oxygenated blood is recirculated to the lungs

  f. Resistance in the ductus to the shunting of blood is caused not only by the diameter of the defect but also by its length

  g. A small patent ductus arteriosus (PDA) may have no hemodynamic effects and calcify with aging

  h. With larger PDAs, LV workload increases (handles both normal CO and shunt flow), but right-sided heart flow is not increased

   i. Increased blood return to the LA and LV overloads the left side of the heart. LV compensates by enlarging, and symptoms of left-sided HF develop.

   ii. Pulmonary hypertension may develop over time

    i. Large shunts can result in equal pressure in the systemic and pulmonary systems (Eisenmenger syndrome with irreversible pulmonary hypertension)

    j. Increased pulmonary pressures then lead to increased work for the RV (which enlarges and fails)

    k. If obstructive pulmonary vascular lesions develop, PAP will rise above aortic pressure and the shunt will reverse, becoming right to left. Cyanosis and right-sided HF result. Deoxygenated blood is distributed to the left arm and the lower body below the ductus (causing cyanosis and clubbing of the toes), whereas the upper body receives oxygenated blood with no abnormalities.

    l. All patients with PDAs are at risk for HF and IE. Vegetations may embolize to the lungs, which leads to infarctions and death.

2. **Etiology and risk factors**
   a. Failure of the ductus to close at birth
   b. Associated anomalies: Atrial and ventricular septal defects
   c. Individuals at risk
      i. Infants with congenital rubella (acquired in first trimester)
      ii. Infants with birth hypoxia or respiratory distress, lung disease
      iii. Premature infants (weighing less than 1000 g)
      iv. Infants born at high altitudes (chronic hypoxia)
      v. Females (twice as common as among males)

3. **Signs and symptoms: Shunt size and PVR determine the hemodynamic effects. Asymptomatic in 50% of cases. Moderate-sized PDA may not become symptomatic until LV failure and pulmonary hypertension develop.**
   a. Child
      i. Easy fatigability, irritability, poor feeding that results in poor weight gain
      ii. History of maternal rubella during first trimester
      iii. History of hypoxia at birth
      iv. Failure to thrive; growth and developmental problems
      v. High number of respiratory tract infections
   b. Physical findings can include
      i. Dyspnea on exertion, tachypnea, hemoptysis
      ii. Angina-like pain, tachycardia, syncope, signs and symptoms of HF
      iii. Deafness, cataracts
      iv. Hoarseness (compression of the laryngeal nerve)
      v. Clubbing, mild cyanosis possible in the left fingers (because of the entry of unsaturated blood into the left subclavian artery); cyanosis in the lower parts of the body and clubbing of the toes (if right- to left-shunting); leg fatigue
      vi. Palpation
         (a) Hyperdynamic precordium: Distinct LV impulse (overload)
         (b) Bounding, brisk peripheral pulses (especially with large defects)
         (c) Prominent apical impulse
         (d) Possible systolic thrill in the second left intercostal space
      vii. Auscultation
         (a) Loud, rough, continuous machinery-like murmur is indicative of a PDA; peaks at S_2, heard in more than 50% of patients
            (1) Is loudest high, at left upper sternal border (pulmonic area), left infraclavicular area
            (2) Caused by pressure gradient between the aorta and the pulmonary artery

(3) Possible mitral flow rumble at the apex

(b) Wide pulse pressure

4. **Diagnostic study findings**

   a. Radiologic: Chest radiograph

     i. LA and LV enlargement (in large left-to-right shunts)

     ii. Increased pulmonary vascular markings, pulmonary edema in failure

     iii. Enlarged aorta; prominent ascending aorta and aortic knob

     iv. Central pulmonary artery enlarged

   b. ECG (normal in small- and medium-sized PDAs)

     i. LV hypertrophy with left axis deviation

     ii. LA enlargement

   c. Transthoracic echocardiography: Detects the PDA, reveals enlarged chambers, shows flow from the aorta to the pulmonary system in diastole. Color-flow Doppler study helps visualize small shunts and associated congenital defects.

   d. TEE: To delineate the PDA

   e. Cardiac catheterization: Not usually necessary

     i. Establishes the aortopulmonary communication and shunt size and direction

     ii. Assesses pulmonary pressures and resistance

     iii. Increased pressures will be evident in the pulmonary artery with right-to-left shunts

5. **Interprofessional collaboration: See ACS**

6. **Management of patient care**

   a. Anticipated patient trajectory: Patients with PDA are at risk of endocarditis, HF, and possibly shortened life span unless the congenital defect is closed

   b. Goals of care

     i. Duct is closed by transcatheter or surgical techniques

     ii. Prompt, aggressive treatment is provided for symptoms of HF

     iii. IE is prevented

   c. Treatments

     i. Indomethacin may be used to close PDAs in infancy, otherwise, surgical correction is needed.

     ii. Infection control: Antibiotic prophylaxis for IE or endarteritis until surgical repair, generally not needed after closure

     iii. Nutrition: Control of fluid and sodium intake, if HF symptoms are present

     iv. Discharge planning: IE prophylaxis, follow-up care and evaluation

     v. Pharmacology

       (a) Patients are usually asymptomatic and do not require medication (except IE prophylaxis) until PDA closure

       (b) Treatment of HF

     vi. Other interventions

       (a) Pharmacologic closure of PDA with prostaglandin inhibitors, such as indomethacin (effective only in infancy). Complications of the use of indomethacin are increased bleeding risks because of platelet dysfunction, necrotizing enterocolitis.

       (b) Transcatheter closure with a detachable coil closure device deployed in the duct to occlude the shunt is being used for older children and adults

       (c) Surgical ligation of the PDA is the alternative and long-standing treatment. It is primarily performed on large ducts and in young infants.

         (1) Surgery is performed through a small left thoracotomy incision

(2) In adults, calcification and rigidity of the ductus make closure much more difficult. A patch may be needed.

(3) Video-assisted thoracoscopic surgery and robotic techniques are also used

(4) Postoperative nursing care involves the same basic care as for thoracotomy

(d) Heart-lung transplantation may be indicated in cases of fixed pulmonary hypertension and right-to-left shunting

d. Potential complications (see also applicable sections)

  i. IE

  ii. LV HF

  iii. Pulmonary hypertension and Eisenmenger syndrome

  iv. Postoperative complications: Uncommon, include recurrent nerve injury, infections, bleeding, possible hemothorax, pneumothorax, or chylothorax

  v. Complications of the surgical procedures: Failure to close, emboli, vascular complications

7. Evaluation of patient care

a. Patient is free of associated complications from the interventions and HF

b. Complications are promptly identified and treated

COARCTATION OF THE AORTA

> **KEY CONCEPT**
> Medical therapy can be used for management of symptoms; however, surgical repair is the only definitive treatment.

1. Pathophysiology

a. A congenital deformity of the aorta that creates a narrowing of the lumen and, subsequently, decreased flow. Usually located just beyond the left subclavian artery or just distal to the ligamentum arteriosum.

b. In the fetus, the smooth muscle of the ductus arteriosus extends into the aorta. After birth, tissue contracts to close the duct, the aorta is pulled inward, and abnormal infolding or narrowing occurs.

c. Thickening of the aortic medial tissue can form a ridge projecting into the lumen of the aorta, obstructing aortic flow.

d. Fetal development of the aortic arch may also be abnormal, in conjunction with the formation of other cardiac defects (VSD, mitral valve defects, bicuspid aortic valve).

e. Pressure gradient develops: Pressures proximal to the coarctation are increased and pressures distal are decreased.

f. LV pressures increase, as do pressures in all aortic arch vessels.

g. Progressively, the LV dilates, hypertrophies, and can fail because of increased afterload.

h. Cerebral and upper extremity systemic hypertension results from the mechanical obstruction and stimulation of the renin-angiotensin system because of decreased renal blood flow.

i. Collateral circulation develops and supports the lower body and extremities, compensating for the decreased blood flow through the aorta. Collaterals involved include the internal mammary, internal thoracic, scapular, epigastric, intercostal, lumbar, and thyrocervical arteries.

j. If the coarctation is left untreated, death is caused by the consequences of the prolonged hypertension (e.g., strokes, CAD, HF, aortic rupture, or dissection). Other complications include IE, cerebral hemorrhage.

2. **Etiology and risk factors**
   a. Incidence higher in males
   b. Associated with the following disorders: VSD, Turner syndrome, cerebral aneurysms (circle of Willis)
   c. Average life expectancy of an untreated patient with significant coarctation is less than 30 years

3. **Signs and symptoms: Usually diagnosed in childhood. Newborns may have HF and require intervention. After infancy, many patients are asymptomatic until after 20 to 30 years of age. Coarctation is often discovered on routine examinations as a result of hypertension or murmur (e.g., during school physicals for sports).**
   a. Subjective findings: Patient may complain of headaches, visual disturbances, epistaxis, leg cramps or fatigue (with exercise), dizziness, dysphagia
   b. Objective findings: Unremarkable in an asymptomatic patient
      i.   Cyanosis in preductal coarctation, more noticeable in the fingers than in the toes
      ii. Possible irritability, poor feeding, tachypnea in a critically ill infant
      iii. Oliguria
      iv. Metabolic acidosis
      v.   Hypotension
   c. Physical examination
      i.   Inspection
         (a) Forceful thrust may be seen at the apex as a result of LV hypertrophy
         (b) Infants may have lower extremity cyanosis
         (c) Rarely, the upper body may be more developed (athletic) than the lower body, which may be underdeveloped (thin legs, narrow hips)
      ii. Palpation
         (a) Check radial and femoral pulses simultaneously for pulse lag (forceful upper extremity pulses, typically weak and delayed or absent lower extremity pulses). Femoral pulses are absent in about 40% of affected patients (the result of narrow pulse pressure, not of absent flow).
         (b) BP in the lower extremities is less than that in the upper extremities (often by >20 mm Hg). Systolic hypertension is seen in the upper extremities.
         (c) BP may vary in the arms, especially if the coarctation is proximal to the left subclavian artery
         (d) Suprasternal notch thrill
         (e) Apical thrust
      iii. Auscultation
         (a) Systolic ejection murmur, heard best at the right upper sternal border
         (b) Loud S_2 (aortic component)
         (c) S_4 present with left hypertrophy

4. **Diagnostic study findings**
   a. Radiologic: Chest radiograph may be the first means of discovery
      i.   Enlarged LV
      ii. Notching of ribs (inferior margins of the third through eighth ribs), caused by the collateral circulation of the intercostal arteries
      iii. "3" sign: Dilated ascending aorta followed by the constricted area, followed by the poststenotic dilatation

    b. ECG: LV hypertrophy pattern

    c. Echocardiography: LV hypertrophy—screen for other associated aortic stenoses, VSDs

    d. MRI, CT: Confirms the diagnosis safely in pregnant patients (MRI), provides good images of the thoracic aorta and the site of coarctation

    e. Cardiac catheterization: Used to exclude CAD in adults preoperatively. Aortogram shows the location, degree, and character of the aortic lumen narrowing.

5. **Interprofessional collaboration: See ACS**

6. **Management of patient care**

    a. Anticipated patient trajectory: Patients with unrecognized coarctation of the aorta will be exposed to severe hypertension and acceleration of atherosclerosis, which can result in HF, stroke, MI, and early death if the defect is not repaired.

    b. Goals of care

       i. Prompt, aggressive treatment is provided for symptoms of HF

      ii. Hypertension is controlled

    c. Treatments

       i. Infection control: IE antibiotic prophylaxis

      ii. Discharge planning

         (a) Lifelong monitoring for recoarctation, stenosis, hypertension, valvular disease

         (b) Genetic counseling for female patients considering pregnancy

         (c) Pregnancy should be avoided until the repair is accomplished. Close supervision for hypertension issues is necessary.

     iii. Pharmacology: Antihypertensives for BP control with close follow-up monitoring

     iv. Psychosocial issues: Issues regarding contraceptive use and pregnancy are sensitive matters and can cause anxiety and stress in younger patients

      v. Other interventions

         (a) Coarctation is relieved by surgery

           (1) If the patient is asymptomatic, surgery is usually delayed until age 1 to 5 years but should be performed as soon as possible to avoid hypertension

           (2) The older the patient, the higher the risk of death from surgery

           (3) Surgical correction decreases the hypertension and reverses LV failure

         (b) When surgery is undertaken, a left thoracotomy incision is performed

           (1) Postoperative nursing involves the basic care for a thoracotomy patient

           (2) Record BP in both arms

           (3) Assess brachial and femoral pulses simultaneously

         (c) Percutaneous transluminal angioplasty, with or without balloon-expandable endovascular stents, is used more often, especially with recoarctation

    d. Potential complications

       i. IE

      ii. Common causes of death from coarctation in older patients are spontaneous aortic rupture, HF, IE, and cerebral hemorrhage

     iii. Postoperative complications are recoarctation, paradoxical or persistent systemic hypertension, aortic dissection or rupture, HF, and stroke; 20% of patients have transient postoperative abdominal pain and/or distention (probably because of restoration of normal pulsatile blood flow and pressure)

     iv. Paradoxical systolic hypertension may occur for the first 24 to 36 hours after surgery; caused by increased levels of circulating catecholamines; treated with sodium nitroprusside, β-blockers, ARBs

v. Complications after percutaneous transluminal angioplasty for restenosis include aneurysms, rupture, recoarctation, stroke

vi. Pregnancy: Increased risk of aortic dissection

HYPERTENSIVE CRISES

> **KEY CONCEPT**
> Hypertensive crises are potentially life-threatening elevations in BP necessitating emergency treatment to prevent severe end organ damage and death. Urgent pharmacologic therapy is needed to prevent death.

1. **Pathophysiology**
   a. Hypertensive pathophysiology and its effects on the heart, brain, and kidneys (Table 4.15)
   b. Hypertensive emergency is defined as a severe elevation in blood pressure with an SBP over 180 mm Hg and/or a diastolic BP (DBP) over 120 mm Hg associated with new or worsening end organ damage. Hypertensive urgencies are a subset of hypertensive emergencies where there is not yet evidence of acute end organ damage.
   c. Hypertensive encephalopathy: Sudden, excessive elevation of the BP (>250/150 mm Hg) → dysfunction of cerebral autoregulation → vasospasm → ischemia → increased capillary pressure and permeability → cerebral edema, hemorrhage
2. **Etiology and risk factors**
   a. Untreated or uncontrolled hypertension
   b. Poor compliance with antihypertensive medication regimen
   c. Renal dysfunction (acute glomerulonephritis, acute or chronic renal failure, renal tumors, renovascular hypertension caused by acute renal artery occlusion)
   d. Preeclampsia of pregnancy

TABLE 4.15	**Sequelae of Hypertension: Its Effects on End Organs That May Lead to Hypertensive Crisis**	
HYPERTENSION		
Enhanced sympathetic stimulation Effects of renin-angiotensin system (increased fluid retention, increased systemic vasoconstriction) Necrosis of arterioles Decreased blood flow to end organs		
Heart	Brain	Kidney
Tachycardia	Loss of autoregulatory mechanisms	↓ Renal perfusion
↑ Cardiac output	Arterial spasm and ischemia → TIAs	↓ Ability to concentrate urine
↓ Perfusion→angina→MI	Weakened vessels→ aneurysms→ hemorrhage→CVA	↑ BUN, creatinine levels
CAD		↑ Proteinuria
LV hypertrophy		Kidney failure
LV failure		Uremia
Angina		

→, Leading to; *BUN*, blood urea nitrogen; *CAD*, coronary artery disease; *CVA*, cerebrovascular accident; *LV*, left ventricular; *MI*, myocardial infarction; *TIA*, transient ischemic attack.

From Victor, R.G. (2015). Systemic hypertension. In D.L. Mann, D.P. Zipes, P. Libby, R.O. Bonow, E. Braunwald, editors: *Braunwald's heart disease: a textbook of cardiovascular medicine*, 10th ed. (pp 934–952). Philadelphia, Elsevier.

e. Adrenergic crisis: Seen with a sharp rise in catecholamine levels caused by medication reactions (monoamine oxidase [MAO] inhibitor interactions, β-adrenergic agonist ingestion, abrupt withdrawal from antihypertensive therapy), pheochromocytoma

f. Postoperative complications: CABG surgery, renal transplantation, peripheral vascular surgery

g. Pituitary tumors

h. Adrenocortical hyperfunction

i. Severe burns

j. Risk factors: Diabetes, obesity, smoking, hyperlipidemia, oral contraceptives, history of hypertension with pregnancy, alcohol abuse

3. **Signs and symptoms: Patient may be unable to respond to questions; significant other may need to answer history inquiries (e.g., complaints of severe headache, epistaxis) (Fig. 4.18)**

a. History

  i. Chronic hypertension

  ii. Positive family history of hypertension

  iii. Medication history positive for MAO inhibitors, oral contraceptives, appetite suppressants, pressor agents, street drugs

  iv. History of any etiologic factor mentioned

  v. History of CAD, renal dysfunction

b. Clinical picture in hypertensive encephalopathy

  i. BP exceeding 250/150 mm Hg

  ii. Retinopathy

  iii. Papilledema of the optic disc

  iv. Severe headache

  v. Vomiting

  vi. Altered level of consciousness (obtunded, comatose)

  vii. Transitory focal neurologic signs (e.g., nystagmus)

  viii. Seizures

  ix. Signs and symptoms of HF

  x. Increased MAP

4. **Diagnostic study findings**

a. Laboratory

  i. BUN and creatinine values elevated in patients with renal disease

  ii. Electrolyte levels: Hypocalcemia, hyponatremia, hypokalemia

  iii. Enzyme levels for MI

b. Radiologic: Chest radiograph may show LV enlargement

c. ECG: LV hypertrophy may be seen

d. Echocardiogram: Impairment of diastolic function, LV hypertrophy, wall motion abnormalities

e. MRI or CT: To exclude stroke or hemorrhage when neurologic symptoms present. Shows diffuse brain edema with hypertensive crisis.

f. Renal ultrasonography: To identify renal artery stenosis

5. **Interprofessional collaboration: See ACS**

6. **Management of patient care**

a. Anticipated patient trajectory: Immediate BP reduction is essential for the prevention or minimization of end organ damage.

b. Goals of care

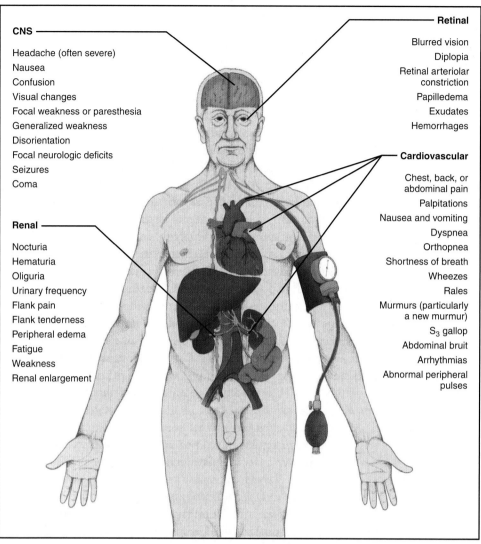

CNS

Headache (often severe)
Nausea
Confusion
Visual changes
Focal weakness or paresthesia
Generalized weakness
Disorientation
Focal neurologic deficits
Seizures
Coma

Renal

Nocturia
Hematuria
Oliguria
Urinary frequency
Flank pain
Flank tenderness
Peripheral edema
Fatigue
Weakness
Renal enlargement

Retinal

Blurred vision
Diplopia
Retinal arteriolar
constriction
Papilledema
Exudates
Hemorrhages

Cardiovascular

Chest, back, or
abdominal pain
Palpitations
Nausea and vomiting
Dyspnea
Orthopnea
Shortness of breath
Wheezes
Rales
Murmurs (particularly
a new murmur)
S_3 gallop
Abdominal bruit
Arrhythmias
Abnormal peripheral
pulses

Fig. 4.18 Symptoms and signs associated with target-organ damage in hypertensive crisis. *CNS,* Central nervous system. (From Antman, E.M., (ed). (2013). *Cardiovascular therapeutics: a companion to Braunwald's heart disease,* 4th ed. Philadelphia: Elsevier.)

     i. Rapid, life-preserving treatment of elevated BP is provided

    ii. For patients with preeclampsia/eclampsia or pheochromocytoma crisis, SBP should be reduced to under 140 mm Hg in the first hour; for patients with aortic dissection, SBP should be reduced to under 120 mm Hg in the first hour

   iii. For other patients, SBP is lowered no more than 25% in the first hour; then, if stable to 160/100 mm Hg in the next 2 to 6 hours, then to normal in the next 24 to 48 hours

   iv. BP is lowered in small decrements to avoid causing hypotension, oliguria, and/ or mental changes from renal, coronary, or cerebral ischemia

    v. Cause of the hypertension is identified and treated

  c. Treatments

    i. Nutrition

      (a) Obtain accurate intake and output measurements, along with daily weights

(b) NPO initially, later a sodium-restricted diet

(c) Dietary consult: For education on weight control, sodium restriction

ii. Discharge planning: Patient education regarding the following:

(a) Importance of BP control: High risk for renal, cerebral, coronary problems with uncontrolled hypertension. Compliance with medication regimen essential.

(b) Need for follow-up to assess the effectiveness of medications and to check for potential side effects from therapy

(c) Lifestyle modification: Limitation of sodium intake, smoking cessation, moderation in alcohol use, walking program, weight control

iii. Pharmacology

(a) No strong evidence preferring one agent over another; however, two smaller trials have shown nicardipine to be better than labetalol at achieving short-term goals

(b) Nicardipine (calcium channel blocker): Better safety profile and similar antihypertensive effect compared with nitroprusside

(1) Dose: 5 mg/h; titrated to a max dose of 15 mg/h

(2) Half-life 3 to 6 hours

(3) Limitations include longer onset of action (5–10 minutes), longer half-life

(c) β-blockers: Block the effects of increased adrenergic tone, reduce mortality and morbidity

(1) Metoprolol: 5 mg IV every 5 minutes up to 15 mg total

(2) Labetalol

   a) Medication of choice for intracranial hemorrhage

      1) Dosage: 20-mg IV bolus, then 20 to 80 mg every 10 minutes or IV infusion

   b) An α- and β-adrenergic blocking agent, used especially for adrenergic crisis. Does not increase heart rate (good in CAD).

(3) Esmolol: 500 mg/kg/min for 4 minutes, then 50 to 300 mg/kg/min IV

(d) Nitroprusside: Medication of choice for hypertensive encephalopathy, cerebral infarction or bleeding, dissecting aortic aneurysm. Contraindicated in pregnancy (can cause fetal renal impairment).

(1) 0.25 to 0.5 mcg/kg/min IV. Titrate every 5 minutes (maximum dose 8–10 mcg/kg/min). Titrate to lowest dose for therapeutic effects

(2) Medication acts in seconds, is quickly reversed by stopping infusion (medication action lasts 1–5 minutes)

(3) Protect bag and lines from light

(4) Watch for cyanide toxicity (blurred vision, confusion, tinnitus, seizures), especially after 48 hours of therapy or with renal insufficiency. Thiocyanate blood level should be measured at 48 hours. Level should not exceed 1.7 mmol/L.

(5) Closely monitor the patient's response to therapy by frequent assessments of BP, hemodynamics. Titrate IV medications to the patient's responses per established parameters.

(e) Fenoldopam (selective dopamine receptor agonist): Very potent vasodilator; as effective as nitroprusside in lowering BP

(1) Dose: 0.1 mcg/kg/min; titrated every 15 minutes to response

(2) Half-life is 10 minutes

(3) Side effects include hypokalemia, headache, flushing, dizziness, reflex tachycardia

(4) Increases intraocular pressure (contraindicated with glaucoma)

(f) ACE inhibitors

(1) Medication of choice for LV failure and pulmonary edema

(2) Enalapril: 1.25 to 5 mg IV every 6 hours

(3) Onset of action: 10 to 15 minutes

(g) IV NTG for hypertension because of cardiac causes (acute MI, failure)

(h) Loop diuretics (torsemide, furosemide, ethacrynic acid) for LV failure, pulmonary edema. Watch for volume depletion.

iv. Psychosocial issues

(a) Reassure the patient and family

(b) Create a calm, quiet atmosphere, conducive to ample rest for the patient

(c) If the patient has been nonadherent with the medication regimen and has not addressed known risk factors, explore the reasons for noncompliance

(1) Make sure the patient knows the rationales for medications and the consequences of inaction

(2) BP medications are expensive. Help the patient find resources— financial services, medication programs for the indigent, use of pill splitters (buying larger doses and splitting the pills may be more economical), purchase of generics

v. Other interventions

(a) Ensure that the patient has adequate IV access; prepare for central line insertion, if needed

(b) Patient should undergo continuous arterial monitoring while medications are being titrated and the condition is unstable

(c) Adjust antihypertensive IV medications promptly by titration, depending on the patient's response. Watch for side effects of medications.

(d) Accurately monitor fluid and electrolyte status. Observe for abnormalities in laboratory test results (e.g., electrolyte levels).

(e) If symptoms of tissue ischemia develop, reduce the speed with which BP is lowered. *Note:* Most problems that occur in hypertensive crisis occur when treatment is too aggressive for the patient to tolerate.

d. Potential complications (see Fig. 4.18)

i. Cerebral dysfunction: Hypertensive encephalopathy, intracerebral or subarachnoid hemorrhage, head injuries, intracranial masses, embolic brain infarction

(a) Mechanism: Increased intracranial pressure (from cerebral edema)

(b) Management: Watch for changes in mentation or vision, headaches, nausea, vomiting. Intracranial pressure monitoring may be needed.

ii. Cardiac or vascular dysfunction

(a) Mechanism: Caused by LV failure, dissecting aortic aneurysm, acute MI, UA, coarctation of the aorta, arrhythmias

(b) Management: Monitor the ECG, observe for T-wave inversions that occur with rapid BP reductions; ischemia is rare. Sudden chest pain may indicate aortic dissection.

iii. Renal failure

(a) Mechanism: Can be a cause or a result of severely elevated BP

(b) Management: Close monitoring, BP control; dialysis may be required

AORTIC AND PERIPHERAL ARTERIAL DISEASE

> ### KEY CONCEPT
> Diseases of the aorta, cerebral arteries, and peripheral arteries have consequences that include aneurysm formation, dissection, or ischemia in their respective perfusion beds.

1. **Pathophysiology**
   a. Aortic aneurysm (Fig. 4.19)
      i. Focal or diffuse weakness of the aortic wall
      ii. Atherosclerosis is the most common cause
      iii. Dilatation, increased pressures, and thinning of the wall all increase wall stress, further weakening and dilating the vessel and producing an aneurysm
      iv. Rupture and death are likely when the diameter exceeds 6 cm for the thoracic aorta or 5 cm for the abdominal aorta
      v. Common sites for aneurysms

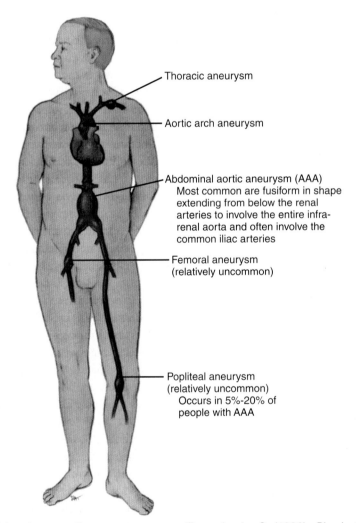

Thoracic aneurysm

Aortic arch aneurysm

Abdominal aortic aneurysm (AAA)
Most common are fusiform in shape extending from below the renal arteries to involve the entire infra-renal aorta and often involve the common iliac arteries

Femoral aneurysm
(relatively uncommon)

Popliteal aneurysm
(relatively uncommon)
Occurs in 5%-20% of people with AAA

Fig. 4.19 Peripheral artery disease: aneurysms. (From Jarvis, C. (1996). *Physical examination and health assessment*, 2nd ed. Philadelphia: Elsevier.)

    (a) Abdominal aortic aneurysm: Location between the renal and iliac arteries is the most common site

    (b) Thoracic aortic aneurysm

       (1) Ascending, transverse, or descending aorta

       (2) Most common in men aged 60 to 70 years or older

    (c) Aneurysms of the iliac, femoral, and popliteal arteries

b. Aortic dissection

    i. Intima of the ascending and/or descending aorta weakened by atherosclerosis or congenital disease of the media

    ii. Hypertension causes or contributes to the injury in 80% of cases

    iii. Tear develops through the intima and is propagated up and down the aorta by a dissecting column of blood

    iv. False channel is created

    v. Some organs may be perfused by the true lumen and some by the false lumen

    vi. Occasionally, a dissection of the ascending aorta extends to the aortic valve, and aortic insufficiency and even bleeding into the pericardium can result

    vii. End organ ischemia and injury can occur

    viii. Classified by either the Debakey or Stanford Classification (Fig. 4.20)

c. Peripheral artery disease (Fig. 4.21)

    i. Atherosclerotic disease develops from the same risk factors and process as those for CAD

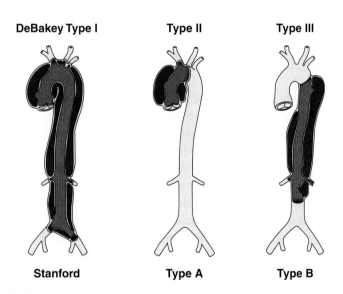

DeBakey Type I **Type II** **Type III**

Stanford **Type A** **Type B**

DeBakey
Type I   Originates in the ascending aorta, propagates at least to the aortic arch and often beyond it distally
Type II   Originates in and is confined to the ascending aorta
Type III Originates in the descending aorta and extends distally down the aorta or, rarely, retrograde into the aortic arch and ascending aorta

Stanford
Type A   All dissections involving the ascending aorta, regardless of the site of origin
Type B   All dissections not involving the ascending aorta

Fig. 4.20 Common classifications of thoracic aortic dissection. (From Topol, E.J., Teirstein, P.S. (2020). *Textbook of interventional cardiology*, 8th ed. Philadelphia: Elsevier.)

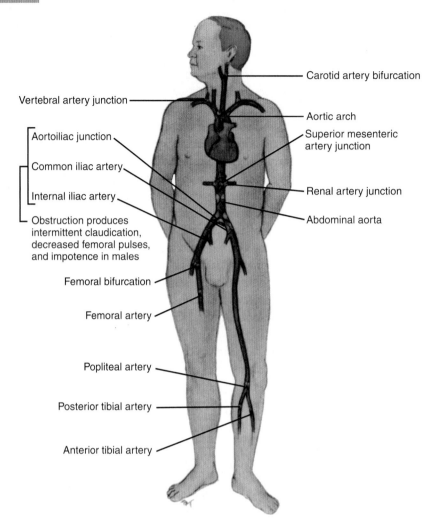

Fig. 4.21 Peripheral artery disease: occlusions. (From Jarvis, C. (1996). *Physical examination and health assessment*, 2nd ed. Philadelphia: Elsevier.)

  ii. Stenosis and hypoperfusion result, culminating in ischemia, occlusion, and infarction (unless supported by collateral circulation)
 iii. Occluded lesions generally occur at bifurcations
 iv. Occlusions can also result from thrombus or embolus
  v. Common sites for peripheral artery disease include the carotid, renal, popliteal, aortoiliac, and femoral arteries (but any artery including the mesenteric can be involved); approximately 70% are located in the infrainguinal area (femoral, popliteal)
2. **Etiology and risk factors**
   a. Atherosclerosis
   b. Congenital abnormalities (cystic medial necrosis, Marfan syndrome)
   c. Trauma: Blunt trauma can create tears in the intima of the thoracic aorta (causing dissecting aneurysm)
   d. Severe hypertension
   e. Arteritis
   f. Raynaud disease
   g. Risk factors are the same as for CAD (smoking, hypertension, diabetes, hyperlipidemia, family history)

3. **Signs and symptoms: Manifestations usually occur at age 60 years or older**
   a. Signs and symptoms vary with the location of the aneurysm or occlusion
      i. Aneurysm (most common): Often asymptomatic, found on routine examination
         (a) Abdominal aortic aneurysm
             (1) Pulsation in the abdominal area
             (2) Dull abdominal or low back pain or ache (impending rupture)
             (3) Nausea and vomiting (pressure against the duodenum)
             (4) Severe, sharp, sudden abdominal pain: Continuous, radiates to back, hips, scrotum, pelvis (rupture)
             (5) Abdominal tenderness, if an inflammatory process
             (6) Syncope, hypovolemic shock
         (b) Thoracic aortic aneurysm
             (1) Sudden, tearing chest pain radiating to the shoulders, neck, and back
             (2) Cough, hoarseness, weak voice from pressure against the recurrent laryngeal nerve
             (3) Dysphagia because of pressure on the esophagus
      ii. Aortic dissections
         (a) Marked by acute severe and instantaneous chest pain (in 90% of cases), radiating to the back, neck, jaw, or abdomen, associated with an absence of the affected pulses and evidence of end organ injury
         (b) "Ripping," "tearing" sensations described
         (c) Pain may be differentiated from that of acute MI by its instantaneous, severe onset and the absence of pulses
         (d) Neurologic symptoms present in 15% of cases
      iii. Peripheral arterial disease
         (a) Intermittent claudication
             (1) Cramping, aching pain with exertion
             (2) Pain in the calf (most often) but may also be in the buttocks
             (3) Reproduced after walking a predictable distance
             (4) Relieved with rest, standing still
         (b) Nonhealing ulcers
         (c) Impotence
         (d) Severe pain in the extremities, pallor, absence of pulses, paresthesias, paralysis (seen in acute thrombosis of an abdominal aortic aneurysm)
         (e) Carotid arteries: Transient ischemic attacks, monocular visual disturbances, sensory or motor deficits, expressive or receptive aphasia, stroke
         (f) 50% of patients with occlusive arterial disease involving the lower extremities are asymptomatic
   b. History
      i. History of atherosclerosis (CAD, CVA) and hypertension
      ii. Risk factors for atherosclerosis
      iii. Trauma: Blunt, deceleration type
      iv. History of impotence (seen in severe aortoiliac disease)
   c. Physical examination: Manifestations depend on the organ perfused (e.g., cerebral vascular disease, renal vascular disease, ischemic or infarcted bowel, ischemic extremities)
      i. Aneurysms: Often asymptomatic except for rupture, when the patient is in obvious severe pain
         (a) Hypertension or hypotensive

      (b) Obvious discomfort with rupture or expansion

      (c) Stridor, hoarseness, dysphagia (pressure on the esophagus, trachea, pharyngeal nerve)

      (d) Bruits: Abdominal aorta; femoral, renal, popliteal artery

      (e) Murmur of aortic insufficiency, if the aneurysm involves the aortic ring

  ii. Aortic dissection

      (a) Hypertension or hypotension

      (b) Dyspnea

      (c) Stridor, hoarseness, dysphagia (pressure on the esophagus, trachea, pharyngeal nerve)

      (d) Palpation: Wide pulse pressure, absence of various peripheral pulses and pressures (50% of cases)

      (e) Auscultation: Murmur of aortic insufficiency (heard in 50% of cases)

  iii. Peripheral arterial disease

      (a) Pain on elevation of the extremities

      (b) Pale, mottled extremities on elevation; rubor on dependence of the extremities

      (c) Ulcers, gangrene in the extremities

      (d) Skin changes because of impaired circulation (hair loss, thin and shiny skin)

      (e) Retinal arterial emboli (carotid disease)

      (f) Weak or absent peripheral pulses

      (g) Cool skin

      (h) Sluggish capillary refill

      (i) Pulsatile mass in the popliteal fossa (popliteal aneurysm)

      (j) Auscultation: Bruits

4. Diagnostic study findings

  a. Laboratory

    i. CBC: Decreased HCT (anemia)

    ii. Elevated BUN and creatinine levels, proteinuria, hematuria (compromised kidneys)

  b. Radiologic

    i. Chest radiograph: For thoracic aortic aneurysm/dissection, increased aortic diameter, right deviation of the trachea, pleural effusions, widened mediastinum

    ii. Abdominal films (anteroposterior, lateral views): For abdominal aneurysm

    iii. Provides anatomic information

  c. Doppler duplex ultrasonography: To assess peripheral, cerebrovascular blood flow and velocity

  d. ABI: Ankle systolic pressure is divided by the systolic pressure at the brachial artery to derive an index. Used to evaluate for the presence and severity of disease.

    i. Normal ABI = 0.9 to 1.4 (pressure normally higher in the ankle)

    ii. ABI less than 0.9 = positive for peripheral artery disease

    iii. ABI less than 0.4 = indicates severe ischemia

  e. CT: Assesses lumen diameter, wall thickness, aneurysm size, mural thrombi, and origin and extent of dissection, including the blood supply to end organs. Three-dimensional CT with angiography gives vivid three-dimensional views of the vascular system.

  f. MRA: Defines the arterial anatomy, shows the presence and severity of the occlusion.

g. TEE: Assesses for the presence of dissection in the aortic root, proximal ascending aorta, or descending thoracic aorta; aortic insufficiency; pericardial effusion. Used intraoperatively to determine the effectiveness of surgery.

h. Peripheral angiography: Defines the anatomy and severity of lesions and their suitability for intervention

i. Aortography: Origin and extent of dissection seen

5. **Interprofessional collaboration: See ACS; also vascular specialist, primary care physician, stroke team**

6. **Management of patient care**

a. Anticipated patient trajectory: Aortic aneurysms and dissections are the most frequently missed preventable causes of sudden cardiac death

b. Goals of care

   i. Patient has no pain at rest or with activity

   ii. Perfusion to affected extremities is adequate

   iii. No interventional complications are experienced

   iv. BP is controlled at the systolic goal set for the patient

   v. Patient understands medications, follow-up requirements, any limitations on activities, proper diet, when to call for medical help, what symptoms to report

c. Treatments

   i. Pain management: Relieve pain by administering ordered analgesics

   ii. Skin care: Meticulous attention to the skin because of poor circulation and tissue perfusion. Assess for pressure points, reddened or inflamed areas.

      (a) Frequent repositioning. Turn at least every 2 hours

      (b) Heel protection: Off bed on pillows or foam pads, or in protective boots; elevated

      (c) Ointments, skin barriers as needed

   iii. Nutrition: Dietary consult—assess nutritional status

   iv. Discharge planning: Teach the patient and significant others about the disease process (aneurysm, peripheral arterial occlusive disease), including the following:

      (a) Risk factor modification (e.g., smoking cessation, BP control, diabetes control)

      (b) Discussion of a walking program, identification of resources to help with follow-up

      (c) Good foot care: Daily washing, nail trimming, use of well-fitting shoes, prompt professional attention to corns, calluses, ulcers

      (d) Weight reduction, if overweight

   v. Pharmacology

      (a) β-blockers (e.g., esmolol, labetalol) to lower BP and decrease heart rate— especially important to reduce torque in cases of dissection

      (b) Simultaneous use of nitroprusside to further lower BP and to decrease contractility and sheer force

      (c) Antiplatelet agents: Aspirin daily (to lower the risk of CVA, MI). May also prevent reocclusions

      (d) Cilostazol: For claudication pain, helps activity tolerance (contraindicated in HF)

      (e) Lipid-lowering agents (statins)

   vi. Treatments

      (a) Dissections: Distal dissections (distal to the left subclavian artery) are usually managed medically. Ascending dissections are treated with medications but require surgery

  (b) Acute aortic dissections: Surgical emergency
   (1) Goals: Stabilize emergently, prevent complications from rupture. Control systemic BP (100–120 mm Hg systolic is the goal).
   (2) Prepare the patient for surgery: Resection, replacement, and/or reconstruction of involved arteries
    a) Continuous BP monitoring
    b) Intubation may be necessary, if the patient's condition is unstable
    c) Assess peripheral pulses and BP, comparing both sides. Pressure differences exceeding 20 mm Hg in the upper extremities indicate possible dissection or occluded subclavian, innominate, brachial, or axillary arteries. Pulses may be impossible to assess by palpating and difficult or impossible to assess with Doppler ultrasonographic studies.
    d) Observe for symptoms of shock
   (3) Proximal dissections carry a high (80%) mortality rate, but survival rate with surgery is also high
   (4) Postoperative nursing care for dissection
    a) Monitor hemodynamics
    b) Watch urinary output, mentation
  (c) Surgery for descending dissections performed only if the patient's condition continues to be unstable after medical therapy, with aortic rupture or Marfan syndrome
  (d) Endovascular stent grafts are being deployed successfully to cover the descending dissections as a less invasive alternative
  (e) Endovascular revascularization interventions are widely used before surgery in peripheral arterial disease
   (1) Percutaneous transluminal angioplasty is used to open occluded arteries, particularly in proximal lesions (iliac, renal)
   (2) Excimer laser technology has also been used to debulk atherosclerotic material
   (3) Stents are used to reduce restenosis in both native arteries and grafts
   (4) Patients with acute arterial occlusions may be eligible for low-dose catheter-directed thrombolytic therapy (e.g., t-PA)
   (5) Mechanical thrombolysis or catheter-directed thrombectomy may also be performed for rapid thrombus removal
   (6) Watch for signs of bleeding, especially if the patient has received thrombolytic therapy
  (f) Femoral-popliteal bypass
   (1) Used in cases of longer lesions, chronic total occlusions, and other cases when endovascular repair is not possible
   (2) Patient's own saphenous vein is most commonly used as the new conduit; in cases where the saphenous is not available (e.g., already used in CABG) or otherwise unsuitable (e.g., poor quality, inadequate size, history of phlebitis), prosthetic graft may be used
   (3) Most common postoperative complications are wound infection, graft infection, postoperative hemorrhage, edema, and occlusion; higher rates of morbidity than in endovascular repair (37% vs. 17%)
   (4) Mortality rate is low (2.3%) and comparable to endovascular repair (3%)

d. Potential complications
  i. Aortic aneurysm: Dissection, embolization of thrombus, end-organ compromise
  ii. Large abdominal aneurysms: DIC is an associated problem
  iii. Ascending aortic dissections: MI, hemorrhagic cerebral infarct, tamponade, AR, death
  iv. Postoperative complications with ascending dissections: Death, CVA, end-organ compromise
  v. Postoperative complications with descending dissections: Ischemia of the spinal cord, paralysis, end-organ compromise
  vi. Postprocedure complications with endovascular intervention: Small bowel infarcts, gangrene

SHOCK

1. **In shock, tissue perfusion to vital body organs is inadequate (see Ch. 10, Sepsis and Septic Shock)**

KEY CONCEPT

Shock is the state of inadequate oxygen supply to meet oxygen demand. It may be the result of a number of pathologic processes, although management is largely similar. The goal of shock treatment is restoring adequate circulation through volume replacement, optimization of hemodynamics, and improving the pumping ability of the heart.

---

2. **Pathophysiology (Table 4.16)**
  a. Diminished tissue perfusion deprives cells of oxygen, nutrients, and energy. Cellular dysfunction and potential cell necrosis ensue because of the lack of oxygenation and resulting acidosis.
  b. Cellular dysfunction is reversible at first but leads to organ damage if untreated
  c. Compensatory mechanisms: To support BP, vasoconstriction is the homeostatic response of the body to hypotension and shock. This response is appropriate for, and probably evolved from, the need to respond to hemorrhagic shock. It is completely inappropriate and detrimental in the management of cardiogenic shock.
  d. Major organs begin to malfunction as they are deprived of oxygen, as a result of hypoxemia and metabolic acidosis (respiratory failure, renal failure, decreased cerebral perfusion, and DIC may be seen)
3. **Etiology and risk factors**
  a. Cardiogenic shock: Impaired tissue perfusion as a result of severe cardiac dysfunction
    i. MI, especially if large and/or anterior
    ii. Myocardial ischemia (left main artery disease, multivessel CAD)
    iii. Papillary muscle rupture, acute valvular dysfunction (acute mitral regurgitation, aortic insufficiency)
    iv. HF, cardiac tamponade
    v. Arrhythmias
    vi. Cardiomyopathy
    vii. Other severe forms of myocardial injury (trauma)
    viii. Risk factors: Peripheral vascular disease, decreased LV EF, diabetes
  b. Hypovolemic shock: Impaired tissue perfusion resulting from severely diminished circulating blood volume

TABLE 4.16 Pathophysiology and Clinical Presentations of Shock

Type of Shock	Forward Cardiac	Central Venous Pressure	Pulmonary Artery Occlusion Pressure	Systemic Vascular Resistance	Clinical Examination	Comments
CARDIOGENIC SHOCK						
Pump failure						
LV MI	↓↓↓	↑↑	↑↑↑	↑↑	+ S$_3$, + S$_4$	Extensive infarct (>40% LV)
RV MI	↓↓	↑↑↑	↔ or ↓	↑	Right sided + S$_3$, + S$_4$	Concomitant inferior wall MI common, consider if elevated right-sided filling pressures with normal or low PAOP or hypotension with clear lung fields
Non-CAD cardiomyopathy	↓↓↓	↑↑	↑↑↑	↑↑	+ S$_3$, + S$_4$	Includes myocarditis, idiopathic, inflammatory causes
Allograft failure	↓↓↓	↑↑	↑↑↑	↑↑	+ S$_3$, + S$_4$	Includes cellular and humoral rejection
Infiltrative disease (late)	↓↓↓	↑↑	↑↑↑	↑ or ↔	+ S$_4$ (early)	Characteristic echocardiographic appearance
Trauma	↓↓	↑ or ↔	↑↑	↑ or ↔	Variable	Site involved: RA–RV >LA–LV; May see combined shock (e.g. hypovolemic vs. obstructive with pump failure)
Mechanical Causes						
Acute aortic regurgitation	↓↓	↕	↑↑ or ↑↑↑	↑↑	EDM	Endocarditis most common cause
Native or prosthetic	↓ or ↔	↑ or ↔				IABP contraindicated
Acute mitral regurgitation	↓↓	↑ or ↔	↑↑↑↑	↑↑	ESM	Prominent PAOP V wave
Native or prosthetic	↓ or ↔	↑ or ↔				IABP very effective
Aortic stenosis	↕	↑ or ↔	↑↑	↑↑		Symptoms may become manifest with increased metabolic demand (e.g., pregnancy, exercise, thyrotoxicosis, sepsis)
Mitral stenosis	↕	↑ or ↔	↑↑↑	↑↑		
VSD (acute post-MI)	↓ or ↓↓	↑ or ↑↑	↑ or ↑↑	↑↑	HSM, thrill	May be 3–5 days s/p MI, uncommon event but high mortality
Free wall rupture (post-MI)	↓ or ↓↓	↑ or ↑↑	↑ or ↑↑	↑	Silent	Catastrophic presentation 1–3 days s/p MI, earlier presentation with lytics

TABLE 4.16 Pathophysiology and Clinical Presentations of Shock—cont'd

Type of Shock	Forward Cardiac	Central Venous Pressure	Pulmonary Artery Occlusion Pressure	Systemic Vascular Resistance	Clinical Examination	Comments
Obstructive Shock						
Pericardial tamponade	↓↓ (LV)	↑↑↑	↑↑	↑↑	Silent	Pressure equalization: RA mean, RV EDP, PA diastolic, PAOP within 5 mm Hg
Pulmonary embolism	↓↓ (RV)	↑↑↑	↑	↑ or ↑↑	RV S$_3$ or S$_4$, RV lift	RV dysfunction, moderate increase in PA pressure (40–50 mm Hg)
Hypovolemic Shock						
Blood or volume loss	↓	↓↓↓	↓↓↓	↑ or ↔	Silent	Look for source of blood or volume loss
Distributive Shock						
Septic shock	↑ or ↑↑	Initial ↓↓	↓↓	↓↓↓	Hyperdynamic precordium	Provide early antibiotics, supportive care, identify occult source (e.g., abscess)
Anaphylactic shock	↔ or ↑	↓↓↓	↓↓	↓↓↓	None	Document antigen exposure
Treatment is epinephrine						
Combined Shock (Precise Hemodynamics Often Difficult to Predict)						
Septic + cardiogenic	↓↓	↓ or ↔	↑↑	↓ or ↓↓	Variable; Infection (e.g., pneumonia) after MI	Common settings: Sepsis-induced LV dysfunction
Cardiogenic + hypovolemic	↓↓↓	↓ or ↔	↑ or ↑↑	↑↑↑	Variable	Free wall rupture after MI, GI bleeding with thrombolytics after MI
Hypovolemic + obstructive	↓↓	↓ or ↔	↓↓	↑↑↑	Quiet precordium	Ruptured aortic dissection with tamponade

↔, Unchanged; *CAD*, coronary artery disease; *EDM*, early diastolic pressure; *EDP*, end-diastolic pressure; *ESM*, early systolic murmur; *GI*, gastrointestinal; *HSM*, holosystolic murmur; *IABP*, intraaortic balloon pump; *LA*, left atrium; *LV*, left ventricle; *MI*, myocardial infarction; *PA*, pulmonary artery; *PAOP*, pulmonary artery occlusive pressure; *RA*, right atrium; *RV*, right ventricle; *s/p*, status post; *VSD*, ventricular septal defect.
From Longo, D.L., Fauci, A.S., Kasper, D.L., et al. (2013). Shock. In D.L. Longo, A.S. Fauci, D.L. Kasper, et al., editors. *Harrison's manual of medicine*, 18th ed. New York: McGraw-Hill.

4   Cardiovascular System

i. Hemorrhage: Loss of blood, plasma, and body fluids because of surgery, trauma, gastrointestinal bleeding

ii. Hypovolemia from fluid shifts (e.g., burns)

iii. Severe dehydration (vomiting, diarrhea, diabetic ketoacidosis, diabetes insipidus, heat stroke)

iv. Internal, extravascular fluid loss: Resulting from third-spacing in interstitial space, ascites, ruptured spleen, pancreatitis, hemothorax

v. Adrenal insufficiency

c. Obstructive shock: Impaired tissue perfusion resulting from some obstruction to blood flow

i. PE (see Ch. 3, Pulmonary System)

ii. Aortic dissection

d. Anaphylactic shock: Impaired tissue perfusion resulting from antigen-antibody reaction that releases histamine into the bloodstream. Capillary permeability increases, and arteriolar dilatation occurs. SVR falls. Blood return to the heart is decreased dramatically. Hypotension results.

i. Contrast media

ii. Medication reactions

iii. Blood transfusion reactions

iv. Food allergies

v. Insect bites or stings

vi. Snake bites

e. Septic shock: Sepsis-induced state with hypotension requiring vasopressor support, despite adequate volume resuscitation along with perfusion abnormalities, including a serum lactate over 2 mmol/mL (18 mg/dL). (See Ch. 10, Sepsis and Septic Shock.)

f. Neurogenic shock: Impaired tissue perfusion caused by damage to or dysfunction of the sympathetic nervous system. This type of shock is rare and may be associated with trauma, anesthesia, or spinal shock.

4. **Signs and symptoms: History and assessments must be done rapidly so that immediate life-preserving therapy can be initiated; information is often obtained from significant others or previous records (e.g., bleeding, trauma, symptoms, fever, medications, exposure)**

a. Clinical picture of cardiogenic shock

i. Inspection

(a) Hypotension: SBP lower than 90 mm Hg by cuff, lower than 80 mm Hg by arterial line

(b) Patient confused, restless, or obtunded

(c) Shallow, rapid respirations

(d) Distended neck veins (RV MI, tamponade, PE)

(e) Large differences in extremity pressures

(f) Oliguria

ii. Palpation

(a) Cold, clammy extremities (vasoconstricted)

(b) Peripheral pulses: Thready, rapid, or absent

(c) Low temperature

iii. Auscultation

(a) Crackles (pulmonary edema)

(b) S_3: Gallop

(c) Systolic murmur (heard with acute mitral regurgitation, VSD, aortic stenosis)

Cardiovascular System

4

(d) Diastolic murmur of aortic insufficiency may be heard (short in acute aortic insufficiency)

(e) Heart sounds distant in tamponade

iv. Hemodynamics

(a) Elevated CVP with neck vein distention (in RV MI, tamponade, massive PE)

(b) Decreased CO, CI (<2 L/min)

(c) Elevated PAOP

(d) Elevated SVR

b. Clinical picture of hypovolemic shock

i. Inspection

(a) Anxiety, irritability

(b) Decreased level of consciousness

(c) Poor capillary refill

(d) Pale, gray skin

(e) Increased heart rate

(f) Hypotension

(g) Collapsed neck veins

(h) Tachypnea

(i) Urinary output decreased or absent

ii. Hemodynamics

(a) Decreased CVP, filling pressures, PAP, PAOP, CO, CI

(b) Increased PVR, SVR

c. Clinical picture of anaphylactic shock

i. Inspection

(a) Altered mental status, headache

(b) Stridor, tachypnea, wheezing

(c) Increased heart rate, decreased BP

(d) Hives; itching; flushed, warm skin

(e) Abdominal cramping, nausea, vomiting, diarrhea

(f) Chills

ii. Hemodynamics

(a) Decreased CVP

(b) Decreased PAOP

(c) Decreased SVR

(d) Variable CO

d. Clinical picture of septic shock (see Ch. 10, Sepsis and Septic Shock)

i. Inspection

(a) Confusion, decreased level of consciousness

(b) Fever, chills

(c) Tachycardia and dyspnea

(d) Tachypnea

(e) Warm skin

(f) Cyanosis, decreased capillary refill

(g) Decreased urinary output

ii. Hemodynamics

(a) Decreased CVP

(b) Decreased PAOP

(c) Decreased SVR

(d) Increased CO

e. Clinical picture of neurogenic shock
- i. Inspection
  - (a) Mentation changes (restlessness, confusion)
  - (b) Warm, dry skin
  - (c) Bradycardia
  - (d) No sweating (temperature-regulating center altered): Risk for overheating, chilling
  - (e) Paralysis
  - (f) Apnea, tachypnea, diaphragmatic breathing
  - (g) Profound hypotension
  - (h) Nausea, vomiting
  - (i) Decreased urinary output
- ii. Hemodynamics
  - (a) Decreased CVP
  - (b) Decreased PAOP
  - (c) Decreased SVR
  - (d) Decreased CO, CI
  - (e) Decreased oxygen saturations by pulse oximetry

5. **Diagnostic study findings**
  a. Laboratory
  - i. ABG levels
    - (a) Cardiogenic shock: Metabolic acidosis on ABG testing (hypocapnia, hypoxemia)
    - (b) Hypovolemic shock: Respiratory alkalosis, metabolic acidosis
  - ii. HCT: Decreased with hemorrhage
  - iii. Leukocytosis (bacteremia in septic shock)
  - iv. Elevated lactate level (bacteremia in septic shock)
  - v. Positive blood culture results (bacteremia in septic shock)
  - vi. Thrombocytopenia (DIC, septic shock)
  - vii. Abnormal electrolyte levels: Check potassium, sodium, chloride, magnesium
  - viii. Troponin levels elevated in acute MI
  b. Radiologic findings: Chest radiograph for
  - i. Cardiomegaly
  - ii. Pulmonary congestion
  - iii. Dilated aortic arch (see Aortic Dissection and Peripheral Arterial Disease)
  - iv. Pleural effusion
  - v. Cervical and thoracic spinal evaluation (for neurogenic shock)
  c. ECG
  - i. Ischemia, infarction
    - (a) RV infarction: ST elevation in RV leads (lead V_4R)
    - (b) Anterior MI commonly associated with cardiogenic shock
    - (c) Prior MI
  - ii. Arrhythmias, conduction defects
  - iii. New right axis deviation: With tachycardia, PE
  d. Echocardiography
  - i. LV and RV dysfunction (abnormal wall motion, chamber sizes)
  - ii. Tamponade, pericardial effusions
  - iii. Valvular disease
  - iv. Hypovolemia (small, hyperdynamic chamber)
  - v. VSD

e. Bedside right-sided heart catheterization: To assess hemodynamics (e.g., CO, CI, SVR, PAOP), monitor volume status; evaluate the effectiveness of vasoactive agents and other therapies

f. TEE: To look for aortic dissection, valvular disease, VSD

g. Cardiac catheterization: Assesses
   i. CAD severity
   ii. LV function
   iii. Valvular function
   iv. Hemodynamics
   v. Shunts
   vi. Aortography: Dissection, aortic regurgitation

6. **Interprofessional collaboration: See ACS; also critical care and infectious disease specialist**

7. **Management of patient care**
   a. Anticipated patient trajectory: Initial management of all forms of shock start with the ABC of airway, breathing and circulation. Rapid identification and treatment of the cause(s) will help avoid end organ damage and death.
   b. Goals of care
      i. SBP is increased to adequately perfuse tissues and vital organs. BP and pulse are within normal limits for the patient.
      ii. Sufficient oxygenation is provided
      iii. Pulmonary congestion is decreased
      iv. Fluid and electrolyte balances are maintained
      v. Intake and output are balanced
   c. Treatments
      i. Positioning: Placing the patient in Trendelenburg's position for severe drop in BP has been shown to be of no value. Legs can be elevated while the patient is lying flat to shift blood volume from the lower periphery to the central organs as a temporary measure.
      ii. Nutrition: Patient will need to receive parenteral or enteral nourishment if on NPO status for a prolonged period
      iii. Infection control: If septic shock, the causative microorganism must be identified and properly treated
      iv. Pharmacology
         (a) Cardiogenic shock
            (1) Inotropic agents: Dobutamine, dopamine, norepinephrine, milrinone, nesiritide
            (2) Vasopressors
            (3) Anticoagulants and antiplatelet agents: Heparin, aspirin, GPIIb/IIIa inhibitors
            (4) Avoid negative inotropic agents
            (5) Diuretics, if pulmonary edema present
         (b) Hypovolemic shock
            (1) Administer emergency infusions of volume replacement fluids, blood products
            (2) Observe for and identify symptoms associated with volume overload, especially if the patient has received large amounts of replacement fluids
         (c) Anaphylactic shock: IV epinephrine, steroids

(d) Septic shock: Appropriate antibiotics, volume replacement fluids, vasopressors

(e) Neurogenic shock: Volume replacement fluids, vasopressors, steroids, atropine (for bradycardia)

v. Other interventions

(a) Treat hypoxemia and acidosis

(1) Give the patient oxygen to maintain the oxygen saturation at 92% or higher

(2) Monitor ABG levels, report abnormalities, correct acidotic states: Ensure adequate ventilation

(3) Hyperventilation with mechanical ventilator may be used to raise pH

(4) Aggressive respiratory care when the patient is intubated to avoid the complication of pneumonia (especially with neurogenic shock)

(5) Arterial line may be required

(b) Treat hypovolemia (inadequate LV filling volumes)

(1) Ensure that the patient has good IV access: Two patent, large-bore IV lines available and/or a central line

(2) Give 250 mL normal saline as a trial. May need to repeat the amounts decided upon with the physician. Closely monitor the patient's response to avoid being too aggressive with fluid replacement. Hemodynamic monitoring is helpful to identify fluid status, patient response. If PAOP is less than 15, volume is needed, especially with RV MI (CVP > 2 mm Hg preferred).

(3) Record vital signs at least every hour, more often as warranted

(4) Monitor heart rate, BP, MAP, CVP, PAOP to evaluate the patient's response to therapy

(5) Maintain a strict hourly record of all intake and output

(6) Analyze laboratory results: BUN level, HCT, electrolyte levels; notify the physician of abnormal findings

(7) Watch for changes in level of consciousness

(8) Observe skin condition: Color, turgor, temperature

(c) Early reperfusion in acute MI is vital: Patient will need to be prepared for emergent angiography and coronary revascularization efforts, such as primary PCI, thrombolysis, CABG

(d) IABP can rapidly correct low CO, decreasing afterload and myocardial oxygen demands while assisting in increasing myocardial oxygen supply

(e) LV or biventricular assist devices can be used as a bridge to potential transplantation

d. Potential complication: Death. Prevention, rapid identification, and appropriate treatment of shock states are vital. Vigilance is the best management for the prevention of death.

MECHANICAL CIRCULATORY SUPPORT DEVICES

KEY CONCEPT

Mechanical circulatory support (MCS) devices provide support to a failing heart, either long or short term. Many require the patient to be in the ICU, although some allow the patient to be discharged home.

1. **IABP: May be necessary to stabilize the patient as a bridge to other interventions. Patient and significant others should be prepared for this procedure.**
   a. Indications/goals of IABP
      i. Decrease afterload
      ii. Decrease myocardial oxygen demands
      iii. Increase coronary perfusion
      iv. Increase CO and tissue perfusion
      v. Prevent cardiogenic shock, limit size of infarctions
      vi. Limit myocardial ischemia
   b. Uses of IABP
      i. Support in acute MI with cardiogenic shock
      ii. Circulatory support after CABG
      iii. Support in high-risk cardiac catheterizations
      iv. In severe ischemia, as a bridge to revascularization
   c. Placed percutaneously via the femoral or subclavian arteries into the descending thoracic aorta
   d. Inflation and deflation of the balloon are synchronized with the patient's ECG or arterial pressure waveform (Figs. 4.22 and 4.23)
      i. During ventricular diastole, the balloon is inflated. Augments diastolic pressures and increases coronary blood flow. Myocardial oxygen supply and contractility improve.
      ii. Just before ventricular systole, the balloon is deflated. Reduces afterload. Myocardial oxygen demand is decreased.
   e. Contraindications
      i. Aortic insufficiency
      ii. Severe aortic disease
      iii. Severe peripheral vascular disease in affected limb
   f. Complications
      i. Ischemia of limb distal to insertion site: Caused by mechanical occlusion of the artery or thromboembolism
      ii. Dissection of the aorta
      iii. Thrombocytopenia
      iv. Septicemia
      v. Infection at the insertion site
   g. Key concepts in the nursing care of patients with IABPs are given in Box 4.7 (see Fig. 4.23)
2. **VAD: May be external or implanted device (in either or both ventricles) that bypasses the affected ventricle, takes over its pumping action, and allows the heart to rest and recover, thus preventing end organ failure. May be implanted as bridge to transplant, bridge to recovery, or destination therapy (Fig. 4.24).**
   a. LVAD: Blood is diverted from the LV, is sent to the pump, and returns to the patient via cannulation of the ascending aorta
   b. Indications
      i. Cardiogenic shock
      ii. Inability to be weaned from cardiopulmonary bypass during cardiac surgery
      iii. Bridge to transplantation: In patients waiting for transplantation
      iv. Destination therapy: In patients not eligible for transplantation, device implanted for the remainder of the patient's life

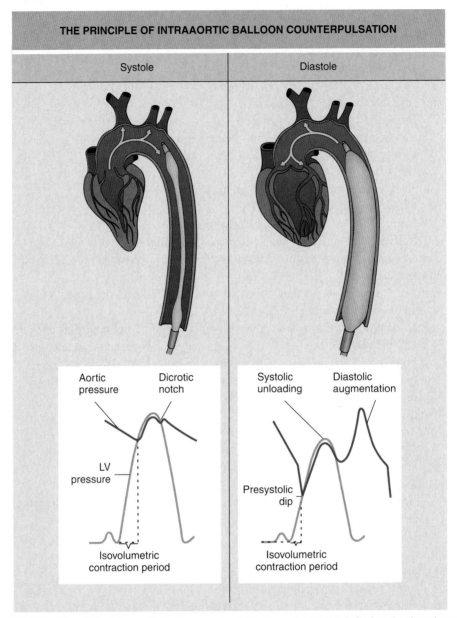

Fig. 4.22 Principle of the intraaortic balloon pump. Initiation of balloon inflation is timed to the arterial dicrotic notch, which produces an augmentation in proximal aortic diastolic pressure. Deflation of the balloon is timed to begin just before the onset of the next ventricular systole, which produces the systolic unloading effect (presystolic dip). *LV*, Left ventricular. (From Crawford, M.H., DiMarco, J.P., Paulus, W.J. (eds.) (2010). *Cardiology*, 3rd ed. Philadelphia: Mosby. Ltd)

    v. Bridge to recovery: Used with medical management to enable recovery of LV function (reverse remodeling) to the point that the patient can do without the device and avoid transplantation
  c. Contraindications
    i. Prolonged cardiac arrest with severe neurologic damage
    ii. No prospect of being weaned from the VAD: Irreversible, extensive organ damage (renal, hepatic, respiratory)

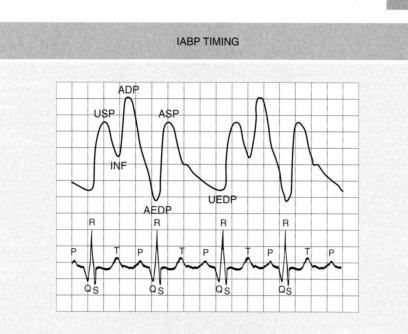

Fig. 4.23 Optimal timing of an intraaortic balloon pump *(IABP)*. Arterial pressure tracing from a patient with an IABP. The balloon was set at 2:1 to evaluate timing. Inflation *(INF)* was timed to the dicrotic notch to follow aortic valve closure. There is augmentation of diastolic pressure *(ADP)* and lowering of the end-diastolic pressure with augmented beats *(AEDP)* compared with the unaugmented end-diastolic pressure *(UEDP)*. The augmented systolic pressure *(ASP)* is often lower than the unaugmented systolic pressure *(USP)* as well. (From Crawford, M.H., DiMarco, J.P., Paulus, W.J. (eds) (2010). *Cardiology*, 3rd ed. Philadelphia: Mosby.)

BOX 4.7   Key Concepts in the Nursing Care of Patients With an Intraaortic Balloon Pump

1. Monitor all vital signs.
2. Monitor arterial pressures closely and watch volume status; improvement should occur with use.
3. Monitor closely for arrhythmias (especially irregular), which can hamper intraaortic balloon pump (IABP) efficacy.
4. Look for signs of improved, effective cardiac output and improved mental status (if patient is not sedated), urinary output, skin color and warmth, capillary refill.
5. Assess peripheral pulses of bilateral upper and lower extremities; document presence and changes from baseline. Watch for changes in color, sensation, and temperature.
6. Keep a close watch on insertion site for signs of bleeding, hematomas.
7. Do not elevate head of bed beyond 15 degrees; patient must keep affected limb straight.
8. Assess pulses in upper extremities, especially left arm. Catheter can migrate up and occlude subclavian artery.
9. If patient is on heparin, watch for side effects from anticoagulation: abnormal laboratory coagulation results, positive results on guaiac stool test, or nasogastric secretions and petechiae.
10. Be knowledgeable about IABP controls, safeguards, and protocols for use.
11. Be alert to signs of infection locally or systemically. Prevent infections by following unit protocols for dressing changes and other precautions.
12. Prevent complications from immobility (e.g., skin breakdown, respiratory compromise).

From Turi, Z.G., Topalian, S.K. (2014). Intra-aortic balloon counterpulsation. In J.E. Parrillo, P. Dellinger, editors. *Critical care medicine: principles of diagnosis and management in the adult*, (pp 90–109), Philadelphia: Elsevier.

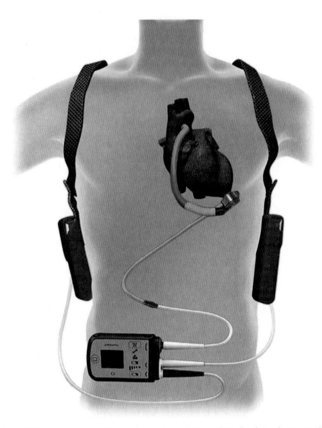

Fig. 4.24 HeartMate 3 is a nonpulsatile left ventricular assist device that works in parallel with the native heart to support systemic circulation. (HeartMate and HeartMate 3 are trademarks of Abbott or its related companies. Reproduced with permission of Abbott, © 2021. All rights reserved.)

  d. Complications of VAD use
   i. Thromboembolism
   ii. Bleeding
   iii. Infections
   iv. Pump thrombosis or malfunction
  e. Nursing care for patients with VADs
   i. Be knowledgeable about VAD operation and protocols of use; cardiac perfusionists are great resources and may be involved in care
   ii. Frequently assess vital signs, hemodynamics, CO, intake and output, circulation. *Note:* Patients with nonpulsatile VADs may not have a pulse, and only a single BP value (mean) can be determined.
   iii. Monitor for arrhythmias and treat promptly
   iv. Patient discharged with an LVAD will need a thorough knowledge of the device and its management in the home setting
 3. ECMO: Cannulas are inserted into large veins or arteries (see Types, in the following text) and blood is pumped from the patient through a membranous oxygenator and is returned to the patient. Once used as a last means of survival, ECMO is becoming more and more common as a means of temporary support. Although these patients typically remain fairly immobile, newer cannulation techniques and more compact pumps and oxygenators now allow for ambulation of certain patients while on ECMO (Fig. 4.25).

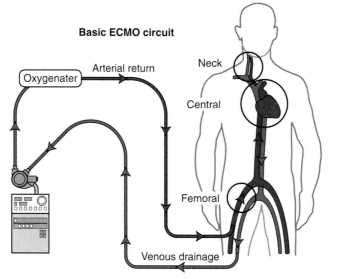

Basic ECMO circuit

Oxygenater

Arterial return

Neck

Central

Femoral

Venous drainage

Fig. 4.25 Illustration of the blood pathway of an extracorporeal membrane oxygenation (*ECMO*) circuit. Blood drains through the circuit to a blood pump, which pushes it through an artificial lung oxygenating the blood and removing carbon dioxide (CO_2) before returning the blood to the body. (From Kacmarek, R.M., Stoller, J.K., Heuer, A. (2021). *Egan's fundamentals of respiratory care*, 12th ed. St. Louis: Elsevier.)

a. Types
   i. Venoarterial (VA): Used for cardiac support, bypasses both heart and lungs; cannulas inserted peripherally (drains from femoral vein, returns to femoral artery) or centrally (drains from IVC, returns to aortic arch)
   ii. Venovenous (VV): Used for pulmonary support, bypasses lungs only; requires functional heart; cannulas may be single lumen (inserted in either internal jugular [IJ] and femoral vein or bilateral femoral veins) or double lumen (inserted in IJ or subcutaneous [SC] vein); double lumen cannula drains from one lumen and returns through the second eliminating the need for multiple cannulas
b. Indications
   i. VA
      (a) Cardiogenic shock
      (b) Inability to wean from cardiopulmonary bypass
      (c) Postheart transplant (graft failure)
      (d) Bridge therapy (to decision, transplant, or to long-term support)
   ii. VV
      (a) ARDS
      (b) Postlung transplant (graft failure)
      (c) Bridge therapy (to decision or transplant)
      (d) Extracorporeal assistance to provide lung rest (e.g., pulmonary contusion, smoke inhalation)
      (e) Status asthmaticus
      (f) Pulmonary hemorrhage
c. Contraindications
   i. Absolute
      (a) Futile treatment without chance of recovery (e.g., end-stage heart disease not eligible for transplant or destination VAD, known severe brain injury, unwitnessed cardiac arrest)

       (b) Unrepaired aortic dissection

       (c) Severe aortic regurgitation

       (d) PVD in peripheral VA ECMO

       (e) Cardiac failure in VV ECMO

    ii. Relative

       (a) Anticoagulation, coagulopathy

       (b) Advanced age

       (c) Obesity

  d. Complications of ECMO use

    i. Hemolysis

    ii. Bleeding

    iii. Thromboembolism

    iv. Heparin-induced thrombocytopenia (HIT)

    v. Neurologic complications (e.g., CVA, seizures)

    vi. Infection

  e. Nursing care for patients on ECMO

    i. Be knowledgeable about ECMO operation and protocols of use; cardiac perfusionists are great resources and are involved in care

    ii. Frequently assess vital signs, hemodynamics, CO, intake and output, circulation

    iii. Monitor for arrhythmias and treat promptly, many ECMO patients are volume dependent and may need volume administration and/or blood transfusion; make sure there are units of packed red blood cells crossmatched in the blood bank at all times

    iv. Monitor free hemoglobin daily for signs of hemolysis, values over 10 should be reported to the provider

END-STAGE HEART DISEASE: CARDIAC TRANSPLANTATION

> **KEY CONCEPT**
> When cardiac disease has advanced to a point at which all possible medical or surgical interventions have been exhausted and life expectancy is less than 24 months. The primary treatment of heart transplantation or implantation of an LVAD as destination therapy is becoming an increasingly common option (see Mechanical Circulatory Support).

1. **Pathophysiology**
   a. Severe LV dysfunction with CO; EF is less than 25%
   b. See Pathophysiology subsection under Heart Failure
2. **Etiology and risk factors**
   a. Ischemic heart disease and CAD
   b. DCM: Idiopathic or secondary to pregnancy or viral infections
   c. Valvular disease
   d. Medication-related myocardial injury
   e. Congenital heart disease
   f. Infection (Chagas disease)
3. **Signs and symptoms: The number of candidates for transplantation far exceeds the number of donor hearts. Careful assessment and selection are necessary to determine who can potentially return to a functional life after transplantation, as well as to ensure that all conventional remedies have been exhausted.**
   a. Subjective findings: Complaints of dyspnea, angina, low exercise tolerance (bed-to-chair existence, bedridden)

    b. Physical findings
       i. Severe HF necessitating frequent hospitalizations
      ii. Cardiac cachexia: Anorexia, weight loss
     iii. Life-threatening arrhythmias
4. **Diagnostic study findings**
    a. See Heart Failure. Follow-up studies to evaluate disease progression and treatment effectiveness and to prevent complications.
    b. Right-sided heart catheterization: Used to guide therapy
       i. Assess PVR
          (a) Irreversible pulmonary hypertension is a cause of perioperative mortality
          (b) Donor heart cannot generate pressure high enough to maintain a sufficient pulmonary flow
          (c) Patients with irreversible pulmonary hypertension may be candidates for heart-lung transplantation
          (d) Pharmacologic agents (e.g., sildenafil) may be used to evaluate the potential for reversibility of increased PVR
      ii. Assess PAP, PAOP, CO
    c. Cardiac arteriography: Pretransplantation to ascertain the degree of CAD and the potential for revascularization
    d. Cardiac biopsy: To rule out amyloidosis and identify patients with sarcoidosis or myocarditis for possible immunosuppressive therapy
    e. EPS: To assess the effectiveness of antiarrhythmic therapy
5. **Interprofessional collaboration: See Heart Failure section, plus transplant coordinator, and psychologist**
6. **Management of patient care**
    a. Anticipated patient trajectory: Heart transplantation is the standard of care and is performed on patients of all ages from newborn to 65 years. Mortality rate is as low as 4% from heart transplantation; average survival time is longer than 5 years.
    b. Goals of care
       i. Balanced fluid status, intake, and output are maintained
      ii. Patient and family participate in identifying lifestyle changes and support required in coping with transplantation
     iii. Patient tolerates the new heart (successful transplantation)
    c. Treatments
       i. Positioning: Head of bed elevated for patient comfort and ease of breathing
      ii. Nutrition
          (a) Assess nutritional status: To optimize the potential for posttransplantation success and facilitate the healing process
          (b) Restrict diet to less than 2 g sodium, 1000 to 1500 mL fluid
     iii. Infection control
          (a) Observe for and prevent infections (from IV drips, central lines, immunosuppressive therapies). Screen visitors for communicable illnesses because of the patient's suppressed immune system. (Have visitors use masks, wash hands, limit contact.)
          (b) Administer antimicrobial prophylaxis used to prevent nosocomial infections
      iv. Discharge planning
          (a) Discuss with the patient and family the following aspects of the transplantation process:
              (1) Body image changes with the new heart

    (2) Importance of family support

    (3) Unknown waiting period

    (4) Cost: Huge financial burden; insurance coverage

    (5) Frequency of checkups, tests; stress need for regular examinations

    (6) Possibility of failure to be accepted as a transplantation candidate

    (7) Possibility of rejection reaction after transplantation

    (8) Dependency issues

    (9) Arrange for the patient and family to talk with transplantation survivors

(b) Home oxygen: May be required for dyspnea, pulmonary congestion

(c) Home health care: Includes IV therapy

(d) Information on the use of indwelling catheters: For home-based IV therapy to reduce infection risks

(e) Hospitalizations: Patient and significant others need to be instructed with regard to the following:

    (1) Possible need for frequent hospital visits for "tune-ups," medication changes, close observation

    (2) Need for hemodynamic monitoring

    (3) Need for high-dose medications

    (4) Use of mechanical assists: IABP, VAD, ventilators

v. Pharmacology: See also Heart Failure

(a) Preload reduction: Diuretics, nitrates

(b) IV inotropic medications (e.g., milrinone, dobutamine to increase CO, improve renal perfusion)

(c) Afterload reduction

(d) Antiarrhythmic therapy

(e) Anticoagulation: For risk of thromboembolism

(f) Immunosuppressive protocols (e.g., cyclosporine, tacrolimus, steroids)

(g) Statin therapy: Lowering lipid levels shows positive effects on cardiac allograft rejection; immunosuppressive medications can cause hyperlipidemia

(h) Antibiotic prophylaxis

vi. Psychosocial issues

(a) Prepare the patient for the rigors of waiting for transplantation and the care before and after

(b) Assess emotional status: Psychiatric history, motivational issues. Transplantation is a major stressful undertaking.

(c) Assess the support system: Strong family, friends, and medical support are needed

(d) Assess financial issues: Insurance coverage for costly procedure, medications, follow-up care

(e) Determine alcohol and illicit drug use history

(f) Assess the ability to comply with a complex lifelong medical regimen: Frequent follow-up examinations (include endomyocardial biopsies, strict medication protocols, rejection issues). Transplantation requires active patient participation.

(g) Determine dependency issues. Formulate a plan with the patient and significant others.

    (1) Allow the patient to do what he or she can

    (2) Family is included in care in the hospital

(3) Home services are arranged

(4) Need for immediate readiness is emphasized. When a donor heart becomes available, ischemic time (time from cross-clamp [donor] to cross-clamp [recipient]) is ideally less than 5 hours (or the heart is not usable); therefore the patient must not travel.

vii. Other interventions

(a) Patient refractory to IV inotropic therapy should be transported to a facility with a cardiac transplantation program

(b) AICD may need to be placed to prevent sudden death

(c) Extracorporeal devices (e.g., LVAD): Used as a bridge to transplantation or therapy for patients (see Mechanical Circulatory Support)

(d) Heart transplantation

(1) Recipient native RA may be left in place; this may cause the appearance of two p-waves on ECG

(2) Heart is denervated during the procedure; bradycardia is a common problem postoperatively, as many as 15% of transplant patients will require a permanent pacemaker

(3) Patients will require immunosuppression for life

(4) In patients with insulin-dependent diabetes, steroid therapy after transplantation can increase blood glucose levels

(5) In patients with renal disease, cyclosporine therapy is nephrotoxic

(6) Current research using ex-vivo organ preservation devices has shown promise in extending the time between procurement of the donor heart and implantation beyond 5 hours

(e) Teaching points for immediately postoperative cardiac transplantation care are similar to those for CABG care

viii. Potential complications

(a) Related to ventricular dysfunction: Arrhythmias, HF, cardiomyopathy

(b) Postoperative complications include those associated with CABG and additional transplantation complications, which include the following:

(1) Allograft rejection

(2) RV failure from high PVR

(3) Bradycardia: Pacemaker may be needed; isoproterenol may be used. Atropine will not help denervated transplanted heart.

(4) Immunosuppressive therapy complications

(5) Increased susceptibility to infection

(6) Adverse effects can include nephrotoxicity, hypertension, hyperlipidemia, seizures

(7) Malignancies (skin and other)

CARDIAC TRAUMA

(See Ch. 11, Multisystem Trauma.)

References and bibliography information are available at http://evolve.elsevier.com/AACN/corecurriculum/.

Neurologic System

Patricia A. Blissitt, PhD, ARNP-CNS, CCRN, CNRN, SCRN, CCNS, CCM, ACNS-BC

CROSSWALK

- **Quality and Safety in Nursing Education (QSEN):** Patient-centered care, Teamwork and collaboration, Evidence-based practice, Quality improvement, Safety, Informatics
- **National Patient Safety Goals:** Identifies patients correctly, Use medicines safely, Uses alarms safely, Prevents infection, Identify patient safety risks
- **American Nurses Association (ANA) standards for Professional Nursing Practice:** Standard 1. Assessment, Standard 2. Diagnosis, Standard 3. Outcomes identification, Standard 4. Planning, Standard 5. Implementation, Standard 6. Evaluation, Standard 9. Communication, Standard 10. Collaboration, Standard 13. Evidence-based practice and research, Standard 14. Quality of practice, Standard 15. Professional practice evaluation
- **AACN Scope and Standards for Progressive and Critical Care Nursing Practice Standard 1. Quality of practice, Standard 2. Professional practice evaluation, Standard 3. Education, Standard 4. Communication, Standard 5. Ethics, Standard 6. Collaboration, Standard 7. Evidence-based practice/research/clinical inquiry**
- **AACN Standards for Establishing and Sustaining Healthy Work Environments (HWE):** Skilled communication, True collaboration, Effective decision-making
- **PCCN content:** Neurology—All items
- **CCRN content:** Neurology—All items

SYSTEMWIDE ELEMENTS

ANATOMY AND PHYSIOLOGY REVIEW

KEY CONCEPT
Knowledge of anatomic and clinical correlation is vital to complete a strong neurologic assessment. Early recognition of neurologic deficits with consideration for anatomic and clinical correlation may facilitate emergent response and promote optimal patient outcomes.

1. **Brain**
   a. Coverings
      i. Scalp
         (a) Skin: Thick dermal layer that includes hair follicles, and sweat and sebaceous glands
         (b) Subcutaneous connective tissue (fascia): Dense fibrous fatty layer between the skin and galea that contains arteries, veins, and nerves
         (c) Galea aponeurotica: Inelastic tendinous tissue; covers the vertex of the skull and is continuous with the frontal, temporal-parietal, and occipital fascia; absorbs the force of external trauma

(d) Subaponeurotic or subgaleal tissue: Loose areolar tissue below the galea: Connective tissue that contributes to the mobility of the scalp

(e) Periosteum (pericranium): Thin layer of tissue that covers the external surface of the skull

ii. Cranium

(a) The part of the skull that contains and protects the brain (Fig. 5.1)

(b) Bones: Frontal, sphenoid, ethmoid, occipital, two temporal and two parietal bones

(c) Divisions: Supratentorial space (above the tentorium cerebelli) and infratentorial space (below the tentorium cerebelli)

(d) Basilar skull: Base of the skull has three depressed compartments: The anterior fossa, middle fossa, and posterior fossa (Fig. 5.2)

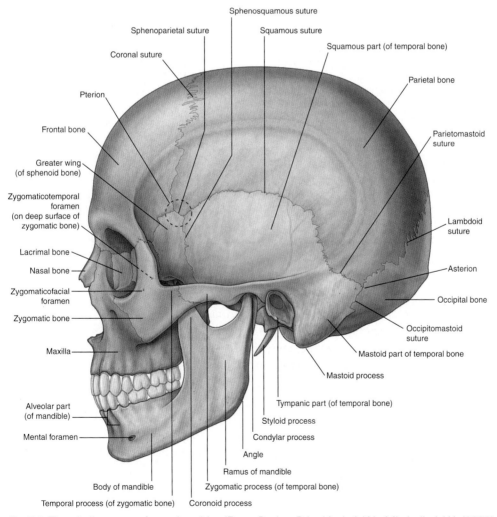

Fig. 5.1 The skull as seen from the side. (From Drake, R.L., Vogl, A.W., Mitchell, A.W. (2020). *Gray's anatomy for students*, 4th ed. Philadelphia: Elsevier.)

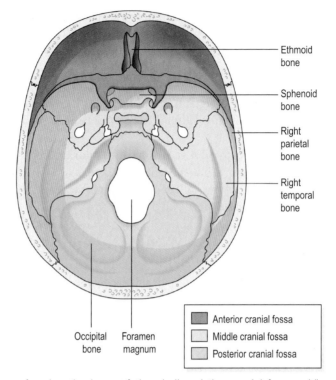

Fig. 5.2 The bones forming the base of the skull and the cranial fossae. Viewed from above. (From Waugh, A., Grant, A. (2018). *Ross & Wilson anatomy and physiology in health and illness*, 13th ed. Philadelphia: Elsevier.)

EXPERT TIP

Basilar skull fractures commonly result in periorbital bruising, mastoid bruising, cerebrospinal fluid (CSF) leaks, rhinorrhea, and otorrhea. CSF leaks increase the risk of meningitis and contribute to headache. Do not insert anything into the ear or nose as this may increase the risk of infection. CSF leaks may heal spontaneously or may require a lumbar drain or surgical repair.

---

   iii. Meninges (Fig. 5.3)
      (a) Dura mater: Meningeal membrane closest to the skull
         (1) Outermost covering of the brain; consists of two layers of tough fibrous tissue, periosteal layer and meningeal layer
         (2) Periosteal layer, the outer layer of the dura mater that forms the periosteum of the internal surface of the skull
         (3) Meningeal layer: The inner layer of the dura mater that folds to form the falx cerebri, tentorium cerebelli, falx cerebelli, and diaphragma sella
         (4) The inner and outer layers of the dura mater are closely connected except where they separate to form the dural sinuses.
         (5) Meningeal arteries and venous sinuses lie in clefts formed by the inner and outer layers of the dura mater.
         (6) Epidural space: A potential space between the internal surface of the skull and the dura mater
         (7) Subdural space: A potential space between the innermost surface of the dura mater and the arachnoid mater; bridging veins lie in the subdural space

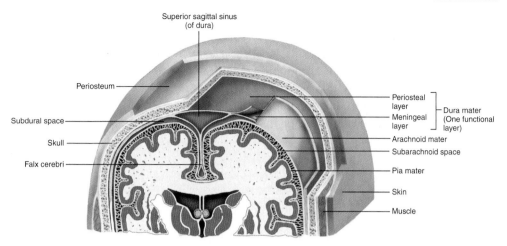

Fig. 5.3 Coverings of the brain. (From Patton, K. (2022). *Anatomy and physiology*, 11th ed. St. Louis: Elsevier.)

(b) Arachnoid mater
  (1) Fine, fibrous, elastic web-like layer between the dura mater and pia mater
  (2) Subarachnoid space
    a) Lies between the arachnoid mater and pia mater; expanded areas of the subarachnoid space form cisterns, widened spaces between the arachnoid mater and the pia mater at the base of the brain
    b) Contains blood vessels including the circle of Willis

EXPERT TIP

The circle of Willis is the site of subarachnoid hemorrhage (SAH); blood mixes with the CSF in the subarachnoid space. The presence of blood in the CSF in contact with the outside of the cerebral blood vessels is thought to be responsible for delayed cerebral ischemia (DCI) after aneurysmal SAH.

---

    c) Contains CSF, which completely surrounds the brain and spinal cord; acts as a shock absorber
    d) Contains the arachnoid villi or granulations: Projections of the arachnoid mater that absorb circulated CSF into the venous system for removal from the CSF pathway
  (c) Pia mater
    (1) Delicate vascular layer that covers the brain surface, following the sulci and gyri, the grooves and folds of the cerebral hemisphere
    (2) Surrounds surface blood vessels and emerging nerves
    (3) Blood vessels of the pia mater form the choroid plexus lining the ventricles
  b. Divisions of the brain
    i. Cerebrum
      (a) Telencephalon: The two cerebral hemispheres including the cerebral cortex, subcortical white matter, and basal ganglia
      (b) The two cerebral hemispheres are separated by a longitudinal fissure, also called the sagittal or interhemispheric fissure; the two cerebral hemispheres are joined by the corpus callosum.

(1) Corpus callosum: Commissural fibers that transfer learned discriminations, sensory experiences, and memory from one cerebral hemisphere to corresponding parts of the other hemisphere

(2) Functional localization is present in the cerebral cortex including cerebral dominance. The cerebral hemispheres consist of the bihemispheric frontal lobe, bilateral temporal and parietal lobes, and a bihemispheric occipital lobe (Table 5.1).

EXPERT TIP

Approximately 90% of people are left brain dominant, including all right-handed and some left-handed people. A patient who experiences a left middle cerebral artery (MCA) stroke is likely to experience aphasia related to the location of the language center in the left hemisphere and correlation with MCA blood flow.

---

(3) Basal ganglia (basal nuclei; Fig. 5.4)

    a) Masses of gray matter including the caudate nucleus, putamen, and globus pallidus (collectively termed the corpus striatum), and, functionally, the subthalamic nucleus in the diencephalon and the substantia nigra nucleus in the midbrain

---

TABLE 5.1 Functional Localization in the Cerebral Cortex

Lobe	Functions
Frontal	Higher mental functions Abstract thinking Behavior and tactfulness Memory Affect Voluntary motor function Concentration Foresight and judgment Inhibition Personality Conjugate eye movements Motor control of speech (dominant hemisphere[a])
Temporal	Hearing Comprehension of spoken language (dominant hemisphere[a]) Visual, olfactory, and auditory perception Memory Learning and intellect Emotion
Parietal	Sensory perception of touch, pain, temperature, position, pressure, and vibration Body awareness Sensory interpretation
Occipital	Visual perception and interpretation Control of some visual and ocular movement reflexes

[a]Cerebral dominance: In right-handed and most left-handed people, the left cerebral hemisphere is dominant for language, mathematical, and analytic functions. The opposite nondominant hemisphere is thought to be concerned with nonverbal, geometric, spatial, visual, and musical functions.
From VanPutte, C.L., Regan, J.L., Russo, A.F., editors. (2020). *Seeley's anatomy and physiology*, 12th ed. New York: McGraw-Hill.

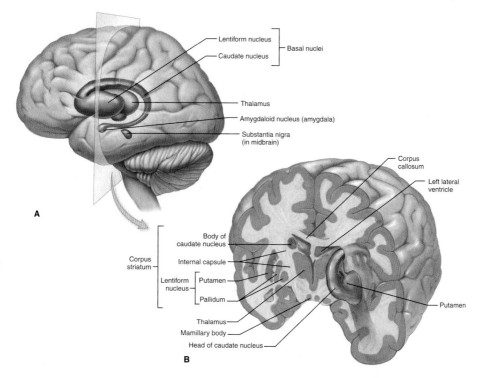

Fig. 5.4 Basal ganglia or basal nuclei. **A**, As seen through the cortex of the left cerebral hemisphere. **B**, As seen in a frontal (coronal) section of the brain. (From Patton, K. (2022). *Anatomy and physiology*, 11th ed. St. Louis: Elsevier.)

b) Functions: Exert regulating and controlling influences on the coordination of voluntary motion, motor integration, movement initiation, muscle tone, and postural reflexes; a major center of the extrapyramidal motor system

> **EXPERT TIP**
> The basal ganglia and substantia nigra are the sites of dysfunction in Parkinson disease. In addition to the classic Parkinson disease motor symptoms of bradykinesia, rigidity, and tremor, nonmotor symptoms consist of depression, cognitive impairment, hallucinations and psychosis, pain, bowel and bladder dysfunction, and orthostatic hypotension.

> **EXPERT TIP**
> Some medications may cause extrapyramidal symptoms. or worsen Parkinson disease including haloperidol, metoclopramide, prochlorazine, promethazine, chlorpromazine, and droperiodol.

(c) Diencephalon: The thalamus, hypothalamus, subthalamus, and epithalamus (Fig. 5.5)

   (1) Thalamus: Bilateral ovoid masses of gray matter adjacent to the lateral walls of the third ventricle; subdivided into several nuclei

      a) Sensory nuclei receive, integrate, and process sensory input for relay to the cerebral cortex; a relay station

      b) Other nuclei, motor, limbic, multimodal, intralaminar, and reticular, participate in affective aspects of brain function; are functionally related to the association areas of the cortex; or have

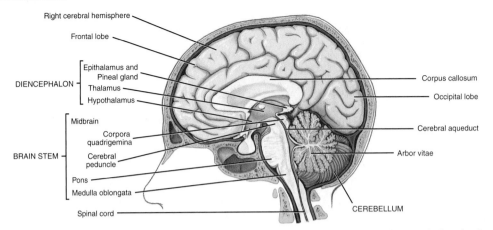

Fig. 5.5 Midsagittal section of the brain showing the major portions of the diencephalon, brainstem, and cerebellum. (From Applegate, E.J. (2011). *The anatomy and physiology learning system*, 4th ed. St. Louis: Elsevier.)

a role in conscious pain, temperature, and touch awareness, motor function, and the ascending reticular activating system (RAS).

(2) Hypothalamus: Below the thalamus; regulates
  a) Body temperature
  b) Hunger
  c) Thirst (water balance)
  d) Behavior: Part of the limbic system; concerned with aggressive and sexual behavior; elicits physical expressions associated with emotions (rage and anger)
  e) Circadian rhythm
  f) Autonomic responses: Control center for the autonomic nervous system (ANS); controls numerous visceral and somatic activities (e.g., heart rate, pupil constriction, and dilation)
  g) Hormonal secretion of the pituitary gland; the hypothalamus provides input to the pituitary by sending hormones (posterior pituitary) or inhibiting and releasing factors (anterior pituitary) through the infundibulum (pituitary stalk; see Ch. 7, Endocrine System)

> **EXPERT TIP**
> Hypothalamic injury may result in variations in temperature unresponsive to temperature management interventions. Hypothalamic injury may result in decreased production of antidiuretic hormone (ADH). Injury to the posterior pituitary may (neurohypophysis) result in decreased release of ADH. In either case, the patient may develop diabetes insipidus.

1) Posterior pituitary gland (neurohypophysis): Stores and releases ADH and oxytocin, produced by the hypothalamus. ADH causes vasoconstriction and increases renal water reabsorption. Oxytocin stimulates uterine contraction and milk ejection.
2) Anterior pituitary gland (adenohypophysis): The anterior pituitary produces and secretes prolactin (PL), growth hormone (GH), thyroid stimulating hormone (TSH), adrenocorticotropic hormone (ACTH), follicle stimulating hormone (FSH), and luteinizing hormone (LH). Hormonal

secretion is under the control of releasing and inhibiting factors produced in the hypothalamus. These releasing and inhibiting factors are transported to the anterior pituitary via the infundibulum (pituitary portal system) to regulate secretion of hormones from the pituitary as needed (see Ch. 7, Endocrine System).

EXPERT TIP

Pituitary tumors may be hormone releasing or inhibiting. Resection of a pituitary tumor may temporarily or permanently worsen hormonal imbalances including but not limited to vasopressin (ADH).

---

       (3) Subthalamus: Functionally related to the basal ganglia (connects to the globus pallidus); participates in motor control

       (4) Epithalamus: Dorsal part of the diencephalon

          a) Contains the pineal gland, which is responsible for the secretion of melatonin and is thought to regulate circadian rhythm.

    (d) Limbic system (Fig. 5.6)

       (1) Composed of the limbic cortex, the cingulate gyrus (superior to the corpus callosum), and parahippocampal gyrus (located in the temporal lobe)

       (2) The limbic cortex is anatomically and functionally connected to other structures, such as the amygdala and hippocampus (both located in the temporal lobe), fornix (hippocampal outflow tract), hypothalamus, olfactory cortex, and thalamus.

       (3) Responsible for homeostasis including autonomic and neuroendocrine control in conjunction with the hypothalamus; smell (olfactory cortex); memory and learning (hippocampal formation); and emotions and basic instinctual drives (amygdala)

  ii. Brainstem (see Figs. 5.5 and 5.7)

    (a) Midbrain (mesencephalon): Located between the diencephalon and pons

       (1) Contains nuclei of cranial nerve (CN) III (oculomotor) and CN IV (trochlear) nuclei

       (2) Contains motor and sensory pathways

       (3) Includes respiratory control centers

       (4) Tectal region (inferior and superior colliculi): Concerned with the auditory and visual systems

       (5) Tegmentum: Consists of ascending tracts from the spinal cord to the brain: Lateral spinothalamic (pain and temperature) and the medial lemniscus (vibration, two-point discrimination, and pressure sensation)

       (6) Connects to the cerebellum via the superior cerebellar peduncles (right and left)

       (7) Includes substantia nigra and red nuclei: Part of the basal ganglia; involved in muscle tone and coordination of movement

       (8) Contains a portion of the reticular formation: Includes the RAS responsible for arousal and consciousness

---

EXPERT TIP

Injury to the RAS may result in coma and persistent vegetative state. The Glasgow Coma Scale is an invalid assessment of level of consciousness (LOC) for a patient in persistent vegetative state. Spontaneous eye opening in persistent vegetative state does not reflect awareness of the surrounding environment.

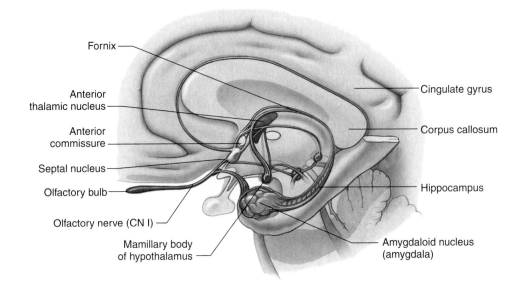

Fig. 5.6 Lateral view of the limbic system within the brain. (From Kelley, L.L., Peterson, C.M. (2018). *Sectional anatomy for imaging professionals*, 4th ed. St. Louis: Elsevier.)

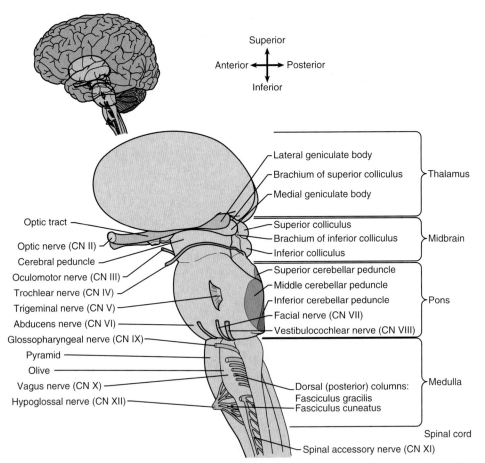

Fig. 5.7 A lateral view of the anatomic structures of the brainstem. (Redrawn from Beck, R.W. (2011). *Functional neurology for practitioners of manual medicine*, 2nd ed. London, UK: Churchill Livingstone.)

(b) Pons (metencephalon): Between the midbrain and medulla
  (1) Contains nuclei of CN V (trigeminal), VI (abducens), and VII (facial), and CN VIII (auditory or acoustic; formally called vestibulocochlear) nuclei
  (2) Middle cerebellar peduncles (right and left) on the basal surface of the pons provide extensive connections between the cerebral cortex and cerebellum, ensuring maximal motor efficiency.
  (3) Contains motor and sensory pathways
  (4) Includes respiratory control centers that help modulate breathing patterns
  (5) Contains a portion of the reticular foramen (RF)
(c) Medulla (myelencephalon): Between the pons and spinal cord
  (1) Contains nuclei of CN IX (glossopharyngeal), X (vagus), XI (accessory), and XII (hypoglossal)
  (2) Motor and sensory tracts of spinal cord continue into the medulla
  (3) Attaches to the cerebellum via the inferior cerebellar peduncles (right and left)
  (4) Includes respiratory, cardiac, and vasomotor control centers
  (5) Contains a portion of the RF

EXPERT TIP

The vomit center is located in the medulla. Vomiting may be a sign of increased intracranial pressure (ICP) which may worsen when the patient's head is lowered. Raising the head of the bed of the patient with increased ICP may lessen the ICP and vomiting.

(d) RF (Fig. 5.8): Diffuse cellular network in the brainstem, with axons projecting to the thalamus and into the cortex; receives input from the cerebrum, spinal cord, other brainstem nuclei, and the cerebellum; has a role in the control of autonomic and endocrine functions, skeletal muscle activity, and visceral and somatic sensation. The RAS is part of the RF.
  (1) Ascending RAS is essential for arousal from sleep, alert wakefulness, focusing of attention, and perceptual association.
  (2) Descending RAS may inhibit or facilitate motor neurons controlling the skeletal musculature.
iii. Cerebellum: Lies in the posterior fossa behind the brainstem and is posterior to the fourth ventricle; separated from the cerebrum by the tentorium cerebelli; two hemispheres; separated by the vermis; communicates with the rest of the brain and spinal cord through the cerebellar peduncles
  (a) Influences muscle tone in relation to equilibrium, locomotion, posture, and nonstereotyped movements
  (b) Important in the synchronization of muscle action to enable coordinated movement
  (c) Receives input from the spinal cord, brainstem, vestibular system, and cerebrum; provides output to the brainstem and thalamus; influences spinal and cerebral activities
c. Cerebral circulation (Fig. 5.9)
  i. Arterial system: Supplied by the internal carotid and vertebral arteries
    (a) Circle of Willis: Anastomosis of arteries at the base of the brain formed by a short segment of the internal carotid arteries (ICA) and anterior carotid arteries (ACA) and posterior cerebral arteries (PCA), which are

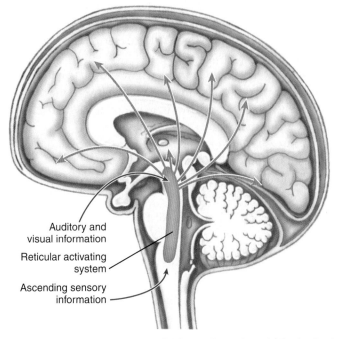

Fig. 5.8 Reticular activating system (RAS). The RAS consists of nuclei in the brainstem reticular formation plus fibers that conduct sensory information to the nuclei and fibers that conduct from the nuclei to widespread areas of the cerebral cortex. Functioning of the reticular activating system is essential for consciousness. (From Huether, S., McCance, K., Brashers, V.L. (2020). *Understanding pathophysiology*, 7th ed. St. Louis: Elsevier.)

connected by an anterior communicating artery (Acomm) and posterior communicating arteries (Pcomm). This anastomosis may permit collateral circulation if a carotid or vertebral artery becomes occluded.

(b) Internal carotid system: ICAs arise from the common carotid arteries, which receive their blood supply on the right from the innominate (brachiocephalic) artery and on the left from the aorta. The MCAs arise directly from the ICAs and extend laterally. Table 5.2 shows the branches of this system and the areas they supply.

(c) Branches of the ICA, external carotid artery, and vertebral arteries (e.g., anterior, middle, posterior meningeal arteries) provide blood supply to the meninges. The external carotid arteries also supply blood to the external head, neck, face, and scalp.

(d) Vertebral system: Vertebral arteries arise from the subclavian arteries and join at the lower pontine border to form the basilar artery (BA). Branches of this system and the areas they supply are summarized in Table 5.2.

(e) Basilar artery: The BA gives rise to the PCAs, and branches of the BA supply the brainstem and portions of the cerebellum. Branches of the vertebrobasilar system and the areas they supply are summarized in Table 5.2.

ii. Cerebral blood flow (CBF)

(a) Normal CBF averages 50 mL/100 g of brain tissue per minute; gray matter (neuronal cell body) CBF is typically higher as it is more metabolically active.

(b) Cerebral perfusion pressure (CPP) and intrinsic regulatory mechanisms affect CBF

Neurologic System

5

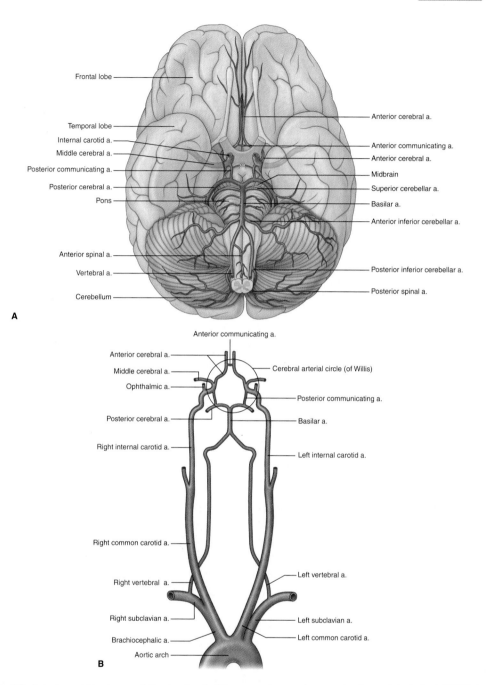

Frontal lobe

Temporal lobe
Internal carotid a.
Middle cerebral a.
Posterior communicating a.
Posterior cerebral a.
Pons

Anterior cerebral a.
Anterior communicating a.
Anterior cerebral a.
Midbrain
Superior cerebellar a.
Basilar a.
Anterior inferior cerebellar a.

Anterior spinal a.
Vertebral a.
Cerebellum

Posterior inferior cerebellar a.
Posterior spinal a.

A

Anterior communicating a.

Anterior cerebral a.
Middle cerebral a.
Ophthalmic a.

Cerebral arterial circle (of Willis)

Posterior cerebral a.

Posterior communicating a.

Basilar a.

Right internal carotid a.

Left internal carotid a.

Right common carotid a.

Right vertebral a.

Left vertebral a.

Right subclavian a.

Brachiocephalic a.

Aortic arch

Left subclavian a.

Left common carotid a.

B

Fig. 5.9 Arteries at the base of the brain. **A**, Diagram shows the cerebral arterial circle (of Willis) and related structures on the base of the brain. Note the arterial anastomoses. **B**, Origins of blood vessels that form the cerebral arterial circle. (From Patton, K. (2022). *Anatomy and physiology*, 11th ed. St. Louis: Elsevier.)

    (1) CPP: Pressure gradient that drives blood into the brain; calculated as the difference between the mean arterial pressure (MAP) and the ICP. CPP = MAP−ICP; CPP ranging from approximately 60 to 150 mm Hg has an insignificant effect on CBF.

    (2) Regulatory mechanisms influence the diameter of the cerebral vasculature

TABLE 5.2   **Major Cerebral Arteries and Areas They Supply**

Artery	Area of the Brain Supplied
INTERNAL CAROTID ARTERY BRANCHES	
Anterior cerebral artery (ACA)	Medial aspect of the frontal and parietal lobes; part of the cingulate gyrus and corpus callosum; via the recurrent artery of Heubner supplies part of the basal ganglia and a portion of the internal capsule
Anterior communicating artery (Acomm)	Connects the right and left anterior cerebral arteries
Middle cerebral artery (MCA) (largest branch of the internal carotid artery)	Most of the lateral surfaces of the frontal, temporal, and parietal lobes; via the lenticulostriate artery, supplies the majority of the basal ganglia and internal capsule
Posterior communicating artery (Pcomm)	Connects the posterior cerebral artery with the internal carotid artery; connects the carotid with the vertebrobasilar circulation
VERTEBRAL ARTERY BRANCHES	
Anterior spinal artery	Anterior one-half to three-quarters of the spinal cord
Posterior inferior cerebellar artery (PICA)	Undersurface of the cerebellum; choroid plexus of the fourth ventricle; medulla
BASILAR ARTERY BRANCHES	
Posterior cerebral artery (PCA)	Occipital lobes and the inferior and medial portion of the temporal lobes; thalamus and part of the hypothalamus; choroid plexuses of the lateral and third ventricles; midbrain
Superior cerebellar artery (SCA)	Upper surface of the cerebellum; midbrain
Anterior inferior cerebellar artery (AICA)	Inferior surface of the cerebellum; portion of the pons

From Hickey, J.V., Strayer, A.L. (editors). (2020). *The clinical practice of neurological and neurosurgical nursing*, 8th ed. Philadelphia: Wolters Kluwer; VanPutte, C.L., Regan, J.L., Russo, A.F., editors. (2020). *Seeley's anatomy and physiology*, 12th ed. New York: McGraw-Hill.

     a)   Pressure or myogenic autoregulation: Alteration in the diameter of the brain's resistance vessels (arterioles) that maintains a constant CBF over a range of MAPs between 50 and 150 mm Hg or a range of CPPs between 60 and 160 mm Hg (accounting for ICP). Chronic hypertension can increase the upper and lower limits for an acceptable range of autoregulation. If cerebral autoregulation is impaired, CBF is dependent on systemic blood pressure (BP). Cerebral autoregulation may be globally or focally impaired.

     b)   Elevated arterial partial pressure of carbon dioxide ($PaCO_2$) and hypoxemia (arterial partial pressure of oxygen [PaO_2] of <50 mm Hg) cause vasodilatation and may increase CBF; decreased $PaCO_2$ causes vasoconstriction and may reduce CBF.

     c)   Metabolic autoregulation: CBF varies with metabolic activity; factors that increase the metabolic rate (e.g., seizures, fever, agitation, pain) increase CBF; reduced metabolic requirements (e.g., hypothermia, barbiturate coma) decrease CBF.

   (3) Inadequate CBF results in brain tissue *ischemia* (CBF <18–20 mL/100 g/min) and brain tissue death, *infarct* (CBF <8–10 mL/100 g/min).

   (4) CBF higher than metabolic demand is called *hyperemia*.

  iii. Venous system: Venous blood from the scalp, skull, and meninges drains into the dural venous sinuses; venous blood from the interior cerebrum drains into the great cerebral vein (vein of Galen) beneath the corpus callosum and then the

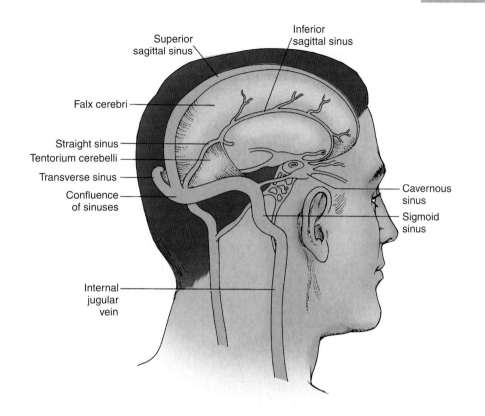

Fig. 5.10 Diagram showing the pattern of distribution of the major dural venous sinuses and their connection to the internal jugular veins. (Redrawn from Barker, E. (2002). *Neuroscience nursing: a spectrum of care*, 2nd ed. St. Louis: Elsevier.)

venous sinuses (Fig. 5.10). Cerebral veins have no valves and not parallel to the cerebral arteries.

(a) Veins empty into venous sinuses between dural layers (Table 5.3).

(b) Internal jugular veins collect blood from the large dural venous sinuses and return blood to the heart.

(c) Scalp veins connect to diploic veins in the skull and dural venous sinuses; emissary veins connect scalp veins and skull veins with the dural venous sinuses.

iv. Blood-brain barrier (BBB): Specialized permeability of the brain capillaries that limits transfer of certain substances from blood into brain tissue. A barrier is formed by tight junctions between brain capillary endothelial cells, reducing the transport mechanisms of these cells. Footlike projections from the astrocytes encase the capillaries.

EXPERT TIP

The BBB provides some protection by decreasing the brain's exposure to toxins. The BBB may also interfere with the effectiveness of intravenous (IV) chemotherapy for brain tumors. Temolazide, a standard chemotherapeutic agent for glioblastoma multiforme, taken orally, crosses the blood-brain barrier.

(a) Water, carbon dioxide, oxygen, glucose, and lipid-soluble substances cross the cerebral capillaries with ease. Uptake of other substances, such as contrast media and ions (e.g., Na^+, K^+), are much slower.

TABLE 5.3	Major Venous Drainage Structures, Their Locations, and Areas Drained
Venous Structure	**Location and Area Drained**
Superior (longitudinal) sagittal sinus	Courses along the midline at the superior border of the falx cerebri; superior cerebral veins empty into it
Straight sinus	Lies in the midline attachment of the falx cerebri and the tentorium; drains the system of internal cerebral veins (including the inferior sagittal sinus and great cerebral vein of Galen)
Transverse sinus	Lies in the bony groove along the fixed edge of the tentorium cerebelli; drains the straight sinus and the superior sagittal sinus
Sigmoid sinus	Lies on the mastoid process of the temporal bone and jugular process of the occipital bone; receives blood from the transverse sinuses and empties into the internal jugular veins
Inferior (longitudinal) sagittal sinus	Lies along the free inferior border of the falx cerebri just above the corpus callosum; receives blood from the medial aspects of the hemispheres
Cavernous sinus	Lies on the inferior surface of the brain, including the eye orbit
Emissary veins	Connect the dural sinuses with veins outside the cranial cavity

From Hickey, J.V., Strayer, A.L. (editors). (2020). *The clinical practice of neurological and neurosurgical nursing*, 8th ed. Philadelphia: Wolters Kluwer.

    (b) Regulates the entry or removal of various substances to maintain a homeostatic environment for the central nervous system (CNS)

    (c) Clinically significant in treating and diagnosing CNS disease. BBB disruption and increased permeability occurs with brain injury, tumors, infections, and stroke.

  d. Ventricular system and CSF (Fig. 5.11)

    i. Ventricles: Four cavities containing CSF

      (a) Lateral ventricles: Largest ventricles, one in each cerebral hemisphere. The anterior (frontal) horns lie in the frontal lobes; the bodies of the lateral ventricles extend back through the parietal lobes to the posterior (occipital) horns, which project into the occipital lobes; the inferior (temporal) horns lie in the temporal lobes. The lateral ventricles connect to the third ventricle via the intraventricular foramen (foramen of Monro).

      (b) Third ventricle: Midline between the two lateral ventricles and between the left and right thalamus and hypothalamus, surrounded by the diencephalon. CSF drains from the third ventricle inferiorly via the cerebral aqueduct.

      (c) Fourth ventricle: In the posterior fossa bordered by the pons, medulla, and superior cerebellar peduncles; continuous with the cerebral aqueduct (aqueduct of Sylvius) superiorly and the central spinal canal inferiorly.

    ii. CSF functions

      (a) Cushions the brain and spinal cord from injury

      (b) Provides support and buoyancy for the brain, decreasing its effective weight on the skull

      (c) Its displacement out of the cranial cavity into the perioptic subarachnoid space and lumbar subarachnoid space (and, to an extent, its increased reabsorption) compensates for increases in intracranial volume and pressure.

      (d) Regulates the nervous system chemical environment to preserve homeostasis

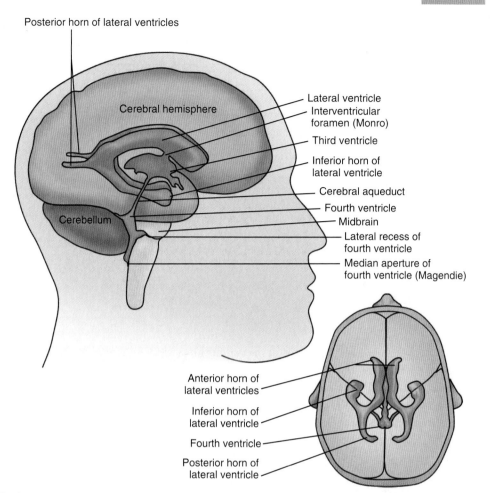

Fig. 5.11 Ventricular system, lateral and superior views. (Redrawn from Odom-Forren. (2018). *Drain's perianesthesia nursing*, 7th ed. St. Louis: Elsevier.)

(e) Enables water-soluble metabolites to diffuse from the brain

(f) Serves as a channel for neurochemical communication within brain

iii. CSF properties: (Table 5.4)

iv. CSF formation

(a) Rate of synthesis is estimated to be 500 mL/day or 20 to 22 mL/h.

(b) Choroid plexus: Tuft of capillaries in the pia mater covered by ependymal epithelial cells found in the lining of all ventricles; responsible for CSF production; lateral ventricles produce the most CSF

(c) Small amounts of CSF are produced by the blood vessels of the brain and meningeal linings.

v. Circulation and absorption of CSF (see Fig. 5.11)

(a) CSF circulates from the lateral ventricles through the interventricular foramina (foramina of Monro) to the third and fourth ventricle via the aqueduct of Sylvius; CSF then circulates to the subarachnoid space of the brain bilaterally via the foramen of Luschka (lateral aperture) and inferiorly to the subarachnoid space and central canal of the spinal cord via the foramen of Magendie (median aperture).

(b) Most CSF is absorbed via the arachnoid villi (granulations) into the dural sinuses.

TABLE 5.4	Normal Properties of Cerebrospinal Fluid
Characteristic	**Normal Finding**
Appearance	Clear, colorless
Specific gravity	1.00
Glucose level	50–75 mg/dL or approximately 60% of serum glucose level
Protein level	Lumbar: 15–45 mg/dL (up to 70 mg/dL in older adults) (*Note:* Increases when blood is present in CSF)
Cells	White blood cells: 0–5/mm³ Red blood cells: 0/mm³
Lactate level	10–25 mg/dL
Pressure	70–180 mm H_2O or <20 cm H_2O, measured at the lumbar level, with the patient in the lateral decubitus position
Volume	Ventricular system and subarachnoid space contain ~125–150 mL of CSF

CSF, Cerebrospinal fluid.
From Pagana, K.D., Pagana, T.J. (2018). *Lumbar puncture and cerebrospinal fluid examination. Mosby's manual of diagnostic and laboratory tests*, 6th ed. St. Louis: Elsevier.

(c) When CSF pressure exceeds venous pressure, CSF is absorbed through the unidirectional valves of the arachnoid villi.

vi. Blood-CSF barrier: Choroid plexus epithelium imposes a barrier analogous to the BBB; permits selective transport of substances from the blood into the CSF.

e. Brain metabolism

i. The brain has high metabolic energy requirements; energy primarily used for neuronal conductive and metabolic activities.

ii. At rest, the brain consumes 25% of body glucose and 20% of body oxygen. The brain receives about 15% of the cardiac output. Normal CBF in adults averages 50 mL/100 g/minute.

iii. CBF is normally coupled to cerebral metabolic rate (CMR); uncoupling may result in ischemia or hyperemia.

iv. The brain uses glucose as its principal energy source.

v. Minimal storage of oxygen and glucose in the brain necessitates a constant supply for normal neuronal function.

vi. Anaerobic glucose metabolism (glycolysis) yields insufficient adenosine triphosphate (ATP) to meet cerebral energy demands. Rate of glycolysis increases markedly during hypoxia in an attempt to maintain functional neuronal activity.

vii. Within seconds to minutes of anoxia, the energy-dependent sodium-potassium pump fails; cytotoxic cerebral edema results.

viii. Hypoglycemia causes neuronal dysfunction and may lead to convulsions, coma, and death.

EXPERT TIP

Although the optimal blood glucose is not known in the presence of brain injury, hypoglycemia may be injurious as well by depriving the brain of the energy needed for normal cerebral metabolism. Although the exact optimal glucose is not known for the individual patient, evidence supports maintaining a blood glucose slightly higher than normal (but <200 mg/dL) for the patient with a brain injury or insult to provide adequate glucose for brain metabolism.

f. Cells of the nervous system
  i. Neuron: Basic functional unit of the nervous system; transmits nerve impulses
    (a) Components of each cell (Fig. 5.12)
      (1) Cell body (soma): Carries out the metabolic functions of the cell; contains a nucleus, cytoplasm, and organelles (e.g., mitochondria) surrounded by a lipoprotein cell membrane
      (2) Dendrites: Short branching extensions of the cell body; conduct impulses toward the cell body
      (3) Axon hillock: Thickened area of the cell body from which the axon originates
      (4) Axon: Long extension of the cell body; conducts impulses away from the cell body; usually myelinated. In the peripheral nervous system (PNS), axons are also covered with neurilemma a layer of Schwann cells. Axons branch into several processes at the terminal end.
      (5) Myelin sheath: White lipoprotein complex that surrounds some axons; formed by oligodendrocytes in the CNS and by Schwann cells in the PNS

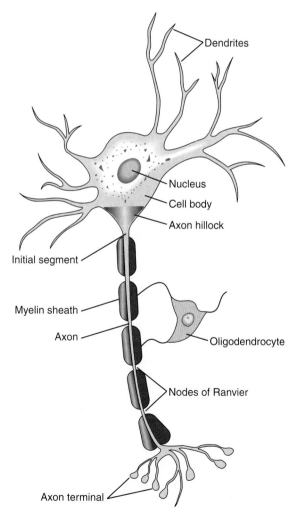

Fig. 5.12 Diagram of a typical neuron showing the cell body, axon, and dendrites. Neurons have many shapes and sizes. (From Banasik, J., Copstead, L.E. (2019). *Pathophysiology*, 6th ed. St. Louis: Elsevier.)

EXPERT TIP

Multiple sclerosis is the result of demyelination of the CNS whereas Guillain-Barré is the result of demyelination of the PNS. The time required for remyelination during recovery from Guillain-Barré accounts for a slower recovery time than the initial onset and progression of the disease.

---

      (6) Nodes of Ranvier: Periodic interruptions in the myelin covering along the axon. Impulses are conducted from node to node (saltatory conduction), which makes conduction more rapid and efficient.

      (7) Synaptic knobs or buttons: At the terminal ends of the axon; contain vesicles that store neurotransmitters (e.g., acetylcholine [ACh])

    (b) Functions of neurons

      (1) Receive input from other neurons, primarily via the dendrites and cell body

      (2) Conduct action potentials or impulses along the axon

      (3) Transfer of signals by synaptic transmission to other neurons, muscle cells, or gland cells

  ii. Neuroglial cells: Support, nourish, and protect the neurons of the CNS; about 5 to 10 times as numerous as neurons. Four types:

    (a) Microglia: Phagocytize tissue debris when nervous tissue is damaged

    (b) Oligodendroglia: Responsible for myelin formation on axons in the CNS

    (c) Astrocytes: Contribute to the structure of the BBB. Provide nutrients for neurons. Constitute the structural and supporting framework for nerve cells and capillaries. Remove excess potassium and neurotransmitters. Contribute to scar formation in response to neuronal cell injury or death.

    (d) Ependyma: Line the ventricles of the brain and the central canal of the spinal cord. Readminister flow of CSF from these cavities into the brain. Aid in CSF production.

g. Synaptic transmission of impulses: Unidirectional conduction of an impulse from a presynaptic neuron across a junction or synapse to a postsynaptic neuron; communication of one neuron with another

  i. Neurotransmitters (Table 5.5): Chemicals secreted by presynaptic knobs or vesicles (usually located at the axon terminal) that excite, inhibit, or modify the response of a postsynaptic neuron. When an action potential reaches the synaptic knob, calcium channels are opened, allowing Ca^{++} influx into the knob, which triggers neurotransmitter release.

    (a) Transmitter diffuses across the synapse and binds with postsynaptic membrane receptors, which causes certain ion channels to open.

    (b) Excitatory neurotransmitters: Open sodium and potassium channels, which result in postsynaptic membrane depolarization

2. **Spine and spinal cord**

  a. Vertebral column (Fig. 5.13)

    i. Composed of 33 vertebrae

    (a) Cervical: Seven vertebrae

      (1) Support the head and neck; smallest vertebrae

      (2) Atlas (first cervical vertebra): Supports the head; articulates with the occipital bone superiorly and the axis inferiorly

      (3) Axis (second cervical vertebra)

        a) Odontoid process (dens): Projection of the axis that protrudes upward through the anterior arch of atlas

        b) Allows for rotation of the head

TABLE 5.5	**Major Neurotransmitters: Type, Location, and Action**	
Neurotransmitter	**Location**	**Action[a]**
Acetylcholine	Distributed throughout the body, including concentrations in the following locations: • Many areas of the brain (e.g., motor cortex, some basal ganglia cells, hypothalamus) • Motor neurons innervating muscles or glands • Cholinergic fibers of the autonomic nervous system (ANS)	Usually excitation Inhibitory effect on some of the parasympathetic nervous system (PNS; e.g., vagus nerve on the heart) Primary neurotransmitter of the PNS
BIOGENIC MONOAMINES		
Norepinephrine	Distributed throughout the central nervous system (CNS) In the brain, produced by neurons with cell bodies in the pons (in the locus ceruleus nuclei) and medulla, which send axons to all areas of the CNS, including the brainstem, spinal cord, cerebellum, cortex, hypothalamus, and thalamus Found in the adrenergic fibers of the ANS	Excitation and inhibition Primary neurotransmitter of the sympathetic nervous system (SNS); regulates SNS effectors Implicated in numerous functions, including motor control, emotional responses, mood, feeding behavior, temperature regulation, and sleep
Dopamine	Produced by neurons of the substantia nigra and distributed throughout the CNS, particularly the basal ganglia Found in the ANS	Mostly inhibition Regulates motor control Also involved in other functions, including emotions, mood, behavior control, and mental functions
Serotonin	Produced in the raphe nuclei of the brainstem that project to several regions in the CNS, including the hypothalamus, brainstem, spinal cord, cortex, basal ganglia, and cerebellum	Mostly inhibition Implicated in a number of functions, including sensory processing, control of body heat, behavior, hunger, emotions, and sleep
AMINO ACIDS		
Gamma-aminobutyric acid (GABA)	Distributed over much of the CNS including neuron terminals in the spinal cord, cerebellum, basal ganglia, and some areas of the cortex	Inhibition
Glutamate	Found in many areas of the CNS High concentrations in the cortex, particularly the hippocampus and basal ganglia Released in large amounts when brain cells are injured by trauma or hypoxia ischemia; hypoxic ischemic changes are attributed in part to glutamate, which affects the hippocampus in particular	Excitation Excessive glutamate receptor stimulation opens ionic channels, causing neuronal disintegration from calcium influx through N-methyl-D-aspartate (NMDA) receptors and cellular swelling from influx of sodium and water

[a]Action is determined by the postsynaptic receptor rather than the neurotransmitter.
Data from VanPutte, C.L., Regan, J.L., Russo, A.F., editors. (2020). *Seeley's anatomy and physiology*, 12th ed. New York: McGraw-Hill.

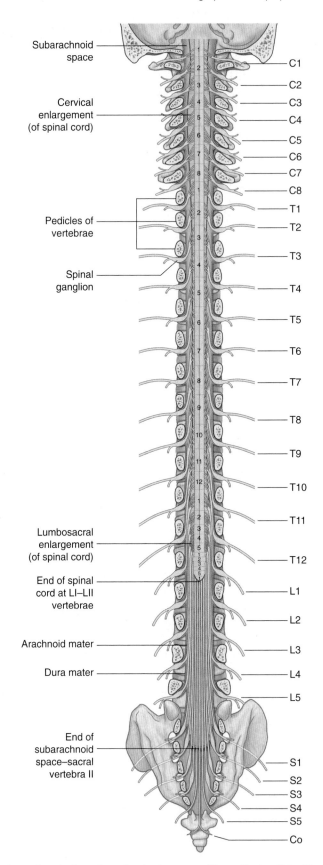

Fig. 5.13 Vertebral canal, spinal cord, and spinal nerves. (From Drake, R.L., Vogl, A.W., Mitchell, A.W. (2020). *Gray's anatomy for students*, 4th ed. Philadelphia: Elsevier.)

    (b) Thoracic: Twelve vertebrae; articulate with the ribs; support the chest muscles

    (c) Lumbar: Five vertebrae; support the lower back muscles; the largest and strongest vertebrae

    (d) Sacral: Five fused vertebrae; form a large triangular bone, the sacrum

    (e) Coccygeal: Four fused rudimentary vertebrae

  ii. Anatomic features of a typical vertebra

    (a) Body (corpus): Flat round, solid portion; lies anteriorly

    (b) Arch: Posterior part of the vertebra. Consists of:

        (1) Pedicles: Two short bony projections that extend posterior from the body

        (2) Lamina: Join each pedicle and fuse posteriorly at the midline to complete the arch; processes project from the laminae

        (3) Spinous process: Midline projection protruding posteriorly from the laminae

        (4) Transverse processes: Projections from the laminae on each side of the vertebrae

        (5) Articular processes (facets): Projections from the laminae that protrude upward or downward (superior or inferior articulating processes); inferior processes articulate with the superior processes of the vertebra directly below

    (c) Intervertebral foramina: Openings between the vertebrae through which bilateral spinal nerves pass

    (d) Spinal foramina (canal): Opening between the arch and the body through which the spinal cord passes

  iii. Intervertebral disks

    (a) Fibrocartilage layer between the bodies of adjoining vertebrae

    (b) Act as shock absorbers

    (c) Composed of the annulus fibrosus (tough outer layer) and nucleus pulposus (gelatinous inner layer)

EXPERT TIP

Intervertebral disks may compress motor and sensory nerve roots and, less often, the spinal cord. The compression of the sensory nerve root accounts for the radiculopathy experienced in herniated nucleus pulposus.

---

  iv. Spinal ligaments: Hold the vertebrae and disks in alignment; prevent excessive spinal flexion or extension

b. Spinal cord

  i. Extends from the superior border of the atlas to the first or second lumbar vertebra in adults

    (a) Continuous with the medulla oblongata

    (b) Conus medullaris: Caudal end of the spinal cord

EXPERT TIP

Conus medullaris and cauda equina injuries or compression may result in bowel, bladder, and sexual dysfunction. Sacral sparing in incomplete spinal cord injury preserves bowel, bladder, and sexual function.

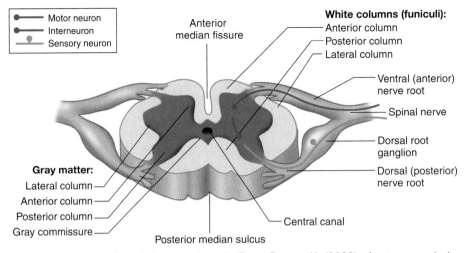

Fig. 5.14 Transverse section of the spinal cord. (From Patton, K. (2022). *Anatomy and physiology*, 11th ed. St. Louis: Elsevier.)

(c) Central canal: In the center of the spinal cord; contains CSF and is continuous with the fourth ventricle

(d) Filum terminale: Nonneural filament that extends downward from the conus medullaris and attaches to the coccyx; helps maintain the position of spinal cord during trunk movement

ii. Meninges: Continuous with the layers covering the brain; includes dura mater, (adjacent to inner surface of the vertebral column), arachnoid mater, and pia mater (layer closest to the spinal cord)

iii. Gray matter (Fig. 5.14)

(a) An H-shaped, internal mass of gray substance surrounded by white matter; consists of cell bodies

(b) Anterior gray column (anterior/ventral horn): Contains cell bodies of efferent motor fibers

(c) Posterior gray column (posterior/dorsal horn): Contains cell bodies of afferent sensory fibers

(d) Lateral column: Contains preganglionic fibers of the sympathetic motor neurons of the ANS, between T1 and L2 spinal cord segments

iv. White matter (see Fig. 5.14)

(a) Composed of three longitudinal columns (funiculi): Anterior, lateral, and posterior

(b) Contains mostly myelinated axons

(c) Funiculi contain tracts (fasciculi): Composed of axons with similar origin, course, and termination; perform specific functions; clinically significant tracts are summarized in Table 5.6; classified as follows (Fig. 5.15):

(1) Ascending/afferent or sensory tracts: Pathways to the brain for impulses that enter the cord via the dorsal/posterior roots of the spinal nerves

(2) Descending/efferent or motor tracts: Transmit impulses from the brain to the motor neurons of the spinal cord that exit via the ventral/anterior root of the spinal nerves

(d) Most tracts are named to indicate the column in which the tract travels, the location of its cells of origin, and the location of axon termination

TABLE 5.6   Major Spinal Cord Tracts

Name	Origin	Termination	Cross	Function
ASCENDING (AFFERENT/SENSORY) TRACTS				
Posterior dorsal columns: Fasciculus gracilis and fasciculus cuneatus	Fasciculus gracilis: Spinal cord at the lumbar and sacral levels	Medulla → thalamus → sensory strip of the cerebral cortex	Ascend in the posterior funiculus and cross over in the lower medulla	Conveys position and vibratory sense, joint and two-point discrimination, tactile localization, pressure and discriminating touch
	Fasciculus cuneatus: Spinal cord at the cervical and thoracic levels			Fasciculus gracilis: Carries impulses from the lower body
				Fasciculus cuneatus: Carries impulses from the upper body
Lateral spinothalamic tract	Posterior horn	Thalamus → cerebral cortex	Crosses over in the spinal cord to the contralateral anterolateral funiculus before ascending	Conveys pain and temperature sensation
Anterior spinothalamic tract	Posterior horn	Thalamus→ cerebral cortex	Crosses over in the spinal cord to the contralateral anterolateral funiculus before ascending	Conveys light touch and pressure sensation
Posterior spinocerebellar tract	Posterior horn	Cerebellum	Ascends uncrossed in the lateral funiculus	Conveys proprioceptive data that influence muscle tone and synergy necessary for coordinated muscle movements
Anterior spinocerebellar tract	Posterior horn	Cerebellum	Mostly crosses in the spinal cord before ascending in the lateral funiculus	Conveys proprioceptive data that influence muscle tone and synergy necessary for coordinated muscle movements
Spinotectal tract	Posterior horn	Tectum (roof) of the midbrain	Ascends crossed in the lateral funiculus	Conveys general sensory information that influences head and eye movement in response to stimuli
DESCENDING (EFFERENT/MOTOR) TRACTS				
Rubrospinal tract	Red nucleus of the midbrain	Anterior horn	Crosses in the midbrain and descends in the lateral funiculus	Conveys impulses to control muscle tone and synergy and to maintain posture
Lateral corticospinal tract	Cerebral cortical motor areas	Anterior horn	Up to 90% crosses in the medulla and descends in the lateral funiculus	Carries impulses for voluntary movement
Anterior corticospinal tract	Cerebral cortical motor areas	Anterior horn	Descends in the anterior funiculus and crosses in the cord at the level at which it terminates	Carries impulses for voluntary movement
Tectospinal tract	Superior colliculus of the midbrain	Anterior horn in the cervical spinal cord	Crosses in the midbrain and descends in the anterior funiculus	Mediates optic and auditory reflexes (e.g., reflexive head turning in response to visual or auditory stimuli)

From Hickey, J.V., Strayer, A.L. (editors). (2020). *The clinical practice of neurological and neurosurgical nursing*, 8th ed. Philadelphia: Wolters Kluwer; VanPutte, C.L., Regan, J.L., Russo, A.F., editors. (2020). *Seeley's anatomy and physiology*, 12th ed. New York: McGraw-Hill.

5   Neurologic System

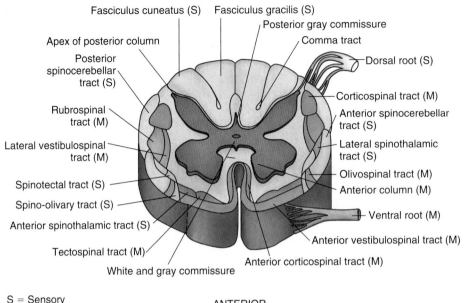

Fig. 5.15 Major ascending and descending tracts of the spinal cord. (Redrawn from Odom-Forren. (2018). *Drain's perianesthesia nursing,* 7th ed. St. Louis: Elsevier.)

(e.g., spinothalamic tract, afferent; responsible for pain and temperature sensation; corticospinal tract, efferent, responsible for voluntary motor function)

    v. Upper and lower motor neurons (UMNs and LMNs)

       (a) UMNs: Located completely in the CNS; regulate LMN activity. UMN lesions are associated with weakness, spastic paralysis, clonus, increased tone, hyperactive reflexes, Babinski's sign.

       (b) LMNs: Spinal and cranial motor neurons in the PNS that directly innervate muscles. LMN lesions cause weakness, flaccid paralysis, muscular atrophy, decreased tone; hypoactive to absent reflexes.

    vi. Reflexes: A reflex arc requires a receptor, sensory (afferent) neuron, motor (efferent) neuron, and effector (e.g., muscle or gland). Reflex arc requires a receptor, sensory (afferent) neuron, motor (efferent) neuron, and effector (e.g., muscle or gland; Fig. 5.16).

3. PNS

  a. Spinal nerves

    i. Thirty-one symmetrically arranged bilateral pairs of nerves, each possessing a sensory (dorsal/posterior) root and a motor (ventral/anterior) root: eight cervical, 12 thoracic, five lumbar, five sacral, and one coccygeal pair (see Fig. 5.13)

    ii. Fibers of the spinal nerves

       (a) Motor fibers: Originate in the ventral/anterior gray column of the spinal cord, form the ventral root of the spinal nerve, and pass to skeletal muscles

       (b) Sensory fibers: Originate in the spinal ganglia of the dorsal/posterior roots; peripheral branches distribute to visceral and somatic structures as mediators of sensory impulses to the CNS

       (c) Autonomic fibers

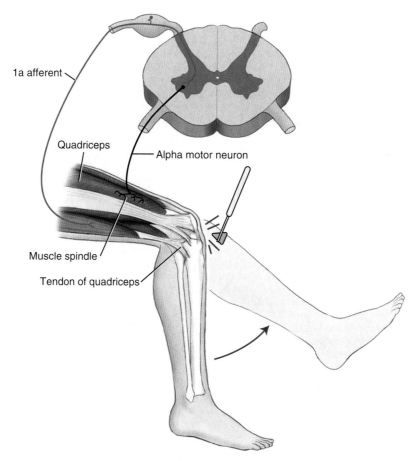

Fig. 5.16 Patellar reflex arc. Forward knee jerk is elicited by tapping of the tendon of the quadriceps. (From Heuer, A.J., Scanlan, C.L. (2018). *Wilkins' clinical assessment in respiratory care*, 8th ed. St. Louis: Elsevier.)

(1) Sympathetic (thoracolumbar division)
    a) Originate from cells between the posterior and anterior gray columns from thoracolumbar, T1 to L2 spinal cord segments
    b) Innervate the viscera, blood vessels, glands, and smooth muscle
(2) Parasympathetic (craniosacral division)
    a) Sacral innervation arises from sacral spinal cord segments, S2 to S4
    b) Pass to the pelvic and abdominal viscera
(d) Cauda equina: An elongated thick bundle of lumbosacral spinal nerve roots below the conus medullaris of the spinal cord, floating freely in CSF at the terminal end of the spinal canal within the lumbar cistern
  iii. Dermatomes (Fig. 5.17): Skin areas supplied by the dorsal root (sensory fibers) of a given spinal nerve; adjacent dermatomes overlap
  iv. Plexuses: Network of spinal nerve roots (Table 5.7)
b. Neuromuscular transmission (Fig. 5.18)
  i. Physiologic anatomy at the neuromuscular junction
    (a) Motor end plate: Distal end of motor axon loses its myelin sheath and flattens out at the end lying close to the muscle fiber membrane (sarcolemma).
    (b) Synaptic cleft: Space between the motor endplate of the axon and the muscle fiber membrane

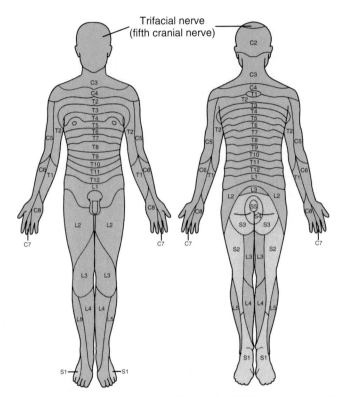

Fig. 5.17 Dermatomes. (From Nagelhout, J.J., Elisha, S. (2018). *Nurse anesthesia*, 6th ed. St. Louis: Elsevier.)

	Spinal Nerve Anterior Branches That Comprise	**Location of**	**Important Nerves**	
Name	**Plexus**	**Plexus**	**That Emerge**	**Areas of Innervation**
Cervical	C1–C4	Deep within the neck	Portion of the phrenic nerve	Muscles and skin of a portion of the head, neck, and upper shoulders; diaphragm
Brachial	C5–C8 and T1	Deep within the shoulder	Phrenic, circumflex, musculocutaneous, ulnar, median, and radial nerves	Shoulder, arm, and hand; diaphragm
Lumbar	L1–L4	Lumbar region of the back	Femoral cutaneous, femoral and genitofemoral branches	Anterior abdominal wall and genitalia; thigh and leg
Sacral	L4 and L5 and S1–S4	Inner surface of the posterior pelvic wall	Tibial, common peroneal, sciatic, and pudendal nerves	Skin of the leg; muscles of the posterior thigh, leg, and foot

TABLE 5.7 **Plexuses and Their Locations and Areas of Innervation**

From Hickey, J.V., Strayer, A.L. (editors). (2020). *The clinical practice of neurological and neurosurgical nursing*, 8th ed. Philadelphia: Wolters Kluwer; VanPutte, C.L., Regan, J.L., Russo, A.F., editors. (2020). Seeley's anatomy and physiology, 12th ed. New York: McGraw-Hill.

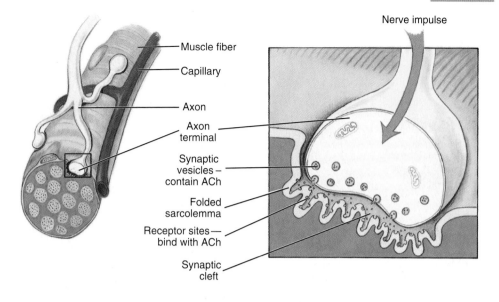

Fig. 5.18 Neuromuscular junction. *ACh*, Acetylcholine. (From Applegate, E.J. (2011). *The anatomy and physiology learning system*, 4th ed. St. Louis: Elsevier.)

    (c) Synaptic gutter: Invagination of the muscle fiber membrane where numerous folds increase the surface area available for neurotransmitter to act

    (d) Vesicles: Nerve terminal structures that store and release the neurotransmitter ACh

  ii. When an action potential reaches the neuromuscular junction, vesicles release ACh into the synaptic cleft. Amount released depends on the magnitude of the action potential and the presence of calcium. ACh attaches to receptor sites on the postjunctional muscle membrane and increases its permeability to Na^+, K^+, and other ions.

  iii. Endplate potential: Motor nerve action potential that is local (e.g., nonpropagated) and graded, rather than all or nothing

  iv. Muscle contraction: Action potentials subsequently form on either side of the endplate and conduct in both directions along the muscle fiber, initiating a series of events that result in muscle contraction.

  v. Acetylcholinesterase: Catalyzes the hydrolysis (degradation) of ACh to choline and acetic acid and thus limits the duration of ACh action on the endplate, which ensures production of only one action potential

c. Cranial nerves: 12 pairs (right and left) of nerves considered part of PNS and the parasympathetic (craniosacral) division of the ANS; motor, sensory or mixed in function (Fig. 5.19 and Table 5.8)

d. ANS (Fig. 5.20)

  i. Structure

    (a) Composed of two neuron chains: presynaptic/preganglionic and postsynaptic/postganglionic

    (b) Preganglionic cell bodies are located within the lateral gray column of the spinal cord or brainstem nuclei.

    (c) Most preganglionic axons are myelinated and synapse on the cell bodies of postganglionic neurons outside the CNS.

    (d) Axons of postganglionic neurons terminate on visceral effectors (e.g., smooth and cardiac muscle, glandular epithelium).

Neurologic System

5

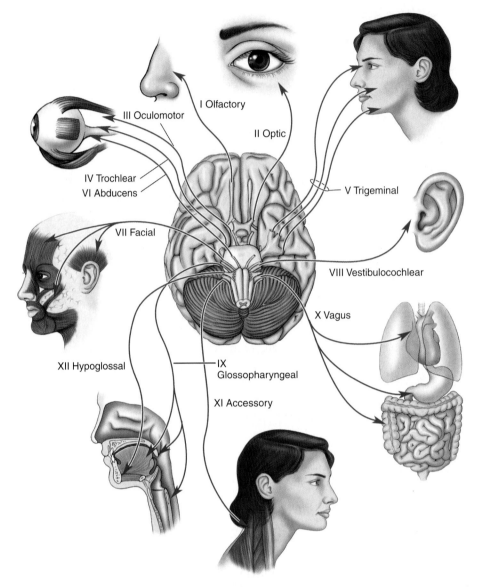

Fig. 5.19 Cranial nerves. (From Herlihy, B. (2022). *The human body in health and illness*, 7th ed. St. Louis: Elsevier.)

    ii. Divisions

        (a) Sympathetic (thoracolumbar)

            (1) Preganglionic axons emerge from cell bodies within the lateral horn of the spinal cord gray matter at the thoracic and upper two lumbar levels. Axons leave the spinal cord via the ventral/anterior roots and pass to:

                a) Paravertebral sympathetic ganglion chain via white rami communicates, ending on cell bodies of postganglionic neurons

                b) Collateral ganglia, ending on postganglionic neurons closer to the viscera

                c) Adrenal medulla, ending on modified postganglionic neurons that are secretory endocrine cells

            (2) Postganglionic axons pass to:

                a) Viscera via the sympathetic nerves

TABLE 5.8 Cranial Nerve Function, Assessment, and Anticipated Deficits

Cranial Nerve	Function	Assessment in Conscious Patient	Assessment in Unconscious or Uncooperative Patient	Anticipated Deficit
Olfactory (I)	Smell	Test each nostril separately. Ask the patient to identify familiar nonirritating odors, such as coffee or peppermint.	Unable to assess	Loss of sense of smell (*anosmia*)
Optic (II)	Vision	1. Inspect the optic disc (fundus), macula, and blood vessels with an ophthalmoscope. 2. Test visual acuity with a Snellen chart or printed material; test each eye individually. 3. Determine visual field using the confrontation test. Have the patient cover one eye and fixate on you with the other. Position yourself about 24 inches directly in front of the patient and close your eye that is opposite the patient's covered eye. With your finger halfway between yourself and the patient, bring your finger from the periphery into the patient's field of vision, evaluating the upward, downward, nasal, and temporal fields. Compare your visual field with the patient's. Repeat the test with the other eye.	Evaluate the pupillary light reflex (provides the sensory limb for this reflex) as part of the assessment with CN III described in the following text.	1. Papilledema (optic disc swollen and distorted with a reddish hue), which is indicative of increased intracranial pressure 2. Decrease or loss of central vision; blindness 3. Visual field defect
Oculomotor (III)	Levator palpebrae innervation raises the upper eyelid Innervates extraocular muscles to move the eye as follows: • Inferior rectus: moves eye downward and outward • Medial rectus: Moves eye medially	1. Evaluate the width and symmetry of the palpebral fissures and eyelid position. 2. Assess pupil shape, size, and equality. Describe size in millimeters. 3. Test the direct light reflex (constriction of the pupil when stimulated by light). This tests the afferent limb of CN II and the efferent limb of CN III. Describe the reflex as brisk, sluggish, or nonreactive.	1. Assess pupil shape, size, equality, and reactivity to light as was done for a conscious patient. 2. Evaluate extraocular movement as described later.	1. Eyelid droop (*ptosis*) 2. Irregularly shaped pupils can be caused by direct trauma, cataracts, or other ocular dysfunction; an irregularly shaped or oval pupil may accompany tentorial herniation that compresses CN III. 3. Disruption or compression of parasympathetic fibers from CN III and/or the nucleus (e.g., from a mass lesion or tentorial herniation) cause the ipsilateral pupil to dilate, which results in unequal pupils (*anisocoria*).

Continued

TABLE 5.8 **Cranial Nerve Function, Assessment, and Anticipated Deficits—cont'd**

Cranial Nerve	Function	Assessment in Conscious Patient	Assessment in Unconscious or Uncooperative Patient	Anticipated Deficit
	• Superior rectus: Moves eye upward and outward • Inferior oblique: Moves eye upward and inward Pupil constriction +10	4. Test the consensual light reflex (constriction of the opposite pupil when light stimulates one eye). Differentiates CN II and CN III lesions. Reflex is "present" or "absent." 5. Test the accommodation reflex: Have the patient look at an object (e.g., finger, pen) positioned 2 to 3 feet in front of the patient; as the object is moved toward the patient, the patient's eyes converge toward the midline, pupils constrict, and the lenses thicken. 6. Assess extraocular movement as part of the assessment for CN IV and VI described in the following text.		4. The direct light reflex is lost with oculomotor (parasympathetic) or optic nerve injury but retained with sympathetic disruption. 5. A blind eye (CN II lesion) does not have a direct light reflex; it has a consensual light reflex if CN III and midbrain connections are intact; cortical blindness does not affect either direct or consensual reflexes. 6. The accommodation reflex is lost.
Oculomotor (III), trochlear (IV), and abducens (VI) (Typically assessed together in regard to extraocular movements [EOMs])	Extraocular movements Oculomotor (III) See previous text Trochlear (IV) Supplies the superior oblique muscle, which moves the eye downward and inward Abducens (VI) Supplies the lateral rectus muscle which abducts the eye horizontally	1. Check the range of EOMs by having the patient's eyes follow your finger through all fields of gaze. Observe for nystagmus at rest and during ocular movements. 2. Ask the patient whether double vision is experienced in any visual field.	In patients who open their eyes, determine whether they can move both their eyes medially (CN III), laterally outward (CN VI), or up and down (more difficult to elicit) in response to a verbal or noxious stimulus. Evaluate whether the eyes move together (conjugate movement).	1. Impairment of EOM • Inability to move eye(s) downward and outward, medially, upward and inward, or upward and outward indicates CN III involvement • Impaired downward and inward movement indicates CN IV involvement • Inability to move the eye(s) horizontally outward indicates CN VI involvement 2. Diplopia

Trigeminal (V)	Three sensory divisions 1. Ophthalmic branch provides sensation to the forehead, upper eyelid, cornea, conjunctiva, nose, and part of the nasal mucosa 2. Maxillary branch provides sensation to the lower eyelid, upper jaw, teeth, gums and lip, upper cheek, hard and soft palates, some of the nasal mucosa, and the lower side of the nose 3. Mandibular branch provides sensation to the lower jaw, teeth, gums and lip, buccal mucosa, tongue, part of the external ear, and auditory meatus All three divisions contribute sensory fibers to the meninges. Motor fibers innervate the muscles of mastication	Sensory examination 1. Test the forehead, cheeks, and jaw on each side of the face. To evaluate light touch sensation, use a wisp of cotton; to evaluate temperature sensation, use test tubes of warm and cold water 2. Corneal reflex: Touch the cornea of each eye with a wisp of cotton. Observe for reflex blinking This tests the afferent limb of CN V and the efferent limb of CN VII. Motor examination 1. Ask the patient to clench his or her teeth and palpate the masseter and temporal muscles. Assess the symmetry and strength of muscle contraction. Assess the strength of the masseter muscles by pushing down on the mandible (chin) against the patient's resistance 2. Assess the patient's ability to chew	Test the corneal reflex	1. Absent, unequal, or uncomfortable sensation when the face is stimulated 2. Absence or weakness of blink response to corneal stimuli 3. Weakness of masseterand/or temporal muscles
Facial (VII)	Motor portions of the nerve innervate all muscles of facial expression Sensory portion conveys taste from the anterior two-thirds of the tongue Parasympathetic fibers innervate the salivary and lacrimal glands	1. Ask the patient to raise his or her eyebrows, frown, smile, and open the eyes against resistance. Note the strength and symmetry of facial movement. 2. Test taste on the anterior two-thirds of the tongue by applying salt and then sugar to both sides of the tongue. Ask the patient to identify the taste before closing the mouth 3. Assess the corneal reflex. This tests the afferent and efferent limb.	Test the corneal reflex	1. Weakness on one or both sides of the upper and/or lower face; if only the lower portion of the face is weak the cause is an upper motor neuron lesion (e.g., stroke) on the contralateral side of the facial weakness; weakness of the entire side of the face is caused by an ipsilateral lower motor neuron lesion of the facial nerve 2. Loss of taste sensation 3. Absence or weakness of the corneal reflex

Continued

TABLE 5.8 **Cranial Nerve Function, Assessment, and Anticipated Deficits—cont'd**

Cranial Nerve	Function	Assessment in Conscious Patient	Assessment in Unconscious or Uncooperative Patient	Anticipated Deficit
Auditory/ Acoustic (vestibulo-cochlear) (VIII)	Cochlear nerve: hearing Vestibular nerve: Aids in maintaining equilibrium or balance and coordinating head and eye movements	Cochlear (hearing) 1. Hearing acuity: Cover one ear, and test the other with a watch or a whisper 2. Weber's test: Place the stem of a vibrating tuning fork on the midline vertex of the skull. Ask the patient if the sound is heard equally in both ears or more on one side. Normally, there is no lateralization of sound. 3. Rinne's test: Place the stem of a vibrating tuning fork on the mastoid bone. When sound is no longer heard, invert the tuning fork and place it in front of the ear. Ask the patient to tell you when sound is no longer heard Vestibular (balance) 1. Assess the patient for complaints of vertigo, nausea, anxiety, nystagmus, postural deviation, and vomiting. All may indicate vestibular nerve dysfunction 2. Observe gait 3. Evaluate balance	The vestibular portion of CN VIII and its connections via the medial longitudinal fasciculus with CN III, IV, and VI provide information regarding the integrity of the brainstem; can be tested by the oculocephalic or oculovestibular reflex. 1. Oculocephalic reflex (doll's eye test): In a comatose patient who has had a cervical spine injury ruled out, turn the patient's head quickly from side to side while holding open the patient's eyes and noting the direction of eye movement. With intact connections between CN VIII and CN III and VI, the eyes move bilaterally in the opposite direction of the head movement. This is described as "doll's eyes present"	1. Impaired hearing 2. Negative result on Weber's test: When sound is referred to the better-hearing ear, decreased hearing is caused by impaired function of the cochlear nerve 3. Negative result on Rinne's test: Because air conduction is normally greater than bone conduction, middle ear disease is suspected in a patient who can hear the tuning fork as well or better when it is placed on the mastoid bone than near the ear 4. Presence of complaints seen with vestibular dysfunction 5. Imbalance 6. Abnormal oculocephalic reflex: There is no eye movement or the eyes move asymmetrically in response to head rotation 7. Abnormal oculovestibular reflex (showing the brainstem pathways to be impaired): The eyes stay in midposition when the ear is irrigated

	Assessment technique	Abnormal findings
	4. Perform the caloric irrigation test (to test the oculovestibular reflex): Position the patient with the head of the bed elevated 30 degrees. After checking to ensure an unoccluded ear canal and intact tympanic membrane, irrigate the canal with cold water. In the awake patient, when the pathway from the vestibular portion of CN VIII through the brainstem to CN III and CN VI is intact, the response will consist of slow conjugate eye deviation toward the irrigated ear and then rapid eye movement away from the irrigated ear. The cerebral cortex controls the fast phase. Awake patients may also experience vertigo, nausea, and vomiting.	2. Oculovestibular reflex (caloric irrigation test): Tested the same as described for a conscious patient Conjugate eye deviation toward the irrigated ear indicates that the pathway from the vestibular portion of CN VIII to CN III and VI is intact. (When the cerebral cortex is depressed, the fast eye deviation is lost.)

Glossopharyngeal (IX) and Vagus (X) (Typically assessed together)
 	
Sensory fibers provide sensation to the pharynx, soft palate, and posterior third of the tongue.
 	
They also supply special receptors in the carotid body and carotid sinus, which are concerned with reflex control of respirations, blood pressure and heart rate.
 	
Motor fibers participate with the vagus nerve in swallowing.
	1. Ask the patient to open his or her mouth and say, "Ahh." Observe for symmetric elevation of the palatal arch and midline uvula.
	2. Test for the gag reflex: Stroke the palatal arch with a tongue blade. The palate should elevate, and the patient should have a gag response. This tests the afferent limb of CN IX and the efferent limb of CN X.
	3. Appraise articulation and voice quality.
	4. Assess the ability to swallow.
	5. Evaluate the ability to taste salt and sugar placed on the posterior third of the tongue.
		1. Test by evaluating the gag and cough reflexes, usually accomplished by observing the patient's response to suctioning or movement of the endotracheal tube or to direct stimulation of the palatal arch.
		2. Evaluate the patient's ability to handle oral secretions by swallowing.
		
		1. Deviation of the uvula to the unaffected side
		2. Palate does not rise on the affected side
		3. Absent gag reflex
		4. Difficulty with vocalization (dysphonia):
		  • No voice
		  • Hoarseness related to vocal cord paralysis; laryngoscopic examination may be indicated
		  • Whisper, nasal-sounding voice indicates soft palate paralysis
		5. Difficulty swallowing (dysphagia)
		6. Loss of taste sensation on the posterior third of the tongue

Continued

TABLE 5.8   Cranial Nerve Function, Assessment, and Anticipated Deficits—cont'd

Cranial Nerve	Function	Assessment in Conscious Patient	Assessment in Unconscious or Uncooperative Patient	Anticipated Deficit
Spinal accessory (XI)	Vagus (X) sensory fibers convey sensation from the palate and larynx (along with IX) and from the larynx, external auditory meatus, and thoracic and abdominal viscera. Motor fibers innervate muscles of the palate, pharynx (along with IX) and larynx. Provides parasympathetic function to the abdominal and thoracic organs. Supplies the trapezius muscle to enable shoulder elevation and the sternocleidomastoid muscle, which allows the head to tilt, turn, and be thrust forward.	1. Assess the sternocleidomastoid (SCM) and trapezius muscles for size, symmetry, and spasticity. 2. Ask the patient to turn his or her head to one side. Place one hand on the patient's cheek and the other on the patient's shoulder for stability. Instruct the patient to resist your attempt to forcibly turn the head back to midline. Repeat on other side. 3. Ask the patient to push the head forward against your hand. Assess the strength of both SCM muscles. 4. Ask the patient to shrug his or her shoulders upward against the resistance of your downward pressure on the shoulders. Note the strength of the trapezius muscles.	Not typically assessed in the unconscious patient.	1. Atrophy or spasticity of the SCM or trapezius muscles 2. Weakness or inability to turn or lift the head or shrug the shoulder
Hypoglossal (XII)	Innervates muscles to tongue.	1. Inspect the tongue for atrophy or fasciculation with the patient at rest. 2. Have the patient protrude the tongue and assess for alignment and symmetry. 3. Ask the patient to move the tongue to the right and left and then press the tongue against the inside of the cheek while you assess its strength. 4. Note articulation.	Not typically assessed in the unconscious patient.	1. If unilateral hypoglossal lesion, the tongue deviates to the paralyzed side. 2. Tongue movement weakness or paralysis 3. Dysarthria

From Vilensky, J.A., Robertson, W.M., Suarez-Quian, C.A. (2015). *The clinical anatomy of the cranial nerves.* Hoboken, New Jersey: Wiley Blackwell.

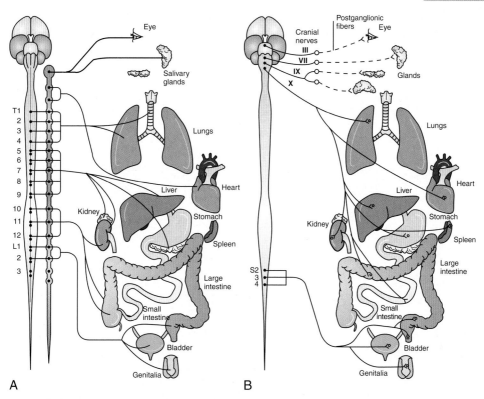

Fig. 5.20 A, The sympathetic portions of the autonomic nervous system. **B,** The parasympathetic portions of the autonomic nervous system with the vagus nerve distribution to the enteric devices. (From Fritz, S., Fritz, L.A. (2021). *Mosby's essential sciences for therapeutic massage,* 6th ed. St. Louis: Elsevier.)

       b) Gray rami communicantes, which return to the spinal nerve and are distributed to autonomic effectors in areas supplied by these nerves

   (3) Functions: (Table 5.9)

       a) Come into widespread activity under emergency conditions ("fight or flight")

       b) In general, antagonistic to parasympathetic activity; assist in maintenance of homeostasis

       c) Synapse with many postganglionic fibers

  (b) Parasympathetic (craniosacral; see Table 5.9):

   (1) Preganglionic cell bodies are located in brainstem nuclei and the lateral gray columns of the middle three sacral spinal cord segments (S2 to S4)

   (2) Preganglionic fibers end on short postganglionic neurons located on or near visceral structures

   (3) Supplies visceral structures in the head via the oculomotor (III), facial (VII), and glossopharyngeal (IX) cranial nerves and those in the thorax and upper abdomen via the vagus (X) nerve

   (4) Sacral outflow supplies the pelvic viscera via the pelvic branches of S2 to S4

   (5) Produces localized reactions rather than the mass action of sympathetic stimulation; assists in maintenance of homeostasis

  iii. Chemical mediation: ANS is divided into *cholinergic* and *adrenergic* divisions based on the neurotransmitter released.

TABLE 5.9	**Autonomic Nervous System Effects on Various Effector Sites**		
Effector Organ		**Sympathetic Influence**	**Parasympathetic Influence**
Eyes	Pupils	Dilation (mydriasis)	Constriction (miosis)
Glands	Lacrimal	Decreased	Increased
	Nasal	Decreased	Increased
	Salivary	Decreased	Increased
	Sweat	Increased	None
Heart		Increased rate	Decreased rate
		Increased conduction velocity	
		Increased contractility	Decreased contractility
Blood vessels	Coronary	Vasodilation	Minimal dilation
	Skeletal	Vasodilation	None
	Abdominal viscera	Vasoconstriction	None
	Cutaneous	Vasoconstriction	None
Blood pressure		Increased	Decreased
Lungs		Bronchodilation	Bronchoconstriction
Gastrointestinal system	Motility	Decreased peristalsis	Increased peristalsis
	Sphincter	Increased tone	Relaxation
	Secretions	Inhibition	Stimulation
Bladder		Decreased detrusor tone	Increased detrusor tone
Sex organs		Ejaculation	Erection
Skin	Pilomotor muscles	Excited (contraction)	None

From Hickey, J.V., Strayer, A.L. (editors). (2020). *The clinical practice of neurological and neurosurgical nursing*, 8th ed. Philadelphia: Wolters Kluwer; VanPutte, C.L., Regan, J.L., Russo, A.F., editors. (2020). *Seeley's anatomy and physiology*, 12th ed. New York: McGraw-Hill; Waxman, S.G. (2017). *The autonomic nervous system, clinical neuroanatomy*, ed 28. New York: McGraw Hill Lange.

    (a) Cholinergic neurons release ACh and include:
        (1) All preganglionic neurons
        (2) Parasympathetic postganglionic neurons
        (3) Sympathetic postganglionic neurons to the sweat glands and skeletal muscle blood vessels (vasodilation)
    (b) Adrenergic neurons release norepinephrine (NE) and include:
        (1) Sympathetic postganglionic endings, except as noted earlier
        (2) Constrictor fibers of the skeletal muscle blood vessels
4. **Physiology of pain (see Ch. 20, Pain)**

ASSESSMENT
1. **History**
    a. Current health issues
        i. Current symptoms including chronologic sequence of onset, duration, location, and frequency, reason for visit
        ii. Factors that relieve or exacerbate symptoms
        iii. Difficulties performing activities of daily living (ADLs)
    b. Patient health history: Significant medical and surgical history including traumatic injury and childhood diseases, and any sequelae

c. Medication history: Use of over-the-counter and prescription medications, nutritional and herbal supplements including amount, frequency, duration, last dose, effectiveness, adverse response. Especially note use of analgesics, antiepileptic medications (AEMs), tranquilizers, sedatives, anticoagulants, platelet aggregation inhibitors, stimulants, antihypertensives, and cardiac medications.

d. Allergies: Medication, food, environmental

e. Family history: Note history of disease that may affect current illness [e.g., cardiac disease, stroke, aneurysm, arteriovenous malformation (AVM), seizure, migraine, dementia, autoimmune disorder]

f. Social history and habits
   i. Significant others affected by the patient's illness
   ii. Support systems available to assist the patient and family
   iii. Alcohol and tobacco use: Past and present, amount, duration
   iv. Any illicit medication use or abuse
   v. Type of work; effect of symptoms on work
   vi. Hobbies, recreational activities
   vii. Current dwelling including layout and number of stairs

g. Functional health history/patterns
   i. Nutrition
   ii. Sleep pattern and hygiene
   iii. Sexuality
   iv. Coping/stress management
   v. Self-esteem/self-concept
   vi. Values and beliefs
   vii. Social, environmental
   viii. Health perception

2. **Physical examination**
   a. Physical examination data
      i. ABCs: Evaluate *a*irway patency, sufficiency of *b*reathing and *c*irculation
      ii. Evidence of acute (neurologic) deficit or disability
      iii. Inspection then palpation of the head, face, and spine: Shape, symmetry, bony contour, coloration, and skin integrity; irregularities may indicate injury, ventricular shunt, previous surgery, or congenital abnormality. Note nares or ear drainage
      iv. Auscultation: Heart for murmurs and clicks; carotid arteries and over eyes for bruit
      v. Assessment of neurologic function
         (a) LOC (Box 5.1)
         (b) Glasgow Coma Scale (GCS; Table 5.10): Used to assess LOC; total score also used to classify severity of brain injury. GCS ranges from 3 (worst score) to 15 (best score); a score of 8 or under signifies severe neurologic injury or illness. Limitations include inability to assess eye opening in patients with periorbital swelling; verbal response in intubated patients; or tetraplegia. Hypoxia, hypotension, hypothermia, medication intoxication, postictal state, and administration of sedatives, analgesics, or paralytic agents can interfere with GCS responses. Presence of any confounding variable should be noted when reporting score. Neurologic deterioration that affects only one side of the body may not be reflected in GCS score.
         (c) The Full Outline of Unresponsiveness Score (FOUR Score): Also used to assess LOC. In addition to eye and motor responses, includes brainstem

BOX 5.1 Assessment of Level of Consciousness

Consciousness is an awareness of self and the environment. A disturbance in consciousness is a sensitive indicator of neurologic dysfunction.

Arousal refers to the type of stimulus (e.g., verbal, noxious, central painful) necessary to elicit a response.

Awareness or the content of consciousness reflects higher cortical functions; can be assessed via the following:
- General behavior and appearance; appropriateness to the situation
- Attention span (distractibility), long- and short-term memory, insight, orientation, and calculation
- Intellectual capacity appropriate for educational level, judgment
- Emotional state, affect
- Thought content: Illusions, hallucinations, delusions
- Execution of planned motor activity: *Apraxia* is the inability to perform these movements
- Recognition and interpretation of sensations
- Language: Fluency, clarity, content, comprehension of written and spoken word, ability to name objects and repeat phrases, patient's awareness of a language disorder

Aphasia: Difficulty in the expression of language (Broca's, expressive or nonfluent aphasia) or understanding of language (Wernicke's, receptive or fluent aphasia) indicates dominant hemisphere dysfunction

Motor speech apraxia: Inability to perform the mouth movements to produce the sounds for the intended words; a motor speech programming disorder indicates a lesion in Broca's speech area

Dysarthria: Difficulty with articulation because impaired movement of the speech musculature may result from dysfunction of cranial nerves V, VII, IX, X, or XII or cerebellar dysfunction that interferes with the coordination of the muscles innervated by these nerves; represents speech impairment without a language deficit.

TABLE 5.10 Glasgow Coma Scale

Response	Score
BEST EYE OPENING	
"Spontaneously": Patient opens eyes without stimulation	4
"To voice": Patient opens eyes when spoken to	3
"To pain": Patient opens eyes when a noxious stimulus is applied	2
"None": Patient does not open eyes to any stimulus	1
BEST VERBAL RESPONSE	
"Oriented": Patient can state his or her name, where he or she is, and the date	5
"Confused": Patient speaks words but cannot state either who he or she is, where he or she is, or the date	4
"Inappropriate words": Patient speaks words with no specific intent at communicating	3
"Incomprehensible sounds": Patient grunts, groans, or makes other sounds	2
"None": Patient makes no attempt to vocalize	1
BEST MOTOR RESPONSE	
"Obeys": Follows commands	6
"Localizes": Attempts to remove noxious stimulus	5
"Withdraws": Pulls away from noxious stimulus	4
"Abnormal flexion": Decorticate posturing[a]	3
"Abnormal extension": Decerebrate posturing[b]	2
"No response": No motor movement of any kind to any stimulus	1
SCORING	

The patient's responses are graded and the best scores achieved for the eye opening, verbal, and motor categories are summed.

Total score ranges from 3–15, with 15 being normal; ≤8 is indicative of severe neurologic injury or illness

[a]Rigid flexion, internal rotation, and adduction of the upper extremity; extension, internal rotation, and plantar flexion of the lower extremity.

[b]Rigid extension, adduction, and internal rotation of the upper extremity; extension, internal rotation, and plantar flexion of the lower extremity.

From Jarvis, C. (2020). *Physical examination and health assessment*, ed 8. St. Louis: Elsevier.

BOX 5.2   Comparison of the Full Outline of Unresponsiveness (FOUR) Score With the Glasgow Coma Scale

FOUR Score	Glasgow Coma Scale
EYE RESPONSE	**EYE RESPONSE**
4 = eyelids open or opened, tracking, or blinking to command	4 = eyes open spontaneously
3 = eyelids open but not tracking	3 = eye opening to verbal command
2 = eyelids closed but open to loud voice	2 = eye opening to pain
1 = eyelids closed but open to pain	1 = no eye opening
0 = eyelids remain closed with pain	**MOTOR RESPONSE**
MOTOR RESPONSE	6 = obeys commands
4 = thumbs-up, fist, or peace sign	5 = localizing pain
3 = localizing to pain	4 = withdrawal from pain
2 = flexion response to pain	3 = flexion response to pain
1 = extension response to pain	2 = extension response to pain
0 = no response to pain or generalized myoclonus status	1 = no motor response
BRAINSTEM REFLEXES	**VERBAL RESPONSE**
4 = pupil and corneal reflexes present	5 = oriented
3 = one pupil wide and fixed	4 = confused
2 = pupil or corneal reflexes absent	3 = inappropriate words
1 = pupil and corneal reflexes absent	2 = incomprehensible sounds
0 = absent pupil, corneal, and cough reflex	1 = no verbal response
RESPIRATION	
4 = not intubated, regular breathing pattern	
3 = not intubated, Cheyne–Stokes breathing pattern	
2 = not intubated, irregular breathing	
1 = breathes above ventilator rate	
0 = breathes at ventilator rate or apnea	

From Wijdicksm, E.F.M., Bamlet, W.R., Maramattom, B.V., et al. (2005). Validation of a new coma scale: the FOUR score. *Annals of Neurology*, 58(4), 585–593.

---

reflexes and breathing pattern. Similar to GCS, additional cranial nerves and respiratory pattern (Box 5.2). Score ranges from 0 to 16 (16 being best).

  (d) Motor function

      (1) Assess size and contour of muscles: Note atrophy, hypertrophy, asymmetry, and joint malalignments

      (2) Observe for involuntary movements, such as fasciculations, tics, tremors (resting versus intention), abnormal positioning, tonic-clonic seizures

      (3) Determine motor response to stimuli

         a) Ability to follow simple commands, such as "Hold up two fingers." Patient should not be asked to squeeze hand because this may be a reflex response to palmar stimulation.

         b) Localization: Able to locate a noxious stimulus (e.g., deep pain stimulus) and attempt to remove it; indicates cortical dysfunction

            1) Noxious stimuli: Central noxious stimuli, such as trapezius squeeze, earlobe squeeze, supraorbital pressure (in the absences of facial fractures), or suctioning preferred; peripheral noxious

TABLE 5.11	**Muscle Groups, Associated Level of Spinal Cord Innervation, and Method of Testing**	
Muscle(s) Tested	**Primary Level(s) of Spinal Nerve Innervation**	**Method of Testing**
Deltoids	C5	Raising of arms
Biceps	C5	Flexion of elbow
Wrist extensors	C6	Extension of wrist
Triceps	C7	Extension of elbow
Hand intrinsics	C8-T1	Hand squeezing, finger flexion, finger abduction
Iliopsoas	L1, L2	Hip flexion
Hip adductors	L2–L4	Adduction of hips (squeezing legs together)
Hip abductors	L4, L5, S1	Abduction of hips (separating hips)
Quadriceps	L3, L4	Knee extension
Hamstrings	L5, S1, S2	Knee flexion
Tibialis anterior	L4, L5	Dorsiflexion of foot
Extensor hallucis longus	L5	Extension of great toe
Gastrocnemius	S1	Plantar flexion of foot

From American Spinal Cord Injury Association: Classification of Spinal Cord Injury (ISNCSCI) *(website)*. https://asia-spinalinjury. org/wp-content/uploads/2019/10/ASIA-ISCOS-Worksheet_10.2019_PRINT-Page-1-2.pdf. (Accessed May 2020); www. asiaspinalinjury.org/elearning/International%20Stds%20Diagram%20Worksheet%2011.2015%20opt.pdf. (Accessed November 2015); VanPutte, C.L., Regan, J.L., Russo, A.F., editors. (2020). *Seeley's anatomy and physiology*, 12th ed. New York: McGraw-Hill; Waxman, S.G. (2017). *The autonomic nervous system, clinical neuroanatomy*, 28th ed. New York: McGraw Hill Lange.

stimuli (nailbed pressure) may elicit reflexive response/ withdrawal; avoid noxious stimuli that traumatizes tissue (e.g., sternal rubs)

c) Withdrawal reflex: Pulls limb(s) away from painful stimuli with normal flexor movement; indicates extensive cortical damage

d) Abnormal flexion (decorticate) posturing (Table 5.11): Associated with lesions to the corticospinal tract just above the brainstem near or in the cerebral hemispheres, in the area of the diencephalon

e) Abnormal extensor (decerebrate) posturing: Extensor (decerebrate) posturing: Indicates damage to the midbrain or upper pons

f) No response: Associated with lower brainstem or high spinal cord dysfunction

(4) Strength testing (if the patient is able to follow commands)

a) Evaluate the integrity and function of UMNs and LMNs that innervate a specific muscle or muscle group (see Table 5.11)

b) Grade strength on a 0 to 5 scale (Table 5.12)

c) Note whether weakness follows a distribution pattern (proximal-distal, right-left, or upper-lower extremity)

d) Pronator drift may detect more subtle upper extremity weakness (patient places both upper extremities in front, shoulder height with palms up; arms must remain in place for 10 seconds without difficulty, maintaining level and/or pronation); the ability to sustain each lower extremity for 5 seconds, one at a time, may also be used to assess lower extremity weakness.

TABLE 5.12 Muscle Strength Grading Scale

Score	Muscle Function
0	Absent, no muscle contraction
1	Contraction of muscle felt or seen
2	Movement through full range of motion with gravity removed
3	Movement through full range of motion against gravity
4	Movement against resistance but can be overcome
5	Full strength against resistance

From Jarvis, C. (2020). *Physical examination and health assessment,* ed 8. St. Louis: Elsevier.

(5) Strength testing for a patient unable to follow commands:
  a) Observe which extremities move spontaneously or to noxious stimuli
  b) *Hemiparesis* or *hemiplegia* may be detected by lifting both arms off the bed and releasing them simultaneously. The limb on the hemiparetic side will fall more quickly and more limply than that on the normal side.
(6) Muscle tone: State of muscle tension assessed by palpating muscles at rest and during passive range-of-motion (ROM) movement; possible abnormalities include:
  a) *Rigidity:* Increased muscular resistance throughout passive ROM movement; seen with a basal ganglia lesion (e.g., Parkinson disease)
  b) *Spasticity:* Increased muscular resistance to joint movement, often followed by release of resistance; increased tone indicates corticospinal tract lesion
  c) *Hypotonia* (flaccidity): Decreased muscle tone associated with LMN lesions, cerebellar dysfunction, or spinal shock related to acute spinal cord injury
(7) Deep tendon reflex (DTR) or muscle stretch reflexes: Elicited by percussing the tendon with a reflex hammer, which causes stretching of the muscle spindles and subsequent contraction of muscle fibers when the monosynaptic reflex arc is intact. Compare responses side to side.
  a) Hyperreflexia usually indicates UMN lesion.
  b) Reflexes may be diminished or absent initially after an acute intracranial injury because of neuronal injury or after an acute spinal cord injury below the level of spinal cord injury because of spinal shock.
  c) Hyporeflexia or areflexia most often because of LMN lesions (e.g., brachial plexus injury)
  d) DTRs commonly tested (Table 5.13)
  e) Grade deep tendon reflexes on a 0 to 4 scale (Table 5.14)
(8) Superficial reflexes: Tested by stroking the skin with a moderately sharp object (abdominal; Table 5.15). These reflexes are lost or abnormal with UMN or LMN lesions.
(9) Pathologic reflexes (Box 5.3)
(10) Abnormal movements (see Box 5.3)
(11) Balance and coordination (see Box 5.3)

TABLE 5.13   **Deep Tendon or Muscle Stretch Reflexes and Level of Spinal Cord Innervation**

Reflex	Level of Spinal Cord Innervation
Biceps	C5, C6
Brachioradialis	C5, C6
Triceps	C7, C8
Quadriceps (patellar)	L2–L4
Achilles (ankle jerk)	S1, S2

From Jarvis, C. (2020). *Physical examination and health assessment*, ed 8. St. Louis: Elsevier.

TABLE 5.14   **Grading Scale for Strength of Deep Tendon Reflexes**

Score	Reflex Response
4 +	Hyperreactive, clonus
3 +	Very brisk
2 +	Normal, average
1 +	Diminished
0	No response, flaccid

From Jarvis, C. (2020). *Physical examination and health assessment*, ed 8. St. Louis: Elsevier.

TABLE 5.15   **Superficial Reflexes, Level of Spinal Nerve Innervation, and Method for Assessment**

Reflex	Spinal Nerve Innervation	Stimulus	Normal Response
Upper abdominal	T8–T10	Stroke upper abdomen	Abdominal wall contraction that causes umbilicus to move toward the stimulus
Lower abdominal	T10–T12	Stroke lower abdomen	Abdominal wall contraction that causes umbilicus to move toward the stimulus
Cremasteric	L1, L2	Stroke medial thigh	Testicular elevation
Bulbocavernous	S3, S4	Apply pressure to glans penis	Contraction of the anus
Perianal	S3–S5	Stroke perianal area	Contraction of the external anal sphincter

From Jarvis, C. (2020). *Physical examination and health assessment*, 8th ed. St. Louis: Elsevier.

   (e) Sensory function
      (1) In an awake, cooperative patient able to understand and follow commands, a complete sensory assessment can be performed. Test with the patient's eyes closed and compare one side of the body with the other.
      (2) In an unresponsive or uncooperative patient, a cursory sensory examination is performed by noting the patient's response to painful stimuli applied while performing various interventions (e.g., venipuncture).

BOX 5.3   **Assessment of Pathologic Reflexes, Abnormal Movements, Balance, and Coordination**

Pathologic reflexes
- Primitive reflexes are present in infants but normally absent in adults; may reappear in association with frontal lobe impairment. Examples include the following:
  - Grasp reflex: In response to palmar stimulation
  - Sucking reflex: In response to lip stimulation
  - Rooting reflex: Mouth opens, head deviates toward a stimulus applied to the lower lip or cheek
- Babinski reflex
  - Stroking the lateral aspect of the sole of the foot from the heel upward and across the ball causing abnormal dorsiflexion of the great toe and extensor fanning of the other toes is a positive Babinski reflex.
  - In an adult, a positive Babinski reflex indicates a lesion of the corticospinal tract anywhere from the motor cortex to the anterior horn of the spinal cord.

Abnormal movements: The distribution, rate, duration, and relationship to activity of any involuntary movements, such as the following should be noted:
- Seizures (refer to Seizures under Specific Patient Health Problems)
- Tremors: Rhythmic trembling movement of muscles
- Clonus: Abrupt onset of brief jerking movements of a muscle or muscle group (e.g., oscillation of the foot between flexion and extension with sudden passive extension of the foot)

Balance and coordination: Primarily evaluates cerebellar function; and is tested in patients able to perform voluntary movements
- Romberg test: Patient stands erect with the feet together, first with the eyes open and then with the eyes closed. A positive Romberg test result indicating posterior column or cerebellar dysfunction occurs when the patient loses balance and sways or falls when the eyes are closed.
- Swaying while sitting indicates cerebellar dysfunction.
- Evaluation for *dystaxia* or *ataxia* (muscle incoordination with volitional movements) and *dysmetria* (inability to halt a movement at a desired point), indicates cerebellar dysfunction.
  - The patient first touches the examiner's finger, positioned at the length of patient's arm from the face, and then touches his or her nose.
  - The patient slaps the thigh first with the palm and then with the back of the hand in quick, alternating movements.
  - The patient runs the heel from the opposite knee down the shin.
- Gait
  - The gait and tandem (heel-to-toe) walking is observed.
  - A wide-based, staggering gait and the inability to perform tandem walking indicate cerebellar dysfunction.
  - Gait disturbances with different clinical characteristics can be correlated with other specific neurologic or muscular dysfunction (e.g., spastic hemiparesis following an upper motor neuron lesion causes the patient to walk with the arm flexed close to the body and the spastic leg to move outward and forward in a semicircle, often with the toe dragged).

From Jarvis, C. (2020). *Physical examination and health assessment*, ed 8. St. Louis: Elsevier.

---

    (3) Sensory function is scored using a 0 to 2 scale (Table 5.16).

    (4) When possible, delineate sensory impairments based on dermatome distribution (see Fig. 5.16).

    (5) Spinothalamic tracts (Box 5.4)

    (6) Posterior columns (see Box 5.4)

EXPERT TIP

Posterior (dorsal) columns are responsible for proprioception (position sense), vibratory sensation, and discriminatory touch. Anterior cord syndrome spares the posterior dorsal columns but results in motor dysfunction and sensory impairment in regard to pain, temperature, and light touch.

---

    (7) Cortical discriminatory sensation (see Box 5.4)

  (f) Cranial nerves (see Table 5.8 and Fig. 5.21)

  (g) Eye and pupil signs: In addition to cranial nerve assessment, other findings may include the following:

TABLE 5.16 Sensory Function Scoring

Score	Sensory Function
0	Absent
1	Impaired or hyperesthetic
2	Normal or intact

Classification of Spinal Cord Injury (ISNCSCI) *(website)*. https://asia-spinalinjury.org/wp-content/uploads/2019/10/ASIA-ISCOS-Worksheet_10.2019_PRINT-Page-1-2.pdf. (Accessed May 2020).

BOX 5.4 Assessment of Spinothalamic Tracts, Posterior Columns, and Cortical Discriminatory Sensation

Lesions or dysfunction of the peripheral nerves, ascending nerve tracts, or sensory perceptive areas of the cerebral cortex (e.g., parietal lobe) may impair sensory function.

SPINOTHALAMIC TRACTS (ANTERIOR AND LATERAL)
- Either pain *or* temperature sensation may be assessed because both functions are carried in the same lateral spinothalamic tracts.
- Pain: The patient distinguishes sharp from dull stimuli randomly applied; gently touch the skin using a sterile subcutaneous needle or broken cotton applicator for sharp sensation and using a blunt edge (head of pin or cotton end of applicator) for dull sensation.
- Temperature: The patient distinguishes between hot and cold stimuli when randomly touched with test tubes filled with hot or cold water.
- Light touch: The patient identifies light touch as a wisp of cotton is stroked across the skin.

POSTERIOR COLUMNS (FASCICULUS GRACILIS AND FASCICULUS CUNEATUS)
- Either proprioception (position sense) *or* vibration sense may be assessed because both are carried in the same tracts.
- Vibration: A vibrating tuning fork is applied to bony prominences; the patient is asked to report when vibration is felt; the vibrating tuning fork is applied first to the distal aspect of each extremity and then moved proximally.
- Proprioception (position sense): The patient closes the eyes and reports whether a finger or toe is being moved up or down; in all four extremities. The finger or toe is held on the sides, not on the top and bottom.

CORTICAL DISCRIMINATORY SENSATION

In addition to the sensory pathways, the association portions of the cortex (e.g., the parietal lobe) are assessed. Deficits are called *agnosias* (not knowing). Examples include the following:
- *Stereognosis:* The patient, without the aid of vision, is asked to identify familiar objects placed in his or her hand. The inability to identify objects is *astereognosia*.
- *Graphesthesia:* The patient is asked to identify numbers or letters traced on the palm. The inability to discern what is written is *agraphesthesia*.
- *Simultaneous double stimulation:* With the patient's eyes closed, the patient's limbs are touched on both sides of the body in corresponding locations. The patient can detect the number and location of stimuli. Inability to identify that he or she is being touched on both sides of body simultaneously is *tactile inattention*. Inability to locate a single touch sensation is *atopognosia*.

From Jarvis, C. (2017). *Physical examination and health assessment*, ed 7. St. Louis: Elsevier.

---

 (1) Pupil abnormalities (Table 5.17)
 (2) Gaze deviation or gaze preference: Horizontal or vertical gaze deviations indicate a cortical or brainstem lesion
  a) Eyes deviate toward the side of a destructive hemispheric lesion (e.g., brain tumor) affecting the frontal gaze centers
  b) Gaze deviates away from irritative foci (seizures) affecting the frontal gaze centers

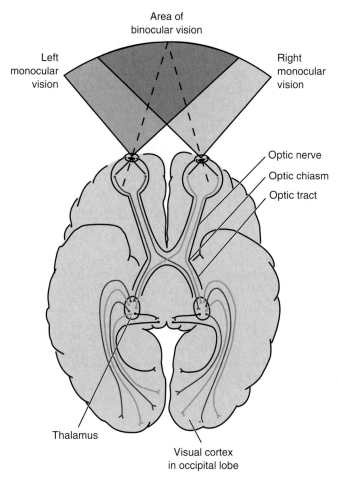

Fig. 5.21 Visual pathways. (From Applegate, E.J. (2011). *The anatomy and physiology learning system*, 4th ed. St. Louis: Elsevier.)

> c) Inability to gaze upward is associated with dorsal midbrain lesions (Parinaud's syndrome).
>
> d) Eyes deviate away from the side of a unilateral pons lesion
>
> (3) Nystagmus (rhythmic, oscillatory eye movements)
>
> a) Detected by having the patient follow your finger through the fields of gaze
>
> b) Because of lesions of the cerebellum, vestibular system, or brainstem pathways, or toxic-metabolic/medication-induced disorders; clinical features vary with the part of the pathway affected
>
> c) Nystagmus may be described as gaze-evoked, optokinetic, convergence-retraction, see-saw, downbeat, horizontal, vestibular, toxic, and ocular bobbing.

EXPERT TIP

Pathologic eye movements may assist in localization of the intracranial lesion. Ocular bobbing is associated with brainstem injury. Rotary nystagmus is associated with supratentorial (hemispheric) lesions.

> (h) Vital signs
>
> (1) Temperature

TABLE 5.17	Pupil Abnormalities Associated With Specific Areas of Brain Dysfunction
Pupil Finding	**Related Brain Dysfunction**
Small, equal, reactive	Bilateral diencephalic damage that affects the sympathetic innervation originating from the hypothalamus; metabolic dysfunction
Nonreactive, midpositioned	Midbrain damage
Fixed and dilated	Ipsilateral oculomotor (cranial nerve III) compression or injury, uncal transtentorial herniation at the late diencephalon level
Bilateral fixed and dilated	Brain anoxia and ischemia; bilateral cranial nerve III compression, central herniation at the medullary level
Pinpoint, nonreactive	Pons damage, often from hemorrhage or ischemia that interrupts the sympathetic nervous system pathways
One pupil is smaller than the other, but both reactive to light; associated with ptosis and an inability to sweat on the same side as the smaller pupil (Horner syndrome)	Interruption of ipsilateral sympathetic innervation that can be caused by a lesion of the anterolateral cervical spinal cord or lateral medulla, damage to the hypothalamus, or occlusion or dissection of the internal carotid artery

From Hickey, J.V. (2020). Comprehensive neurological examination and neurological assessment. In J.V. Hickey, A.L. Strayer (editors). *The clinical practice of neurological and neurosurgical nursing*, 8th ed. Philadelphia: Wolters Kluwer; Hickey, J.V., Baumann, J.J. (2020). Intracranial hypertension: theory and management of increased intracranial pressure. In J.V. Hickey, A.L. Strayer (editors). *The clinical practice of neurological and neurosurgical nursing*, 8th ed. Philadelphia: Wolters Kluwer; Jarvis, C. (2020). *Physical examination and health assessment*, 8th ed. St. Louis: Elsevier.

    a) Hyperthermia increases cerebral oxygen consumption by 10% for every 1.8° F (1° C) elevation. Higher metabolic demand increases the risk for CNS ischemia. *Neurogenic fever* can be caused by damage to the hypothalamus, where the thermoregulation center is located.

    b) Hypothermia, if extreme, can lead to cardiac dysrhythmias, coagulopathies, electrolyte shifts, pneumonia, and other complications. Hypothermia is seen with hypothalamic lesions, spinal cord injury with autonomic dysfunction, and metabolic or toxic encephalopathy.

(2) Respirations: Respiratory dysrhythmias often correlate with lesions at specific locations in the brain, although effects may vary and may be influenced by other factors (Table 5.18; also consider FOUR score)

(3) Pulse and BP

    a) Both are notoriously unreliable parameters in detecting CNS disease or neurologic deterioration. May change late in the course of increased ICP and thus are of limited clinical use.

    b) Cardiac dysrhythmias may be seen with neurologic disorders, particularly with blood in the CSF, after posterior fossa surgery with increased ICP, or with stroke in certain locations.

    c) Tachycardia and hypertension may be seen with injury or compression of the hypothalamus that results in sympathetic nervous system stimulation.

    d) Cushing's response (late sign of central herniation syndrome) occurs when intracranial hypertension causes compression of the medullary vasomotor center. Features of Cushing's response include an increase in systolic BP widening of the pulse pressure,

TABLE 5.18	**Respiratory Patterns Associated With Specific Areas of Brain Dysfunction**	
Breathing Pattern	**Description**	**Location of Brain Lesion or Type of Dysfunction**
Cheyne-Stokes	Regular cycles of respirations that gradually increase in depth to hyperpnea and then decrease in depth to periods of apnea	Usually bilateral lesions deep within the cerebral hemispheres, basal ganglia, or diencephalon: metabolic disorders
Central neurogenic hyperventilation	Deep, rapid respirations	Midbrain, upper pons
Apneustic	Prolonged inspiration followed by a 2- to 3-second pause; occasionally, may alternate with an expiratory pause	Lower pons
Cluster	Cluster of irregular breaths followed by an apneic period lasting a variable amount of time	Lower pons or upper medulla
Ataxic or irregular	Irregular, unpredictable pattern of shallow and deep respirations and pauses	Medulla

From Hickey, J.V., Strayer, A.L. (editors). (2020). *The clinical practice of neurological and neurosurgical nursing*, ed 8. Philadelphia: Wolters Kluwer.

and bradycardia. The term *Cushing's triad* is sometimes used to include respiratory changes associated with medullary ischemia.
    (4) Pain (see Ch. 20)
  b. Monitoring data: The term *multimodality monitoring* is used in reference to multiple monitoring methods in the care of the critically ill neuroscience patient but may include data from the physical assessment (observational data), as well as information from physiologic parameters (physiologic data).

KEY CONCEPT
Worsening of the neurologic assessment is often seen before changes obtained with multimodality monitoring. The critical care nurses' bedside neurologic assessment may detect early subtle changes earlier than multimodality monitoring.

---

    i. ICP and CPP monitoring: See specific patient health problems for greater detail
      (a) Principle: Based on the Monro-Kellie Hypothesis (Monroe-Kellie Doctrine), ICP monitoring looks at the composite pressure from brain, blood, and CSF in the cranium. CPP is a derived parameter (MAP-ICP) that provides a measure of the pressure gradient that drives blood flow through the brain; an indirect indicator of CBF (see Cerebral Blood Flow discussed previously). An intracranial catheter may be placed in the ventricle, parenchyma, subdural, or epidural space. ICP can be measured via ventricular catheters coupled with an external strain gauge transducer or a fiberoptic transducer tipped catheter.
      (b) Clinical uses: Measurement of ICP and CPP in a number of intracranial conditions including traumatic brain injury (TBI), hemorrhagic stroke, brain tumor, CNS infection, and encephalopathy; normal ICP is 0 to 15 mm Hg; treatment is typically initiated for greater than 20 to 22 mm Hg.
      (c) Periprocedural care: Aseptic technique; monitor for infection; synchronization of ICP monitor to bedside monitor for central alarm
      (d) Advantages: May be placed at bedside for continuous monitoring of ICP/CPP; assists in guiding ICP/CPP management

(e) Disadvantages: Does not reflect global ICP/CPP related to compartmental constraints (cerebral falx, tentorium cerebelli); inconsistency in practice regarding measurement of CPP (leveling of external strain gauge transducer for ICP and MAP); fiberoptic catheters associated with drift with increased duration of use. The optimal range of ICP/CPP is not known; increased risk of infection with ventricular catheters; risk of overdrainage with ventricular catheters

ii. Jugular venous oxygen saturation (SjO_2)

(a) Principle: Assesses the coupling or uncoupling of cerebral blood flow (CBF) and cerebral oxygen consumption (metabolism). Placement of a fiberoptic oximetry catheter into the jugular bulb allows for continuous measurement of SjO_2 and intermittent jugular venous blood gas sampling. Reflects a global view of cerebral oxygenation.

(b) Clinical uses: May detect episodes of uncoupling between CBF and metabolism indicating cerebral ischemia (CBF is less than the metabolic demand) or hyperemia (CBF exceeds the metabolic demand). Factors that decrease cerebral oxygen supply (e.g., hypoxemia, anemia, insufficient cerebral perfusion) or increase cerebral metabolic demand (e.g., seizures, hyperthermia) lower SjO_2 and can cause ischemia. Factors that increase oxygen supply (e.g., increased CBF, hyperoxia) or reduce cerebral oxygen demand (e.g., large area of cerebral infarction, hypothermia) raise SjO_2 and can cause hyperemia (oxygen supply exceeds demand).

(1) Normal SjO_2 is 55% to 75%; SjO_2 below 55% is indicative of global ischemia and warrants treatment; SjO_2 above 75% indicates hyperemia.

(2) Cerebral extraction of oxygen (CEO_2): Calculated by subtracting SjO_2 from arterial oxygen saturation (SaO_2). Normal = 24% to 42%; lower than 24% indicates hyperemia; higher than 42% indicates cerebral oxygen supply insufficient for demand.

(3) When jugular venous and arterial blood gas levels are analyzed simultaneously, arteriovenous oxygen difference ($AJVDO_2$) can be calculated. Abbreviated formula: $AJVDO_2 = 1.34 (SaO_2 - SjO_2)$ hemoglobin/100. Normal $AJVDO_2$ is 5.0 to 7.5 mL/dL (or volume %); less than 5.0 mL/dL indicates hyperemia and more than 7.5 mL/dL (or volume %) indicates cerebral oxygen supply insufficient for demand.

(4) Knowledge of uncoupling between cerebral oxygen delivery and demand can prompt implementation of interventions to improve the balance and prevent ischemia or hyperemia.

EXPERT TIP

Retrograde jugular oxygenation may guide safe lowering of the PCO_2 in cerebral hyperemia to decrease vasodilation and lower ICP. However, lowering the PCO_2 below 35 mm Hg increases vasoconstriction and may increase the risk of cerebral ischemia and must be done cautiously based on knowledge of the patient's intracranial dynamics.

(c) Periprocedural care: After insertion, lateral cervical radiograph confirms location of the catheter tip. Calibrate the continuous SjO_2 monitor. Because readings may be inaccurate because of poor catheter position or improper calibration, a strategy for troubleshooting any abnormal value should be established.

(d) Advantages: Continuous monitoring of global brain oxygenation which can be used to guide management of oxygenation and lowering of $PaCO_2$ to lessen hyperemia.

(e) Disadvantages: Difficulty maintaining optimal position; if distal to jugular bulb, SjO_2 may be artificially high related to facial vein blood; potential complications include infection, bleeding, vascular injury, and thrombosis.

iii. Partial pressure of brain tissue oxygen ($PbtO_2$)

   (a) Principle: Oxygen-sensing probe inserted into brain parenchyma continuously monitors $PbtO_2$ around the tip. Provides data regarding the balance between oxygen delivery to the cerebral extracellular space and oxygen consumption by cerebral tissue. $PbtO_2$ values lessened with systemic hypoxia and hypotension, fever, shivering, pain, agitation, increased ICP/decreased CPP, seizures

   (b) Clinical uses: Normal $PbtO_2$ varies depending on the brand of monitor used. Depth and duration of low $PbtO_2$ correlate with a poorer outcome from brain injury. When cerebral hypoxia is recognized, interventions to improve cerebral oxygen delivery and minimize cerebral oxygen consumption can be instituted. Use of the device may be beneficial for patients with severe TBI, stroke, tumor, or SAH and cerebral vasospasm.

   (c) Postprocedure care: Observe for potential complications, including infection, hemorrhage; respond to $PbtO_2$ under 20 mm Hg urgently

   (d) Advantage: Continuous monitoring of localized brain tissue oxygenation for rapid response to ischemia

   (e) Disadvantage: Controversial; lack of consensus regarding optimal position; not magnetic resonance imaging (MRI) compatible

iv. Near-infrared cerebral spectroscopy (NIRS)

   (a) Principle: Sensor placed on the scalp emits near-infrared light that penetrates the scalp and skull to measure oxygen saturation in underlying brain tissue.

   (b) Clinical uses: Normal values are ill-defined but changes in trends may indicate alterations in regional cerebral oxygen saturation (rSO_2).

   (c) Periprocedural care: Monitor for skin breakdown under sensors

   (d) Advantage: Noninvasive

   (e) Normal values not known; may be used for trending data. Measurements may be unreliable because of stray light, sensor disruption, drift, movement artifact, temperature changes, or contamination from extracranial circulation.

v. Continuous electroencephalographic (EEG) monitoring

   (a) Principle: Continuously monitors electrical activity of the brain by means of electrodes attached to the scalp

   (b) Clinical uses: Identifies the onset of seizures or cerebral ischemia so appropriate interventions can be initiated. Monitors burst activity in patients in medication-induced coma for refractory increased ICP and status epilepticus so that the minimal amount of barbiturate or propofol to achieve the desired burst suppression is administered. Continuous EEG with scalp or intracranial electrodes may also be used to determine the epileptogenic focus in epilepsy patients.

   (c) Periprocedural care: Move the patient carefully to avoid dislodging the electrodes; EEG readings are influenced by electrical, environmental, movement, and biologic artifacts.

(d) Advantage: Scalp electrodes are noninvasive.

(e) Disadvantage: Results nonspecific in regard to neuropathology; scalp electrodes may fail to capture some electrical activity compared with intracranial electrode strips or grids. Most electrodes must be removed before computed tomography (CT) scan and are not MRI compatible; interpretation difficult; compressed spectral array not widely available for easier interpretation.

vi. Evoked potentials (EPs; somatosensory, auditory, and visual):

(a) Principle: Specialized recording of electrical potentials from the cerebral cortex, brainstem, spinal cord, and PNS to determine integrity of neural pathway

(b) Application: Prognostication; guidance during surgical procedures

(c) Periprocedural care: Move the patient carefully to avoid dislodging the electrodes; EEG readings are influenced by electrical, environmental, movement, and biologic artifacts.

(d) Advantage: Noninvasive

(e) Disadvantage: EP readings are influenced by electrical, environmental, movement, and biologic artifacts

vii. EEG-derived sedation monitoring: Bispectral index (BIS) and Patient State Index (PSI)

(a) Principle: EEG-derived technology that quantifies features of the EEG waveform using computerized algorithms; sensors are placed over the forehead to determine a numeric value along with muscular artifact (electromyography [EMG]).

(b) Application: Monitoring LOC during sedation and general anesthesia

(c) Suppression ratio monitoring during chemically induced coma (e.g., barbiturate-induced coma)

(d) To determine level of sedation when neuromuscular blocking agents are in use

(e) Periprocedural care: Prepare skin; apply sensors; monitor for skin breakdown

(f) Advantage: Noninvasive

(g) Disadvantage: Although BIS and PSI both range from 0 to 100, they are not interchangeable values. There is lack of agreement in regard to target BIS and PSI values. EMG artifact may affect reading.

viii. Transcranial Doppler ultrasonography (TCD)

(a) Principle: Probe positioned over thin areas of the cranium emits a low-frequency pulsed ultrasonic signal to measure the direction and velocity of blood flow through underlying major vessels.

(b) Clinical uses: High velocities correlate with cerebral vasospasm or hyperemia. If MCA velocity is more than 120 cm/s, the ratio of MCA to ICA velocity can be calculated (Lindegaard ratio/hemispheric index). A ratio of 3 or more is associated with cerebral artery vasospasm and less than 3 suggests hyperdynamic flow. Can detect emboli, stenotic or occluded vessels, and other vascular anomalies. May reveal blood flow alterations indicating ICP elevations. May also be used to evaluate cerebral autoregulation and as an ancillary test of brain death.

(1) Advantages: Noninvasive, portable, relatively inexpensive, can be safely repeated often or used continuously to monitor changes

(2) Disadvantages: Absolute velocities vary depending on many factors—age, hematocrit, $PaCO_2$, cardiac output, and the metabolic activity

of the brain tissue supplied by the artery being insolated. Difficult to distinguish anatomic variations of arteries from arterial disease; does not detect bilaterally symmetric disease, long regions of vasoconstriction or stenosis, or distal artery disease. Poor sonographer interrater reliability may weaken the validity of the results; hyperostosis may not permit adequate bone windows.

(c) Preprocedure and postprocedure care: No specific care required; no known complications related to ultrasound; as low (ultrasound setting) as reasonably allowed (ALARA) principle is used with all ultrasound.

ix. Continuous CBF monitoring

(a) Principle: Sensor placed on the surface of the brain continuously measures regional CBF

(1) Thermal diffusion flowmetry: Temperature variation between two plates on a brain surface sensor provides an inverse measure proportional to CBF.

(2) Laser Doppler flowmetry: Laser Doppler probe positioned on the brain surface or in the parenchyma measures CBF.

(b) Clinical uses: Provides a continuous measure of regional CBF that can be used to evaluate autoregulation and detect local brain ischemia. Can guide therapy to avoid or reduce cerebral ischemia.

(c) Advantages: Measures regional CBF, not a derived parameter.

(d) Disadvantages: Invasive; may require frequent recalibration. Lack of agreement regarding treatment parameters.

(e) Periprocedural care: Observe for potential complications, including infection or CSF leakage. Troubleshoot abnormal values; data may be unreliable if the probe loses contact with the brain surface or comes in contact with large blood vessels. Alterations in hematocrit, strong external light, or probe movement artifact can influence laser Doppler measurements.

x. Pupillometry

(a) Principle: A handheld device that uses infrared technology to quantify pupil size and rate of reactivity to light as well as a number of other parameters.

(b) Application: Demonstrates trends in pupil sizes and reactivity in neurologic injury and illness

(c) Clinical uses: Supplements subjective observation of pupillary reactivity. Trend changes in pupil size and reactivity may reflect intracranial pathology.

(d) Advantages: Noninvasive and objective

(e) Disadvantages: The Neurologic Pupil index (NPi) is a proprietary parameter that is not fully described.

xi. Cerebral microdialysis

(a) Principle: A catheter with a semipermeable membrane is placed in the interstitial (extracellular) tissue of the brain; isotonic fluid similar in composition to the interstitial fluid is perfused in the catheter's semipermeable membrane. This allows molecules of greater concentration in the interstitial fluid to flow into the catheter for sampling. Samples are collected in a microvial and analyzed with a calibrated bedside microdialysis machine as often as hourly.

(b) Application: Primarily research; measures biomarkers that reflect brain injury, hypoxia/ischemia excitotoxicity, neuronal dysfunction present in severe intracranial pathology, including lactate, pyruvate, glutamate, glycerol, and glucose

   (c) Clinical utility has not been determined: Used to monitor severe TBI; severe aneurysmal SAH, aneurysmal SAH vasospasm

   (d) Advantages: May reflect changes in neuronal function before changes in clinical presentation

   (e) Disadvantages: Invasive; typically placed adjacent to ICP and $PbtO_2$ catheter; labor intensive, requires trended data for interpretation

   (f) Postprocedure care: Hourly attainment of laboratory samples; obtaining results of laboratory samples with a bedside analyzer; routine calibration of the microdialysis analyzer with known quantities

  c. Appraisal of patient characteristics: Patients in critical care units with acute neurologic problems have conditions that vary in complexity. During their hospitalization, their clinical status may move along the continuum of care from improvement to deterioration in a nonlinear fashion. This potential for gradual or abrupt changes in clinical condition with possibly life-altering effects creates barriers in the ability to monitor life-sustaining functions with precision. Clinical attributes of patients with acute neurologic disorders that the nurse needs to assess include the following: Resiliency, vulnerability, stability, complexity, resource availability, participation in care and decision-making, and predictability.

DIAGNOSTIC STUDIES

  a. Laboratory

    i. Complete blood count (CBC) and differential

    ii. Blood glucose level

    iii. Blood chemistry tests including osmolality, electrolyte levels

    iv. Clotting profile including prothrombin time (PT), international normalized ratio (INR), partial thromboplastin time (PTT), D-dimer levels, fibrinogen levels, prothrombotic states (ischemic stroke), platelet function and aggregation

    v. Arterial blood gas (ABG) levels

    vi. Toxicology screen

    vii. Urinalysis

    viii. CSF analysis: Compare with normal values and request a culture and sensitivity test

  b. Radiologic

    i. Skull series: In the absence of CT scans, skull radiographs may be useful in diagnosing skull abnormalities (e.g., fractures, erosion, penetrating injuries), noting shift of the pineal gland, and detecting intracranial air or abnormal calcifications

    ii. Spine series: Assesses vertebral integrity and alignment to diagnose fractures, dislocations, bony defects, or degenerative processes; CT (Box 5.5) and MRI (Box 5.6 and Table 5.19) often used to further delineate abnormalities

    iii. CT scan (see Box 5.5)

    iv. Perfusion CT (see Box 5.5)

    v. CT angiogram (CTA)

    vi. MRI of brain, spine (see Box 5.6)

    vii. MRA (MRI angiography)

    viii. Myelography, the contrast agent may cause headache and seizures.

    ix. Cerebral angiography

BOX 5.5 Computed Tomographic Studies

COMPUTED TOMOGRAPHY (CT)

Technique
- X-ray beam is projected through narrow section of brain or spine; detectors at opposite side measure attenuation of radiation after it passes through tissues. Readings are fed into a computer that derives absorption of x-rays by tissues in path of beam. Computer-generated images are printed as serial thin slices of adjacent anatomy.
- Hyperdense tissue (e.g., bone) absorbs more x-rays and appears whiter on final image. Hypodense features (e.g., air, fluid) absorb fewer x-rays and appear darker.
- Scan may be repeated after patient has received intravenous (IV) contrast agent to delineate vasculature and enhance tissues where there is disruption of blood-brain barrier.

Clinical Uses
- Brain: Valuable in detection of intracranial hemorrhage, especially subarachnoid hemorrhage, cerebral edema, contusions, hydrocephalus, larger mass lesions, and evidence of probable increased intracranial pressure. Bone windows provide exquisite detail of skull architecture. Limitations include poor visibility of posterior fossa, base of brain, and brainstem.
- Spine: Provides clear look at bony structures to better visualize vertebral fractures, dislocations, degenerative changes, canal stenosis, congenital abnormalities, and surgical fixation; may identify mass lesions.
- CT angiogram: Postcontrast CT scan reconstructed to outline cerebral vasculature. Useful in screening for vascular lesions (e.g., aneurysm, arteriovenous malformation). Sometimes helpful in delineating architecture of aneurysm before surgical clipping or endovascular intervention.
- Agitated patients may require sedation to optimize image quality.
- If contrast enhancement used, assess for allergy to contrast medium, secure informed consent. Patients with renal insufficiency are at risk for contrast-induced nephropathy.

PERFUSION COMPUTED TOMOGRAPHY

Technique
- CT scan performed during IV bolus administration of iodinated contrast material.
- Computer calculations provide measures of regional cerebral blood volume, mean transit time, and regional cerebral blood flow.

Clinical Uses
- Used in acute stroke and other cerebrovascular diseases to identify infarcted and marginally perfused areas.

Periprocedural Care
- Same as for computed tomography.

From Pagana, K.D., Pagana, T.J. (2018). *Mosby's manual of diagnostic and laboratory tests*, 6th ed. St. Louis: Elsevier; Van Leeuwen, A.M., Bladh, M.L. (2019). *Davis's comprehensive handbook of laboratory and diagnostic tests*, ed 8, Philadelphia: F.A Davis.

    x. Spinal angiography: Used to diagnose the source of bleeding, vessel injuries, and vascular abnormalities (e.g., AVMs) in or around the spinal cord. See the description of cerebral angiography earlier for further information.

   xi. Nuclear medicine studies (Box 5.7)

      (a) Radioisotope brain scan

      (b) Single photon emission computed tomography (SPECT): Used in the detection of early ischemia related to cerebral ischemia and also after a seizure to localize the seizure

      (c) Positron emission tomography (PET): Measures cerebral metabolism

 c. Electrophysiologic studies (see Box 5.7)

    i. Electromyography

   ii. Nerve conduction velocity

  iii. EEG

  iv. Evoked potentials

BOX 5.6   **Magnetic Resonance Imaging**

TECHNIQUE
- Magnetic fields and radiofrequency waves create signals that generate an image.
- Factors that contribute to image can be manipulated to emphasize different characteristics of normal and abnormal tissue.
- Gadolinium, a contrast agent, may be used to enhance some lesions.

CLINICAL USES
- Brain: Tissue contrast resolution is superior to that of computed tomography (CT); MRI generally better detects contusions, tumors, infection, edema, subacute and chronic hemorrhage, ischemia or infarction, vascular abnormalities, and degenerative diseases. Better visualizes tissues in posterior fossa, basilar skull, and brainstem; better differentiates gray and white matter. Gadolinium enhances areas of increased vascularity or blood-brain barrier disruption.
- Spine: MRI is far superior to CT in visualizing soft tissues and defining lesions, such as cysts, vascular abnormalities, contusions, tumors, edema, hemorrhage, ischemia or infarction of spinal cord, and degenerative processes (e.g., intervertebral disk disease, stenosis).

PERIPROCEDURAL CARE
- All metal objects must be removed from patient before scanning.
- MRI is contraindicated in patients with metallic implants, such as cardiac pacemakers or ferromagnetic aneurysm clips. MRI safety guidelines recommended for other implanted devices must be followed. Cerebrospinal fluid shunts will need to be assessed for settings and reprogrammed on return from MRI.
- Patient must be able to tolerate removal from metallic life-support devices (e.g., ventilator, intravenous infusion pump) or nonmetallic alternatives may be used during the study.
- Inform patient that he or she will need to lie very still, will be in a small, confined space, and will hear a loud, clunking noise. Patient may need sedation if claustrophobic or agitated.
- Nephrogenic systemic fibrosis may occur with exposure to gadolinium for MRI in patients with renal insufficiency.

See Table 5.19 for other MRI technology.

From Pagana, K.D., Pagana, T.J. (2018). *Mosby's manual of diagnostic and laboratory tests*, 6th ed. St. Louis: Elsevier; Van Leeuwen, A.M., Bladh, M.L. (2019). *Davis's comprehensive handbook of laboratory and diagnostic tests*, 8th ed. Philadelphia: F.A Davis.

---

    d. Lumbar puncture (LP)
       i. Principle: Needle placed into the subarachnoid space below the conus medullaris, usually at L3 to L4 or L4 to L5 interspace
      ii. Clinical application:
         (a) Obtain CSF for laboratory examination
         (b) Measure or reduce CSF pressure
         (c) Administer medication
         (d) Prepare for other diagnostic studies (e.g., myelography)
    e. Brain biopsy

PATIENT CARE

1. **Inability to establish or maintain a patent airway secondary to decreased LOC or impaired protective airway reflexes (e.g., gag, cough, and swallow: see Ch. 3, Pulmonary System)**
2. **Impaired respiratory gas exchange related to respiratory muscle weakness or paralysis, cerebral pathology, or associated neurologic deficits (see Ch. 3, Pulmonary System)**
3. **Myocardial repolarization abnormalities, cardiac arrhythmias because of ANS disruption or catecholamine release (see Ch. 4, Cardiology System)**
4. **Fluid and electrolyte imbalance associated with intracranial pathology secondary to inadequate fluid intake, use of diuretics to treat increased ICP, or disorders of**

Neurologic System

5

TABLE 5.19 Some Types of Magnetic Resonance Imaging Technology and Their Clinical Uses

Magnetic Resonance Imaging Technology	Clinical Uses
Diffusion-weighted imaging	Detects small movements of water; visualizes acute ischemic lesions and cytotoxic edema; useful in the early diagnosis of ischemic stroke
	Enables immediate assessment of stroke-related vasospasm and neurovascular changes
	Differentiates acute from chronic lesions and irreversible from reversible infarction
Perfusion-weight imaging	Assesses abnormally low cerebral blood flow in areas of viable brain tissue, the ischemic penumbra
Fluid-attenuated inversion recovery (FLAIR) imaging	Suppresses signals from certain fluids, such as cerebrospinal fluid, and provides a high signal for brain tissue lesions
	Superior capability in detecting hemorrhage, stroke, infections and white matter lesions that abut the ventricles; excellent for visualizing cerebral edema
Echoplanar imaging	Uses ultrafast imaging technology to assist with diagnosis of quickly evolving cerebrovascular disease
Functional MRI	Detects changes in the brain's oxygen consumption and blood flow in response to sensory stimuli or performance of a motor activity
	Provides functional data in addition to anatomic information for brain mapping and identifying disease, such as brain tumors, arteriovenous malformations, and language lateralization preepilepsy surgery
Magnetic resonance spectroscopy	Provides neurochemical data related to tissue metabolism, including brain pH, levels of metabolites and some neurotransmitters
	May aid in determining tumor malignancy, differentiating tumors from treatment-related necrosis and other brain lesions, and locating epileptogenic foci
Magnetic resonance angiography (MRA)/ magnetic resonance venography (MRV)	Flowing blood affects radiofrequency signals emitted during MRI and these effects are manipulated to create an image of the cerebral and extracranial vasculature; less risk-prone alternative to cerebral angiography, although not as sensitive; assesses patency, stenosis and occlusion of cerebral vessels
	Used for visualizing larger vessels, screening neck vessels for abnormalities (although it typically overemphasizes degree of stenosis), evaluating patency of major veins and venous sinuses, and identifying vascular malformations (e.g., aneurysms)
Diffusion tensor imaging	Measures diffusion of water in the brain tissue to enable visualization of anatomic substructures, particularly white matter fiber tracts
	Can detect disruption or damage to white matter tracts from injury/disease
	Used in the presurgical mapping of brain tumors

From Bautista, C., Livesay, S.L. (2016). Diagnostics for stroke. In J.V. Hickey, S.L. Livesay, editors. *The continuum of stroke care*, Philadelphia: Lippincott Williams & Wilkins; Saindane, A.M. (2015). Recent advances in brain and spine imaging. *Radiology Clinics of North America*, 53, 477–496.

sodium, syndrome of inappropriate antidiuretic hormone (SIADH), cerebral salt wasting (CSW), or diabetes insipidus (DI).
   a. Description of problem: May occur with:
      i. DI: Intracranial pathologic condition affecting hypothalamic or posterior pituitary system can impede or stop the production or secretion of ADH from the hypothalamus or posterior pituitary, respectively, causing diabetes insipidus (Table 5.20; see Ch. 7, Endocrine System).
      ii. SIADH: CNS pathology impairs feedback mechanism responsible for ADH suppression; ADH continues to be released in the presence of normal renal

---

BOX 5.7 Nuclear Medicine and Electrophysiologic Studies

NUCLEAR MEDICINE STUDIES

Radioisotope Brain Scan

Technique
- Radioactive substance introduced into blood before brain scanning
- In some disorders, radioisotope accumulates in abnormal areas of brain, probably owing to blood-brain barrier breakdown or increased vascularity of lesion.

Clinical Uses
- Used to screen for brain tumors and evaluate cerebrovascular disease, some infectious processes

Periprocedural Care
- Radioisotope injected at varying time intervals before scanning. Agitated patients may require sedation.

Single Photon Emission Tomography (SPECT)

Principle
- Rotating gamma camera system detects disintegration of single-photon-emitting radioisotopes, such as technetium-99m, thallium-201, iodine-123, or hexamethylpropyleneamine oxime (HMPAO), administered to patient
- Delineates regional brain perfusion because tracer distribution depends on blood flow

Clinical Uses
- Adjunct measurement or a primary modality if other blood flow techniques not available
- May be used to detect tumors or seizure foci or to determine effects of stroke or brain injury

Periprocedural Care
- Radioisotope may be administered at varying times before scanning. Patient must lie still during study

Positron Emission Tomography (PET)

Principle
- Positron-emitting radiopharmaceuticals of carbon, fluorine, nitrogen, or O_2 administered and gamma rays emitted are recorded by pairs of detectors around head
- Provides high-sensitivity quantitative measurements of regional cerebral blood flow, oxygen metabolism, glucose uptake and metabolism, and blood volume

Clinical Uses
- Identifies abnormalities in brain's functional metabolism that precede structural alterations associated with disease
- Provides information about seizures, tumors, neurodegenerative disease, cerebrovascular disease, and brain injury. Limited availability because of expense of equipment

Periprocedural Care
- Patient should take nothing by mouth for prescribed period before testing
- Study may last over 1 hour and requires patient to lie still

ELECTROPHYSIOLOGIC STUDIES

Electromyography (EMG)

Principle
- Needle electrodes inserted into skeletal muscle record electrical potentials from resting and contracting muscle fibers and display them on oscilloscope

Clinical Uses
- Aids in diagnosis of lower motor neuron disease, neuromuscular junction, and muscle disorders
- Differentiates lesions of muscles, peripheral nerves, and anterior horn cells

Periprocedural Care
- No risk to patient, although needle electrodes can be painful
- Muscle damage from needle electrodes may elevate creatine phosphokinase level postprocedure

Nerve Conduction Velocity (NCV)

Principle
- Large motor nerve stimulated at two or more locations; response is measured in muscle innervated by that nerve. Nerve conduction velocity and amplitude of muscle response can be determined
- Pure sensory fiber may be stimulated and response recorded along course of same nerve

Continued

BOX 5.7 Nuclear Medicine and Electrophysiologic Studies—cont'd

Clinical Use
- Diagnoses peripheral neuropathies and nerve compression or trauma

Periprocedural Care
- No risk to patient, although needle electrodes are uncomfortable

Electroencephalography (EEG)

Principle
- Electrodes attached to scalp are used to record electrical activity of brain
- Amplitude, frequency, and characteristics of brain electrical impulses are evaluated

Clinical Uses
- Most helpful in diagnosis of seizures
- May detect changes associated with space-occupying lesions, infectious processes, dementia, medication intoxication, or brain injury
- May be used to verify absence of electrocerebral activity to support diagnosis of brain death

Periprocedural Care
- Preprocedure care varies, depending on the institution and type of EEG. Verify whether certain medications should be withheld from patient.
- Postprocedure: Wash conductive paste from hair. No risks.

Evoked Potentials (EPs)

Principle
- Electrodes are placed on scalp in locations appropriate for type of evoked response (potential) tested: Brainstem auditory evoked response (BAER), visual evoked response (VER), or somatosensory evoked response (SER).
- Stimulus is applied (e.g., clicking noise for BAER, strobe light or pattern shift for VER, and electrical stimulation of a peripheral nerve for SER) and evoked responses are measured and recorded by computer, which calculates an average curve. Evoked potential latencies and amplitudes are compared with normal responses and compared for the two sides of the body.

Clinical Uses
- Evaluates functional integrity of sensory pathways
- Useful in determining prognosis in severe head injury
- BAER is useful in determining brainstem function
- VER is useful index of hemispheric function; helps diagnose optic nerve disorders
- SER may demonstrate lesions of peripheral pathways, spinal cord, or brainstem
- May aid in detecting lesions, disease, or injury that affects specific sensory path
- May be used during intracranial or spinal surgery to monitor patient's response to procedure

Periprocedural Care
- No specific care needed

From Pagana, K.D., Pagana, T.J. (2018). *Mosby's manual of diagnostic and laboratory tests*, 6th ed. St. Louis: Elsevier; Van Leeuwen, A.M., Bladh, M.L. (2019). *Davis's comprehensive handbook of laboratory and diagnostic tests*, ed 8, Philadelphia: F.A Davis.

and adrenal function and normovolemia (see Table 5.20 and Ch. 7, Endocrine System); a dilutional hyponatremia. Other etiologies for SIADH include medications, pulmonary, and oncologic disease.

   iii. CSW: Excessive sodium excretion with subsequent diuresis associated with acute CNS disease. Thought to be caused, at least in part, by impaired sodium reabsorption from the proximal tubules because of an increase in circulating natriuretic peptides (produced in the brain). As a result, vasodilation, natriuresis, diuresis, and suppression of the renin-angiotensin II-aldosterone axis occurs. Brain natriuretic peptide (BNP) has been found in the hypothalamus; edema, ischemia, or infarction of the hypothalamus may trigger its release. Increased sympathetic nervous system activity related to brain injury or aneurysmal SAH may also contribute to renal sodium excretion, a true hyponatremia (see Table 5.20).

TABLE 5.20 Manifestations and Treatment of Neurogenic Diabetes Insipidus, Syndrome of Inappropriate Secretion of Antidiuretic Hormone, and Cerebral Salt Wasting

Parameter	Diabetes Insipidus	Syndrome of Inappropriate Secretion of Antidiuretic Hormone	Cerebral Salt Wasting
Urine specific gravity	Low	Elevated	Elevated
Urine osmolality	Low	Increased	Increased
Urine sodium level	Low in relation to serum	Elevated	More elevated
Serum osmolality	Elevated	Decreased	Decreased
Serum sodium level	Elevated	Decreased	Decreased
Clinical manifestations	Hypovolemia, dehydration Intensive thirst (if mechanism is not impaired) Large volumes of dilute urine (specific gravity <1.010) Urine osmolality increases in response to administration of aqueous pitressin	Euvolemia or hypervolemia Usually low urine output, low blood urea nitrogen (BUN) level Muscle cramps, weight gain without edema, lethargy, confusion, personality change, irritability, sluggish deep tendon reflexes, seizures, cerebral edema, coma, and death	Hypovolemia, dehydration Increased BUN levels, high urine output, net sodium loss
Treatment	Administer fluid to replace urine output and insensible losses Administer exogenous antidiuretic hormone (ADH): • Aqueous pitressin—often used in critical phase • Pitressin tannate in oil • 1-Deamino-8-D-arginine vasopressin (DDAVP; desmopressin) • Nasal lysine vasopressin	Restrict fluids For severe symptoms: • Give hypertonic saline solution • Diurese with furosemide • Give demeclocycline hydrochloride to produce renal resistance to ADH Vasopressin 2 Receptor Antagonists: conivaptan (Vaprisol); tolvaptan (Samsca)	Replete salt and fluid volume Give fludrocortisone acetate (Florinef) to increase renal tubule sodium reabsorption Do *not* use Vasopressin 2 Receptor Antagonists

From Edwards, J., Lee, K. (2015). Endocrine disorders in neurocritical care. In J.C. Hemphill, A.A. Rabenstein, O.B. Samuels, editors. *The practice of neurocritical care*, Minneapolis: Neurocritical Care Society; Gahart, B.L., Nazareno, A.R., Ortega, M.O. (2020). *Gahart's 2020 Intravenous medications*, 36th ed. St. Louis: Elsevier; Skidmore-Roth, L. (2020). *Mosby's 2020 nursing drug reference*, 33rd ed. St. Louis: Elsevier.

 b. Goals of care
  i. Vital signs and neurologic status remain stable
  ii. Electrolyte levels, osmolality, and intravascular volume are maintained within the desired ranges
 c. Interprofessional collaboration: Nurse, physician, advanced practice provider, laboratory personnel.
 d. Interventions
  i. Monitor vital signs, neurologic status, input and output, and hemodynamics at least hourly until condition is stable
  ii. Monitor serum and urine electrolyte levels, osmolality, fluid balance, and daily weight; report abnormal values; do not allow a sodium increase greater than 8 to 12 mEq/L in 24 hours (risk of central pontine myelinolysis)

iii. Provide prescribed fluid and electrolyte replacements and pharmacologic agents to correct imbalances; observe for any adverse effects (see Table 5.20)

5. **Infection related to invasive lines, monitoring and therapeutic devices, and traumatic and surgical wound**
6. **Seizures: See Seizures under Specific Patient Health Problems**
7. **Potential for gastrointestinal ulceration and bleeding secondary to ANS disruption, stress, lack of enteral nutrition, possible steroid use: See Ch. 9, Gastrointestinal System**
8. **Dysphagia**
   a. Description of problem: Dysphagia can occur secondary to dysfunction of the muscles used for mastication and swallowing or to deficits in CN V, VII, IX, X, XI, and XII involved in swallowing. May lead to aspiration and inadequate oral food intake.

> **EXPERT TIP**
> Weak or absent cough reflex may result in silent aspiration. The cough reflex is a protective reflex. The cough reflex may be temporarily impaired after an anterior approach to the cervical spine and the patient may need a swallow evaluation by speech therapy before oral intake.

   b. Goals of care
      i. Nutritional and fluid intake are adequate.
      ii. No aspiration occurs.
   c. Interprofessional collaboration: Nurse, physician, advanced practice provider, speech therapist, dietician
   d. Interventions
      i. Involve a dietician to identify the patient's caloric needs and the best diet to achieve nutritional goals
      ii. Ensure that swallow function is intact before starting oral food intake; follow hospital-specific nurse initiated swallow screen protocols.
      iii. If dysphagia is present, request a speech therapy consult to evaluate swallow and recommend food consistency and feeding techniques to minimize aspiration risk.
      iv. Until dysphagia resolves (or if oral diet modification is not possible), provide nutrition via an enteral route. In the acute phase, a gastric or postpyloric feeding tube may be used. If dysphagia is likely to persist, a feeding tube may be inserted by endoscopy, interventional radiology, or surgically.
      v. An initial swallow screen or assessment may be performed by the nurse: take precautions to avoid aspiration (see Ch. 3, Pulmonary System)
         (a) If patient is at risk for aspiration related to dysphagia, initiate strict NPO status until patient is evaluated by the speech therapist.
         (b) Keep suction readily available.
         (c) Elevate the head of the bed (HOB) at least 30 degrees during tube feeding unless contraindicated; discontinue tube feedings if head-down position needed.
         (d) Secure the feeding tube to prevent dislodgement.
         (e) Regularly assess for proper feeding tube placement using evidence-based methods, such as external length and radiographic confirmation initially and as needed
         (f) During oral feeding: Have the patient sit up with the head forward; place food on the unaffected side of the oral cavity; encourage small mouthfuls

and thorough chewing; ensure that the mouth is clear of food after each bite; do not leave the patient unattended while the patient is eating; minimize distractions, follow the speech therapist's recommendations, assess the mouth for pocketing and provide oral care before leaving the patient. Maintain upright position after the meal, especially if patient is prone to gastroesophageal reflux or a history of vomiting.

9. **Pain (see Ch. 20)**

10. **Corneal abrasion secondary to impaired corneal reflex**
    a. Description of problem: Impaired corneal reflex caused by CN V (afferent limb), CN VII (efferent limb), or brainstem dysfunction makes the cornea vulnerable to injury
    b. Goals of care: Eyes are protected from corneal injury
    c. Interprofessional collaboration: Nurse, physician, advanced practice provider.
    d. Interventions
        i. Assess corneas for abrasions, irritation, or drainage
        ii. Cleanse exudate from eyes at least once a shift
        iii. Apply lubricant to the eyes as prescribed
        iv. Protect the eyes from injury; in some cases, the eyes may be taped closed or protective shields may be used, avoiding dry abrasive gauze.

11. **Inability of the patient to communicate needs effectively**
    a. Description of problem: Barriers to effective communication may include endotracheal (ET) intubation, decreased LOC, expressive or receptive dysphasia, motor speech apraxia, or dysarthria
    b. Goals of care: Effective communication is maintained so the patient's needs can be met.
    c. Interprofessional collaboration: Nurse, physician, advanced practice provider, speech therapist.
    d. Interventions
        i. Collaborate with a speech therapist to assess the patient's comprehension and expression of written and spoken language and to identify the best interventions.
        ii. Explain the nature of and reason for communication deficits to the patient and family; encourage patience with communication difficulties
        iii. Speak slowly in a normal tone. Use short phrases. If the patient has a hearing loss, speak to the patient on the unaffected side; repeat or rephrase, as necessary.
        iv. Stand so the patient can see your lip movements and nonverbal expressions. Allow time for the patient to respond.
        v. Use alternative strategies for communicating (e.g., gestures, yes or no questions, pointing, pictures, alphabet board)
        vi. Communicate for short periods to avoid tiring and frustrating the patient; be supportive and understanding of the patient's frustrations
        vii. Involve the family in using effective communication techniques

12. **Weakness or paralysis of one or more extremities**
    a. Description of problem: Neurologic disorders can decrease muscle strength, control, mass, or endurance. Loss of motor function leaves the patient unable to perform purposeful activities, including repositioning, transfers, and ambulation. Skin breakdown, contractures, and venous thromboembolism (VTE)/deep venous thrombosis (DVT) may occur as a result. Spasticity, which often occurs in body areas affected by UMN lesions, may also reduce ROM and further impair functional mobility.

   b. Goals of care
- i. Full joint ROM is maintained
- ii. If possible, muscle strength is regained
- iii. Patient demonstrates how to compensate for weakness or paralysis so independence is regained
- iv. Patient exhibits no evidence of complications, such as contractures, skin breakdown, or VTE/DVT
- v. Problematic spasticity is controlled

   c. Interprofessional collaboration: Nurse, physician, advanced practice provider, physical therapist, occupational therapist, pharmacist.

   d. Interventions
- i. Assess motor strength every shift
- ii. Use pressure-relief devices as appropriate
- iii. Reposition the patient frequently if he or she is not on a rotational bed. Assess skin integrity while turning. Maintain functional anatomic alignment; protect bony prominences; keep head and trunk straight to normalize posture and tone and to encourage symmetry.
- iv. Position hemiplegic patients in opposition to spastic adduction and flexion in the arm and extension in the leg.
- v. Position proximal joints (pelvis, shoulders) correctly to reduce tone in extremities.
- vi. Follow the recommendations of an occupational therapist and physical therapist on how to move and position the patient, and use splints, braces, and elastic gloves; teach ROM and transfer techniques.
- vii. If necessary, administer prescribed antispasmodic medication (e.g., dantrolene sodium, baclofen, diazepam).
- viii. Perform ROM exercises to joints; progress from passive to active as tolerated. Do not pull on a paretic limb.
- ix. Encourage progressive independent activity as tolerated; encourage movement toward the paretic side.
- x. Place items within reach of the unaffected arm.
- xi. Involve the family in therapy as appropriate.

13. Sensory and perceptual deficits

   a. Description of problem: Brain pathology can result in a number of sensory deficits, including:
- i. Decreased awareness of pain, temperature, light touch, discriminatory touch
- ii. Decreased vision: Monocular, binocular, visual field cuts, such as homonymous hemianopsia, bitemporal hemianopsia
- iii. Decreased smell and taste
- iv. Decreased ability to respond to internal and external environment: Perceptual deficits (apraxia and neglect)

   b. Goals of care
- i. Patient regains sensory and perceptual function or learns compensatory measures
- ii. Patient responds to the environment appropriately and safely
- iii. Patient maintains adequate nutritional intake (related to loss of smell and taste)

   c. Interprofessional collaboration: Nurse, physician, advanced practice provider, occupational, physical, and speech therapists.

    d. Interventions
       i. Teach compensatory measure (e.g., assess warmth and coolness of objects using extremities with normal sensation; protective positioning of paretic extremities; and visual scanning to compensate for visual field deficits).
      ii. Use intact sensory modalities as alternatives to maneuver in environment
     iii. Reinforce teaching strategies used by the therapists

14. Cognitive deficits
    a. Description of problem: Brain pathology can cause a number of cognitive deficits including the following:
       i. Disorientation to time, place, person, and situation
      ii. Diminished attention span and problem-solving abilities, impulsiveness, poor judgment, belligerence
     iii. Memory loss and lack of sequential thought (e.g., inability to recall events in the order in which they occurred)
     iv. Inability to follow requests or instructions
      v. Inability to recognize deficits
    b. Goals of care
       i. Patient responds to the environment appropriately
      ii. Patient organizes thoughts and uses appropriate judgment to carry out ADLs with minimal assistance
     iii. Patient is able to compensate for cognitive deficits
     iv. Patient does not injure self
    c. Interprofessional collaboration: Nurse, physician, advanced practice provider, speech therapist.
    d. Interventions
       i. In an unresponsive patient, increase environmental awareness by providing familiar stimulation to all five senses. Provide only one stimulus at a time for brief periods to avoid sensory overload.
      ii. Orient to the environment frequently
        (a) Call the patient by name; tell the patient your name
        (b) Inform the patient about time and location
        (c) Provide tools to help maintain orientation (e.g., calendar, clock, newspapers, radio, television, use of dry erase board in room, family photos)
        (d) Keep the patient's items in the same place
     iii. Establish and maintain a predictable schedule
     iv. Provide simple instructions frequently in a calm tone
      v. With therapists, teach ADLs using cues and drills
     vi. Protect the patient from injury (e.g., use restraints only if necessary, keep side rails up and call light within reach, locate the patient near the nurses' station)
     vii. Remove unnecessary or aggravating stimuli; provide prescribed pharmacologic agent(s) to control agitation
    viii. Teach and involve the family in care as appropriate

15. Situational crisis for the patient secondary to neurologic deficits causing loss of control and independence, and a change in role (see Ch. 2, Psychosocial Aspects of Critical Care)

16. Situational crisis for the family secondary to disruption of the usual family roles, burden of care, and concern about the family member's pathologic condition and deficits (see Ch. 2, Psychosocial Aspects of Critical Care)

SPECIFIC PATIENT HEALTH PROBLEMS

INCREASED INTRACRANIAL PRESSURE OR INTRACRANIAL HYPERTENSION

> **KEY CONCEPT**
> ICP may vary between compartments of the brain, such as right versus left hemisphere, and supratentorial versus infratentorial. Increased ICP compromises CPP. Elevation of the MAP with vasopressors may maintain the desired CPP with a slightly elevated ICP and lessen the risk of cerebral ischemia.

1. **Pathophysiology**
   a. Nondistensible intracranial cavity is filled to capacity with brain tissue (80%), CSF (10%), and intravascular blood (10%).
   b. Monro-Kellie hypothesis/doctrine: If the volume of one of the intracranial constituents increases, a reciprocal decrease in the volume of one or both of the others must occur or ICP will increase.
   c. Principal spatial buffers that resist elevations in ICP with volume increases include displacement of CSF from the cranial vault to the perioptic subarachnoid space and the lumbar subarachnoid space and compression of the low-pressure venous system. Decreased CSF production and increased CSF absorption may also contribute to spatial compensations.
      i. The volume of fluid that can be displaced for spatial compensation is finite; when intracranial volume exceeds the amount of fluid (CSF and venous blood) displaced, ICP rises.
      ii. The relationship between ICP and volume can be plotted as a volume-pressure response curve that depicts the effects of increasing intracranial volume on ICP (Fig. 5.22). Flat portion of the curve reflects the phase in which spatial buffers compensate for increases in intracranial volume so there is little change in ICP. Brain compliance, a measure of the brain's adaptive capacity, is high at this portion of the curve. Once compensatory mechanisms are exceeded, the curve turns sharply upward, which indicates that small increases in volume then cause significant ICP elevations. At this point on the curve, brain compliance is low. Patient response to changes in intracranial volume depends, in part, on the effectiveness of the patient's innate compensatory mechanisms or clinical interventions to control intracranial volume as indicated on the volume-pressure response curve.
   d. As ICP increases and approaches the MAP, CPP decreases. When CPP falls below a critical point (<60–70 mm Hg), autoregulation becomes impaired and CBF gradually falls, which leads to cerebral ischemia.
   e. Herniation syndromes: ICP elevations cause displacement of brain structures (Fig. 5.23)
      i. *Cingulate* or *subfalcine* herniation: Unilateral cerebral lesion shifts brain tissue laterally across the midline, which causes distortion of the cingulate gyrus under the falx cerebri.
      ii. *Uncal transtentorial* herniation: Expanding lesion forces the uncus of the medial temporal lobe over the edge of the tentorium.
      iii. *Central transtentorial* herniation: Midline, bilateral, or unilateral cerebral lesions displace one or both hemispheres, the diencephalon, and the midbrain downward through the tentorial notch, which causes midbrain compression; can progress to tonsillar herniation.

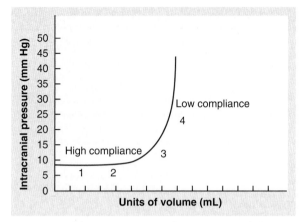

Fig. 5.22 Intracranial pressure (ICP)-volume curve. The concept of the pressure-volume curve can be used to represent the stages of increased ICP. At stage 1 on the curve, there is high compliance. The brain is in total compensation, with accommodation and autoregulation intact. An increase in volume (brain tissue, blood, or cerebrospinal fluid) does not increase the ICP. At stage 2, the compliance is beginning to decrease, and an increase in volume places the patient at risk of increased ICP and secondary injury. At stage 3, there is significant reduction in compliance. Any small addition of volume causes a great increase in ICP. Compensatory mechanisms fail, there is a loss of autoregulation, and the patient exhibits manifestations of increased ICP (e.g., headache, changes in level of consciousness or pupil responsiveness). With a loss of autoregulation, the body attempts to maintain cerebral perfusion by increasing systolic BP. However, decompensation is imminent. The patient's response is characterized by systolic hypertension with a widening pulse pressure, bradycardia with a full and bounding pulse, and altered respirations. This is known as Cushing's triad and is a neurologic emergency. As the patient enters stage 4, the ICP rises to lethal levels with little increase in volume. Herniation occurs as the brain tissue is forcibly shifted from the compartment of greater pressure to a compartment of lesser pressure. In this situation, intense pressure is placed on the brainstem, and if herniation continues, brainstem death is imminent. (From Lewis, S.L., Bucher, L., Heitkemper, M.M., et al. (2017). *Medical-surgical nursing: assessment and management of clinical problems*, 10th ed. St. Louis: Elsevier.)

    iv. *Tonsillar* herniation: Posterior fossa contents, particularly the cerebellar tonsils, are displaced through the foramen magnum, which causes brainstem distortion.

    v. *Upward transtentorial* herniation: The cerebellum herniates upward when the pressure in the infratentorial space is greater than the pressure in the supratentorial space.

    vi. *Transcalvarial* herniation: Brain protrudes out of a cranial defect, such as a fracture or decompressive craniectomy (surgical site in which the bone is removed).

2. Etiology and risk factors

  a. Rate and extent of ICP elevation depends on

    i. Amount of volume (blood, brain, and/or CSF) increase

    ii. Rate of volume change (e.g., the faster the volume increases, the greater the rise in ICP)

    iii. Total volume within the intracranial cavity

    iv. Intracranial compliance (e.g., the capacity for compensation)

  b. Increases in brain volume are caused by:

    i. Mass lesions: Any space-occupying lesion

      (a) Hematomas: Subdural, epidural, intracerebral

      (b) Abscesses

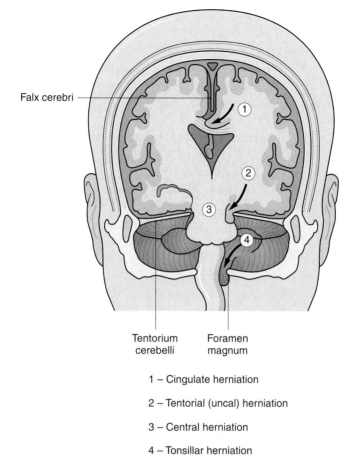

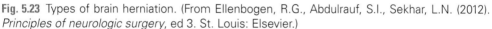

Falx cerebri

Tentorium
cerebelli

Foramen
magnum

1 – Cingulate herniation

2 – Tentorial (uncal) herniation

3 – Central herniation

4 – Tonsillar herniation

Fig. 5.23 Types of brain herniation. (From Ellenbogen, R.G., Abdulrauf, S.I., Sekhar, L.N. (2012). *Principles of neurologic surgery*, ed 3. St. Louis: Elsevier.)

    (c) Tumors: May be spherical, well delineated, and encapsulated or diffuse and infiltrating masses. May enlarge because of cell proliferation, necrosis, edema, or hemorrhage. Cause neurologic symptoms because of compression, invasion, or destruction of brain tissue.

  ii. Cytotoxic edema (intracellular edema): Intracellular swelling of neurons, glia, and endothelial cells, in gray and white matter, caused by cellular hypoxia or acute hypoosmolality (water intoxication). Hypoxia depletes cellular ATP and breaks down the ATP-dependent sodium-potassium pump in the cell membrane, which leads to intracellular accumulation of sodium and water and cellular swelling. Acute extracellular hypoosmolality causes water to move into the cell via osmosis. Seen in early stages of infarction.

 iii. Vasogenic cerebral edema: Direct or hypoxic injury, severe hypertension, endotoxins, or inflammatory mediators break down the BBB; this allows osmotically active molecules such as proteins to leak into the interstitium, which draws water from the vascular system and cells into the interstitial space. Seen around late states of infarction, contusions, tumors, or abscesses or generalized, as with meningitis or diffuse brain injury.

 iv. Interstitial edema: High intraventricular pressure (e.g., obstructive or communicating hydrocephalus) causes fluid to extravasate into tissues around the ventricles.

c. Increases in cerebral blood volume (CBV) may be caused by:

   i. Venous outflow obstruction

     (a) Head rotation, neck hyperextension or hyperflexion, or a tight cervical collar or tracheal tube securement device can compress the jugular veins, diminish venous return, and cause venous engorgement.

     (b) Thrombus or another venous lesion may block the outflow of intracranial blood.

     (c) Raised intrathoracic and/or intraabdominal pressure may impede venous return.

   ii. Hyperemia: CBF exceeds metabolic demand.

     (a) Increased ICP can reduce CPP and CBF, causing vasodilation, increasing CBV, and further elevating ICP.

     (b) Autoregulation may be impaired, globally or regionally, by cerebral injury or insult. When impaired, arterioles passively dilate with elevated arterial BP, increasing CBF and CBV.

     (c) BP that exceeds the limits of autoregulation can increase CBV.

     (d) Increased $PaCO_2$ and PaO_2 lower than 60 mm Hg cause cerebral vasodilatation, resulting in greater CBF.

     (e) Certain anesthetics (e.g., halothane, nitrous oxide) and other medications (e.g., nitroprusside, nitroglycerin) cause cerebral vasodilatation, which increases CBV. These should be used cautiously with neurosurgical patients.

d. Increases in CSF volume (hydrocephalus)

   i. Increased production of CSF (an uncommon cause)

   ii. Decreased reabsorption of CSF

     (a) Obstruction of CSF circulation (see Fig. 5.11) because of a mass lesion, edema, hemorrhage, or inflammatory process in or near the ventricular system or on the convexity of the brain blocking the subarachnoid space (*noncommunicating hydrocephalus*)

     (b) Impaired reabsorption of CSF from the subarachnoid space into the venous system because of meningeal inflammation or the obstruction of arachnoid villi by debris (e.g., blood cells, infectious matter; *communicating hydrocephalus*)

3. **Signs and symptoms**

a. Change in LOC

b. ICP monitoring data show elevated ICP

c. Clinical presentation may show little or no change if the cause is a slow, progressive pathologic condition (e.g., slow-growing tumor)

d. Papilledema may be the initial sign if ICP rises gradually but is a late sign with acute ICP elevations

e. More commonly, deterioration in LOC; motor strength and movement; pupillary size, shape, and reactivity; cranial nerve function; and vital signs will indicate possible ICP elevations over time. Cushing's triad including bradycardia, increased systolic BP and widened pulse pressure, is typically a late sign or may not be exhibited at all. The respiratory changes associated with Cushing's triad may be inhibited by mechanical ventilation settings.

   i. LOC changes may present as restlessness, agitation, disorientation, confusion, or lethargy, which may progress to less responsive or comatose states, or coma may be evident at the outset.

   ii. Increased ICP can exert pressure on the motor and sensory nerve tracts, leading to impairment or loss of function, usually on the side contralateral

to the compression. Sometimes ipsilateral hemiparesis or hemiplegia is seen if brain tissue is displaced laterally and the contralateral cerebral peduncle is compressed *(Kernohan's notch phenomenon)*. See section on motor function under Patient Assessment for a description of other abnormal motor responses.
  iii. Pupil abnormalities are described in Table 5.17.
  iv. Other cranial nerve abnormalities: Cranial nerves involving extraocular movements, III, IV, and VI (especially), may be impaired with increased ICP, as well as occasionally cranial nerve VII (facial). The impaired extraocular movements (EOMs) may manifest as impaired lateral gaze. Dysconjugate gaze or diplopia.
  v. See also section on vital signs under Patient Assessment
  f. Other findings suggesting ICP elevation must be evaluated in light of the history and clinical presentation
  i. Increasing headache, blurred vision
  ii. Seizures
  iii. Vomiting: May result from lesions that involve the vestibular nuclei, impinge on the floor of the fourth ventricle, or produce medullary compression. The vomit center of the brain is in the medulla.
  iv. Hiccups: May result from brainstem compression, the medulla, and vagal nerve
  v. Abnormal respiratory patterns (see Table 5.18)
4. **Diagnostic study findings**
  a. CT scan: Brain CT without contrast shows indications of mass effect and probable increased ICP.
  i. Shift of the ventricles and falx away from the mass
  ii. Effacement (visual obliteration) of the sulci and ventricles
  iii. Compressed or absent basal cisterns
  b. ICP monitoring: Direct measurement of ICP
  i. Indications: Patients who present with:
      (a) Severe TBI (GCS score ≤8) and abnormal admission CT scan of the head; an abnormal CT consists of the presence of contusions, hematomas, swelling, herniation, or compressed basal cisterns
      (b) Severe TBI (GCS score ≤8) with a normal CT scan of the head on admission but with 2 or more of the of the following clinical features: Age older than 40 years, unilateral or bilateral motor posturing, or a systolic BP less than 90 mm Hg
  ii. External strain gauge transducers are commonly used when monitoring ICP; the placement of an external ventricular drain into one of the lateral ventricles with the catheter attached to an external strain gauge transducer and CSF drainage system is the most common form of ICP monitoring in the United States (Fig. 5.24).
  iii. Normal ICP is 0 to 15 mm Hg. Thresholds for treating sustained ICP elevations vary, but 20 to 25 mm Hg is the upper limit beyond which intervention is recommended in patients with TBI. Pressure variations may exist between different intracranial compartments (e.g., supratentorial and infratentorial regions). Patients vary in the tolerance to ICP parameters. CPP should consistently be considered in conjunction with ICP.
  iv. ICP waveform is produced by vascular (primarily arterial) pulsations (Fig. 5.25). The ICP waveform may also reflect venous and respiratory input. Normal ICP waveform has three characteristic peaks of decreasing amplitude:
      (a) P_1 (percussion wave) has a fairly consistent amplitude.

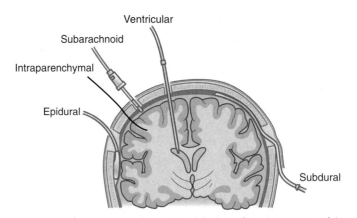

Fig. 5.24 Coronal section of brain showing potential sites for placement of intracranial pressure monitoring devices. (From Harding, M.M., Kwong, J., Roberts, D., et al. (2020). *Lewis's medical-surgical nursing: assessment and management of clinical problems*, 11th ed. St. Louis: Elsevier.)

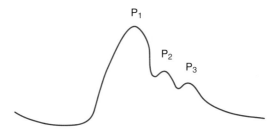

Fig. 5.25 Components of the intracranial pressure wave. (From McQuillan, K.A., Makic, M.B.F. (2020). *Trauma nursing: From resuscitation through rehabilitation*, 5th ed. St. Louis: Elsevier.)

   (b) P_2 (tidal wave) has variable amplitude.
   (c) P_3 (dicrotic wave) tapers to baseline.
   v. Different intracranial conditions can alter the waveform configuration. Elevated P_2 (P_2 of greater amplitude than P_1) is thought to reflect reduced brain compliance and impaired autoregulation, which indicates a greater likelihood that the patient's ICP will sustain an exaggerated increase in response to stimuli (e.g., turning, coughing). However, elevation of P_2 does not consistently reflect a deterioration in neurologic status.

> **EXPERT TIP**
> Often, only a P_1 and P_2 component of the ICP waveform are seen. Occasionally, a P_4 may be seen. Elevation of P_2 of greater amplitude than P1 does not consistently reflect decreased compliance.

   vi. ICP monitoring has not been conclusively proven to improve patient outcomes. The patient's clinical presentation may reflect deterioration before ICP monitoring.
5. **Goals of care**
   a. ICP remains below 20 to 22 mm Hg, CPP remains 60 to 70 mm Hg or as ordered, and, if monitored, cerebral oxygenation ($PbtO_2$, SjO_2, or rSO_2) or CBF remains within the desired range.
   b. No complications occur as a result of ICP monitoring.
   c. Patient's neurologic status improves.

6. **Interprofessional collaboration: Nurse, physician, advanced practice provider, pharmacist, respiratory therapist.**
7. **Management of patient care**
   a. Anticipated patient trajectory: As the volume in the intracranial compartment is reduced, the patient's ICP will decrease to within normal levels, and recovery from the precipitating event will run its course.
      i. Positioning
         (a) Facilitate venous return.
            (1) Elevate the HOB to a level that minimizes ICP and optimizes CPP (and, if monitored, CBF and oxygenation), usually 30 degrees
            (2) Avoid hyperextension, flexion, or rotation of the head and neck
            (3) Ensure that the tracheal tube securement devices are not wrapped too tightly around the head or neck
            (4) If a cervical collar is used, ensure proper fit and placement
         (b) Avoid sharp hip flexion
         (c) With each patient position change, ensure that the external transducer and intraventricular catheter drainage chamber are appropriately positioned.
      ii. Pain management: Short-acting or easily reversible analgesics (e.g., morphine sulfate, fentanyl) may be used to control pain and reduce ICP. Give cautiously to patients not on a ventilator; avoid causing hypotension; monitor effectiveness of analgesia.
      iii. Seizure control: Prophylactic antiepileptic medications (AEMs) are not routinely recommended. However, if a seizure occurs, the seizure may increase ICP.
      iv. Normothermia; no shivering during temperature management

---

EXPERT TIP

Shivering increases the metabolic demand and may increase ICP and risk of secondary neuronal injury. Normothermia is more effectively achieved in the absence of shivering.

---

      v. Infection control: Strict sterile technique, including face mask, must be used during monitor insertion and when accessing the intraventricular catheter system (e.g., to obtain CSF specimens) or zero-balancing an external strain-gauge system.
      vi. CSF drainage: Overdrainage may result in increased headache, formation of subdural hematoma, pneumocephalus, or herniation. In general, drainage of 20 mL/h is safe (~22 mL/h is made hourly). There are no randomized trials demonstrating a sustained benefit from CSF drainage. Sustained elevations in ICP may require pharmacotherapy (e.g., mannitol or hypertonic saline) or surgical intervention (hemicraniectomy).
      vii. ICP/CPP measurement: Maintain an ICP monitoring system with an external strain-gauge system and CSF drainage reference at a consistent anatomic reference point (e.g., external auditory meatus, tragus). To ensure accuracy in ICP monitoring, turn the drainage system off to the ventricular drain before determining the ICP. A corresponding waveform should be present when documenting the ICP.
      viii. Transport: Ensure that the ventriculostomy system is properly leveled or turned off to drainage during transport to prevent excessive CSF outflow. A ventriculostomy remaining open during transport must be continuously monitored to avoid overdrainage. Zero-balance external strain-gauge system again after moving the patient.
      ix. Pharmacology (Box 5.8)

BOX 5.8 Pharmacologic Management of Increased Intracranial Pressure

- Supplemental oxygen: To prevent hypoxia and insufficient cerebral oxygen delivery, which can cause or worsen brain ischemia and increase increased intracranial pressure (ICP).
- Prescribed fluids: To maintain euvolemic state, normal electrolyte levels, and desired cerebral perfusion pressure (CPP) (usually 50–70 mm Hg). Typically, isotonic crystalloids (e.g., normal saline) are administered. Hypotonic and glucose-containing solutions are generally avoided. Hypertonic saline solutions, and, if indicated, blood products may also be used.
- Vasoactive and inotropic agents: May be used to support blood pressure and CPP once hemodynamic parameters confirm that patient is euvolemic.
- Analgesia and sedation management: May be effective in reducing ICP, in restless or agitated patients. Short-acting or easily reversible agents preferred (e.g., midazolam, propofol, dexmedetomidine). Other physiologic causes of agitation that require different treatment (e.g., hypoxia, electrolyte imbalance) should be ruled out. Sedation should be given cautiously if patient is not on ventilator support. Hypotension is to be avoided.
- Neuromuscular blocking agents (e.g., vecuronium, atracurium, cisatracurium, vecuronium): along with sedation may be used to lower ICP if other therapies (e.g., cerebrospinal fluid drainage, sedation) are ineffective and patient is still agitated, has increased muscle tone, resists ventilator, or is shivering. Neuromuscular blocking agents do not stop EEG-documented seizure activity.
- Diuretics: Ensure adequate hydration before administration; replace fluids to avoid dehydration and hypotension resulting in a low CPP.
  Mannitol: Osmotic diuretic administered as bolus (0.25–1.0 g/kg) to reduce ICP by creating osmotic gradient that pulls fluid from brain tissue into the intravascular space; expands plasma volume, which reduces blood viscosity. A serum osmolality above 310–320 mmol/osm should be avoided to minimize risk of mannitol-induced renal failure.
  Loop diuretics (e.g., furosemide, acetazolamide): May lower ICP by reducing sodium and water transport into brain, causing diuresis, and decreasing cerebrospinal fluid production
- Hypertonic saline solutions lower ICP by pulling interstitial fluid from brain tissue into intravascular space, expanding intravascular volume, and may modify injury-induced inflammatory response. Hypertonic saline concentrations of 2% or 3% are given as continuous infusions. Hypertonic saline 23.4% is given as a 30-mL bolus over 15–30 minutes. A central venous catheter is recommended for concentrations of 3% or greater. The serum sodium is monitored every 4–6 hours.
- High-dose barbiturates (commonly pentobarbital [Nembutal] or propofol [Diprivan]) are used to induce therapeutic coma for refractory intracranial hypertension. High dose barbiturates and propofol lower ICP by suppressing cerebral metabolism to decrease CBF and volume, inhibiting free radical-mediated lipid peroxidation, and altering vascular tone.
  Administration: Ensure patient is euvolemic and hemodynamically stable before initiating therapy. Typical loading dosage for pentobarbital is 3–10 mg/kg intravenously (IV) over 30 minutes to 3 hours, followed by an infusion of 0.5 mg/kg/h to 3 mg/kg/h maintenance.
  Propofol dosage is 10 mcg/kg/min IV, then titration to desired effect. Doses up to 200 mcg/kg/min have been recommended for therapeutic coma.
  Monitoring: Closely monitor hemodynamic status. Vasopressors often required to maintain blood pressure and CPP. Monitor EEG; titrate pentobarbital or propofol to achieve burst suppression on continuous EEG; 80% burst suppression frequently prescribed.
  Potential side effects: Hypotension and myocardial depression are of particular concern because they can further compromise CPP and lead to cardiovascular collapse.
- Glucocorticoids: Not recommended for reducing ICP or improving outcome in traumatic brain injury or stroke; may be used to reduce edema and ICP associated with intracranial tumors, spinal cord tumors, and bacterial meningitis.

From Human, T., Tesoro, E., Peacock, S. (2020). Pharmacotherapy pearls for emergency neurologic life support. *Emergency Neurologic Life Support Version 4.0* (pp. 196–218). Chicago, Neurocritical Care Society; Gahart, B.L., Nazareno, A.R., Ortega, M.O. (2020). *Intravenous medications*, ed 36. St. Louis: Elsevier; Harring, T.R., Deal, N.S., Kuo, D.C. (2014). Disorders of sodium and water balance. *Emergency Medical Clinics of North America*, 32(2), 379-401; Elsevier; Skidmore-Roth, L. (2020). *Mosby's 2020 nursing drug reference*, 33rd ed. St. Louis: Elsevier.

    x. Skin care: Provide meticulous care to prevent breakdown in patients with sensory or motor deficits

    xi. Psychosocial issues: Research findings are inconsistent. Family presence may reduce or may increase ICP. Help alleviate the family's fear and anxiety by providing information and encouraging the use of appropriate coping mechanisms and support systems

    xii. Treatments

(a) Noninvasive
  (1) Eliminate any unnecessary noxious stimuli that may elevate ICP.
  (2) Maintain normothermia. Use antipyretic agents and other cooling methods to reduce hyperthermia, which increases the CMR. An increase in body temperature of 1.8° F (1° C) increases the CMR 5% to 10%, and thereby raises ICP. Also avoid shivering which increases the cerebral metabolic requirements and may result in increased ICP and secondary ischemia. Controlled temperature management with hypothermia may be used in refractory increased ICP when other options have been exhausted.
  (3) Note the effects of various interventions (e.g., suctioning) on ICP, CPP, and other parameters. If the patient evidences poor brain compliance, provide prescribed sedation before performing interventions or space activities to minimize ICP elevations.
  (4) Suction only when clinically indicated to avoid excessive ICP elevations; limit the number of suction catheter passes (1 or 2 times); pass the catheter for 10 seconds or less; hyperoxygenate with 100% fraction of inspired oxygen (FiO_2); may require sedative, or neuromuscular blocking agent before procedure.
  (5) Hyperventilation causes vasoconstriction, reducing CBF and CBV, which lowers ICP. However, lowering the $PaCO_2$, reduces CBF and exacerbates cerebral ischemia. Decrease $PaCO_2$ only in an emergent (e.g., central herniation) situation or in conjunction with advanced monitoring ($PbtO_2$, SjO2, rSO_2, CBF).
  (6) Maintain normoglycemia. Hypoglycemia or hyperglycemia can worsen cerebral edema and outcome from brain insult.
  (7) Decompress the gut and bladder to prevent increased intraabdominal pressure, which can raise ICP.
  (8) Avoid patient straining, coughing, vomiting or using the Valsalva maneuver, which raises ICP via increased intrathoracic pressure and impeding of cerebrovenous outflow; a bowel regimen with stool softener may help.
(b) Invasive
  (1) ET intubation and ventilatory support may be required for adequate ventilation.
  (2) Intracranial monitoring (see ICP Monitoring under Diagnostic Study Findings): Assess neurologic status, ICP, CPP, CBF, and oxygenation parameters (SaO_2, SpO_2, $PbtO_2$, SjO_2, and CBF as available) and record hourly and when changes occur. Consider all intracranial and extracranial parameters (e.g., vital signs, ABG levels) in treatment decisions. Notify the physician if parameters are outside the acceptable range. If the ICP waveform dampens, readings may be inaccurate. Troubleshoot the monitoring system when changes occur in waveform, readings, or drainage; notify the neurosurgeon if the problem cannot be rectified. Secure the monitoring device to the patient to prevent dislodgement.
  (3) CSF drainage: Drain continuously or intermittently as ordered; ensure that the air-fluid interface is properly positioned at the prescribed level at or above the foramen of Monro. Close the drainage system to obtain accurate ICP readings. Note the character and volume of drainage

at least hourly. Notify the physician if there is no CSF drainage or excessive drainage, or if drainage character changes (e.g., more bloody or cloudy).

    (4) Surgical interventions to reduce ICP

        a) Removal of a mass lesion, débridement of necrotic brain tissue, resection of a portion of the brain

        b) Unilateral or bilateral decompressive craniectomy (e.g., removal of a portion of the cranium and opening of the dura) allows room for the edematous brain to control refractory ICP elevations. (Patient will need protective helmet when ICP stabilized and patient mobilizing before return of the bone flap to the remaining cranium.)

        c) Placement of a ventricular shunt for long-term CSF removal

    xiii. Ethical issues: May discuss halting further treatment or withdrawing therapy with the family when the patient has refractory ICP elevations and concurrent findings that indicate a poor prognosis

  b. Potential complications

    i. Intracranial infection: Meningitis, ventriculitis, abscess

      (a) Mechanism: ICP monitoring devices and surgical interventions provide an entry portal for organisms

      (b) Management: See Infection Control under Management of Patient Care earlier and Intracranial Infections: Bacterial Meningitis and Intracranial Infections including encephalitis and brain abscess

    ii. Hemorrhage at ICP monitor insertion site

      (a) Mechanism: Disruption of blood vessels during insertion of ICP monitor

      (b) Management: Normalize coagulation parameters before ICP monitor placement. Monitor neurologic status closely before and after insertion; notify the physician of changes in neurologic status. CT scan can identify hemorrhage; surgical evacuation of hematoma may be necessary.

    iii. Brain ischemia and death

      (a) Mechanism: Uncontrolled intracranial hypertension compromises CPP and CBF leading to brain ischemia; irreversible brain death ensues when CBF ceases. Organ donation is a consideration with brain death. See Brain Death section.

      (b) Management: Interventions to minimize ICP and optimize CPP and oxygenation to prevent ischemia. Once brain death occurs, the family should be notified and organ donation considered.

STROKE
Intracranial Aneurysms

> **KEY CONCEPT**
> Aneurysmal SAH is one category of stroke designated for management in a comprehensive stroke center. Prevention of rebleed, management of hydrocephalus, securement of the aneurysm, and strategies to effectively treat DCI associated with cerebral vasospasm are key components of care. Administration of nimodipine, induced hypertension with normovolemia to slight hypervolemia, and cerebral angioplasty are strategies used to lessen the risk of secondary neuronal injury from DCI.

1. Pathophysiology

  a. Localized dilatation of an artery resulting from weakness of the vessel wall

b. In adults, 85% occur in the anterior circulation, usually at bifurcations in the anterior circle of Willis. Anterior circulation aneurysms most commonly occur at the bifurcations of the Acomm, Pcomm, or MCA. Common sites in the posterior circulation include the apex of the basilar artery, where the basilar artery bifurcates into the posterior cerebral arteries, extending laterally; basilar artery junctions with the adjoining vertebral artery (VA), anterior inferior cerebellar artery (AICA), or superior cerebellar artery (SCA); and the vertebral and posterior inferior cerebellar artery (PICA) bifurcations.

c. Most intracranial aneurysms are berry or saccular shaped with a neck/stem and sac/dome. Fusiform aneurysms are cylindrical elongated outpouchings of the arterial wall without a neck or stem.

d. Approximately 10% to 30% of patients have multiple aneurysms.

e. Aneurysm growth is not thoroughly understood but is affected by hemodynamic factors and arterial wall integrity. As the aneurysm enlarges, it can compress surrounding nerves and brain tissue, causing neurologic deficits.

f. Enlargement further weakens the vessel wall, so rupture can occur. Rupture most often causes SAH and less frequently intracerebral, intraventricular (common with anterior communicating artery aneurysms), or subdural hemorrhage. After aneurysmal rupture, the risk of an untreated aneurysm rebleeding is greatest the first 24 hours. Aneurysmal SAH is responsible for about 3% of all strokes.

g. Nonaneurysmal causes of SAH
   i. Trauma is the most common cause of SAH (see Ch. 11, Multisystem Trauma). Aneurysmal rupture is the most common cause of spontaneous aneurysmal SAH.
   ii. AVM (discussed later)
   iii. Perimesencephalic SAH is a venous bleed in the basal cisterns anterior to the midbrain of the brainstem. It is typically benign.

2. **Etiology and risk factors**
   a. Etiology of most aneurysms is unclear. Although they were once thought to be caused primarily by congenital defects, research indicates that the likely cause is multifactorial including genetic, hemodynamically induced degenerative changes, localized inflammation, and perhaps remodeling of the arterial wall.
   b. Familial association is a risk factor found in some patients, but causes are not known. Risk of aneurysm-related SAH (aSAH) increases if a first-degree family member has had an aSAH. Risk of aSAH increases with age (highest incidence in 40- to 60-year age group), systemic hypertension, atherosclerosis, smoking, heavy alcohol consumption, and sympathomimetic substance (amphetamines and cocaine) abuse.
   c. A higher risk of aneurysm formation and rupture is found in association with female gender, ischemic heart disease in women, cigarette smoking, and diseases, such as adult polycystic kidney disease and Ehlers-Danlos syndrome.
   d. Traumatic aneurysm: An aneurysm forms as a result of injury to the cerebrovascular wall.
   e. Mycotic aneurysm: Bacterial or fungal infections release septic emboli that attach to the cerebral vessel wall and weaken it.
   f. Atherosclerotic aneurysm: Deposition of atheromatous material damages vessel walls, which causes formation of fusiform aneurysms.

3. **Signs and symptoms**
   a. Before rupture, most patients are asymptomatic.
   b. Large aneurysms may compress nearby brain tissue causing focal neurologic symptoms. Examples of focal symptoms include the following:
      i. CN deficits, especially CN III, IV, or VI dysfunction (pupil dilation, ptosis, impaired EOMs)

TABLE 5.21 Hunt and Hess Classification of Aneurysmal Subarachnoid Hemorrhage

Grade	Description
I	Asymptomatic, or mild headache and slight nuchal rigidity
II	Cranial nerve palsy (e.g., III and VI), moderate to severe headache, nuchal rigidity
III	Mild focal deficit, lethargy, or confusion
IV	Stupor, moderate to severe hemiparesis, early decerebrate rigidity
V	Deep coma, decerebrate rigidity, moribund appearance. Add one grade for serious systemic disease (e.g., hypertension, chronic obstructive pulmonary disease) or severe vasospasm on angiography.
MODIFIED CLASSIFICATION ADDS THE FOLLOWING	
0	Unruptured aneurysm
1a	No acute meningeal or brain reaction, but with fixed neurologic deficit

From Barrett, K.M., Meschia, J.F. (2013). Appendix. Practical clinical stroke scales. In *Stroke. Neurology in practice series*, Sussex, UK: Wiley-Blackwell.

    ii. Pain behind or above the eye
    iii. Localized headache
  c. A patient usually presents for treatment with signs of intracranial hemorrhage (usually SAH) from aneurysmal rupture. Specific signs and symptoms vary with the severity and location of the hemorrhage. Aneurysmal SAH is graded most commonly using the Hunt and Hess scale (Table 5.21). Good outcomes are correlated with Hunt and Hess scores of I to II and worse outcomes with scores of IV and V. (The World Federation of Neurologic Surgeons scale is another tool that may be used to grade aSAH. It combines features of the Hunt Hess and GCS.)
  d. Other signs and symptoms of aSAH
    i. Presenting complaint: "Worst headache of my life" also referred to as a *thunderclap headache*. A sentinel or warning headache may occur if the aneurysm leaks.
    ii. Nausea, vomiting, dizziness
    iii. Usually brief loss of consciousness but may be prolonged if the hemorrhage is large or causes hydrocephalus or brain edema
    iv. Symptoms of meningeal irritation
      (a) *Nuchal rigidity:* Resistance to flexion of the neck
      (b) *Brudzinski's sign:* Flexion of the hip and knee as the examiner flexes the patient's neck
      (c) *Kernig's sign:* Resistance or hamstring pain and spasm when the patient's hip is flexed and the knee is extended
      (d) Headache, photophobia
    v. Cranial nerve deficits (pupillary and eye movement dysfunction)
    vi. Motor deficits (e.g., hemiparesis, decerebrate posturing)
    vii. Alterations in vital signs may be seen
  e. Evidence of intracerebral/intraparenchymal hemorrhage (ICH/IPH) or SDH because of rupture
  f. Evidence of stroke syndrome (see Ischemic Stroke, ICH/IPH Stroke)
  g. Evidence of increased ICP (see Increased Intracranial Pressure)
4. Diagnostic study findings
  a. CT scan (initial study of choice) reveals ICH, SDH, intraventricular blood, amount and distribution of SAH, and hydrocephalus. Density of SAH and risk of vasospasm are graded using the Fisher Scale (Table 5.22). Greater density of SAH, especially

Grade	Blood Seen on Computed Tomographic Scan
0	Unruptured
I	No blood seen on scan
II	Diffuse subarachnoid blood or vertical layers <1 mm thick
III	Dense subarachnoid blood (clot) in the fissures and basal cisterns and/or vertical layers ≥1 mm thick
IV	Intracerebral or intraventricular clot with diffuse or no subarachnoid blood

TABLE 5.22 Fisher Grading Scale for Aneurysmal Subarachnoid Hemorrhage

From Barrett, K.M., Meschia, J.F. (2013). Appendix. Practical clinical stroke scales. In *Stroke. Neurology in practice series*, Sussex, UK: Wiley-Blackwell.

    around the base of the brain, correlates with high incidence and severity of cerebral vasospasm.

  b. CTA

  c. MRI reveals evidence of hemorrhage and hydrocephalus but is not the study of choice.

  d. MRA may diagnose aneurysms 4 mm or more.

  e. TCD may reveal vasospasm/DCI (most often related to cerebral vasospasm).

  f. LP performed in patients with suspected SAH for whom there is no evidence of blood on CT scan and no signs of increased ICP.

5. Goals of care

  a. Brain ischemia is minimized to optimize neurologic outcomes.

  b. Rebleeding, vasospasm with DCI, hydrocephalus, increased ICP, seizures, hyponatremia (from CSW), neurogenic pulmonary edema or respiratory insufficiency, and catecholamine-induced cardiac arrhythmias (stunned myocardium) are prevented or, if they occur, are recognized and appropriately managed.

  c. Patient and family are prepared for interventions, possible complications, and outcomes.

6. Interprofessional collaboration: See Intracranial Aneurysms.

7. Management of patient care

  a. Anticipated patient trajectory: Numerous factors influence the clinical course and outcome, including the location and extent of hemorrhage; the occurrence and severity of complications; age (e.g., cerebral vasospasm/DCI); and preexisting disorders. Anticipated patient trajectory for ICP is also relevant if aneurysm rupture precipitates intracranial hypertension (see section on Increased ICP, especially external ventricular CSF drainage). Other care needs specific to patients with aneurysms include the following:

    i. Positioning: Elevate the HOB 30 degrees, as tolerated, to promote cerebral venous outflow and arterial inflow. Consideration for degree of head elevation must also include CPP and degree of clinically significant cerebral vasospasm/DCI.

    ii. Pain management: Administer prescribed analgesics for headache and surgical incision pain. Short-acting or easily reversible agents preferred. Give cautiously to patients not on ventilatory support; avoid hypotension; monitor effectiveness of pain management.

    iii. Nausea and vomiting: Administer antiemetics as prescribed; monitor effectiveness of antiemetics.

    iv. Attain and maintain normothermia; avoid shivering

    v. Nutrition: Maintain normoglycemia. If LOC or dysphagia precludes oral intake, use alternative methods of feeding early; aspiration precautions as indicated (see Dysphagia under Patient Care).

vi. Fluid and electrolytes: Maintain normovolemia to slight hypervolemia; monitor electrolytes, particularly sodium for decrease related to CSW; manage hyponatremia with sodium replacement (tablets, IV sodium, or hypertonic saline), avoiding increases in sodium greater than 8 to 12 mEq/dL every 24 hours; once goal sodium obtained, wean hypertonic saline gradually and continue to monitor for repeated decreases in hyponatremia.

vii. Bowel and bladder elimination: May require indwelling catheter for accurate intake and output and to avoid retention; bowel regimen to prevent straining and facilitate evacuation.

viii. Infection control: See Increased Intracranial Pressure if a ventriculostomy tube is placed; monitor for infection related to any invasive devices (indwelling urinary catheter, intubation, vascular access, procedural and surgical sites).

ix. Skin care: See Increased Intracranial Pressure

x. Discharge planning: LOC may improve over time allowing patient to be transferred to rehabilitation unit after critical care and acute care stay; otherwise may require skilled nursing facility or home health.

xi. Pharmacology
   (a) Supplemental oxygen to prevent hypoxia and insufficient cerebral oxygen delivery; intubation and mechanical ventilation as needed to prevent hypoxia
   (b) Administer prescribed fluids and antihypertensives (e.g., labetalol, nicardipine) before aneurysm securement or vasopressors (typically phenylephrine or NE) during vasospasm/DCI to maintain BP at the desired level; carefully avoid even transient occurrences of hypotension. In general, before aneurysmal repair, the desired systolic BP less than 140 mm Hg or a mean BP less than 110 mm Hg is desirable to minimize the risk of rebleed; after repair, pharmacologically induced hypertension is recommended for patients with DCI. Goal is to keep CPP above 60 mm Hg. Use measurements from an arterial line, minimally invasive hemodynamic monitors, serial TCDs, CT perfusion/SPECT scans, and clinical presentation to guide therapy.
   (c) IV antifibrinolytic therapy (e.g., aminocaproic acid [Amicar] or tranexamic acid [TXA]) may be administered short-term to lessen the risk of rebleed before aneurysm securement; however, this may place the patient at increased risk for thrombotic complications.
   (d) Cerebroselective calcium channel blocker (e.g., nimodipine) for vasospasm may require changing 60 mg every 4 hours to 3 mg every 2 hours to lessen systemic hypotension.
   (e) Sedation may be prescribed to control agitation, which can elevate BP and ICP.
   (f) Stool softeners may be prescribed to prevent straining, which can elevate BP and ICP.
   (g) Prophylactic anticonvulsants may be prescribed, at least in the acute phase or if seizure occurs.
   (h) Antibiotics may be prescribed for mycotic aneurysm.
   (i) DVT/VTE prophylaxis: Sequential compression devices to lower extremities and heparin or low molecular weight heparinoids after aneurysmal securement

xii. Psychosocial issue: Intervene to help alleviate the patient's and family's fear and anxiety by providing information and encouraging the use of appropriate coping mechanisms and support systems

xiii. Treatments
   (a) Noninvasive

(1) SAH patients in poor neurologic and medical condition may be managed medically until status improves.

(2) Before aneurysm repair, avoid BP elevations, which increase the risk of rupture: Manage pain; have the patient avoid straining and performing the Valsalva maneuver; minimize coughing and vomiting; exercise caution if gastric tube must be inserted; provide a quiet environment.

(3) Before aneurysm repair, administer nimodipine, antihypertensives, and antifibrinolytic agents as prescribed. After aneurysm repair administer nimodipine, antihypertensives as needed and antiplatelet agents postcoiling with or without stenting. Maintain euvolemia to slight hypervolemia

(4) Monitor neurologic status closely and report changes to the physician.

(b) Invasive

(1) Adequate ventilation may require ET intubation and ventilatory support.

(2) Ventriculostomy tube is placed for high-grade SAH (e.g., Hunt and Hess grade of ≥III), hydrocephalus, or increased ICP. Before aneurysm repair avoid CSF overdrainage, which may relieve tamponade on the aneurysm and cause rebleeding.

(3) Cerebral oxygenation or CBF monitor may be placed to assist in management.

(4) Surgical or endovascular interventions may be performed to seal off the aneurysm and prevent bleeding or rebleeding. Early securement of the ruptured aneurysm, within the first 24 to 48 hours after rupture, improves outcome. Once the aneurysm is obliterated, vasospasm and other complications can be treated more aggressively.

(5) Surgical repair

a) Clipping of the aneurysm neck to obliterate the aneurysm. Complications include rupture during placement of the clip, incomplete placement of the clip across the stem of the aneurysm, and trapping of the parent artery which may result in secondary stroke.

b) Aneurysms not amenable to clipping may be resected or wrapped to reinforce the vessel wall; the parent artery may be sacrificed infrequently.

(6) Interventional neuroradiologists may insert devices, such as coils, detachable balloons, and/or stents to occlude the aneurysm. Postcoiling and stent placement; antiplatelet agents will be indicated to prevent cerebroembolic strokes.

(c) Complications of coiling include intraarterial rupture, arterial dissection, coil migration, prolapse, malfunction, or compaction and aneurysm reformation

(1) Selective cerebral angioplasty for DCI secondary to clinically significant vasospasm.

(d) Complications of cerebral angioplasty include arterial rupture or dissection

xiv. Ethical issues: Halting further treatment or withdrawing current therapy may be considered with the family when diagnostic study findings and neurologic examination indicate a dismal prognosis.

b. Potential complications: See Box 5.9; also see health problems under Patient Care

BOX 5.9   Potential Complications of Intracranial Aneurysms

REBLEEDING

Mechanism

- Most common during first 24 hours to 2 weeks after rupture when aneurysm is not repaired
- Peak incidence is first 24–28 hours and at 7–10 days after initial subarachnoid hemorrhage (SAH).
- Typically causes sudden severe headache, nausea, vomiting, and neurologic deterioration
- Associated with significant mortality and morbidity

Management

- Early surgical or endovascular repair is most effective intervention to prevent rebleed
- Any coagulopathy that may be present should be corrected
- Avoidance of abrupt changes in systemic blood pressure and systemic hypertension before aneurysmal repair is recommended. The specific blood pressure parameter is unclear. A systolic blood pressure of <160 mm Hg has been recommended.

VASOSPASM AND DELAYED CEREBRAL ISCHEMIA (DCI)

Mechanism

- Sustained arterial contraction reduces distal CBF and may cause brain ischemia, delayed cerebral ischemia (DCI) or infarct
- Commonly occurs 3–14 days after rupture, but may occur up to 3 weeks (21 days) after SAH
- Incidence and degree are directly related to amount of blood in subarachnoid space
- Neurologic symptoms may not occur or there may be subtle or dramatic deterioration in neurologic function
- Signs and symptoms may include the following:
  - Headache, change in level of consciousness, focal neurologic signs (e.g., speech impairment, hemiparesis), seizures; hypotension and hypovolemia can worsen ischemia and exacerbate neurologic deficits.
  - TCD, usually done daily during the peak vasospasm period after SAH, may detect vasospasm (blood flow velocity >120 cm/s indicates vasospasm, flow velocities >200 cm/s are diagnostic of severe spasm; a ratio of the middle cerebral artery velocity to internal carotid artery velocity (Lindegaard ratio or Hemispheric Index) >3 indicates cerebral vasospasm rather than hyperemia; a ratio >6 indicates severe vasospasm)
  - Cerebral angiography is used to diagnose or confirm vasospasm
  - $PbtO_2$ (brain tissue partial pressure of oxygen) or CBF decreases if the catheter is located in region fed by the spastic vessel; $PbtO_2$ is a local measure of brain tissue oxygenation

Management

- Immediately following SAH diagnosis, a cerebroselective calcium channel blocker (e.g., nimodipine) is given prophylactically to protect the neurons in the area of ischemia and to improve long-term outcomes. Dosage is 60 mg every 4 hours or, if hypotension occurs, 30 mg every 2 hours for 21 days. Nimodipine is to be administered orally or per gastric tube, not sublingual.
- After aneurysm repair, euvolemia to slight hypervolemia and blood pressure augmentation are used to enhance cerebral perfusion. Before aneurysm repair a modified version of this intervention may be used. Fluids, vasopressors, and inotropic agents are used to maintain systolic blood pressure above a pressure at which delayed cerebral ischemia (DCI) related to vasospasm subsides.
- Goals are to maintain cerebral perfusion pressure between 60 and 70 mm Hg. Minimally invasive hemodynamic monitors may be preferable to central venous catheters for hemodynamic monitoring. Therapeutic goals for hemodynamic status vary depending on neurologic, pulmonary, and cardiac status. Neurologic, hemodynamic, pulmonary, and fluid and electrolyte status require close monitoring during vasospasm therapy so that complications (pulmonary edema, heart failure, myocardial ischemia, stroke, electrolyte imbalance) can be prevented or minimized. Hypovolemia has been shown to increase the likelihood of DCI during vasospasm.
- Endovascular intervention may be used to treat confirmed vasospasm unresponsive to nimodipine, and euvolemia and blood pressure augmentation.
  - Balloon angioplasty may be performed to enlarge a stenotic vessel.
- A vascular smooth muscle relaxant (e.g., papaverine [Papacon], milrinone, nicardipine) may be injected into a spastic artery during angiography to relax and dilate the vessel. Effects may be temporary and may cause intracranial pressure (ICP) elevation.

Continued

BOX 5.9   Potential Complications of Intracranial Aneurysms—cont'd

HYDROCEPHALUS

Mechanism

- Clot formation may obstruct flow of CSF, and blood in subarachnoid space may obstruct arachnoid villi, impeding reabsorption of CSF.
- The onset may be delayed days or weeks after SAH.
- Symptoms may include diminished level of consciousness, ataxia, headache, blurred vision, diplopia, nausea, vomiting, incontinence, and signs of increased ICP.

Management

- Initially ventriculostomy tube is placed to drain CSF until ICP is normal and ventricular and subarachnoid spaces are clear of blood. With less acute onset and no concern for downward central herniation, lumbar drain may be placed to remove CSF.
- Ventricular size is monitored with serial computed tomographic (CT) scans.
- If CSF drainage is required to keep ICP >20 mm Hg and the ventricular system remains enlarged on CT scan, a ventriculoperitoneal shunt inserted for long-term management.

INCREASED INTRACRANIAL PRESSURE AND RELATED COMPLICATIONS

- Refer to Increased Intracranial Pressure under Specific Patient Health Problems.

SEIZURES

- Refer to Seizures under Specific Patient Health Problems.

HYPONATREMIA

Mechanism

- Usually secondary to cerebral salt wasting (CSW), true salt wasting.
- May precede or occur during vasospasm.

Management

- Do not allow patient to become hypovolemic as the risk of cerebral infarction related to cerebral vasospasm is increased.

CARDIAC ARRHYTHMIAS AND REPOLARIZATION ABNORMALITIES

- See Chapter 4, Cardiovascular System

Mechanism

- Stunned myocardium and arrhythmias associated with SAH; may be related to systemic release of catecholamines. Patient may develop Tako-Tsubo cardiomyopathy with left ventricular dysfunction.

Management

- See Chapter 4, Cardiovascular System

From Connolly, E.S., Rabinstein, A.A., Carhuapoma, J.R., et al. (2012). Guidelines for the management of aneurysmal subarachnoid hemorrhage. *Stroke*, 43, 1711–1737; Diringer, M.N., Bleck, T.P., Hemphill, J.C. (2013). Critical care management of patients following aneurysmal subarachnoid hemorrhage: recommendations from the Neurocritical Care Society's Multidisciplinary Conference. *Neurocritical Care*, 15, 211–240. (website); www.neurocriticalcare.org/sites/default/files/pdfs/Critical%20 Care%20Management%20of%20Patients%20Following%20Aneurysmal.pdf; Sayona, J., Meurer, W.J., Qualls, S., Edlow, B.L. (2019). Subarachnoid hemorrhage. In C. Venkatasubramanian, G.A. Lopez, K.H. O'Phelan, editors. *Emergency Neurologic Life Support Version 4.0* (pp. 121–130). Chicago: Neurocritical Care Society. From Edlow, J.A., Figaji, A., Samuels, O. (2015). Emergency neurologic life support: subarachnoid hemorrhage. *Neurocritical Care*, 23(Supp 2):103–109; Webb, A., Owens, S. (2015). Subarachnoid hemorrhage. In J.C. Hemphill, A.A. Rabenstein, O.B. Samuels, editors. *The practice of neurocritical care*, Minneapolis: Neurocritical Care Society.

Arteriovenous Malformation

KEY CONCEPT

AVMs may or may not rupture. AVMs may cause ischemic neurologic injury by shunting blood away from healthy brain tissue.

1. **Pathophysiology:** An AVM is an abnormal vascular network consisting of one or more direct connections between arteries and veins without an intervening capillary network. The complex and abnormal tangled mass of vascular channels (neither arterial, venous, nor capillary) between the arterial and venous circulation is referred to as the nidus. AVMs may be localized or extensive; most often located in the supratentorial structures; commonly involving the cortex. Affected vessels develop thin walls and become passively enlarged. A significant number of patients with AVMs also have aneurysms, usually in major feeding arteries. Brain parenchyma between AVM vessels consists of nonfunctional neuroglia. Brain tissue around an AVM may receive insufficient perfusion because of the diversion of blood to the AVM *(vascular steal* phenomenon). High flow volume and increased venous pressure predispose the fragile vessels of the AVM to rupture, most often causing ICH and, less frequently, IVH, SAH, or SDH. Deep-seated AVMs or those that have a deep venous drainage component are more likely to bleed than more superficial lesions or those with a more superficial venous drainage.

2. **Etiology and risk factors:** AVMs are congenital lesions caused by an embryonic vascular malformation. Cerebral AVMs are sometimes found in association with Sturge-Weber syndrome. AVMs may occur as a result of genetic mutations or posttrauma angiogenesis. Signs and symptoms may be caused by the mass effect of the vascular malformation, inadequate perfusion to adjacent brain tissue, venous hypertension, or hemorrhage from the lesion.

   a. An AVM may be found incidentally during diagnostic tests.

   b. Many are not symptomatic until adulthood.

   c. Clinical signs and symptoms associated with hemorrhage into the parenchyma (see ICH/IPH), subdural space, ventricles, or subarachnoid space (see Intracranial Aneurysms) are the most common presentation; other signs and symptoms depend on the extent and location of bleeding.

   d. Seizures: Common presenting sign; more common initial symptom in patients with large AVMs

   e. Headache: Recurrent, unresponsive to traditional therapy

   f. Pulsatile tinnitus

   g. Progressive neurologic deficits; depend on the area of the brain affected

   h. AVMs are commonly graded according to the Spetzler-Martin AVM grading scale (Table 5.23). Higher grade of lesion correlates with increased morbidity with surgical intervention. Other grading scales exist.

3. **Imaging**

   a. CT: Noncontrast scan

   b. CTA

   c. Cerebral angiography

   d. MRI

   e. MRA

4. **Goals of care**

   a. AVM is obliterated without hemorrhage or brain tissue injury

   b. Patient's neurologic status remains normal or improves

   c. Complications, such as hemorrhage, cerebral edema, hydrocephalus, increased ICP, and seizures are prevented or minimized

   d. Patient and family are prepared for interventions, possible complications, and outcomes

5. **Interprofessional collaboration: See Intracranial Aneurysms**

6. **Management of patient care**

TABLE 5.23 **Spetzler-Martin Grading Scale for Arteriovenous Malformations**	
Feature	Grade
SIZE	
0–3 cm	1
3.1–6.0 cm	2
>6 cm	3
LOCATION[a]	
Noneloquent	0
Eloquent	1
DEEP VENOUS DRAINAGE	
Not present	0
Present	1

[a]Eloquent refers to anatomic areas of the brain known to control important neurologic functions, such as the sensorimotor cortex, thalamus, and brainstem.
From Oglivy, C.S., Stieg, P.E., Awad, I., et al. (2013). Recommendations for the management of intracranial arteriovenous malformations: a statement for healthcare professionals from a special writing group of the stroke council, American Stroke Association. *Stroke*, 32, 1468–1471.

a. Anticipated patient trajectory: Numerous factors influence the clinical course and outcome including the location, size, and characteristics of the AVM; the occurrence and severity of complications (e.g., ruptured AVM vs. intact); the effectiveness of interventions to obliterate the lesion; the patient's age; and the presence of comorbidities. If the AVM ruptures, the patient is managed similarly to other patients with intracranial hemorrhage (refer to Intracranial Aneurysms and ICH/ IPH). Morbidity, mortality, and risk of vasospasm are lower from AVM hemorrhage than from aneurysmal hemorrhage. Clinically significant cerebral vasospasm/DCI is less likely.

   i. Nausea and vomiting: Administer antiemetics as prescribed; monitor effectiveness of antiemetics
   ii. Attain and maintain normothermia; avoid shivering
   iii. Nutrition: Maintain normoglycemia. If LOC or dysphagia precludes oral intake, use alternative methods of feeding early; aspiration precautions as indicated (see Dysphagia under Patient Care)
   iv. Fluid and electrolytes: Maintain normovolemia to slight hypervolemia; monitor electrolytes, particularly sodium; manage hyponatremia with sodium replacement (tablets, IV normal saline, or hypertonic saline), avoiding increases in sodium greater than 8 to 12 mEq/dL every 24 hours; once goal sodium obtained, wean hypertonic saline gradually and continue to monitor for repeated decreases in hyponatremia
   v. Bowel and bladder elimination: May require indwelling urinary catheter for accurate intake and output and to avoid retention; bowel regimen to prevent straining and facilitate evacuation
   vi. Infection control: See Increased Intracranial Pressure if a ventriculostomy tube is placed; monitor for infection related to any invasive devices (indwelling urinary catheter, intubation, vascular access, procedural and surgical sites)
   vii. Pain management and nutrition: See Intracranial Aneurysms
   viii. Skin care: See Increased Intracranial Pressure
   ix. Discharge planning: See Increased Intracranial Pressure

x. Pharmacology
   (a) IV fluids to maintain normovolemia
   (b) Antihypertensives to maintain BP in the desired range
   (c) Antiepileptic medications to prevent or treat seizures
xi. Psychosocial issues: See Intracranial Aneurysms
xii. Treatments: May include conservative management, a single treatment, or a combination of interventions. Choice of treatment depends on AVM size, location, and characteristics; the patient's clinical condition, preexisting comorbidities, and age; and the specialization and experience of the physicians
   (a) Noninvasive: Radiosurgery (e.g., gamma knife, proton beam): Uses stereotactic-directed radiation to initiate vessel wall inflammation, which causes thickening (sclerosis) and eventually thrombosis and obliteration of the AVM vessels. Obliterates or shrinks AVMs up to 3 cm in diameter with little collateral damage to normal brain tissue. AVM is vulnerable to hemorrhage until vessels thrombose (takes 1–3 years).
   (b) Invasive
       (1) Craniotomy and microsurgery to resect the AVM: Spetzler-Martin grade 1 and 2 (and some grade 3) lesions usually amenable to surgical resection. Grade 4 to 5 lesions are more complex, have higher treatment-associated morbidity, and therefore may require multifaceted treatment approach.
       (2) Embolization: Flow-directed and flow-assisted microcatheters are navigated through the vasculature to the pathologic area, where a solid or liquid embolic agent is delivered to obliterate some or all of the AVM. May be curative, palliative, or an adjunct to surgery or radiosurgery, preprocedure, to diminish the size of the AVM and reduce the risk of hemorrhage during surgery or after radiosurgery.
xiii. Ethical issues: See Intracranial Aneurysms
b. Potential complications
   i. Rebleeding
      (a) Mechanism: Increased risk for rebleed after initial hemorrhage; causes sudden neurologic deterioration
      (b) Management
          (1) Obliteration of the AVM; treatment is generally elective unless an ICH or SDH requires urgent intervention
          (2) Maintain BP within the ordered range
          (3) Monitor neurologic status and BP; maintain BP within prescribed parameters
   ii. Seizures (see Seizures section): AVM obliteration may reduce the incidence of seizures
   iii. Hydrocephalus
      (a) Mechanism: May occur from SAH, IVH, or compression of the ventricle or aqueduct of Sylvius by the AVM
      (b) Management: See Potential Complications under Intracranial Aneurysms
   iv. Postoperative cerebral edema and hemorrhage
      (a) Mechanism: May result from normal reperfusion as a result of the shunting of high-pressure arterial blood into low-pressure veins. Usually occurs early in the postoperative period; may be complicated by hypertension. Neurologic deterioration, especially a change in LOC, typically signals onset.

(b) Management: Monitor neurologic status and BP; maintain BP within prescribed parameters

v. Hemorrhage or ischemia with endovascular therapy
    (a) Mechanism: Vessel rupture or a thromboembolic event may occur during or after an endovascular procedure
    (b) Management
        (1) Administer prescribed heparin therapy to prevent thromboembolism and maintain coagulation within the desired range. If hemorrhage occurs, heparin reversal indicated.
        (2) See Management under Postoperative Cerebral Edema and Hemorrhage Complication for AVMs

vi. Increased ICP
    (a) Mechanism: Cerebral edema, intracranial hemorrhage, venous outflow obstruction, and hydrocephalus can all increase ICP.
    (b) Management: See Increased Intracranial Pressure

KEY CONCEPT

Effective management of the ischemic stroke patient includes attention to critical time goals, appropriate interventions, and focused aftercare. Delays in care are typically associated with increased risk of hemorrhagic transformation. Hemorrhagic transformation can happen with or without IV thrombolytic agents (e.g., alteplase or tenecteplase) or mechanical thrombectomy. Best practice strategies include maintaining the BP within prescribed parameters and avoiding abrupt changes in the BP.

Ischemic Stroke

1. **Pathophysiology: Approximately 85% of all strokes are ischemic. A cerebral artery becomes narrowed or occluded, interrupting CBF and oxygen delivery and causing brain ischemia in that vascular territory. Lack of oxygen and glucose halts ATP energy-dependent cell functions, which renders neurons inactive. Depending on the degree of CBF reduction, nonfunctional, ischemic neurons may remain viable and recover function. If the energy supply remains insufficient or is further reduced, numerous intracellular biochemical and molecular cascades are triggered (e.g., ionic shifts [calcium influx]; excessive lactic acid production; accumulation of excitatory neurotransmitters [e.g., glutamate]; activation of proteases, endonucleases, and phospholipases; increased free radical formation), which produces cytotoxic edema, disruption of the cell membrane and neuronal death (apoptosis). A core area of brain infarction forms surrounded by a marginally perfused dysfunctional but viable ischemic tissue called the *ischemic penumbra*. Tissue in the penumbra is vulnerable to cell death if CBF and oxygen delivery are not quickly restored or if secondary insults occur (e.g., hypoxia, hypotension, metabolic derangements). Mechanisms include the following:**
   a. Thrombosis (most common cause of stroke)
       i. Atherosclerosis of large cerebral vessels causes injury and plaque formation along the vessel wall. Platelets aggregate with fibrin and a thrombus forms. Progressive vessel narrowing occurs, eventually occluding the vessel or preventing adequate perfusion.
       ii. Plaques may embolize and occlude smaller vessels.
   b. Embolus
       i. Emboli may originate from atherosclerotic plaques in the extracranial or large intracranial vessels; a diseased heart; cardiac arrhythmia (e.g., atrial fibrillation), right to left intracardiac shunt (patient foramen ovale), infection; particulate

matter, fat, or air that gains access to the vasculature; hypercoagulability; or clots caused by vascular injury.

   ii. Emboli usually lodge at arterial bifurcations, where blood flow is the most turbulent and atherosclerotic narrowing is more common. Tiny emboli or fragments may become lodged in smaller vessels.

  c. Small vessel disease (lacunar strokes)

    i. Lipohyalinosis (hyaline-lipid material lines small penetrating arteries, causing vessel wall thickening) and microatheroma occlude small penetrating arteries that perfuse deep cerebral white matter. Affected brain tissue softens and sloughs away, forming a small cavity or lacune.

    ii. Lacunar strokes are most prevalent in the basal ganglia, thalamus, and white matter of the pons and internal capsule.

    iii. Chronic hypertension, diabetes mellitus, and smoking are primary risk factors.

  d. Other less common mechanisms: Hematologic diseases (e.g., sickle cell anemia, polycythemia vera, and prothrombotic states), prolonged systemic hypotension or hypoxia, migraine or vasospasm, arteritis, arterial dissection (spontaneous or traumatic), and infection

    i. Cerebral venous thrombosis (CVT) is thrombosis of the venous sinuses or jugular vein with decreased venous drainage and decreased absorption of CSF. Increased ICP results. Secondary effects include cortical vein thrombosis, cerebral infarct with hemorrhage, and seizures. Etiologies include prothrombotic states, infection, inflammatory disease, oral contraceptives, hormone replacement, pregnancy, and malignancy.

EXPERT TIP

A current management strategy for CVT is heparinization with a therapeutic PTT. Hemorrhage is not an absolute contraindication to heparinization.

---

  e. Cryptogenic stroke are those in which a diagnostic workup fails to identify the stroke origin.

2. **Etiology and risk factors**

  a. Previous stroke or transient ischemic attack (TIA)

  b. Family history of stroke

  c. Age: Risk doubles every 10 years after age 55 years.

  d. Gender: Males have a higher incidence than females but greater stroke-related mortality.

  e. Race: Black Americans have a higher incidence of stroke and nearly twice the risk of death compared with White Americans.

  f. Hypertension, hypercholesterolemia, diabetes mellitus

  g. Hypercoagulable states, such as polycythemia vera, sickle cell anemia, pregnancy

  h. Vascular inflammatory processes, vasospasm, migraine, cerebral artery atherosclerosis, carotid artery stenosis

  i. Cardiac disease: Atrial fibrillation (most common source of cardioemboli), coronary artery disease, heart failure, valvular disease, myocardial infarction, patent foramen ovale with atrial septal aneurysm, left atrial or ventricular thrombi

  j. Behavioral risk factors include smoking, heavy alcohol use, illicit medication use, sedentary lifestyle, obesity, and medication noncompliance

  k. Medication history

    i. Oral contraceptive use, especially in women over 35 years of age who smoke

    ii. Nonaspirin nonsteroidal antiinflammatory drugs (NSAIDs) can interfere with the antiplatelet effects of medications, such as aspirin, clopidogrel, and aspirin with dipyridamole.

3. **Signs and symptoms**

  a. Report of a prior TIA: Ischemic event that results in a reversible, short-lived neurologic deficit. Deficits are the same as for stroke but are short-lived; the highest risk of stroke is within 24 hours of a TIA, so emergent patient evaluation and treatment for secondary prevention are important to avoid a disabling stroke. The ABCD2 scale (age, BP, clinical presentation, duration, and diabetes) score can be used to predict 2-, 7-, and 90-day likelihood of stroke after TIA.

  b. Onset of focal neurologic deficits that correlate with a known vascular territory and persist for over 24 hours

  c. Clinical presentation varies, depending on the area of the brain involved and the extent of injury (Tables 5.24 and 5.25).

  d. Headache may or may not be present.

  e. Spontaneous BP elevations are common after acute stroke, although low-normal BP may be seen with stroke affecting the entire anterior circulation or if coronary artery events occur simultaneously.

  f. National Institutes of Health Stroke Scale (NIHSS): Routinely used to measure neurologic function after acute ischemic stroke. Scores range from 0 to 38, the higher the score indicates greater neurologic impairment. NIHSS score greater than 20 represents severe stroke with poor prognosis. Used to determine stroke severity and to guide decisions about thrombolytic use. (Scale available at https://www.ninds.nih.gov/sites/default/files/NIH_Stroke_Scale_Booklet.pdf) The NIHSS has also been validated in hemorrhagic strokes (spontaneous aneurysmal SAH and ICH/IPH).

4. **Diagnostic study findings**

  a. Laboratory

    i. Serum glucose level, hemoglobin A1C, electrolyte levels, CBC, liver and renal function studies, lipid panel, tests for prothrombic states (e.g., the presence of factor V Leiden, antiphospholipid antibody and lupus anticoagulant; deficiencies in protein C and protein S, and antithrombin III; and increased levels of von Willebrand factor, and plasma fibrinogen): To assess stroke risk factors, identify imbalances that warrant treatment, and rule out conditions that mimic stroke.

    ii. Platelet count, PT, PTT, INR: To check adequacy of coagulation

    iii. Toxicology screen: May identify medication (e.g., cocaine) that precipitated stroke

  b. Radiologic

    i. CT scan without contrast is performed to exclude hemorrhage or mass lesions as the cause of deficits. Ischemia and infarctions are not often seen for 24 hours or more after the occlusive event, whereas hemorrhage is seen immediately. By ruling out intracranial hemorrhage, CT scan without contrast is one component in the identification of eligibility for thrombolytic administration. Ideally, the CT scan is completed within 25 minutes of arriving at the door and the CT is interpreted within 20 minutes of scan completion.

      (a) Alberta Stroke Program Early CT Score (ASPECTS) quantifies the severity of the MCA territory ischemic stroke (Fig. 5.26). Each area of gray white loss deducts one point from the total score. The scores range from 0 to 10;

TABLE 5.24	Signs and Symptoms of Stroke Syndromes Associated With Specific Vessel Involvement
Occluded Vessel	**Signs and Symptoms[a]**
Internal carotid artery	Contralateral face, arm, and leg paralysis and sensory deficits
	Homonymous hemianopsia (loss of half of field of vision)
	Transient monocular blindness (amaurosis fugax) because of retinal artery emboli
	Ipsilateral Horner syndrome
	Headache behind ipsilateral eye
	Dominant hemisphere: Aphasia
	Nondominant hemisphere: Neglect and/or agnosia
Anterior cerebral artery (ACA)	Motor and sensory deficits in contralateral lower extremity with distal weakness (e.g., foot) worse; impaired gait
	Possible mild contralateral upper extremity weakness
	Abulia (slowness to react)
	Cognitive impairment: Perseveration, amnesia
	Apraxia
	Personality changes, flat affect, easy distractibility, lack of initiative
	Urinary incontinence
Middle cerebral artery (MCA)	Contralateral paralysis and sensory loss in arm with leg spared or with less deficit
	Contralateral lower face paralysis
	Homonymous hemianopsia
	Dominant hemisphere: Aphasia, dyslexia, agraphia (inability to express thoughts in writing), acalculia (inability to do simple math)
	Nondominant hemisphere: Constructional apraxia (inability to reproduce or complete a drawing, drawing left half incomplete), dressing apraxia (inability to dress self), loss of sense of spatial relationships, autotopagnosia (inability to recognize parts of body)
Vertebral artery	Wallenberg syndrome (see posterior inferior cerebellar artery)
	Ipsilateral facial weakness and numbness, facial and eye pain
	Clumsiness, ataxia, dizziness or vertigo
	Nystagmus
	Dysphagia, dysarthria
Basilar artery	Nausea and vomiting
	Progressive decline in level of consciousness
	Impaired ocular movement, conjugate gaze paralysis, diplopia
	Pupillary changes: Pupils miotic (pontine) or large and less light responsive (midbrain)
	Facial sensory loss; facial, pharyngeal, and lingual muscle weakness
	Dysarthria, dysphagia
	Alternating hemiparesis
	Pons: Possible "locked-in syndrome" (no movement except extraocular movement; consciousness but cortical function, including sensation, are preserved)
	Dysmetria
	Ataxia, vertigo
	Acute deafness

Continued

TABLE 5.24	**Signs and Symptoms of Stroke Syndromes Associated With Specific Vessel Involvement—cont'd**
Occluded Vessel	**Signs and Symptoms[a]**
Posterior cerebral artery (PCA)	Manifestations can vary widely: • Homonymous hemianopsia; visual deficits—loss of depth perception, blindness, visual hallucinations • Memory loss • Thalamus involvement: Contralateral sensory loss (all modalities), hemiparesis, intention tremors, spontaneous pain • Cerebral peduncle involvement: Weber syndrome (contralateral hemiplegia with ipsilateral cranial nerve III palsy) [a]Midbrain stroke: Parinaud syndrome: impaired upward gaze, presence of downward gaze, and nystagmus
Posterior inferior cerebellar artery	Nausea and vomiting
	Dysphagia, impaired gag reflex and swallowing
	Dysarthria
	Nystagmus, diplopia
	Hiccups
	Vertigo, ataxia
	Wallenberg syndrome (lateral medullary syndrome): Ipsilateral facial numbness and Horner's syndrome and loss of pain and temperature sensation over contralateral trunk and extremities

[a]Some or all of the deficits may be evident when a particular vessel is occluded; syndromes frequently overlap.
From Campbell, W.W., Barohn, R.J. (2020). DeJong's the neurologic examination, 8th ed. Philadelphia: Wolters Kluwer. Hickey, J.V., Strayer, A.L. (editors). (2020). *The clinical practice of neurological and neurosurgical nursing*, 8th ed. Philadelphia: Wolters Kluwer.

no involvement of the MCA territory is 10; 7 or under is associated with a worse outcome.

   ii. CT scan with contrast

   iii. CTA

   iv. Perfusion CT scan: computer software (e.g., RAPID) may be used to calculate the volume of the perfused lesion to the volume of ischemic core. A mismatch of more than 1.8 (volume of perfusion greater than volume of ischemic core) has been used to predict the benefit of endovascular reperfusion.

   v. Cerebral angiography: A modified Thrombolysis in Cerebral Infarction (mTICI) score may be assigned after completion of endovascular therapy as an indicator of reperfusion (Table 5.26).

   vi. MRI

   vii. Diffusion-weighted MRI

   viii. MR angiogram (MRA)

   ix. PET scan

   x. SPECT scan

  c. 12 electrocardiogram (ECG), continuous ECG monitoring

  d. Echocardiogram

  e. Carotid duplex

  f. TCD

  g. LP

  h. Once the patient is stable, additional diagnostic tests to identify the underlying disease that contributed to stroke may be performed.

TABLE 5.25	**Signs and Symptoms of Stroke Syndromes Associated With Specific Stroke Location**
Location	**Signs and Symptoms**
Right (nondominant) hemisphere	Left hemiparesis and sensory loss
	Left visual field deficit
	Right gaze preference
	Dysarthria
	Flat affect
	Spatial perception deficits
	Constructional and dressing apraxia
	Neglect of left side (inattention to objects in the left visual field and to left auditory stimuli)
Left (dominant) hemisphere	Anosognosia (unawareness or denial of deficits on affected side)
	Right hemiparesis and sensory loss
	Right visual field deficit
	Left gaze preference
	Acalculia, agraphia
	Aphasia (expressive, receptive or global)
	Apraxia of left limbs
	Finger agnosia (inability to identify the finger touched)
	Right-left disorientation
Brainstem, cerebellum	Diplopia
	Dysmetria
	Hemiparesis or quadriparesis
	Hemisensory loss or sensory loss in all four limbs and face
	Ocular movement abnormalities
	Acute hearing loss
	Nausea and vomiting, oropharyngeal weakness, dysarthria
	Vertigo, tinnitus, ataxia

From Campbell, W.W., Barohn, R.J. (2020). *DeJong's the neurologic examination*, 8th ed. Philadelphia: Wolters Kluwer. Hickey, J.V., Strayer, A.L. (editors). (2020). *The clinical practice of neurological and neurosurgical nursing*, 8th ed. Philadelphia: Wolters Kluwer.

5. **Goals of care**
   a. Adequate brain perfusion is maintained to minimize ischemia
   b. Optimal recovery of neurologic function occurs
   c. Potential complications are prevented or are recognized and appropriately managed
   d. Patient and family are prepared for interventions, possible complications, and outcomes
6. **Interprofessional collaboration: See Intracranial Aneurysms**
7. **Management of patient care**
   a. Anticipated patient trajectory: Patient's clinical course and outcome are influenced by the location and extent of brain ischemia and infarction; the neurologic deficits that result; the occurrence and severity of complications; age; and preexisting health problems. Specific needs for patients with ischemic stroke in the acute care setting include the following:
      i. Transport: When possible, the stroke victim should be rapidly transported to the emergency department for quick assessment and diagnostic studies. If CT

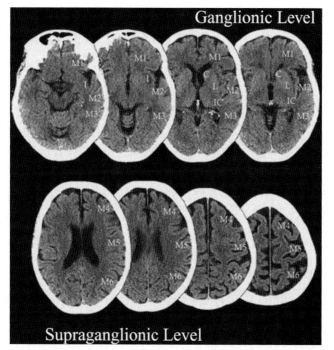

Fig. 5.26 Axial noncontrast head computed tomography (CT) demonstrating middle cerebral artery territory regions defined by the Alberta Stroke Program Early CT Score (ASPECTS). *C,* Caudate; *I,* insular ribbon; *IC,* internal capsule; *L,* lentiform nucleus; *M1,* anterior MCA cortex; *M2,* MCA cortex lateral to insular ribbon; *M3,* posterior MCA cortex; *M4,* anterior MCA territory immediately superior to M1; *M5,* lateral MCA territory immediately superior to M2; *M6,* posterior MCA territory immediately superior to M3. (From Jankovic, J., Mazziotta, J.C., Pomeroy, S.L., et al. (2022). *Bradley and Daroff's neurology in clinical practice*, 8th ed. Philadelphia: Elsevier.)

TABLE 5.26	**Modified Thrombolysis in Cerebral Infarction**
Score	**Cerebral Angiography Criteria**
0	No perfusion
1	Minimal flow past the occlusion with little to no perfusion
2a	Antegrade partial perfusion of less than half of the downstream ischemic territory
2b	Antegrade partial perfusion of half of greater of the downstream ischemic territory
3	Antegrade complete perfusion of the downstream ischemic territory

Perfusion signifies capillary opacification or blush angiographically.
Modified from Yoo, A.J., Simonsen, C.Z., Prabhakaran, S., et al. (2013). Refining angiographic biomarkers of revascularization: improving outcome prediction after intra-arterial therapy. *Stroke,* 44(9), 2509–2512.

scanning is unavailable, the patient's condition should be stabilized and the patient should be transferred to an appropriate facility, preferably an accredited Primary or Comprehensive Stroke Center.

ii. Monitor oxygenation status and report deterioration immediately; maintain SpO$_2$ greater than 94%

iii. Monitor cardiac status for at least 24 hours

iv. Monitor neurologic status and report deterioration immediately; maintain BP within prescribed parameters; too low may be just as detrimental as too high;

BOX 5.10   Recommendations for the Intravenous Administration of Intravenous Alteplase (tPA) for Acute Ischemic Stroke[a]

INDICATIONS (CLASS I: STRONGLY RECOMMEND)

- Within 3 hours of onset of signs and symptoms of ischemic stroke (last known well)
- Within 3 hours of onset of signs and symptoms of ischemic stroke and age 18 to 80 years old
- Within 3 hours of onset of signs and symptoms of ischemic stroke severity from mild but disabling to severe
- Within 3 to 4.5 hours of onset of signs and symptoms of ischemic stroke (last known well) in those patients 18 to 80 years of age, without history of both diabetes mellitus and prior stroke, NIHSS score ≤25, not taking oral anticoagulants, and without evidence of ischemic injury involving one-third or more of the middle cerebral artery territory
- Patient with signs and symptoms of acute ischemic stroke with a blood pressure that can be safely lowered ≤185/110 mm Hg with antihypertensive agents before administration of alteplase
- Signs and symptoms of stroke with an initial blood glucose >50 mg/dL
- Early mild to moderate ischemic stroke changes on noncontrast computed tomography (CT) without obvious hypodensity
- Currently taking antiplatelet therapy (single or dual) before stroke signs and symptoms
- Signs and symptoms of acute ischemic stroke in end-stage renal disease on hemodialysis and a normal activated partial thromboplastin time (aPTT)

CONTRAINDICATIONS (CLASS III: NOT RECOMMENDED; NO BENEFIT OR RISK GREATER THAN BENEFIT)

- Unclear time of onset of signs and symptoms of stroke, unwitnessed onset, and last known well >4.5 hours, including those with stroke on awakening
- Acute intracranial hemorrhage on CT
- Extensive regions of hypoattenuation/hypodensity on CT
- Prior ischemic stroke within 3 months
- Severe head trauma within 3 months
- Intracranial/intraspinal surgery within 3 months
- History of intracranial hemorrhage
- Signs and symptoms of subarachnoid hemorrhage
- Gastrointestinal malignancy or bleed within 21 days
- Coagulopathy with platelets <100,000/mm³, international normalized ratio (INR) >1.7, aPTT >40 seconds, or prothrombin time (PT) >15 seconds
- Low molecular weight heparin within the previous 24 hours
- Currently taking direct thrombin inhibitors or direct factor Xa inhibitors unless aPTT, INR, platelet count, ecarin clotting time, thrombin time or direct factor Xa activity assays are normal or >48 hours has passed since the last dose taken
- Concurrently on glycoprotein IIb/IIIa receptor inhibitors
- Infective endocarditis
- Aortic arch dissection
- Intra-axial intracranial neoplasm

[a]Additional recommendations, class II, not listed here, are of moderate to weak strength.
Modified from Powers, W.J., Rabinstein, A.J., Ackerson, T., et al. (2019). Guidelines for the early management of patients with stroke: 2019 update to the 2018 guidelines for the early management of acute ischemic stroke. *Stroke, 50*, e344–418.

---

    notify provider immediately; monitor for signs and symptoms suggestive of hemorrhagic transformation

    (a) If a thrombolytic is given (IV or intraarterial) or thrombectomy is performed, maintain systemic BP less than 180/105 mm Hg for the first 24 hours, monitoring vital signs and neurologic status every 15 minutes for the first 2 hours; every 30 minutes for the next 6 hours; and every hour for the next 16 hours (Box 5.10).

    (b) If neither thrombolytics nor thrombectomy are used, permissive hypertension up to 220/120 mm Hg is acceptable during the first 24 hours.

  v. Positioning

    (a) Maintain HOB at 30 to 45 degrees to minimize risk of aspiration and ventilator-associated pneumonia, and promote venous outflow. If patient has a critical cerebral artery stenosis that is responsive to a lower position, maintain HOB in lower position. Monitor response to BP at various head of bed positions; maintain HOB congruent with prescribed BP parameters. Get the patient out of bed as early as possible while assessing neurologic status and BP. Collaborate with physical and occupational therapy.

(b) Use protective positioning to protect the patient's extremities on affected side related to paralysis, impaired sensation, and neglect during positioning.

(c) Position patient items in the unaffected visual field initially; gradually moving objects to the affected side and encouraging the patient to attend to that side.

vi. Attain and maintain normothermia; avoid shivering; fever in acute stroke has been demonstrated to worsen outcome.

vii. Nutrition: Maintain normoglycemia. If LOC or dysphagia precludes oral intake, use alternative methods of feeding early; aspiration precautions as indicated (see Dysphagia under Patient Care).

viii. Fluid and electrolytes: Maintain normovolemia; monitor electrolytes, particularly sodium for decrease related to SIADH; manage hyponatremia with sodium replacement (tablets, IV sodium, or hypertonic saline), avoiding increases in sodium greater than 8 to 12 mEq/dL every 24 hours; once goal sodium obtained, wean hypertonic saline gradually and continue to monitor for repeated decreases in hyponatremia.

ix. Bowel and bladder elimination: May require indwelling urinary catheter for accurate intake and output and to avoid retention; bowel regimen to prevent straining and facilitate evacuation; remove indwelling catheter as soon as possible; monitor postvoided residuals for retention.

x. Pain management: See Increased Intracranial Pressure

xi. Communication, cognition, and swallow: Collaborate with speech therapist

xii. Skin care: See Increased Intracranial Pressure

xiii. Discharge planning: LOC may improve over time allowing patient to be transferred to rehabilitation unit after critical care and acute care stay; otherwise may require skilled nursing facility or home health

xiv. Discharge planning: See Intracranial Aneurysms

xv. Pharmacology (Box 5.11)

xvi. Psychosocial issues (see Intracranial Aneurysms): Depression is common after stroke (estimated at 30%–60% of all stroke patients) and if present should be treated with appropriate pharmacotherapy and supportive care. Ensure that the possibility of developing depression is discussed with the patient and family before discharge.

xvii. Patient education: Risk factors pertinent to that patient with emphasis on the modifiable risk factors identified for the patient.

xviii. Treatments

(a) Noninvasive

(1) Monitor neurologic status closely and report changes to the physician

(2) Attain and maintain normothermia; use of hypothermia remains controversial

(3) Initiate occupational, physical, and speech therapy early

(b) Invasive

(1) Intubation and mechanical ventilation may be required for adequate ventilation; monitor oxygen saturation; avoid $PaCO_2$ lower than 35 mm Hg

---

BOX 5.11   **Pharmacologic Therapy for Ischemic Stroke**

- Supplemental oxygen is administered to maintain adequate systemic and brain tissue oxygenation; maintain oxygen saturation (SpO_2) >94%.
- Alteplase (tPA)
  - tPA is a thrombolytic agent that breaks up clot-causing vessel occlusion, thereby restoring cerebral blood flow to ischemic tissues and improving neurologic outcome.
  - Intravenous (IV) tPA administration considered if within 3 hours of stroke symptom onset (e.g., last known well) and patient meets recommended criteria (see Box 4.11); the dose is 0.9 mg/kg to a maximum dose of 90 mg; 10% of dose is given over 1 minute and the remaining 90% over 1 hour via infusion pump. Alteplase may be given up to 4.5 hours based on established criteria and clinical judgment.
  - Intraarterial administration may be beneficial in carefully selected patients who have undergone a major ischemic stroke within 6 hours of symptom onset; caused by an occlusion of the middle cerebral artery. Or for a carefully selected few that have undergone a major ischemic stroke who have contraindications for IV Tenecteplase.
- Antihypertensives are used to maintain the blood pressure (BP) within desired range. Hypotension must be avoided to prevent worsening ischemia.
  - When no thrombolytic agent is used, aggressive treatment of hypertension is deferred unless acute myocardial infarction, aortic dissection, hypertensive encephalopathy, or severe left ventricular failure is present or BP exceeds 220 mm Hg systolic, or 120 mm Hg diastolic; use IV labetalol or nicardipine to achieve BP control.
  - For patients who are candidates for thrombolytic administration, systolic BP must be maintained below 180 mm Hg and diastolic below 105 mm Hg from the initiation of infusion and through the first 24 hours to reduce risk of hemorrhage; IV labetalol, nicardipine infusion, or hydralazine may be used to control BP.
- Isotonic crystalloids without glucose (e.g., normal saline) are prescribed to maintain hypervolemia or normovolemia.
- Vasoactive or inotropic agents are prescribed if necessary to maintain desired BP.
- Insulin is given as necessary to maintain blood glucose level below 200 mg/dL; hyperglycemia can increase infarct size and cerebral edema.
- Antiplatelet agents, such as aspirin, clopidogrel, and extended-release dipyridamole and aspirin (Aggrenox) to inhibit platelet aggregation and prevent recurrent stroke should be initiated once hemorrhage is ruled out. In patient not receiving thrombolytics, initiation of the antiplatelet agent may be purposely delayed 24 hours if tPA is given.
- If the stroke is the result of a cardioembolic mechanism, anticoagulation is indicated. However, anticoagulation may not be started for several days to minimize risk of hemorrhagic transformation. IV heparin or warfarin (oral) may be used for both valvular and nonvalvular atrial fibrillation. The newer direct thrombin inhibitor (DTI; dabigatran) or direct acting Xa inhibitor agents (apixaban, rivaroxaban) are only indicated for nonvalvular atrial fibrillation patients. Serial blood level monitoring with the DTI or Xa inhibitor agents is not available. The newer DTI or Xa inhibitor agents increase the risk of hemorrhage with renal failure.

From Demaerschalk, B.M., Kleindorfter, D.O., Adeoye, O.M., et al. (2016). Scientific rationale for the inclusion and exclusion criteria for intravenous alteplase in acute ischemic stroke, *Stroke*, 47, 581–641; Powers, W.J., Rabinstein, A.J., Ackerson, T., et al. (2019). Guidelines for the early management of patients with stroke: 2019 update to the 2018 guidelines for the early management of acute ischemic stroke. *Stroke*, 50, e344–e418.

---

   (2) Avoid any invasive procedures in patients who are candidates for thrombolytic therapy. If invasive devices, such as an indwelling catheter, are needed wait at least 30 minutes after thrombolytic infusion is complete.

   (3) CBF or oxygenation monitor may be placed to guide therapy

   (4) Interventional radiology

      a) Mechanical thrombectomy using stent-retrieval devices have been shown to be the most effective strategy for clot removal in large vessel occlusions (LVOs).

      b) Angioplasty via balloon inflation may be used at the site of stenosis of a cerebral vessel (typically large vessel).

      c) Intravascular large vessel stenting (e.g., carotid) is used with angioplasty to maintain vessel patency; stents are prothrombotic and will require antiplatelet therapy.

d) Intraarterial thrombolytics may be delivered to the site of the occlusion; efficacy is less than with mechanical thrombectomy and less commonly performed.

e) Thrombolysis in cerebral infarction (TICI) Score: quantifies reperfusion after thrombolysis with alteplase, tenecteplase, or mechanical thrombectomy

(5) Surgical interventions to prevent stroke

a) Carotid endarterectomy removes atherosclerotic plaque and clot from the intraarterial lumen.

b) Extracranial-intracranial bypass (EC-IC bypass) is used selectively to provide collateral circulation for patients with severe major vessel stenosis in Moyamoya disease; the graft vascular may be superficial temporal artery, femoral or saphenous vein, or ulnar or radial artery.

c) Decompressive craniectomy for large territory ischemic stroke (e.g., MCA) to minimize risk of herniation from increased ICP

xix. Ethical issues: See Intracranial Aneurysms

b. Potential complications (Box 5.12)

KEY CONCEPT

Reversal of systemic coagulopathy (if present), BP control, and supportive interventions are key to the care of the spontaneous intracerebral/intraparenchymal hemorrhage, ICH/IPH patient. Chronic hypertension is the most common etiology for spontaneous intracerebral hemorrhage. Posthemorrhage, a systolic BP of 140 mm Hg, systolic is considered adequate to maintain cerebral perfusion yet minimize an increase in the hemorrhage size.

Intracerebral /Intraparenchymal Hemorrhagic Stroke

1. Pathophysiology

a. Rupture of a blood vessel within the cranium. Includes ICH, and IVH. ICH compresses and irritates cerebral tissues, causing ischemic cellular responses, cerebral edema, increased ICP, and CPP compromise. Functional loss and death of neurons result. IVH blocks the outflow of CSF from the ventricles resulting in increased ICP.

b. ICH may occur deep within the cerebral hemispheres, in the thalamus, basal ganglia or internal capsule; in the brainstem or cerebellum; but also lobar.

c. ICH is associated with chronic hypertension; typically involves small, deep penetrating arteries. ICH that is associated with cerebral amyloid angiopathy (CAA) usually occurs in the more superficial cortical arteries.

d. ICH/IPH strokes account for approximately 10% of all strokes.

2. Etiology and risk factors

a. Hypertensive vascular disease is a major risk factor in 60% to 70% of all spontaneous intracerebral/intraparenchymal hemorrhages

b. CAA is the result of β-amyloid protein deposits in small meningeal and cortical blood vessel walls. CAA makes the blood vessel walls more friable.

c. Ischemic stroke with a hemorrhagic conversion

d. Vasculitis, vascular brain tumor, venous infarction (e.g., CVT); use of anticoagulants or platelet aggregation inhibitors; systemic hemorrhagic disorders and diathesis; hepatic failure; disseminated intravascular coagulation (DIC)

BOX 5.12 Potential Complications of Ischemic Stroke

HEMORRHAGE

Mechanism
- Energy depletion and acidosis in tissue surrounding infarction can allow red blood cell extravasation, creating hemorrhagic infarction.
- Risk is increased if thrombolytics, anticoagulants, or antiplatelet agents given or if severe hypertension occurs.

Management
- Hold anticoagulants and antiplatelet agents for 24 hours after administration of tissue plasminogen activator.
- Monitor vital signs and neurologic status frequently.
  - With thrombolytic therapy monitor vital signs and neurologic status every 15 minutes for 2 hours, every 30 minutes for 6 hours, hourly for 16 hours, then every 2 to 4 hours
- The thrombolytic agent should be stopped or held if the neurologic condition changes. Changes must be reported to the physician emergently. The patient should be prepared for computed tomography (CT) scan. If CT excludes hemorrhage, thrombolytics may be resumed.
- Bleeding at puncture sites, sclera, oropharynx, nares, gastrointestinal and genitourinary tracts may occur and must be monitored.
- The BP and coagulation parameters must be maintained within the desired ranges.
- The coagulation parameters (platelet count, prothrombin time, partial thromboplastin time, international normalized ratio, fibrinogen), and complete blood count must be monitored.

REPERFUSION INJURY

Mechanism
- Restoration of perfusion to ischemic tissue causes activation of oxygen free radicals that further injure compromised cells. May occur hours to weeks after initial stroke; new or same stroke symptoms may appear.

Management
- The neurologic status must be monitored closely after reperfusion is established (e.g., after thrombolytic therapy).

SECONDARY INJURY
- Following ischemic stroke, normothermia must be attained and maintained. Fever has been associated with worse outcomes after acute ischemic stroke.

RECURRENT STROKE

Mechanism
- Most recurrences occur within hours to days of first ischemic stroke; highest risk is within first 30 days.

Management
- The modifiable individual risk factors that contributed to the stroke must be identified and treated.
- Antiplatelet and antithrombotic therapy must be administered as prescribed.
- Patient and family education about lifestyle changes are provided specific to the patient's and family's risk factors.

INCREASED INTRACRANIAL PRESSURE

Mechanism
- Cerebral edema (usually peaks 2–5 days after stroke) and intracerebral hemorrhage can increase intracranial volume and pressure.
- Acute ischemic strokes including one-third of the cerebral hemisphere or greater are at risk for massive cerebral edema with herniation. A decompressive craniectomy is indicated.

Management
- Refer to Increased Intracranial Pressure under Specific Patient Health Problems.

SEIZURES
- Refer to Seizures under Specific Patient Health Problems.

TABLE 5.27 **Distinguishing Signs and Symptoms Associated With Hemorrhagic Stroke**

Deep Subcortical Structure	Distinguishing Signs and Symptoms[a]
Cerebellum	Dizziness
	Vertigo
	Ataxia
	Occipital headache
	Nystagmus, ipsilateral gaze deficit
	Dysarthria
Pons	Contralateral hemiparesis and, with more extensive hemorrhage, quadriparesis and "locked-in" syndrome
	Impaired lateral eye movement
	Small, poorly reactive pupils
	Possible abnormal respiratory patterns (see Table 5.20)
Thalamus	Contralateral hemiparesis and sensory loss, equal in the face, arm, and leg; or hemisensory loss alone
Putamen (often involving the internal capsule)	Contralateral hemiparesis and sensory loss dysarthria

[a]In addition to these distinguishing features, signs and symptoms of increased intracranial pressure will likely be present.
From Lam, A.M., Singh, V., O'Meara, A.M.I. (2019). Intracerebral hemorrhage. In C. Venkatasubramanian, G.A. Lopez, K.H. O'Phelan, editors. *Emergency neurologic life support version 4.0* (pp. 106–120). Chicago: Neurocritical Care Society.

   e. Increased age and race; Black Americans, Hispanic, and Asian peoples have a higher incidence than White Americans of the same age.
   f. Use of illicit medications, particularly sympathomimetics (e.g., cocaine, amphetamines)
3. **Signs and symptoms**
   a. Sudden, spontaneous onset; may progress in minutes to hours
   b. Specific clinical presentation varies, depending on the location, extent, and rate of bleeding. Symptoms may include severe headache, decreased LOC, nausea and vomiting, ataxia, seizures, hemiplegia or hemiparesis (arm, leg, or both), aphasia, cranial nerve dysfunction, impaired swallowing, and gaze deviation.
   c. Table 5.27 shows distinguishing signs and symptoms of hemorrhagic stroke into deeper intracranial structures.
   d. The ICH score ranges from 0 to 6 (worst score) and may be used to assess severity and predict prognosis with consideration for GCS size of ICH, location, age, and ventricular involvement (Table 5.28).
4. **Diagnostic study findings (also see Ischemic Stroke for studies used in generic stroke evaluation)**
   a. Laboratory
      i. Clotting profile (platelet count, PT, PTT, INR): other less commonly used laboratory tests may include platelet aggregation assay, activated clotting time, thrombin time, ecarin clotting time, and DIC panel
      ii. CBC, sedimentation rate: Sedimentation rate may indicate cause related to infection, inflammation, or malignancy
      iii. Serum glucose and electrolyte levels
      iv. Toxicology screen: To identify medications that may have precipitated ICH

Component	Intracerebral Hemorrhage Score Points
TABLE 5.28 Determination of the Intracerebral Hemorrhage Score	
GCS SCORE	
3–4	2
5–12	1
13–15	0
ICH VOLUME, CM³	
≥30	1
<30	0
IVH	
Yes	1
No	0
INFRATENTORIAL ORIGIN OF ICH	
Yes	1
No	0
AGE, YEARS	
≥80	1
<80	0
Total ICH Score	0–6

GCS, Glasgow coma scale; *ICH*, intracerebral hemorrhage; *IVH*, intraventricular haemorrhage.
From Hemphill, III J.C., Bonovich, D.C., Besmertis, L., et al. (2001). The ICH score: a simple, reliable grading scale for intracerebral hemorrhage. *Stroke*, 2001;32(4), 891–897.

   b. Radiologic
      i. CT scan
     ii. MRI
    iii. CT angiography, MRA, cerebral angiography
   c. LP: For suspected SAH with no evidence of blood on CT scan and no signs of increased ICP. If hemorrhagic stroke extends into the ventricle or SAH exists, the CSF contains red blood cells (RBCs) and appears xanthochromic. CSF protein and white blood cells (WBC) levels are elevated. CSF pressure may be elevated.

5. Goals of care
   a. Attain and maintain systolic BP of approximately 140 mm Hg
   b. Increased ICP is controlled (<20 mm Hg); adequate CPP (70 mm Hg) and oxygenation are maintained to minimize brain ischemia.
   c. Recovery of neurologic functions is optimal.
   d. Potential systemic and neurologic complications are prevented or recognized and appropriately managed.
   e. Patient and family are prepared for interventions, possible complications, and outcomes.

6. Interprofessional collaboration: See Intracranial Aneurysms

7. Management of patient care
   a. Anticipated patient trajectory: Numerous factors influence the clinical course and outcome, including the location and extent of the hemorrhage, the occurrence and severity of complications; age; and preexisting health problems. Hemorrhagic stroke carries much higher mortality and morbidity than ischemic stroke. Anticipated

patient trajectory for increased ICP is relevant for these patients (see Increased Intracranial Pressure). Other needs specific to patients with hemorrhagic stroke in the acute care setting include the following:

i. Monitor neurologic status and vital signs; notify providers of neurologic deterioration; maintain vital signs as prescribed

ii. Pain management and nutrition: See Intracranial Aneurysms

iii. Positioning: Maintain the HOB at 30 degrees to promote cerebral venous outflow, minimize risk of aspiration and ventilator associated pneumonia (VAP); maintain ICP/CPP within acceptable limits

iv. Nausea and vomiting: Administer antiemetics as prescribed; monitor effectiveness of antiemetics.

v. Attain and maintain normothermia; avoid shivering

vi. Nutrition: Maintain normoglycemia. If LOC or dysphagia precludes oral intake, use alternative methods of feeding early; aspiration precautions as indicated (see Dysphagia under Patient Care).

vii. Fluid and electrolytes: Maintain normovolemia to slight hypervolemia; monitor electrolytes, particularly sodium; manage hyponatremia with sodium replacement (tablets, IV normal saline, or hypertonic saline, avoiding increases in sodium >8–12 mEq/dL every 24 hours); once goal sodium obtained, wean hypertonic saline gradually and continue to monitor for repeated decreases in hyponatremia.

viii. Bowel and bladder elimination: May require indwelling urinary catheter for accurate intake and output and to avoid retention; bowel regimen to prevent straining (with possible intracranial) rebleed and facilitate evacuation

ix. Infection control: See Increased Intracranial Pressure if a ventriculostomy tube is placed; monitor for infection related to any invasive devices (indwelling urinary catheter, intubation, vascular access, procedural and surgical sites)

x. Skin care: See Increased Intracranial Pressure

xi. Discharge planning: See Intracranial Aneurysms

xii. Pharmacology
   (a) IV fluids to maintain normovolemia
   (b) Antihypertensives to maintain BP in the desired range
   (c) Anticonvulsants to prevent or treat seizures

xiii. Psychosocial issues: See Intracranial Aneurysms

xiv. Transport: See Ischemic Stroke

xv. Discharge planning: See Intracranial Aneurysms

xvi. Pharmacology
   (a) Provide supplemental oxygen; may require intubation and mechanical ventilation
   (b) Administer prescribed IV fluids, typically isotonic nonglucose-containing solutions; administer hypertonic saline as needed for hyponatremia
   (c) Administer prescribed antihypertensives; generally IV labetalol or nicardipine used initially. A systolic BP of 140 mm Hg is recommended. Avoid hypotension and CPP less than 70 mm Hg.
   (d) Vasoactive or inotropic agents may be used to maintain BP and CPP.
   (e) Fresh frozen plasma, platelets, and/or vitamin K, prothrombin complex concentrate (PCC), recombinant activated clotting factor 7 may be used to correct coagulopathy. New anticoagulants (DTIs, factor Xa inhibitors may respond to PCC, rVIIa, activated charcoal, hemodialysis; a U.S. Food and Drug Administration (FDA)-approved antidote to dabigatran

is now available as idarucizumab. An FDA-approved antidote to apixaban and rivaroxaban is now available as andexanet. Transfusion of platelets and vasopressin have been used for clopidogrel and aspirin with variable success.

(f) Sedation may be prescribed for agitation, which can elevate BP and ICP, and potentially increase the risk of rebleed.

xvii. Psychosocial issues: See Ischemic Stroke; there is some evidence that postponing a Do Not Attempt Resuscitation discussion with family may result in an improved prognosis.

xviii. Treatments

(a) Noninvasive: See Ischemic Stroke

(b) Invasive

(1) Intubation and mechanical ventilation may be required for adequate ventilation; avoid $PaCO_2$ of less than 35 mm Hg.

(2) Surgical or stereotactically guided evacuation of the hematoma may be performed to decompress the brain.

(3) An intraventricular catheter may be necessary to alleviate hydrocephalus, monitor and manage increased ICP.

(4) Cerebral oxygen or blood flow monitor may be used to guide therapy.

xix. Ethical issues: See Intracranial Aneurysms

b. Potential complications (see also health problems described under Patient Care)

i. Increased ICP (see Increased Intracranial Pressure section)

ii. Hydrocephalus

(a) Mechanism: Ventricular extension of the bleed can impair CSF flow or reabsorption. Cerebral edema and clot formation can obstruct CSF flow. (See Intracranial Aneurysms for signs and symptoms.)

(b) Management: See Intracranial Aneurysms

Intraventricular Hemorrhage

> **EXPERT TIP**
> Intraparenchymal hemorrhage associated with ventricular bleeding increases mortality and morbidity. Increased ICP may result in sudden herniation if the ventricular catheter becomes occluded.

1. Pathophysiology

a. Bleeding from a parenchymal intracerebral hemorrhage causes erosion of the ventricular wall and rupture into the ventricle.

b. Local vessels in the ventricle in the subependymal area are distended and some are occluded by thrombus.

c. The initial event may be ependymal erosion or it may occur as a result of the presence of intraventricular blood. Parenchymal hemorrhagic infarcts may also occur at the ventricular edge.

d. Neuronal injury occurs as a result of

i. Obstructive hydrocephalus

ii. Damage to adjacent structures, such as the diencephalon (thalamus) by compression, edema, and inflammation

iii. Blood breakdown products and inflammatory mediators in the CSF cause inflammation and fibrosis resulting in nonobstructive hydrocephalus

2. **Etiology and risk factors**
   a. Spontaneous intracerebral hemorrhage is the most common cause followed by aneurysmal SAH.
   b. Other common causes include TBI, AVM, venous sinus thrombosis, and Moyamoya disease.
   c. Risk factors for spontaneous related IVH include older age, baseline ICH volume at a higher level, a MAP greater than 120 mm Hg, and the location of the primary ICH close to the ventricles.
   d. Primary IVH, nontraumatic ICH confined to the ventricular system and parenchymal ependymal lining is rare. Possible etiologies include choroid plexus AVM and dural AVMs.
3. **Signs and symptoms**
   a. Obstructive hydrocephalus (large ventricles)
   b. Increased ICP
   c. Decreased LOC; coma
   d. Herniation
4. **Diagnostic and study findings**
   a. Brain CT, cerebral angiography, CT angiography
   b. Ventricular blood mixed with CSF from ventricular catheter
   c. Clotting profile (platelet count, PT, PTT, INR): other less commonly used laboratory tests may include platelet aggregation assay, activated clotting time, thrombin time, ecarin clotting time, and DIC panel
   d. The amount of blood may be quantified using a modified Graeb scale with scores assigned to each of the four ventricles, as well as the right and left temporal and occipital horns
5. **Goals of care: Similar to ICH**
   a. Attain and maintain systolic BP of approximately 140 mm Hg
   b. Increased ICP is controlled (>20 mm Hg); adequate CPP (70 mm Hg) and oxygenation are maintained to minimize brain ischemia.
   c. Recovery of neurologic functions is optimal.
   d. Potential systemic and neurologic complications are prevented or recognized and appropriately managed
   e. Patient and family are prepared for interventions, possible complications, and outcomes.
6. **Interdisciplinary collaboration. See Intracranial Aneurysms**
7. **Management of patient care**
   a. Anticipated patient trajectory: Numerous factors influence the clinical course and outcome, including the location and extent of the hemorrhage, the occurrence and severity of complications; age; and preexisting health problems. Hemorrhagic stroke, particularly with IVH, carries much higher mortality and morbidity than ischemic stroke. Anticipated patient trajectory for increased ICP is relevant for these patients (see Increased Intracranial Pressure). Other needs specific to patients with hemorrhagic stroke in the acute care setting include the following:
      i. Monitor neurologic status and vital signs; notify providers of neurologic deterioration; maintain vital signs as prescribed
      ii. Pain management and nutrition: See Intracranial Aneurysms
      iii. Positioning: Maintain the HOB at 30 degrees to promote cerebral venous outflow, minimize risk of aspiration and VAP; maintain ICP/CPP within acceptable limits

    iv. Nausea and vomiting: Administer antiemetics as prescribed; monitor effectiveness of antiemetics.

    v. Attain and maintain normothermia; avoid shivering

    vi. Nutrition: Maintain normoglycemia. If LOC or dysphagia precludes oral intake, use alternative methods of feeding early; aspiration precautions as indicated (see Dysphagia under Patient Care).

    vii. Fluid and electrolytes: maintain normovolemia to slight hypervolemia; monitor electrolytes, particularly sodium; manage hyponatremia with sodium replacement (tablets, IV normal saline, or hypertonic saline, avoiding increases in sodium >8–12 mEq/dL every 24 hours); once goal sodium obtained, wean hypertonic saline gradually and continue to monitor for repeated decreases in hyponatremia.

    viii. Bowel and bladder elimination: may require indwelling urinary catheter for accurate intake and output and to avoid retention; bowel regimen to prevent straining (with possible intracranial) rebleed and facilitate evacuation

    ix. Infection control: See Increased Intracranial Pressure if a ventriculostomy tube is placed; monitor for infection related to any invasive devices (indwelling urinary catheter, intubation, vascular access, procedural and surgical sites)

    x. Skin care: See Increased Intracranial Pressure

    xi. Discharge planning: See Intracranial Aneurysms

    xii. Pharmacology

        (a) IV fluids to maintain normovolemia

        (b) Antihypertensives to maintain BP in the desired range

        (c) Anticonvulsants to prevent or treat seizures

    xiii. Psychosocial issues: See Intracranial Aneurysms

    xiv. Transport: See Ischemic Stroke

    xv. Discharge planning: See Intracranial Aneurysms

    xvi. Pharmacology

        (a) Provide supplemental oxygen; may require intubation and mechanical ventilation

        (b) Administer prescribed IV fluids, typically isotonic nonglucose-containing solutions; administer hypertonic saline as needed for hyponatremia

        (c) Administer prescribed antihypertensives; generally IV labetalol or nicardipine used initially. A systolic BP of 140 mm Hg is recommended. Avoid hypotension and CPP less than 70 mm Hg.

        (d) Vasoactive or inotropic agents may be used to maintain BP and CPP.

        (e) Fresh frozen plasma, platelets, and/or vitamin K, PCC, and recombinant activated clotting factor 7 may be used to correct coagulopathy. New anticoagulants (DTIs, factor Xa inhibitors) may respond to PCC, rVIIa, activated charcoal, hemodialysis; an FDA-approved antidote to dabigatran is now available as idarucizumab. An FDA-approved antidote to apixaban and rivaroxaban is now available as andexanet. Transfusion of platelets and vasopressin have been used for clopidogrel and aspirin with variable success.

        (f) Sedation may be prescribed for agitation, which can elevate BP and ICP, and potentially increase the risk of rebleed.

    xvii. Psychosocial issues: See Ischemic Stroke; there is some evidence that postponing a Do Not Attempt Resuscitation discussion with family may result in an improved prognosis.

xviii. Treatments
  (a) Noninvasive: See Ischemic Stroke
  (b) Invasive
    (1) Intubation and mechanical ventilation may be required for adequate ventilation; avoid $PaCO_2$ of less than 35 mm Hg.
    (2) Surgical or stereotactically guided evacuation of the hematoma may be performed to decompress the brain.
    (3) An intraventricular catheter may be necessary to alleviate hydrocephalus, monitor and manage increased ICP.
    (4) Cerebral oxygen or blood flow monitor may be used to guide therapy.
xix. Ethical Issues: See Intracranial Aneurysms
b. Potential complications (see also health problems described under Patient Care)
  i. Increased ICP (see Increased Intracranial Pressure section)
  ii. Hydrocephalus
    (a) Mechanism: Ventricular extension of the bleed can impair CSF flow or reabsorption. Cerebral edema and clot formation can obstruct CSF flow. (See Intracranial Aneurysms for signs and symptoms.)
    (b) Management: In additional to intraventricular drainage which may require serial irrigations and aspirations by neurosurgery to maintain patency of the intraventricular catheter, intraventricular thrombolysis has also been trialed with some success. Preservative-free intraventricular alteplase has been shown to be safe with no increase in ventriculitis or rebleeding but its efficacy is and long-term prevention of shunting has not been established.

EXPERT TIP

Patient with unresolved hydrocephalus may require permanent CSF diversion, such as a ventricular shunt. A patient with a shunt may undergo a brain MRI; however, the settings must be checked upon completion of the MRI as they can be altered or turned off by the magnetic environment.

BRAIN TUMOR

KEY CONCEPT

Care of the neurooncology patient includes a multifaceted, interprofessional approach. Craniotomy for brain tumor or decompressive spine surgery for spinal tumor is just the beginning to the management of the patient with a CNS tumor. Patients can have extensive edema with neurologic deterioration including herniation, coma, and death if corticosteroids are decreased too quickly or abruptly stopped.

---

1. **Pathophysiology: A brain tumor is a space-occupying lesion inside the cranium composed of abnormal cells. As the cells divide and the tumor enlarges, surrounding structures are compressed, stretched, or torn. Brain tumors may be primary or metastatic. Primary tumors are the supporting tissue of the brain, not neurons, including tumors of the meninges (meningioma), astrocytes (grade IV astrocytoma, glioblastoma multiforme), oligodendrocytes (oligodendroglioma), and ependymal (ependymoma) cells. Brain tumors rarely metastasize outside the CNS. Common primary brain tumors that metastasize to the brain are lung, breast, colon, renal, melanoma (skin), thyroid, and uterine. Brain tumors may be "malignant" by location (e.g., brainstem), aggressiveness (grade I through IV with IV being the most aggressive), histology, or patient factors (preexisting morbidity). Intracranial neoplasms may also have a cystic component, necrosis, as well as metabolically active cells, and marked angiogenesis. Vasogenic edema is common.**

Brain tumor patients have variable rates of survival, depending on location, histology, and tumor management.

2. **Etiology and risk factors**
   a. The cause of most brain tumors remains unknown
   b. The only known modifiable risk factor is exposure to ionizing radiation
   c. Genetic predisposition (e.g., neurofibromatosis)
   d. Unknown environmental risks
   e. Risk factors associated with primary tumors when brain tumor is metastatic (e.g., lung cancer and smoking)
3. **Signs and symptoms: Brain tumor signs and symptoms may be:**
   a. Localized: Anatomic and clinical correlation (e.g., frontal lobe and primary motor strip involvement)
   b. Generalized: Decreased LOC, seizures, cognitive-behavioral deterioration, fatigue
   c. Associated with increased ICP: Headache, vomiting, decreased LOC, papilledema, edema of the optic disk (CN II)
4. **Diagnostic study findings**
   a. Radiologic
      i. Head CT with and without contrast
      ii. MRI with and without contrast: Identifies tumor location, mass effect
         (a) Fluid-attenuated inversion recovery (FLAIR): Removes fluid (CSF) for better visualization of tissue
         (b) Multimodality MRI, includes diffusion- and perfusion-weighted imaging, diffusion tensor imaging: Delineates perfusion, metabolism, angiogenesis, and grading of tumor
      iii. Magnetic resonance spectroscopy (MRS): Assess metabolites to determine growth rate of tumor
      iv. PET: Quantifies metabolism of tumor as an indicator of aggressiveness, tumor recurrence, or residual tumor
      v. Cerebral angiogram
      vi. Systemic workup: Identify primary tumor if metastases is suspected; typically includes chest, abdominal, pelvic CT; bronchoscopy or biopsy of primary site
   b. Laboratory endocrine workup: Identify neuroendocrine involvement (e.g., pituitary adenoma, craniopharyngioma) by laboratory analysis including ACTH, cortisol, LH, FSH, PL, TSH, thyroid profile (T3, T4), and GH
   c. Visual: Computerized visual field testing and ophthalmoscopic examination to assess for papilledema, impaired EOMs (dysconjugate gaze, gaze paresis, diplopia)
   d. Audiometry: Hearing deficits (e.g., acoustic neuroma)
5. **Goals of care**
   a. Optimal neurologic function
   b. Potential symptoms of brain tumors are managed optimally
   c. Potential complications of tumor and management of tumor are recognized and appropriately managed
   d. Patient and family are prepared for intervention, possible complications, and outcomes
6. **Interprofessional collaboration: Nurse, physician (may include neurosurgeon, interventional neuroradiologist, oncologists, neuroophthalmologist, endocrinologist, internal medicine), advanced practice provider, neuropsychologist, speech, occupational and physical therapists, palliative care, social worker, case manager, chaplain.**
7. **Management of patient care**

a. Anticipated patient trajectory: Patient's clinical course and outcome are influenced by the location and extent of brain tumor; the neurologic deficits that result; the occurrence and severity of complications; age; and preexisting health problems. Specific needs for patients with brain tumor in the acute care setting include the following:

   i. Monitor neurologic status and report deterioration immediately; maintain BP within prescribed parameters

   ii. Pain: Headache related to tumor mass effect, invasive procedure, metastatic disease

   iii. Positioning

   (a) Maintain HOB at 30 degrees to minimize risk of aspiration, VAP, and promote venous outflow. Get the patient out of bed as early as possible while assessing neurologic status and BP. Collaborate with physical and occupational therapy.

   (b) Use protective positioning to protect the patient's extremities on affected side related to paralysis, impaired sensation during positioning.

   (c) Position patient items in the unaffected visual field initially; gradually moving objects to the affected side and encouraging the patient to attend to that side.

   iv. Symptom management:

   (a) Vasogenic edema: Administration of corticosteroids; monitor and manage side effects (skin breakdown, fluid and electrolyte imbalance, hyperglycemia, gastrointestinal irritation); taper steroids as prescribed; do not abruptly stop; may require increased dosage immediately postoperatively or with additional treatment

---

EXPERT TIP

Patients with brain tumors may also have increased edema with chemotherapy and radiation, requiring an increase in corticosteroid therapy. The cerebral edema associated with brain tumors is vasogenic. Corticosteroids decreases vasogenic cerebral edema. Abrupt withdrawal of corticosteroids may result in brain herniation related to massive rebound edema.

   (b) Seizures: Prophylactic anticonvulsants; monitor levels; adverse effects; fall risk

   (c) VTE (DVT and PE): Malignancy increases tendency toward thrombosis; prophylaxis: intermittent sequential compression devices; anticoagulation

   (d) Nausea and vomiting: Related to corticosteroids, chemotherapy, radiation, management with antiemetics; dietary adjustment; proton pump inhibitors

   (e) Fatigue: Allow rest between ADLs; sleep

   (f) Consider palliative care consult

   v. Infection control: Hand hygiene; infection control precautions; investigate source of fever aggressively and treat infections aggressively (may be at increased risk of sepsis related to altered immune status resulting from corticosteroids, radiation, and chemotherapy); may require meds to boost immune system, treat neutropenia

   vi. Nutrition: Monitor dietary intake. Maintain normoglycemia. If LOC or dysphagia precludes oral intake, use alternative methods of feeding early; aspiration precautions as indicated (see Dysphagia under Patient Care).

   vii. Fluid and electrolytes: Maintain normovolemia; monitor electrolytes, particularly sodium for decrease related to SIADH; manage hyponatremia with sodium replacement (tablets, IV normal saline or hypertonic saline), avoiding increases in sodium greater than 8 to 12 mEq/dL every 24 hours; once goal sodium obtained, wean hypertonic saline gradually and continue to monitor for repeated decreases in hyponatremia. Observe for diabetes insipidus in patients with neuroendocrine tumors (urine output >200–250 mL/h for 2 consecutive hours, urine specific gravity <1.005, urine osmolality <200 mOsm/kg, thirst, hypernatremia); attain and maintain euvolemia with fluid replacement and hormonal (ADH/vasopressin) replacement

  viii. Bowel and bladder elimination: May require indwelling urinary catheter for accurate intake and output and to avoid retention; bowel regimen to prevent straining and facilitate evacuation; remove indwelling catheter as soon as possible; monitor postvoided residuals for retention

  ix. Communication, cognition, and swallow: Collaborate with speech therapist

  x. Skin care: Increased risk of breakdown related to corticosteroids and radiation therapy

  xi. Discharge planning: Follow-up care; placement in rehabilitation, skilled nursing, home, outpatient speech therapist (ST)/physical therapist (PT)/occupational therapist (OT); patient and family education regarding medications, possible complications, additional treatment

  xii. Psychosocial issues: Frustration related to neurologic dysfunction, depression, uncertain prognosis, distress related to potential for increased disability and death, body image

  xiii. Treatments:
   (a) Surgery
    (1) Biopsy (open procedure or stereotactic): for tissue diagnosis, primary or secondary
    (2) Craniotomy for debulking, gross total removal and tissue diagnosis; may be performed awake (after skull and dura opened) to monitor patient's neurologic status
    (3) Shunt: tumor obstructing CSF pathway or increased production of CSF (e.g., ependymoma)
    (4) CSF leak treatment: CSF leak precautions (avoid coughing, sneezing, Valsalva); lumbar drain; or surgical closure of the leak
    (5) Cranioplasty to replace skull bone after cerebral edema subsides
   (b) Radiation
    (1) External beam
    (2) Whole brain
    (3) Stereotaxic radiosurgery (Gamma Knife)
    (4) Proton therapy
    (5) Interstitial brachytherapy: Implanted at tumor site
   (c) Chemotherapy
    (1) IV: Bevacizumab, carmustine, lomustine, cisplatin, carboplatin, vincristine, etoposide, methotrexate
    (2) In situ: Biodegradable carmustine impregnated wafer placed at surgical site during craniotomy
    (3) Oral (e.g., temozolomide for glioblastoma multiforme)
   (d) Surgery related to primary sites outside the cranium

  xiv. Ethical issues: End-of-life care considerations

  xv. Potential complications: See health problems described under Patient Care

SPINAL AND SPINAL CORD TUMORS

> **KEY CONCEPT**
> The first indication of metastatic disease from lung, breast, and prostate tumors may be spinal cord compression resulting in constipation and urinary retention.

1. **Pathophysiology:** A spinal tumor is a space-occupying lesion either: (1) extradural, outside the spinal cord in the vertebral bodies or epidural tissue; (2) intradural/extramedullary in the arachnoid or pia mater tissue; or (3) intramedullary, in the spinal cord itself, encroaching on tracts and gray matter. Spinal tumors may be primary or metastatic. Examples of primary intradural (extradural) tumors include schwannomas, neurofibromas, and ependymomas. Astrocytomas and ependymomas are found intramedullary. Spinal and spinal cord tumors may be located in the various regions of the spinal column. As the cells divide and the tumor enlarges, surrounding structures, such as the nerve roots, meninges, and spinal cord are compressed, stretched, or torn. Spinal tumors rarely metastasize outside the CNS. Common primary tumors that metastasize to the spine are lung, breast, and prostate. Metastatic spinal cord tumors are typically extradural. Hemorrhage and cyst may occur as well. Vasogenic edema is common. Spinal and spinal cord tumor patients have variable rates of survival depending on location, histology, and tumor management.

2. **Etiology and risk factors**
   a. The cause of most primary spinal tumors remains unknown
   b. The only known modifiable risk factor is exposure to ionizing radiation
   c. Genetic predisposition (e.g., neurofibromatosis)
   d. Unknown environmental risks
   e. Risk factors associated with primary tumors when brain tumor is metastatic (e.g., lung cancer and smoking)

3. **Signs and symptoms of a spinal or spinal cord tumor may be:**
   a. Radicular pain: A radiating pain that follows a dermatomal pattern or pain that may increase when lying down
   b. Motor weakness: Paralysis of the extremities, difficulty walking, clumsiness falling; spasticity
   c. Impaired sensation; paresthesias, dysesthesias
   d. Loss of bowel or bladder function: Urinary retention, constipation

4. **Diagnostic studies**
   a. Radiologic
      i. Plain spine x-ray
      ii. MRI with and without contrast
      iii. Myelogram
      iv. CT with and without contrast
      v. Spinal angiogram
      vi. Systemic workup: Identify primary tumor if metastases is suspected; typically includes chest, abdominal, pelvic CT; bronchoscopy or biopsy of primary site (e.g., prostate)

5. **Goals of care**
   a. Optimal neurologic function
   b. Symptoms of spinal cord tumors are minimized
   c. Potential complications of tumor and management of tumor are recognized and appropriately managed

    d. Patient and family are prepared for intervention, possible complications, and outcomes

6. **Interprofessional collaboration: See Intracranial Aneurysms.**

7. **Management of patient care**

    a. Anticipated patient trajectory: Patient's clinical course and outcome are influenced by the location and extent of spine or spinal cord tumor; the neurologic deficits that result; the occurrence and severity of complications; age; and preexisting health problems. Specific needs for patients with spine or spinal cord tumor in the acute care setting include the following:

        i. Monitor neurologic status and report deterioration immediately; maintain BP within prescribed parameters and notify provider immediately

        ii. Pain or discomfort related to tumor mass effect, invasive procedure, metastatic disease; administer analgesics and muscle relaxers as prescribed

        iii. Positioning

            (a) Maintain bed position as prescribed; if spine is considered unstable or has not been definitively treated, may require spine precautions (no flexion of the bed, logroll, orthotics, as needed)

            (b) Use protective positioning to protect the patient's extremities on affected extremities related to paralysis, impaired sensation during positioning

        iv. Symptom management:

            (a) Vasogenic edema: Administration of corticosteroids; monitor and manage side effects (skin breakdown, fluid and electrolyte imbalance, hyperglycemia, gastrointestinal irritation); taper steroids as prescribed; do not abruptly stop; may require increased dosage immediately postoperatively or with additional treatment

            (b) VTE (DVT and PE): Malignancy increases tendency toward thrombosis; prophylaxis: intermittent sequential compression devices; anticoagulation

            (c) Nausea and vomiting: Related to corticosteroids, chemotherapy, radiation, management with antiemetics; dietary adjustment; proton pump inhibitors

            (d) Fatigue: Allow rest between ADLs; sleep

            (e) Consider palliative care consult

        v. Infection control: Hand hygiene; infection control precautions; investigate source of fever aggressively and treat infections aggressively (may be at increased risk of sepsis related to altered immune status resulting from corticosteroids, radiation, and chemotherapy); may require medication to boost immune system/WBC count; manage neutropenia

        vi. Nutrition: Monitor dietary intake. Maintain normoglycemia. If LOC or dysphagia precludes oral intake, use alternative methods of feeding early; aspiration precautions following anterior surgical approaches to the cervical spine, cervical orthoses, or special positioning related to spine instability.

        vii. Fluid and electrolytes: Maintain normovolemia; monitor electrolytes, attain and maintain euvolemia with fluid replacement and hormonal replacement

        viii. Bowel and bladder elimination: May require indwelling urinary catheter for accurate intake and output and to avoid retention; bowel regimen to prevent straining and facilitate evacuation; remove indwelling catheter as soon as possible; avoid overdistension; monitor postvoided residuals for retention

        ix. Skin and mucous membrane care: Increased risk of breakdown related to corticosteroids and radiation therapy

        x. Discharge planning: Follow-up care; placement in rehabilitation, skilled nursing, home, outpatient PT/OT; patient and family education regarding medications, possible complications, additional treatment

    xi. Psychosocial issues: Frustration related to neurologic dysfunction, depression, distress related to potential for increased disability and death, body image

    xii. Treatments:

      (a) Surgery

        (1) Biopsy (open procedure or stereotactic): For tissue diagnosis, primary or secondary

        (2) Surgical decompression for debulking, gross total removal and tissue diagnosis; may be performed for palliation primarily; may also include fixation/stabilization with instrumentation/hardware; interventional neuroradiology may perform embolization to the feeder vessels of the tumor before surgery to lessen hemorrhage during surgery

        (3) Vertebroplasty

        (4) CSF leak treatment: Lumbar drain or surgical closure of the leak

      (b) Radiation

        (1) External beam

        (2) Stereotactic body (spine) radiosurgery

      (c) Chemotherapy

    xiii. Ethical issues: End-of-life care considerations

    xiv. Potential complications: See health problems described under Patient Care

---

KEY CONCEPT

The BBB and brain-CSF barrier lessens the effectiveness of IV antimicrobial agents in the management of CNS infections. Intraventricular or intrathecal administration may increase the effectiveness of antimicrobial therapy. The patient must tolerate clamping of the ventricular drain after instillation of the preservative-free antimicrobial agent for optimal efficacy.

INTRACRANIAL INFECTIONS
Bacterial Meningitis

KEY CONCEPT

Neisseria meningitidis (meningococcal meningitis) may initially present with flulike symptoms; however, CNS and other symptoms may progress rapidly with increased mortality and morbidity. Meningococcal meningitis is highly contagious.

---

1. **Pathophysiology: Bacterial organisms gain access to the subarachnoid space, CSF, and pia mater and arachnoid mater layers of the meninges. Once access is gained, bacteria proliferate because immune defense mechanisms are limited. Bacterial exudate forms in the subarachnoid space and meningeal inflammation occurs, which can obstruct CSF flow. Cerebral capillaries become permeable, which leads to vasogenic edema and increased ICP results. Progressive involvement may include the following:**

  a. Vasculitis; ischemia or infarction of neuronal tissue

  b. Inflammation of the ependymal cells lining the ventricles (ependymitis) and development of purulent intracranial effusions (pyocephalus)

  c. Petechial hemorrhage within the brain

  d. Cranial nerve inflammation

  e. Scar tissue formation and fibrotic changes in the arachnoid layer, which contribute to the development of hydrocephalus

  f. Subdural empyema or brain abscess

2. **Etiology and risk factors**
   a. Infecting organisms: Organisms vary with the primary cause. Two organisms account for the majority of bacterial meningitis in adults: *Neisseria meningitides* (meningococcal meningitis) and *Streptococcus pneumoniae* (pneumococcal meningitis). Other causative bacteria include *Haemophilus influenzae, Listeria monocytogenes, Mycobacterium tuberculosis*, staphylococci—usually *Staphylococcus aureus*, but also *Staphylococcus epidermidis* (most common after neurologic surgery), and gram-negative enteric bacilli (e.g., *Escherichia coli*).
   b. Sources of infection
      i. Neurologic surgery or invasive procedures, monitoring devices (ventricular or lumbar CSF drain); ventricular shunt infections, penetrating head injury, basilar skull fracture with dural tear
      ii. Otitis media; sinusitis; mastoiditis; osteomyelitis of the skull or vertebrae; dental abscess, recent dental work
      iii. Exposure to infectious organisms (e.g., *N. meningitides);* crowded conditions (school dormitory, military barracks); infection elsewhere in the body with bacteremia or septic emboli
      iv. IV medication use
   c. Immunosuppression increases susceptibility
3. **Signs and symptoms**
   a. Headache that becomes progressively worse
   b. General signs of infection: Malaise, fever, tachycardia, chills
   c. Rash: Patients with meningococcal meningitis (*N. meningitides*) develop red or purple petechiae progressing to purpura or ecchymosis over the trunk, legs, conjunctiva, and mucous membranes; does not fade when compressed
   d. Neurologic: Irritability, confusion; progressive decrease in LOC; focal neurologic signs (hemiparesis, hemiplegia), skin hypersensitivity, seizures, cranial nerve deficits
   e. Meningeal irritation: Headache, photophobia, nuchal rigidity, Brudzinski's sign, Kernig's sign
   f. Nausea and vomiting
4. **Diagnostic study findings**
   a. Laboratory
      i. Cultures: CSF, blood, drainage from sinuses or wounds, nasopharynx, sputum, and rash aspirate to identify causative organism
      ii. Serology tests (e.g., latex agglutination antigen test, counter immunoelectrophoresis, radioimmunoassay, enzyme-linked immunosorbent assay) to identify antibodies or antigens associated with specific disease or organism; polymerase chain reaction (PCR) detects deoxyribonucleic acid (DNA) to identify causative organism; CSF lactate before administration of antibiotics
   b. Radiologic
      i. CT scan usually normal in acute uncomplicated meningitis; may show meningeal enhancement, hydrocephalus, cerebral edema, cortical infarcts, and cerebral abscesses
      ii. Skull radiographs: May visualize infected sinuses or basilar skull fracture
   c. EEG: May show generalized slow-wave activity over both hemispheres
   d. LP: May be done if no evidence of increased ICP or coagulopathy
   e. ICP may be severely elevated in bacterial meningitis
      i. Head CT should be done before LP to minimize risk of herniation
      ii. Opening pressure may be elevated

  iii. CSF analysis: cell count and differential, protein, glucose, gram stain, bacterial cultures. CSF glucose less than two-thirds of the blood glucose is indicative of bacterial infection. The CSF may be cloudy with elevation of WBC count.

5. Goals of care
 a. Infection and neurologic deficits resolve
 b. ICP is controlled (<20–22 mm Hg)
 c. Patient expresses relief from pain
 d. Potential systemic and neurologic complications are avoided or minimized

6. Interprofessional collaboration: See Intracranial Aneurysms.

7. Management of patient care
 a. Anticipated patient trajectory: Aggressive treatment, initiated early, may completely resolve signs and symptoms. Amount of brain damage caused by infectious process, resulting neurologic deficits, and incidence and severity of complications will determine the clinical course. Anticipated patient trajectory for increased ICP may also be relevant (see Increased Intracranial Pressure). Other needs specific to patients with intracranial infection in the acute care setting include the following:
  i. Monitor neurologic status including vital signs. Notify physician of neurologic deterioration
  ii. Positioning: Raise the HOB at least 30 degrees to control headache and ICP, minimize risk of aspiration and VAP (if intubated and mechanically ventilated)
  iii. Pain management
   (a) Administer analgesics to treat headache, preferably short-acting or easily reversible agents; give cautiously if the patient is not on ventilator support; avoid inducing hypotension
   (b) Monitor pain relief and neurologic status
   (c) Dim lights to promote rest, relieve photophobia
  iv. Nutrition: See Intracranial Aneurysms
  v. Infection control: A presumptive diagnosis of some infectious organisms (e.g., *N. meningitides)* will require patient isolation until confirmed or ruled out. Some infections must be reported to state health agencies, federal health agencies, or both. Names of individuals in recent physical contact with the patient may be requested and prophylaxis given to exposed contacts.
  vi. Discharge planning: Patient usually discharged home, unless neurologic deficits persist that require rehabilitation or care in a skilled nursing facility
  vii. Pharmacology
   (a) Antibiotics are given to cover the known or suspected causative organisms at the first suspicion of bacterial meningitis. Antibiotic therapy should not be delayed and may be initiated even before obtaining a CSF sample if LP is delayed. If necessary, antibiotic(s) can be modified after the causative organism is confirmed.
   (b) In suspected community-acquired bacterial meningitis, dexamethasone 10 mg IV may be given before or with the first antibiotic dose to stabilize the BBB and decrease the resistance to CSF outflow and then continued every 6 hours for 4 days. Provide gastrointestinal prophylaxis. Monitor for adverse effects of corticosteroids.
   (c) IV fluids (typically isotonic solutions) to maintain euvolemia; if necessary, vasoactive and inotropic agents for cardiovascular support
   (d) Antipyretics to maintain normothermia
   (e) Anxiolytics to alleviate anxiety and sedation to manage ICP
   (f) Anticonvulsants to control seizures

       viii. Treatments
- (a) Noninvasive
  - (1) Monitor neurologic status and vital signs frequently
  - (2) Institute temperature management measures; avoid patient shivering
- (b) Invasive
  - (1) Intubation, mechanical ventilation if needed
  - (2) ICP monitoring

  b. Potential complications (see health problems described under Patient Care)
- i. Waterhouse-Friderichsen syndrome (adrenal hemorrhage)
  - (a) Mechanism: May be seen in fulminant meningococcal meningitis. Results in adrenal insufficiency, subsequent hypotension, respiratory distress, and circulatory collapse.
  - (b) Management: Immediate adrenal corticosteroid replacement, supportive therapy
- ii. Disseminated intravascular coagulation
  - (a) Mechanism: Associated primarily with meningococcal meningitis
  - (b) Management (see Ch. 8, Hematologic and Immune Systems)
- iii. Brain abscess, subdural effusions, encephalitis
  - (a) Mechanism: Extension of bacterial infection into the parenchyma or subdural space
  - (b) Management: Antibiotics for brain abscess or encephalitis. Abscess may need surgical decompression.
- iv. Hydrocephalus
  - (a) Mechanism: Purulent exudate and meningeal fibrosis in the subarachnoid space can obstruct CSF flow and reabsorption
  - (b) Management: See Management of Hydrocephalus in Box 5.1
- v. Increased ICP
  - (a) Mechanism: Accumulation of purulent exudates, hydrocephalus, and cerebral edema
  - (b) Management: See Increased Intracranial Pressure
- vi. Seizures: See Seizures section
- vii. Fluid and electrolyte imbalance: Patient may develop SIADH. See the section on fluid and electrolyte imbalances under Patient Care
- viii. Skin care: See Increased Intracranial Pressure

Viral Meningitis

1. **Pathophysiology: Viral organisms gain access to the subarachnoid space, CSF, and pia mater and arachnoid mater layers of the meninges. Once access is gained, viruses proliferate because immune defense mechanisms are limited. Lymphocytes infiltrate meninges.**
   a. Viral meningitis is also known as aseptic meningitis. Viral meningitis is more common than bacterial meningitis and typically less severe.
   b. The most common cause of viral meningitis are enteroviruses (cocksackie, echo, and polio). Arboviruses, herpes, mumps, varicella zoster, influenza, cytomegalovirus, Epstein-Barr, and West Nile may be causative organisms and tend to be seasonal. Human immunodeficiency virus (HIV) may present as aseptic meningitis at the time of seroconversion.
2. **Etiology and risk factors**
   a. Exposure to viruses
   b. Immunosuppression

3. **Signs and symptoms:**
   a. Similar to bacterial meningitis, symptoms include: headache, low-grade fever, nuchal rigidity, photophobia, malaise, and symptoms of systemic of upper respiratory viral infection.
   b. Unlike bacterial meningitis, patients with viral meningitis do not typically have changes in LOC or seizures.
4. **Diagnostic study findings**
   a. CT if focal neurologic deficits or increased IC
   b. LP: CSF is typically clear; cultures negative for bacterial infection; normal glucose; increased WBC count; PCR positive for enteroviruses if present
5. **Goals of care**
   a. Infection and neurologic deficits resolve
   b. ICP is controlled (<20–22 mm Hg)
   c. Patient expresses relief from pain
   d. Potential systemic and neurologic complications are avoided or minimized
6. **Interprofessional collaboration: Nurse, physician (including infectious disease), advanced practice provider, clinical, pharmacist, respiratory, therapist, dietician**
7. **Management of patient care**
   a. Symptomatic and supportive
      i. Bed rest with HOB elevated 30 degrees, quiet dark environment
      ii. Symptom management: nausea, fever, pain
      iii. Monitor fluid and electrolyte status and replace as needed
      iv. No routine antiviral pharmacotherapy

Fungal Meningitis

1. **Pathophysiology: Fungal organisms gain access to the subarachnoid space, CSF, and pia mater and arachnoid mater layers of the meninges. Once access is gained, fungi proliferate because immune defense mechanisms are limited. Fungal exudate forms in the subarachnoid space and meningeal inflammation occurs; common fungal infections include cryptococcus and candida.**
2. **Etiology and risk factors**
   a. Immunosuppression: Patients who are immunosuppressed related to HIV+ status (especially with a CD4 count <100); chemotherapy; transplant recipients (antirejection medication); immunosuppressive for autoimmune disorders (rheumatoid arthritis, multiple sclerosis, lupus erythematosus); and uncontrolled diabetes
   b. Patients who have undergone neurosurgical procedures and have CNS shunts
   c. Patients with cryptococcal lung infections or candida mucosal membrane infections
3. **Signs and symptoms**
   a. Nuchal rigidity, fever, malaise, photophobia, and vomiting
4. **Diagnostic study findings**
   a. Head CT before LP to rule out increased ICP
   b. LP: CSF analysis for cell count, glucose, protein and Cryptococcus antigen, India ink, PCR, enzyme immunoassay, latex agglutination, Candida, beta-D-glucan assay
   c. Brain MRI: multiple cerebral abscesses
5. **Goals of care**
   a. Infection and neurologic deficits resolve
   b. ICP is controlled (<20–22 mm Hg)

    c. Patient expresses relief from pain

    d. Potential systemic and neurologic complications are avoided or minimized

6. **Interprofessional collaboration: See Intracranial Aneurysms.**

7. **Management of patient care**

    a. Supportive care: Management of increased ICP, externalization of CSF drainage, fever, fluid and electrolyte status, analgesics

    b. Antifungal agents: amphotericin B and flucytosine

    c. Management of compromised immune status

Viral Encephalitis

> **KEY CONCEPT**
> Changes in the temporal lobe may be noted on MRI with viral encephalitis. Temporal lobe seizures are common.

1. **Pathophysiology: Inflammation of brain tissue caused by viruses that enter the body, colonize, then migrate through the choroid plexus, cerebral capillaries, or along peripheral nerves into the CNS. Viruses attack susceptible neurons, causing brain tissue inflammation and necrosis; may also inflame the meninges.**

2. **Etiology and risk factors**

    a. Increased risk with immunosuppression

    b. Caused by viruses such as:

        i. Herpes simplex virus is the most common type of fatal endemic encephalitis in the United States.

        ii. Enterovirus; cytomegalovirus; measles, mumps, varicella, lymphocytic choriomeningitis viruses; Epstein-Barr virus; rabies virus

        iii. Arboviruses: Transmitted by arthropods (e.g., mosquito or tick acquires the viral infection after biting an infected host [e.g., horse, bird]; the infected arthropod vector then bites and infects a human). Examples: Eastern equine, Western equine, West Nile, St. Louis, and California encephalitis are all transmitted by mosquitoes. Transmission may also occur via blood transfusion or transplant from an infected donor. Some arboviruses have specific seasonal and geographic prevalence; primarily afflict humans of distinct age groups (e.g., risk of severe neurologic disease with West Nile virus increases significantly in those aged ≥60 years), and immunosuppressed.

3. **Signs and symptoms**

    a. Symptom onset and progression varies with the pathogen and the area of the brain involved.

    b. Common findings: Headache, fever, altered LOC, nuchal rigidity

    c. Possible findings: Cranial nerve dysfunction, focal deficits, aphasia, motor deficits, involuntary movements, ataxia, nystagmus, seizures

    d. Herpes simplex virus: Fever, headache, nausea and vomiting, altered LOC, and seizures develop over days. Frontal and temporal lobe damage from the virus may cause strange behavior, personality changes, hemiparesis, aphasia, temporal lobe seizures, hallucinations, signs of increased ICP, and eventually temporal lobe (uncal) herniation.

    e. Arthropod-borne encephalitis: Gradual onset of flu-like symptoms (e.g., fever, chills, malaise, headache, myalgia, nausea and vomiting). Lymphadenopathy and erythematous rash may also accompany the onset of West Nile virus infection. Then changes in LOC, meningeal signs, seizures, tremors, ataxia, abnormal reflexes, muscle weakness, and possibly motor and cranial nerve deficits appear. West Nile encephalitis may manifest with severe muscle weakness or flaccid paralysis.

4. **Diagnostic study findings**
   a. Laboratory findings
      i. CSF cultures: To identify the causative organism
      ii. LP: See Intracranial Infections: Bacterial Meningitis for indications.
         (a) Increased WBCs, primarily lymphocytes; RBCs present with cerebral hemorrhage
         (b) Viral cultures
         (c) Immunoglobulin (Ig)M antibodies by PCR
      iii. Serologic tests: See Intracranial Infections: Bacterial Meningitis
   b. Radiologic
      i. CT scan
      ii. MRI: Initial studies may be normal; later studies may reveal abnormalities (e.g., hemorrhage, edema) in the affected areas (e.g., inferior frontal and temporal areas with herpes simplex encephalitis; thalamus, midbrain, and other gray matter structures with West Nile encephalitis); more sensitive to tissue changes than CT
   c. EEG
   d. Brain tissue biopsy
5. **Goals of care: See Intracranial Infections: Bacterial Meningitis**
6. **Interprofessional collaboration: See Intracranial Infections: Bacterial Meningitis**
7. **Management of patient care**
   a. Anticipated patient trajectory: See patient trajectory for Intracranial Infections: Bacterial Meningitis. Other acute care needs for patients with viral encephalitis include the following:
      i. Positioning: See Intracranial Infections: Bacterial Meningitis
      ii. Pain management: See Intracranial Infections: Bacterial Meningitis
      iii. Nutrition: See Intracranial Aneurysms
      iv. Skin care: See Increased Intracranial Pressure
      v. Infection control: See Intracranial Infections: Bacterial Meningitis
      vi. Discharge planning: See Intracranial Infections: Bacterial Meningitis
      vii. Pharmacology
         (a) Antiviral agents as prescribed (e.g., acyclovir [Zovirax]) for treatment of herpes types 1 and 2 and varicella-zoster virus. Early treatment helps reduce mortality and morbidity.
         (b) Prescribed IV fluids (typically isotonic solutions) to maintain euvolemia; if necessary, vasoactive and inotropic agents to support cardiovascular function
         (c) Prescribed antipyretics to maintain normothermia
         (d) Anxiolytic for anxiety and sedation for increased ICP
         (e) Anticonvulsants to control seizures
      viii. Treatments: See Intracranial Infections: Bacterial Meningitis
   b. Potential complications (see also health problems described under Patient Care)
      i. Increased ICP
         (a) Mechanism: Brain inflammation and cerebral edema
         (b) Management: See Increased Intracranial Pressure

    ii. Seizures: See Seizures section

    iii. Fluid and electrolyte imbalance: See Fluid and Electrolyte Imbalance under Patient Care

---

EXPERT TIP

The pathophysiology of both Guillain-Barré and myasthenia gravis (MG) includes an autoimmune component. Both respond to IV Immunoglobulin G (IVIg) and plasmapheresis (plasma exchange). Deterioration of ventilatory effort may be life-threatening if intervention is delayed. Although bilevel positive airway pressure (BiPAP) can be considered before intubation in MG crisis, it is not recommended before intubation in Guillain-Barré.

NEUROMUSCULAR/AUTOIMMUNE DISEASE
Guillain-Barré Syndrome

EXPERT TIP

Avoid unnecessary movement and passive range-of-motion (PROM) exercises early during the onset and progression of Guillain-Barré. Movement exacerbates pain associated with demyelination.

---

1. **Pathophysiology: Acute inflammatory polyneuropathy. Myelin sheath of inflamed and edematous peripheral nerves is destroyed by macrophages and lymphocytes, which causes loss of saltatory conduction. Myelin destruction is patchy. Varied amounts of axonal damage may also worsen outcomes. Remyelination gradually transpires. Four variations of Guillain-Barré syndrome (GBS) exist:**
   a. Acute inflammatory demyelinating polyneuropathy (most common)
   b. Acute motor-sensory axonal neuropathy
   c. Acute motor axonal neuropathy without sensory loss
   d. Miller Fisher syndrome: Uncommon, more benign
2. **Etiology and risk factors**
   a. Exact etiology is unclear; thought to be caused by an autoimmune response, likely related to an acute infection (e.g., respiratory or gastrointestinal)
   b. Approximately 50% of patients who develop GBS have an infection, usually viral, within 28 days before the onset of symptoms; *Campylobacter jejuni* infection and cytomegalovirus (CMV) are frequently associated with GBS.
   c. Influenza and rabies vaccination may trigger GBS.
   d. Surgery and renal transplantation may precede onset.
   e. May occur with Hodgkin disease or systemic lupus erythematosus
3. **Signs and symptoms**
   a. History of acute infection within 4 weeks before in more than half of all patients
   b. Acute onset; symptoms progress rapidly over hours to 3 weeks
   c. Progressive symmetric weakness, usually starting in the legs and ascending to the trunk, arms, and cranial nerves
   d. Ineffective ventilation if the respiratory muscles (especially the diaphragm) are involved
   e. Decreased or absent deep tendon reflexes
   f. Sensory loss usually mild but may be severe or not present; paresthesias common, often affecting the hands and feet
   g. Pain may include dysesthesia, muscle aches, or cramps; back pain often an early symptom
   h. Cranial nerve dysfunction; CN VII most commonly affected
   i. Autonomic dysfunction: BP variation, arrhythmias, ileus, diaphoresis or loss of sweating, urine retention

j. Miller Fisher syndrome: Ophthalmoplegia, ataxia, areflexia, typically without sensory loss, rarely affecting the respiratory muscles

4. **Diagnostic study findings**
   a. EMG or nerve conduction velocity testing
   b. LP: CSF with albumin cytologic dissociation with less than 10 WBCs and elevated CSF
   c. Serial respiratory parameters: Vital capacity (VC), negative inspiratory force (NIF), maximal inspiratory pressure (MIP), and maximal expiratory pressure (MEP), ABG as guides for intubation

5. **Goals of care**
   a. Neurologic function returns to normal
   b. Pain is relieved
   c. Complications are prevented or effectively managed
   d. Patient and family are prepared for interventions

6. **Interprofessional collaboration: See Increased Intracranial Pressure**

7. **Management of patient care**
   a. Anticipated patient trajectory: Symptoms usually start to subside about 2 weeks after maximal weakness and gradually resolve; most recovery occurs within the first 6 months. Long-term outcome depends on the location and extent of axonal damage; approximately 30% of patients have persistent deficits ranging from fatigue to lower extremity paralysis. Other acute care needs for patients with GBS include the following:
      i. Monitor neurologic status and vital signs, especially respiratory status; notify provider immediately of increased weakness, difficulty breathing; assess functional vital capacity (FVC), NIF, and MEP every 4 to 6 hours.
      ii. Positioning: Position in good body alignment with the head of the bed raised at least 30 degrees to avoid aspiration; and alleviate pressure on vulnerable peripheral nerves.
      iii. Pain management
         (a) NSAIDs and nonnarcotic analgesics may be tried but are typically ineffective; gabapentin or amitriptyline may be used for neuropathic pain; use narcotics cautiously in unprotected airway.
         (b) Promote comfort via repositioning or applying warm or cool compresses; PROM may be pain-inducing initially
      iv. Nutrition: If dysphagia precludes oral intake, use alternative feeding methods early in the disease course. Patient at risk for aspiration. See recommendations for Dysphagia under Patient Care.
      v. Skin care: See Increased Intracranial Pressure
      vi. Discharge planning: Discharge destination determined in large part by persisting motor and sensory deficits
      vii. Pharmacology
         (a) Supplemental oxygen as needed to maintain adequate oxygenation
         (b) IVIg: In divided doses over 2 to 5 days to modulate the immune system and neutralize or modify detrimental immune factors
         (c) Steroids are not indicated and may worsen condition.
         (d) Anticoagulants for DVT/VTE prophylaxis
      viii. Psychosocial issues (see Intracranial Aneurysms): Educate the patient and family regarding the clinical course of GBS and the interventions provided. Reassure that function will likely return. Establish effective means for patient communication. See interventions for Inability of Patient to Communicate Needs Effectively under Patient Care.

ix. Treatments
    (a) Noninvasive: Monitor neurologic status closely for worsening or resolving deficits
    (b) Invasive
        (1) Therapeutic plasma exchange or plasmapheresis: When IVIg is not used, plasmapheresis may be performed daily for 5 days or every other day for 10 days (for a total of five treatments) to remove detrimental circulating immune factors. There is no added benefit to simultaneous therapeutic plasma exchange and IVIg.
        (2) Intubation may be required to maintain a patent airway, remove secretions, and enable mechanical ventilatory support. Elective intubations are preferred over emergency intubations. The threshold for elective intubations may be FVC under 20 mL/kg, NIF weaker than −30 cm H_2O, MEP under 40 cm H_2O, and hypercapnia. In acute neuromuscular respiratory failure related to GBS, noninvasive positive pressure ventilation (NIPPV) should not be used.

b. Potential complications (see health problems described under Patient Care)
  i. Respiratory failure
    (a) Mechanism: Weakness of the muscles used for ventilation and secretion clearance; cranial nerve deficits can impair protective airway reflexes; hypoventilation, secretion retention, atelectasis, and pulmonary infection can occur
    (b) Management: See Ch. 3, Pulmonary System
  ii. Autonomic dysfunction: Typically benign cardiac arrhythmias—unrelated to hypoxia, gastroparesis, urinary retention
    (a) Mechanism: Because of ANS involvement
    (b) Management
        (1) Continuous ECG monitoring to detect arrhythmias; monitor BP frequently
        (2) Treat arrhythmias, hypertension, or hypotension as appropriate
        (3) Sit patient up slowly to prevent orthostatic hypotension
        (4) Use a urinary catheter to relieve retention
        (5) Gastric tube should be inserted if ileus occurs
  iii. SIADH: See Fluid and Electrolyte Imbalance under Patient Care and Ch. 7, Endocrine System
  iv. Sleep deprivation
    (a) Mechanism: Pain, autonomic dysfunction, and other factors can disrupt the sleep-wake cycle
    (b) Management
        (1) Relieve pain and anxiety
        (2) Provide uninterrupted time, the patient-desired environment, and prescribed medication to enhance sleep
        (3) Change patient position gently; movement during worsening and plateau phase (during flaccidity) is painful

Myasthenia Gravis

> **EXPERT TIP**
>
> Cholinergic crisis (precipitated by an increased dose of cholinesterase inhibitor) may be differentiated from myasthenia crisis by diarrhea and abdominal cramps seen in cholinergic crisis but not myasthenia crisis.

1. Pathophysiology: A chronic and sometimes progressive neuromuscular disease, MG is the result of defect at the neuromuscular junction. Normally, the neurotransmitter ACh transmits the neuronal impulse from the axon of the neuron, across the synaptic cleft to the end plate of the muscle, and the result is muscle contraction. The defect at the neuromuscular junction is ACh antibodies on the receptors of the postsynaptic neuromuscular junction (the muscle side of the neuromuscular junction) for 85% of the patients with MG. The ACh antibodies block the stimulating effect of ACh on the muscle. Other receptor antibodies include muscle-specific tyrosine kinase (MuSK) and possibly lipoprotein receptor-related protein 4 (LRP4). In MG, the defect at the neuromuscular junction results in weakness and fatigue, particularly with repetitive movement.

2. Etiology and risk factors
   a. Exact etiology is unclear; thought to be caused by an autoimmune response
   b. Genetics; familial predisposition
   c. Tumor or dysplasia of the thymus gland
   d. Increased likelihood of MG in patients with other autoimmune disorders including thyroid disease, diabetes mellitus type 1, rheumatoid arthritis, lupus erythematosus, and CNS demyelinating diseases.

3. Signs and symptoms
   a. Muscle weakness, particularly of the ocular, facial, swallowing (bulbar), respiratory, neck, and extremity muscles
   b. Muscles weaken and fatigue easily with repetitive use
   c. Variable course; may be limited to ocular symptoms including ptosis and diplopia; patient may experience exacerbations, remissions, and instability; complete or permanent remissions are rare
   d. Respiratory insufficiency which may require mechanical ventilation

4. Diagnostic study findings
   a. Serologic testing for ACh receptor antibodies and MuSK antibodies. MuSK antibodies are not reliable in ocular MG
   b. IV acetylcholinesterase inhibitor (edrophonium chloride, [Tensilon]) testing; administered IV, muscle weakness temporarily improves if patient has MG (may cause bradycardia, asystole, and bronchoconstriction; have atropine available)
   c. Serial respiratory parameters: Vital capacity, negative inspiratory force, MIP, MEP, ABG as guides to determine need for intubation. The threshold for elective intubations may be FVC under 20 mL/kg, NIF weaker than -30 cm H_2O, MEP under 40 cm H_2O, and hypercapnia.
   d. Electrodiagnostic testing: Repetitive nerve stimulation; single-fiber EMG
   e. Ice pack on the eyelids for 2 to 5 minutes with temporary improvement of ptosis
   f. CT or MRI of the thymus

5. Goals of care
   a. Neurologic function is maximized
   b. Complications of muscle impairment are prevented or effectively managed
   c. Patient and family are prepared for interventions
   d. Patient/family knowledgeable about disease

6. Interprofessional collaboration: Nurse, physician, advanced practice provider, pharmacist, physical and occupational therapist.

7. Management of patient care
   a. Anticipated patient trajectory: Once diagnosed, patient's condition will be stabilized on anticholinesterase agents. Patient will have minimal exacerbations. Exacerbations may be related to physical illness, surgery, infection, or other medications that have

been demonstrated to worsen MG. Patient will not experience myasthenia crisis or cholinergic crisis, the latter related to too much anticholinesterase medication. Patient will not experience complications related to disease, such as aspiration and falls with injury.

    i. Monitor neurologic status and vital signs, especially respiratory status; notify provider immediately of increased weakness, difficulty breathing

    ii. Pharmacology

        (a) Anticholinesterase inhibitors: Pyridostigmine; received on time and adequate dosage. During myasthenia crisis requiring intubation, administration of anticholinesterase inhibitors are controversial as they may increase secretions. They may be restarted with weaning of mechanical ventilation and use of NIPPV.

        (b) Glucocorticosteroids for short- (during exacerbations) or long-term use; high-dose prednisone is considered first-line treatment for myasthenia crisis

        (c) Targeted immunosuppressive such as azathioprine, cyclosporine, mycophenolate mofetil, cyclophosphamide, and tacrolimus for long-term use

        (d) Supplemental oxygen as needed to maintain adequate oxygenation; intubation and mechanical ventilation as required during disease-related crises

        (e) Avoidance of pharmacologic agents that may worsen MG (current list maintained at http://www.myasthenia.org/)

        (f) IVIg: Divided doses over 3 to 5 days to modulate the immune system and neutralize or modify detrimental immune factors.

    iii. Positioning: Position in good body alignment with the HOB raised at least 30 degrees to avoid aspiration; alleviate pressure on vulnerable peripheral nerves

    iv. Nutrition: If dysphagia precludes oral intake, use alternative feeding methods early in the disease course. Patient at risk for aspiration. See recommendations for Dysphagia under Patient Care.

    v. Skin care: See Increased Intracranial Pressure

    vi. Discharge planning: Discharge destination

    vii. Psychosocial issues (see Intracranial Aneurysms): Educate the patient and family regarding the clinical course of MG and the interventions provided. Long-term management with medications

    viii. Treatments

        (a) Noninvasive: Monitor neurologic status closely for worsening or resolving deficits

        (b) Invasive

            (1) Therapeutic plasma exchange or plasmapheresis: When IVIg is not used, plasmapheresis may be performed every other day for 8 to 12 days; removes detrimental circulating immune factors. There is no added benefit to simultaneous therapeutic plasma exchange and IVIg. Both have a transient effect of about 2 weeks. If response to one is inadequate, follow-up with the other may provide benefit.

            (2) Intubation may be required to maintain a patent airway, remove secretions, and enable mechanical ventilatory support. Elective intubations are preferred. NIPPV (e.g., BiPAP) may decrease the need for intubation if administered before hypercapnia. Late signs of respiratory failure include hypoxia, hypercapnia with normalization of respiratory alkalosis, and paradoxical breathing.

      (3) Thymectomy, if thymoma or thymic hyperplasia, may stop worsening of MG

b. Potential complications (see health problems described under Patient Care)
  i. Respiratory failure
    (a) Mechanism: Weakness of the muscles used for ventilation and secretion clearance; cranial nerve deficits can impair protective airway reflexes; hypoventilation, secretion retention, atelectasis, and pulmonary infection can occur; aspiration
  ii. Cholinergic crisis: Muscular weakness similar to MG crisis but also with diarrhea and cramping; hold anticholinesterase inhibitors until symptoms subside.
  iii. Sleep deprivation: Related to neuromuscular weakness, mechanical ventilation
    (a) Mechanism: Pain, autonomic dysfunction, and other factors can disrupt the sleep-wake cycle
    (b) Management
      (1) Relieve anxiety and discomfort
      (2) Provide uninterrupted rest and sleep time

Cerebral Palsy

> **EXPERT TIP**
> Although movement disorders, including spasticity are among the most common sign and symptom of cerebral palsy, CP impacts other body systems as well.

1. **Pathophysiology**
  a. Most CP is related to periventricular white matter damage, leukomalacia, associated with perinatal ischemia-hypoxia and neuroinflammatory insults.
  b. The initial brain insult is considered a static process whereas the clinical manifestations that occur over a lifetime as the brain ages are dynamic.
  c. Anatomic patterns of brain abnormality are heterogenous.
  d. The injury may occur in utero, at the time of birth, shortly after, or during the first 2 years

2. **Risk factors**
  a. Birth at less than 27 weeks gestational age
  b. Low birth weight, less than 1500 grams
  c. Full-term birth risk factors include placenta abnormalities, birth defects, low birth weight, meconium aspiration, birth asphyxia, neonatal seizures, hypoglycemia, neonatal infection, emergency cesarean section, and respiratory distress.
  d. Maternal risk factors include malnutrition (e.g., iodine deficiency), infection (e.g., rubella), multiple births, fetal demise of a twin, and artificial reproduction therapies.
  e. Genetic disorders

3. **Signs and symptoms (motor dysfunction and associated comorbidities)**
  a. Movement disorders including spasticity, dystonia, choreoathetosis, tremors, ataxia, myoclonus singly or in combination. Spasticity is most common.
  b. Epilepsy
  c. Cognitive impairment
  d. Speech impairment (aphasia, dysarthria, mutism, oral motor dysfunction, drooling)
  e. Somatosensory deficits
  f. Chronic pain and other sensory deficits (e.g., vision and hearing impairment)

g. Pulmonary disorders (e.g., aspiration, respiratory muscle incoordination)

h. Gastrointestinal disorders (e.g., constipation, gastroesophageal reflux disease, vomiting, dysphagia)

i. Urinary disorders (e.g., enuresis, frequency, urgency, and stress incontinence)

j. Complications include orthopedic deformity (scoliosis, hip dysplasia, foot deformities, and disuse complications related to decreased mobility

4. **Diagnostic study findings**

a. MRI abnormalities: white matter changes; combination gray and white matter changes; may identify structural changes that have a genetic basis; genetic and metabolic testing are not routinely recommended.

b. Diagnosis made primarily by clinical observation and history. Abnormal neurologic findings include poor neck and trunk control; posturing and thrusting movements, abnormal gait (walking on toes, impaired balance, scissoring of legs), abnormal muscle tone (e.g., clonus), and primitive reflexes.

c. Other related to comorbidities: EEG (to identify seizures) and hearing and vision assessment

5. **Goals of care: Anticipated trajectory**

a. Dependent on gross motor function: Improved motor control, gait, independent self-care, optimal mobility, sitting balance, prevention of orthopedic complications, comfort, and decreased care burden.

6. **Interdisciplinary collaboration: See Intracranial Aneurysms.**

7. **Management**

a. Anticipated patient trajectory: Maintain or improve prehospitalization mobility status, respiratory, gastrointestinal, and urinary function, nutrition, and communication status.

   i. Mobility: Reinforce physical, occupational, and speech therapy strategies

   ii. Pharmacology

   (a) Administer and monitor effects of antispastic medications, such as baclofen (oral or intrathecal), tizanidine, diazepam, botulinum toxin injections

   (b) Administer and monitor effects of medications for comorbid conditions, such as epilepsy, drooling (anticholinergic medication), and pain

   iii. Nutrition

   (a) Assess nutritional status

   (b) Administer nutrition as prescribed

   iv. Respiratory status

   (a) Assess oxygenation status

   (b) Aspiration precautions; collaborate with speech therapy as needed for dysphagia and modification of diet

   (c) Respiratory therapy as needed; oral care

   v. Surgical management: Monitor for improvement of symptoms and potential complications

   (a) Dorsal rhizotomy, selective surgical resection of lumbar-sacral dorsal nerve roots for management of spasticity

   (b) Implantation of intrathecal baclofen pump for spasticity

   vi. MRI precautions: Follow manufacturer's guidelines regarding compatibility; may be incompatible, and MRI cannot be done. If MRI conditional, pump may need to be emptied before MRI, turned off before MRI, and/or reprogrammable post-MRI.

   (a) Gastrostomy

Muscular Dystrophies

> **KEY CONCEPT**
> Muscular dystrophies (MDs) may start early or later in life as a teen or adult. Some patients with MD are at risk for malignant hyperthermia. Dantirum must be readily available as an antidote.

1. **Pathophysiology**
   a. A heterogenous group of muscle disorders with dystrophic pathologic features seen on muscle biopsy. MD is associated with progressive weakness and loss of muscle mass.
   b. Genetic mutations interfere with the protein production (dystrophin) in the formation of healthy muscle tissue.
2. **Etiology and risk factors**
   a. Genetic predisposition
      i. Duchenne muscular dystrophy (DMD): X-linked recessive gene: most common; associated with frequent falls, difficulty moving to a sitting position, trouble running and jumping, waddling gait, walking on toes; begins in early childhood
      ii. Becker muscular dystrophy (BMD): X-linked recessive gene; milder than DMD; signs similar to DMD; begins in teens to 20 years
      iii. Myotonic muscular dystrophy (MMD, DMI): autosomal dominant; inability to relax muscles after contractions, initially facial and neck muscles.
      iv. Facioscapulohumeral dystrophy (FSHD): autosomal dominant: muscle weakness in the face, hip, and shoulders initially; may begin from teens to 50 years
   b. Unknown carrier without prenatal workup
3. **Signs and symptoms**
   a. Onset of signs and symptoms vary from birth to adulthood. Limb girdle MD in early childhood or adolescence after independence in ambulation has been established. Some become apparent in adulthood. Males more commonly affected than females
   b. A common feature of all MD is skeletal muscle weakness; however, the degree, distribution, and progressive nature may differ among subtypes
   c. Ambulation may never be achieved, achieved and lost early, or achieved and lost later
   d. Muscle atrophy or hypertrophy, joint contractures, and myotonia
   e. May have minimal to severe respiratory impairment including impaired airway clearance and secretion management, nocturnal hypoventilation preceding daytime dyspnea, atelectasis, mucous plugging, pneumonia, dysphagia, and respiratory failure.
   f. Cardiac abnormalities cardiomyopathy
   g. Pulmonary problems: may deteriorate to a need for mechanical ventilation
   h. Dysphagia: at risk for aspiration, pneumonia
4. **Diagnostic studies**
   a. Laboratory tests: creatinine kinase
   b. Genetic testing
   c. EMG
   d. Muscle biopsy
   e. Other testing: ECG, echocardiogram, pulmonary function
5. **Diagnostic findings**
   a. CK elevation, myoglobinuria

    b. EMG with myopathy, myotonic discharges

    c. Muscle biopsy with variation in fiber size, fibrin splitting, hypertrophic or atrophic fibers, increased nuclei, inflammation

6. **Goals of care**

    a. Maintain muscle strength and mobility for as long as possible, including respiratory and cardiac function

    b. Minimize risk of injury and complications

    c. Minimize pain and discomfort

7. **Interprofessional collaboration: Nurse, physician, advanced practice provider, pharmacist, respiratory therapist, dietician, occupational, physical, and speech therapists, clinical psychologist.**

8. **Management**

    a. Maintain or improve prehospitalization mobility status, cardiac and respiratory function, nutrition, and communication.

    b. Pharmacology;

        i. Prednisone may be used to slow muscular weakness and increase muscle mass

        ii. Cardiac meds for prolonged QRS, AV block, BBB, and possible pacing

        iii. Analgesics

        iv. DMD, BMD, and MMD subtypes are associated with malignant hyperthermia. Avoid amitriptyline, digoxin, propranolol, quinine, sedatives, and specific anesthetics: thiopentone, halothane, suxamethonium, neostigmine. Administer Dantrium as emergency rescue agent.

    c. Monitor and manage respiratory status

        i. Aspiration precautions

        ii. Respiratory therapy

    d. Impaired mobility: PT and OT for stretching exercises, braces during ambulation

    e. Surgical intervention

        i. Heel cord straightening to decrease contractures

KEY CONCEPT

Prolonged seizures may become increasingly more difficult to stop. Antiepileptic medications are prescribed based on seizure type. Correction of a treatable underlying cause will lessen recurrence. A seizure that persists beyond 5 minutes is status epilepticus.

SEIZURE DISORDERS

EXPERT TIP

Status epilepticus of any type (e.g., tonic-clonic versus subclinical) is a neurologic emergency and must be stopped as soon as possible to prevent neuronal injury.

---

1. **Pathophysiology**

    a. *Seizures* are paroxysmal episodes of desynchronized and excessive electrical discharges from neurons that result in a sudden transient alteration in brain function.

    b. Epilepsy is a chronic seizure disorder consisting of recurrent unprovoked seizures.

    c. Aura is the initial warning or awareness at the beginning of the seizure. The patient may experience similar sensory or visceral experiences including taste, smell, visual, or auditory changes each time.

d. Ictus refers to the actual seizure and postictal is the time period immediately after the seizure

e. Seizures increase cerebral metabolic demand and can deplete high-energy phosphates (e.g., ATP), causing failure of energy-dependent functions (e.g., sodium-potassium-ATPase pump).

f. CBF can increase to three to five times the normal level.

g. Aspiration and trauma may occur during a seizure. Prolonged seizures can cause cerebral edema, neuronal dysfunction and injury, hyperthermia, metabolic derangements, arrhythmias, rhabdomyolysis, fractures, and death.

h. Seizures that occur in the acute phase of a neurologic insult can worsen neurologic outcome.

i. In *status epilepticus*, the brain's excitatory and inhibitory circuits become altered, which allows prolonged or frequently recurring seizures. The longer status epilepticus lasts, the more difficult it is to control.

j. Seizures lasting more than 5 minutes or recurrent seizures without complete recovery, status epilepticus, promote an imbalance of excitatory and inhibitory neurotransmitters. Glutamate, the principal excitatory neurotransmitter, is released which in turn results in calcium influx with a decrease in inhibitory gamma-aminobutyric acid (GABA) receptors and an increase in N-methyl-D-aspartate (NMDA) and AMPA excitatory receptors.

2. **Etiology and risk factors**

a. Inadequate levels of or withdrawal from anticonvulsant therapy

b. Acute withdrawal from the chronic use of sedatives or depressants (e.g., alcohol, benzodiazepines, barbiturates)

c. Medication toxicity or adverse medication reaction (e.g., cefepime, ibupropion, baclofen withdrawal)

d. Metabolic disorders (e.g., acidosis uremia, liver failure, hypoglycemia, electrolyte disorders, fever)

e. Neurologic pathologic conditions, such as TBI, CNS infections, brain tumors, cerebral edema, stroke, cerebral anoxia, hypertensive encephalopathy, AVM, increased ICP

f. Congenital/genetic

g. Idiopathic

3. **Signs and symptoms**

a. *Tonic-clonic seizure.* A generalized seizure involving the entire or large areas of both cerebral hemispheres. Loss of consciousness is followed by brief period of muscle rigidity (tonic phase) and then rhythmic muscle jerking (clonic phase) bilaterally. In the tonic phase, apnea may occur momentarily and cyanosis may develop. Hyperventilation may accompany the clonic phase or occur as the seizure terminates. Incontinence, profuse salivation, and diaphoresis are common during the seizure, which usually lasts 1 to 5 minutes. Headache, amnesia for the seizure, confusion, myalgia, and fatigue are common in the postictal phase.

b. *Myoclonic seizure:* Sudden, brief muscular contractions that may occur singly or repetitively; usually involve the extremities or face, but can be generalized.

c. *Partial or focal seizure:* A seizure localized in an area of one hemisphere. Partial seizures may be simple or complex. If the patient remains conscious, the seizure is referred to as a *simple partial seizure*. If the patient has loss of awareness during the seizure and amnesia for the event, it is referred to as a *complex partial seizure or focal impaired awareness*. Partial seizures may progress and secondarily generalize to include both cerebral hemispheres with loss of consciousness. The clinical presentation is related to the area of the brain affected.

   i. Motor events, such as face twitching or limb jerking
   ii. Automatisms (e.g., lip smacking, fidgeting, blinking): Common with complex partial seizures
   iii. Sensory events: Numbness or tingling; visual, auditory, gustatory, or vertiginous symptoms
   iv. Psychic events (e.g., hallucinations, illusions)
   v. Autonomic events (e.g., diaphoresis, vomiting)

 d. Todd's paralysis: Todd's paralysis is temporary focal weakness or paralysis after a partial or generalized seizure most likely related to neuronal exhaustion. Todd's paralysis may last up to 24 hours but other etiologies, such as stroke should be considered with prolonged weakness.

 e. *Status epilepticus:* Seizures occur for a prolonged period (>5 minutes) or repetitively without full recovery between ictal episodes. May be generalized convulsive, nonconvulsive (without visible movement), or, less commonly, focal motor seizures. Status epilepticus may be clinical or subclinical (the patient is unresponsive to all stimuli; the eyes may deviate away from the side of the seizure focus, and the EEG demonstrates seizure activity).

   i. Refractory status epilepticus: Status epilepticus that continues despite first-line therapy (benzodiazepines) and second-line therapy (anticonvulsants)
   ii. Super refractory status epilepticus: Status epilepticus that continues beyond 24 hours despite third-line therapy (e.g., drug-induced coma)

 f. Sudden unexplained death from epilepsy (SUDEP): sudden unexpected, nontraumatic death in an individual with epilepsy without anatomic or toxicologic cause.

4. **Diagnostic study findings**
 a. Laboratory
   i. Electrolyte or metabolic abnormalities (e.g., sodium imbalance, hypomagnesemia, hypoglycemia/hyperglycemia, and hypoxemia, hypercapnea) may precipitate or result from seizures.
   ii. Other: liver function tests (LFTs), ammonia, blood urea nitrogen, creatinine, lactate
   iii. Infectious disease workup: urine, blood, bronchoscopy, and wound cultures, cultures, chest x-ray, other)
   iv. Serum enzyme levels, particularly creatine phosphokinase levels, elevated after seizures
   v. Myoglobinuria is common after prolonged seizures
   vi. Anticonvulsant levels (e.g., free and total phenytoin levels)
   vii. Other tests (e.g., toxicology screen) may reveal disorders that precipitated the seizure
 b. Radiologic: To determine precipitating or complicating cause, for example, head CT, MRI
 c. EEG: Identifies seizure activity and localizes the foci; monitoring may be intermittent or continuous (cEEG)
 d. LP: cell count, protein, glucose, gram stain, bacterial and viral cultures

5. **Goals of care**
 a. Oxygenation and ventilation are maintained.
 b. Hemodynamic stability is maintained.
 c. Seizure activity is controlled.

d. No injuries or other complications result from the seizures.

e. No toxic effects are experienced from AEMs

6. **Interprofessional collaboration: Nurse, physician (may include neurologist and infectious disease specialist), advanced practice provider, EEG technician, respiratory therapist, pharmacist.**

7. **Management of patient care**

a. Anticipated patient trajectory: Seizures are controlled and, if identified, the precipitating factor is effectively treated. Specific needs of patients with seizures may include the following:

    i. Positioning: During or after the seizure (if possible), turn the patient on his or her side to prevent aspiration.

    ii. Protect and assess for injury.

    iii. Discharge planning: After seizures and precipitating factors are controlled and metabolic responses to seizure are resolved, the patient can typically be discharged to home. Unresolved neurologic impairment from seizures may require discharge to a rehabilitation center or skilled nursing care facility.

    iv. Pharmacology

      (a) Supplemental oxygen

      (b) Prescribed IV fluids to maintain euvolemia

      (c) Anticonvulsant(s) to control seizures. Monotherapy preferred, but if one anticonvulsant is not effective, another may be added. Monitor and maintain therapeutic plasma levels, observe for toxic effects.

        (1) Benzodiazepines are generally used to control acute seizures. An anticonvulsant medication (usually phenytoin [Dilantin] or fosphenytoin [Cerebyx] is given simultaneously to prevent recurrent seizures; Table 5.29).

        (2) Valproic acid (Depakene) or levetiracetam (Keppra) may be added for seizures refractory to phenytoin.

        (3) If seizure activity is not halted with these medications in the usual dosages, high-dose pentobarbital, propofol, or midazolam infusions may be used (see Table 5.29).

    v. Management of status epilepticus

      (a) Pharmacologic

        (1) First-line/emergent therapy: benzodiazepines: (IV lorazepam or diazepam; IM midazolam)

        (2) Second-line/urgent therapy: anticonvulsants (fosphenytoin, valproic acid, levetiracetam; alternatives include phenobarbital and lacosamide)

        (3) Third-line therapy: ET intubation if it has not occurred before third-line therapy (continuous infusions of midazolam, propofol, barbiturates (e.g., pentobarbital), ketamine, lidocaine, or inhaled anesthetic agents (e.g., isoflurane)

      (b) Other, such as ketogenic diet per feeding tube

      (c) cEEG: cEEG as soon as possible with a goal of burst suppression (percentage as determined by provider)

    vi. Psychosocial issues: Depression and social isolation may occur; ensure provision of counseling and support for dealing with seizures and potentially necessary life changes

    vii. Treatments

      (a) Noninvasive

TABLE 5.29 **Anticonvulsants Commonly Used to Treat Status Epilepticus**

Medication	Typical Dosage	Onset	Desired Medication Level	Major Adverse Effects
Lorazepam	4 mg (0.1 mg/kg) intravenously (IV) at 2 mg/min; maximum 4 mg per dose	Usually around 5–20 minutes	Not typically assessed	Sedation; respiratory depression (more common with use of diazepam); may cause hypotension Contains propylene glycol which may cause metabolic acidosis and paradoxical agitation
Diazepam	0.15 mg/kg IV: maximum 10 mg/dose IV, per single dose: May repeat every 5 minutes	As early as 10–20 seconds; onset 1–3 minutes	Not typically assessed	Sedation; respiratory depression, hypotension may occur
Midazolam	For refractory seizures: 0.2 mg/kg IV (rate 2 mg/min) initial: Infusion: 0.05–2 mg/kg/h	1–5 minutes	Not typically assessed	Sedation, neuromuscular block, respiratory depression and arrest, hypotension
Phenytoin	20 mg/kg IV, no faster than 50 mg/min in saline solution: then 300–400 mg/day in divided doses; do not give intramuscularly (a vesicant); filter for IV infusion; not compatible in dextrose-containing IV solutions	30–60 minutes	Total level: 10–20 mcg/mL; Free level 12 mcg/mL	Dysrhythmias (e.g., bradycardia); cardiovascular collapse; use cautiously in patients with heart block or Stokes-Adams syndrome; hypotension may occur. Purple glove syndrome or Stevens-Johnson (toxic epidermal necrolysis)
Fosphenytoin (Cerebyx)	Dosed as phenytoin equivalents (PE), 20 mg/kg PE IV at 150 mg PE/min; can be given faster than phenytoin IV; maximum 1500 mg/PE/dose; may be given intramuscularly; converted to phenytoin; compatible in standard IV solutions, including those with glucose	Conversion to phenytoin half-life is 15 minutes	Same as for phenytoin (actually assess phenytoin levels)	Same as for phenytoin
Valproic acid (Depakote)	20–40 mg/kg IV; may give additional 20 mg/kg	Oral immediate-release CMax: 4 hours	50–100 mcg/mL	Sedation, tremors, hepatic toxicity, thrombocytopenia, gastrointestinal disturbance, alopecia
Levetiracetam (Keppra)	1000–3000 mg IV, 2–5 mg/kg/min IV rate; maximum dose 3000 mg/day	Oral immediate-release CMax: 1 hour Oral controlled-release CMax: 4 hours	Not typically assessed	Sedation, weakness, incoordination, behavioral abnormalities, leukopenia

Drug	Dosing	Onset/Peak	Level	Adverse effects
Lacosamide (Vimpat)	50 mg twice daily PO; may increase 100 mg/day every week up to 150–200 mg twice daily (adjust for renal or hepatic disease)	Peaks in 30 minutes to 1 hour (IV formulation)	Not typically assessed	Diplopia, dizziness, headache, agitation, nausea, anemia, neutropenia, agranulocytosis
Phenobarbital (Luminal)	20 mg/kg/dose IV up to a dose of 50–100 mg/minute; maintenance 1–3 mg/kg/day in 2–3 doses daily	Onset: 5 minutes. Peak: 15 minutes	20–40 mcg/mL	Sedation, hypotension, respiratory depression may occur
Pentobarbital (Nembutal)	Typical loading dose is 5–15 mg/kg IV, rate ≤50 mg/min, followed by an infusion of 0.5 mg/kg/h to 5 mg/kg/h maintenance	3–5 minutes	10–50 mcg/mL	Hypotension, myocardial and respiratory depression, immune suppression, and CNS depression, which obscures the neurologic examination
Propofol (Diprivan)	Initial 1–2 mg/kg/IV over 3–5 minutes; repeated boluses every 3–5 minutes (maximum 10 mg/kg load; initial rate 20 mcg/kg/min; maintenance 30–200 mcg/kg/min)	<1 minute	Not typically assessed	Hypotension, respiratory depression and arrest; propofol infusion syndrome— metabolic acidosis, cardiac failure, rhabdomyolysis, hyperkalemia, and renal failure
Ketamine	1.5 mg/kg IV push over 3–5 minutes; repeat until seizures stop; maximum total loading dose of 4.5 mg/kg. Infusion rate: 1.2 mg/kg/h; maintenance range: 0.3–10 mg/kg/h	1–5 minutes	Not typically assessed	Hypertension, hypersalivation, hallucinations, cardiac ischemia

From Hemphill, J.C., Rabinstein, A.A., Samuels, O.B. (2015). *The practice of neurocritical care*. Minneapolis: Neurocritical Care Society; Gahart, B.L., Nazareno, A.R., Ortega, M.O. (2020). *Intravenous medications*, 36ᵗʰ ed. St. Louis: Elsevier; Glauser, T., Shinnar, S., Gloss, D., et al (2016). Evidence-based guideline: treatment of convulsive status epilepticus in children and adults: report of the Guideline Committee of the American Epilepsy Society. *Epilepsy Current*, 16(1), 48–61; Elsevier, Skidmore-Roth, L. (2020). *Mosby's 2020 nursing drug reference*, 33ʳᵈ ed. St. Louis: Elsevier.

(1) If the patient has a neurologic disease or injury that puts the patient at high risk for seizures, implement seizure precautions: Maintain the bed in a low position with side rails up and padded; ensure that harmful objects are out of reach; keep suction and airway equipment readily available

(2) Facilitate repeat EEG or provide cEEG monitoring to detect subclinical seizures and evaluate the effectiveness of anticonvulsant therapy

(3) Observe, record, and report seizures including the body parts involved, the order of involvement, and the nature of movements; eye deviation, nystagmus, and pupil size change; respiratory pattern and function; neurologic status throughout the seizure and postictal phase; the duration of each phase

(4) Maintain a patent airway; ensure adequate ventilation and circulation during and after a seizure; suction airway as necessary

(5) Prevent injury during seizures: Stay with the patient; never force anything into the patient's mouth; do not restrain the patient; remove harmful objects from the vicinity; loosen tight clothes; if the patient is out of bed, lower the patient to the floor; padded siderails and head and footboard

(6) Reorient the patient after the seizure

(7) Investigate and treat the underlying cause

(8) Educate the patient and family about seizures, actions to take for another seizure, planned diagnostic tests and interventions, prescribed anticonvulsants

  (b) Invasive: Intubation and ventilator support if necessary

b. Potential complications

  i. Metabolic complications may include acidosis, hypoxemia, hypoglycemia, electrolyte imbalances, including fluctuations in glucose, potassium sodium, magnesium, calcium, phosphate, and pH

    (a) Mechanism: Seizures cause increased metabolic demands and imbalances

    (b) Management: Identify and correct imbalances

  ii. Cerebral edema, ischemia, and brain dysfunction

    (a) Mechanism: Seizures increase the CMR; if cerebral oxygen delivery does not keep up with metabolic demand, brain ischemia, edema, neuronal dysfunction, and death can occur. Hyperemia from increased CMR encourages vasogenic edema. Initial hyperglycemia may be followed by hypoglycemia after glycogen stores are exhausted; which may potentially increase secondary neuronal injury.

    (b) Management: Control seizures. Monitor neurologic status. Avoid hypoxia. Optimize cerebral oxygen delivery.

  iii. Increased ICP

    (a) Mechanism: Cerebral edema and hyperemia

    (b) Management: See Increased Intracranial Pressure

  iv. Renal failure (acute tubular necrosis)

    (a) Mechanism: Myoglobinuria from muscle breakdown, rhabdomyolysis, during prolonged seizure activity can lead to acute renal failure.

    (b) Management (see Ch. 6, Renal System)

  v. Hyperthermia

    (a) Mechanism: Seizures increase the metabolic rate and muscle activity, which elevates body temperature

(b) Management: Antipyretics, cooling measures as warranted

    vi. Cardiovascular: Hypertension, hypotension, myocardial infarction, arrhythmias

   vii. Pulmonary: Hypoxia, neurogenic or cardiogenic PE, aspiration, pneumonia; ventilator dependence, acute respiratory distress syndrome

  viii. Infectious disease: Invasive device associated infection (ET tube, urinary catheter, sepsis); impaired immune status on barbiturate therapy

    ix. Musculoskeletal: Bone fractures, joint dislocations, muscular wasting with drug-induced coma

     x. Integumentary: Oral mucosa injury; device-related pressure injury; impaired mobility

    xi. Hypothermia associated with barbiturate coma (decreased metabolism)

KEY CONCEPT

Effective management of the underlying cause of encephalopathy is the key to treatment. The exact etiology of specific-types of encephalopathies is not entirely understood. In hepatic encephalopathy, ammonia levels are not necessarily considered diagnostic and do not correlate with the severity of hepatic encephalopathy.

ENCEPHALOPATHY

1. **Pathophysiology: Encephalopathy is not a disease in itself but results from other systemic or brain disorders. Global mental status dysfunction caused by one or more of the following direct or indirect pathologic conditions affecting the brain: Buildup of toxins, metabolic imbalance, alterations in CBF, changes in the structure or electrical activity of the brain, changes in the supply or utilization of neurotransmitter substances, or other cellular changes that alter neurologic functioning.**

  a. Hepatic

    i. The exact pathophysiology is unknown.

    ii. Hepatic encephalopathy is thought to be multifactorial including neurotoxins mediated by retention of ammonia; impairment of neural transmission resulting in an imbalance between excitatory and inhibitory signaling; systemic inflammatory response syndrome (SIRS); alterations in brain metabolism and the BBB; and bacterial overgrowth

  b. Infectious/septic

    i. The exact pathophysiology is not completely understood.

    ii. Infectious encephalopathy is multifactorial and not likely related to microorganism or toxins in the cerebral tissue. The release of proinflammatory cytokines, chemokines, and prostaglandins occurs. Current hypotheses include changes in brain cell function and signaling with abnormalities of brain perfusion and oxygenation. This may be worsened with renal or hepatic dysfunction, abnormal glucoses, fever, and medications.

  c. Ischemic: Posterior reversible encephalopathy syndrome (PRES) is one subtype.

    i. The pathophysiology of PRES is controversial. A rapid increase in systemic BP may in part explain PRES. However, additional mechanisms include impaired cerebral autoregulation with increased CBF and endothelial dysfunction with cerebral hypoperfusion.

  d. Anoxic: Anoxic encephalopathy, also referred to as *hypoxic-ischemic brain injury* (*HIBI*) or *hypoxic ischemic encephalopathy* (*HIE*) results from a critical decline or loss of CBF, oxygen, and nutrients. Particularly vulnerable areas of the brain include the CA-1 area of the hippocampus, caudate, putamen, and neocortex. The brainstem is typically spared. A cellular injury cascade consists of imbalance of inhibitory and excitatory neurotransmitter with neurotoxicity for elevated excitatory neurotransmitters, calcium influx, development of oxygen free radicals, oxidative stress, cytotoxic edema, with neuronal necrosis and apoptosis.

   e. Metabolic: Metabolic encephalopathy is a result of the nonstructural disruption of the brain chemistry including electrolytes, water, amino acids, excitatory and inhibitory neurotransmitters, and metabolic substrates

   f. Uremic: Accumulation or uremic neurotoxins is responsible for uremic encephalopathy. The uremic neurotoxins may in turn cause hormonal disturbances, alterations in metabolism, and an imbalance between excitatory and inhibitory transmitters.

2. **Etiology and risk factors**
   a. Numerous disorders in various body systems can lead to encephalopathy, such as severe systemic hypertension, hypoxia, infection, sepsis, vascular disease, liver or kidney dysfunction, hypoglycemia, hyperglycemia, lead toxicity, concussive brain injury.

   b. Systemic diseases are often in their end stage when encephalopathy becomes apparent (e.g., uremic or hepatic encephalopathy)

   c. Hepatic: Acute liver failure; portosystemic bypass shunting, chronic alcoholism, hepatitis; triggers include; infections/sepsis, excessive use of diuretics, gastrointestinal bleeding, dehydration, electrolyte imbalance, CNS depressants, failure to comply with hepatic encephalopathy treatment (lactulose)

   d. Infectious/septic: Infection with a resultant overwhelming inflammatory response with at least one organ dysfunction; risk factors include immunosuppression, older age, multiple comorbid diseases, and cardiovascular dysfunction associated with tissue hypoxia

   e. Ischemic (subtype PRES): Systemic hypertension, preeclampsia/eclampsia, posttransplant, infection, sepsis, and shock, immune suppression, autoimmune disease, oncologic chemotherapy, metabolic disorders (e.g., hypercalcemia, hypomagnesemia), tumor lysis syndrome, dialysis/erythropoietin, ephedra overdose, IVIg, and idiopathic.

   f. Anoxic ischemic encephalopathy/HIE: Cardiac arrest related to cardiac disease; respiratory neurologic and metabolic conditions; trauma intoxication; and metabolic conditions. Also asphyxia, lack of airflow related to hanging, drowning, strangulation, suffocation, and chocking.

   g. Metabolic: Electrolyte abnormalities including hyper-/hyponatremia, hyper-/hypoglycemia, hyper-/hypocalcemia, hyper-/hypomagnesemia, hypophosphatemia; recreational drugs and drugs of abuse, thiamine deficiency associated with alcoholism, malnutrition (Wernicke's encephalopathy)

3. **Uremic: Renal failure with elevation of blood urea nitrogen (BUN). Signs and symptoms:**
   a. Vary widely, from memory problems to behavioral disorders and depressed LOC; neurologic changes are consistent with the cause of the encephalopathy

   b. Family history: Relevant in degenerative or hereditary disorders that lead to encephalopathy

   c. Social history: May suggest precipitating cause (e.g., chronic alcohol abuse leads to thiamine deficiency and Wernicke's encephalopathy)

   d. Medical history: Consistent with neurologic changes that correlate with the cause of the encephalopathy

e. Hepatic: Mental status changes may range from mild confusion to comatose. In stage I, mild confusion, difficulty with simple math and easily distracted; in stage II, lethargy, disorientation, change in personality; in stage III, somnolence to obtundation and gross disorientation; and stage IV, nonresponsive to pain, comatose: motor signs, such as asterixis, hypertonia, hyperreflexia, and extrapyramidal (EPS) symptoms

f. Infectious/sepsis: Mental status changes may range from mild confusion and lethargy to severe cognitive dysfunction and coma; delirium; muscle rigidity, tremors, and seizures

g. Ischemic (PRES): Headache, impaired visual acuity or visual field deficits, confusion, focal neurologic deficits, decline in LOC, and seizures; most often reversible

h. Anoxic/hypoxic-ischemic: Early HIE neurologic signs and symptoms include coma, seizures and myoclonus, and dysautonomia. Delayed signs and symptoms include seizures, persistent vegetative state, movement disorders, cognitive impairment, posttraumatic stress disorder (PTSD), depression, and dysautonomia.

i. Metabolic: Altered mental status from confusion to comatose state, seizures Wernicke's encephalopathy is associated with mental status changes, as well as oculomotor dysfunction, and gait ataxia.

j. Uremic: Symptoms include fatigue, apathy, emotional lability, irritability, perceptual errors, delirium delusion, hallucinations, tremors, seizure, and varying levels of consciousness. Symptomatology may vary related to rapidity of rise of BUN and age or other comorbidities. Symptoms may be alleviated by dialysis or renal transplantation.

4. **Diagnostic study findings: Vary, depending on the cause**
   a. Imaging: CT, MRI, SPECT, PET
   b. Serum chemistries, toxicology screen, cultures
   c. LP for CSF analysis once CT is read and does not show evidence of significant increased ICP.
   d. EEG
   e. Hepatic: Diagnosis is primarily based on clinical presentation; a diagnosis of exclusion after ruling out other causes of changes in mental status demonstrated on neuropsychologic testing; ammonia levels are not necessarily considered diagnostic for hepatic encephalopathy and do not correlate with the severity of hepatic encephalopathy; other labs should be performed to rule out other causes of encephalopathy, CT scan to rule out intracranial lesion, such as ICH.
   f. Infectious/septic: Diagnosis is primarily based on clinical presentation; EEG may detect subtle changes in cortical function associated with sepsis, as well as seizures associated with sepsis; biomarkers, such as neurospecific enolase (NSE) and S100 B may be seen in septic shock. Imaging may be unremarkable; however, vasogenic edema and leukoencephalopathy may be seen on MRI in comatose septic patients.
   g. Ischemic (PRES): Clinical presentation plus radiologic features on MRI FLAIR, diffusion-weighted imaging (DWI), and anoxic encephalopathy demonstrate vasogenic edema in the parietal-occipital region; punctate, ICH, and SAH may be seen as well. CT scan may show vasogenic edema with a bihemispheric distribution.
   h. Hypoxic-ischemic: Neurologic presentation. There are no tests specific to HIE. Brain biomarkers for neuronal injury, such as NSE, protein s100-ß, and neurofilament heavy chain (NfH) proteins are elevated in serum and CSF. Imaging: CT may be initially normal but MRI will later show tissue injury in areas of vulnerability. EEG diagnostic for seizures. SSEP provides prognostication.
   i. Metabolic: Diagnosis made by laboratory values and clinical presentation; may be diagnosis of exclusion

j. Uremic laboratory analysis of BUN. EEG changes may correlate with uremic encephalopathy. Imaging to rule out other causes of encephalopathy or neurologic disorders

5. **Goals of care**
   a. Cause of encephalopathy is determined or resolved
   b. Neurologic status returns to baseline or improves

6. **Interprofessional collaboration: See Increased Intracranial Pressure; also other team members, depending on the cause.**

7. **Management of patient care: Relates to the primary cause of encephalopathy**
   a. Anticipated patient trajectory: Etiology of encephalopathy will be determined. Risk factors will be eliminated or controlled. Patient will return to baseline neurologic status.
   b. Hepatic: Care of the patient with hepatic encephalopathy depends on the severity of the encephalopathy. If patient has difficulty maintain airway, may require ET intubation, management of precipitating causes, and correction of hyperammonemia. Rifaximin may potentiate the effect of lactulose to maintain remission of the encephalopathy. Provide appropriate nutrition.
   c. Infectious/septic: Care of the patient with infectious/septic encephalopathy depends on early treatment of the sepsis and supportive care for the failing organs. Withdrawal of any benzodiazepines, strategies to reduce delirium, dexmedetomidine may have neuroprotective effects. Antipsychotic drugs be effective.
   d. Ischemic (PRES): No specific treatment regimen is available other than management of hypertension and elimination of the underlying cause. Antiepilepsy drugs may be needed for seizures. Magnesium levels should be maintained at high normal values.
   e. HIE: Medical stabilization emergency, targeted temperature management (hypothermia vs. normothermia), management or prevention of shivering, management of myoclonus, hemodynamic stabilization, ventilator support during targeted temperature management, ICP management, other system support (renal, endocrine, hematologic, and gastrointestinal).
   f. Metabolic: Correction of underlying electrolyte disorders. Removal of toxins.
   g. Uremic: Correction of uremia with dialysis or renal transplantation. Correction of underlying electrolyte disorders. Management of seizures if present.

KEY CONCEPT

The underlying cause of the coma is critical to coma treatment or reversal. Reversible conditions, such as hypothermia, metabolic abnormalities, and medications, may confound the neurologic examination.

COMA

1. **Pathophysiology: The patient in a coma is unresponsive to the environment of self and shows no evidence of arousal (wakefulness, vigilance) to any stimuli, lasting more than 1 hour. There is a disturbance of the cerebral cortex and/or the RAS. Causes may be primary or secondary, structural or metabolic. A coma may also be induced pharmacologically. The patient typically presents with closed eyes with only reflexive, nonpurposeful movements and an inability to interact or respond to their external environment.**

2. **Etiology and risk factors**
   a. Brain trauma
   b. Stroke
   c. CNS infections

    d. Brain tumors

    e. Seizure

    f. Anoxic-ischemic encephalopathy

    g. Metabolic disorders: Liver, renal, sepsis, electrolyte disturbances, carbon dioxide narcosis, adrenal failure

    h. Medications: Opioids, alcohol, cocaine, amphetamines, sedative-hypnotics, aspirin, acetaminophen, antiepileptic medications, antidepressants

    i. Environmental causes: Hypothermia, carbon monoxide

    j. History suggestive of the previously described risk factors

3. **Signs and symptoms**

    a. State of unresponsiveness, GCS or FOUR Score

    b. Abnormal breathing patterns

    c. Pathologic reflexes: Decorticate or decerebrate posturing, positive Babinski reflex in an adult; presence of an oculocephalic reflex; presence of an oculovestibular reflex

    d. Pupil abnormalities

    e. Absence of purposeful movements

4. **Diagnostic study findings**

    a. Laboratory analysis including serum chemistries, hematologic panel, ABGs, toxicology, cultures

    b. Imaging: CT, CTA, CT perfusion, MRI

    c. LP

    d. EEG

5. **Goals of care**

    a. Cause of coma is resolved

    b. Neurologic status returns to baseline or improves

6. **Interprofessional collaboration: See Increased Intracranial Pressure; also other team members, depending on the cause.**

7. **Management of patient care: Relates to the primary cause of coma and prevention of nosocomial injury**

KEY CONCEPT

Determination of brain death must be a systematic stepwise approach each and every time. The $PaCO_2$ must rise to at least 60 mm Hg and 20 mm Hg above patient's baseline $PaCO_2$ to stimulate the brainstem without the patient taking a breath to declare brain death by clinical examination.

BRAIN DEATH

1. **Pathogenesis: Brain death is the irreversible absence of brain function. The criteria for brain death in an adult include unresponsiveness and lack of movement (spinal reflexes may persist); and absence of cranial nerve function (pupillary, oculocephalic, oculovestibular, corneal, cough, and gag reflexes) and absence of spontaneous respirations. The presence of a known irreversible cause for coma, masking neuromuscular or sedative agents; metabolic or endocrine abnormality; and hypothermia must be excluded.**

2. **Etiology and risk factors**

    a. Brain trauma

    b. Stroke

    c. CNS infections

    d. Brain tumors

    e. Seizures

    f. Anoxic-ischemic injury

    g. Metabolic disorders: Liver, renal, sepsis, electrolyte disturbances, carbon dioxide narcosis, adrenal failure

    h. Medications: Opioids, alcohol, cocaine, amphetamines, sedative- hypnotics, aspirin, acetaminophen, antiepileptic medications, antidepressants

    i. Environmental causes: Hypothermia, carbon monoxide

    j. History suggestive of the previously discussed risk factors

3. **Signs and symptoms: Clinical bedside examination supportive of brain death**

    a. Clinical examination demonstrates state of unresponsiveness, GCS of 3 or FOUR score of 0.

    b. Absence of spontaneous breathing

    c. Absence of pupillary response; corneal, cough, and gag reflexes; absence of oculocephalic and oculovestibular reflexes

    d. Absence of purposeful movement

4. **Diagnostic study findings**

    a. Absence of reversible causes of coma: Hypothermia, electrolyte abnormalities (hypoglycemia, hyperglycemia, hyponatremia), and negative toxicology screen

    b. Apnea test: Absence of spontaneous breath when PCO_2 is allowed to rise sufficiently to stimulate the brainstem to initiate a spontaneous breath; during testing patient is maintained on FiO_2 100% without other ventilatory support; $PaCO_2$ rises 20 mm Hg above baseline and greater than 60 mm Hg; patient is observed for any spontaneous respiratory effort. Absence of any respiratory effort supports brain death.

    c. Ancillary tests

        i. Cerebral angiogram: Absence of CBF

        ii. Nuclear medicine cerebral flow study: Absence of cerebral flow

        iii. TCD: Absence of cerebral flow

        iv. Absence of electrical activity on EEG

        v. Evoked potentials show disruption of pathway (SSEP)

5. **Goals of care**

    a. Brain death is either established or ruled out

    b. Organ donation is considered if patient is brain dead

    c. Neurologic status returns to baseline or improves if patient is not declared brain dead

6. **Interprofessional collaboration: Nurse, physician (may include neurologist, neurointensivist, and neurosurgeon), advanced practice provider, EEG technician, respiratory therapist, pharmacist, Interprofessional Ethics Committee.**

7. **Management of patient care**

    a. Eliminate all reversible causes of comatose state

    b. Collaborate with team depending on outcome of brain death determination

    c. Provide support to family

NEUROSURGICAL PROCEDURES

> **KEY CONCEPT**
> Once the skull and dura are opened under anesthesia, the patient may be awakened just before resection of a brain tumor or epilepsy focus to allow changes in the patient's neurologic examination to guide the neurosurgeon in removal of as much disease tissue as possible yet spare the patient any additional neurologic deficits.

1. **Craniotomy**
   a. Description: Opening the skull during surgery to access intracranial contents. Skull bone is removed and replaced at the end of the procedure or preserved for later replacement. A subgaleal drain may be placed at the end of the procedure to facilitate healing. A craniotomy may be performed asleep or awake.
   b. Indications: Removal of a brain tumor, placement of a clip on an aneurysm, evacuation of a blood clot or abscess, or foreign object, resection of an AVM or perform a cerebrovascular bypass and epilepsy surgery.
   c. Complications: Neurologic injury, seizures, blood loss, intracranial clot formation, cerebral edema, herniation, hydrocephalus, CSF leaks, pneumocephalus, complications related to positioning and proning in surgery, infection (bone flap, meningitis, brain abscess)
   d. Management of patient care
      i. Monitor neurologic status
      ii. Monitor incision for blood loss initially and infection; monitor subgaleal drainage for the amount of blood and the presence of any CSF
      iii. Administer antiepileptic drugs, corticosteroids, and antibiotics as prescribed
2. **Craniectomy**
   a. Description: Removal of part of the skull bone without replacement. It may or may not be replaced depending on the size and location.
   b. Indications: Decompression after TBI with cerebral edema, large vessel territory stroke with actual or potential edema, postcraniotomy infection
   c. Complications: neurologic injury, seizures, blood loss, intracranial clot formation, cerebral edema, extracranial or paradoxical herniation, hydrocephalus, CSF leaks, pneumocephalus, complications related to positioning and proning in surgery, infection (meningitis, brain abscess), and headaches, impaired memory, dizziness, mood/behavior disturbances related to sunken brain/trephine syndrome.
   d. Management of patient care:
      i. Monitor neurologic status
      ii. Monitor incision for blood loss initially and infection; monitor subgaleal drainage amount of blood, presence of CSF, tension or depression at site
      iii. Initially avoid dependent positioning; monitor tension; helmet to protect brain when out of bed
      iv. Administer antiepileptic drugs, corticosteroids, and antibiotics as prescribed
      v. Cranioplasty care after bone flap replaced or synthetic materials used to repair skull defect
3. **Burr holes**
   a. Small ovals of skull bone are removed as the initial stage of performing a craniotomy or to access small areas of the intracranial content.
   b. Indications: Removal of epidural and subdural hematomas (intracranial blood clots), stereotaxic brain biopsy, epilepsy surgery
   c. Management of patient care
      i. Monitor neurologic status
      ii. Monitor incision for blood loss initially and infection; monitor drainage amount of blood and presence of CSF

References and bibliography information are available at http://evolve.elsevier.com/AACN/corecurriculum/.

CHAPTER 6

Renal System

Bryan Boling, DNP, AG-ACNP, CCRN-CSC, CEN

SYSTEMWIDE ELEMENTS

ANATOMY AND PHYSIOLOGY REVIEW

1. Process of urine formation: Urine formation occurs in the renal nephron and involves four processes—filtration, reabsorption, secretion, and excretion
    a. Anatomic structures of the kidney: Most humans are born with two kidneys; a small number are born with one. The kidneys are located in the retroperitoneal space above the pelvis (Fig. 6.1).
        i. Cortical (outermost) layer
            (a) Metabolically active portion of the kidney where aerobic metabolism occurs and where ammonia and glucose are formed
            (b) Metabolic needs are more than satisfactorily met by an abundant oxygen supply
            (c) Contains all glomeruli and portions of the proximal and distal tubules
        ii. Medullary (middle) layer
            (a) Region of active glycolytic metabolism; supplies energy for active transport
            (b) Metabolism demands high oxygen consumption, yet oxygen supply limited

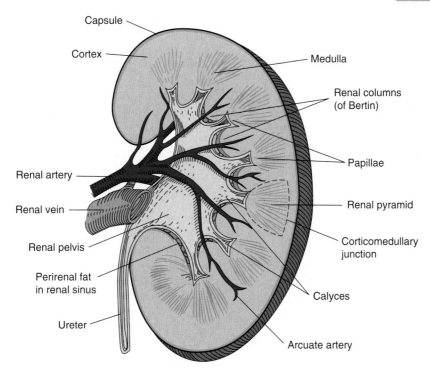

Fig. 6.1 Major structures of the kidney shown in a diagram of the cut surface of a bisected kidney. (From Yu, A.S., Chertow, G.M., Luyckx, V.A., et al. (2020). *Brenner and Rector's the kidney*, 11ᵗʰ ed. Philadelphia: Elsevier.)

In the figure, the following structures are labeled: Capsule, Cortex, Medulla, Renal columns (of Bertin), Renal artery, Papillae, Renal vein, Renal pyramid, Renal pelvis, Corticomedullary junction, Perirenal fat in renal sinus, Calyces, Ureter, Arcuate artery.

      (c) Plays role in concentration of urine

      (d) Composed of 6 to 10 renal pyramids, formed by collecting ducts and extending into the renal pelvis

      (e) Site of the deepest part of the long loops of Henle and the collecting ducts of the nephron

  iii. Renal sinus, pelvis, and collecting system

      (a) Papillae: Rounded projections of renal tissue located at the apical ends of the renal pyramids positioned with the base facing the cortex and the apices facing renal pelvis; the apical portion opens into the minor calices

      (b) Corticomedullary junction: Point of division between the cortex and the medulla formed by the base of the pyramids

      (c) Renal lobe: Composed of a pyramid plus the surrounding cortical tissue

      (d) Calix

         (1) Minor calix wraps around the papilla; receives urine from the collecting duct

         (2) Major calix channels urine from the renal sinus to the renal pelvis

         (3) Urine flows from the renal pelvis to the ureter

  iv. Nephron: Anatomic microscopic structure (Fig. 6.2)

      (a) Structural and functional unit of the kidney

      (b) Approximately 1 million in each kidney

      (c) Compensates for a significant degree of nephron destruction by:

         (1) Filtering a greater solute load

         (2) Hypertrophy of the remaining functional nephrons

      (d) Types of nephrons, based on location and function

         (1) Cortical nephrons located in the outer region of the cortex; contain short loops of Henle with a low capacity for sodium reabsorption

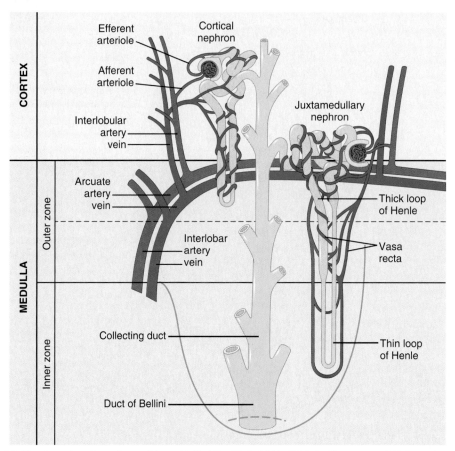

Fig. 6.2 The functional nephron. (From Hall, J.E., Hall, M.E. (2021). *Guyton and Hall textbook of medical physiology*, 1st ed. Philadelphia: Elsevier.)

    (2) Juxtamedullary nephrons located in the inner cortex adjacent to the medulla; have long loops of Henle that penetrate deep into the medulla and have a greater capacity for concentration of urine because they are sodium-retaining nephrons

  (e) Functional segments of the nephron

    (1) Renal corpuscle

      a) Bowman's capsule: Specialized portion of the proximal tubule that supports the glomerulus

      b) Glomerulus: Capillary bed with semipermeable membrane

        1) Normally permeable to water, electrolytes, nutrients, wastes; relatively impermeable to large protein molecules, albumin, erythrocytes

        2) Composed of three cellular layers: Fenestrated endothelial layer, basement membrane, and epithelium podocyte cells that contribute to characteristic semipermeability of this membrane

        3) Characteristics of cellular layers: Endothelial cells contain fenestrations 50 to 100 nm wide, favoring the movement of water and solute; remaining layers are less porous with openings 1500 nm-thick, which may explain the impedance of macromolecules

        4) Major factor influencing filtration is molecular size

5) Ionic charge also affects filtration
  a) Electrical potential of the glomerular membrane possesses a negative charge, which favors the passage of positively charged molecules and impedes negatively charged molecules, such as albumin
  b) Loss of membrane electrical potential in glomerular disease is reason for proteinuria
(2) Renal tubules
  a) Segmentally divided into the proximal convoluted tubule, descending loop of Henle, ascending loop of Henle, distal convoluted tubule, and collecting duct
  b) Each segment has a specific cellular structure and function
b. Physiologic processes

KEY CONCEPT
The kidneys filter the blood and create urine as a means to eliminate waste products, maintain electrolyte balance, and excrete excess fluid volume.

---

i. Glomerular ultrafiltration is the first step in the formation of urine
  (a) Characteristics of glomerular filtrate
    (1) Normal: Protein-free and red blood cell (RBC)-free, plasmalike substance with a specific gravity (SG) of 1.010. Filtrate contains water, electrolytes, glucose, amino acids, acid-base components, wastes, and other solutes. Pharmaceutical agents can also be included in filtrate.
    (2) Small and middle-sized molecules (up to 60–75 kilodalton [kD]) pass freely through the glomerular membrane (e.g., inulin 5 kD passes, albumin >60 kD does not pass)
    (3) Abnormal: Increased permeability of the glomerular membrane allows erythrocytes and protein to be filtered into urine. SG of urine may artificially increase because of the presence of protein or glucose.
    (4) Filtration of osmotically active substances (glucose, urea): Can cause diuresis
  (b) Filtration is determined by the glomerular pressure and presence of a normal semipermeable glomerular membrane
    (1) Glomerular hydrostatic pressure is 50 mm Hg and favors filtration; this capillary hydrostatic pressure reflects cardiac output
    (2) Colloid osmotic pressure of 25 mm Hg and Bowman's capsule hydrostatic pressure of 10 mm Hg oppose hydrostatic pressure and thus oppose filtration
      a) Colloid osmotic pressure results from oncotic pressure of plasma proteins in the glomerular blood supply
      b) Bowman's capsule pressure reflects renal interstitial pressure
    (3) Net filtration pressure is derived using the following formula:

Glomerular hydrostatic pressure(facilitates):	+50 mm Hg
Colloid osmotic pressure(opposes):	−25 mm Hg
Bowman's capsule pressure(opposes):	−10 mm Hg
Net pressure favoring filtration:	+15 mm Hg

  (c) Glomerular filtration rate (GFR)

(1) Clinical assessment tool to determine renal function; not measured directly in clinical practice, estimated GFR (eGFR) is derived using one of several equations (see the following section)

(2) Definition: Volume of plasma cleared of a given substance per minute (may be determined by using endogenous creatinine)

(3) GFR equation

$$GFR = \frac{(U_x \times V)}{P_x}$$

where

x = a substance freely filtered through the glomerulus and not secreted or reabsorbed by tubules (e.g., creatinine)

P = plasma concentration equation of x

V = urine flow rate (mL/min)

U = urine concentration of x

(4) eGFR calculation: Most commonly use Cockcroft-Gault equation (Table 6.1); however, this equation does not take into account obesity and was developed before the use of standardized creatinine assays. It tends to overestimate creatinine clearance (C_{Cr}) and thus GFR by 10% to 40%. The National Kidney Foundation recommends using the Chronic Kidney Disease Epidemiology Collaboration (CKD-EPI) Creatinine Equation (2009) to estimate GFR (see Table 6.1).

(5) Normal adult GFR: 125 mL/min or 180 L/day

(6) Normal adult urine volume: 1 to 2 L/day, reflecting greater than 99% reabsorption of filtrate

(7) Factors affecting GFR

    a) Changes in glomerular hydrostatic pressure

        1) Secondary to changes in systemic blood pressure (BP)

        2) Caused by variation in afferent or efferent arteriolar tone; increased afferent arteriole resistance decreases GFR; increased efferent arteriole tone increases GFR

    b) Alterations in oncotic pressure because of dehydration, hypoproteinemia, or hyperproteinemia

    c) Alterations in Bowman's capsule pressure because of urinary tract or nephron destruction, or interstitial edema of kidney

ii. Tubular functions of reabsorption, secretion, and excretion comprise the following steps in urine formation:

TABLE 6.1	Formulas for Estimation of Creatinine Clearance Without Urine Specimen
Cockcroft-Gault Formula	
Male	C_{cr} (in mL/min) = ([140 − age in years] × weight in kg) ÷ (P_{cr} in mg/dL × 72)
Female	C_{cr} (in mL/min) = ([140 − age in years] × weight in kg) ÷ (P_{cr} in mg/dL × 72) × 0.85
CKD-EPI CREATININE EQUATION (2009)	
GFR = 141 × min (Scr/κ,1)^α × max (Scr/κ, 1)$^{-1.209}$ × 0.993^{Age} × 1.018 [if female] × 1.159 [if black]	

C_{cr}, Creatinine clearance; *CKD-EPI*, Chronic Kidney Disease Epidemiology Collaboration; *GFR*, glomerular filtration rate; P_{cr}, plasma creatinine level.

From Cockcroft, D.W., Gault, M.H. (1976). Prediction of creatinine clearance from serum creatinine. *Nephron*, 16(1), 31–41; Kidney Disease: Improving Global Outcomes (KDIGO) Acute Kidney Injury Work Group. (2012). KDIGO Clinical practice guideline for acute kidney injury, *Kidney International Supplements*, 3 (Suppl 2013), 1–150.

(a) Conversion of 180 L of plasma filtered per day to 1 to 2 L of excreted urine
(b) Absorption and secretion by two processes:
   (1) Passive mechanisms: Solute moves without the expenditure of metabolic energy
       a) Diffusion: Solute following either a concentration or an electrical gradient
           1) A solute moves from a solution of higher concentration through a semipermeable membrane to a solution of lower concentration
           2) Selectivity of the membrane's permeability and electrical gradient determine diffusion of the solute
           3) The electrical gradient causes a solute to passively migrate to the oppositely charged compartment (e.g., Na^+, a positive ion, migrates to a negatively charged compartment, whereas Cl^-, a negative ion, moves toward a positively charged compartment)
       b) Osmosis: Water following an osmotic gradient
           1) Water normally moves from an area of low concentration to an area of higher concentration
           2) An osmotic agent, such as sodium or mannitol, normally remains within a single compartment
   (2) Active mechanisms:
       a) Ion transport requires energy: Adenosine triphosphate (ATP) permits ions to move *against* the concentration gradient
       b) Maximal tubular transport capacity: Active reabsorption mechanisms in the tubule have limited capacity for reabsorption of certain substances, such as glucose. Plasma glucose level of 375 mg/min (transport maximum [Tm]) results in no excretion in urine; plasma glucose level above 375 mg/min results in glucose excretion in urine. Tm for glucose can vary from one nephron to another; as a result, glucose can sometimes spill into the urine at lower serum levels.
(c) Proximal convoluted tubule
   (1) Reabsorbs approximately 65% of filtered sodium and water and a slightly lower percentage of filtered chloride
   (2) Major function is active reabsorption of sodium chloride (NaCl) with passive reabsorption of water
   (3) Also reabsorbs glucose, amino acids, phosphates (PO_4^{3-}), uric acid, potassium ion (K^+)
   (4) Regulates acid-base balance through reabsorption of carbonic acid (H_2CO_3) and bicarbonate (HCO_3^-), and secretion of hydrogen ions (H^+)
   (5) Secretes K^+, ammonium ion (NH_4^+), organic acids, bases, foreign substances (e.g., medications)
(d) Loop of Henle
   (1) Variations in length depend on the type of nephron (e.g., juxtamedullary with long loops or cortical with short loops)
   (2) Has two distinct segments
       a) Descending segment, the thin limb, is permeable to water and impermeable to Na^+
       b) Ascending segment, the thick limb, has active NaCl pump and is impermeable to water; target site for loop diuretics

(3) Major function is concentration or dilution of urine, accomplished by a countercurrent mechanism that maintains hyperosmolar concentration in the interstitium of the renal medulla

(e) Distal convoluted tubule

(1) Receives hyposmotic (or hypotonic) urine from the ascending loop of Henle

(2) Major functions

a) Reabsorption of water, NaCl, and sodium bicarbonate

b) Secretion of K^+, NH_4^+, and H^+ ions

c) Regulation of composition, tonicity, and volume

(3) Water permeability here is controlled by antidiuretic hormone (ADH); Na^+ reabsorption is determined by aldosterone

(f) Collecting duct

(1) Receives urine, which is isotonic to plasma, from the distal convoluted and collecting tubules

(2) Functions with the distal convoluted tubule; affected by ADH and aldosterone

(3) Final urinary adjustments for composition, tonicity, and volume made here before urine enters the renal pelvis and progresses to the ureter and bladder

2. **Renal hemodynamics: Normal blood flow patterns**

a. Renal vasculature

i. Specialized arrangement of renal blood vessels reflects interdependence of blood supply with kidney function

ii. Pathway of blood supply

(a) Kidney: Aorta→segmented renal arteries→interlobar artery→arcuate artery→interlobular artery→(nephron)→interlobular vein→arcuate vein→interlobar vein→renal vein→inferior vena cava

(b) Nephron: Afferent arteriole→glomerular capillary→efferent arteriole→peritubular capillary→vasa recta adjacent to tubules→interlobular vein→renal vein→inferior vena cava

iii. Juxtaglomerular apparatus: Site of renin synthesis

(a) Specialized cells composed of juxtaglomerular cells and macula densa

(1) Juxtaglomerular granular cells: Smooth muscle cells containing granules of inactive renin

(2) Macula densa: Portion of the distal tubule making contact with afferent arterioles of its respective glomerulus

(b) Responds to arterial BP in afferent and efferent arterioles and to sodium in distal tubule

b. Renal blood flow (RBF) parameters

i. Kidney receives 20% to 25% of cardiac output or 1200 mL/min

ii. RBF is

(a) Higher in males than in females

(b) Increased with increasing age (until maturity), in the supine position, and in the afternoon

(c) Decreased in the older adult, at night, and with exercise

iii. Distribution of RBF

(a) Cortex: Metabolically active region, receives most (85%–90%) of the blood supply

(b) Medulla: Site of anaerobic metabolism, receives 10% to 15% of blood supply

   c. Intrarenal autoregulation: General principles
      i. GFR remains relatively constant; a change in arterial pressure from 70 mm Hg to 180 mm Hg results in a GFR change of less than 10%
      ii. Major site of autoregulation is the afferent arteriole
      iii. Increase in the renal arterial pressure causes afferent vasoconstriction; decrease causes efferent vasoconstriction, producing an increased GFR/RBF ratio
      iv. Changes in vascular tone of the efferent arteriole (primarily vasoconstriction) complement efforts to maintain GFR by compensating for reduced blood flow
   d. Neural control
      i. Route of nerve supply is along renal blood vessels; renal neurologic intervention is vasoconstrictive
      ii. Hypotension decreases systemic arterial pressure, stimulating the carotid sinus and aortic arch baroreceptors to trigger the sympathetic response (release of epinephrine), which decreases RBF and GFR by vasoconstricting both afferent and efferent arterioles
      iii. Other factors that stimulate increased sympathetic tone are stress, fear, and exercise
      iv. This neuronal effect is not the primary factor in autoregulation; a denervated kidney can be transplanted and still be able to compensate for changes in BP
   e. Hormonal modulation of RBF (see Renal Regulation of Blood Pressure)
      i. Renin-angiotensin-aldosterone system: A mechanism to sustain systemic BP and plasma volume
         (a) Responds to a decreased afferent arteriolar pressure by increasing angiotensin II levels
         (b) Angiotensin II vasoconstricts renal blood vessels, particularly the efferent artery, which reduces RBF but increases GFR
      ii. Renal prostaglandins: Modulate the effects of vasoactive substances, such as angiotensin II, on the kidney by causing vasodilatation
   f. Pharmacologic effects
      i. Epinephrine and norepinephrine: Cause efferent arterioles to vasoconstrict, which leads to a rise in the filtration fraction and a dose-related decrease in RBF
      ii. Dopamine: Pharmacologic action on RBF is dose-related for renal vasodilatation and increased sodium excretion. In general, has a vasodilatory effect on renal vasculature at dosages between 1 and 4 mcg/kg/min intravenously (optimal dosage, 3 mcg/kg/min); dosages above 10 mcg/kg/min cause renal vasoconstriction, decreasing RBF and GFR. Dopamine therapy has no effect on the prevention of acute tubular necrosis.
      iii. Furosemide and mannitol: Increase GFR initially by increasing blood flow to the kidney and later by decreasing intratubular pressure
      iv. Calcium channel blockers: Relax renal arteriole and ameliorate renal failure related to renal transplantation and nephrotoxicity because of radiocontrast dyes or cyclosporine
      v. Atrial natriuretic factor (atrial natriuretic peptide, or ANP): Improves function in oliguric acute kidney injury (AKI), but no change in outcome
3. **Body water regulation**
   a. Thirst: Regulator of water intake
      i. Thirst center is located in the anterior hypothalamus
      ii. Neuronal cells are stimulated by intracellular dehydration, which causes sensation of thirst
      iii. Role is maintenance of satiety state (e.g., drinking exact amount of fluid to return body to normal hydration state)

b. ADH: Sodium osmoreceptor mechanism for control of extracellular fluid (ECF) osmolality and sodium concentration

   i. ADH is synthesized in the paraventricular and supraoptic nuclei of the hypothalamus and travels along the axons of the supraoptico-hypophyseal tract for storage or release from the posterior pituitary. The supraoptic area of the hypothalamus may overlap with the thirst center, providing integration of the thirst mechanism, osmolality detection, and ADH release.

   ii. Release of ADH occurs with the following:
      (a) Increased serum osmolality stimulates osmoreceptor cells in the hypothalamus that transmit along the neurohypophysial tracts, leading to ADH release from the posterior pituitary; normal serum osmolality is 285 to 295 mOsm/L
      (b) Volume contraction states reverse the inhibitory effect on ADH release; controlled by stretch receptors in the left atrium that activate the ADH mechanism

   iii. In the presence of ADH, water reabsorption occurs in the distal tubule and collecting ducts, which results in a hypertonic urine, hypotonic medullary interstitium, and eventual correction of contracted ECF

   iv. ADH secretion is inhibited when serum osmolality decreases (water intoxication). When this occurs, the distal tubule and collecting duct become relatively impermeable to water, so that large volumes of hypotonic filtrate are delivered to the collecting duct; this results in dilute urine and excess water loss (compared with extracellular solute concentration), which returns serum osmolality to normal limits.

c. Countercurrent mechanism of the kidney: Mechanism for the concentration and dilution of urine

   i. Isotonic glomerular filtrate leaves the proximal tubule and enters the loop of Henle

   ii. Descending limb of the loop of Henle is permeable to water only. Water is gradually drawn into the hypertonic medullary interstitium, which gradually increases the osmolality of the filtrate as it becomes dehydrated. At the hairpin turn of the loop, osmolality is dramatically increased by the removal of water and NaCl pump action; osmolality can reach 1000 to 1200 mOsm/L. Concurrently, the medullary interstitium becomes hypotonic.

   iii. Thick ascending limb of the loop of Henle is permeable to NaCl but impermeable to water. The medullary interstitium becomes more hypertonic as its sodium concentration is increased by pumping action at the ascending limb.

   iv. A dilute filtrate reaches the distal tubule. If ADH is absent, dilute filtrate is excreted unchanged, which results in dilute urine with water excretion in excess of solute. If ADH is present, the collecting duct reabsorbs water and concentrated urine is excreted.

4. **Electrolyte regulation**

a. Sodium regulation: Normal serum concentration is 136 to 145 mEq/L solute

   i. Na^+ is the major extracellular cation and osmotically active solute. Because variation in body sodium can be associated with an exchange of water between intracellular and extracellular compartments, sodium affects ECF volume.

   ii. Renal reabsorption sites: Normal percentages of reabsorbed filtered sodium
      (a) Proximal tubule: 60% of filtered Na^+
      (b) Loop of Henle: 30%
      (c) Distal tubule and collecting duct: 10%

iii. Major factors that influence Na$^+$ excretion include GFR, the sympathetic nervous system, aldosterone, the renin-angiotensin-aldosterone system, vasopressin (ADH), and ANP (a peptide hormone that plays a role in regulating and monitoring fluid, electrolyte, and cardiovascular balance)

iv. Sodium reabsorption increases at the renal tubules under the following conditions:

   (a) Decreased GFR secondary to renal hypoperfusion (e.g., shock): Less sodium is delivered to the renal tubules, and less is excreted

   (b) Secretion of aldosterone (a mineralocorticoid secreted by the adrenal cortex)

      (1) Major effects are to increase renal tubular reabsorption of Na$^+$ and to control selective renal excretion of K$^+$

      (2) Increases Na$^+$ in ECF, which promotes water reabsorption; at the same time, K$^+$ is secreted into the distal tubule and collecting duct to be excreted

      (3) Regulated by K$^+$ concentration in the ECF, the renin-angiotensin-aldosterone mechanism, total body sodium, and adrenocorticotropic hormone (ACTH)

   (c) ANP action: Causes natriuretic, diuretic, and hypotensive effects secondary to its potent vasodilatory properties; the increased urinary excretion of Na$^+$ is matched by an accompanying loss of K$^+$ and PO$_4^{3-}$

v. Sodium reabsorption decreases at the renal tubules under the following conditions:

   (a) Increased GFR (excess ECF volume): Increases renal perfusion and GFR; more sodium is delivered to the renal tubules and more is excreted in urine

   (b) Inhibition of aldosterone secretion, which results in renal Na$^+$ excretion

   (c) Secretion of ANP and ADH, administration of diuretics, especially loop-affecting diuretics

b. Potassium regulation: Normal serum concentration is 3.5 to 5.5 mEq/L

   i. Potassium is a major intracellular cation (K^+) necessary for the maintenance of osmolality and electroneutrality of cells

   ii. Renal transport sites: K^+ is actively reabsorbed in the proximal tubule (50%–70%) and thick ascending loop; active and passive secretion in the distal tubule and collecting duct maintain the electroneutrality of urine. This electrical gradient is determined primarily by reabsorption of Na$^+$ from urine.

   iii. Factors enhancing K^+ excretion

      (a) Increase in cellular potassium via increased exchange with Na$^+$ (K^+ excreted in urine whereas Na$^+$ is reabsorbed) or via acute metabolic or respiratory alkalosis (causes movement of K$^+$ ions into cells)

      (b) High-volume tubular flow rates in the distal portion of the nephron: Increase the number of available K$^+$ ions and thus increase the excretion of potassium

      (c) Aldosterone (provides feedback mechanism for maintenance of K^+ in ECF)

         (1) Elevation of serum potassium stimulates the secretion of aldosterone

         (2) Aldosterone acts on the distal nephrons and collecting ducts, enhancing the retention of Na$^+$ and excretion of K^+

         (3) Excretion of excess K^+ eventually returns levels to normal

      (d) Hydrogen ions: Alkalemia (associated decrease in H^+) stimulates K^+ secretion

    (e) Diuretics: Loop and thiazide diuretics block NaCl and waste reabsorption, increasing tubular flow and secretion of K^+

c. Calcium regulation: Normal serum concentration is 8.5 to 10.5 mg/dL or 2.20 to 2.60 mmol/L

  i. Major functions of calcium ions (Ca^{2+}): Generation of cardiac action potential and pacemaker function, contraction of cardiac and vascular smooth muscle, transmission of nerve impulses, blood coagulation, formation of bones and teeth, and maintenance of cellular permeability

  ii. Total serum Ca^{2+}: 40% bound to protein, 50% ionized, and 10% combined with carbonate, phosphate, citrate, and various ions

  iii. Renal transport sites: 98% to 99% of filtered Ca^{2+} is reabsorbed. Reabsorptive pathways are similar to those for sodium transport. Most active reabsorption occurs in the proximal tubule. Other sites include the loop (20%–25%) and the distal tubule (10%).

  iv. Factors influencing Ca^{2+} reabsorption:

    (a) Parathyroid hormone (PTH)

      (1) Decrease in serum calcium stimulates secretion of PTH

      (2) PTH stimulates tubular reabsorption of Ca^{2+} at the distal portion of the nephron, stimulates increased phosphate excretion, and mobilizes calcium and phosphate from bone

    (b) Vitamin D: Calcium absorption from the small intestine depends on the presence of activated vitamin D (1,25-dihydroxycholecalciferol)

      (1) Activation process: Absorption of ultraviolet light converts 7-dehydrocholesterol in skin to cholecalciferol. The liver hydroxylates vitamin D to form 25-hydroxycholecalciferol. The kidney further hydroxylates to the final activated form of vitamin D (1,25-dihydroxycholecalciferol) in the proximal tubule. PTH stimulates this activation process.

      (2) Decreased serum calcium level reduces urinary Ca^{2+} excretion, so activated vitamin D must be available to absorb Ca^{2+} from the small intestine to maintain adequate serum calcium levels.

    (c) Corticosteroid effect: Large doses decrease Ca^{2+} absorption in the intestines; may influence the activation of vitamin D in the liver

    (d) Diuretic effect: Diuretics can cause Na^+ and Ca^{2+} excretion. Ultimate effect of reduced serum calcium is decreased excretion. A decrease in total body fluid volume leads to diminished GFR and reduced calcium excretion.

d. Phosphate regulation: Normal serum concentration is 3.0 to 4.5 mg/dL

  i. About 85% of phosphate is found in bone, 14% to 15% in cells, and <1% in ECF spaces. Phosphates (PO_4^{3-}) play a significant role in intracellular energy production and may also influence deoxyribonucleic acid (DNA), ribonucleic acid (RNA), and genetic code information. Phosphates are used by the kidneys to buffer H^+.

  ii. Renal transport sites: Reabsorption of phosphate is an active process that occurs in the proximal tubule and requires Na^+. Factors influencing phosphate excretion include the following:

    (a) PTH secretion: Inhibits phosphate reabsorption (and thus promotes its excretion)

    (b) Alterations in GFR: Increased GFR decreases reabsorption of plasma phosphates and vice versa

e. Magnesium regulation: Normal serum concentration is 1.5 to 2.2 mEq/L

i. The magnesium ion (Mg^{2+}) is the second major intracellular cation and is a significant factor in cellular enzyme systems and biochemical reactions

ii. Although Mg^{2+} may have a role in the management of acute myocardial infarction (MI), overall evidence does not recommend routine Mg^{2+} administration in MI; one large trial showed that magnesium administration decreases the mortality rate in MI by 25%; however, two more recent trials showed no benefit over placebo.

iii. Renal transport site: The reabsorptive process is similar to that of Ca^{2+} and is linked to Na^+ reabsorption along the renal tubules.

iv. Factors influencing reabsorption include the availability of sodium (Na^+ is necessary for reabsorption) and the availability of PTH (has minimal effect on Mg^{2+} reabsorption)

f. Chloride regulation: Normal serum concentration is 96 to 106 mEq/L

i. Renal transport sites: Reabsorbed with Na^+ at all Na^+ absorptive sites in the nephron

ii. Factors influencing excretion include acidosis (HCO_3^- reabsorbed whereas Cl^- excreted to maintain electrochemical balance) and alkalosis (HCO_3^- excreted as Cl^- reabsorbed)

5. **Excretion of metabolic waste products: Excretion is a primary renal function. The kidney excretes more than 200 metabolic waste products. The products measured for interpretation of renal function are blood urea nitrogen (BUN) and serum creatinine.**

a. Urea: Nitrogen waste product of protein metabolism filtered and reabsorbed along the entire nephron

i. Is an unreliable indicator of GFR, because urea excretion is influenced by:

(a) Urine flow (decrease in urine flow rate may allow for reabsorption of urea)

(b) Extrarenal factors (e.g., hypoperfusion states or medications such as corticosteroids)

(c) Gastrointestinal (GI) bleeding or catabolic states, such as fever or infection

(d) Changes in protein intake or metabolism

ii. Elevation in BUN level without an associated rise in creatinine level ($>20:1$ ratio) suggests:

(a) Volume depletion, low renal perfusion pressure

(b) Severe catabolic process or trauma with massive muscle injury (e.g., burns)

(c) GI bleeding with blood collection in intestines

iii. Elevated levels of both BUN and creatinine (at a $10:1$ ratio) indicate renal disease

b. Creatinine: A waste product of muscle metabolism

i. Most commonly used marker for detection of AKI; elevated serum creatinine level is correlated with deterioration in renal function

ii. Creatinine is freely filtered, so its production normally equals its excretion, which makes it a reasonably reliable indicator of kidney function

iii. Diagnostic use is limited, however; recent studies indicate that serum creatinine may not increase until 48 to 72 hours following AKI despite increase in GFR

iv. In addition, a number of nonrenal factors (e.g., body weight, muscle metabolism, medications, dietary intake) can influence levels

6. **Renal regulation of acid-base balance: The kidneys regulate acid-base balance by minimizing wide variations in body fluid balance in conjunction with retaining or excreting hydrogen ions. Acid-base balance is also regulated by the lungs and the body buffers (serum bicarbonate, blood, and plasma proteins).**

a. Bicarbonate (HCO_3^-) reabsorption
  i. Primarily occurs in the proximal tubule with less in the distal tubule; occurs with reabsorption of Na^+
  ii. Occurs if the filtrate contains more than 28 mEq/L (Tm) as in acidemia, volume contraction
b. Hydrogen ion secretion
  i. Passive secretion occurs in the proximal tubule; active secretion occurs distally in exchange for Na^+
  ii. Acid is buffered by ammonia (NH_3^+) or phosphate (HPO_4^{2-}) before excretion, which provides for hydrogen (H^+) excretion without lowering pH
  iii. H^+ secretion is increased during acidemia and decreased during alkalemia
c. Renal buffers of hydrogen ions
  i. Buffers that are filtered by the glomerulus
    (a) HCO_3^- is completely reabsorbed (up to 28 mEq/L)
    (b) Phosphate (PO_4^{3-}) is secreted and then reacts with hydrogen
    (c) $H^+ + HPO_4^{2-} = H_2PO_4^-$
  ii. Buffers produced by the kidney tubule
    (a) HCO_3^- can be synthesized in the distal tubule when H^+, excreted into urine as HCO_3^-, is delivered by ECF with Na^+. H^+ and HCO_3^- both come from the distal tubule cell as a result of ionization of carbonic acid (H_2CO_3); thus

$$H_2CO_3 \overset{CA}{\leftrightarrow} H^+ + HCO_3^-$$

where CA is carbonic anhydrase.
    (b) Carbonic acid comes from hydration of carbon dioxide (CO_2) via CA:

$$H_2O + CO_2^+ \overset{CA}{\leftrightarrow} H_2CO_3^-$$

    (c) CO_2 is derived from either cellular metabolism or dissolved CO_2 in venous blood; thus new HCO_3^- can be made in the distal tubule from extraurinary sources
    (d) Complete equation

$$H_2O + CO_2^+ \overset{CA}{\leftrightarrow} H_2CO_3^- \overset{CA}{\leftrightarrow} H^+ + HCO_3^-$$

d. Summary of renal responses to acidemia
  i. H^+ secretion is increased at the distal tubule with increased excretion of titratable acids (HPO_4^{2-})
  ii. All HCO_3^- is reabsorbed in the proximal tubule
  iii. Ammonium is produced to accommodate H^+ excretion:
    $$NH_3^+ + H^+ \rightleftarrows NH_4^+$$
  iv. Urinary pH can be as low as 4.5 for excretion of a more acid urine in the presence of acidemia
e. Summary of renal responses to alkalemia
  i. H^+ secretion in the distal tubule is decreased
  ii. Excess HCO_3^- is excreted
  iii. Production of NH_4^+ is decreased
  iv. Urine is alkaline with a pH over 7
7. **Renal regulation of BP: Renal regulation of BP involves five mechanisms:**
  a. Maintenance of volume and composition of ECF
    i. Normal plasma volume is essential for control of BP
    ii. Alterations in plasma volume eventually affect BP. Reduction of plasma volume lowers arterial BP, leading to compensation by vasoconstriction. Expansion

of plasma volume increases cardiac preload and, in accordance with Starling's curve, raises BP.

b. Aldosterone—body sodium balance, which determines ECF volume: Aldosterone stimulates renal tubular reabsorption of Na^+ in exchange for excretion of primarily K^+ ions

c. Renin-angiotensin-aldosterone system: Preserves BP and avoids serious volume reduction

    i. Juxtaglomerular apparatus: Granular cells contain inactivated renin. Factors that trigger juxtaglomerular cells to release renin reflect diminished GFR (e.g., reduced arterial BP in afferent and efferent arterioles, reduced Na^+ content or concentration at distal tubule, sympathetic stimulation of kidneys).

    ii. Renin, an enzyme, is released from juxtaglomerular cells into the afferent arteriole.

    iii. Upon entering the circulation, renin acts on angiotensinogen to split away the vasoactive peptide angiotensin I and convert it to angiotensin II. Requires the presence of angiotensin-converting enzyme (ACE), found primarily in the lung and liver but also in the kidney and all blood vessels. Angiotensin II is a potent systemic vasoconstrictor.

    iv. Circulatory effect of angiotensin II on arterial BP

       (a) Significant peripheral arteriole constriction with moderate venous constriction occurs, which results in the reduction of vascular volume

       (b) Renal arteriolar constriction results in the renal retention of sodium and water; this expands ECF volume, thus increasing arterial BP

    v. Fluid volume response to angiotensin II restores effective circulating volume in the following ways:

       (a) Angiotensin II stimulates aldosterone release, which enhances Na^+ reabsorption

       (b) Vasoconstriction to further decrease GFR leads to Na^+ reabsorption

       (c) The thirst mechanism is stimulated

d. Renal prostaglandins: Modulating effect

    i. Major renal prostaglandins are prostaglandins E_2, D_2, I_2 (vasodilators), and A_2 (vasoconstrictor)

    ii. Physiologic role is modulation, amplification, and inhibition. Vasoactive substances (angiotensin, norepinephrine, bradykinins) stimulate the synthesis and release of prostaglandins. Prostaglandins modulate the action of the vasoactive substances.

    iii. Prostaglandins diminish arterial BP and increase RBF by arterial vasodilation and inhibition of the distal tubules' response to ADH. Suppressed ADH response leads to sodium and water excretion, which ultimately decreases the effective circulatory volume.

    iv. Pharmacologic prostaglandin inhibitors are the nonsteroidal antiinflammatory drugs (NSAIDs). In cases of compromised renal function, avoid the use of NSAIDs (e.g., salicylic acid, ibuprofen [Motrin], indomethacin [Indocin], and naproxen [Naprosyn]).

    v. Loop diuretics stimulate prostaglandin secretion, which leads to vasodilation and decreased preload

e. Kallikrein-kinin system: Renal kallikreins are proteases that release kinins and are excreted in the urine. Kinins stimulate both the renin-angiotensin and prostaglandin systems, appearing to link renal hemodynamics and fluid-electrolyte excretion.

8. **RBC synthesis and maturation**
   a. Erythropoietin secretion: Stimulates the production of erythrocytes in the bone marrow and prolongs the life of erythrocytes
   b. Mechanism of erythropoietin synthesis and secretion
      i. Renal cortical interstitial cells produce erythropoietin, a glycosylated, 165-amino-acid protein
      ii. Renal erythropoietin production accounts for 90% of RBC production; the remaining 10% is produced by the liver
      iii. Hypoxia stimulates renal erythropoietin production; the liver is not as responsive to hypoxia and therefore cannot support erythropoiesis in renal failure
   c. Erythropoietin deficiency: Primary cause of anemia in chronic kidney disease (CKD); bleeding is the second most common cause
9. **Aging kidney**
   a. Age-related changes include a decrease in renal mass and volume and a progressive decrease in the percentage of glomeruli. In general, renal function is diminished by 10% at age 65 years; may diminish further with aging.
   b. Renal response in the older adult (see Ch. 16, Older Adult Patients)
      i. Decreased renal mass associated with a diminished number of nephrons
      ii. Decreased GFR; diminished RBF secondary to age-related changes in vasculature
      iii. Diminished creatinine production ($10\,mL/min/1.73\,m^2$ per decade) and diminished ability to excrete creatinine; therefore change in serum creatinine level may not be evident. Uric acid levels are slightly increased.
      iv. Decreased serum renin and aldosterone levels reduce the ability to conserve sodium, impair urinary water excretion, and limit urinary concentration

ASSESSMENT

1. **History**
   a. Patient health history
      i. Previous health problems: Indicate the presence of or predisposition to renal disease
         (a) Kidney and/or urinary tract disease
         (b) Cardiovascular disease
            (1) Hypertension: BP control and treatment may prevent or halt renal damage
            (2) Hypotension resulting in diminished renal perfusion (e.g., shock, heart failure)
            (3) Atherosclerosis
         (c) Diabetes mellitus: Renal disease caused by vascular disease alterations, infection, or neuropathy
         (d) Immunologic disorders, recent infections (streptococcal)
         (e) Pulmonary disease (Goodpasture syndrome)
         (f) Allergies, recent blood transfusions (history of incompatibility reaction)
         (g) Other: Toxemia of pregnancy, renal transplantation, anemia, recent surgery, dialysis, exposure to medications and toxins, renal calculi, azotemia, hematuria, exposure to chemicals or poisons
      ii. History of specific signs and symptoms
         (a) Signs and symptoms of urinary tract disorders
            (1) Dysuria
            (2) Abnormal appearance of urine

a) Hematuria (grossly bloody)
b) Pyuria (cloudy)
c) Biliuria or bilirubinuria (orange)
d) Myoglobinuria (usually clear; red-brown urine)

(3) Urine frequency, urgency, incontinence, hesitancy; nocturia
(4) Polydipsia
(5) Patterns of urine output
a) Normal volume: 0.5 to 1 mL/kg/h
b) Oliguria: Less than 400 mL/24 h
c) Anuria: Less than 50 mL to no output over 24 hours
d) Polyuria: Excessive output exceeding 24-hour intake
e) Nonoliguria: Normal or excess urine volume in the presence of AKI

KEY CONCEPT

It is important to note that the old standard of 30 mL/h may be inadequate depending on the size of the patient. Adequacy of urine output should be assessed based on body weight

---

(6) Fever
(7) Pain in costovertebral angle, flank, or groin
(8) Pattern of weight gain or loss; dry weight is the ideal weight that minimizes symptomatology for a patient with renal failure as achieved by a dialysis treatment

b. Family health history: Genetic renal disease accounts for about 30% of azotemia. A family history of the following disorders may indicate a higher risk for renal disease:
  i. Cardiovascular disease, hypertension
  ii. Diabetes mellitus
  iii. Gout
  iv. Malignancy
  v. Polycystic kidney disease and medullary cystic disease
  vi. Hereditary nephritis (Alport syndrome)
  vii. Renal calculi

c. Social history and habits
  i. Social history: Sexual activity before renal disease and sexual dysfunction related to renal disease
  ii. Habits
    (a) Dietary habits
      (1) Dietary and fluid restrictions; compliance or noncompliance with these restrictions
      (2) Dietary intake: Number and nutritional value of meals
    (b) Exercise
    (c) Frequency, type, quantity of caffeine, tobacco, alcohol, or illicit medications

d. Medication history

KEY CONCEPT

Over-the-counter medications, such as NSAIDs and certain dietary supplements and weight loss drugs need to be included as both can lead to renal disease.

    i. Nephrotoxic agents: Radiocontrast dye and antibiotic therapy (tetracyclines, aminoglycosides, gentamicin, amphotericin B)

    ii. Diuretics, antihypertensives

    iii. Cardiac glycosides (digoxin), antiarrhythmic agents

    iv. Electrolyte replacement therapy

    v. Immunosuppressive agents:

      (a) Corticosteroids

      (b) Azathioprine, cyclophosphamide, antithymocyte globulin (ATG), cyclosporine, monoclonal antibody (OKT3), tacrolimus (FK-506)

    vi. Analgesics, such as meperidine (Demerol)

2. Physical examination

  a. Physical examination data

    i. Inspection

      (a) Diminished level of consciousness (lethargy, coma)

      (b) Skin

        (1) Abnormal color: Grayish tinge from anemia, yellowish tinge if retained carotenoids or urochrome pigments in uremia

        (2) Capillary integrity: Easily bruised

        (3) Skin turgor

        (4) Purpura lesions: Present in some forms of renal failure

      (c) Eye: Cataracts, periorbital edema

      (d) Ear: Nerve deafness (Alport syndrome)

      (e) Edema

        (1) Significance depends on amount of water and Na^+ retained

        (2) Edema of renal failure often related to hypoalbuminemia

      (f) Respiration: May see rate and pattern similar to Kussmaul's respirations

      (g) Muscle tremors, weakness, weight loss with uremic syndrome

      (h) Tetany: Positive Chvostek's and Trousseau's signs; rarely observed; result from severe hypocalcemia or very rapid correction of acidosis

      (i) Asterixis: Indicates progressive uremic state

        (1) Ask the patient to face the examiner and raise the upper extremities in a fixed hyperextension position

        (2) Palms (fingers separated) must be visible to the examiner

        (3) Positive sign—irregular movements of the wrists, flapping movements of the fingers—occurs within 30 seconds

      (j) Fatigue: Occurs with activities of daily living and exercise, and at rest

      (k) Mobility: Extent and strength with ambulation

      (l) Nutritional status

        (1) Anemia: Pale skin, weakness, shortness of breath

        (2) Tolerance of diet: Nausea and vomiting; likes and dislikes

        (3) Weight loss

      (m) Arteriovenous access: Type, patency, signs of infection

    ii. Palpation: To determine size and shape of the kidney and to check for tenderness, cysts, and masses

      (a) Right kidney is easier to palpate because it is lower in the abdomen

      (b) Palpate the bladder for urinary distention because of obstruction

      (c) Palpate the flank area to elicit tenderness or pain

      (d) Palpate pulses for a baseline reading and to determine abnormalities

    iii. Percussion

      (a) At costovertebral angles to elicit pain or tenderness associated with:

(1) Pyelonephritis

(2) Calculi

(3) Renal abscess

(4) Intermittent hydronephrosis

(b) At abdomen for the presence of ascites

    iv. Auscultation: Listen for aortic and renal artery bruits (heard in flanks or intercostal regions of anterior abdomen)

  b. Monitoring data: Intake and output (I&O), hemodynamics, body weight, central venous pressure (CVP), and/or pulmonary artery occlusion pressure to determine relationship between cardiac filling pressures and hydration status; correlate findings with daily weight

3. **Appraisal of patient characteristics: Patients with acute, life-threatening renal problems come to acute care settings with a wide range of biochemical, metabolic, and psychosocial clinical characteristics. During their stay, their clinical status may significantly improve or deteriorate, slowly or abruptly change, involve one or all life-sustaining functions, and be readily or nearly impossible to monitor with precision. Some attributes of patients with acute renal disorders that the nurse needs to assess are the following: resiliency, vulnerability, stability, complexity, resource availability, participation in care and decision-making, and predictability.**

DIAGNOSTIC STUDIES

  a. Laboratory

    i. Blood

      (a) Complete blood count: Reduced hematocrit and hemoglobin levels may reflect bleeding or a lack of erythropoietin

      (b) Serum creatinine: To estimate GFR (normal level, 0.6–1.2 mg/dL)

        (1) Creatinine excretion is proportional to its production

        (2) A significant elevation in creatinine level is associated with renal disease and correlates with percentage of nephrons damaged

      (c) BUN: Normal level, 10 to 20 mg/dL (Table 6.2)

        (1) Prerenal problem: Ratio of BUN to serum creatinine equal to or greater than 20:1 suggests extrarenal problem (dehydration, catabolic state). Elevation in both BUN and creatinine results from decreased GFR.

        (2) Renal failure: Caused by nephron damage

      (d) Serum chemistry tests (calcium, phosphate, alkaline phosphatase, bilirubin, uric acid, sodium, potassium, chloride, carbon dioxide, magnesium, glucose, cholesterol)

      (e) Baseline arterial blood gas (ABG) levels, clotting profile

      (f) Serum osmolality, total protein and albumin

TABLE 6.2	**Interpretation of Blood Urea Nitrogen and Serum Creatinine Levels**		
Condition	**Ratio of Blood Urea Nitrogen to Creatinine**	**Blood Urea Nitrogen**	**Serum Creatinine**
Normal	20:1	10–20 mg/100 mL	0.6–1.2 mg/100 mL
Prerenal disease	≥25:1	↑	Normal or slight elevation
Renal disease (acute or chronic)	10:1	↑	↑

From Sharfuddin, A.A., Weisbord, S.D., Palevsky, P.M., Molitoris, B.A. (2016). Acute kidney injury. In B.M., Brenner (editor), *Brenner and Rector's the kidney*, 10th ed, Philadelphia, Elsevier.

　　ii. Urine
　　　　(a) Visual examination for color and clarity
　　　　　　(1) Clear and colorless in hyposthenuria
　　　　　　(2) Cloudy when infection is present
　　　　　　(3) Foamy when albumin is present
　　　　(b) Osmolality (50–1200 mOsm/kg for random specimen)
　　　　(c) SG: Wide range of normal values (1.003–1.030); provides reasonable
　　　　　　estimate of urinary osmolality; actually measures density
　　　　　　(1) Low normal (<1.010): Suspect diabetes insipidus, volume overload, or
　　　　　　　　heart failure
　　　　　　(2) Above normal (>1.030): Occurs in proteinuria, glycosuria, severe
　　　　　　　　dehydration, presence of x-ray contrast medium
　　　　(d) Creatinine clearance (C_{cr}): 24-hour urine collection
　　　　　　(1) Purpose: To determine the presence and progression of renal disease,
　　　　　　　　estimate percentage of functioning nephrons, or determine specific
　　　　　　　　medication dosages
　　　　　　(2) In 24 hours, the following occurs:

$$\frac{(U_{cr} \times V)}{P_{cr}} = C_{cr}$$

where
U_{cr} = amount of urinary creatinine excreted
V = urine volume per minute
P_{cr} = plasma creatinine level
　　　　　　(3) In average-size patients, a satisfactory 24-hour urine collection always has
　　　　　　　　approximately 1 g of creatinine, regardless of the degree of renal function
　　　　　　(4) Cockcroft-Gault formula or CKD-EPI Creatinine Equation for
　　　　　　　　estimation of C_{cr} (see Table 6.1)
　　　　(e) Culture and sensitivity: Evaluate for infection
　　　　(f) pH (normal range, 4.5–8; average value, 6); alkaline urine is
　　　　　　frequently seen with infection; in absence of infection, possibly
　　　　　　indicates renal tubular acidosis if both alkaline urine and systemic
　　　　　　acidosis are present
　　　　(g) Glucose: In urine when renal threshold for glucose exceeded
　　　　(h) Acetone: In urine with starvation or diabetic ketoacidosis; a false-positive
　　　　　　result can occur in patients taking salicylates
　　　　(i) Protein: Expressed quantitatively as 1 + to 4 +; diagnostic for the presence
　　　　　　of glomerular membrane disease (nephritic syndrome) and allows the
　　　　　　detection of myeloma proteins causing renal failure
　　　　(j) Spot urine electrolytes
　　　　　　(1) Measure urinary concentrations of Na^+, K^+, Cl^-
　　　　　　(2) Screening test for tubular function; assess the kidney's ability to
　　　　　　　　conserve sodium and concentrate urine
　　　　(k) Urinary sediment
　　　　　　(1) Casts: Precipitations of protein in the kidney that take the shape of the
　　　　　　　　tubules in which they are formed
　　　　　　　　a) Hyaline casts: Entirely protein; small amounts are normal in urine;
　　　　　　　　　if large amounts, suspect significant proteinuria, such as albumin
　　　　　　　　　or myeloma protein in urine
　　　　　　　　b) Erythrocyte casts: Diagnostic for active glomerulonephritis or
　　　　　　　　　vasculitis

       c) Leukocyte casts: Indicative of an infectious process and intrarenal inflammation

       d) Granular casts: Small number, possibly the result of degenerating erythrocyte or leukocyte casts indicative of an infectious process or an allergic interstitial nephritis

       e) Fatty casts: Abundant in nephrotic syndrome

       f) Renal tubular casts: Seen in AKI

    (2) Bacteria: Presence determined by Gram stain

    (3) Erythrocytes: Small numbers normal; in abundance during active glomerulonephritis, interstitial nephritis, malignancies, and infection

    (4) Leukocytes: Small numbers normal; present in infection and interstitial nephritis

    (5) Renal epithelial cells: Rarely seen; present in abundance during ATN, nephrotoxic injury, and allergic reaction in the kidney

    (6) Crystals: Seen in diseases of stone formation or following certain intoxications

    (7) Eosinophils: Indicate allergic reaction in the kidney

  iii. Novel Biomarkers

    (a) Serum and urine biomarkers

      (1) Plasma and/or urine Cystatin C

      (2) Plasma and/or urine neutrophil gelatinase-associated lipocalin (NGAL)

      (3) Interleukins

      (4) Kidney injury molecule-1 (KIM-1)

    (b) These may lead to earlier detection of AKI, as well as better prognostication

    (c) May be better in combination as a panel than as individual tests

    (d) Cystatin C is becoming more common in clinical practice, but generally, use of these tests is not widespread in acute care

b. Radiologic

  i. Plain abdominal x-ray study: Determines position, shape, and size of the kidney and identifies calcification in the urinary system

  ii. Diagnostic ultrasonography: Identifies hydronephrosis, differentiates solid and cystic tumors, localizes cysts or fluid collections

  iii. Computed tomography (CT): Identifies tumors and other pathologic conditions that create variations in body density (e.g., abscess or lymphocele); used in renal trauma to determine reason for acute flank pain

  iv. Magnetic resonance imaging (MRI)

    (a) Provides better tissue characterization than CT; provides direct imaging in several planes for detection of renal cystic disease, inflammatory processes, and renal cell carcinoma

    (b) Detects alterations in blood flow (e.g., slow or absent flow)

    (c) Identifies morphologic changes in renal transplant

  v. Chest radiography: Identifies pulmonary edema, cardiomegaly, left ventricular hypertrophy, uremic lung, Goodpasture disease, and infection

  vi. Intravenous pyelography (IVP)

    (a) Visualizes the urinary tract for diagnosing partial obstruction, renovascular hypertension, tumor, cyst, congenital abnormality

    (b) Complications include allergic reaction to dye, dehydration

    (c) Contraindicated in the presence of the following:

      (1) Poor renal function: Because of the dehydrating effect contrast dye and nephrotoxicity may further compromise function.

(2) Multiple myeloma: Contrast dye may precipitate myeloma protein in the kidney.

(3) Pregnancy: Abdominal irradiation should be avoided.

(4) Heart failure: Osmotic effect of dye can compromise cardiac function by expanding vascular volume.

(5) Diabetes mellitus

(6) Sickle cell anemia: The contrast creates an elevated renal oncotic pressure can promote renal tissue sickling, infarction.

vii. High-excretion tomography: Indicated when kidneys cannot be readily visualized on IVP

viii. Renal scan: Determines renal perfusion and function; can provide information about obstructions and renal masses. Radioactive dye is taken up by normal kidney tubule cells. A decrease in uptake indicates hypoperfusion. Often used to assess renal transplants.

ix. Retrograde pyelography: Used to examine upper region of collecting system

x. Retrograde urethrography: Used to examine the urethra

xi. Cystoscopy: Detects bladder or urethral pathology

xii. Renal arteriography (angiography): Identifies tumors and distinguishes type of renal or renovascular disease. Potential complications can be serious:

(a) Allergic reaction to dye can cause same complications seen with contrast dye.

(b) Puncture of a peripheral artery, with consequent hematoma, embolism, or thrombus formation, is the greatest technical risk.

xiii. Voiding cystourethrography: Identifies abnormalities of lower urinary tract, urethra, bladder to detect reflux and residual urine

xiv. Magnetic resonance urography: A form of magnetic imaging that offers results similar to those of contrast dye

c. Kidney biopsy: The most common invasive diagnostic tool

i. For renal disease that cannot be definitively diagnosed by other means

ii. Determines cause and extent of lesions; helpful in planning treatment

iii. Percutaneous renal biopsy (PRB) is the most common type

iv. Other types of biopsy

(a) CT-guided: Performed by radiologist; similar to PRB; useful for obese patients

(b) Transjugular renal biopsy: Useful in patients with bleeding disorders, mechanical ventilation, hypertension, morbid obesity; technically complicated and reserved for very high-risk patients

(c) Open: For severe anatomic deformities or if a "deep specimen" is needed for diagnosis; contraindications to open biopsy include bleeding tendency, hydronephrosis, hypertension, cystic disease, and neoplasms

(d) Laparoscopic renal biopsy: Surgical procedure using either a retroperitoneal or transperitoneal approach

v. Nursing care

(a) Patient must lie flat for 6 to 8 hours following procedure

(b) Hematuria, flank, or abdominal pain should prompt call to provider for immediate evaluation

(c) Complications include bleeding, infection, injury to other abdominal organs, renin-mediated hypertension

PATIENT CARE

1. **Volume overload: A state in which an individual experiences fluid retention and edema because kidneys are unable to excrete excess body water**
   a. Description of problem
      i. Intake greater than output
      ii. Weight gain with oliguria or anuria, low SG ($\leq$1.015), dilute urine
      iii. Elevated BP, bounding pulses, neck vein distention; elevated CVP, pulmonary artery pressure (PAP), and pulmonary artery occlusive pressure (PAOP), and muffled heart sounds
      iv. Edema: Peripheral, anasarcal, ascitic, periorbital, pulmonary
      v. Dyspnea, orthopnea, crackles on auscultation, pulmonary congestion
      vi. Decreased (diluted) hemoglobin, hematocrit, and electrolyte values
      vii. Anxiety, restlessness, stupor (seen with water intoxication)
   b. Goals of care
      i. Patient maintains dry weight
      ii. BP, CVP, PAP, and PAOP are normal
      iii. Patient is free of edema
      iv. Breath sounds are clear bilaterally
      v. I&O are balanced
   c. Interprofessional collaboration: Nurse, physician, advanced practice provider, respiratory therapist, case manager, dietitian, nephrologist, hemodialysis nurse (if dialysis indicated).
   d. Interventions
      i. Identify presence of common causes of fluid volume excess
         (a) Expanded total body water volume secondary to renal failure with oliguria or anuria
         (b) Expanded blood volume because of renal sodium retention
         (c) Lower plasma oncotic pressure because of loss of plasma proteins
         (d) Increased capillary permeability
      ii. Document I&O; compare with daily weight; consider insensible losses—fluid losses via lungs, skin, and bowel (600–800 mL/day)
      iii. Assess renal function
         (a) Urine volume, urinalysis, creatinine clearance, and BUN/creatinine ratio
         (b) Spot electrolytes, urine concentration (SG, osmolality)
         (c) 24-hour urine collection for protein evaluation
      iv. Restrict fluids in volume overload associated with impaired renal function, impaired cardiac function, or syndrome of inappropriate secretion of ADH (SIADH)
      v. Administer diuretics (preferably loop) if patient has a GFR of 25 mL/min or higher
      vi. Consider acute dialysis with ultrafiltration for rapid volume removal
2. **Dehydration: A state in which an individual experiences vascular, cellular, or intracellular volume depletion because of active fluid loss. Dehydration may occur in the diuretic phase of AKI or as a result of aggressive diuretic therapy.**
   a. Description of problem
      i. Output greater than intake
      ii. Weight loss with elevated SG (>1.020), concentrated urine, variable urinary output (UOP)
         (a) Polyuric phase: Large volume of dilute urine with low SG
         (b) Dehydration with normal renal function: Oliguria, concentrated urine with an elevated SG

    iii. Hypotension, increased pulse, decreased CVP

    iv. Thirst, dry skin and mucous membranes, poor skin turgor

    v. Increased body temperature

    vi. Weakness, stupor (seen with severe hypovolemia)

  b. Goals of care

    i. Patient's weight is normal and stable

    ii. Vital signs and hemodynamic parameters are normal

    iii. Fluid balance and urine output are within normal limits (WNL)

  c. Interprofessional collaboration: See Volume Overload

  d. Interventions

    i. Identify common causes of fluid deficit

      (a) Renal water losses

        (1) Diuretic abuse

        (2) Salt-wasting nephropathies

        (3) Diabetes insipidus (nephrogenic, central)

        (4) Osmotic or postobstruction diuresis

      (b) GI losses

        (1) Diarrhea, vomiting, nasogastric suction

        (2) Fistula and wound drainage

        (3) GI bleeding

      (c) Skin: Insensible losses

      (d) Third-spacing (ECF) phenomena

    ii. Document I&O; compare with daily weight

    iii. Administer fluid therapy

      (a) Fluid challenge to increase RBF and urinary excretion

      (b) Caution for fluid challenge: Monitor for pulmonary edema and renal failure unresponsive to volume expansion (e.g., no increase in UOP)

      (c) Follow with replacement fluid therapy until volume goal achieved, then proceed to maintenance fluid regimen

    iv. Assess renal function

      (a) Urine volume, creatinine clearance, BUN/creatinine ratio

      (b) Urinalysis; urine concentration (SG, urine osmolality), spot electrolytes

      (c) 24-hour urine collection for protein evaluation

3. Malnutrition

  a. Description of problem: Malnutrition is associated with increased morbidity in CKD, especially in the presence of hypoalbuminemia. Dietary protein intake is restricted to preserve kidney function in early stages of chronic kidney disease. Protein restriction can contribute to malnutrition.

  b. Goals of care

    i. Patient's intake meets nutritional requirements

    ii. Patient maintains stable baseline weight and adequate muscle mass

    iii. Serum protein and albumin, BUN, and creatinine levels are normal

  c. Interprofessional collaboration: See Volume Overload

  d. Interventions

    i. Identify cause of inadequate nutritional intake; direct care there

    ii. Teach appetite-enhancing measures

      (a) Provide oral hygiene before meals

      (b) Give small, frequent meals

      (c) Identify preferred foods, especially those high in complex carbohydrates and essential amino acids

   iii. Teach the necessary elements of the renal patient's diet

      (a) Essential amino acids, adequate calories, vitamin and iron supplements (folic acid, multivitamins) as warranted

      (b) Adjusted protein and electrolyte intake (Na^+ and K^+) to avoid uremic symptoms and electrolyte imbalances. Excessively diminished protein intake causes use of protein stored in muscles, which leads to body muscle wasting. Providing increased calories can help avoid this situation.

   iv. Monitor pattern of changes in weight and nutritional intake

   v. Assess for nonadherence with dietary instructions

4. Hypertension

  a. Description of problem

    i. In renal failure, the hypertensive state (diastolic BP >90 mm Hg, systolic BP >140 mm Hg) is usually created by fluid retention and/or stimulation of the renin-angiotensin mechanism; preexisting hypertension is common

    ii. Clinical findings (see Ch. 4, Cardiovascular System)

  b. Goals of care (see Ch. 4, Cardiovascular System)

    i. Goal in patients aged 60 years or older without albuminuria (urinary albumin excretion <30 mg/24 hours) is systolic BP 140 mm Hg or under and diastolic BP 90 mm Hg or higher

    ii. Goal in patients aged 60 years or older without albuminuria is systolic BP 150 mm Hg or under and diastolic BP 90 mm Hg or under

    iii. Goal in patients over 70 years old with albuminuria (urinary albumin excretion >30 mg/24 hours) is systolic BP under 140 mm Hg and diastolic BP under 90 mm Hg

  c. Interprofessional collaboration: Nurse, physician, advanced practice provider, case manager, dietitian, nephrologist, cardiologist, hemodialysis nurse (if dialysis indicated).

  d. Interventions (see Ch. 4, Cardiovascular System): A combination of lifestyle modification and pharmacologic therapy should be used to treat hypertension; therapy should be increasingly aggressive depending on the severity of the hypertension, comorbidities present, and the age of the patient

    i. Lifestyle modification

      (a) Achieve and maintain a healthy weight (body mass index 20–25 kg/m²)

      (b) Limit sodium intake to less than 2 g/day

      (c) At least 30 minutes of cardiovascular exercise 5 times/week

      (d) Limit alcohol consumption to 2 or less standard drinks (30 mL of spirits, 100 mL of wine, 285 mL of full-strength beer, or 425 mL of light beer) per day for men and 1 or less standard drink/day for women

      (e) Smoking cessation

    ii. Pharmacologic therapy general principles

      (a) Most patients will require two or more agents to achieve target goals

      (b) Recommendations include the use of ACE inhibitors or angiotensin receptor blockers in patients with CKD, otherwise, no particular medication is favored

    iii. Administer antihypertensive agents as ordered (see Ch. 4, Cardiovascular System)

    iv. Administer diuretics, as ordered, to treat edema and hypertension

      (a) General characteristics of diuretics

        (1) Inhibit the active transport of sodium or chloride, resulting in an increase in urine output

        (2) The diuretic effect reduces effective plasma circulating volume, thereby lowering BP

(b) Complications
    (1) Volume depletion
    (2) Hypokalemia, hyponatremia, hypochloremia
    (3) Hyperkalemia, hyperuricemia, azotemia
    (4) Metabolic alkalosis
    (5) Hypertensive crisis (see Ch. 4, Cardiovascular System)
(c) Types of diuretics: Used as single therapy to treat hypertension or with other antihypertensive agents to enhance their therapeutic effect
    (1) Thiazides
        a) Sodium reabsorption inhibited in the ascending loop of Henle and the beginning portion of the distal tubule
        b) Increased potassium excretion occurs with a weak carbonic anhydrase inhibitory effect
        c) Side effects: Rashes, leukopenia, thrombocytopenia, hypercalcemia, and acute pancreatitis
    (2) Loop diuretics: The most potent diuretics available. The primary site of action is the thick segment of the medullary ascending loop of Henle.
        a) Block the reabsorption of NaCl, thus contributing to a large diuresis of isotonic urine; potassium excretion also enhanced
        b) Increase RBF by stimulating increased secretion of prostaglandin, which exerts a vasodilatory effect on renal vasculature leading to reduction in preload
        c) Vasodilatory effect of loop diuretics can be minimized, if the cardiovascular effect is negative, by the administration of ACE inhibitors
        d) Increase GFR even with a decrease in ECF volume because the tubuloglomerular feedback mechanism is blocked
        e) Side effects: Volume depletion, agranulocytosis, thrombocytopenia, transient deafness, abdominal discomfort, hypokalemia, hypomagnesemia, metabolic alkalosis, and hyperglycemia
        f) Prolonged use without electrolyte replacement results in all other electrolyte imbalances
    (3) Potassium-sparing diuretics: Aldosterone inhibitors
        a) Promote Na^+ secretion into the distal tubule and K^+ reabsorption; cause mild diuresis and protect K^+ level
        b) Usually selected for patients receiving digoxin and diuretic therapy who cannot tolerate low serum K^+ levels or when a mild diuretic effect is desirable
        c) Side effects: Hyperkalemia, hyponatremia, headache, rash, nausea, diarrhea, urticaria, and gynecomastia or menstrual disturbances
    (4) Osmotic diuretic: A nonabsorbable solute (mannitol)
        a) Exerts an osmotic effect, causing water diuresis in excess of NaCl
        b) Side effects: Blurred vision, rhinitis, rebound plasma volume expansion, thirst, urinary retention, and fluid and electrolyte imbalance
    (5) Carbonic anhydrase inhibitors (acetazolamide sodium)
        a) Inhibit the enzyme carbonic anhydrase
        b) Increase the excretion of Na^+ by interfering with HCO_3^- reabsorption. Sodium bicarbonate is lost in the urine, which creates a hyperchloremic metabolic acidosis.

c) Are beneficial when an alkaline urine is desirable, such as with metabolic alkalosis

d) Side effects: Hyperchloremic acidosis, renal calculi, rash, nausea, vomiting, anorexia, diminished renal function

(6) Other agents: Pharmacologic agents that increase both cardiac output and GFR contribute to diuresis (e.g., xanthines [theophylline, aminophylline] and digoxin)

(d) General nursing considerations in the administration of diuretics

(1) Collaborate with the physician to determine the weight and fluid balance desired at the conclusion of diuretic therapy

(2) Observe for fluid, electrolyte, and acid-base disorders

(3) Maintain I&O records; correlate with daily weights

(4) Monitor serum K^+ levels, especially if the patient is taking digoxin (hypokalemia increases risk of digitalis toxicity)

(5) Administer potent or high doses of diuretics in the early morning or afternoon unless a urinary catheter is in place

(6) Monitor BP during aggressive diuresis because hypotension can indicate dehydration and impending circulatory collapse

(7) Advise the patient to report the onset of side effects, such as difficulty hearing

(8) Be aware that a diminished response to diuretics may be related to electrolyte imbalances, particularly hyponatremia, hypochloremia, and hypokalemia

5. **Metabolic acidosis: A condition commonly associated with renal failure caused by the inability of the kidney to excrete hydrogen ions (see Ch. 3, Pulmonary System)**

6. **Anemia: In renal disease, anemia is related primarily to a lack of erythropoietin synthesis and secretion by the kidney but can also be caused by actual blood loss (e.g., stress ulcer).**

a. Description of problem (see Ch. 8, Hematologic and Immunologic Systems)

b. Goals of care (see Ch. 8, Hematologic and Immunologic Systems)

c. Interprofessional collaboration: See Volume Overload; include hematology consult if the patient is unresponsive to therapies.

d. Interventions

i. Identify common causes of anemia associated with renal failure

(a) Suppression of erythropoietin synthesis and secretion

(b) Blood loss

(c) Uremic syndrome

ii. Treat chronic anemia associated with renal failure

(a) Oral or intravenous (IV) iron unless the patient has excess body iron stores

(b) Folic acid and pyridoxine (vitamin B_6): Important, especially in dialysis patients, because these are dialyzable vitamins

(c) Epogen (recombinant human erythropoietin): Stimulates erythrocyte production and prevents the anemia of CKD; effect does not begin until 2 to 6 weeks with peak results in 3 months after administration; as a result, it is not used in AKI

7. **Uremic syndrome**

a. Description of problem: Uremic state results from the kidney's inability to excrete toxic waste products; uremic symptoms usually occur at BUN levels above 100 mg/dL or at a GFR below 10 to 15 mL/min (Table 6.3)

TABLE 6.3   **Clinical Findings in Uremic Syndrome**

Uremic syndrome affects every organ, producing a constellation of symptoms that can occur in any combination

System	Findings
Neurologic	Sensorium changes (loss of attention span, lethargy, fatigue, coma)
	Headache
	Peripheral neuropathy
	Tremors
	Uremic seizures
Skin	Pale yellow tinge
	Pruritus
	Dryness
	Ecchymoses
	Edema
	Uremic frost (rare)
Hematologic and immunologic	Bleeding secondary to platelet dysfunction Diminished immune response
	Anemia secondary to erythropoietin loss or bleeding
Gastrointestinal	Nausea and/or vomiting
	Anorexia, weight loss
	Stomatitis
	Uremic fetor
	Dysgeusia (metallic, unpleasant taste)
	Gastritis, colitis (rare)
	Constipation
Metabolic	Carbohydrate intolerance
	Hyperkalemia
	Hyponatremia or hypernatremia
	Hypocalcemia
	Hyperphosphatemia
	Hypermagnesemia
Musculoskeletal	Renal osteodystrophy—soft tissue calcification
	Bone pain
	Diminished mobility with decreased strength and change in gait
	Muscle atrophy and weakness to paralysis
Genitourinary	Flank pain
	Hematuria
	Proteinuria
	Dysuria, urinary frequency, polyuria
	Normal urine volume to oliguria or anuria
	Urinary tract infections
	Sexual dysfunction

Continued

TABLE 6.3   Clinical Findings in Uremic Syndrome—cont'd

Uremic syndrome affects every organ, producing a constellation of symptoms that can occur in any combination

System	Findings
Cardiac	Pericarditis
	Heart murmurs
	Increased rate of atherosclerosis
	Hypertension
	Pulse: normal, bradycardia, or tachycardia secondary to uremia or electrolyte imbalance
	12-Lead electrocardiogram changes consistent with uremic pericarditis, hyperkalemia, or hypocalcemia
	Chest pain—pleuritic, pericardial, or caused by ischemic heart disease
Endocrine	Hyperparathyroidism (secondary)
Pulmonary	Pleuritis
	Pulmonary edema
	Deep, rapid respirations; Kussmaul's respirations
	Recent respiratory infections (Goodpasture syndrome or recent streptococcal infection), antineutrophil cytoplasmic antibody-related or Wegener granulomatosis
Psychosocial	Altered self-image
	Diminished body image
	Depression to suicidal ideation
Other	Deafness (Alport syndrome)

From Meyer, T.W., Hotstetler, T.H. (2016). The pathophysiology of uremia. In B.M. Brenner (editor), *Brenner and Rector's the kidney*, 10th ed, Philadelphia, Elsevier.

Renal System

6

    b. Goals of care: BUN level is maintained below 100 mg/dL or at a level that minimizes uremic symptoms

    c. Interprofessional collaboration: See Volume Overload

    d. Interventions: Based on minimizing azotemia and preventing dehydration

       i. Restrict oral protein intake

      ii. Remove blood if it is present in the GI tract because this is another protein source that can be metabolized to ammonia and urea. These metabolites cannot be handled by diseased kidneys.

     iii. Consider dialysis to maintain BUN level below 100 mg/dL. In each patient, uremic symptoms develop at individual levels of BUN and creatinine. Identify these values, then strive to maintain BUN and creatinine below those levels.

8. Infection

    a. Description of problem: Major cause of mortality and morbidity in patients with AKI and can seriously compromise patients with CKD (see Ch. 8, Hematologic and Immunologic Systems)

    b. Interventions (see Ch. 8, Hematologic and Immunologic Systems)

       i. Keep in mind: Patients with renal failure have an impaired immune response from uremic toxins and reduced phagocytosis by the reticuloendothelial system

    ii. Use "CAUTI bundles" of educational and procedural interventions to reduce the risk of catheter-associated urinary tract infection (CAUTI)

      (a) Restrict use of urinary catheters for appropriate indications, including acute urinary retention or outlet obstruction, accurate measurement of UOP in critically ill patients, patients undergoing urologic surgery, presence of open sacral or perineal wounds in patients with urinary incontinence, prolonged immobilization (e.g., unstable spinal or pelvic fractures), end-of-life care

      (b) Leave catheters in place only as long as are needed; postoperative patients should ideally have catheter removed within 24 hours unless there are appropriate indications for continued use

      (c) Use aseptic technique when inserting catheters

      (d) Maintain a closed drainage system (e.g., if system is interrupted, replace entire catheter/drainage system using sterile technique, obtain urine samples aseptically)

      (e) Maintain unobstructed urine flow (e.g., do not allow drainage tubing or catheter to kink, keep drainage bag below the level of the bladder, do not allow drainage bag to sit on the floor, empty drainage bag at regular intervals)

    iii. Use alerts or reminders to remove catheters, stop orders, and/or nurse-driven protocols for catheter removal if certain criteria are met

    iv. Consider alternatives to indwelling urinary catheters (e.g., condom catheters, routine use of ultrasonic bladder scanning to detect urinary retention, external female catheters (e.g., Purewick catheters)

9. **Bone disease—osteomalacia, osteitis fibrosa: Chronic hypocalcemia can precipitate hyperparathyroidism, which leads to the mobilization of calcium from the bone and results in softening of the bone (osteomalacia)**

  a. Description of problem

    i. History of chronic hypocalcemia, hyperparathyroidism, or both

    ii. Bone pain, fractures, and radiologic examination of the skull, hands, and feet revealing signs of demineralization

    iii. Activity intolerance with ambulation

  b. Goals of care

    i. Hypocalcemia remains within an asymptomatic range

    ii. No fractures or bone pain is present

  c. Interprofessional collaboration: See Volume Overload

  d. Interventions: See Electrolyte Imbalances—Calcium Imbalance; Hypocalcemia and Electrolyte Imbalances—Phosphate Imbalance; Hyperphosphatemia later in this chapter

10. **Altered metabolism and excretion of pharmacologic agents related to renal failure**

  a. Description of problem

    i. Kidneys unable to metabolize or excrete pharmacologic agents

    ii. Unusual untoward effects may include enhanced sensitivity to medications

    iii. Active or toxic metabolites of a medication retained

    iv. Increased azotemia because of elevation in metabolic wastes from medication usage

  b. Goals of care

    i. Patient tolerates pharmacologic therapy with no untoward medication effects

    ii. Prescribed serum medication levels are adequate

  c. Interprofessional collaboration: See Volume Overload; also Pharmacologist

  d. Interventions

    i. Recognize alterations in the body's use of medications during renal failure

      (a) Distribution of medications in a uremic state

        (1) Decreased stores of body fat affect distribution of lipid-soluble medications

        (2) Low cardiac output states reduce renal metabolism or excretion of medications

        (3) Acidemia alters tissue uptake of medications

        (4) Increased body water has a dilutional effect

        (5) Decreased protein binding causes competition by various medications for tissue binding sites, leading to a higher concentration of unbound medications

      (b) Uremic effects that can alter medication absorption

        (1) Decreased GI motility and altered gastric pH

        (2) Electrolyte imbalances, which may affect GI tract

        (3) Inability of the kidney to excrete or metabolize medications

        (4) Diminished protein binding

   ii. Follow general principles for medication administration during renal insufficiency

      (a) Reduce medication dosage

      (b) Increase intervals between doses

      (c) Question orders for nephrotoxic agents (e.g., NSAIDs)

      (d) Closely observe patients to recognize toxicity because of medication accumulation

      (e) Report any untoward signs, especially elevated serum creatinine level, so the medication can be reconsidered, reduced in dosage, or discontinued

      (f) Monitor serum medication levels, especially in situations requiring a specific medication concentration (e.g., antibiotics, digoxin)

      (g) To ensure a more stable serum concentration, administer initial loading doses of medications that have a long half-life (e.g., digoxin)

11. Ineffective patient and family coping (See also Ch. 2, Psychosocial Aspects of Critical Care)

  a. Description of problem

    i. Insufficient, ineffective, or compromised support, comfort, assistance, or encouragement, usually by a supportive primary person (family member or close friend). The patient may need to manage adaptive tasks related to the stress of renal failure on the patient and the family.

    ii. Signs of maladaptive patient coping

      (a) Verbalization of the inability to cope or to ask for help

      (b) Inability to meet role expectations and solve problems

      (c) Diminished communication and socialization

      (d) Destructive behavior toward self or others (e.g., suicide attempt)

      (e) Failure to comply with the treatment regimen

   iii. Signs of maladaptive family coping

      (a) Patient communicates concern about the family's response to his or her disease

      (b) Family members demonstrate preoccupation with their own personal reactions—fear, anticipatory grief, guilt, anxiety

      (c) Family has inadequate understanding of the patient's condition or therapy interferes with effective supportive behaviors

      (d) Family withdraws from communication with the patient or demonstrates overprotective or underprotective behaviors

   b. Goals of care
      i. Patient demonstrates increased functional independence, adherence with treatment regimen, and participation in programs that enhance quality of life (e.g., exercise or rehabilitation program)
      ii. Patient appropriately expresses ideas, feelings, and needs, participates in family activities, and accepts family support, as appropriate
      iii. Patient and family adjust to any necessary role changes
      iv. Patient resumes employment
   c. Interprofessional collaboration: See Volume Overload
      i. Psychiatrist or psychologist
      ii. Social worker, palliative care
   d. Interventions
      i. Identify common causes of stress in the patient and family
         (a) Life-threatening nature of renal disease
         (b) Inability to perform activities of daily living
         (c) Restrictions caused by a shunt, a fistula, or a Tenckhoff catheter; demands of dialysis schedule and other treatments
         (d) Reversal in family roles, effects on sexual behavior and sexuality, and questions regarding ability to maintain or return to work
      ii. Recognize that psychologic consequences of renal disease and its treatment include denial, depression, and dependency, and that the suicide rate among patients maintained with hemodialysis is believed to be 100 times that of the general population
      iii. Assess the patient's ability to cope with renal disease
      iv. Specific nursing interventions to support adaptation of the patient with renal failure
         (a) Teach the patient about the various treatment alternatives and encourage participation in selection of the treatment method
         (b) Link with support systems
            (1) Visits with successfully adjusted patients
            (2) Support for family members; patients with supportive families tend to have fewer physical complications, survive longer, and adjust more readily

SPECIFIC PATIENT HEALTH PROBLEMS

RENAL TRAUMA

(See Ch. 11, Multisystem Trauma)

ACUTE KIDNEY INJURY

1. **Definition**
   a. AKI (formerly Acute Renal Failure) is the preferred terminology as it better reflects the extended spectrum of renal impairment. AKI affects 5% to 7% of all hospitalized patients and 20% of the critically ill. Oliguria with AKI is associated with a 50% mortality rate in high acuity patients and a 50% to 70% mortality rate in trauma or postoperative patients. Nonoliguria with AKI carries a better prognosis and a lower mortality rate of 26%. A mortality rate of 87% is seen in patients with AKI 24 hours after cardiogenic shock because of acute MI. These mortality rates in the critically ill have not improved in the last 45 years, so prevention of AKI remains the best intervention.

> **KEY CONCEPT**
> AKI is common in high-acuity patients and can seriously affect patient outcomes. AKIs can be classi-
> fied as prerenal, intrarenal, or postrenal.

2. **Pathophysiology**
   a. Prerenal conditions
      i. Physiologic states diminish renal perfusion without renal tubular damage
      ii. Effects of diminished kidney perfusion
         (a) Decreased renal arterial pressure
         (b) Decreased afferent arterial pressure (<100 mm Hg), which diminishes
            forces favoring filtration
   b. Intrarenal conditions
      i. Cortical involvement of vascular, infectious, or immunologic processes
         (a) Causes renal capillary swelling and cellular proliferation, which eventually
            decrease the GFR
         (b) Edema and cellular debris obstruct the glomeruli, which results in oliguria
      ii. Medullary involvement after prolonged ischemia or hypoperfusion or
         nephrotoxic injury to the tubular portion of the nephrons
         (a) Medullary hemodynamics: Hypoperfusion states and oxygen insufficiency
            disrupt the fine balance between limited oxygen supply and high oxygen
            consumption in the outer medullary region; may contribute to AKI from
            hypoxic medullary damage.
            (1) Conditions predisposing to hypoperfusion
               a) Presence of endotoxin
               b) Rhabdomyolysis
               c) Hypercalcemia
               d) NSAID use
               e) Exposure to radiologic contrast agents
               f) Antibiotic use (e.g., amphotericin)
            (2) Pharmacologic agents can also alter medullary hemodynamics,
               especially if administered in absence of volume depletion (e.g.,
               furosemide, mannitol, dopamine). Other substances suspected
               of improving medullary hemodynamics are nitric oxide, which is
               normally produced by the macula densa to control glomerular blood
               flow and renin release, and ANP, an endogenous vasodilator.
         (b) Tubular necrosis produced as localized damage in a patchy pattern (actual
            necrosis) or in apoptosis as disruption of cellular function (usually in
            the distal tubules): Extent of the damage differs in nephrotoxic injury,
            ischemia or hypoperfusion, sepsis-associated states, and multiple organ
            failure
            (1) Nephrotoxic injury affects the epithelial cellular layer (can
               regenerate)
            (2) Ischemia and hypoperfusion alter renal tubular cells and damage the
               tubular basement membrane (cannot regenerate)
               a) Cellular injury may involve several factors: ATP depletion,
                  oxygen-free radical formation, loss of epithelial cell polarity, and
                  increased calcium levels; apoptosis causes DNA fragmentation and
                  cytoplasmic condensation

    b) ATP depletion: Begins 30 seconds after the kidney is hypoperfused; normal homeostatic benefits of cellular ATP (preservation of cellular volume, ionic composition, membrane integrity) are lost

    c) Oxidative metabolism produces oxygen-free radicals

       1) Because these substances are highly reactive and volatile, intracellular mechanisms (enzyme systems and antioxidants) exist for their rapid breakdown and destruction

       2) Left unopposed, as during ischemic events, these radicals disrupt cellular functioning (e.g., during ischemia, the renal cell is unstable and unable to protect itself from oxygen-free radicals, which results in renal cell injury)

    d) Loss of epithelial cell polarity: Ischemia alters the passage of water, electrolytes, and other charged elements through the tubule's epithelial wall, which leads to a concentration defect

    e) Increased calcium levels: Ischemic and hypoperfusion states lead to a rise in intracellular calcium levels that causes renal vasoconstriction and a decrease in GFR

  (3) Systemic inflammatory response syndrome (SIRS): Released endotoxins significantly reduce renal perfusion, and renal vasoactive substances alter renal cellular metabolism and constrict renal vasculature (see Ch. 10, Sepsis and Septic Shock)

  (4) Multiorgan dysfunction syndrome results in rapid and progressive deterioration of renal function

(c) Phases of recovery: Classic form of AKI has four phases, whereas nonoliguric form has only three; the nonoliguric phase seems to be synonymous with the diuretic phase, which suggests that nonoliguric AKI reflects less tubular damage, so recovery is more rapid.

(d) Onset, or initial phase, precedes the actual necrotic injury and correlates with a major alteration in renal hemodynamics.

  (1) Associated with a decrease in RBF and GFR

  (2) Most important factor altering RBF is decrease in cardiac output

  (3) Other mechanisms contributing to decreased renal perfusion are increased sympathetic activity and renal vascular resistance

  (4) A consistent increase in cardiac output during this phase will maintain an increase in RBF and protect the patient from impending AKI

(e) Oliguric phase reflects four processes.

  (1) Obstruction of tubules by cellular debris, tubular casts, or tissue swelling

  (2) Reabsorption or back-leak of urine filtration through the damaged tubular epithelium and into circulation

  (3) Tubular cell damage with development of necrotic, patchy areas; the cell leaks ATP and K^+, edema is present, mitochondria are altered, and calcium leaks into the cell

  (4) Renal vasoconstriction continues and may contribute to the decreased GFR

(f) Nonoliguric phase reflects less tubular damage; symptomatology resembles that of the diuretic phase.

  (1) Urine output may exceed 1 L/h

  (2) Solute present in urine at approximately 350 mOsm/L

  (3) Creatinine clearance is as high as 15 mL/min, and Na^+ excretion is low

  (4) Hyperkalemia remains a significant problem

  (5) Phase of short duration; recovery phase reached in 5 to 8 days

(g) Diuretic phase: Signifies that tubular function is returning
    (1) Tubular obstruction relieved, but cellular edema remains as scar tissue forms on necrotic areas
    (2) Large daily urine output, sometimes exceeding 3 L; output because of the osmotic-diuretic effect of elevated BUN level and impaired ability of tubules to conserve Na^+ and water
    (3) Recovery phase
        a) Occurs after gradual improvement of kidney function extending over a 3- to 12-month period
        b) Residual renal impairment in GFR may result with serum creatinine level remaining higher than previously

  c. Postrenal conditions: Associated with obstruction of the urinary collecting system
    i. Partial obstruction: Can increase renal interstitial pressure, increasing opposing forces of glomerular filtration; result is diminished urine output
    ii. Complete obstruction: Impediment to urine flow accompanies bilateral kidney involvement; the "backup" pressure of urine compresses the kidneys
  d. Clinical problems
    i. Uremic syndrome
    ii. Volume overload and dehydration
    iii. Electrolyte imbalances
    iv. Metabolic acidosis
    v. Pericarditis
    vi. Pulmonary edema
    vii. Altered metabolism and excretion of pharmacologic agents related to renal failure
  e. Classification
    i. RIFLE
      (a) Risk: Increased creatinine × 1.5 or UOP < 0.5 mL/kg/h × 6 hours
      (b) Injury: Increased creatinine × 2 or UOP < 0.5 mL/kg/h × 12 hours
      (c) Failure: Increased creatinine × 3 (or ≥4 mg/dL) or UOP < 0.3 mL/kg/h × 24 hours or anuria × 12 hours
      (d) Loss: Complete loss of renal function more than 4 weeks
      (e) ESRD: End-stage renal disease
    ii. Acute Kidney Injury Network (AKIN)
      (a) Modification of Risk, Injury, Failure, Loss, and End-stage Renal disease (RIFLE)
      (b) Stage 1: Increased creatinine × 1.5 (or >0.3 mg/dL) or UOP < 0.5 mL/kg/h × 6 hours
      (c) Stage 2: Increased creatinine × 2 or UOP <0.5 mL/kg/h×12 hours
      (d) Stage 3: Increased creatinine × 3 (or ≥4 mg/dL) or UOP < 0.3 mL/kg/h × 24 hours or anuria × 12 hours or undergoing renal replacement therapy

3. Etiology and risk factors: Table 6.4
4. Signs and symptoms
  a. Malaise, fatigue, lethargy, confusion
  b. Twitching and/or weakness secondary to metabolic acidosis
  c. Impaired mobility
  d. Change in urine color and/or volume: Oliguria (<400 mL/24 h); nonoliguria (excess, dilute urine); anuria (no urine output or <100 mL/24 h); or hematuria
  e. Cardiac involvement
    i. Dysrhythmias secondary to electrolyte imbalance or heart failure
    ii. Change in pulse rate (either tachycardia or bradycardia)

TABLE 6.4	**Common Causes of Acute Kidney Injury**
Type of Renal Failure	**Causes**
Prerenal failure	Hypovolemia secondary to hemorrhage, gastrointestinal losses, third-spacing phenomena
	Excessive use of diuretics Impaired myocardial contractility (such as heart failure, pericardial tamponade)
	Sepsis, such as gram-negative shock with vasodilatation
	Increased renal vascular resistance from anesthesia or surgery
	Bilateral renal vascular obstruction caused by embolism or thrombosis
Intrarenal failure Cortical involvement	Acute poststreptococcal glomerulonephritis
	Acute cortical necrosis
	Systemic lupus erythematosus (lupus nephritis)
	Goodpasture syndrome, antineutrophil cytoplasmic antibody disease, such as Wegener granulomatosis
	Bilateral endocarditis
	Pregnancy (e.g., abruptio placentae and abortion)
	Malignant hypertension
	Human immunodeficiency virus—related nephropathy
Medullary involvement	Nephrotoxic injury: occurs after exposure to nephrotoxic agents; the effects are accentuated by dehydration, which leads to more extensive tubular damage; nephrotoxic damage may also compound the clinical picture of any type of existing renal deterioration
	• Antibiotics: aminoglycosides, tetracyclines, penicillins, cephalosporins, pentamidine • Antiviral agents: acyclovir • Nonsteroidal antiinflammatory medications • Immunosuppressive medications: cyclosporine, tacrolimus • Angiotensin-converting enzyme inhibitors or angiotensin II receptor blockers • Carbon tetrachloride (found in cleaning agents) • Heavy metals: lead, arsenic, mercury, uranium • Pesticides and fungicides • Radiocontrast dye (e.g., in angiography or computed tomography) • Chemotherapeutic agent toxicity (e.g., cisplatin, uric acid crystals)
	Ischemic injury: during ischemia injury may occur if mean arterial pressure drops below 60 mm Hg for over 40 minutes; causes include massive hemorrhage, transfusion reaction (tubules are obstructed with hemolyzed erythrocytes), and cardiogenic shock Multiple organ dysfunction syndrome: triggered by the inflammatory or immune response, leading to the progressive deterioration of organs with the kidneys as a prime target
	Systemic inflammatory response syndrome: renal injury can result from endotoxins, an inflammatory or immune response, or renal hypoperfusion
Postrenal failure	Ureteral obstruction (e.g., stone, tumor, fibrosis, or clot)
	Abscess
	Prostate hypertrophy
	Crystal deposition (e.g., uric acid, calcium oxalate, acyclovir)

From Kidney Disease: Improving Global Outcomes (KDIGO) Acute Kidney Injury Work Group. (2012). KDIGO Clinical practice guideline for acute kidney injury, *Kidney International Supplements*, 2(1):1–138.

iii. Hypertension

iv. Cardiac friction rub, indicative of pericarditis

f. Skin changes: Dry skin, edema, pallor, bruising, uremic frost (rare), pruritus

g. Flank pain

h. Local or systemic infection presenting with shaking, chills, and fever

i. Abdominal distention secondary to enlarged bladder, obstruction

j. Uremic signs and symptoms: See Table 6.3

5. **Diagnostic study findings**

a. Noninvasive study findings

i. Prerenal

(a) Urinalysis

(1) Urinary sodium level less than 10 mEq/L

(2) SG greater than 1.020

(3) Minimal or no proteinuria

(4) Normal urinary sediment

(5) Urine osmolality higher than 400 mOsm/kg

(b) Serum BUN/creatinine ratio higher than 25 : 1

(c) Fraction of excreted sodium (FENa) <1%

$$FENa = \frac{urine\ sodium \times plasma\ creatinine}{plasma\ sodium \times urine\ creatinine} \times 100$$

(d) Fraction of excreted urea (FEUrea) <1%; FENa is not accurate in patients receiving diuretic therapy, use FEUrea instead

$$FEUrea = \frac{urine\ sodium \times plasma\ urea}{plasma\ sodium \times urine\ urea} \times 100$$

ii. Intrarenal—cortical disease

(a) Urinalysis

(1) Urinary sodium level less than 10 mEq/L

(2) SG variable

(3) Moderate to heavy proteinuria

(4) Hematuria

(5) Urinary sediment with erythrocyte casts, leukocytes

(6) Urine osmolality less than 350 mOsm/kg

(b) Serum BUN and creatinine levels elevated but remain in 10 : 1 ratio

(c) FENa (or FEUrea) over 2%

iii. Intrarenal—medullary disease

(a) Urinalysis

(1) Urinary sodium level greater than 20 mEq/L

(2) SG 1.010

(3) Minimal to moderate proteinuria

(4) Urinary sediment with numerous renal tubular epithelial cells, tubular casts, and a rare erythrocyte

(b) Serum BUN and creatinine levels elevated

(c) FENa (or FEUrea) over 2%

iv. Postrenal

(a) Serum BUN and creatinine levels elevated with complete obstruction

(b) Bacteriologic report showing significant positive results for a specific organism

    v. Special

      (a) Antistreptolysin O titer: To diagnose recent streptococcal infection (may cause poststreptococcal glomerulonephritis)

      (b) Antiglomerular basement membrane titers: To diagnose Goodpasture syndrome, a devastating disease of pulmonary hemorrhage and renal failure

      (c) Antineutrophil cytoplasmic antibody test for pulmonary and renal failure

      (d) Serum studies for complement components: A fall in complement levels is seen in active complement-mediated glomerulonephritis (e.g., lupus nephritis)

      (e) Serum electrophoresis for immunoglobulin levels: Abnormal proteins (as in multiple myeloma) can damage kidneys

      (f) Hepatitis serologic tests: Hepatitis B and C cause kidney disease

  b. Radiologic: To rule out obstruction as a cause of oliguria or anuria because immediate treatment may reverse renal failure. Kidney size provides diagnostic information, because small kidneys imply chronic rather than acute renal failure (see Diagnostic Studies under Patient Assessment).

6. **Interprofessional collaboration: Nurse, physician, advanced practice provider, respiratory therapist, pharmacist, social worker, case manager, dietitian, nephrologist, hemodialysis nurse (if dialysis indicated).**

7. **Management of patient care: Anticipated patient trajectory; patients with AKI experience rapid decline with recovery from 8 days for nonoliguric ATN and from 2 weeks to 3 months for oliguric ATN. Transfer or discharge varies with the stage of renal recovery. Expect patients with AKI to have needs in numerous areas:**

  a. Uremic syndrome (see Patient Care, discussed earlier)

  b. Volume overload and dehydration (see Patient Care, discussed earlier)

  c. Electrolyte imbalances

    i. Mechanism: Inability of kidneys to excrete electrolytes and concentrate urine in AKI

    ii. Management: See later sections on hyperkalemia, hypocalcemia, hyperphosphatemia, and hypermagnesemia, which are the most common imbalances

  d. Metabolic acidosis

    i. Mechanism: Inability of the kidney to secrete hydrogen ions in urine

    ii. Management (see Ch. 3, Pulmonary System)

      (a) Administration of one to three ampules of sodium bicarbonate mixed in 5% dextrose in water or one-half normal saline for a slow drip infusion for acute acidosis; IV push bicarbonate may lead to intracellular acidosis or hypervolemia

      (b) Dialysis to correct or minimize acidosis

  e. Pericarditis

    i. Mechanism: Uremic toxins on myocardium result in pericarditis with or without pericardial effusion

    ii. Management (see Ch. 4, Cardiovascular System)

      (a) Daily continuous dialysis to maintain BUN levels below 80 mg/dL

      (b) Consider pericardiocentesis for large effusions over 250 mL

      (c) Pericardiectomy necessary for repeated episodes or those causing cardiac tamponade

  f. Pulmonary edema

    i. Mechanism

      (a) Volume overload resulting from volume retention secondary to AKI or excess IV fluids administered to prevent AKI

    (b) Uremic cardiac effects, such as left ventricular hypertrophy, uremic pericarditis

  ii. Management (see Ch. 3, Pulmonary System, and Ch. 4, Cardiovascular System)

g. Altered metabolism and excretion of pharmacologic agents (see Patient Care, discussed earlier)

h. Skin care: Impaired skin integrity because of uremia, malnutrition, immobility

  i. Assess for uremic effects on skin integrity (see Table 6.3)

  ii. Keep skin clean, dry, and intact to prevent infection

  iii. Use aseptic technique during wound care

i. Nutrition: AKI is associated with accelerated protein catabolism that contributes to negative nitrogen balance and uncontrollably high BUN levels usually indicative of a hypercatabolic state. Repeated elevations of BUN over 100 mg/dL despite routine dialysis correlate with evidence of rapid muscle wasting and indicate the need for higher levels of protein consumption, together with a continuous form of dialysis.

  i. Maintain protein intake at a minimum of 0.6 to 0.8 g/kg of body weight; administer higher amounts of protein during hypercatabolism

  ii. Provide total calories of 30 to 35 kcal/kg/day of a carbohydrate and lipid combination while controlling glucose and triglyceride intake

  iii. Be aware that hyperalimentation and daily dialysis have been associated with increased survival rates in AKI, as well as promotion of renal tubular cell regeneration. Hyperalimentation requirements include consumption of large amounts of both essential and nonessential amino acids.

  iv. Give IV glucose and lipid solution to augment caloric and nutritional intake, thereby reducing the need for protein in hypercatabolic states

  v. Maintain fluid restriction by limiting nonelectrolyte-containing fluids

  vi. Administer water-soluble vitamins. Avoid excessive doses of vitamin C (not >250 mg/day), which may exacerbate AKI. Be cautious with vitamin A, because excessive intake in the absence of renal excretion can lead to vitamin A toxicity.

  vii. Monitor serum protein, albumin, hematocrit, and urea levels and weigh daily to assess the effectiveness of nutritional therapy

j. Infection control: Uremia increases patient susceptibility to infection

  i. Assess for BUN levels over 80 to 100 mg/dL, because these are associated with an increased risk of infection

  ii. Monitor for early signs of septic shock

  iii. Monitor serum protein and albumin levels because inadequate levels have an immunosuppressive effect

k. Sleep pattern disturbance

  i. Mechanism: During AKI, sleep is interrupted by the intensity of care, acute care environment, sleep apnea, and uremic condition (e.g., tremors, restless legs syndrome). Nursing research reveals an increase in the number of recalled nightmares the night before dialysis at the uremic peak, which results in a disturbed sleep pattern. Disruption of sleep interferes with the healing process and quality of life.

  ii. Management

    (a) Obtain a sleep history (e.g., day or night sleeper)

    (b) Organize care to minimize patient interruptions

    (c) Limit noise in the environment

    (d) Provide three to four 90-minute sleep cycles in each 24-hour period

l. Discharge planning

  i. Teach patient and family members or significant others the following:

(a) Etiology and course of the disease

(b) Dietary and fluid restriction requirements

(c) Dialysis procedure, and schedule

(d) Prospects for recovery

ii. Assess and prepare the home for patient care and, if appropriate, for dialysis

iii. Make the patient and family aware of community resources (e.g., national or local kidney foundation [http://www.kidney.org], local dialysis center)

iv. Assist in patient transition to rehabilitation and/or home care

m. Pharmacology

i. Use pharmacologic agents with adequate fluid replacement to reestablish or augment RBF. This does not protect the tubules from damage but may limit the extent of damage, creating nonoliguric ATN.

(a) Renal-dose dopamine: No benefit in treating AKI. Dopamine may actually compromise the kidney by moving oxygen to the renal medulla; can cause tachycardia and mesenteric ischemia and does not decrease mortality.

(b) Diuretics: May be ineffective or even harmful in the treatment of AKI; have an important role in the management of volume overload

(1) Commonly used agents

a) Traditional diuretics (mannitol, loop diuretics): Used to convert oliguria to nonoliguria

b) Mannitol: Protects the kidney by preventing the buildup of cellular debris, reducing tubular obstruction, and augmenting blood flow. Preserves mitochondrial function via osmotic effect; limits recovery ischemia and free radical production. Administer with caution; may precipitate pulmonary edema.

c) Furosemide: Acts as both a diuretic and augments RBF; maximum administration rate should not exceed 4 mg/kg/min

(2) Diuresis encourages removal of sloughed tubular cells, eliminating tubular obstruction

(3) Volume replacement needs to be a priority before administering diuretics; a trial of diuretics can be attempted but should be limited when effectiveness is in question

(4) Monitor and report changes in urine output (onset of oliguria, nonoliguria, or anuria)

(5) Obtain urine and blood specimens, analyze results

ii. Metabolism and excretion of pharmacologic agents may be altered in AKI (see Patient Care)

n. Treatments

i. Prevention modalities for AKI: Remain the best intervention; preservation of renal function is the desired outcome

(a) Identify patients at higher risk for AKI

(1) Hemodynamic instability; blood loss or hypotension in surgical patients

(2) Multiple trauma, multiorgan dysfunction syndrome, rhabdomyolysis

(3) Systemic and/or renal intravascular hemolysis

(4) Receipt of nephrotoxic medications

(b) Monitor for prerenal or onset stage of ATN (see Diagnostic Study Findings for prerenal failure)

(1) Renal hypoperfusion from any cause diminishes the GFR as the MAP drops to 60 mm Hg or below

(2) Hypotension can eliminate renal autoregulation

(c) Correct hypotension and/or renal hypoperfusion by fluid administration and/or pharmacologic agents

(1) Fluid administration: The single best modality for reinstating renal perfusion is to increase cardiac output and volume status through the administration of fluids, especially in preventing radiocontrast-associated AKI

    a) Consider the following fluids: Normal saline, albumin, and/or blood products

    b) Monitor patient response to administration of as much as 1 to 2 L normal saline over 2 or more hours; observe for nonresponse to volume expansion or pulmonary edema

(2) Pharmacologic agents: Include calcium channel blockers, ANP

    a) Dopamine not proven to be clinically useful

    b) Calcium channel blockers vasodilate renal vasculature and augment renal function; found to be useful in AKI secondary to renal transplantation, radiocontrast nephrotoxicity, and cyclosporine use

    c) ANP use associated with improvement in oliguric rather than nonoliguric AKI; beneficial in management of heart failure

    d) Mucomyst (N-acetylcysteine) beneficial in the prevention of AKI secondary to IV radiocontrast nephrotoxicity; consider 600 mg by mouth twice daily

ii. Hemodialysis (Fig. 6.3)

(a) Early initiation of any form of dialysis is beneficial for the prevention and management of acute and chronic renal failure

(b) Indications for which hemodialysis remains the initial treatment of choice

(1) AKI

(2) CKD when medications and diet no longer provide effective therapy

(3) Symptomatic uremia (e.g., acidosis, hyperkalemia, pericardial friction rub)

(4) To keep BUN level lower than 100 mg/dL and improve survival rate

(c) Contraindications

(1) Intolerance to systemic heparinization (e.g., heparin-induced thrombocytopenia); consider nonheparin anticoagulant, such as argatroban

(2) Hemodynamic instability: Labile cardiovascular status incompatible with rapid changes in ECF volume

(d) Principles of hemodialysis: Include osmosis (optional), diffusion, and convection-ultrafiltration

(1) Osmosis: Movement of water across a semipermeable membrane from an area of lesser to an area of greater osmolality

(2) Diffusion: Movement of molecules from area of higher to an area of lower concentration

(3) Ultrafiltration and convection: Movement of particles through a semipermeable membrane by hydrostatic pressure

(e) Hemodynamics: By means of vascular access and a blood pump, about 300 mL of blood travels through an extracorporeal dialyzer, which removes wastes, toxic substances, excess electrolytes, metabolic products, and pharmacologic agents and then returns the blood to the systemic circulation (see Fig. 6.3).

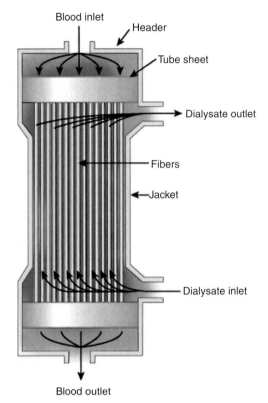

Blood inlet

Header

Tube sheet

Dialysate outlet

Fibers

Jacket

Dialysate inlet

Blood outlet

Fig. 6.3 Hollow-fiber dialyzer, the most common type in clinical use today. (From Crawford, P.W., Lerma, E.V. (2008). Treatment options for end stage renal disease. *Primary Care: Clinics in Office Practice*, 35[3], 407–432.)

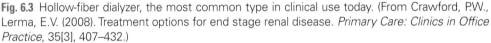

(f) Anticoagulation
  (1) Before the procedure, heparinization is performed to keep blood anticoagulated within the hemodialysis machine (regional heparinization)
  (2) For patients without complications, 5000 units heparin is administered to start and 2000 units/h is given while the patient is on the machine (general heparinization); dosage may be adjusted to meet the needs of the individual patient
  (3) Nonheparin hemodialysis is available at some facilities
  (4) Patient must be monitored closely for signs of bleeding
(g) Vascular access for dialysis
  (1) Central venous access (e.g., dual-lumen internal jugular, femoral, or subclavian catheter): For emergent dialysis or temporarily after failure of a permanent catheter while awaiting repair or replacement
    a) Blood flow must range from 200 to 500 mL/min to accommodate hemodialysis
    b) Double- or triple-lumen catheter requires the use of a large vein, such as the femoral vein, which limits ambulation and carries the risk of dislodgement, infection, and kinking; other sites include the right or left subclavian and right or left jugular vein
    c) Palpate peripheral pulses in the cannulated extremity
    d) Observe for bleeding or hematoma formation; if it occurs, apply pressure dressing and notify the physician

    e) Properly position the catheter to avoid dislodgment during the dialysis procedure

    f) If the femoral vein catheter is to be maintained after dialysis, connect it to a pressurized IV flow system. A low dose of heparin may be considered. Maintain a secure aseptic dressing to minimize the risk of infection. No standing or ambulation is allowed while the catheter is in place.

    g) On removal of a femoral catheter, apply direct pressure to the puncture site for 5 to 10 minutes (or the time needed to stop the bleeding after dialysis and after the period of heparinization). Complete this procedure with the application of a pressure dressing and a period of bed rest.

  (2) Permanent vascular access: An arteriovenous fistula is usually placed in an upper rather than a lower extremity

    a) Surgical procedure with anastomosis of an artery to a vein, or an artificial vascular graft is used

    b) Do not perform venipuncture, start IV therapy, give injections, or take BP with a cuff on the arm with a fistula; post this information on signage above bed

    c) Palpate the thrill or auscultate the bruit to confirm patency

    d) Avoid circumferential dressings and restrictive clothing

    e) Report bleeding, skin discoloration, drainage, and other signs of infection; culture the drainage

    f) For profuse bleeding, apply a pressure dressing

  (3) External permanent vascular access: An arteriovenous shunt is rarely selected

    a) Auscultate for the bruit or palpate for the thrill to assess shunt patency

    b) Promptly report any suspicion of clotting (color change of blood, separation of serum from erythrocytes, absence of pulsations in tubing)

    c) Hydrate adequately to minimize clotting

    d) Change the sterile dressing over the shunt at least daily; reinforce the dressing as necessary

    e) Do not perform venipuncture, give IV therapy, give injections, or take BP with a cuff on the shunt arm

    f) Instruct the patient in the care of the shunt site

(h) Frequency: AKI may require daily dialysis or a one-time dialysis treatment to resolve an acute problem, such as a hyperkalemic episode

(i) Complications

  (1) Muscle cramps, nausea, vomiting

  (2) Bleeding

  (3) Infection (e.g., hepatitis C or infection related to catheter placement or skin flora)

  (4) Hypertension, anaphylactic reactions

  (5) Technical error (dialyzer rupture)

  iii. Continuous renal replacement treatment (CRRT)

    (a) Description

      (1) Form of dialysis specifically developed for the critically ill, hemodynamically unstable patient

(2) May also be selected when both hemodialysis and peritoneal dialysis are contraindicated

(b) Indications

(1) Conditions of fluid overload or cardiovascular instability requiring a continuous method of fluid removal or compensation for azotemia (e.g., ATN)

(2) Ascites, diuretic-resistant edema, acute pulmonary edema

(3) Postcardiac surgery, recent acute MI

(4) Inability to tolerate the cardiovascular effect of rapid fluid losses associated with hemodialysis or failure of a trial of hemodialysis

(c) Contraindications: Rare; hematocrit over 45% is a contraindication for manual forms of CRRT (e.g., continuous arteriovenous hemofiltration, continuous arteriovenous hemodialysis)

(d) Types of CRRT

(1) Slow continuous ultrafiltration

a) Use the principle of ultrafiltration, the exchange of primarily plasma water along with particles (e.g., K^+, BUN, creatinine) by convection

b) Exchange rate depends on membrane area, fiber diameter, hematocrit, plasma protein concentration, pressure gradient, and blood flow rate

(2) Continuous venovenous hemofiltration (CVVH): Most commonly used type of CRRT. The replacement fluid is often electrolyte or bicarbonate based. Uses a blood pump with a venovenous blood access and administration of replacement fluid. Ultrafiltration is the primary principle involved, and solute is removed by convection. No dialysate is used.

(3) Continuous venovenous hemodialysis (CVVHD): Uses a blood pump in conjunction with the dialysate flowing countercurrently to the blood for the ultrafiltration, diffusion, and osmotic dialysis effect. No replacement fluid is used.

(4) Continuous venovenous hemodiafiltration (CVVHDF): Similar to CVVHD; uses a blood pump and dialysate flowing countercurrently to remove and replace high volumes of fluid hourly. Solute removal is via both convection and diffusion. Replacement fluid is used.

(e) Principles: See Principles of Hemodialysis

(f) Anticoagulation

(1) Commonly heparin or citrate; use of citrate as an anticoagulant is off-label

(2) Citrate causes binding of serum calcium; therefore must monitor calcium levels. Calcium administration may be necessary.

(g) Frequency: A continuous dialysis form providing the ability to dialyze 24 hours a day and 7 days a week; the advantage in the critically ill is homeostasis with avoidance of erratic swings in the levels of toxic substances

(h) Overview of the method for CRRT

(1) Prepare the patient: Explain the procedure. Verify orders. Prepare the system. Obtain baseline serum analyses, clotting time, blood chemistry analyses, ABG levels, and complete blood count. Prepare and administer anticoagulant, as prescribed.

(2) Prepare the hemofilter, apply the blood pump if initiating CVVH or CVVHD, and connect to the vascular access properly

(3) Determine the blood flow through the hemofilter and the resulting ultrafiltration rate, and begin fluid replacement therapy

(4) Monitor fluid replacement according to the patient's condition and desired rate of filtrate output to prevent circulatory collapse

(5) Regulate BP, oncotic pressure, and ultrafiltration compartment to optimize the amount of filtrate (according to the prescribed dialyzing device)

(6) Maintain accurate hourly total body I&O records

(7) Potential complications include clotting, hypotension, air entry, blood leak

  iv. Peritoneal dialysis (PD): Effective in the critically ill for maintaining homeostasis; however, if hemodialysis is contraindicated, CRRT is generally used (CVVH); a combination of PD (for solute removal) and hemodialysis (for ultrafiltration) is also effective in AKI (Fig. 6.4)

    (a) Indications

      (1) Fluid overload

      (2) Electrolyte or acid-base imbalance

      (3) Acute or chronic renal failure

      (4) Intoxication from dialyzable medications and poisons

      (5) Pericarditis

      (6) Unavailability of vascular access for hemodialysis

    (b) Contraindications: Bleeding disorder, abdominal adhesions, recent peritoneal surgery

    (c) Principles of PD: Primarily osmosis and diffusion

    (d) Description: Dialysate is instilled into the peritoneal cavity through a catheter, allowed to "pool" (usually for a minimum of 30 minutes), then drained. New dialysate is infused, which initiates the next cycle.

    (e) Anticoagulation: Minimal amount of heparin required

    (f) Frequency: Continuous form of dialysis; dialysis sessions can last 3 to 4 days or longer depending on the needs of the patient

    (g) Hemodynamics: No direct effect on hemodynamics

    (h) Complications

      (1) Bladder or bowel perforation secondary to catheter placement

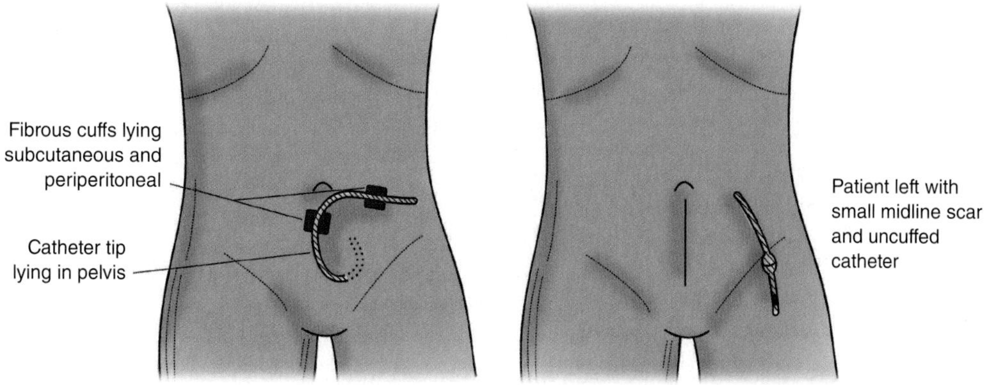

Fibrous cuffs lying subcutaneous and periperitoneal

Catheter tip lying in pelvis

Patient left with small midline scar and uncuffed catheter

Fig. 6.4 Permanent peritoneal catheter. (From Mitchell, D.C., Neary, W.D. [2013]. Principles of renal access surgery. *Surgery*, 31[5], 246–50.)

(2) Peritonitis, abdominal bleeding

(3) Respiratory impairment secondary to increased abdominal size

CHRONIC KIDNEY DISEASE

1. **Definition**

   a. CKD is a slowly progressive renal disorder present for more than 3 months, culminating in ESRD. The decline in kidney function correlates with the degree of nephron loss.

KEY CONCEPT

CKD may be present in high acuity patients. They may require renal replacement therapy, such as CRRT if they are not stable enough for their usual treatment regimens. In addition, CKD may affect medication clearance, requiring alterations in dosing and titration of continuous infusions.

---

2. **Pathophysiology: Systemic changes occur when overall renal function is less than 20% to 25% of normal.**

   a. The kidney has a unique ability to compensate and preserve homeostasis despite a significant (80%) loss of nephron function. During CKD, injury occurs to the nephrons in a progressive manner. The remaining intact nephrons compensate for loss of functioning nephrons by cellular hypertrophy, which enables these nephrons to accept larger blood volumes for clearances and results in excretion of more solute.

   b. Stages of CKD: CKD is classified based on cause, GFR, and albuminuria.

      i. Diminished renal reserve: 50% nephron loss

         (a) Kidney function is mildly reduced, but the excretory and regulatory functions are sufficiently maintained to preserve a normal internal environment; the patient is usually problem free

         (b) The serum creatinine value usually doubles; a normal value of 0.6 mg/dL rises to 1.2 mg/dL, which is still WNL

      ii. Renal insufficiency: 75% nephron loss

         (a) Evidence of impaired renal capacity appears in the form of mild azotemia, slightly impaired urinary concentrating ability, increasing serum phosphorus level, anemia, decreasing serum calcium and bicarbonate levels; hyperkalemia may occur

         (b) Factors that exacerbate renal disease at this stage by increasing nephron damage are infection, dehydration, medications, cardiac failure, and instability of the primary disease

         (c) Serum creatinine level usually ranges from 4.0 to 9.9 mg/dL

      iii. ESRD: 90% of nephrons damaged; GFR is usually less than 15 mL/min

         (a) Renal function has deteriorated so that persistent abnormalities exist

         (b) Patient requires artificial support to sustain life (dialysis or transplantation)

         (c) Serum creatinine level is 10 mg/dL or higher

      iv. Uremic syndrome: Complete nephron loss

         (a) The body's systemic responses to the buildup of uremic waste products and the results of the failed organ system

         (b) Usually described as the constellation of signs and symptoms exhibited in renal failure

         (c) Symptoms may be avoided or diminished by the initiation of early dialysis treatment or renal transplantation

3. **Etiology and risk factors: Table 6.5**
4. **Signs and symptoms of uremia: See Table 6.3**
5. **Diagnostic study findings: See Diagnostic Studies under Patient Assessment**
    a. Noninvasive Study findings
        i. Urinalysis: The following abnormalities may be the first indicators of renal disease. See later for specific findings for CKD.
            (a) Proteinuria: May exceed 3 g/24 h in patients with glomerulonephropathies and nephrotic syndrome
            (b) Leukocyte casts and pyuria: Indicate infection in the urinary tract; suspect renal disease when pyuria occurs in conjunction with hematuria, casts, and proteinuria
            (c) Eosinophiluria: May occur in allergic interstitial nephritis
            (d) Epithelial cells: Renal tubular cells with lipid droplets in the cytoplasm suggest nephrotic syndrome; large numbers of these cells are present in glomerulonephritis and pyelonephritis
            (e) Casts: Provide important diagnostic clues (see section on casts in Diagnostic Studies under Patient Assessment)
                (1) Mixed leukocyte and erythrocyte casts may be prominent in acute exudative glomerulonephritis
                (2) Fatty casts are seen in glomerular diseases in conjunction with moderate to heavy proteinuria
                (3) Waxy, broad casts are seen in the final stages of renal failure
            (f) Urine osmolality: Varies with the stage of CKD
            (g) Creatinine clearance or GFR
                (1) A decrease of 10 to 50 mL/min or a renal reserve of 25% is associated with the onset of renal insufficiency

TABLE 6.5 Common Causes of Chronic Kidney Disease	
Disorder	**Underlying Cause**
Tubulointerstitial disease or interstitial nephritis	Chronic pyelonephritis (most common cause) Analgesic-abuse nephropathy
	Immunologic mechanisms (transplant rejection, allergic response, hypersensitivity)
Glomerulonephropathies	Focal glomerulosclerosis
	Crescentic glomerulonephritis (rapid and progressing)
	Chronic glomerulonephritis
	Systemic lupus erythematosus (lupus nephritis)
	Bacterial endocarditis
Nephrotic syndrome Renal vascular disorders	Glomerular disease
	Systemic vasculitis (e.g., polyarteritis nodosa, hypersensitivity vasculitis)
	Scleroderma
	Coagulopathies, such as hemolytic uremic syndrome
	Thromboembolic renal disease
	Sickle cell nephropathy
	Hypertensive nephrosclerosis: benign, malignant, or accelerated
Renal cancer	Renal cell carcinoma, the most common renal neoplasm

From Kidney Disease: Improving Global Outcomes (KDIGO) Acute Kidney Injury Work Group. (2012). KDIGO Clinical practice guideline for acute kidney injury, *Kidney International Supplements*, 3(Suppl 2013):1–150.

(2) A creatinine clearance of 10 to 15 mL/min is consistent with ESRD
  ii. Serum studies
    (a) Creatinine: An inverse relationship exists between serum creatinine level and GFR, and the stage of CKD
      (1) Diminished renal reserve: A 50% nephron loss is reflected by either a normal creatinine level of 1.4 mg/dL or a twice-normal creatinine level of 2.8 mg/dL.
      (2) Renal insufficiency: A 75% nephron loss causes the serum creatinine level to quadruple.
      (3) ESRD: A 90% nephron loss correlates with a serum creatinine value of 10 mg/dL or higher.
      (4) Uremic syndrome: A creatinine value of 10 mg/dL or higher is maintained by some form of dialysis.
    (b) BUN: In CKD, BUN levels above 100 mg/dL are usually associated with uremic symptoms; therefore BUN level is used to determine the frequency and duration of dialysis treatments.
    (c) Uric acid: Increased serum levels may suggest gout or gouty nephropathy when the elevation is out of proportion to the degree of renal failure
    (d) Serum triglyceride level: May be elevated
    (e) Glucose tolerance test: Identifies the presence of carbohydrate intolerance
    (f) Serum protein and albumin levels: Decreased values indicate malnutrition associated with a restricted-protein diet, anorexia, or chronic infection
  b. Invasive study findings
    i. IVP
      (a) Small kidneys, or one atrophied and one normal-sized kidney, may indicate bilateral disease; unilateral disease always causes compensatory hypertrophy of the contralateral kidney
      (b) Enlarged kidneys suggest polycystic disease or obstruction
      (c) Scarring and altered calices can suggest chronic pyelonephritis or analgesic nephropathy
    ii. Ultrasonography: Identifies renal parenchymal disease and rules out obstruction; generally lacks the ability to differentiate between renal diseases
    iii. CT: May reveal renal perfusion defects, pyelonephritis, renal cystic disorders, or renal colic
    iv. MRI: Used to diagnose renovascular lesions
    v. Special: Baseline motor nerve conduction velocity studies and long bone x-ray films of the skull, hands, and feet identify the development of uremic neuropathy and bone disease
6. **Interprofessional collaboration: See AKI—include consultation with a cardiologist and/or renal transplant surgeon.**
7. **Management of patient care**
  a. Anticipated patient trajectory: Patients with CKD, especially ESRD, face complex self-care expectations on discharge and the need for lifelong compliance with an intricate healthcare regimen. Throughout the course of recovery and discharge, patients with CKD may be expected to have needs in the following areas:
    i. Skin care (see Management of Patient Care under AKI)
    ii. Nutrition: Critical element in care; modification of diet in renal disease is implemented during the early stages of CKD for prevention and prolongation of renal health and in ESRD for moderation of uremic symptoms

(a) General CKD diet: Restricted-protein diet of 0.6 to 0.8 g protein/kg/day with a total caloric intake of 35 mg/kcal/kg body weight and 2 g each of sodium and potassium. High-quality biologic protein (such as eggs, fish, meat) should account for two-thirds of daily total protein intake.

(b) Dietary modifications for CKD: In the early stages of CKD, 0.6 g protein/kg/day plus 0.3 g protein/kg/day of high-quality biologic protein

(c) Dietary modifications for ESRD: 0.8 g protein/kg/day with a caloric intake of 35 mg/kcal/kg body weight

(d) Adjustments are made to the standard CKD diet depending on the type of dialysis and appetite; in many instances, protein intake is increased

    (1) Hemodialysis or PD: Increased protein requirements. Hemodialysis patients need 1.1 to 1.2 g protein/kg/day; PD patients, 1.3 to 1.4 g protein/kg/day.

    (2) Continuous ambulatory peritoneal dialysis (CAPD): 1.1 to 1.4 g protein/kg/day

    (3) CRRT: Requirements have not been substantiated; however, increased amino acid losses necessitate higher protein supplementation, approximately 1.5 to 2.5 g protein/kg/day

    (4) Diminished appetite: Administer unlimited-protein diet to prevent malnutrition

(e) Be aware that the presence of hypoalbuminemia is associated with increased mortality in CKD

(f) Low BUN value is another predictor of mortality because it suggests reduced protein intake, reduced muscle mass, chronic illness, and cachexia

(g) Sodium: Restrict to minimize hypertension, thirst, and weight gain

(h) Potassium: Restrict for most hemodialysis patients, but PD patients may not require restriction

(i) Lipids: Hyperlipidemia occurs in 40% to 50% of CKD patients

    (1) Most common types

        a) Hypertriglyceridemia

        b) Elevated levels of low-density lipoproteins

        c) Normal or reduced levels of high-density lipoproteins

    (2) Increased risk of atherosclerosis

    (3) Current guidelines recommend the use of statins in all adults over 50 years with nondialysis dependent CKD and in adults 18 to 49 with known coronary artery disease, diabetes mellitus, prior ischemic stroke, or estimated 10-year risk of coronary death or nonfatal MI greater than 10%

(j) Vitamins: Water-soluble vitamins (e.g., vitamin B complex and C) are prescribed specifically for dialysis patients

iii. Infection control: Risk of bacterial infection increases with decline in GFR

(a) Common infections include peritonitis secondary to PD catheterization and infection at hemodialysis vascular catheter site. Septicemia related to these infections is associated with a high mortality rate.

(b) Immunocompromise accompanies uremia (see Patient Care)

(c) All adults with CKD should be offered annual influenza vaccinations unless otherwise contraindicated; patients with stage 4 or 5 CKD should be vaccinated against hepatitis B and pneumococcal pneumonia

iv. Discharge planning

(a) General patient and family teaching: Be aware that the uremia of CKD impairs cognition and memory. In addition, the complexity of the renal replacement therapies demands multiple patient and family teaching sessions. Patient compliance is essential to minimize uremic symptoms, as well as to ensure patient safety.

(1) Assess knowledge related to CKD, treatments, medications

(2) Assess the effects of uremia on the patient's learning abilities (e.g., decreased attention span and memory, altered cognition)

(3) Develop a teaching plan including reinforcement, self-care activities, treatment, and compliance expectations

(4) Instruct the patient and family or significant others about all aspects of CKD

    a) Normal renal function and renal disease state

    b) Management of diet, fluids, medications, skin, rest

    c) Avoidance of infection

    d) Treatment alternatives and benefits and disadvantages of each; support the patient's and family's decision

(5) Instruct the patient and family about general features and elements of care for dialysis treatments

    a) Dynamics of hemodialysis or PD

    b) Special diet and fluid allowances

    c) Care of the dialysis access

    d) Need for weight control

    e) Signs and symptoms of complications, such as an electrolyte imbalance

    f) Transportation to the dialysis center

(b) Outcomes specific to various renal replacement therapies (Box 6.1)

  v. Pharmacology (see also Renal Transplantation)

(a) CKD patients take an average of 8 to 10 medications

(b) Effect of CKD on pharmacologic agents: See Patient Care

(c) Compliance necessary to receive optimal effect of pharmacologic therapy; nonadherence is associated with exaggerated uremic symptoms, exacerbation of coexisting disease (e.g., cardiac disease, diabetes, hypertension), and increased morbidity

  vi. Psychosocial issues: ESRD and dialysis or transplantation require adaptation and coping; adjustment is difficult and may contribute to depression

(a) Body image disturbance: Results from the effects of uremia, dependency on treatments, and primary illness other than renal disease (see Ch. 2, Psychosocial Aspects of Critical Care)

(b) Sexual dysfunction: An experience of change in sexual function viewed as unsatisfying, unrewarding, or inadequate; results from uremia, its complications, and/or its treatment

  vii. Treatments: Renal replacement therapies include hemodialysis, PD, and renal transplantation. CRRT is usually reserved for critically ill AKI patients but is an option for the CKD patient in the ICU (see Treatments under Acute Renal Failure).

(a) Chronic hemodialysis

(1) Patient usually has hemodialysis treatment 3 times a week (3–5 hours per treatment) via a permanent or temporary vascular access

(2) Dialysis temporarily replaces renal function; thus the patient must be compliant with diet and fluid restrictions

(3) Anticoagulation (heparin) usually required. A minimum heparin dosage can be used for patients at risk (e.g., postoperatively). In rare

Renal System

6

BOX 6.1 Outcomes of Renal Replacement Therapies

HEMODIALYSIS

- Circulatory access is maintained.
- Patient has hemodialysis treatment, usually 3 times a week (3–5 hours for each treatment).
- Patient complies with rigid diet and fluid restrictions.

CHRONIC PERITONEAL DIALYSIS

Follows same principles and procedures as acute peritoneal dialysis; differences relate to patient expectations and use of automated peritoneal dialysis machine.

- Patient expectations for peritoneal dialysis:
  - Maintenance of Tenckhoff catheter
  - Use of aseptic technique throughout the procedure
  - Treatment 3 to 4 times a week for 10 hours each treatment in hospital or 7 days, 4 times per day or every night with cycler
  - Adherence to dietary and fluid restrictions
- Expectations for home peritoneal dialysis:
  - Proper environment: treatment requires space and storage area for equipment
  - Cardiovascular stability: Not as necessary for home peritoneal dialysis because rapid fluid shifts and dramatic cardiovascular effects are not associated with this treatment
  - Family support systems: Helpful but not essential because most patients use dialysis at night, and the family routine may not be disrupted
  - Cognitive ability: Moderate technologic skill is required, but aseptic technique is essential

CONTINUOUS AMBULATORY PERITONEAL DIALYSIS (CAPD)

- Patient demonstrates ability to perform procedure.
- Patient recognizes that exchanges are 4 times a day, 7 days a week. Each exchange is 4 to 8 hours.
- Patient completes a rigorous training program.
- Patient demonstrates proper care of the Tenckhoff catheter.
- Patient adheres to the treatment schedule.
- Patient stores the dialysis equipment appropriately.
- Patient demonstrates measures to avoid complications, such as peritonitis, back strain, visceral herniation, obesity, fluid excess.

RENAL TRANSPLANTATION

(See Treatment under End-Stage Renal Conditions section)
- Patient and family demonstrate knowledge of diet and fluid regimen, signs and symptoms of rejection.
- Patient demonstrates ability to obtain and record daily weight and administer medications.
- Patient reports for frequent clinic and other follow-up outpatient visits.
- Patient adheres to activity limitations and rehabilitation program.

From National Kidney Foundation. (2015). KDOQI clinical practice guideline for hemodialysis adequacy: 2015 update. *American Journal of Kidney Disease*, 66(5), 884–930; Kidney Disease: Improving Global Outcomes (KDIGO) Transplant Work Group. (2009). KDIGO clinical practice guideline for the care of kidney transplant recipients, *American Journal of Transplantation* 9(Suppl 3), S1–S157.

---

situations (e.g., patient has coagulopathy), heparin-free hemodialysis may be possible. For heparin-induced thrombocytopenia, use a nonheparin anticoagulant, such as argatroban.

    (4) Availability of chronic hemodialysis: Hospital, satellite center, or home performed by a surrogate or the patient

  (b) Chronic PD: Follows the same principles and procedures as acute PD; differences relate to the patient's expectations and the use of an automated PD machine

    (1) Frequency of treatment varies with the PD approach

      a) Hospital based or at home: Usually dialyze 4 times per week for 10 hours

      b) Nighttime home PD: Dialyze all night every night

c) CAPD: A continuous form; dialyze 24 hours a day, 7 days a week

(2) A peritoneal catheter is permanent access placed surgically

(3) Dietary and fluid restrictions vary

(4) Anticoagulation performed using heparin (low dose)

(c) CRRTs: See Treatment under Acute Renal Failure

b. Potential complications: Table 6.6

ELECTROLYTE IMBALANCES—POTASSIUM IMBALANCE: HYPERKALEMIA

The serum potassium level in hyperkalemia is above 5.5 mEq/L

KEY CONCEPT

Electrolyte imbalances are common in high acuity patients, even in those without CKD. Nurses should be careful to monitor patients for signs of electrolyte disturbances and treat them as ordered.

---

1. Pathophysiology
   a. Inability of the kidney tubules to excrete K^+ because of tubular damage, salt depletion, or increased potassium load from injured tissues; or may be induced by medications, such as potassium-sparing diuretics (e.g., spironolactone), which inhibit aldosterone, or amiloride and triamterene, which block the sodium channel and thereby inhibit Na^+ reabsorption and promote K^+ retention
   b. Reduction in K^+ excretion caused by decreased renal perfusion because less Na^+ is available for exchange with K^+ (e.g., in cardiac failure)
   c. Alteration in K^+ release (rhabdomyolysis) or distribution (insulin deficiency)

TABLE 6.6 Potential Complications of Chronic Kidney Disease

Potential Complication	Mechanism/Description	Management
Hypervolemia	See Volume Overload under Patient Care	See Volume Overload under Patient Care
Electrolyte imbalance	Accompanies the inability to concentrate urine; there is risk of imbalance of any electrolyte during ESRD, but the most common imbalances are hyperkalemia, hypocalcemia, and hyperphosphatemia (see sections on specific imbalances)	See section on specific electrolyte imbalance
Metabolic acidosis	See Patient Care	Keep in mind that the dialysis controls metabolic acidosis • Acetate or lactate found in a hemodialysis and peritoneal dialysis bath is to be absorbed into the body and enters the Krebs cycle, where it is converted to bicarbonate; conversion requires the presence of oxygen at the tissue level • Bicarbonate bath: Available with some adjusted hemodialysis machines that dialyze with a bath containing bicarbonate (35–36 mEq/L), which obviates the need for the metabolic conversion expected with acetate or lactate

Continued

TABLE 6.6 Potential Complications of Chronic Kidney Disease—cont'd

Potential Complication	Mechanism/Description	Management
Anemia (see also Patient Care)	Production of erythropoietin is decreased	Assess dosage of epoetin alfa (DNA recombinant-engineered erythropoietin; Epogen, Procrit) on a routine basis, maintaining prescribed HCT value (33%–36%); dose at approximately 80 to 120 units/kg/wk in 1 to 3 doses/wk
		Epoetin alfa is an effective replacement agent for erythropoietin
		• Takes 3 months to produce a near-normal HCT associated with a mild to moderate improvement in exercise tolerance and work capacity, increased aerobic performance, and improved oxygen transport • Cardiac output and ejection fraction also improve • Side effects: Increased blood viscosity and HCT may lead to problems, such as shortened life of the fistula, hypertension, increased clotting tendencies, limited reuse of dialyzers; these effects are minimized when HCT is maintained in the lower normal range; seizures and hypertension also are potential effects • Darbepoetin alfa is a longer-acting erythropoietin substitute than can be used every 2 weeks; as effective as epoetin alfa
Uremic syndrome Cardiac involvement (major cause of death in ESRD)	Volume-pressure overload results in LV hypertrophy and heart failure	General: See Ch. 4 for heart failure, LV hypertrophy, CAD, hypertension uremic pericarditis: See Potential Complications under Acute Renal Failure
	CAD—primary CAD is present in about half of hemodialysis patients and is exacerbated in ESRD, especially with dialysis	
	Uremic pericarditis—caused by the accumulation of uremic toxins; may progress to pericardial effusion and, if untreated, cardiac tamponade	
	Symptomatic hyperkalemia—leads to delayed cardiac conduction that may result in asystole	
	Hypertension (essential or nonessential)—underlying cause of ESRD or occurs as a result of ESRD because of hypervolemia, vascular disease	
Pulmonary involvement	Uremic toxins may cause uremic pneumonitis and pleural effusion; in severe cases, fluid overload may mimic clinical picture of ARDS	Initiate frequent dialysis Provide antibiotics as necessary Administer oxygen, provide pulmonary care Monitor progress with ABG analysis and chest radiography
	Depressed immunity results in increased susceptibility to infection; increased risk of pneumonia	

Renal System

6

Continued

TABLE 6.6 **Potential Complications of Chronic Kidney Disease—cont'd**

Potential Complication	Mechanism/Description	Management
Neurologic involvement (as uremic encephalopathy)	Neurologic presentations include • Restless legs syndrome • Peripheral neuropathy 　• "Burning" sensation of the feet progressing to paresthesia and intense pain on the dorsal and ventral surfaces of the feet 　• Foot drop and diminished muscle strength 　• Impaired gait and possibly paralysis 　• Slowing of nerve conduction velocity and a segmental demyelination of the nerves • Intellectual and memory impairment • Acute postdialysis dementia (e.g., dialysis disequilibrium) • Dialysis dementia (rare)—associated with chronic dialysis and long-term exposure to aluminum-containing substances • Seizures • Uremic encephalopathy	Intensify dialysis treatments; increase time and/or frequency Treat seizures with anticonvulsants Administer vitamin replacement therapy, because a deficit may further compromise neurologic function Eliminate aluminum hydroxide gels, which are associated with aluminum accumulation and toxicity and are believed to be responsible for dialysis dementia Correct electrolyte imbalances (hypocalcemia) Orient the patient as necessary
Endocrine and metabolic involvement	Accumulation of uric acid leads to hyperuricemia manifested as gout with joint pain and inflammation, low-grade fever hypertension Secondary hyperparathyroidism: Combination of hypercalcemia and demineralization of bone with metastatic calcifications Hyperlipidemia: An increase in LDL levels and triglycerides is common in CKD Carbohydrate intolerance: Manifested as moderate levels of hyperglycemia and elevated insulin levels	Initiate dietary therapy for elevated LDL levels; monitor serum lipid profile (total cholesterol, triglycerides, LDL, HDL) Lipid-lowering agents often necessary High LDL levels may accelerate progression to ESRD Institute dialysis to minimize uremia and improve glucose tolerance Administer allopurinol for gout and monitor uric acid level Administer low-dose corticosteroids to decrease serum lipid levels
Gastrointestinal involvement	Uremic toxins affect gastrointestinal tract, producing • Uremic bowel: Diarrhea or constipation, malabsorption syndrome, weight loss, and fatigue • Peptic ulcer disease: Gastric pain and possibly bleeding	Minimize or alleviate uremia via dialysis Administer a protein-restricted diet Administer zinc to improve taste Use nonmagnesium-containing antacids or H_2 blockers (ranitidine) or proton pump inhibitors (omeprazole) for gastrointestinal irritation

Continued

TABLE 6.6	**Potential Complications of Chronic Kidney Disease—cont'd**	
Potential Complication	**Mechanism/Description**	**Management**
Coagulopathy	Platelet adhesiveness is diminished, which is sometimes associated with mild thrombocytopenia	Initiate dialysis to minimize the uremic effect on platelet function Give iron and folic acid supplements
	Bleeding tendency may be increased, leading to bruising and purpura	Testosterone, other androgens may reverse anemia (rarely used)
Musculoskeletal involvement	Hypocalcemia and, if present, secondary hyperparathyroidism may lead to reciprocal hyperphosphatemia	Monitor serum calcium level, administer calcium tablets Administer activated vitamin D (1,25-dihydroxychocalciferol) with phosphate-binding therapy
	Bone pain, impaired growth, and pathologic fractures may occur	
Sexual dysfunction	Amenorrhea, abnormal menstruation, infertility, increased prolactin may occur	Administer estrogen replacement therapy Assess for zinc deficiency, which may be responsible for male impotence
	Diminished testosterone, decreased libido, impotence may be seen	Review current medications (e.g., β-blockers) for contribution to sexual dysfunction Renal transplantation may restore sexual function and fertility Assess for depression and need for an antidepressant

ABG, Arterial blood gas; *ARDS*, acute respiratory distress syndrome; *CAD*, coronary artery disease; *CKD*, chronic kidney disease; *DNA*, deoxyribonucleic acid; *ESRD*, end-stage renal disease; *HCT*, hematocrit; *HDL*, high-density lipoprotein; *LDL*, low-density lipoprotein; *LV*, left ventricular.

From Kidney Disease: Improving Global Outcomes (KDIGO) Acute Kidney Injury Work Group. (2012). KDIGO Clinical practice guideline for acute kidney injury, *Kidney International Supplements*, 3(Suppl 2013):1–150.

d. Clinical problems
   i. Cardiac arrhythmia: Bradycardia to asystole
2. **Etiology and risk factors**
   a. Acute and chronic renal failure or renal disease associated with distal tubule dysfunction (e.g., sickle cell anemia)
   b. Increased cellular destruction with potassium release, such as occurs in burns, trauma, crash injuries, severe catabolism, acute acidosis, intravascular hemolysis, rhabdomyolysis, and thrombocytosis
   c. Excessive administration or ingestion of potassium chloride
   d. Adrenal cortical insufficiency: Hypoaldosteronism or Addison disease
   e. Aldosterone deficiency
   f. Low cardiac output or sodium depletion
   g. Metabolic acidosis: Precipitates the movement of intracellular K^+ to the extracellular space
   h. Certain medications
      i. Potassium-sparing diuretics, which block Na^+ reabsorption, thereby facilitating K^+ retention
      ii. The antibiotics pentamidine and trimethoprim, which also promote K^+ retention via the same mechanism
      iii. Medications that inhibit aldosterone production (e.g., ACE inhibitors, NSAIDs, heparin, cyclosporine, tacrolimus) and angiotensin II antagonists

    iv. Medications that inhibit extrarenal K⁺ disposal (nonselective β-blockers, propranolol, nadolol, timolol)

    v. Release of K⁺ from injured cells: Seen in cocaine ingestion, rhabdomyolysis, and chemotherapy-induced tumor lysis syndrome

3. **Signs and symptoms: Detection of electrolyte imbalances is difficult. Suspect imbalances with renal or endocrine disease with excessive loss of body fluids (e.g., vomiting, diarrhea), in some medication intoxications (e.g., indiscriminate use of electrolyte replacement, hormonal therapy, or vitamins), and with acute changes in mental status (confusion, agitation, coma; Table 6.7).**

4. **Diagnostic study findings**
   a. Laboratory: Serum potassium level exceeds 5.5 mEq/L
   b. Electrocardiogram (ECG): Progressive changes reveal peaked and elevated T waves→widened QRS→prolonged PR interval→flattened or absent P wave and ST segment depression→idioventricular rhythm→asystole cardiac arrest

TABLE 6.7	**Signs and Symptoms of Potassium Imbalance**	
System	**Hyperkalemia**	**Hypokalemia**
Cardiovascular	Bradycardia	Diminished, irregular pulses
	Dysrhythmias	Increased myocardial excitability or irritability
	Hypotension	Dysrhythmias: Premature atrial contractions, premature ventricular contractions, sinus bradycardia, paroxysmal atrial tachycardia, atrioventricular blocks, atrioventricular or ventricular tachycardia
		Enhanced digoxin effect to the point of digoxin toxicity
Neurologic	Lethargy	Drowsiness to coma, malaise, and confusion
	Apathy	Muscle cramping (commonly in calf muscle)
	Confusion	Muscular weakness progressing to paralysis
Pulmonary	Deep rapid respiration (Kussmaul's respirations) when hyperkalemia accompanied by acidosis	Shallow respirations secondary to muscle weakness
	Shallow respirations if muscle paralysis present	
Gastrointestinal	Abdominal cramping and diarrhea	Vomiting Paralytic ileus
Musculoskeletal	Irritability to flaccid paralysis and numbness of extremities	Pain in calf similar to that of deep venous thrombosis
	Fatigue associated with diminished exercise tolerance	
	Diminished mobility to paralysis	
Genitourinary	Oliguria	Polyuria

From Mount, D.B. (2016). Disorders of potassium balance. The pathophysiology of uremia. In B.M. Brenner (editor), *Brenner and Rector's the kidney*, 10th ed, Philadelphia, Elsevier.

5. Interprofessional collaboration: Nurse, physician, advanced practice provider, dietitian, nephrologist, hemodialysis nurse (if dialysis indicated)
6. Management of patient care
    a. Anticipated patient trajectory: Patients with acute symptomatic hyperkalemia face a life-threatening condition requiring urgent intervention and resolution. Recovery requires compliance with a treatment plan to prevent repeat episodes.
7. Goals of care
    a. Symptomatic hyperkalemia is eliminated
    b. Cardiac function is restored to WNL for the patient
8. Patients may be expected to have needs in the following areas:
    a. Positioning: Position to promote comfort; hyperkalemia can cause fatigue, muscle irritability, numbness, and flaccid paralysis
    b. Nutrition: After K^+ stabilized to a safe, asymptomatic level, restrict dietary potassium (e.g., orange juice, cola, banana)
    c. Discharge planning: Include discharge teaching to promote dietary adherence to avoid hyperkalemia
    d. Pharmacology
        i. Provide cardiac monitoring before and during pharmacologic therapy; monitor potassium levels frequently
        ii. In emergency situations (e.g., if serum K^+ >6.5 mEq/L or ECG change indicates symptomatic hyperkalemia)
            (a) Administer regular insulin and dextrose IV with β-agonist inhalant to temporarily shift K^+ into cells
                (1) Insulin can rapidly lower serum potassium level
                (2) Dextrose must accompany insulin; patients who lack endogenous insulin production can experience a paradoxical increase in potassium or hypoglycemia
            (b) Administer a β-agonist (albuterol in a concentrated form) by inhalation; observe medication action in 30 minutes; effect is complementary to the potassium lowering created by insulin
            (c) Use sodium bicarbonate IV when severe metabolic acidosis complicates the hyperkalemia
            (d) Consider IV calcium chloride or calcium gluconate (IV push) to stabilize the cardiac membrane; contraindicated in patients taking digoxin; if no improvement in ECG, can repeat calcium bolus in 3 to 5 minutes
            (e) Essential to follow aforementioned temporary measures with a therapeutic measure to permanently remove potassium from the body (e.g., sodium polystyrene sulfonate [SPS; Kayexalate], hemodialysis)
            (f) SPS with sorbitol administered orally or rectally for the exchange of Na^+ into the intestinal cell and K^+ into the bowel space; when administered in combination with sorbitol, enhances a diarrhea stool for actual K^+ loss
                (1) With SPS, Na^+ ion is exchanged 1:1 for a K^+ ion in the bowel cell wall; therefore assess the amount of sodium retained, as well as the potassium loss
                (2) Ensure that the SPS and sorbitol mixture is expelled, especially postoperatively, because retained SPS can cause bowel obstruction and perforation
                (3) Rectal route of administration is rapid and produces a predictable outcome

e. Treatment: Hemodialysis is a rapid form of treatment for serum potassium reduction (see Acute Kidney Injury and Chronic Kidney Disease)

ELECTROLYTE IMBALANCES—POTASSIUM IMBALANCE: HYPOKALEMIA

The serum potassium level in hypokalemia is below 3.5 mEq/L

1. **Pathophysiology**
   a. Potassium loss exceeding intake
   b. Alkalosis: Stimulates the secretion of K^+ in the distal tubule
   c. Intracellular shifting of K^+

2. **Etiology and risk factors**
   a. Alkalosis: Causes K^+ to shift into the cell
   b. Abnormal GI losses: Nasogastric suction and drainage, laxative abuse, diarrhea, prolonged episode of vomiting
   c. Starvation or malnutrition (including hyperalimentation without adequate potassium replacement)
   d. Diuretic therapy (loop diuretics, thiazides, acetazolamide), renal tubular acidosis
   e. Increased adrenal corticosteroid secretion or corticosteroid therapy
   f. Liver disease
   g. Bartter syndrome: Hypokalemia, hyponatremia, hypomagnesemia, metabolic alkalosis, and hyperreninemia
   h. Severe stress (K^+ shifts into cells)

3. **Signs and symptoms: See Table 6.7**

4. **Diagnostic study findings**
   a. Laboratory: Serum potassium levels below 3.5 mEq/L
   b. ECG: Depressed ST segments, flat or inverted T wave, presence of U wave, and ventricular dysrhythmias

5. **Interprofessional collaboration: See Electrolyte Imbalances—Potassium Imbalance: Hyperkalemia**

6. **Management of patient care**
   a. Anticipated patient trajectory: Patients with acute hypokalemia face serious cardiac symptomatology that requires immediate resolution in the clinical setting. Recovery and discharge require compliance with a treatment regimen that prevents repeated episodes.

7. **Goals of care**
   a. Cardiac arrhythmias
      i. Mechanism: Hypokalemia depresses myocardial contractility and conductivity
      ii. Management: Treat hypokalemia; if warranted, institute cardiopulmonary resuscitation for asystolic cardiac arrest

8. **Patients may be expected to have needs in the following areas:**
   a. Positioning: Place in a position of comfort to minimize muscle cramping and weakness, as well as to promote adequate respirations
   b. Nutrition: Provide foods containing potassium (e.g., orange juice, raisins, milk, green vegetables, etc.)
   c. Discharge planning: Include discharge teaching to promote sufficient potassium intake and compliance with the dietary regimen
   d. Pharmacology: Provide cardiac monitoring before and during pharmacologic therapy
      i. Administer oral potassium supplements when indicated; dilute to prevent GI irritation and to facilitate absorption

    ii. Observe for ECG changes and the presence of dysrhythmias

   iii. Monitor serum potassium levels

   iv. Record the amount of urine output and other drainage (gastric aspirate, diarrhea) to aid in calculating total body potassium balance

    v. Recognize and treat signs of alkalosis

   vi. Never give IV potassium chloride rapidly; large concentrations can precipitate hyperkalemia, producing necrosis of the vessel wall, and possibly inducing ventricular fibrillation. Never administer as an IV push.

   vii. Determine whether the patient is receiving digitalis or diuretics; correct potassium losses, because these can precipitate digitalis toxicity and decrease the effectiveness of most diuretics

  viii. Emergency treatment

      (a) Slowly administer IV potassium chloride while the patient is monitored with ECG for dysrhythmias

      (b) Monitor for signs and symptoms of hyperkalemia

      (c) Maintain a record of serum potassium levels to assess the adequacy of replacement therapy

   ix. Follow-up: If the patient is receiving digitalis and diuretics, consider the use of potassium chloride supplements or potassium-sparing diuretics

  e. Potential complications

     i. Digoxin toxicity

      (a) Mechanism: Hypokalemia enhances the effect of digoxin

      (b) Management: IV potassium on medication pump with cardiac monitoring

    ii. Dysrhythmias

      (a) Mechanism: Hypokalemia decreases the cardiac threshold, increasing the risk of dysrhythmia

      (b) Management: IV potassium on medication pump with cardiac monitoring

ELECTROLYTE IMBALANCES—SODIUM IMBALANCE: HYPERNATREMIA

The serum sodium level in hypernatremia is above 145 mEq/L

1. **Pathophysiology**

  a. Increased ECF volume: Sodium and water retention

  b. Decreased ECF volume: Sodium retention without water retention; greater water loss compared with sodium loss (e.g., diuresis of water without excretion of equal amounts of sodium)

2. **Etiology and risk factors**

  a. Normal kidneys: Lack of ADH or neurohypophyseal insufficiency (e.g., diabetes insipidus, water loss in excess of sodium loss)

     i. Potassium depletion: Creates a concentrating defect in the kidney, causing polyuria

    ii. Hypercalcemia: Polyuria and dehydration

   iii. Medications (e.g., osmotic diuretics or sodium bicarbonate, or NaCl solution); also mineralocorticoids, laxatives, and antacids

   iv. Excessive adrenocortical secretion

    v. Loss of the thirst mechanism (e.g., in a comatose patient)

   vi. Uncontrolled diabetes mellitus with osmotic diuresis because of hyperglycemia

   vii. Head injury

  viii. Postcentral nervous system surgery: Causes fluctuation (increase and decrease) in ADH release

    b. Impaired renal function: Inability of renal tubules to respond to ADH (e.g., nephrogenic diabetes insipidus)

3. **Signs and symptoms: Findings relate to "edematous states" and/or hypoproteinemia (Table 6.8)**

4. **Diagnostic study findings**
    a. Serum Na^+ level above 145 mEq/L, elevated hematocrit with volume depletion
    b. Serum osmolality greater than 295 mOsm/L
    c. Urine SG may be greater than 1.030, except in diabetes insipidus, in which SG can be as low as 1.005
    d. Urine osmolality 800 to 1400 mOsm/L; lower with diabetes insipidus
    e. Urine Na^+ level higher than 40 mEq/L when hypernatremia is caused by sodium excess and normal to low value during a water deficit

TABLE 6.8	**Signs and Symptoms of Sodium Imbalance**	
System	**Hypernatremia**	**Hyponatremia**
General	Excessive weight gain	Weight loss or gain
	Dehydration—extreme thirst, fever, decreased urine output, dry mucous membranes	Malaise Headache Gait disturbances in older adults
		Decreased hematocrit and blood urea nitrogen level (dilutional effect)
Cardiovascular	Weak, thready pulse with increased extracellular fluid (ECF) Tachycardia with decreased ECF often progressing to bradycardia	Rapid pulse with volume overload Hypotension or hypertension Decreased central venous pressure and jugular venous pressure with volume overload
	Hypertension with increased ECF	
	Hypotension with or without postural changes with decreased ECF	
Neurologic	Restlessness	Confusion to coma
	Irritability	Muscle weakness
	Lethargy	
	Confusion to coma	
	Twitching to seizures	
	Muscle tension	
Pulmonary	Labored breathing (dyspnea) associated with pulmonary edema	Dyspnea with crackles Pulmonary edema
Gastrointestinal	Anorexia	Abdominal cramps
	Edematous tongue	Nausea
Musculoskeletal	Muscle weakness	
Integumentary	Dry, flushed skin	Poor skin turgor
	Dry mucous membranes	
	Pitting edema	
Genitourinary	Oliguria or anuria with dehydration	Thirst
	Polyuria with osmotic diuresis	Normal urine output to polyuria
		Urine sodium level <20 mEq/L

From Slotki, I.N., Skorecki, K.L. (2016). Disorders of sodium balance. The pathophysiology of uremia. In B.M. Brenner (editor), *Brenner and Rector's the kidney*, 10th ed, Philadelphia, Elsevier.

5. Interprofessional collaboration: See Electrolyte Imbalances—Potassium Imbalance: Hyperkalemia
6. Management of patient care
   a. Anticipated patient trajectory: Patients with hypernatremia are experiencing a hyperosmolar state usually secondary to a serious previously existing condition. Both conditions need to be treated and resolved before discharge. Recovery and discharge require compliance with a treatment regimen that prevents repeat episodes.
7. **Goals of care**
   a. Serum and urine Na^+ levels are in a normal range or in a high, asymptomatic range
   b. Normal fluid status is maintained
8. **Patients may be expected to have needs in the following areas:**
   a. Positioning: Initiate fall prevention protocol if patient exhibits neurologic signs and symptoms
   b. Skin care
      i. Dehydration: Hydrate patient and lubricate skin
      ii. Volume overload: Protect bony prominences; change position often
   c. Nutrition: Dietary and fluid restrictions with restricted sodium; I&O
   d. Pharmacology: Medication adjustments
      i. Avoid laxatives and antacids (e.g., sodium bicarbonate) containing high-sodium ingredients
      ii. Use diuretics: Promote a greater loss of water than Na^+
      iii. Administer corticosteroids to stimulate reabsorption of Na^+ and excretion of K^+
   e. Treatments
      i. Monitor serum sodium levels, serum osmolality, urine osmolality, I&O, and body weight
      ii. Perform neurologic assessments and correlate with serum Na^+ levels
      iii. Administer water in excess of sodium if the patient requires volume expansion (5% dextrose in water or 0.45 normal saline or both)
      iv. Avoid rapid correction of sodium level, because this may precipitate acute pulmonary edema or cerebral edema; reduce sodium level gradually by encouraging Na^+ losses via diuretics or administration of fluids
      v. Determine precipitating factors and treat as ordered
      vi. For patients in renal failure, treat via dialysis
   f. Potential complications
      i. Dyspnea, labored respirations related to pulmonary edema
      ii. Seizures
         (a) Mechanism: Disruption of sodium pump dynamics in cerebral tissues, which leads to electrical instability
         (b) Management: Seizure precautions and correction of hypernatremia

ELECTROLYTE IMBALANCES—SODIUM IMBALANCE: HYPONATREMIA

The serum sodium level in hyponatremia is below 136 mEq/L
1. **Pathophysiology**
   a. Excess of water relative to the amount of sodium in the body, producing a dilutional effect on the sodium concentration
   b. Na^+ loss exceeds water loss
2. **Etiology and risk factors**
   a. Water excess: Excessive water intake without sodium intake; SIADH

b. Sodium depletion
   i. Abnormal losses via diaphoresis, diuretics, nasogastric suction, diarrhea
   ii. Hyperglycemia (glucose-induced diuresis)
   iii. Salt-losing renal diseases: Interstitial nephritis
   iv. Bartter syndrome (hyponatremia, hypokalemia, hypomagnesemia, metabolic alkalosis, and hyperreninemia)
c. Heart failure and cirrhosis of the liver: Decreased cardiac output increases water retention by the kidneys

3. **Signs and symptoms: Permanent neurologic changes with a serum sodium level below 110 mEq/L, monitor for gait disturbances in the older adult (see Table 6.8)**

4. **Diagnostic study findings**
   a. Serum Na^+ level below 136 mEq/L and low hematocrit caused by water excess
   b. Urine volume and SG can be normal
   c. Urine Na^+ level less than 20 mEq/L (if caused by Na^+ deficit) and normal to elevated (if caused by water excess)
   d. Serum osmolality below 280 mOsm/L

5. **Interprofessional collaboration: See Electrolyte Imbalances—Potassium Imbalance: Hyperkalemia**

6. **Management of patient care**
   a. Anticipated patient trajectory: Patients with hyponatremia experience a hypoosmolar condition. Recovery requires compliance with a treatment plan that prevents repeat episodes.

7. **Goals of care**
   a. Serum sodium level is WNL or at an asymptomatic level
   b. Normal fluid status is maintained

8. **Patients may be expected to have needs in the following areas:**
   a. Skin care: See Electrolyte Imbalances—Sodium Imbalance: Hypernatremia
   b. Nutrition and fluid balance
      i. For sodium and water losses: Provide high-sodium diet and adequate fluid intake
      ii. For water intoxication: Restrict fluid intake (limit of 500 mL/day)
      iii. For water intoxication related to SIADH: Restrict water intake, because decreased sodium is caused by the inability to excrete water normally
   c. Pharmacology
      i. Discontinue medications that cause loss of Na^+ (e.g., diuretics, laxatives)
      ii. Administer NaCl tablets orally as indicated
      iii. Administer diuretics to treat water intoxication
   d. Treatments
      i. Monitor neurologic signs
      ii. For Na^+ and water losses:
         (a) Replace fluids with normal (0.9%) or hypertonic (3%) saline
         (b) Administer hypertonic saline via an infusion pump; measure serum sodium levels frequently; observe for pulmonary edema; monitor I&O
         (c) Monitor effectiveness of nutrition and other therapies by measuring serum and urine sodium levels and osmolality concentrations
      iii. For water intoxication:
         (a) Restrict fluid intake
         (b) Monitor serum sodium levels to determine whether sodium replacement is indicated

(c) Do not give normal saline in SIADH; normal saline does not correct the basic cause of SIADH

    iv. Monitor for fall risk in the older adult

  e. Potential complications: See Electrolyte Imbalances—Sodium Imbalance: Hypernatremia

ELECTROLYTE IMBALANCES—CALCIUM IMBALANCE: HYPERCALCEMIA

The serum calcium level in hypercalcemia is above 10.5 mg/dL

1. **Pathophysiology**
   a. Increased mobilization of calcium from bone
   b. Increased intestinal reabsorption of calcium ion (Ca^{2+}): May occur with large dietary intake or excessive vitamin D supplementation, or in granulomatous disease (e.g., sarcoidosis)
   c. Altered renal tubular reabsorption of Ca^{2+}

2. **Etiology and risk factors**
   a. Primary hyperparathyroidism: Causes increased tubular reabsorption of Ca^{2+} and Ca^{2+} release from bone
   b. Metastatic carcinoma with "osteolytic lesions" that release calcium into plasma and multiple myeloma
   c. Prolonged bed rest: Causes calcium to be mobilized from the bones, teeth, and intestines
   d. Alkalosis: Increases calcium binding to protein; decreases serum calcium levels
   e. Thyrotoxicosis
   f. Excessive intake of vitamin D: Increases Ca^{2+} reabsorption from intestines
   g. Medications: Thiazide diuretic therapy inhibits Ca^{2+} excretion
   h. Renal tubular acidosis

3. **Signs and symptoms: Table 6.9**

4. **Diagnostic study findings**
   a. Laboratory
      i. Serum calcium level: Above 10.5 mg/dL
      ii. Other serum studies: Thyroid-stimulating hormone, PTH, PTH-related peptide, vitamin D levels
      iii. Sulkowitch's urine test for calcium
   b. Radiologic
      i. Nephrocalcinosis: Calcium deposits in renal parenchyma, renal calculi
      ii. Calcium deposits visible on bone films
   c. ECG: Shortening of the ST segment

5. **Interprofessional Collaboration: See Electrolyte Imbalances—Potassium Imbalance: Hyperkalemia**

6. **Management of patient care**
   a. Anticipated patient trajectory: Clinical course, recovery, and discharge planning for patients with hypercalcemia vary depending on whether the condition is acute or chronic.

7. **Goals of care**
   a. Calcium stays WNL or in an asymptomatic range
   b. Cardiac and neurologic function is normal

8. **Patients may be expected to have needs in the following areas:**
   a. Nutrition: Restrict dietary calcium (e.g., milk, cheese, yogurt)

TABLE 6.9	**Signs and Symptoms of Calcium Imbalance**	
System	**Hypercalcemia**	**Hypocalcemia**
Cardiovascular	Hypertension (33% of all cases)	Dysrhythmias
		Irregular pulse
Neurologic	Lethargy	Lethargy
	Increased fatigue	Generalized tonic-clonic seizures
	Confusion to coma	
	Subtle personality changes	
Pulmonary		Labored and shallow breathing
		Wheezing
		Bronchospasm when respiratory muscles involved
Gastrointestinal	Anorexia	Paralytic ileus with absent bowel sounds
	Nausea and vomiting	Constipation with or without distended abdomen or diarrhea
	Abdominal pain and constipation	
Renal	Acute or chronic renal failure	Oliguria or anuria
	Renal vascular constriction	
	Polyuria	
	Renal calcium deposits	
	Flank and thigh pain associated with renal calculi	
Musculoskeletal	Hypotonicity and weakness of muscles	Positive Chvostek's and Trousseau's sign
	Pathologic fractures	
	Metastatic calcifications	Functional and physical limitations on ambulation and exercise
	Bone pain	Bone pain and fractures

From Smorgorzewski, M.J., Stubbs, J.R., Yu, A.S.L. (2016). Disorders of calcium, magnesium, and phosphate balance. The pathophysiology of uremia. In B.M. Brenner (editor), *Brenner and Rector's the kidney*, 10th ed, Philadelphia, Elsevier.

    b. Discharge planning: Teach the patient how to comply with the dietary regimen to avoid hypercalcemia

    c. Pharmacology

       i. Administer digitalis cautiously; hypercalcemia enhances the action of digitalis and toxicity can result

       ii. Administer NaCl infusion and diuretics to reduce Ca^{2+} absorption

      iii. Be aware that corticosteroids reduce GI absorption of Ca^{2+}

      iv. Institute mithramycin therapy to stimulate bone uptake of calcium

      v. Consider the administration of bisphosphonates (e.g., pamidronate), calcitonin, or corticosteroids for the treatment of moderate to severe hypercalcemia associated with malignancy to reduce the rate of bone turnover

    d. Treatments

       i. Monitor I&O status and renal function parameters

      ii. If the patient is in renal failure, use dialysis

      iii. Administer bisphosphonates

e. Potential complications
  i. Cardiac arrest
    (a) Mechanism: Enhanced digoxin effect, dysrhythmias (particularly atrioventricular blocks) may progress to cardiac arrest
    (b) Management: Cardiopulmonary resuscitation

ELECTROLYTE IMBALANCES—CALCIUM IMBALANCE: HYPOCALCEMIA

The serum calcium level in hypocalcemia is below 8.5 mg/dL

1. **Pathophysiology**
   a. Excessive GI losses of calcium secondary to diarrhea, diuretic use, and increased levels of lipoproteins
   b. Malabsorption syndromes, such as vitamin D deficiency and hypoparathyroidism
2. **Etiology and risk factors**
   a. Hypoparathyroidism or hypomagnesemia (Mg^{2+} needed for effective action of PTH)
   b. CKD
     i. Hyperphosphatemia because of CKD: Potentiates the peripheral deposition of calcium
     ii. Vitamin D deficiency because of CKD, hepatic failure, rickets: Lack of activated vitamin D (1, 25-dihydroxycholecalciferol or 25 hydroxycholecalciferol) necessary for Ca^{2+} absorption
   c. Vitamin D resistance: Inability to absorb Ca^{2+} from the intestine; vitamin D mediated
   d. Chronic malabsorption syndrome resulting from magnesium depletion, gastrectomy, high-fat diet (fat impairs Ca^{2+} absorption), small bowel disorder that prevents absorption of vitamin D
   e. Increased thyrocalcitonin: Stimulates osteoblasts to prevent Ca^{2+} entry into serum
   f. Malignancy
     i. Osteoblastic metastasis: Calcium is consumed for abnormal bone synthesis
     ii. Medullary carcinoma of the thyroid: Secretion of thyrocalcitonin is abnormal
   g. Acute pancreatitis: Calcium precipitates in an inflamed pancreas
   h. Hyperphosphatemia: Calcium and phosphate bind together and precipitate in tissues
     i. Cytotoxic medications (cytolysis of bone)
     ii. Increased oral intake of phosphates
     iii. CKD (decreased excretion of phosphate)
3. **Signs and symptoms: See Table 6.9**
4. **Diagnostic study findings**
   a. Serum calcium level below 8.5 mg/dL
   b. ECG: Prolonged ST segment and QT interval
   c. Trousseau's sign:
     i. Apply a BP cuff to the upper arm and inflate
     ii. If carpopedal spasm occurs, the test result is positive
     iii. If no spasm appears in 3 minutes, the test result is negative
     iv. Remove the cuff and tell the patient to hyperventilate (30 times per minute)
     v. Respiratory alkalosis that develops can also produce a carpopedal spasm (a positive result if it occurs)
   d. Chvostek's sign: Tap on the supramandibular portion of the parotid gland; observe for twitches in the upper lip on the side tapped; muscle spasm indicates a positive test result

5. Interprofessional collaboration: See Electrolyte Imbalances—Potassium Imbalance: Hyperkalemia
6. Management of patient care
    a. Anticipated patient trajectory: Patients with hypocalcemia face a life-threatening condition requiring urgent pharmacologic intervention. Recovery and discharge focus on preventing repeat episodes.
7. Goals of care
    a. Serum calcium level is WNL, and the patient is asymptomatic
    b. There is no evidence of complications from hypocalcemia
8. Patients can be expected to have needs in the following areas:
    a. Nutrition
        i. Assess for a history of starvation, abuse of diet aids, or malabsorption
        ii. Administer a diet high in calcium
    b. Discharge planning
        i. Provide discharge teaching to promote dietary intake of calcium
        ii. Instruct on the warning signs of tetany or seizures
    c. Pharmacology
        i. Administer 10% calcium gluconate or calcium chloride slowly IV (1 mL/min) for emergency intervention; monitor for decreased cardiac output, enhanced digitalis effects, and dysrhythmias
        ii. Chronic hypocalcemia necessitates daily oral doses of calcium, usually administered in the range of 1.5 to 3 g/day
        iii. Administer correct vitamin D supplement (1,25-dihydroxycholecalciferol or 25-hydroxycholecalciferol) as ordered
        iv. With phosphate deficiency, replace phosphates before administering calcium; hyperphosphatemia usually accompanies hypocalcemia
    d. Treatments
        i. Monitor serum calcium and phosphate levels
        ii. Institute cardiac monitoring; monitor therapeutic effectiveness via Chvostek's and Trousseau's signs plus ECG
        iii. Implement seizure precautions; provide a quiet environment
        iv. Monitor respiratory function; bronchospasm may precipitate respiratory arrest
        v. In renal failure, use dialysis and activated vitamin D
    e. Potential complications
        i. Tetany, seizures
            (a) Seizure precautions
            (b) Calcium bolus at bedside
            (c) Treat cause of hypocalcemia; replace calcium

ELECTROLYTE IMBALANCES—PHOSPHATE IMBALANCE: HYPERPHOSPHATEMIA

The serum phosphate level in hyperphosphatemia is above 4.5 mg/dL
1. Pathophysiology
    a. Inability to excrete phosphate (HPO_4^-) via the kidney because of a decrease in GFR to one-tenth of normal or because of renal failure
    b. Excessive intake because of diet, or cathartic abuse or medications (cytotoxic agents)
2. Etiology and risk factors
    a. Acute or chronic renal failure (inability to excrete HPO_4^-)
    b. Hypoparathyroidism: PTH causes hypophosphatemia and lowers body phosphate levels

TABLE 6.10 Signs and Symptoms of Phosphate Imbalance

System	Hyperphosphatemia	Hypophosphatemia
General	Vague, like those of hypocalcemia	Fatigue
Neurologic	Seizures	Confusion and malaise
Musculosketal	Muscle cramping, joint pain, pruritus	Muscle weakness and wasting with or without impaired ambulation
Gastrointestinal		Lack of appetite, changes in weight
Pulmonary		Dyspnea
Cardiovascular		Tachycardia, hypotension
Renal		Decreased urine output

From Smorgorzewski, M.J., Stubbs, J.R., Yu, A.S.L. (2016). Disorders of calcium, magnesium, and phosphate balance. The pathophysiology of uremia. In B.M. Brenner (editor), *Brenner and Rector's the kidney*, 10th ed, Philadelphia, Elsevier.

   c. Cathartic abuse or use of phosphate-containing laxatives or enemas

   d. Use of cytotoxic agents for neoplasms: Serum phosphate level increases as a result of cytolysis

   e. Overadministration of IV or oral phosphates

3. **Signs and symptoms: Vague symptomatology similar to that of hypocalcemia (Table 6.10)**

4. **Diagnostic study findings**

   a. Laboratory: Serum phosphate level higher than 4.5 mg/dL

   b. ECG: Changes comparable with those seen in hypocalcemia

5. **Interprofessional collaboration: See Electrolyte Imbalances—Potassium Imbalance: Hyperkalemia**

6. **Management of patient care**

   a. Anticipated patient trajectory: Patients with hyperphosphatemia differ in clinical course depending on whether it is an acute or chronic problem. Recovery and discharge focus on preventing repeat episodes.

7. **Goals of care**

   a. Phosphate level stays WNL or within a safe asymptomatic range

   b. There are no episodes of tetany or seizures

8. **Patients may be expected to have needs in the following areas:**

   a. Nutrition: If hypocalcemia accompanies hyperphosphatemia, administer a diet high in calcium and low in phosphorus

   b. Discharge planning (a) Provide discharge teaching to promote dietary compliance to avoid hyperphosphatemia (e.g., adherence with use of HPO_4^- binders)

      i. Instruct on the warning signs of seizures

   c. Pharmacology

      i. Administer phosphate binders, which act on the intestines to limit phosphate absorption, thereby reducing the serum phosphate level (e.g., calcium carbonate)

      ii. Administer acetazolamide to increase urinary phosphate excretion via the normal kidney

      iii. Monitor serum phosphate and calcium levels to determine the effectiveness of therapy

   d. Treatment: Institute dialysis for rapid correction of hyperphosphatemia

   e. Potential complications: See Electrolyte Imbalances—Calcium Imbalance: Hypocalcemia

ELECTROLYTE IMBALANCES—PHOSPHATE IMBALANCE: HYPOPHOSPHATEMIA

The serum phosphate level in hypophosphatemia is below 3.0 mg/L

1. **Pathophysiology**
   a. Increased cell uptake to form sugar phosphates: Occurs during hyperventilation or glucose administration
   b. Decreased phosphate absorption from the bowel
   c. Renal phosphate wasting (loss of proximal tubular function): Seen in Fanconi syndrome and vitamin D-resistant rickets
2. **Etiology and risk factors**
   a. Inadequate phosphate intake (seen in chronic alcoholism)
   b. Chronic phosphate depletion: Occurs in osteomalacia and rickets
   c. Long-term hyperalimentation without adequate phosphate replacement; glucose phosphorylation uses phosphate and can lead to phosphate depletion if no replacement is available
   d. Hyperparathyroidism: Causes renal phosphaturia
   e. Malabsorption syndrome
   f. Abuse or overadministration of phosphate-binding gels
   g. Fanconi syndrome: Loss of phosphates in urine leading to osteomalacia (adults)
3. **Signs and symptoms: Vague presentation (see Table 6.10)**
4. **Diagnostic study findings**
   a. Laboratory
      i. Serum phosphate level below 3.0 mg/dL, low serum alkaline pyrophosphate level, and high serum pyrophosphate level
      ii. Hypercalcemia and hypophosphatemia: Indicators of acute phosphate depletion in hyperparathyroidism; PTH increases the serum calcium level by promoting the release of Ca^{2+} from bone and decreases serum phosphate level by promoting excretion of HPO_4^- into urine
   b. Radiologic: Skeletal abnormalities resembling osteomalacia (e.g., pseudofractures characterized by thickened periosteum and new bone formation over what appears to be an incomplete fracture)
5. **Interprofesssional collaboration: See Electrolyte Imbalances—Potassium Imbalance: Hyperkalemia**
6. **Management of patient care**
   a. Anticipated patient trajectory: Patients with hypophosphatemia differ in their clinical course depending on whether the condition is acute or chronic. The treatment regimen aims to prevent repeat episodes.
7. **Goals of care**
   a. Serum phosphate level is in an asymptomatic range
   b. No neuromuscular signs of hypophosphatemia are present
8. **Patients may have needs in the following areas:**
   a. Nutrition: If hypercalcemia accompanies hypophosphatemia, use a calcium-restricted diet
   b. Discharge planning
      i. Provide teaching to promote the proper use of phosphate binders
      ii. Instruct on the warning signs of seizures; numbness and tingling around the mouth can occur immediately before a seizure
   c. Treatments
      i. Treat the primary cause of hypophosphatemia
      ii. Monitor phosphate and calcium levels
      iii. Administer oral phosphate (potassium phosphate) or IV phosphorus

    iv. Dialysis is an option in renal failure for acute episodes and/or for maintenance once the imbalance is corrected

  d. Potential complications: See Electrolyte Imbalances—Calcium Imbalance: Hypocalcemia

ELECTROLYTE IMBALANCES—MAGNESIUM IMBALANCE: HYPERMAGNESEMIA

The serum magnesium level in hypermagnesemia is above 2.5 mEq/L

1. **Pathophysiology**
   a. Mg^{2+} regulates nerve and muscle tone by preventing their activation by Ca^{2+}. Elevated level of Mg^{2+} can lead to excessive relaxation of nerves and muscles, including the myocardium and respiratory muscles.
   b. Magnesium is required for more than 300 enzymes to work, including those involved in protein, fat, and carbohydrate metabolism. Elevated Mg^{2+} levels can disrupt numerous metabolic interactions.
2. **Etiology and risk factors**
   a. Renal failure: Decreases excretion of Mg^{2+}
   b. Adrenal insufficiency
   c. Excessive intake or administration of Mg^{2+}-containing antacid gels or laxatives
   d. Acidotic states (e.g., diabetic ketoacidosis)
3. **Signs and symptoms: Vague presentation (Table 6.11)**
4. **Diagnostic study findings**
   a. Laboratory: Serum magnesium level over 2.5 mEq/L
   b. ECG: Peaked T wave similar to that seen in hyperkalemia
5. **Interprofessional collaboration: See Electrolyte Imbalances—Potassium Imbalance: Hyperkalemia**
6. **Management of patient care**
   a. Anticipated patient trajectory: Patients with acute hypermagnesemia have a clinical course complicated by dramatic shifts in neurologic status. Emergent therapies are followed by preventive measures before discharge. Patients may have needs in the following areas:
      i. Nutrition: Eliminate or avoid magnesium-containing nutritional supplements (e.g., total parenteral nutrition, tube feeding, or oral protein drinks)
     ii. Discharge planning: Teach dietary and pharmacologic restrictions
    iii. Pharmacology
       (a) Teach the patient to avoid medications containing magnesium (e.g., laxatives, antacids)

TABLE 6.11	**Signs and Symptoms of Magnesium Imbalance**	
System	**Hypermagnesemia**	**Hypomagnesemia**
General	Lethargy to coma	Dizziness
Neurologic	Fatigue, muscle weakness with or without loss of deep tendon reflexes	Lethargy, confusion to psychosis, muscle weakness or tremors to tetany, seizures
Pulmonary	Decreased respiration to apnea	
Cardiovascular	Bradycardia, hypotension secondary to depressed myocardial contractility, may lead to cardiac arrest	Irregular pulse Dysrhythmias Enhanced digitalis effect Normal to decreased blood pressure

From Smorgorzewski, M.J., Stubbs, J.R., Yu, A.S.L. (2016). Disorders of calcium, magnesium, and phosphate balance. The pathophysiology of uremia. In B.M. Brenner (editor), *Brenner and Rector's the kidney*, 10th ed, Philadelphia, Elsevier.

   (b) If renal function is normal, administer diuretics or induce diuresis with saline to encourage magnesium loss
   (c) Consider calcium gluconate administration to minimize symptoms of increased magnesium
   iv. Treatments
   (a) Determine the primary cause of hypermagnesemia and intervene
   (b) Consider dialysis if excesses are caused by renal failure
   (c) Monitor ECG and neurologic signs
   (d) Monitor serum magnesium levels
   b. Potential complications: See Electrolyte Imbalances—Potassium Imbalance: Hyperkalemia

ELECTROLYTE IMBALANCES—MAGNESIUM IMBALANCE: HYPOMAGNESEMIA

The serum level in hypomagnesemia is below 1.5 mEq/L

1. **Pathophysiology**
   a. Decreased intake, diminished intestinal reabsorption, or excess losses of magnesium in urine, wounds, or extracellular drainage
   b. Diminishes ability to relax muscular and neural tone
   c. Disrupts numerous physiologic and metabolic enzyme reactions
2. **Etiology and risk factors**
   a. Starvation, malabsorption syndrome, hypocalcemia, prolonged hyperalimentation without adequate Mg^{2+} replacement; excessive fistula or GI losses of Mg^{2+} (e.g., severe diarrhea, nasogastric suction) without sufficient replacement
   b. Bartter syndrome
   c. Excessive diuretic therapy or excessive corticosteroid administration
   d. Chronic alcoholism
   e. Alkalotic states (in some instances)
   f. Hypocalcemia, hypoparathyroidism, hyperaldosteronism, hyperthyroidism
   g. Medications: Cisplatin, cyclosporine, amphotericin, gentamycin
   h. Acute or chronic pancreatitis
3. **Signs and symptoms: Vague presentation (see Table 6.11)**
4. **Diagnostic study findings**
   a. Laboratory: Serum magnesium levels below 1.5 mEq/L
   b. ECG: Flat or inverted T waves, possible ST segment depression, and prolonged QT interval
5. **Interprofessional collaboration: See Electrolyte Imbalances—Potassium Imbalance: Hyperkalemia**
6. **Management of patient care**
   a. Anticipated patient trajectory: Patients with acute hypomagnesemia can experience serious neuromuscular symptoms. Emergent therapies are followed by a preventive regimen.
7. **Goals of care**
   a. Serum magnesium level returns to normal
   b. There are no significant cardiac or neuromuscular symptoms
8. **Patients may be expected to have needs in the following areas:**
   a. Nutrition
      i. Provide magnesium-containing supplements (e.g., seafood, green vegetables, whole grains, nuts)
      ii. Observe for coexisting electrolyte imbalances (e.g., hypocalcemia)

b. Discharge planning
   i. Teach dietary measures to increase magnesium intake
   ii. Teach diuretic regimen
c. Pharmacology
   i. Administer magnesium sulfate intramuscularly or IV
   ii. Calcium gluconate may be given when replacing with large boluses of magnesium, because calcium retards the effects of a sudden reversal to hypermagnesemia
   iii. If hypokalemia occurs simultaneously with hypomagnesemia, correct the magnesium deficit first
   iv. Be aware that hypomagnesemia enhances digitalis toxicity
d. Treatments
   i. Establish seizure precautions
   ii. Correct alkalosis if present
   iii. Monitor ECG changes
   iv. Monitor serum magnesium levels
e. Potential complications: See Electrolyte Imbalances—Potassium Imbalance: Hypokalemia

RHABDOMYOLYSIS

1. **Pathophysiology**
   a. Injury of the skeletal muscle results in release of intracellular components into the circulation
   b. High concentrations of muscle cell contents including potassium, calcium, creatine kinase (CK), and myoglobin are absorbed into the bloodstream
   c. High levels of myoglobin result in nephrotoxicity. Proposed mechanisms include tubular obstruction, oxidant injury, and vasoconstriction.
2. **Etiology and risk factors**
   a. Anything that causes muscle damage can lead to rhabdomyolysis
   b. Most common causes are medication and alcohol abuse, medications (e.g., statins, certain psychiatric agents), trauma, and immobility
3. **Signs and symptoms**
   a. Classic triad of myalgia, weakness, and reddish-brown (or tea-colored) urine; however, only reported in less than 10% of cases.
   b. Urine myoglobin concentrations greater than 100 mg/dL lead to staining of urine.
   c. More than 50% of patients do not complain of muscle pain or weakness.
   d. May present with tachycardia, malaise, fever, nausea and vomiting
   e. Signs and symptoms of AKI may appear as syndrome progresses.
4. **Diagnostic study findings**
   a. Laboratory testing
      i. Plasma CK—no standard value, but 5× reference range is commonly accepted; more than 5000 is associated with increased risk for kidney injury
      ii. Serum and urine myoglobin levels are not useful in diagnosis because of short half-life and lack of sensitivity
      iii. Additional testing is needed to determine the cause and potential complications
         (a) Electrolyte imbalances are common; early hypocalcemia progressing to hypercalcemia, hypokalemia, hyperkalemia, hypophosphatemia
         (b) Blood alcohol levels, urine medication screen may provide clues to etiology

      (c) Coagulation profile may show evidence of disseminated intravascular coagulation

    b. ECG: May show P-R prolongation, peaked T waves, widened QRS complex in setting of hyperkalemia

5. **Interprofessional collaboration: See Electrolyte Imbalances—Potassium Imbalance: Hyperkalemia**

6. **Management of care**
    a. Anticipated patient trajectory: Outcomes vary depending on the patient population, severity, and complications with mortality ranging from 1.6% to 46%. Outcomes are generally worse for patients who develop AKI (33% of patients).

7. **Goals of care**
    a. Prevent or correct AKI
      i. Aggressive IV fluid therapy; no specific rate shown to be superior, generally 2 to 5 mL/kg/h is a reasonable goal
      ii. Target UOP 200 to 300 mL/h
      iii. Diuresis with azetazolamide 5 mg/kg and/or mannitol 0.5 g/kg bolus then 0.1 g/kg/h may be helpful in patients with inadequate UOP despite adequate volume resuscitation
      iv. CRRT needed in anuric patients
    b. Alkalinization of urine
      i. Common intervention despite lack of clear evidence
      ii. Administration of sodium bicarbonate infusion in urine pH over 7
    c. Correct and/or maintain electrolyte imbalances

END-STAGE RENAL CONDITION: RENAL TRANSPLANT

1. **Renal transplantation: Promotes primary disease management by minimizing complications, slowing the progression of the primary disease process, and decreasing the mortality rate (Fig. 6.5)**

KEY CONCEPT
Renal transplantation is the definitive treatment for CKD. Posttransplant, patients will need to be on antirejection medication for life. Nurses should monitor for signs of rejection including a flu-like prodrome and signs and symptoms of renal failure.

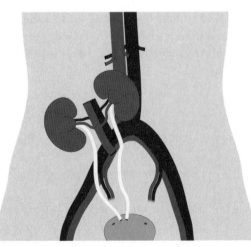

Fig. 6.5 Kidney transplantation. (From Mahendran, A.O., Barlow, A.D. (2013). Kidney transplantation. *Surgery*, 32(7), 364–70.)

2. **Grafts: Survival rates have improved**
   a. Living donor transplants have a longer survival rate than cadaveric transplants
   b. One-year rates are 98% for living grafts and 89% for cadaveric grafts
3. **Donors: Wait time for cadaveric donation is about 24 months. Living donors must have ABO blood type compatibility, maximal compatibility in human leukocyte antigen (HLA) type, acceptable serologic cross-match, and optimal health. Intraperitoneal laparoscopic surgery, a minimally invasive procedure, is a common option for living donors.**
4. **Recipient selection criteria: Begins with the presence of irreversible ESRD; few contraindications exist**
   a. Age no longer a definitive barrier; most programs use 70 years as the upper limit but consider physiologic and individual differences in the decision-making process
   b. No preexisting antibodies (to donor kidney) and/or ABO blood type incompatibility
   c. No preexisting infection
   d. No medical or surgical contraindications
   e. Functioning bladder or urinary tract
   f. No psychosis, severe personality disorder, or history of nonadherence with medical regimen
   g. "Last resort" alternative: Patient may be accepted based on the inability to participate in other treatment alternatives; this may be caused by lack of vascular access or physical intolerance of the procedure
5. **Tissue type compatibility**
   a. ABO blood typing: To determine blood type compatibility between donor and recipient
   b. HLA typing: Serologic testing for specification of the HLA-A, HLA-B, and HLA-C locus antigen plus lymphocyte-defined typing of the D locus (includes DP, DQ, and DR antigens)
   c. Mixed lymphocyte culture: Reveals degree of difference between the D loci of donor and recipient
   d. Cross-match for preformed antibody (microlymphocytotoxicity cross-match): Presence of preformed antibodies significantly decreases the viability of any graft
6. **Immunocompetent cells: Two kinds of lymphocytes involved in the rejection processes**
   a. B lymphocytes: Involved in humoral immunity and are precursors to antibody-producing cells; responsible for hyperacute rejection and partially involved in acute and chronic rejection
   b. T lymphocytes: Implicated in cell-mediated immunity, which is involved in acute and chronic rejection; three types—effectors, helpers, and suppressors
7. **Types of rejection**
   a. Hyperacute: Irreversible process; occurs within minutes or hours of surgery
   b. Accelerated: Occurs from the second to fifth day in the immediate postoperative period; physiologic characteristics are similar to those of hyperacute rejection; rarely reversible, involving both humoral and cellular immunity
   c. Acute: Often reversible with high doses of antirejection medication
      i. Occurs most frequently 2 weeks after transplantation but can be seen from the first week postoperatively up to 1 year and beyond
      ii. T cells or cellular immunity is the primary mechanism
      iii. Antigen leaves the graft and enters the serum, where it is recognized and incorporated into macrophage RNA. With reexposure to antigen, the macrophage releases RNA-antigen complexes into the serum, where plasma

lymphocytes manufacture specific antibody. The plasma lymphocytes then travel to the kidney for the immunologic attack.

    d. Chronic: Cannot be reversed; a gradual decline that ultimately leads to organ failure
       i. Usually occurs 1 to 5 years after transplantation
      ii. Involves B-cell or humoral response to antibody
     iii. A slow, chronic immunologic response with gradual deterioration of renal tissue; involves primarily the glomerular basement membrane and endothelial layer of the blood vessels

8. Instruct the patient and family about transplantation as a treatment alternative, including the following:
    a. Survival rates; patient selection criteria; treatment expectations (e.g., antirejection medications); need for frequent clinic visits the first year; and dietary limitations
    b. Benefits: Replacement of renal function, alleviation of most pathophysiologic effects of uremia, and return to many normal life activities
    c. Complications, including rejection; immunosuppressive effects (increased susceptibility to infections, risk of malignancies, esophagitis, peptic ulcer, acute pancreatitis); and surgical complications

9. Provide preoperative teaching
    a. Need to report to the hospital on request
    b. Expected preoperative workup
    c. Surgical procedure
       i. The kidney is transplanted into the iliac fossa
      ii. Revascularization is usually accomplished by anastomosing the renal artery to the hypogastric artery and the renal vein to the external iliac vein (see Fig. 6.5)
     iii. The ureter is anastomosed to the recipient's ureter at the pelvis of the kidney (ureteropelvic anastomosis), or the donor's ureter can be implanted into the host's bladder (ureteroneocystostomy)
    d. Immediate postoperative recovery period care

10. Provide postoperative teaching
    a. How to obtain and record daily I&O, temperature, BP, and weight
    b. Antirejection medication and side effects
    c. Need to report signs and symptoms of rejection
       i. Fever
      ii. Pain, tenderness, redness, and swelling at the site of the graft
     iii. Weight gain
     iv. Decreased urine output
      v. Hypertension
    d. Activity limitations in the first 3 months: Avoidance of lifting or strenuous exercise, avoidance of crowds
    e. Need to report signs and symptoms of infection
    f. Knowledge of diet
    g. Schedule of clinic visits

11. Administer maintenance transplant immunosuppressive therapy as ordered. A single standard of practice for immunosuppressive therapy has not been agreed upon; various combinations of the following medications may be given:
    a. Corticosteroids: Suppress the production of cytotoxic T cells and prevent the production of interleukin-2 (IL-2), which initiates the immunologic response; no agreement on the optimal dosage; begin with a high dosage and taper over the initial few weeks

b. Azathioprine: Begin dosing at 3 to 5 mg/kg/day and decrease gradually to 1 to 3 mg/kg/day to prevent or deter acute rejection episodes

c. Cyclosporine: To inhibit activated T-cell proliferation and IL-2 production; maintenance dosage 3 to 5 mg/kg/day to be continued for the life of the graft

d. Tacrolimus (similar to cyclosporine): A macrolide antibiotic with immunosuppressive effect; inhibits T-cell receptor signals and IL-2; appears to improve long-term graft survival rate; administer 0.15 mg/day in divided doses

e. Mycophenolate mofetil (MMF): An antimetabolite agent that assists as an intervention for acute rejection; a 50% reduction in acute rejection seen in first year with its use

f. Sirolimus: A macrolide antibiotic; blocks T-cell activation at a phase beyond tacrolimus

g. Cyclophosphamide: Used when azathioprine is contraindicated to diminish the production of antibodies and initiate the destruction of circulating lymphocytes

12. **Administer antirejection therapy for treatment of acute or accelerated rejection**

a. Corticosteroids: IV 500 to 1000 mg/day for a maximum of 5 days, followed by oral corticosteroids

b. Antilymphocyte globulin: To deplete circulating T cells and suppress cell-mediated immunity allograft responses; toxicity includes agranulocytosis and hemolytic response and predisposition to infection

c. OKT3: A murine monoclonal antibody administered over 14 days to suppress or inactivate one or two antigen-recognition sites on T cells (T2 or T3); side effects include respiratory distress, fever, and severe immunosuppression

13. **Ethical issues**

a. Living organ donation: A disparity continues to exist between the number of patients waiting for transplantation and the number of available organs

b. Donor mortality rate is about 0.03%; rate of serious donor morbidity is 0.23%

References and bibliography information are available at http://evolve.elsevier.com/AACN/ corecurriculum/.

Endocrine System

Jennifer MacDermott, MS, RN, ACNS-BC, NP-C, CCRN

SYSTEMWIDE ELEMENTS

ANATOMY AND PHYSIOLOGY REVIEW

1. **Definition of a hormone**
   a. Hormones are chemical messengers that are synthesized and secreted by specialized cells and released into the blood, exerting biochemical effects on target cells away from the site of origin
   b. Hormones control metabolism, transport of substances across cell membranes, fluid and electrolyte balance, growth and development, adaptation, and reproduction
2. **Hormones are chemically categorized by physiologic action:**
   a. Peptide or protein hormones: Growth hormone (GH), follicle-stimulating hormone (FSH), luteinizing hormone (LH), adrenocorticotropin hormone (ACTH), calcitonin, glucagon, insulin, oxytocin, somatostatins, thyroid stimulating hormone (TSH), thyrotropin-releasing hormone (TRH)
   b. Steroids: Glucocorticoids, mineralocorticoids, androgens, estrogens, progestins
   c. Catecholamines: Epinephrine, norepinephrine, dopamine
   d. Iodothyronines: Triiodothyronine (T_3), tetraiodothyronine (T_4)
3. **Hormone circulation**
   a. Hormones circulating freely in blood
      i. Responsible for regulation of body metabolism
      ii. Catecholamines, most peptide hormones

  b. Hormones circulating with binding proteins
    i. Provide blood with reservoir of hormone, minimizing abrupt changes in concentrations and increase the half-life of the circulating hormone
    ii. Thyroxine (T_4), triidothyronine (T_3), steroid hormones, GH
4. **Hormone receptors**
  a. Specificity of hormone action is determined by the presence of a specific hormone receptor on or in the target cell
    i. Peptide or protein hormones and catecholamines react with receptors on the cell surface called transmembrane receptors
    ii. Steroid hormones and iodothyronines react with receptors inside the cell referred to as intracellular receptors
  b. Receptors distinguish hormones from each other and translate the hormonal signal into a cellular response
  c. The hormone-receptor complex initiates intracellular events that lead to the biologic effects of the hormone acting on the target cell
5. **Feedback control of hormone production**
  a. Feedback control can be positive (low levels of hormone stimulate the release of its controlling hormone) or negative (high levels of hormone inhibit the release of its controlling hormone)
  b. Feedback control systems allow self-regulation and prevent hormonal overproduction

HYPOTHALAMUS

1. **Location: Base of the forebrain (Fig. 7.1)**
2. **Composition**
  a. Preoptic area: Manufactures gonadotropin-releasing hormone
  b. Lateral, medial, and periventricular zones: Role in feeding, circadian rhythms, maintenance of body temperature, satiety, memory, synthesis of many releasing hormones affecting anterior pituitary
3. **Hormones**
  a. Control secretion of anterior pituitary hormones
  b. Hypothalamic releasing hormones: TRH, corticotropin-releasing hormone (CRH), GH-releasing hormone
  c. Hypothalamic inhibiting hormones: GH inhibitory hormone, gonadotropin-releasing hormone, dopamine or prolactic-inhibiting factor

PITUITARY GLAND (ALSO CALLED HYPOPHYSIS)

1. **Location: Base of forebrain within depression of sphenoid bone; connected to hypothalamus by the pituitary stalk (made up of the infundibulum and pars tuberalis), which links nervous and endocrine systems**
2. **Composition**
  a. Adenohypophysis (anterior pituitary): Hormones controlled by hypothalamic releasing or inhibiting hormones in response to stimuli received in the central nervous system
  b. Neurohypophysis: pars nervosa (posterior pituitary), infundibulus, and pars tuberalis
    i. Hormones controlled by nerve fibers originating in hypothalamus and terminating in posterior pituitary gland
    ii. Hormones synthesized in hypothalamus, stored in posterior pituitary, and released after activation of cell bodies in nerve tract

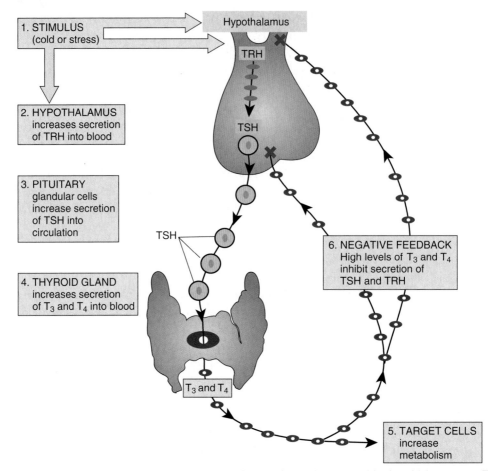

Fig. 7.1 Hypothalamus-pituitary-thyroid gland feedback mechanism with thyroid hormone. T_3, Triiodothyronine; T_4, tetraiodothyronine; *TRH*, thyrotropin-releasing hormone; *TSH*, thyroid stimulating hormone. (From Hubert, R.J., VanMeter, K.C. (2018). *Gould's pathophysiology for the health professions*, ed 6. St. Louis, Elsevier.)

3. **Anterior pituitary hormones**
   a. GH (also called somatotropin)
      i. Primary target cells: liver, muscle, and adipose tissue
      ii. Regulation of secretion
         (a) Stimulation: Growth-releasing hormone (GRH) in response to physical and/or emotional stress, exercise, starvation, hypoglycemia, aging, other protein-depleted states
         (b) Inhibition: Somatostatin, hyperglycemia, obesity, and excess glucocorticoid production, pharmacologic doses of corticosteroids
      iii. Physiologic activity
         (a) Adipose tissue: Decreases glucose uptake and increases lipolysis resulting in decreased adiposity
         (b) Liver: Increases protein synthesis and gluconeogenesis
         (c) Muscle: Decreases glucose uptake, increases amino acid uptake and protein synthesis resulting in increased lean body mass
         (d) Bone: Increases protein synthesis, cell size, and cell number resulting in bone and cartilage growth
         (e) Heart, lung, kidney, pancreas, intestine, skin, connective tissue: Increases protein synthesis, cell size, and cell number resulting in organ growth

(f) Works with insulin, thyroid hormones, cortisol, and sex steroids to promote growth

iv. Disorders resulting from dysfunction

(a) Excess: Gigantism (prepubertal), acromegaly (postpubertal)

(b) Deficiency: Dwarfism (prepubertal)

b. Adrenocorticotropic hormone (ACTH) or corticotropin

   i. Primary target cells: adrenal cortex

   ii. Regulation of secretion

(a) Stimulation: CRH in response to physical or emotional stress, trauma, hypoglycemia, hypoxia, surgery, decreased plasma cortisol levels

(b) Inhibition: Increased plasma cortisol levels exert negative feedback on CRH and thus ACTH

   iii. Physiologic activity

(a) Increases cortisol and adrenal androgen production

(b) Promotes growth of adrenal cortex

   iv. Disorders resulting from dysfunction

(a) Excess: Cushing disease

(b) Deficiency: Adrenal insufficiency (chronic), adrenal crisis (acute)

c. TSH

   i. Primary target cells: thyroid epithelial cells

   ii. Regulation of secretion

(a) Stimulation: TRH in response to low concentration of thyroid hormones

(b) Inhibition: Somatostatin, increased thyroid hormone levels

   iii. Physiologic activity

(a) Increases synthesis and releases stored thyroid hormones

(b) Stimulates iodide uptake into thyroid cells

(c) Increases size, number, and secretory activities of thyroid cells

   iv. Disorders resulting from dysfunction: See Thyroid Gland

d. Other anterior pituitary hormones under hypothalamic control

   i. LH

   ii. FSH

   iii. Prolactin

4. **Posterior pituitary hormones**

a. Antidiuretic hormone (ADH) or vasopressin

   i. Primary target cells: Cells lining the distal renal tubule and principal cells of collecting ducts in kidney

   ii. Regulation of secretion

(a) Stimulation: Increase in plasma osmolality, reduction in blood volume or blood pressure, certain medications (barbiturates, nicotine, opiates), nausea

(b) Inhibition: Decrease in plasma osmolality, cortisol, atrial natriuretic peptide (ANP), alcohol

   iii. Physiologic activity

(a) Increases water and urea permeability in the renal tubule and collecting duct, thereby controlling extracellular fluid osmolality

(b) Release of ADH results in a reduction in urine (antidiuresis) and increased in urine osmolality

(c) Absence of ADH causes urine to increase (diuresis) and reduced urine osmolality

(d) In pharmacologic amounts, constricts arterioles to increase blood pressure

      iv. Disorders resulting from dysfunction
- (a) Excess: Syndrome of inappropriate ADH (SIADH)
- (b) Deficiency: Diabetes insipidus

  b. Oxytocin

THYROID GLAND

1. **Location: Midportion of neck, below cricoid cartilage and anterior to larynx and trachea**
2. **Composition: Two lobes connected by a midventral isthmus**
   a. Follicular cells: Secrete T_3 and T_4; T_4 converted in periphery to T_3
   b. Parafollicular cells (C cells): Secrete calcitonin
3. **T_3 and T_4**
   a. Regulation of secretion
      i. Stimulation: TSH in the anterior pituitary stimulates thyroid hormone release, which is regulated by TRH from the hypothalamus; decreased levels of thyroid hormones stimulate the release of TSH and TRH
      ii. Inhibition: Elevated levels of thyroid hormones inhibit TSH and TRH; somatostatin
   b. Physiologic activity
      i. Increases metabolic activity of cells, which results in increased oxygen consumption, increased rate of chemical reactions, and heat production
      ii. Stimulates carbohydrate, fat, and protein metabolism. Works with insulin, GH, and sex steroids to promote growth.
      iii. Positive chronotropic and inotropic effects, increases stroke volume, increases cardiac output, decreases peripheral vascular resistance
      iv. Increases respiratory rate and minute ventilation in response to hypercapnia and hypoxia; stimulates oxygen use and enhances oxygen supply
      v. Increases erythropoiesis, renal tubular sodium reabsorption, renal plasma flow, and glomerular filtration rate
      vi. Enhances alertness, responsiveness to stimuli, hunger awareness, and learning ability
      vii. Increases speed and amplitude of nerve reflexes
      viii. Increases metabolism and clearance of steroid hormone and insulin
      ix. Critical for fetal neural and skeletal system development
   c. Disorders resulting from dysfunction
      i. Excess: Hyperthyroidism (chronic), thyroid storm (acute)
      ii. Deficiency: Hypothyroidism (chronic), myxedema coma (acute), euthyroid "sick" syndrome (acute)
4. **Calcitonin**
   a. Regulation of secretion
      i. Stimulation: Increase in calcium levels
      ii. Inhibition: Decrease in calcium levels
   b. Physiologic activity
      i. Decreases blood calcium levels by inhibiting calcium mobilization from bone and decreasing calcium resorption in the kidney
      ii. Decreases phosphate levels by inhibiting bone remodeling and by increasing phosphate loss in urine

PARATHYROID GLANDS

1. **Location: Four glands on posterior surface of thyroid gland**
2. **Composition: Chief (or principal) cells secrete parathyroid hormone (PTH)**

3. **Regulation of secretion**
   a. Stimulation: Decrease in serum calcium
   b. Inhibition: Increase in serum calcium and vitamin D metabolites, elevated serum magnesium levels
4. **Physiologic activity**
   a. Kidney
      i. Increases distal nephron reabsorption of calcium
      ii. Decreases proximal tubular reabsorption of phosphate
      iii. Stimulates production of fat-soluble form of vitamin D
   b. Gastrointestinal (GI) tract: Increases calcium (indirectly through vitamin D)
   c. Bone: Increases calcium and phosphate resorption (chronic PTH elevation) and increases bone synthesis (indirectly through vitamin D)
5. **Disorders resulting from dysfunction**
   a. Excess: Hyperparathyroidism
   b. Deficiency: Hypoparathyroidism

ADRENAL GLANDS
1. **Location: Retroperitoneal, superior to each kidney**
2. **Composition: Two endocrine tissues (epithelial and neuronal) that produce distinct hormones**
   a. Cortex: Secretes glucocorticoids, mineralocorticoids, adrenal androgenic steroids
   b. Medulla: Secretes catecholamines epinephrine and norepinephrine
3. **Cortical hormones**
   a. Glucocorticoids (cortisol is major hormone)
      i. Regulation of secretion
         (a) Stimulation: ACTH in anterior pituitary stimulates cortisol release, which is regulated by CRH from hypothalamus
         (b) Inhibition: Cortisol exerts negative feedback on anterior pituitary and hypothalamus
      ii. Physiologic activity
         (a) Increases gluconeogenesis through carbohydrate and protein metabolism
         (b) Decreases glucose uptake in muscle and adipose tissue (insulin-antagonistic effect)
         (c) Decreases protein stores and synthesis in all cells except liver cells
         (d) Increases protein catabolism and promotes lipolysis
         (e) Stimulates erythropoietin synthesis
         (f) Increases tissue responsiveness to other hormones, such as glucagon and the catecholamines
         (g) Antiinflammatory effects
            (1) Decreases production of proinflammatory cytokines
            (2) Stimulates production of antiinflammatory cytokines
            (3) Decreases migration of inflammatory cells to sites of injury
            (4) Prevention of immune response to tissue antigens released by injury
         (h) Increases abdominal and visceral adiposity
         (i) Increases bone resorption, reduced intestinal and calcium absorption and resorption, and inhibits osteoblast function
         (j) Inhibits fibroblast proliferation and collagen formation
         (k) Inhibits ADH secretion and action
         (l) Stimulates appetite

      iii. Disorders resulting from dysfunction

         (a) Excess: Cushing syndrome

         (b) Deficiency: Adrenocortical insufficiency (Addison disease), adrenal crisis (acute)

            (1) Critical illness-related corticosteroid insufficiency may occur in prolonged critical illness and septic shock

   b. Mineralocorticoids (aldosterone is major hormone)

      i. Primary target cells: kidney, colon, salivary glands, sweat glands, and heart muscle

      ii. Regulation of secretion

         (a) Stimulation: Renin-angiotensin system, hyponatremia, elevated ACTH, hyperkalemia, angiotensin II

         (b) Inhibition: Hypokalemia and increased plasma volume or increased ANP

      iii. Physiologic activity

         (a) Increases sodium (Na^+) reabsorption in the distal nephron and colon, indirectly increasing extracellular fluid volume

         (b) Increases potassium and hydrogen excretion

         (c) Increases inflammation and fibrotic effects on cardiovascular system

      iv. Disorders resulting from dysfunction

         (a) Excess: Primary aldosteronism, characterized by potassium depletion, extracellular fluid volume expansion, and nephrosclerotic hypertension

         (b) Deficiency: Adrenocortical insufficiency or Addison disease (chronic), adrenal crisis (acute)

4. Medullary hormones: Epinephrine (or adrenaline), norepinephrine, dopamine

   a. Primary target cells: Vascular smooth muscle (α_1), pancreatic β cells (α_2), heart (β_1), liver (β_2), and adipose (β_3)

   b. Regulation of secretion: Stimulated by fear, anxiety, pain, trauma, exercise, fluid loss, hemorrhage, extremes in temperature, surgery, hypoxia, hypoglycemia, hypokalemia, hypernatremia, hypotension

   c. Physiologic activity

      i. Fight-or-flight (stress) response: Increases heart rate and myocardial contractility, resulting in an increase in cardiac output, stimulation of fuel stores from muscle and fat, piloerection, dilation of pupils, and increased bowel and bladder sphincter tone

      ii. Relaxes bronchial smooth muscle (epinephrine)

      iii. Activates lipolysis in adipose tissue and increases ketogenesis in liver

      iv. Increases serum glucose through glucogenolysis and gluconeogenesis

      v. Decreases visceral smooth muscle energy demand

      vi. Decreases GI and urinary tract smooth muscle motility

   d. Disorders resulting from dysfunction

      i. Excess: Pheochromocytoma (epinephrine and norepinephrine)

      ii. Deficiency: Persons with an intact sympathetic nervous system manifest no clinically significant disability

PANCREAS

1. Location: Lies transversely behind the peritoneum and stomach

2. Composition

   a. Endocrine cells within the islets of Langerhans

      i. alpha (α): Secretes glucagon

      ii. beta (β): Secretes insulin, proinsulin, C peptide, and amylin

      iii. delta (δ): Produces somatostatin

      iv. F cells: Secrete pancreatic polypeptide

3. **Glucagon**
   a. Regulation of secretion
      i. Stimulation: Hypoglycemia, catecholamines, serum amino acids, GI hormones, and glucocorticoids
      ii. Inhibition: Hyperglycemia, somatostatin, and carbohydrate-only meal (stimulates insulin secretion and inhibits glucagon secretion)
   b. Physiologic activity
      i. Increases blood glucose via increased hepatic glycogenolysis and gluconeogenesis and reduced glycolysis and glycogen synthesis
      ii. Stimulation of ketogenesis
      iii. Is a major insulin-antagonistic hormone
4. **Insulin**
   a. Regulation of secretion
      i. Stimulation: Increases in blood glucose, gastrin, secretin, cholecystokinin, and GI hormone levels; β-adrenergic stimulation
      ii. Inhibition: α-adrenergic receptors activated by epinephrine and norepinephrine, catecholamines, fasting, exercise, and medications (including diazoxide, phenytoin, and vinblastine)
   b. Physiologic activity
      i. Maintains blood glucose and free fatty acid levels through:
         (a) Increasing glucose uptake and metabolism and glycogen storage in the skeletal muscle
         (b) Increasing glucose uptake and metabolism and triglyceride synthesis and storage in the adipocytes
         (c) Increasing glucose metabolism, glycogen storage, triglyceride synthesis and storage, and suppressing glucose output in the liver
         (d) Suppressing lipolysis of triglycerides in adipose tissue
         (e) Suppressing very-low-density lipoprotein (VLDL) production in liver
   c. Disorders resulting from dysfunction
      i. Excess: Hypoglycemia
      ii. Deficiency: Type 1 diabetes mellitus, type 2 diabetes mellitus, stress-induced hyperglycemia
5. **Somatostatin**
   a. Present in islet cells, hypothalamus, and GI tract
   b. Physiologic activity: Inhibits secretion of insulin, glucagon, GH, TSH, gastrin, and vasoactive intestinal peptide (VIP)

PINEAL GLAND AND THYMUS GLAND
1. **Typically, does not require critical care intervention**

GONADAL HORMONES (TESTOSTERONE, ESTROGEN, PROGESTERONE)
1. **Typically, does not require critical care intervention**

ASSESSMENT
1. **History**
   a. Patient health history
      i. Presence of pathophysiologic processes that can result in endocrine dysfunction
         (a) Trauma
         (b) Infection, inflammation, thrombotic or autoimmune processes

      (c) Neoplasms and exposure to the chemotherapeutic agents and radiotherapy used to treat the neoplasms

      (d) Infiltrative disorders

      (e) Seizure disorders

      (f) Vascular disorders

      (g) Cardiac disease

      (h) Pulmonary disease

      (i) Renal disease, chronic renal failure

      (j) Chronic liver failure

      (k) Malnutrition

    ii. Pregnancy, postpartum state

    iii. Presence of preexisting chronic endocrine disorder

    iv. Poor compliance with pharmacologic therapy for endocrine disorder

    v. Presence of unrelated critical illness in patient with chronic endocrine disorder

    vi. Presence of prolonged critical illness, sepsis, or other shock disorder

    vii. Positive family history of endocrine disorder

    viii. Use of systemic steroids

    ix. Indicators of altered health patterns (Box 7.1)

  b. Surgical history

BOX 7.1 Indicators of Altered Health Patterns in the Assessment of Endocrine Disorders

COGNITION AND PERCEPTION
- Personality changes
- Lethargy
- Emotional lability
- Attention span deficit
- Memory impairment
- Visual disturbances
- Changes in level of consciousness
- Depression, paranoia, delusions, delirium

NUTRITION AND METABOLISM
- Change in weight (increase or decrease)
- Nausea, anorexia, vomiting
- Polydipsia
- Heat or cold intolerance
- Edema
- Change in hair texture, distribution of hair loss

ELIMINATION
- Diarrhea or constipation
- Polyuria, anuria, oliguria, nocturia
- Excessive perspiration

ACTIVITY AND EXERCISE
- Fatigue
- Weakness
- Impairment in performance of activities of daily living

SLEEP AND REST
- Restlessness
- Inadequate sleep

Continued

BOX 7.1 Indicators of Altered Health Patterns in the Assessment of Endocrine Disorders—cont'd

SEXUAL FUNCTION
- Menstrual irregularities
- Impotence
- Decreased libido
- Infertility

ROLES AND RELATIONSHIPS
- Discord in previously stable relationships
- Physical and emotional inability to engage in usual role activity

COPING AND STRESS TOLERANCE
- Inability to cope
- History of past or present psychiatric disorder

HEALTH PERCEPTION AND MANAGEMENT
- Evidence of noncompliance with prescribed medical regimen

From Ball, J., Dains, J., Flynn, J., et al. (2015). *Seidel's guide to physical examination*, ed 8. St. Louis, Elsevier; Williams, L. (2015). *Understanding medical surgical nursing*, ed 5. Philadelphia, F.A. Davis Company.

   c. Family history: Endocrine disorders in other family members

   d. Social history

      i. Older adults may be at special risk for the development of an endocrine crisis because of changes associated with aging and a diminished thirst mechanism (see Ch. 16, Older Adult Patients)

     ii. Economically disadvantaged persons may be at risk for development of an endocrine crisis because many of the regimens for treating chronic endocrine disorders are costly and necessitate regular medical follow-up

    iii. Teenagers with poor compliance with prescribed medical regimen, particularly diabetic patients, are at increased risk of crisis

   e. Medication history

      i. Use of pharmacologic agents to treat chronic endocrine disorders

     ii. Use of pharmacologic agents that may stimulate or inhibit hormone release, or interfere with hormone action at target tissue

    iii. Exposure to radiographic contrast dyes

2. Physical examination

   a. Physical examination data

      i. Inspection

        (a) Altered level of consciousness, disorientation, irritability, paranoia

        (b) Excessive or diminutive stature

        (c) Fat distribution in relation to gender and maturational level

        (d) Mobility, tremor, hyperkinesis

        (e) Seizure activity

        (f) Sweating, perspiration

        (g) Unusual pigmentation striae or thinning of the skin; petechiae

        (h) Scars, especially in the neck area

        (i) Hair distribution and texture relative to gender and maturation

        (j) Temperature, edema, skin turgor

        (k) Periorbital edema, ptosis, eye protrusion, stare, dry eyes

        (l) Hydration status of oral cavity, enlarged tongue, fruity odor to breath

(m) Goiter

(n) Presence of medical alert identification

ii. Palpation

(a) Abnormal skin temperature or turgor

(b) Enlarged or nodular thyroid gland, often painful

(c) Abdominal pain with palpation

iii. Percussion: Abnormal deep tendon reflexes

iv. Auscultation

(a) Neck: Bruits over the thyroid gland

(b) Heart

(1) Distant heart sounds

(2) Third heart sound

(3) Pericardial and/or pleural friction rub (because of effusion)

(c) Heart rate and rhythm disturbances

(d) Altered respiratory pattern

(e) Altered bowel sounds

b. Monitoring data

i. Electrocardiography

ii. Blood pressure monitoring

iii. Temperature monitoring

iv. Pulse oximetry

3. **Appraisal of patient characteristics**

a. Patients with chronic, acute, or life-threatening endocrine problems enter critical care units with a wide range of clinical characteristics. During their stay, their clinical status may slowly or abruptly improve or deteriorate. Changes in the patient's condition may involve one or all life-sustaining functions, and functions can be easy or nearly impossible to monitor with precision. Examples of clinical attributes that the nurse should assess when caring for a patient with an acute endocrine disorder are the following: resiliency, vulnerability, stability, complexity, resource availability, participation in care and decision making, and predictability.

DIAGNOSTIC STUDIES

a. Laboratory: Blood and urine

i. Serum

(a) Electrolyte levels

(b) Glucose, creatinine, blood urea nitrogen (BUN), cholesterol

(c) Osmolality, creatine phosphokinase (CPK), cholesterol, beta hydroxybutyrate (BHB)

(d) Hemoglobin, hematocrit, white blood cell count with differential

(e) Specific hormone assays as appropriate

ii. Arterial blood gas (ABG)

iii. Urine specific gravity, osmolality, pH

b. Radiologic (to identify precipitating factor)

i. Radiography (skull, chest, abdomen)

ii. Computed axial tomography (CT)

iii. Magnetic resonance imaging (MRI)

iv. Arteriography

v. Bone mineral densitometry

vi. Nuclear medicine imaging

c. Other
    i. Electrocardiography (ECG)
    ii. Visual field testing

PATIENT CARE

1. **Fluid volume deficit (hypovolemia)**
   a. Description of problem
       i. Dry skin and mucous membranes, decreased skin turgor
       ii. Hypotension, orthostasis, tachycardia
       iii. Hypernatremia, increasing BUN with normal creatinine, increasing serum osmolality
       iv. Weight loss
       v. Polyuria, negative intake and output (I&O) balance
       vi. Hemoconcentration
   b. Goals of care
       i. Fluid and electrolyte balance are restored
       ii. Cardiovascular stability is maintained
   c. Interprofessional collaboration: Nurse, physician, advanced practice provider
   d. Interventions
       i. Administer fluids and hormone therapy as prescribed
       ii. Monitor and document I&O, electrolyte levels, vital signs, urine specific gravity, weight, laboratory test results on flow sheet
       iii. Provide oral care and skin care

2. **Fluid volume excess (hypervolemia)**
   a. Description of problem
       i. Intake exceeding output, weight gain
       ii. Deterioration of mental status
       iii. Third heart sound
       iv. Pulmonary congestion and dyspnea
       v. Hemodilution
       vi. Abnormal electrolyte values
       vii. Edema, ascites
   b. Goals of care: Restoration of fluid and electrolyte balance
   c. Interprofessional collaboration: Nurse, physician, advanced practice provider, respiratory therapist
   d. Interventions
       i. Monitor I&O, electrolyte levels, pulmonary status and function
       ii. Use flow sheet to document I&O, vital signs, urine specific gravity, weight, laboratory test results
       iii. Identify patients at risk for fluid overload
       iv. Administer prescribed diuretics

3. **Altered carbohydrate, fat, and/or protein metabolism**
   a. Description of problem
       i. Hyperglycemia with or without ketosis
       ii. Weight loss of 10% to 20%
       iii. Generalized fatigue and weakness
   b. Goals of care
       i. Body weight normalizes
       ii. No evidence of ketosis is present
       iii. Nitrogen balance is positive
   c. Interprofessional collaboration: Nurse, physician, advanced practice provider, dietitian

d. Interventions
  i. Provide sufficient calories and vitamins
  ii. Administer hormone or antihormone therapy as prescribed
  iii. Monitor marker of nutritional status in consultation with dietitian

4. **Need for patient and family education and discharge planning**
  a. Description of problem
    i. Lack of knowledge or skills may seriously compromise self-care
    ii. Patient and/or family is unable to explain or follow instructions correctly
    iii. Patient and/or family raises questions and requests information
  b. Goals of care: Patient demonstrates knowledge and skills needed for providing self-care and contacting healthcare resources
  c. Interprofessional collaboration: Nurse, physician, advanced practice provider, respiratory therapist, diabetes educator, dietitian, care manager
  d. Interventions
    i. Assess patient and family knowledge of health disorder and required care
    ii. Provide appropriate information about health disorder and self-care
    iii. Provide an opportunity for patient and family to demonstrate needed skills
    iv. Provide appropriate resources for additional information and support (e.g., American Diabetes Association https://www.diabetes.org/)

SPECIFIC PATIENT HEALTH PROBLEMS

ALTERED GLUCOSE METABOLISM

1. **Diabetic ketoacidosis (DKA)**
  a. Pathophysiology: Serious metabolic complication of insulin-dependent, or type 1, diabetes (can also occur in type 2). A state of insulin deficiency combined with increase in level of insulin-antagonistic hormones (glucagons, cortisol, catecholamines, and GH). Result is altered metabolism of carbohydrate, fat, and protein and hyperglycemia.
    i. Decreased insulin level with gluconeogenesis and increased insulin resistance result in exaggerated hepatic glucose production
    ii. Ketosis and metabolic acidosis result from increased synthesis of ketones and lactic acidosis
    iii. Fluid and electrolyte imbalance and osmotic diuresis are caused by glycosuria; accompanied by loss of sodium, potassium, and chloride
    iv. Altered mental status results from hyperosmolality, cellular dehydration, acidosis, and possibly impaired oxygen dissociation, because glycosylated hemoglobin binds oxygen more tightly
  b. Etiology and risk factors
    i. Diagnosed diabetes mellitus
      (a) Insufficient exogenous insulin, including poor compliance or insulin pump malfunction
      (b) Infection, trauma, pancreatitis
      (c) Myocardial infarction, cerebrovascular accident
      (d) Poor compliance with established self-care regimen
        (1) Alcohol or cocaine
        (2) Educational deficits
        (3) Psychosocial distress or disease, eating disorders
        (4) Adolescence

      (e) Medications; glucocorticoids, beta-blockers, thiazide diuretics, certain chemotherapeutic agents, atypical antipsychotics (especially olanzapine and risperidone)

  ii. Undiagnosed diabetes mellitus

  iii. Euglycemic DKA is most commonly seen in SGLT2 inhibitor use, pregnancy, decreased caloric intake, heavy alcohol use, and chronic liver disease

c. Signs and symptoms

  i. Blurred vision, diminished level of consciousness, fatigue, weakness

  ii. Nausea, abdominal cramping, vomiting

  iii. Polyuria, polydipsia, weight loss

  iv. Decreased skin turgor, dry mucous membranes

  v. Fruity odor to breath (ketosis)

  vi. Tachycardia, hypotension

  vii. Tachypnea, Kussmaul's respirations

  viii. Seizures

d. Diagnostic study findings

  i. Noninvasive study findings

     (a) Elevated plasma glucose (>250 mg/dL); euglycemia (<250 mg/dL) in 10% of DKA cases

     (b) Metabolic acidosis: Arterial pH less than 7.3; serum HCO_3^- less than 18 mEq/dL

     (c) Positive results for serum and urine ketones

     (d) Anion gap greater than 10 mEq/l ($Na^+ - \{Cl + HCO_3\}$); for accurate calculation Na must be corrected for hyperglycemia; see Pharmacology 2(a))

     (e) Hyponatremia, hypocalcemia, hyperkalemia, hypophosphatemia

e. Interprofessional collaboration: Nurse, physician, advanced practice provider, respiratory therapist, diabetes educator or diabetes case manager, dietitian

f. Management of patient care

  i. Anticipated patient trajectory: DKA can reoccur easily if medication compliance, diet, and sick-day management are not well understood.

g. Goals of care

  i. Acid-base electrolyte and fluid balance is restored

  ii. Blood glucose level normalizes

  iii. Absence of ketosis

  iv. Neurologic and pulmonary status are normalized

  v. Underlying precipitating factor is identified

  vi. Patients with DKA may have needs in the following areas:

     (a) Pharmacology

       (1) Administer intravenous (IV) fluids to correct shock or hypovolemia; administer 1 to 1.5 L of 0.9% sodium chloride solution in first hour

       (2) Once euvolemia is obtained, administer IV fluids based on corrected sodium (Na^+) at a rate of 250 to 500 mL/h and adjust based on the hemodynamic and electrolyte status

         a) Corrected Na^+ = Measured serum Na^+ + ([{Serum glucose in mg/dL − 100}/100]×1.6)

         b) 0.9% NaCl is recommended if the corrected Na^+ level is under 135 mEq/L

         c) 0.45% NaCl is recommended if the corrected Na^+ level is over 135 mEq/L

d) When serum glucose is less than 200 mg/dL, change IV fluids to 0.45% NaCl with 5% dextrose at 150 to 250 mL/h

(3) Administer regular insulin

a) Administer IV regular insulin with bolus 0.1 unit/kg body weight followed by continuous regular insulin at 0.1 unit/kg/h

b) Transition to SQ insulin when serum glucose is less than 250 mg/dL, serum bicarbonate is 18 mEq/L or over, venous pH is over 7.3, and calculated anion gap is 12 mEq/L or less

c) When transitioning to SQ insulin, overlap IV to basal SQ therapy by at least 2 hours to prevent recurrence of ketosis and accelerated hyperglycemia

d) Maintain glucose value between 150 and 200 mg/dL until DKA has resolved

(4) Administer sodium bicarbonate only if life-threatening acidosis with pH under 6.9

(5) Administer potassium replacement to maintain goal potassium value 4 to 5 mEq/L

(b) Treatments

(1) Monitor the serum glucose level every 1 to 2 hours

(2) Monitor electrolyte levels while acidosis and volume deficits are being corrected

(3) Monitor liver enzyme levels, BUN, venous or arterial pH, creatinine

(4) Record I&O, daily weights

(5) Assess pulmonary and neurologic status

(c) Psychosocial issues

(1) For patients with newly diagnosed diabetes, major lifestyle changes required

(2) For patients with preexisting diabetes, address noncompliance or poor compliance with medical regimen

vii. Potential complications

(a) Nonanion gap metabolic acidosis

(b) Dehydration, rhabdomyolysis

(c) Hypoglycemia, hypokalemia

(d) Thromboembolism

(e) Arrhythmias, cardiac arrest

(f) Cerebral edema (more common in children but described in adults up to age 28 years)

viii. Discharge planning

(a) For patients with newly diagnosed diabetes: Education about disease, pathophysiology, and self-care management

(b) For patients with previously diagnosed diabetes: Education about self-care regimen, compliance, and sick-day management

2. **Hyperglycemic Hyperosmolar State (HHS; Hyperglycemic, Hyperosmolar Nonketotic Coma—HHNK)**

a. Pathophysiology: Life-threatening hyperglycemic emergency accompanied by hyperosmolality, severe dehydration, and alterations in neurologic status with or without mild ketosis. Relative insulin deficiency that impairs glucose transport across cell membrane. There may be sufficient insulin present to inhibit lipolysis or ketogenesis in liver but not enough to control hyperglycemia.

    i. Increased gluconeogenesis and glycogenolysis, and insufficient use of glucose by peripheral tissue lead to hyperglycemia

    ii. Hyperosmolality resulting from hyperglycemia and hypernatremia may impair insulin secretion, promote insulin resistance, and inhibit free fatty acid release from adipose tissue

    iii. Fluid shifts from intracellular to extracellular space to offset hyperosmolality

    iv. Osmotic diuresis caused by hyperglycemia results in extracellular fluid volume depletion; fluid deficits usually are greater than those in DKA

    v. Severe electrolyte losses (sodium, chloride, phosphate, magnesium, potassium) occur with osmotic diuresis

    vi. Volume depletion compromises glomerular filtration, diminishing urinary escape of glucose

    vii. Evolves over days to weeks until cellular dehydration results in coma

b. Etiology and risk factors

    i. Inadequate insulin secretion and/or action: Newly diagnosed type 2, or noninsulin-dependent, diabetes

    ii. Inadequate dose or poor compliance with insulin or oral hypoglycemic

    iii. Advanced age and severe dehydration (majority of patients)

    iv. Infection, sepsis

    v. Stroke, myocardial infarction

    vi. Uremia

    vii. Trauma, burns

    viii. GI hemorrhage

    ix. Lack of access to fluids or inability to recognize or express need for fluids

    x. Medications: Corticosteroids, thiazide diuretics, phenytoin, sympathomimetics, and atypical antipsychotics

    xi. Preadmission medication regimen for cardiovascular or renal disease

c. Signs and symptoms

    i. Lethargy, progressive mental status decline, blurred vision, weakness, seizures, coma

    ii. Polydipsia, polyuria

    iii. Flushed skin and dry mucous membranes

    iv. Tachycardia, hypotension

    v. Shallow, rapid respirations

d. Diagnostic study findings

    i. Severely elevated glucose levels (>600 mg/dL)

    ii. No or minimal ketosis

    iii. Plasma hyperosmolality (>320 mOsm/kg)

    iv. Sodium and potassium levels vary with the state of hydration but are often severely depleted as a result of osmotic diuresis

    v. Acidosis, if present, usually caused by lactic acid or renal dysfunction

e. Interprofessional collaboration: Nurse, physician, advanced practice provider, respiratory therapist, diabetes educator, home care coordinator, or discharge planner.

f. Management of patient care

    i. Anticipated patient trajectory: HHS can occur in diabetic patients over a period of days to weeks if medication compliance, diet, and sick-day management are not well understood.

g. Goals of care

    i. Fluid and electrolyte balance is restored

    ii. Blood glucose level is normalized

     iii. Peripheral tissue perfusion is restored

     iv. Underlying precipitating factor is identified

     v. Throughout their course of recovery and discharge, patients with HHS/HHNK may be expected to have needs in the following areas:

      (a) Pharmacology

       (1) Administer IV fluids to correct hypovolemia or shock; administer 1 L of 0.9% sodium chloride solution in first hour

       (2) Once euvolemia is obtained administer IV fluid based on corrected sodium (Na⁺) at a rate of 250 to 500 mL/h and adjust based on the hemodynamic and electrolyte status

        a) Corrected Na^+ = Measured serum Na^+ + ([{Serum glucose in mg/dL – 100}/100] × 1.6)

        b) 0.9% NaCl is recommended if the corrected Na^+ level is under 135 mEq/L

        c) 0.45% NaCl is recommended if the corrected Na^+ level is over 135 mEq/L

        d) When serum glucose is under 300 mg/dL, change IV fluids to 0.45% NaCl with 5% dextrose

       (3) Administer regular insulin

        a) Administer IV regular insulin with bolus 0.1 unit/kg body weight followed by continuous regular insulin at 0.1 unit/kg/h

        b) Transition to SQ insulin when serum glucose is under 300 mg/dL

        c) When transitioning to SQ insulin, overlap IV to basal SQ therapy by at least 2 hours to prevent the recurrence of hyperglycemia

        d) Insulin infusion is usually stopped when serum glucose level is under 300 mg/dL; maintain glucose value between 200 and 300 mg/dL until patient is mentally alert

        e) Utilization of standard paper based or computerized protocol for DKA management has shown improved outcomes

       (4) Administer potassium replacement to maintain goal potassium value 4 to 5 mEq/L

      (b) Treatments

       (1) Monitor the serum glucose level every 1 to 2 hours

       (2) Monitor electrolyte levels while volume deficits are being corrected

       (3) Monitor liver enzyme levels, BUN, venous pH, and creatinine

       (4) Record I&O, daily weights

       (5) Assess neurologic and pulmonary status

     vi. Potential complications

      (a) Heart failure

      (b) Hypoglycemia

      (c) Thromboembolic event

      (d) Dehydration, rhabdomyolysis

3. Hyperglycemia

  a. Pathophysiology: Glucose production outweighs glucose utilization resulting in a serum glucose level of more than 140 mg/dL.

  b. Etiology and risk factors

     i. Type 1 diabetes: β cell destruction that results in absolute insulin deficiency; genetic link, autoimmune disorder

     ii. Type 2 diabetes: Relative deficiency of insulin caused by decreased sensitivity of receptors to insulin, decreased production, premature destruction of insulin or receptors (e.g., insulin resistance), and/or hyperinsulinemia; polygenetic etiologies, dietary link

iii. Stress induced: Critical illness activates of the hypothalamic-pituitary-adrenal axis, sympathetic system, and cytokine release resulting in gluconeogenesis, decreased glucose utilization, and insulin resistance

iv. Administration of hyperglycemia-provoking agents: Glucocorticoids, vasopressors, enteral nutrition, parenteral nutrition

v. Withholding hypoglycemic medications

vi. Hyperglycemia in critical care can occur in known or previously undiagnosed diabetes, be related to hospitalization or physiologic stress, or occur as a result of a combination of factors. Hyperglycemia in nondiabetics is a predictor of mortality.

c. Signs and symptoms: polyuria, polydipsia

d. Diagnostic study findings: Serum glucose level over 140 mg/dL in a hospitalized patient

e. Interprofessional collaboration: Nurse, physician, advanced practice provider, dietician

f. Management of patient care

i. Anticipated patient trajectory: Hyperglycemia occurs frequently in critically ill patients. During acute illness, patients will require close monitoring and appropriate protocolized treatment to maintain goal glucose levels while avoiding high glucose variability.

g. Goals of care

i. Serum glucose maintained between 140 and 180 mg/dL; lower glucose targets may be appropriate in selected patients

ii. Throughout their clinical course, patients with hyperglycemia may be expected to have needs in the following areas:

(a) Pharmacology

(1) Insulin therapy should be instituted for persistent hyperglycemia of 180 mg/dL or more

(2) Continuous infusion of regular insulin IV

a) Allows for rapid dosing adjustment in response to changes in patient status

b) Administered using a validated written protocol or computerized protocol

---

EXPERT TIP

Best practice for hyperglycemia management includes use of a nursing protocol or computerized tool for management.

---

(3) Subcutaneous insulin therapy

a) Basal

b) Prandial: Administration based on carbohydrate ingestion

c) Correction (supplementation): Short- or rapid-acting insulin used to treat blood glucose above goal; usually administered as corrective scale

(4) Noninsulin agent should be used only in select stable patients and are inappropriate for most hospitalized patients

(5) Using subcutaneous correction insulin therapy as a monotherapy only is strongly discouraged in hospitalized patients

  (6) In patients with poor oral intake or NPO, basal insulin plus correction insulin is preferred

  (7) In noncritically ill patients with good nutritional intake, basal insulin with prandial and correction insulin is recommended

 (b) Treatment

  (1) Appropriate blood glucose monitoring

   a) Patients with regular meals should have blood glucose testing before meals and at bedtime

   b) Patients who are NPO or receiving enteral or parenteral nutrition should have blood glucose testing every 4 to 6 hours

   c) Patients receiving IV insulin should have blood glucose testing every 30 minutes to every 2 hours

---

KEY CONCEPT

Capillary samples should be used cautiously in patients with high or low hemoglobin concentrations, hypoperfusion, vasopressor use or presence of interfering substances. If capillary sample value does not correlate with the clinical status of the patient, a serum (venous or arterial) sample should be obtained.

---

  (2) Provide adequate calories to meet metabolic demands

   a) Individualized medical nutrition based on treatment goals, physiologic parameters, and medication use

   b) Consistent carbohydrate meal plans

 iii. Potential complications

  (a) Hypoglycemia

  (b) High glucose variability

  (c) Poor immune response or infection, delayed wound healing

  (d) Inflammation

  (e) Critical illness polyneuropathy (CIP): Associated with stress-induced hyperglycemia

4. **Hypoglycemia**

 a. Pathophysiology: Glucose production (feeding and/or liver gluconeogenesis) lags behind glucose utilization resulting in a serum glucose level under 70 mg/dL

  i. Level 1 hypoglycemia is glucose 54 to 69 mg/dL

  ii. Level 2 hypoglycemia is glucose under 54 mg/dL and threshold that neuroglycopenic symptoms begin to occur

  iii. Level 3 hypoglycemia occurs when patient is altered mentally and/or physical status requires assistance

 b. Etiology and risk factors

  i. Insulin therapy

   (a) Insulin dose greater than the body's current needs

   (b) Sudden rotation of injection sites from a hypertrophied area to one with unimpaired absorption

   (c) Inappropriate timing of insulin related to glucose intake

  ii. Oral hypoglycemic therapy, especially with sulfonylurea agents

  iii. Interruption of glucose source

   (a) New NPO status or enteral feedings or parenteral nutrition stopped

   (b) Reduction in oral intake

   (c) Intake compromised because of nausea, vomiting, or anorexia

iv. Strenuous physical exercise that is not compensated by increased glucose intake or decreased dose of insulin

v. Decreased requirements for exogenous insulin resulting from
   (a) Recovery from physiologic stress (infection, trauma, surgery)
   (b) Weight loss
   (c) Immediate postpartum period
   (d) Decrease in steroid dose

vi. High blood glucose variability

vii. Impaired cognition or altered ability to report hypoglycemia symptoms

viii. Interference with insulin metabolism or counterregulatory hormone response
   (a) Reduced renal function
   (b) Altered hepatic enzyme activity
   (c) Heart failure
   (d) Sepsis, infection, malignancy
   (e) Use of β-adrenergic blocking agents

ix. High severity of illness

x. Excessive alcohol intake

xi. Neuroendocrine tumor of pancreas (most commonly insulinoma), adrenal insufficiency

c. Signs and symptoms

i. Autonomic
   (a) Adrenergic: Palpitations, tachycardia, anxiety, tremors
   (b) Cholinergic: Diaphoresis, warmth, nausea, hunger

ii. Neuroglycopenic
   (a) Weakness, behavioral changes, confusion, dizziness, amnesia, lethargy
   (b) Visual change, dysarthria
   (c) Seizure, loss of consciousness, coma

d. Diagnostic study findings:

i. Hypoglycemia: Serum glucose levels under 70 mg/dL

ii. Severe hypoglycemia: Serum glucose level under 40 mg/dL

e. Interprofessional collaboration: Nurse, physician, advanced practice provider, dietician, diabetes educator

f. Management of patient care

i. Anticipated patient trajectory: Hypoglycemia is a potential complication with a high likelihood of recurrence in patients in whom insulin-food-activity balance either has not been achieved or has been disrupted or in whom diabetes has been newly diagnosed.

g. Goals of care

i. Serum glucose maintained between 140 to 180 mg/dL; however, lower glucose targets may be appropriate in selected patients

ii. Neurologic status is normalized

iii. Throughout their course of recovery and discharge, patients with hypoglycemia may be expected to have needs in the following areas:
   (a) Hypoglycemia treatment protocols should be established to allow nurses to avoid treatment delays

---

EXPERT TIP

Best practice for hypoglycemia management includes use of a nursing protocol to reduce treatment delays.

    (b) Pharmacology
        (1) Discontinue insulin infusion if present
        (2) Administer 15 to 20 g oral glucose (preferred treatment)
            a) Avoid fat-containing foods, which will delay glucose absorption
            b) Add protein source to carbohydrate if patient will not eat meal within 1 hour
        (3) Administer 12.5 to 25 g IV glucose for a patient who is NPO or experiencing severe hypoglycemia; readminister glucose until level is greater than 70 mg/dL
        (4) If the patient experiences recurrent hypoglycemia episodes, consider initiation of continuous IV dextrose-containing infusion
    (c) Treatment
        (1) Remeasure glucose level 15 minutes after treatment
        (2) Consider more frequent ongoing glucose monitoring to evaluate for recurrent hypoglycemia
        (3) Assess neurologic status
        (4) The use of SQ insulin and its absorption may be reduced in a patient with poor perfusion—IV insulin should be considered in patients with low cardiac output states, shock states, or vasopressor therapy
  iv. Avoidance of potential complications
    (a) Ventricular arrhythmias
    (b) Seizures, coma

ALTERED ANTIDIURETIC HORMONE PRODUCTION

1. **Diabetes insipidus (DI)**
  a. Pathophysiology: Occurs when any organic lesion or chemical substance affecting the hypothalamus or posterior pituitary interferes with ADH synthesis and transport or release. Deficiency results in inability to conserve water and excretion of large amounts of dilute urine.
  b. Etiology and risk factors
    i. Central diabetes insipidus (CDI) or neurogenic: ADH deficiency
      (a) Idiopathic (up to 50%): Autoimmune (common), familial (rare)
      (b) Head trauma or surgical injury to hypothalamus or pituitary (most common cause of polyuria after neurosurgery)
      (c) Craniopharyngioma, pituitary tumor, germinomas
      (d) Meningitis, encephalitis, toxoplasmosis, tuberculosis
      (e) Vascular causes not well understood
      (f) Inflammatory/autoimmune disorders: Langerhans cell histiocytosis, sarcoidosis
      (g) Lung cancer, leukemia, lymphoma
      (h) Increased intracranial pressure, brain death
    ii. Nephrogenic diabetes insipidus (NDI): ADH resistance
      (a) Renal: Kidney failure, polycystic kidneys, pyelonephritis, congenital disorder, obstructive nephropathy, myeloma, renal sarcoidosis, amyloidosis
      (b) Metabolic: Hypercalcemia and hypokalemia leading to temporary resistance to vasopressin
      (c) Familial
      (d) Lithium, amphotericin B, ofloxacin, chemotherapy agents
      (e) Obstructive renal disease
    iii. Primary polydipsia: High fluid intake in excess of free water excretion

c. Signs and symptoms
  i. Polydipsia, persistent (may be difficult to recognize in critically ill patient)
  ii. Polyuria (40–50 mL/kg/24 h)
  iii. Decreased skin turgor, dry mucous membranes
  iv. Tachycardia; hypotension if the patient has become dehydrated
  v. CDI symptoms are often abrupt presenting in weeks to months of onset, whereas NDI presents with more insidious onset for months or even years
d. Diagnostic study findings
  i. Noninvasive study findings
    (a) Elevated plasma osmolality (>300 mOsm/kg) and hypernatremia (>145 mEq/L)
    (b) Decreased urine osmolality (<300 mOsm/kg), low specific gravity (1.001–1.005), and low urine sodium
    (c) Two-step water deprivation test
      (1) Water deprivation for 8-hour period
        a) Differentiates psychogenic polydipsia from diabetes insipidus; in diabetes insipidus the kidneys will be unable to concentrate urine
        b) No response occurs in either neurogenic or NDI
      (2) Desmopressin (dDAVP) administered intramuscular or subcutaneous injection and urine osmolality is measured to direct treatment and goals of care
        a) In DI, it demonstrates that the kidneys can concentrate urine with exogenous ADH and urine osmolality over 750 mOsm/kg; corrects CDI
        b) No response in NDI; urine osmolality under 300 mOsm/kg
        c) Low plasma ADH levels in patients with CDI
e. Copeptin concentrations may be used in the future to distinguish between DI and primary polydipsia and may also help to distinguish a central etiology; currently a standard value has not been established for diagnosis but initial research shows improved sensitivity and specificity over water deprivation testing
f. Interprofessional collaboration: Nurse, physician, advanced practice provider, dietician
g. Management of patient care
  i. Anticipated patient trajectory: Patients with DI may experience spontaneous resolution of symptoms or require lifetime medication.
h. Goals of care
  i. ADH deficiency is corrected
  ii. Tissue hypoperfusion is prevented
  iii. Fluid and electrolyte balance is restored
  iv. Throughout their clinical course, patients with DI may be expected to have needs in the following areas:
    (a) Pharmacology
      (1) ADH (CDI)
        a) Aqueous pitressin or vasopressin (intravenous [IV] or subcutaneous [SQ])
        b) Desmopressin acetate (DDAVP)
        c) Lypressin (nasal)
      (2) Thiazide diuretics (NDI): Promotes concentration of urine, improving specific gravity and urine osmolality
      (3) Amiloride (NDI): Adjunctive treatment with thiazide diuretics

          (4) Spironolactone, angiotensin converting enzyme (ACE) inhibitors or angiotensin II receptor blocker (ARB): Modification of renin-angiotensin system

          (5) Hypotonic solutions (most commonly 0.45% saline) administered IV in amounts equivalent to urine output

          (6) Electrolyte replacement

      (b) Treatments

          (1) Management of underlying condition

          (2) Monitor I&O, urine specific gravity and osmolality

          (3) Monitor serum osmolality and electrolytes

          (4) Monitor body weight

          (5) Frequent oral care because of dry mouth

          (6) Hypoosmotic diet: 1 mmol sodium, 2 to 3 mmol potassium, 2 to 3 g protein/kg/day

    v. Potential complications

      (a) Dehydration

      (b) Hypoperfusion

      (c) Electrolyte imbalance

      (d) Brain edema

          (1) Occurs when hypernatremia correction occurs too rapidly in patients with chronic (>48 hours) hypernatremia

          (2) Associated with Na^+ correction greater than 10 mEq over 24 hours

2. SIADH

  a. Pathophysiology: Syndrome characterized by plasma hypotonicity, hyponatremia, and excessive electrolyte excretion that result from abnormally high or continuous secretion of ADH. Dysfunction results in water intoxication and a dilutional hyponatremia.

  b. Etiology and risk factors

    i. Ectopic ADH production

      (a) Malignancy, most commonly lung but also nasopharyngeal, GI, and pancreatic

      (b) Mesothelioma, lymphoma, sarcoma

    ii. Increased ADH release

      (a) Medications: Antidepressants, neuroleptics, clofibrate, carbamazepine, sodium valproate, chlorpropamide, antineoplastic drugs, nonsteroidal antiinflammatory drugs, nicotine, amiodarone, proton pump inhibitors, sulfonylureas, vasopressin analogues

      (b) Pulmonary infections, cystic fibrosis, positive pressure ventilation

      (c) Central nervous system infections, traumatic brain injury, subdural hematoma, subarachnoid hemorrhage, brain tumors, multiple sclerosis

      (d) General anesthesia, stress, pain, exercise

    iii. Idiopathic

  c. Signs and symptoms

    i. Confusion, impaired memory, headache, poor concentration

    ii. Muscle twitching or seizure activity, delayed deep tendon reflexes

    iii. Nausea, vomiting

    iv. Urine output less than 400 to 500 mL in 24 hours

    v. Weight gain

  d. Diagnostic study findings

    i. Noninvasive study findings

       (a) Hyponatremia (<135 mEq/L) and decreased plasma osmolality (<275 mOsm/L)

       (b) Elevated urine sodium (>30 mEq/L) and osmolality (>100 mOsm/kg)

       (c) Low serum sodium and osmolality

       (d) Elevated plasma ADH levels

       (e) Absence of adrenal, thyroid, pituitary, or renal insufficiency

  e. Interprofessional collaboration: Nurse, physician, advanced practice provider

  f. Management of patient care

     i. Anticipated patient trajectory: If the underlying cause of SIADH is treated, the symptoms will resolve. If the precipitating cause cannot be removed or treated, the patient will require ongoing electrolyte monitoring throughout recovery and discharge.

  g. Goals of care

     i. Fluid balance is restored

     ii. Electrolyte balance is restored

     iii. Patients with SIADH may be expected to have needs in the following areas:

       (a) Pharmacology

         (1) Fluid restriction (500–1000 mL over 24 hours)

         (2) Sodium replacement: Recommended correction rate is 8 to 10 mEq in the first 24 hours or 18 mmol/L in the first 48 hours

           a) 3% sodium chloride (only indicated for moderate or severe hyponatremia symptoms) administer 150 mL over 20 minutes, may be repeated if severe neurologic impairment persists

           b) Enteral urea

         (3) Selective vasopressin V_2-receptor antagonist

       (b) Treatments

         (1) Monitor I&O, urine specific gravity and osmolality, and serum osmolality and electrolytes

         (2) Monitor body weight

         (3) Initiate seizure and injury precautions

     iv. Potential complications

       (a) Fluid overload

       (b) Electrolyte imbalance

       (c) Central pontine myelinolysis

         (1) Irreversible demyelination of neurons in pons that occurs when hyponatremia correction occurs too rapidly

       (d) Recommendation to correct sodium 8 to 10 mmol/L in a 24-hour period

         (1) Seizures (usually in patients with serum Na^+ <120 mEq/L)

ALTERED THYROID HORMONE PRODUCTION

1. **Thyroid crisis (thyroid storm)**

  a. Pathophysiology: Life-threatening emergency characterized by an increased action of T_3 and T_4 in a patient with hyperthyroidism

  b. Etiology and risk factors

     i. Toxic adenoma, toxic multinodular goiter, Graves disease

     ii. Poor compliance with antithyroid therapy or thyroxine overdosage

     iii. Radioactive iodine treatment or iodinated contrast dyes

     iv. Infection

     v. Cerebrovascular disease, pulmonary thromboembolism

     vi. Surgery, trauma, burn injury, or intense exercise

vii. Diabetic ketoacidosis

viii. Pregnancy, during labor, during complicated deliveries

ix. Medications: Cytotoxic chemotherapy, aspirin overdosage, organophosphates, lithium, amiodarone

x. Severe emotional stress

c. Signs and symptoms

   i. Altered mental status: Confusion, overt psychosis, paranoia, seizure, coma

   ii. Weakness, lethargy

   iii. Hyperkinesis and tremor, restlessness and agitation

   iv. Warm, moist, flushed, soft skin; hyperthermia

   v. Neck enlargement, palpable goiter

   vi. Tachycardia, atrial fibrillation, palpitations

   vii. Dyspnea, tachypnea

   viii. Nausea, vomiting, diarrhea, jaundice, abdominal pain

   ix. Weight loss, osteoporosis

   x. Embolic events

d. Diagnostic study findings

   i. Elevated total and free T_3 and T_4 levels and subnormal TSH level

   ii. Elevated hepatic aminotransferase level, alkaline phosphate, CPK, lactate dehydrogenase (LDH), bilirubin

   iii. Moderate leukocytosis with mild left shift

   iv. Increased radioiodine uptake (RAIU) with nuclear medicine imaging with iodine-131

   v. Elevated TSH receptor antibodies (TRAb) are diagnostic for Graves disease; TRAb is measured with either third-generation TSH binding inhibition immunoglobulin (TBII) assays or bioassays for thyroid stimulating immunoglobulin (TSI)

   vi. Ultrasound measurement of thyroidal blood flow can distinguish thyroid hyperactivity from destructive thyroiditis

e. Interprofessional collaboration: Nurse, physician, advanced practice provider, respiratory therapist

f. Management of patient care

   i. Anticipated patient trajectory: Once cardiovascular stability is restored and the patient is stabilized, definitive management will include thyroidectomy or pharmacologic termination of thyroid function. These treatments will render the patient hypothyroid, which requires lifelong thyroid hormone replacement.

g. Goals of care

   i. Vital signs, including temperature, are stabilized

   ii. Neurologic, cardiovascular, pulmonary, and renal status are normalized

   iii. Throughout their recovery and discharge, patients with thyrotoxicosis may be expected to have needs in the following areas:

     (a) Pharmacology

       (1) Administer β-adrenergic antagonists:

         a) Propranolol, nadolol: Heart rate control and may block T_4 to T_3 conversion at high doses

         b) Atenolol, metoprolol: Heart rate control

         c) Esmolol infusion: Heart rate control in the intensive care unit setting of severe thyrotoxicosis

       (2) Administer calcium channel blockers verapamil or diltiazem: Effective heart rate control for patients who do not tolerate or are not β-adrenergic antagonists candidates

(3) Administer antithyroid medications

    a) Propylthiouracil, methimazole, or carbimazole: Stops thyroid hormone synthesis

    b) Inorganic iodine: Blocks new thyroid hormone synthesis and thyroid hormone release

(4) Administer antipyretic acetaminophen (do not use salicylates as it inhibits T_4 and T_3 binding, increasing levels of T_4 and T_3)

(5) Administer glucocorticoid hydrocortisone: Blocks conversion of T_4 to T_3

(6) Administer IV fluids for dehydration and electrolytes as appropriate

  (b) Treatments

    (1) Support airway and ventilation

    (2) Monitor cardiovascular, pulmonary, and neurologic status

    (3) Monitor I&O and daily weights

    (4) Institute cooling measures; avoid causing shivering

    (5) Continuous ECG monitoring

    (6) Extracorporeal plasmapheresis, therapeutic plasma exchange

    (7) Radioactive iodine (RAI) therapy

    (8) Thyroidectomy

  iv. Potential complications

    (a) Heart failure, myocardial infarction, arrythmias, cardiac arrest

    (b) Shock

    (c) Hepatic failure

2. **Myxedema (hypothyroid) coma**

  a. Pathophysiology: Hypothyroidism results from a deficiency of thyroid hormones. Myxedema coma is a life-threatening emergency resulting from severe deficiency of these hormones.

  b. Etiology and risk factors

    i. Discontinuation or inadequate dose of thyroid replacement

    ii. Sepsis, infection

    iii. Trauma, exposure to cold, critical illness, other physical stress

    iv. Cerebrovascular accidents, congestive heart failure

    v. GI bleeding

    vi. Acidosis, hypoglycemia, hyponatremia, hypercapnia

    vii. Medications: Lithium carbonate, anesthetics, depressants, sedatives, narcotics, amiodarone, high-dose furosemide, glucocorticoids, metformin

  c. Signs and symptoms

    i. Hypothermia (91°–95° F [32.8°–35.0° C])

    ii. Disorientation, poor memory, depression, hallucination, altered level of consciousness, seizures, comatose

    iii. Macroglossia, hoarse voice, vocal cord edema

    iv. Bradycardia, hypotension, shock

    v. Slow, shallow respirations; hypoventilation

    vi. Urinary retention

    vii. Delayed deep tendon reflexes

    viii. Dry, brittle skin and hair; nonpitting edema

  d. Diagnostic study findings

    i. Noninvasive study findings

      (a) Increased TSH level, decreased T_4 and T_3 levels

      (b) Hyponatremia

      (c) High cholesterol level, hyperlipoproteinemia

      (d) Respiratory acidosis, hypoxemia

(e) Elevated serum lactate dehydrogenase and creatine kinase (CK)

(f) Anemia

(g) Prolonged QTc

(h) Normal or reduced cortisol level

e. Interprofessional collaboration: Nurse, physician, advanced practice provider, respiratory therapist

f. Management of patient care

   i. Anticipated patient trajectory: Once the patient's condition is stabilized, the patient will require lifelong thyroid hormone replacement and compliance with the medical regimen to prevent reoccurrence.

g. Goals of care

   i. Pulmonary, cardiovascular, and neurologic function are normalized

   ii. Temperature and electrolytes are normalized

   iii. Throughout their clinical course, patients with myxedema coma may be expected to have needs in the following areas:

     (a) Pharmacology

      (1) Administer thyroid hormone replacement IV

      (2) Administer empiric IV glucocorticoids (obtain cortisol level before initiation but do not delay administration awaiting result)

      (3) Administer IV fluids if dehydration and electrolytes as appropriate

      (4) Administer hypertonic (3%) saline in the presence of severe symptomatic hypernatremia (105–120 mmol/L), correct at a rate limited to 8 to 10 mmol/L per 24-hour period

     (b) Treatments

      (1) Institute rewarming; monitor temperature

      (2) Support airway and ventilation

      (3) Continuous ECG monitoring

      (4) Prevent infection

   iv. Potential complications

     (a) Severe hypercapnia and hypoxemia, pulmonary edema

     (b) Arrhythmias, myocardial infarction, cardiac tamponade, shock

     (c) Infection

     (d) Coagulopathy, disseminated intravascular coagulation (DIC) associated with sepsis

     (e) Ascites, GI bleeding

     (f) Central pontine myelinolysis

      (1) Irreversible demyelination of neurons in pons that occurs when hyponatremia correction occurs too rapidly

      (2) Associated with Na^+ correction greater than 12 mEq over 24 hours or more than 18 mEq over 48 hours

     (g) Seizures (usually in patients with serum Na^+ <120 mEq/L)

      (1) Euthyroid-sick syndrome (also called nonthyroidal illness syndrome)

       a) Pathophysiology: progressive reduction in circulating T_3 followed by decline in serum T_4 and TSH in a patient with normal thyroid function setting of critical illness

       b) Management of patient care

        1) Anticipated patient trajectory: Believed to be a physiology, adaptive role in illness. Randomized controlled trials are limited but have failed to show benefits to hormone replacement and in some cases have been linked to harm events. Current recommendations do not favor administration of thyroid hormone in this setting.

ACUTE ADRENAL INSUFFICIENCY OR CRISIS

1. **Pathophysiology: Deficiency of glucocorticoid and/or mineralocorticoid production resulting in electrolyte and fluid abnormalities that result in life-threatening cardiovascular collapse**
2. **Etiology and risk factors**
    a. Autoimmune adrenalitis, congenital adrenal hyperplasia, bilateral adrenal hemorrhage, bilateral adrenalectomy
    b. Acute injury or infection of the adrenal glands
    c. Sepsis or other infections (tuberculosis, fungal infection, human immunodeficiency virus)
    d. Tumor, metastasis to adrenal glands, lymphoma
    e. Head trauma
    f. Pituitary surgery, pituitary apoplexy, pituitary infiltration
    g. Infiltrative disease (amyloidosis, hemochromatosis, xanthogranulomatosis)
    h. Drug induced: mitotane, ketoconazole, metyrapone, etomidate, aminoglutethimide, T_4, cytotoxic T-lymphocyte-associated protein 4 [CTLA-4] inhibitors
    i. Long-term exogenous glucocorticoid use or abrupt cessation of corticosteroids
3. **Signs and symptoms**
    a. Confusion, altered mental status, severe weakness, fatigue, dizziness
    b. Tachycardia, volume depletion, severe hypotension, vascular collapse
    c. Nausea, vomiting, constipation, anorexia, abdominal pain, back pain, arthralgia, myalgia
    d. Petechiae, hyperpigmentation (usually seen in chronic adrenal insufficiency)
    e. Fever
4. **Diagnostic study findings**
    a. Hyponatremia, hyperkalemia, hypercalcemia
    b. Hypoglycemia (more severe in children than in adults)
    c. Anemia, eosinophilia, lymphocytosis
    d. Elevated creatinine
    e. Low morning cortisol level (<5 mcg/dL) in the early morning or low cortisol level during state of stress (e.g., postcode, low perfusion states)
    f. Plasma ACTH greater than twofold the upper limit of the reference range
    g. ACTH stimulation test will confirm the diagnosis. However, in the hemodynamically unstable patient, empiric treatment with corticosteroids is recommended before testing.

Note: Additional testing of serum renin and aldosterone should be performed to confirm primary adrenal insufficiency for concomitant mineralocorticoid deficiency

5. **Interprofessional collaboration: Nurse, physician, advanced practice provider, respiratory therapist**
6. **Management of patient care**
    a. Anticipated patient trajectory: If the precipitating event is avoidable (e.g., abrupt withdrawal of steroid use), symptoms will not recur. Any patient requiring continued steroid use will need close monitoring; physiologic stress (illness, surgery) may require increased dosage or cause inadvertent discontinuation of steroid use. Abrupt withdrawal or unmet increased demand will increase symptoms throughout the course of recovery and discharge.
7. **Goals of care**
    a. Blood pressure and tissue perfusion are maintained
    b. Cortisol levels are restored

c. Patients with acute adrenal insufficiency may be expected to have needs in the following areas:
   i. Pharmacology
      (a) Rapid administration of IV fluids and electrolytes if appropriate
      (b) Hormone replacement
         (1) Glucocorticoid (hydrocortisone) administration
         (2) Mineralocorticoid (fludrocortisone) administration if concomitant aldosterone deficiency
      (c) Administration of IV dextrose, as needed for hypoglycemia
   ii. Treatments: Monitor heart rate and rhythm and blood pressure
d. Potential complications: Cardiovascular collapse

ACUTE HYPERPARATHYROIDISM AND HYPOPARATHYROIDISM

1. **Pathophysiology: Parathyroid gland dysfunction resulting in overproduction (hyperparathyroidism) or underproduction (hypoparathyroidism) of PTH which is associated with disturbances in calcium and phosphorus balance and bone metabolism. See Chapter 6, Renal System for further discussion of the pathophysiology of calcium and phosphorus imbalances.**
2. **Etiology and risk factors**
   a. Hyperparathyroidism (hypercalcemia)
      i. Primary hyperparathyroidism (90% of cases): Benign neoplasm or adenoma
      ii. Secondary hyperparathyroidism: Chronic renal failure, intestinal malabsorption syndromes, and vitamin D deficiency
      iii. Humoral hypercalcemia of malignancy
      iv. Medications: Thiazide diuretics, lithium
   b. Hypoparathyroidism: Inadequate PTH with hypocalcemia
      i. Congenital absence of parathyroid glands or other genetic disorder
      ii. Parathyroidectomy or damage to the parathyroid glands during thyroidectomy or radical neck surgery
      iii. Autoimmune disorder, infiltrative diseases, metastatic cancer
      iv. Hypomagnesemia or hypermagnesemia (interferes with PTH secretion)
      v. Idiopathic
3. **Signs and symptoms: See Chapter 6, Renal System**
4. **Diagnostic study findings**
   a. Hyperparathyroidism: Normal serum calcium with elevated intact PTH levels, elevated serum calcium (>14 mg/dL) or ionized calcium (>5.6 mg/dL) with elevated or inappropriate normal intact PTH levels
   b. Hypoparathyroidism: Low serum calcium, elevated serum phosphate levels, low or inappropriately normal serum PTH levels
5. **Interprofessional collaboration: See Chapter 6, Renal System**
6. **Management of patient care**
   a. Hyperparathyroidism
      i. Parathyroidectomy is definitive treatment
      ii. For management of acute hypercalcemia, see Chapter 6, Renal System
   b. Hypoparathyroidism: for management of acute hypocalcemia, see Chapter 6, Renal System

References and bibliography information are available at http://evolve.elsevier.com/AACN/corecurriculum/.

Hematologic and Immunologic Systems

Nicole Brumfield, DNP, APRN, FNP-BC, AG-ACNP-BC

CROSSWALK

- **Quality and Safety in Nursing Education (QSEN):** Patient-centered care, Teamwork and collaboration, Evidence-based practice, Safety, Informatics
- **National Patient Safety Goals:** Identify patients correctly, Improve staff communication, Prevent infection, Identify patient safety risks
- **American Nurses Association (ANA) standards for Professional Nursing Practice:** Standard 1. Assessment, Standard 2. Diagnosis, Standard 3. Outcomes identification, Standard 4. Planning, Standard 5. Implementation, Standard 6. Evaluation, Standard 7. Ethics, Standard 8. Culturally congruent practice, Standard 9. Communication, Standard 10. Collaboration, Standard 11. Leadership, Standard 12. Education, Standard 13. Evidence-based practice and research, Standard 14. Quality of practice
- **AACN Scope and Standards for Progressive and Critical Care Nursing Practice:** Standard 1. Quality of practice, Standard 6. Collaboration, Standard 7. Evidence-based practice/ research/clinical inquiry
- **AACN Standards for Establishing and Sustaining Healthy Work Environments (HWE):** Skilled communication, True collaboration, Effective decision-making
- **PCCN content:** Professional Caring and Ethical Practice- All items
- **CCRN content:** Professional Caring and Ethical Practice- All items

SYSTEMWIDE ELEMENTS

ANATOMY AND PHYSIOLOGY REVIEW

1. **Composition of blood and blood cells**
   a. Blood consists of 55% plasma and 45% cellular elements.
      i. Red blood cells (RBCs, erythrocytes) are the most numerous.
         (a) They contain hemoglobin, which binds to oxygen.
         (b) They carry oxygen to body cells, tissues, and organs.
         (c) They are shaped as biconcave discs, which allows maximum surface area to carry oxygen (O_2) and great flexibility to pass through small vessels.
      ii. White blood cells (WBCs, leukocytes) have many subtypes.
         (a) They have multiple roles in inflammatory and immune responses.
         (b) They are able to leave the blood vessels and travel to sites of injury and inflammation.
      iii. Platelets (thrombocytes) are the smallest blood cells.
         (a) They have multiple roles in blood coagulation.
         (b) They also nurture the vascular endothelium.

2. **The formation and maturation of blood cells**
    a. All blood cells begin as stem cells in the bone marrow (Fig. 8.1). They differentiate into cell lines that produce cells that have different structures and functions.
    b. RBC production is stimulated when kidney cells sense hypoxia.
        i. Erythropoietin is released by the kidney and directs production of RBCs in the bone marrow.
        ii. Iron, folic acid, and vitamin B_{12} are necessary for production.
        iii. Reticulocytes are released into the blood and mature into RBCs.
        iv. RBCs live for an average of 120 days.
            (a) Old and defective RBCs are destroyed by phagocytic cells in the spleen, liver, bone marrow, and lymph nodes.
            (b) As hemoglobin breaks down, heme molecules are converted into bilirubin. The bilirubin must be conjugated by the liver, changing it into a water-soluble substance that can be excreted as bile.
            (c) As RBCs break down, iron is also released, and much of it is recycled for future use.
    c. WBC production is stimulated by cytokines and growth factors that stimulate the development of stem cells and colony-forming units. There are two distinct stem cell lines: the myeloid line and the lymphoid line (see Fig. 8.1).
        i. Myeloid stem cells prompt the development of granulocytes and monocytes, the WBCs that perform phagocytosis.
        ii. Granulocytes, distinguished by granules in their cytoplasm, include neutrophils, eosinophils, and basophils.
            (a) Neutrophils are important in defense against bacteria and other microorganisms. Immature neutrophils are released into the circulation as "bands," where they mature into segmented neutrophils, "segs."
            (b) Eosinophils increase in number and activity during parasitic and allergic responses.
            (c) Basophils are active in allergic responses.
        iii. Monocytes are large phagocytic cells that circulate in the blood.
            (a) They are called macrophages when they migrate into tissues.
            (b) They also serve as antigen presenting cells which activate adaptive immunity.
        iv. The WBCs are particularly important for the immediate immune responses to infection and injury known as *innate immunity*.
            (a) This response occurs immediately and involves activation of inflammation.
            (b) Plasma proteins, such as complement components, enhance the process.
        v. Lymphoid progenitor cells become the T and B lymphocytes that comprise the slower but more specific responses known as *adaptive immunity* (Fig. 8.2).
            (a) T cells are originally processed in the thymus, and B cells are processed in the bone marrow.
            (b) These cells reside in the lymph nodes and spleen.
            (c) When stimulated by an antigen, the T helper cells direct the T and B lymphocytes to mount a specific immune response to the invading antigen.
            (d) T cell cloning takes place, and cytotoxic T cells are released into the circulation to target the antigen.
            (e) B cells are stimulated to become plasma cells, which are able to produce antibodies specifically designed to attack the invading antigen.
            (f) T and B memory cells are produced for future responses to this antigen.

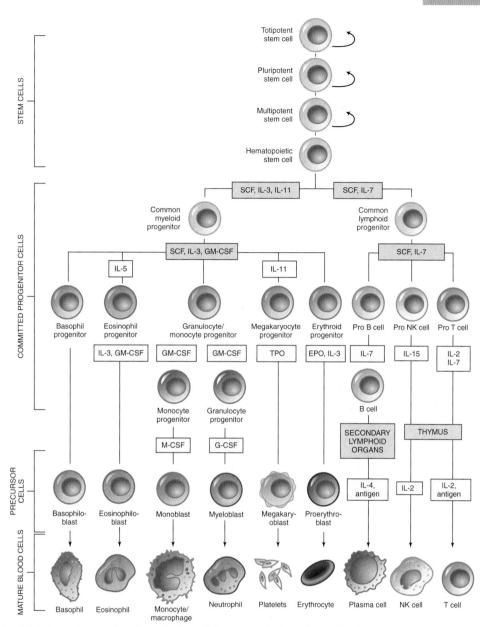

Fig. 8.1 Maturation and differentiation of hematopoietic cells. *EPO,* Erythropoietin; *G-CSF* or *GM-CSF,* granulocyte colony-stimulating factor; *IL,* interleukin; *NK,* natural killer; *SCF,* stem cell factor; *TPO,* thrombopoietin. (From McCance, K.L., et al. (2019). *Pathophysiology: the biology basis for disease in adults and children,* 8th ed, St. Louis, Elsevier.)

vi. The lifespan of a WBC varies according to cell type: Neutrophils live for 4 to 5 days and need to be continually replaced whereas macrophages live for months to years.

d. Platelets (thrombocytes) are fragments of large megakaryocytes.

i. Platelet production is stimulated by a protein called thrombopoietin, which is produced by the liver and kidneys in response to a low platelet count.

ii. Platelets live for about 10 days. They are removed from the circulation by macrophages as they age or become defective.

iii. Hemostasis depends on adequate numbers and function of platelets.

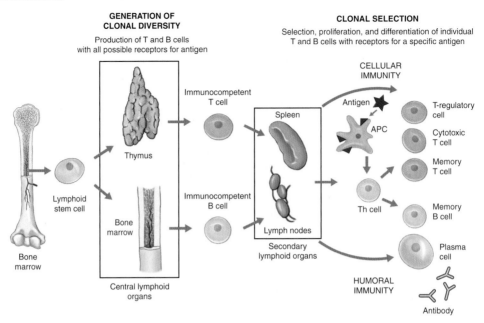

GENERATION OF CLONAL DIVERSITY
Production of T and B cells with all possible receptors for antigen

CLONAL SELECTION
Selection, proliferation, and differentiation of individual T and B cells with receptors for a specific antigen

Fig. 8.2 Overview of the adaptive immune response. *APC*, Antigen presenting cell. (From Huether, S.E., McCance, K.L., Brashers, V.L. (2020). *Understanding pathophysiology*, 7th ed, St. Louis, Elsevier.)

    iv. Platelets contain granules that release substances necessary for blood coagulation. These include phospholipids and enzymes, such as thromboxane A$_2$.

    v. Glycoproteins present on platelet outer membranes, including GPIIb/IIIa, will bind to fibrinogen during the coagulation process.

3. Hemostasis

  a. Blood clotting is initiated when injury or other stimulus leads to exposure of the vascular endothelium (Fig. 8.3).

    i. Platelets begin to adhere to the injured area, binding to glycoproteins.

    ii. The platelets are then activated and adhere to each other forming a platelet plug, a process known as *primary hemostasis*.

    iii. For a small injury, the platelet plug may stop the flow of blood.

    iv. For larger injuries, the platelet plug provides a framework for the formation of a blood clot, a process known as *secondary hemostasis*.

    v. The release of tissue factor from injured tissue begins the process of activating the proenzymes that become the coagulation factors. The process can also be activated by vascular injury.

    vi. The final pathway involves the activation of Factor X, which cleaves prothrombin into thrombin. The thrombin then splits fibrinogen into fibrin that forms the clot.

    vii. The resultant clot consists of fibrin strands that form a meshwork that traps erythrocytes and other particles.

    viii. The clot eventually dissolves as naturally occurring tissue plasminogen activator (tPA) initiates the process of fibrinolysis.

      (a) Once activated, the proenzyme plasminogen is converted into plasmin.

      (b) The plasmin breaks apart the fibrin strands, dissolving the clot.

    ix. The overall process of coagulation is normally confined to an area of injury, with hemostasis controlled by inhibitors of clotting, such as antithrombin.

I. Subendothelial exposure

- Occurs after endothelial sloughing
- Platelets begin to fill endothelial gaps
- Promoted by thromboxane A$_2$ (TXA$_2$)
- Inhibited by prostacyclin I$_2$ (PGI$_2$)
- Platelet function depends on many factors, especially calcium

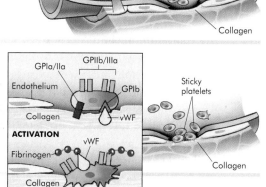

II. Adhesion

- Adhesion is initiated by loss of endothelial cells (or rupture or erosion of atherosclerotic plaque), which exposes adhesive glycoproteins such as collagen and von Willebrand factor (vWF) in the subendothelium. vWF and, perhaps, other adhesive glycoproteins in the plasma deposit on the damaged area. Platelets adhere to the subendothelium through receptors that bind to the adhesive glycoproteins (GPIb, GPIa/IIa, GPIIb/IIIa).

III. Activation

- After platelets adhere they undergo an activation process that leads to a conformational change in GPIIb/IIIa receptors, resulting in their ability to bind adhesive proteins, including fibrinogen and von Willebrand factor.
- Changes in platelet shape
- Formation of pseudopods
- Activation of arachidonic pathway

IV. Aggregation

- Induced by release of TXA$_2$
- Adhesive glycoproteins bind simultaneously to GPIIb/IIIa on two different platelets
- Stabilization of the platelet plug (blood clot) occurs by activation of coagulation factors, thrombin, and fibrin
- Heparin neutralizing factor enhances clot formation

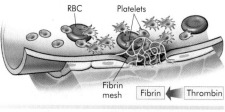

V. Platelet plug formation

- RBCs and platelets enmeshed in fibrin

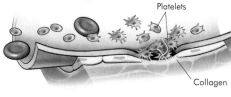

VI. Clot retraction and clot dissolution

- Clot retraction, using large number of platelets, joins the edges of the injured vessel.
- Clot dissolution is regulated by thrombin and plasminogen activators.

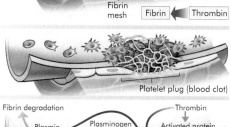

Fig. 8.3 Overview of hemostasis: blood vessel damage, blood clotting, and clot dissolution. *RBC*, Red blood cell. (From McCance, K.L., et al. (2019). *Pathophysiology: the biology basis for disease in adults and children*, 8th ed, St. Louis, Elsevier.)

ASSESSMENT OF HEMATOLOGIC AND IMMUNOLOGIC SYSTEMS

1. **History**
   a. Patient health history
      i. Many times, a hematologic or immunologic problem is identified when the patient seeks medical attention for some other reason.
      ii. Elements of the medical history indicating a potential or existing hematologic or immunologic problem include the following:
         (a) Prolonged bleeding from surgeries, procedures, dental extractions
         (b) Liver disease

    (c) Previous blood transfusions

    (d) Medication use/anticoagulant therapy

    (e) Thromboembolism

    (f) Nutritional deficiency or malabsorption disorder

    (g) Recurrent infection

    (h) Cancer or previous cancer treatment

    (i) Splenectomy

    (j) Human immunodeficiency virus (HIV)

    (k) Family history of hematologic and immunologic disorders

  iii. Review of systems with the patient and/or family for signs and symptoms

    (a) General: Fatigue, weakness, lethargy, malaise, fever, chills, night sweats, dyspnea, restlessness, apprehension, pain, altered mental status, vertigo, dizziness, confusion

    (b) Skin: Pruritus, change in skin color, rash, petechiae, unusual bruising, ulcers or other lesions

    (c) Head and neck: Headache, change in vision, epistaxis, gingival bleeding, sore throat, pain with swallowing, enlarged lymph nodes

    (d) Respiratory: Cough, hemoptysis, dyspnea, orthopnea

    (e) Cardiovascular: Palpitations, dizziness with position changes

    (f) Gastrointestinal (GI): Change in eating habits, anorexia, abdominal pain, nausea, vomiting, hematemesis, change in bowel habits, hematochezia, melena, change in weight

    (g) Genitourinary: Hematuria, pain with urination, menorrhagia, enlarged inguinal lymph nodes

    (h) Musculoskeletal: Swelling of joints, tenderness or pain in the bones or joints

    (i) Endocrine: Heat or cold intolerance

b. Family history indicating a potential hematologic or immunologic problem: Hemophilia, sickle cell anemia, cancer

c. Social/occupational history and habits that may contribute to the diagnosis and treatment of the underlying condition including the following:

  i. Any unusual or excessive exposure to chemicals (e.g., gasoline, benzene, solvents, glues, paints, varnishes) or radiation (e.g., x-rays) at work or in pursuit of a hobby

  ii. Any unusual dietary preferences, pica

  iii. Excessive alcohol consumption

  iv. Sexual history: Including if they are sexually active, gender of partner(s), number of partners, history of sexually transmitted diseases, current contraceptive method, use of safe sex practices

  v. Recreational medication history: Including intravenous (IV) medication use

d. Medication history

  i. Current medications or a recent change in medication. Always ask about over-the-counter and herbal medication use because many of these preparations contain aspirin or nonsteroidal antiinflammatory medications (NSAIDs).

  ii. Many medications used to treat nonhematologic and nonimmunologic problems can affect the hematologic and immunologic systems; examples of these medications are the following:

    (a) Analgesics and antiinflammatory medications

      (1) Aspirin and aspirin-containing medications

      (2) NSAIDs

    (b) Glucocorticoids

    (c) Antibiotics, antifungals, antivirals

(d) Anticoagulants

(e) Antiseizure agents

(f) Antineoplastic chemotherapy agents

(g) Antipsychotic agents

(h) Immunosuppressive agents

2. **Physical examination**

   a. Physical examination data

      i. Inspection

         (a) Temperature: Exceeds 38°C (100.4°F)

         (b) Skin: Pallor, jaundice, flushing, rash, petechiae, purpura, ecchymoses, hematomas, urticaria, altered integrity

         (c) Head and neck: Integrity of mucosal membranes, tongue appearance (e.g., smooth, coated), conjunctival bleeding

         (d) Chest: Shortness of breath, hemoptysis

         (e) Abdomen: Vomiting, hematemesis, hematuria, diarrhea, melena

         (f) Musculoskeletal system: Swelling of joints

      ii. Palpation and percussion

         (a) Skin: Warm to touch

         (b) Neck: Enlarged lymph nodes

         (c) Abdomen: Hepatomegaly, splenomegaly, enlarged lymph nodes in the axilla or groin

         (d) Musculoskeletal system: Pain on palpation

      iii. Auscultation

         (a) Tachycardia

         (b) Hypotension

         (c) Orthostatic changes (systolic blood pressure decreases 20 mm Hg when the patient moves from lying to sitting or standing)

         (d) Tachypnea

         (e) Crackles, rhonchi

   b. Monitoring data

      i. Fatigue related to hypoxemia

      ii. Pulse oximetry

      iii. Skin color

      iv. Skin turgor as an indicator of dehydration

      v. Overt and covert bleeding

      vi. Acute or persistent pain

      vii. Body temperature

3. **Appraisal of patient characteristics: Patients with chronic, acute, or life-threatening hematologic or immunologic problems enter critical care units with a wide range of clinical characteristics. During their stay, their clinical status may slowly or abruptly improve or deteriorate. Changes in the patient's condition may involve one or all life-sustaining functions, and functions can be easy or nearly impossible to monitor with precision. Examples of clinical attributes that the nurse should assess when caring for a patient with an acute hematologic or immunologic disorder are the following: Resiliency, vulnerability, stability, complexity, resource availability, participation in care and decision-making, and predictability.**

DIAGNOSTIC STUDIES

   a. Laboratory: See Tables 8.1 and 8.2 for normal values

      i. Blood testing

TABLE 8.1	**Hematologic and Immune Values**	
Laboratory Test	**Normal Value**	**Description**
RBC	Males: 4.2–5.4 million/μL	Number of erythrocytes available to carry oxygen
	Females: 3.6–5.0 million/μL	
Hgb	Males: 14–17 g/dL	Amount of Hgb available to carry oxygen
	Females: 12–16 g/dL	
Hct	Males: 43%–52%	Percent of blood volume made up of RBCs
	Females: 36%–48%	
RBC indices		Indicators of RBC size and amount of Hgb; used to diagnose types of anemia
MCV	82–98 μm³	
MCH	26–34 pg/cell	
MCHC	32–36 g/dL	
RDW	11.5–14.5%	
Reticulocyte count	0.5–1.5%	Immature RBCs present in the blood
WBC	4500–10,500/μL	Number of leukocytes available to participate in immune function
WBC differential (% of total)		Percent of various types of WBC available to participate in immune function
Neutrophils	50%–70%	
Segmented	56%	
Bands	0%–3%	
Eosinophils	0%–3%	
Basophils	0.5%–1.0%	
Monocytes	3%–7%	
Lymphocytes	25%–40%	
T-cells	800–2500 cells/μL	
T-helper (CD4) cells	600–1500 cells/μL	
Cytotoxic T (CD8) cells	300–1000 cells/μL	
Platelet count	150,000–400,000/μL	Number of thrombocytes available to participate in hemostasis
Erythrocyte sedimentation rate	Males: 0–15 mm/h	Test for inflammation; sed time is faster because of increased plasma proteins
	Females: 0–20 mm/h	

Normal values vary between laboratories. Refer to local laboratory standard values when interpreting test results.
HCT, Hematocrit; *Hgb*, hemoglobin; *MCH*, mean corpuscular hemoglobin; *MCHC*, mean corpuscular hemoglobin concentration; *MCV*, mean corpuscular volume; *RBC*, red blood cell; *RDW*, red cell distribution width; *WBC*, white blood cell.
Data from Fischbach, F.T., Dunning, M.B. (2018). *Manual of laboratory and diagnostic tests*, 10th ed. Philadelphia, Wolters Kluwer.

- (a) Complete blood count
- (b) Coagulation panel
- (c) Indicators of immune competence including quantitative immunoglobins and helper T cell (CD4+) counts
- (d) Liver function testing (LFT) and complete metabolic panel (CMP)
- ii. Sputum culture: Detects and identifies microorganisms in the sputum
- iii. Urine tests
  - (a) Urinalysis can detect gross amounts of blood or protein in the urine
  - (b) Urine cultures detect and identify microorganisms in the urine
  - (c) Urine protein electrophoresis determines the levels of proteins excreted in the urine, particularly the levels of immunoglobulins

TABLE 8.2   Coagulation Values

Laboratory Test	Normal Value	Description
Platelet count	150,000–400,000/µL	Number of thrombocytes available to participate in hemostasis
Bleeding time	3–10 minutes	Time required for primary hemostasis; indicator of platelet function
INR	0.8–1.1	Test of blood clotting time; used to monitor warfarin therapy
Therapeutic anticoagulation	2.0–3.0	
APTT	30–40 seconds	Test of blood clotting time; used to monitor unfractionated heparin therapy
Therapeutic anticoagulation	1.5–2.5 times normal	
ACT	70–120 seconds	Test of blood clotting time; used during cardiac procedures
Therapeutic anticoagulation	150–210 seconds	
Fibrinogen	200–400 mg/dL	Amount of fibrinogen available to form clots
D-dimer	<1.37 nmol/L	Indicator of fibrinolysis
Thromboelastogram (TEG)	Reaction time (R Time) 7.5–15 minutes K Time 3–6 minutes at angle–45 degrees Maximum amplitude (MA) 50–60 mm	Assesses the efficiency of blood coagulation, and thus bleeding and thrombotic risks, as well as monitoring of antithrombotic therapies

Normal values vary between laboratories. Refer to local laboratory standard values when interpreting test results.
ACT, Activated clotting time; *APTT,* activated partial thromboplastin time; *INR,* international normalized ratio.
Data from Fischbach, F.T., Dunning, M.B. (2018). *Manual of laboratory and diagnostic tests*, 10th ed. Philadelphia, Wolters Kluwer.

    iv. Stool occult blood test: Detects microscopic amounts of blood in the stool

  b. Radiologic

    i. Abdominal ultrasound is used to evaluate the kidneys, liver, and spleen.

    ii. A liver-spleen scan uses a radioactive tracer to evaluate the size and function of the liver and spleen.

    iii. A lymphangiogram uses contrast dye to radiologically visualize the lymph system, particularly the size and architecture of lymph nodes.

  c. Biopsy

    i. Bone marrow biopsy includes aspiration of bone marrow fluid and removal of a needle core biopsy sample of the bone marrow tissue for pathologic examination.

    ii. Lymph node biopsy involves the removal of one or more lymph nodes for pathologic examination.

  d. Skin tests: Assess immune functioning, pointing out hyposensitivities or hypersensitivities to a particular antigen. Examples of allergens used in skin testing are allergenic extracts (e.g., dust, pollen, animal dander); purified protein derivative (PPD) for tuberculin skin tests; mumps virus; *Candida albicans* and other skin fungi.

KEY CONCEPT

Older adults may have may a decreased response to skin tests because of changes in the immune system.

PATIENT CARE

1. **Risk for hemorrhage**
   a. Description of problem
      i. Disease and/or treatment creates a potential for bleeding.
      ii. Clinical findings include reports of unusual bruising, prolonged bleeding, hematemesis, hemoptysis, hematochezia, melena, hematuria, and menorrhagia.
   b. Goals of care
      i. Restoration of normal hemostasis with no evidence of spontaneous bleeding
      ii. Maintenance of platelet counts and coagulation panel parameters within an acceptable range
      iii. Patient's and family's verbalization of an understanding of the underlying pathology and bleeding precautions
   c. Interprofessional collaboration: Nurse, physician (including a hematologist), advanced practice provider, pharmacist, blood bank specialist/pathologist
   d. Interventions
      i. Assess incisions, IV sites, and drains for signs of bleeding
      ii. Monitor for signs of shock: Tachycardia, hypotension, low urine output, altered mental status
      iii. Monitor complete blood count (CBC) and coagulation panel results to assess oxygen-carrying capacity and hemostatic function
      iv. Apply local measures (pressure, topical agents) to control bleeding
      v. Stop all anticoagulants
      vi. Restore intravascular volume with fluids, blood, and blood components in patients who are actively bleeding (see Table 8.3 and guidelines for transfusion from the American Association of Blood Banks; Carson et al., 2016)
      vii. Minimize trauma to skin and mucous membranes
      viii. Control environment to prevent hypothermia

2. **Ineffective tissue perfusion**
   a. Description of problem
      i. Anemia is defined as a reduction in RBCs or in the amount of hemoglobin, resulting in decreased oxygen-carrying capacity and inadequate tissue perfusion.
      ii. Clinical findings include fatigue, weakness, pallor, tachycardia, tachypnea, dyspnea, cold skin temperature, signs of overt or covert bleeding, hemoglobin below 12 g/dL.
   b. Goals of care
      i. Stable respiratory status with normal respiratory rate and oxygen saturation (SpO_2)
      ii. Stable cardiovascular status with normal skin temperature and perfusion
      iii. Acceptable tolerance for activity
      iv. Hemoglobin level with acceptable range
   c. Interprofessional collaboration: Nurse, physician (including a hematologist/oncologist), advanced practice provider, pharmacist, blood bank specialist/pathologist
   d. Interventions
      i. Administer supplemental oxygen for SpO_2 less than 92%
      ii. Provide diet rich in iron and B vitamins and oral supplements as ordered
      iii. Administer recombinant erythropoietin as ordered
      iv. Administer blood transfusion as ordered when indicated by patient status and guideline recommendations (see Table 8.3)

TABLE 8.3 Indications and Treatment With Blood Components

Component	Volume	Infusion Time	Indications
Packed red blood cells (PRBCs), leukocyte reduced (standard for transfusion)	300–350 mL	2–4 hours	Medical ICU patients with a hemoglobin <7 g/dL and surgical patients with a hemoglobin <8 g/dL
Platelets, leukocyte reduced apheresis derived (standard for transfusion)	Approximately 200–300 mL per unit	30 minutes	Thrombocytopenia, platelet count <20,000/µL; clients who are actively bleeding with a platelet count <50,000/µL
Fresh frozen plasma	200–300 mL	Infuse within 60 minutes	Deficiency in plasma coagulation factors; reversal of anticoagulation
Cryoprecipitate	10–20 mL/unit, 5 units are pooled in one bag	Infuse within 30 minutes	DIC; fibrinogen levels <100 mg/dL, factor XIII replacement
Granulocytes	200–300 mL	Infuse over 2–4 hours	Neutropenia with documented infection

DIC, Disseminated intravascular coagulation; *ICU,* intensive care unit.
Modified from Lewis, S.L., Dirksen, S.R., Heitkemper, M.M., et al. (2017). *Medical-surgical nursing,* 10th ed. St. Louis, Elsevier.

   v. Monitor patient response to activity
  vi. Plan periods of rest between period of activity and nursing care
 vii. Prioritize and limit routine blood draws to decrease diagnostic blood loss
   (a) Additional blood conservation measures include the use of pediatric tubes for blood collection and acceptance of normovolemic anemia

3. **Susceptibility to infection**
  a. Description of problem
    i. Immunocompromise may arise from various disease processes, medical therapies, poor nutritional status, in the very young or older adult patient, or in the presence of stress, which increases patient risk for infection
    ii. Clinical findings include reports of fever, chills, night sweats, sore throat, cough, malaise, pain with swallowing, pain with urination, pain with defecation, diarrhea, reddened areas, sore areas, and swollen areas (these symptoms may not be present if the patient is neutropenic and unable to mount a WBC response); flushing, lethargy, skin warm to touch; abnormal vital signs—temperature exceeding 38°C (100.4°F), hypotension, tachycardia; WBC count higher than 10,000/µL, WBC count lower than 1500/µL, absolute neutrophil count (ANC) lower than 500/µL.
  b. Goals of care
    i. Vital signs within normal limits for the patient
    ii. Absence of signs or symptoms of active infection
    iii. Maintenance of the WBC count within an acceptable range
    iv. Patient's and family's verbalization of an understanding of the underlying pathology and infection prevention
  c. Interprofessional collaboration: Nurse, physician (including a hematologist/oncologist), advanced practice provider, pharmacist, blood bank specialist/pathologist
  d. Interventions
    i. Monitor patient for signs of infection: Inspect skin, mucous membranes, IV sites, incisions

    ii. Analyze WBC and differential for leukocytosis and leukopenia with granulocytopenia

   iii. Collect cultures, monitor results, and notify provider of results

   iv. Monitor and promote optimal fluid and nutritional intake

    v. Promote handwashing for all individuals with patient contact

   vi. Promote activity by assisting with ambulation, coughing, deep breathing

  vii. Prevent patient contact with anyone who has a communicable/infectious disease

 viii. Provide private room and promote neutropenic precautions according to facility protocol if ordered

   ix. Discontinue lines, tubes, and drains as soon as possible

SPECIFIC PATIENT HEALTH PROBLEMS

THROMBOCYTOPENIA

1. **Pathophysiology**
   a. Thrombocytopenia is defined as a platelet count less than 150,000/μL. A low platelet count increases the risk of bleeding, and a platelet count of less than 20,000 to 50,000/μL can lead to spontaneous bleeding.
   b. Capillary fragility and petechiae also develop when there are not enough platelets to nurture the vascular endothelium.
   c. Thrombocytopenia is commonly seen in acutely and critically ill patients and is associated with increased mortality.
2. **Etiology and risk factors**
   a. Decreased platelet production
      i. Bone marrow infiltration with malignant cells (e.g., leukemia, multiple myeloma, malignant metastases)
      ii. Current or recent treatment with antineoplastic agents
      iii. History of radiation therapy to the bones and marrow in which blood cells are made
   b. Increased platelet destruction
      i. DIC: See Disseminated Intravascular Coagulation section
      ii. Antibody mediated
         (a) Immune thrombocytopenic purpura (ITP)
            (1) Autoimmune disorder results in platelet destruction by antibodies. Autoantibodies bind to platelet glycoproteins. The platelets are then removed by the spleen leading to thrombocytopenia, bleeding, and splenomegaly.
            (2) Associated with acquired immunodeficiency syndrome (AIDS), systemic lupus erythematosus, and other diseases and medications
         (b) Heparin-induced thrombocytopenia (HIT) and thrombosis
            (1) HIT is an immune-mediated reaction to heparin
            (2) Although approximately 10% of patients experience mild thrombocytopenia while receiving heparin, 1% to 5% experience a more serious form.
            (3) In HIT, heparin forms a complex with platelet factor 4, a substance released by active platelets. The resulting complex expresses a new antigen. This stimulates the production of immunoglobulin (Ig) G antibodies, which then form immune complexes. These attach to and activate the remaining platelets, leading to thrombosis.

> **KEY CONCEPT**
> Patients who receive heparin or have received it within the past 2 weeks should be monitored for signs of HIT: Severe thrombocytopenia and clinical evidence of thromboembolism.

         (4) Patients may develop major thromboembolic events, including limb ischemia and pulmonary emboli (PE).

         (5) Monitoring platelets for a drop of more than 50% from baseline even if still above the normal of 150,000

         (6) When HIT is suspected, all heparin is stopped, and confirmatory testing for heparin antibodies is performed

         (7) Treatment includes administration of nonheparin anticoagulants (e.g., argatroban or bivalirudin)

      (c) Alloimmunization after multiple platelet transfusions

    iii. Thrombotic thrombocytopenic purpura (TTP) is an acute form of thrombocytopenia that is related to deficiency of a plasma enzyme. It leads to excessive platelet aggregation and clots that consist mainly of platelets. Patients often have severe thrombocytopenia less than 20,000/µL and may develop organ ischemia.

    iv. Hemolytic uremic syndrome (HUS) is an acute condition that results from bacterial toxins entering the blood. It is associated with infectious colitis caused by specific strains of organisms, such as *E. coli* O151:H7. The toxin enters the blood and is deposited in the glomeruli. Platelets and RBCs are damaged as they circulate through the inflamed capillaries leading to thrombocytopenia and hemolytic anemia.

    v. Sepsis

    vi. Mechanical injury of platelets because of prosthetic heart valve

  c. Sequestration of platelets in the spleen (e.g., with liver disease and portal hypertension)

3. Signs and symptoms

  a. Signs: Petechiae, purpura, ecchymosis, epistaxis; oozing of blood from venipuncture sites, conjunctival bleeding; bleeding from the oropharynx, GI tract, or genitourinary tract; splenomegaly

4. Diagnostic study findings

  a. Laboratory

    i. Blood

      (a) Platelet count less than 50,000/µL

      (b) Additional platelet studies including platelet antibodies are done to diagnose specific disorders, such as HIT.

    ii. Urine: Can test positive for blood

    iii. Stool: Can test positive for blood

  b. Radiologic: Spleen ultrasonography or liver-spleen scan

  c. Bone marrow biopsy to determine whether adequate numbers of platelets are being made in the bone marrow

5. Interprofessional collaboration: Nurse, physician (including a hematologist/ oncologist), advanced practice provider, blood bank specialist/pathologist

6. Management of patient care

  a. Goals of care

    i. Absence of bleeding, ecchymosis, epistaxis

    ii. Prevention of injury

   b. Interventions
     i. Identify and treat the cause of thrombocytopenia
     ii. Platelet transfusion may be considered for patients with active bleeding or potential for hemorrhage to maintain a platelet count of greater than 50,000/μL. The American Association of Blood Banks (AABB) guidelines for platelet transfusion include specific recommendations for patients undergoing invasive procedures or surgery (Kaufman et al., 2015).
     iii. Desmopressin (DDAVP) may be prescribed to enhance platelet function.
     iv. Intravenous immune globulin (IVIG) and glucocorticoids may be prescribed for patients with thrombocytopenia related to immune reaction.
     v. Prevent trauma to skin and mucous membranes; limit use of automatic blood pressure cuffs, use only low suction on mucous membranes
   c. Potential complications
     i. Bleeding following trauma of procedures, surgery
     ii. Thromboembolism with HIT and TTP
   d. Additional nursing considerations
     i. Patients who receive platelet inhibiting medications (e.g., aspirin, clopidogrel) may have adequate numbers of platelets, but they may not be functional, so the risk of bleeding is increased.

DISSEMINATED INTRAVASCULAR COAGULATION

1. **Pathophysiology**
   a. DIC is a unique coagulopathy characterized by both intravascular clotting and bleeding; it is always secondary to another pathologic process.
     i. The multiple disorders that are associated with DIC are thought to damage the vascular endothelium, releasing inflammatory cytokines and initiating coagulation.
     ii. This results in the generation of thrombin and systemic formation of fibrin clots, which are deposited in the microvasculature.
     iii. Small blood vessel occlusion results in tissue and organ ischemia; the process continues as the natural inhibitors of coagulation are overwhelmed.
     iv. Available platelets and clotting factors are eventually depleted, resulting in uncontrolled hemorrhage.
   b. The process results in clots forming where they are not needed (in the microvasculature) and inability to form a stable clot at a bleeding site.
   c. The DIC process also includes abnormal fibrinolysis that leads to release of fibrin degradation products and D-dimers, increasing the potential for more bleeding.
     i. Plasma D-dimer is formed from breakdown of activated coagulation factors and clots.
     ii. Elevated levels of D-dimer in the blood is indicative of thromboembolism. Levels can also be elevated after surgery or injury and may not be accurate in the critically ill.
   d. Diagnosis of DIC in patients with liver failure is challenging because of baseline coagulation panel abnormalities and potential for bleeding.

2. **Etiology and risk factors**
   a. Acute infection, sepsis, and septic shock
   b. Major trauma and extensive surgery, including traumatic brain injury
   c. Obstetric complications, such as abruptio placenta, amniotic fluid embolus
   d. Metastatic cancer; leukemia and solid tumors
   e. Immunologic conditions, transfusion reactions

3. **Signs and symptoms**
   a. Clinical manifestations vary but can be dramatic with a sudden onset of bleeding.
   b. Signs: Occurrence of spontaneous bleeding for no obvious reason, a preceding or concurrent pathologic process that is known to precipitate DIC, petechiae, purpura, ecchymoses, hematomas, epistaxis, and spontaneous or uncontrollable hemorrhage from multiple unrelated sites (e.g., sites of venipuncture, tubes, drains, lines, incisions, and wounds); kidney and other organ dysfunction because of tissue ischemia

---

EXPERT TIP

In a patient with bleeding from multiple sites, a coagulopathy, such as DIC should be suspected.

---

4. **Diagnostic study findings**
   a. Blood
      i. DIC cannot be diagnosed by a single test; a coagulation panel is needed.
      ii. Prolonged international normalized ratio (INR), prolonged partial thromboplastin time (PTT), decreased fibrinogen level, decreased platelet count, increased level of fibrin degradation products and D-dimers
      iii. Thromboelastography (TEG) may be used to assess platelet function and fibrinolytic activity. This technique can be used at the point of care in the emergency department or intensive care unit (ICU) and can yield results faster than a coagulation panel. TEG measures the strength of bonds between platelets and fibrin. Results are displayed as a number and a graph which is indicative of clot formation and strength.
      iv. CBC to assess hemoglobin and hematocrit
   b. Radiologic: Findings are usually noncontributory except to identify the underlying pathologic process.
5. **Interprofessional collaboration: Nurse, physician (including a hematologist/ oncologist), advanced practice provider, pharmacist, blood bank specialist/ pathologist**
6. **Management of patient care**
   a. Goals of care
      i. Identification and treatment of the cause of DIC
      ii. Restoration of adequate tissue perfusion
      iii. Restoration of normal hemostasis and decreased bleeding
   b. Interventions
      i. Facilitate identification of and treatment for the patient's primary disorder
         (a) Halting the process that triggered DIC may prevent further activation of clotting and end the uncontrolled coagulopathy.
         (b) Patients may clinically improve when sepsis or other precipitating conditions are effectively managed.
      ii. Provide general critical care support; fluid volume management, hemodynamic support, support of ventilation and oxygenation
         (a) Hypotension, hypoxia, and acidosis can worsen coagulopathy
         (b) Intubation and mechanical ventilation may be necessary
      iii. Prevent hypothermia
         (a) Hypothermia can worsen coagulopathy as clotting factors are less active below normal body temperature
         (b) Warm patient environment and body surface with warming blanket
         (c) Use warmer and rapid infusion system during massive transfusion

  iv. Transfuse blood and blood components as prescribed (see Table 8.3)

   (a) Packed RBCs

   (b) Fresh frozen plasma

   (c) Cryoprecipitate

   (d) Platelet concentrate

  v. Administer vitamin K to enhance production of clotting components in the liver

  vi. Analyze serial coagulation panel results

  vii. Gently mobilize patient in bed and out of bed with adequate assistance to prevent trauma

  viii. Provide emotional support to patient and family

   (a) DIC in a critically ill patient is associated with high mortality

   (b) Provide information on interventions, laboratory indicators, and patient responses to therapy

 c. Potential complications

  i. Hypovolemic shock

   (a) Lack of clotting components and platelets creates bleeding that is difficult to control, depleting intravascular volume.

   (b) Management: Monitor the patient for a systolic blood pressure of less than 90 mm Hg, heart rate of over 100 beats/min, anxiety, unresponsiveness, diaphoresis, urine output of less than 0.5 mL/kg/h, platelet count of less than 50,000/μL, PTT of longer than 40 seconds, and visible uncontrolled bleeding; anticipate transfusion of blood and blood components

  ii. Multiple organ dysfunction syndrome

   (a) Microvascular thrombi cause tissue ischemia and necrosis in solid organs and peripheral circulation

  iii. Monitor for adverse reaction to transfusion therapy (Table 8.4)

   (a) Transfusion-associated acute lung injury (TRALI)

   (b) Transfusion-associated circulatory overload (TACO)

   (c) Transfusion-associated immune modulation (TRIM)

   (d) Acute febrile and other reactions

 d. Additional nursing considerations

  i. Patients with abnormal coagulation panel results but no clinical bleeding are generally not transfused.

  ii. Patients requiring surgery or invasive procedures may require transfusion to correct laboratory indicators of risk for bleeding.

  iii. As patients recover, serum plasmin helps break down microclots to restore tissue perfusion.

  iv. As patients recover, the liver replaces depleted clotting components, and the bone marrow replaces RBCs and platelets.

MEDICATION-INDUCED COAGULOPATHY

1. **Pathophysiology**

 a. Effective hemostasis depends on the availability of active platelets and adequate levels of procoagulant factors

  i. Antiplatelet agents limit the activation and multiple hemostatic functions of platelets, often for the life span of circulating platelets

  ii. Other anticoagulants limit production of key factors, such as prothrombin and subsequent activation of thrombin, a necessary step in blood clotting

 b. Therapeutic anticoagulation carries with it the risk for bleeding

TABLE 8.4	**Types of Blood Transfusion Reaction**			
Reaction	**Mechanism**	**Signs and Symptoms**	**Time of Occurrence**	**Treatment**
Febrile reaction, nonhemolytic (most common)	Sensitization to donor WBCs, platelets or plasma proteins	Fever (rise of 1° C), chills, flushing, nausea, vomiting	Immediately or up to 4 hours posttransfusion	Stop transfusion Continue normal saline Notify provider and blood bank Give acetaminophen as ordered
Allergic reaction	Recipient sensitivity (IgE antibodies) against donor plasma proteins	Hives, itching, flushing, rash, wheezing, angioedema. Anaphylaxis is possible.	Occurs immediately or up to 4 hours posttransfusion	Stop transfusion Continue normal saline Notify provider and blood bank Give antihistamine as ordered If signs resolve, transfusion may be restarted with physician order
Hemolytic	Transfusion of ABO- or Rh-incompatible blood; antibodies in recipient plasma attach to antigens on donor RBCs leading to hemolysis	Fever, chills, hypotension, chest pain, flank pain, tachypnea, tachycardia, shock or circulatory collapse, hemoglobinuria, DIC	Immediately or may occur up to 24 hours posttransfusion	Stop transfusion Continue normal saline Call Rapid Response if warranted Notify provider and blood bank immediately; provide supportive therapy to maintain blood pressure and urine output
Bacterial	Blood contaminated with organisms	High fever, chills, flushing, tachycardia, shock, DIC, renal failure	Within 30 minutes of the start of the transfusion	Stop transfusion. Notify provider and blood bank; give antibiotics, IV fluids, vasopressors
Transfusion associated circulatory overload (TACO)	Transfusion administered quicker than circulation can accommodate	Dyspnea, cough, crackles, pulmonary edema, tachycardia, hypertension	Anytime during the transfusion	Slow the transfusion Administer O_2 Obtain stat chest x-ray Provide frequent monitoring Administer diuretic as ordered
Transfusion-related acute lung injury (TRALI)	Reaction involving antibodies from donor and recipient WBC antigens	Severe respiratory distress, hypoxia, fever, cyanosis	Occurs immediately or up to 6 hours posttransfusion	Stop transfusion Call rapid response if warranted Notify provider and blood bank Administer O_2 Monitor closely, may require critical care management
Transfusion-related immune modulation (TRIM)	Immune response to transfusion where antibodies form against antigens in the transfused blood	Decreased lymphocytes and immune function; antibodies that can make future transfusion or organ donation difficult	Initial: Decreased lymphocytes; Late: Formation of antibodies	Monitor for signs of infection; continue to restrict transfusion therapy

DIC, Disseminated intravascular coagulation; *Ig*, immunoglobulin; *IV*, intravenous; *RBC*, red blood cell; *WBC*, white blood cell.
Modified from Lewis, S.L., Dirksen, S.R., Heitkemper, M.M., et al. (2017). *Medical-surgical nursing*, 10th ed. St. Louis, Elsevier.

Hematologic and
Immunologic Systems

8

TABLE 8.5 **Antithrombotic Medications**

Medication	Mechanism of Action	Reversal
Abciximab (Reopro)	Glycoprotein IIb/IIIa receptor blocker	Platelet transfusion
Alteplase (tPA)	Thrombolytic (Fibrinolytic)	No specific reversal agent
Apixaban (Eliquis)	Direct Xa inhibitor	Andexanet alpha (ANDEXXA)
Argatroban	Direct thrombin inhibitor	No specific reversal agent
Aspirin	Irreversible inhibitor of cyclooxygenase	Platelets, consider use of desmopressin
Bivalirudin (Angiomax)	Direct thrombin inhibitor	FFP, cryoprecipitate, FVIIa
Clopidogrel (Plavix)	Inhibition of ADP-P2Y12 receptors on platelets	Platelet transfusion
Dabigatran (Pradaxa)	Direct thrombin inhibitor	Idarucizumab (Praxbind)
Eptifibatide (Integrilin)	Glycoprotein IIb/IIIa receptor blocker	Platelets
Fondaparinux (Arixtra)	Inhibition of Xa	No specific reversal agent
Heparin (unfractionated)	Xa and thrombin inhibition	Protamine
Low-molecular-weight heparin	Same as unfractionated heparin; mainly Xa effect	Protamine
Rivaroxaban (Xarelto)	Direct anti-Xa inhibitor	Andexanet alpha (ANDEXXA)
Warfarin (Coumadin)	Vitamin K antagonist	IV vitamin K, PCC, FFP

FFP, Fresh frozen plasma; *PCC*, prothrombin complex concentrate, *tPA*, tissue plasminogen.
From Good, V.S., Kirkwood, P.L. (2018). *Advanced critical care nursing*, 2nd ed. St. Louis, Elsevier.

    i. An increasing number of patients receive anticoagulant medications during hospitalization and as outpatients (Table 8.5)

    ii. Common reasons for anticoagulation include atrial fibrillation, prosthetic heart valves, and prevention/treatment of thromboembolic events

      (a) In patients receiving anticoagulants, excessive bleeding may result from traumatic events, such as a fall or surgery

      (b) Excessive bleeding may occur from known or unknown disorders, such as peptic ulcer disease

    iii. Current practice guidelines recommend anticoagulation for most hospitalized patients unless there is a contraindication, increasing the number of patients at risk of bleeding (see guidelines for hospitalized patients from the American Society of Hematology; Schunemann et al., 2018).

      (a) Excessive bleeding may occur during and following invasive procedures or surgery

      (b) Cardiovascular procedures including coronary angioplasty, percutaneous coronary interventions, and heart surgery use IV anticoagulants during the procedure

  c. Nurses need to be aware of the many classes of medications that have anticoagulant or antiplatelet effects and collaborate with providers to limit the associated risks.

2. Etiology and risk factors

  a. Anticoagulant or antiplatelet agents

  b. Advanced age

  c. Risk for falls and other trauma

  d. Invasive procedure or surgery

3. Signs and symptoms

  a. Prolonged bleeding from incisions and puncture sites; purpura, ecchymoses, hematomas, epistaxis, spontaneous and/or uncontrollable hemorrhage from sites, such as venipuncture, tubes, drains, lines, incisions, and wounds; bleeding from the GI tract

b. New onset of pain in the abdomen, joints, or other sites may indicate occult bleeding

4. **Diagnostic findings**
   a. Blood
      i. INR, PTT, platelet count, and other tests of coagulation may be abnormal
      ii. CBC may show low hemoglobin and hematocrit
   b. Radiologic
      i. X-rays may be performed to look for collections of blood, such as hemothorax
      ii. Computed tomography (CT) scans may reveal collection of blood, such as CT of the abdomen to assess for retroperitoneal hematoma, CT of the head to assess for cerebral bleeding

5. **Interprofessional collaboration: Nurse, physician (including a hematologist), advanced practice provider, pharmacist, blood bank specialist/pathologist**

6. **Management of patient care**
   a. Goals of care
      i. Identify patients at risk of bleeding complications
      ii. Early recognition and control of bleeding
      iii. Prevention of hypovolemic shock, severe anemia, and tissue/organ ischemia and damage
   b. Interventions
      i. Monitor CBC and coagulation profiles
      ii. Carefully review medication records daily to identify anticoagulant and antiplatelet medications and the need to adjust medication dosages and use

> **EXPERT TIP**
> During hospitalization, acute and critical care nurses need to continually assess patients receiving anticoagulants as treatments (e.g., atrial fibrillation, dialysis, extracorporeal membrane oxygenation), changes in other medications, and changes in diet can increase the risk of bleeding.

      iii. Notify provider of overt or suspected bleeding
      iv. Be prepared to reverse anticoagulation with appropriate agents or blood components
         (a) Use of protamine to reverse heparin
         (b) Use of vitamin K, fresh frozen plasma, or prothrombin complex concentrate to reverse warfarin (see Table 8.5)
   c. Potential complications
      i. Hypovolemic shock
      ii. Anemia
      iii. Tissue and organ ischemia and damage
   d. Additional nursing considerations
      i. Educate patients and families about medication actions, doses, and recommended monitoring
      ii. Educate patients and families about how to incorporate bleeding precautions for patients during hospitalization and following discharge

THROMBOEMBOLIC DISORDERS

1. **Pathophysiology**
   a. Hypercoagulable disorders, such as deep venous thrombosis (DVT) and PE occur when the normal mechanisms of hemostasis are stimulated to form thrombi that can occlude blood vessels.

b. Venous thrombosis most commonly occurs within the deep veins of the legs. The clots may or may not cause clear signs and symptoms. As fibrinolysis occurs, the clots break down and can break off. Now emboli, they then follow the flow of blood from the leg veins into the larger inferior vena cava and into the right side of the heart. As the clots flow into the pulmonary vasculature, the vessels narrow and the clots lodge into branches of the pulmonary vessels, leading to infarction of a section or sections of the lung. These PE can be small, large, single, or multiple.

2. **Etiology and risk factors**
   a. Venous stasis caused by bed rest, immobility, venous obstruction, indwelling IV catheters
   b. Hypercoagulability caused by recent surgery, pregnancy, cancer, genetic factors
   c. Vascular trauma caused by surgery or traumatic injury

3. **Signs and symptoms**
   a. Symptoms: Leg tenderness or pain with palpation or movement
   b. Signs: DVT: Sudden painful swelling of one extremity, circumference of one extremity different from that of the other corresponding extremity; fever; PE: Acute onset of dyspnea, tachycardia, chest pain, shock.

> **KEY CONCEPT**
> Some patients do not have obvious clinical manifestations of developing DVT and PE. Subtle signs, such as unilateral leg edema or unexplained tachycardia should be investigated.

4. **Diagnostic study findings**
   a. Laboratory
      i. D-dimer may be done as screening test to determine whether clots have formed and are breaking down through fibrinolysis
      ii. Coagulation values, such as INR, PTT, and CBC may be performed in anticipation of anticoagulation therapy
   b. Radiologic
      i. Ultrasound studies of the lower extremities to identify DVT
      ii. Ventilation-perfusion lung scan to identify probability of PE
      iii. Rapid CT scan of the chest to identify and quantify PE

5. **Interprofessional collaboration: Nurse, physician, advanced practice provider, pharmacist, radiologist**

6. **Management of patient care**
   a. Goals of care
      i. Prevention of additional thrombi and PE
      ii. Stable cardiopulmonary status
      iii. Optimal anticoagulation regimen
      iv. Prevention of ongoing and future thromboembolic events
   b. Interventions
      i. Use ESC Guidelines (Konstantinies & Meyer, 2019) for managing patients with DVT and PE.
      ii. With life-threatening PE, thrombolytic therapy or pulmonary embolectomy may be considered.
      iii. Anticoagulation is instituted with heparin, low-molecular-weight heparin, or oral anticoagulants, such as rivaroxaban.
      iv. In patient with DVT, the patient is placed on bed rest and the entire leg is elevated.

    v. As leg inflammation resolves, ambulation is permitted.

    vi. Anticoagulation with oral agents is continued on an outpatient basis.

  c. Potential complications

    i. Respiratory failure because of decreased lung perfusion from pulmonary infarcts

    ii. Right heart failure and cardiopulmonary collapse because of high pulmonary vascular resistance from pulmonary infarcts

    iii. Chronic venous insufficiency because of destruction of vein valves in leg affected by clots

  d. Additional nursing considerations

    i. Prevention of venous thromboembolism is a major goal of care for hospitalized patients

    ii. Prevention strategies recommended by guidelines from the American Society of Hematology (Schünemann, 2018) include:

      (a) Early ambulation after surgery, childbirth

      (b) Leg exercises to increase venous flow

      (c) Pneumatic compression devices

      (d) Prophylactic anticoagulation

ANEMIA

1. Pathophysiology

  a. Anemia is a reduction in the number of RBCs, the quantity of hemoglobin, or the volume of RBCs.

    i. Anemia results in varying degrees of hypoxia.

    ii. The compensatory response for anemia includes increasing cardiac output and respiratory rate, redistribution of blood to sustain blood supply to the brain and heart through a reduction in blood supply to the skin, bowels, and kidneys, and increasing the kidney's production of erythropoietin to stimulate erythropoiesis.

  b. Acute blood loss from trauma, surgery, or disruption of a major blood vessel dramatically changes the body's hemodynamic status and necessitates emergency intervention. With chronic blood loss occurring over weeks or months, such as in slow GI bleeding or menorrhagia, the body has time to compensate, and thus the symptoms of chronic blood loss may be more insidious.

2. Etiology and risk factors

  a. Inadequate RBC production

    i. Iron deficiency, folate and vitamin B_{12} deficiency

    ii. Chronic kidney disease

    iii. Bone marrow suppression from antineoplastic chemotherapy

    iv. Bone marrow infiltration with malignant cells

    v. History of radiation therapy to bones where blood cells are made

    vi. Hematopoietic stem cell transplantation

    vii. Aplastic anemia

    viii. Certain medications (e.g., zidovudine)

  b. Increased RBC destruction

    i. Hemolytic anemias

      (a) Immune destruction of RBCs, including transfusion reaction

      (b) Splenic destruction

      (c) Damage by artificial heart valve, cardiopulmonary bypass

      (d) Inherited disorders (e.g., sickle cell disease)

    ii. RBC membrane defects (e.g., hereditary spherocytosis)

    c. Acute or chronic blood loss
        i. Trauma, surgery
        ii. Coagulopathy
        iii. Complication of anticoagulation
        iv. Active or slow GI bleeding
        v. Frequent diagnostic blood draws

3. Signs and symptoms
    a. Symptoms: Fatigue, dyspnea, activity intolerance; altered mental status, headache
    b. Signs: Pallor, possible jaundice; possible hepatosplenomegaly with liver disease and some types of malignant disease, tenderness of the liver and spleen with palpation and percussion; tachycardia, hypotension, and orthostatic changes in vital signs, syncope
    c. Clinical manifestations above may not be present until the hemoglobin level is at or below 7 g/dL

> **EXPERT TIP**
> The clinical manifestations of anemia vary depending on the severity and whether the loss of RBCs is acute or chronic.

4. Diagnostic study findings
    a. Laboratory
        i. Blood
           (a) Hemoglobin level of less than 12 g/dL in women and less than 14 g/dL in men
           (b) Other findings vary with the cause of anemia and can include increased reticulocyte count, decreased serum iron level, increased or decreased total iron-binding capacity, decreased ferritin level, increased indirect bilirubin level, positive Coombs' test result
        ii. Urine: Can test positive for blood
        iii. Stool: Can test positive for blood
    b. Radiologic: GI studies may be obtained to detect the source of bleeding
    c. Biopsy: Bone marrow biopsy may be performed to evaluate bone marrow production of RBCs or detect the presence of bone marrow infiltration with malignant cells
    d. Endoscopy: To detect the source of bleeding

5. Interprofessional collaboration: Nurse, physician, advanced practice provider, pharmacist, blood bank specialist/pathologist

6. Management of patient care
    a. Goals of care
        i. Improved oxygen delivery to tissues and organs
        ii. Absence of hypovolemia because of bleeding
        iii. Tolerable level of fatigue
    b. Interventions
        i. Administer supplemental oxygen for SpO_2 less than 92%. Elevate head of bed for shortness of breath.
        ii. Frequently assess vital signs, oxygenation, and indicators of active bleeding.
        iii. Assess patient's ability to tolerate anemia by evaluating vital signs, oxygen, and subjective patient data before and after activity.

iv. Use the guidelines from the AABB (Carson et al., 2016) to determine whether transfusion is indicated. Consider transfusion of RBCs in patients who are symptomatic with hypotension, shortness of breath, tachycardia, and so on.

(a) Patient care during transfusion:

(1) Pretransfusion: Correctly identify patient and verify blood product per hospital policy; check for adequate IV status; obtain vital signs immediately before initiation; start transfusion

(2) Intratransfusion: Continue to monitor vital signs according to blood bank policy; document data as indicated

(3) Posttransfusion: Obtain vital signs, finalize blood bank charting

(4) Leukocyte depleted red blood cell transfusions may be requested in instances for patients who have had prior transfusion reaction, are immunocompromised, or who may require chronic transfusions as in sickle cell disease.

(b) Transfusion reactions (see Table 8.4)

(1) TRALI

(2) TACO

(3) TRIM

(4) Acute febrile and other reactions

> **KEY CONCEPT**
>
> According to the AABB guidelines, patients who have moderate to severe signs and symptoms of anemia should be considered for transfusion of RBCs.

v. Consider transfusion in patients with active bleeding and those requiring surgery or invasive procedures

vi. Provide adequate period of rest between cares and activities

vii. Provide diet or supplements with iron, vitamin B_{12}, and folate. IV iron sucrose may provide needed iron more quickly.

viii. Administer recombinant erythropoietin to stimulate bone marrow production of RBCs

ix. Involve patient and family in decisions regarding treatment of anemia

x. Provide education on taking oral iron preparations with food to prevent peptic ulcers and on managing GI distress including nausea, heartburn, constipation, or diarrhea because of the supplement

c. Potential complications

i. Hemorrhagic shock

(a) Control active bleeding with local pressure and other measures

(b) Provide volume replacement for hypovolemia

(c) Transfusion of packed RBCs may be required

(d) Surgery or interventional radiology procedure may be required

ii. Respiratory failure

(a) Risk because of diminished oxygen-carrying capacity

(b) Place the patient in a position of comfort to ease the work of breathing; oxygen administration and transfusion of packed RBCs may be required

iii. Weakness and fatigue

(a) Inadequate circulating hemoglobin decreases oxygen availability to cells, creating decreased energy stores in the body

    (b) Conserve the patient's energy by assisting with nutrition and the activities of daily living, passive range-of-motion exercises; provide supplemental oxygen if indicated when the patient is out of bed to a chair or is ambulating

  d. Additional nursing considerations for patient receiving blood transfusions

    i. Blood should be infused through a large-bore needle or catheter

    ii. IV solutions other than normal saline will cause hemolysis of RBCs

    iii. Blood is run through standard blood tubing with a filter

    iv. Medications should not be added to the blood infusion

    v. Blood products are double checked with another licensed provider

    vi. The patient is assessed before starting the blood transfusion and frequently during the procedure according to facility protocol

    vii. The patient is observed for adverse reactions (see Table 8.4)

    viii. Premedication with an antihistamine and acetaminophen may be prescribed to prevent a mild hypersensitivity or febrile reaction

    ix. If an adverse reaction is observed during the transfusion, the blood is stopped and the problem reported to the provider and the blood bank

    x. Blood should be infused within 4 hours

    xi. For patients receiving multiple units of blood and components, there are additional considerations

      (a) Packed RBCs may be warmed using a blood warming device to prevent hypothermia and coagulopathy

      (b) IV calcium may be indicated as the citrate added to banked blood may lead to hypocalcemia

SICKLE CELL ANEMIA

1. **Pathophysiology**

  a. Sickle cell anemia is an inherited hemolytic anemia. Abnormal hemoglobin known as hemoglobin S (HbS) is produced instead of hemoglobin A. This results in chronic anemia and multiple clinical manifestations because of the sickling and breakdown of RBCs.

  b. Sickling of the cells may be triggered by illness, infection, cold, hypoxia, acidosis, dehydration, and other stressors

    i. The abnormally rigid RBC membranes burst, leading to hemolysis and hemolytic anemia

    ii. The sickled cells also form clots which lead to blood vessel occlusion

  c. The trait is the result of a point mutation in the β chain of the hemoglobin molecule, where the amino acid valine is substituted for glutamic acid

  d. Those that are homozygous with two genes for HbS are likely to have *sickle cell disease* and major clinical manifestations

  e. Those that are heterozygous with one HbS gene are likely to have *sickle cell trait*, a condition associated with less sickling and fewer manifestations

2. **Etiology and risk factors**

  a. Patients with sickle cell trait commonly identify themselves as African Americans

  b. Exposure to stressors which precipitate increased clinical manifestations and a sickle cell crisis

3. **Signs and symptoms**

  a. Clinical manifestations of sickle cell anemia result in hemolytic anemia, hyperbilirubinemia, and syndromes known as *sickle cell crisis*

  b. Blood vessel occlusion by sickled cells is common and can be precipitated by stressors. This leads to acute, severe pain in the abdomen, chest, bones, and joints.

The sickled cells can infarct vessels which supply the liver, spleen, kidneys, and other organs. The crisis typically lasts between 4 and 6 days.

   c. An aplastic crisis occurs when the patient does not have enough RBCs and becomes severely anemic. This problem develops because of the short half-life of RBCs (10–20 days rather than 120). Sickled cells may also be sequestered in the spleen.

4. Diagnostic study findings

   a. The disease is usually detected by screening of newborns

   b. Hemoglobin S is identified

      i. Treatment for patients with sickle cell anemia includes rest, hydration, supplemental oxygen, analgesia, and antibiotic therapy or blood transfusion as needed

5. Interprofessional collaboration: Nurse, physician/hematologist, advanced practice provider, pharmacist, social worker, psychologist, psychiatrist

6. Management of patient care

   a. Goals of care

      i. Prevention of sickling episodes and crises

      ii. Acceptable hemoglobin levels

      iii. Maintenance of vital organ function

   b. Interventions

      i. Educate patient and family regarding avoidance of situations that can lead to sickling episodes, such as severe physical exertion and cold.

      ii. Educate patient regarding individualized plan to manage symptoms, such as pain.

      iii. Administer hydroxyurea to decrease sickling and prevent crises.

      iv. Administer anticoagulants to decrease incidence of clotting.

      v. Administer blood transfusions as ordered to restore oxygen-carrying capacity.

      vi. During a sickle cell crisis, provide hydration and supplemental oxygen.

      vii. During a crisis, administer opioids, NSAIDs, and topical anesthetic patches for maximal effectiveness.

      viii. Assist patient with information on stem cell transplant as a treatment option when indicated.

EXPERT TIP

Pain management is challenging during a sickle cell crisis, as patients often have a tolerance to opioids and may require high doses. The use of end-tidal CO_2 monitoring enhances safe administration.

---

   c. Potential complications

      i. Sickle cell crisis with acute pain and vascular obstruction requiring hospitalization

      ii. Patients are admitted to ICU when ventilation, oxygenation, or hemodynamics are compromised

      iii. Acute chest syndrome with pulmonary infarction, severe chest pain, and possible respiratory failure require hospitalization and critical care management. Diagnostic criteria include: Fever and/or respiratory symptoms, accompanied by a new pulmonary infiltrate on chest radiograph.

      iv. Injury to the spleen can occur over time as sickled cells are removed from the circulation. This process leads to ischemia, chronic damage, and eventual immunosuppression.

      v. Iron overload may occur because of chronic transfusion therapy.

NEUTROPENIA

1. **Pathophysiology**
   a. Neutropenia is defined as an absolute neutrophil count of less than 1000 cells/μL. The calculation for ANC = segs + bands = WBC divided by 100. A low number of neutrophils puts the patient at increased risk of infection. The longer the patient is neutropenic, the greater the chance of infection. Patients are often admitted to critical care units with a diagnosis, such as sepsis or acute leukemia that is complicated by neutropenia.
   b. Common sites of infection seen in neutropenic patients are the lung (pneumonia), blood (sepsis), skin, urinary tract, and GI tract (mucositis, esophagitis, perirectal lesions). Major gram-positive infections include *Staphylococcus epidermis*, *Staphylococcus aureus*, and streptococci. Gram-negative infections are less common, but infection with organisms, such as *Pseudomonas aeruginosa* can be very serious. Patients with neutropenia may also develop fungal infections including *Candida* and *Aspergillus*, and viral infections including reactivation of *Herpes simplex* 1 and 2 and cytomegalovirus (CMV). Because affected patients do not have adequate numbers of WBCs to mount an immunologic response, the classical signs of infection may be absent. Fever may be the only sign of infection, leading to a diagnosis of *neutropenic fever*.

2. **Etiology and risk factors**
   a. Decreased neutrophil production
      i. Bone marrow infiltration with malignant cells
      ii. Recent history of antineoplastic chemotherapy, especially if high-dose chemotherapy was administered as part of bone marrow transplantation
      iii. History of radiation therapy to bone marrow
      iv. Use of certain medications (e.g., zidovudine, clozapine)
      v. Autoimmune disorder (e.g., systemic lupus erythematosus, rheumatoid arthritis)
   b. Increased neutrophil use: Overwhelming sepsis, viral infection

3. **Signs and symptoms**
   a. Symptoms: Malaise; fever, chills, and night sweats; sore throat; dyspnea; shortness of breath; abdominal pain, sinus pain, headache; confusion; pain with swallowing, urination, or defecation
   b. Signs: Cough, crackles, diarrhea, temperature exceeding 38° C (100.4° F) or fever may not be present, tachycardia, hypotension, loss of integrity of skin and mucous membranes (especially at IV and central venous catheter sites), lymphadenopathy

4. **Diagnostic study findings**
   a. Laboratory: ANC lower than 500/μL
   b. Radiologic: Chest x-ray may show pulmonary infiltrates indicative of infection
   c. Bone marrow biopsy may be done to determine cause

5. **Interprofessional collaboration: Nurse, physician (including oncologist or infectious disease specialist), advanced practice provider**

6. **Management of patient care**
   a. Goals of care
      i. Prevention of infection
      ii. Early detection and intervention to prevent sepsis
   b. Interventions
      i. Use guidelines from the American Society of Clinical Oncology (Tabplitz et al., 2018) to manage care.
      ii. Monitor patient for fever greater than 38° C (100.4° F), pain, and malaise; lack of neutrophils may prevent normal inflammatory response with pulmonary

infiltrates, purulent drainage as WBCs are major components of these signs. Fever may not be present; all signs and symptoms need to be considered.

   iii. Perform cultures of sputum, throat, blood, lesions, wounds, and urine promptly

   iv. Administer prescribed antibiotics as soon as possible; mortality rate increases for patients with an ANC lower than 500/μL. The goal of therapy is to support the patient until his or her own WBCs are available to fight infection.

   v. Institute neutropenic precautions for patients with ANC less than 500/μL

   vi. Provide private room, preferably with high-efficiency particulate air (HEPA) filtration, and do not admit visitors or staff with signs or symptoms of infection

   vii. Assess daily WBC, differential, and ANC

   viii. Assess IV sites, skin for signs of infection

   ix. Monitor nutritional and fluid intake

   x. Administer granulocyte colony-stimulating factor (G-CSF or GM-CSF) to enhance bone marrow production of neutrophils and monocytes

  c. Potential complications

   i. Infection resulting in neutropenic fever

     (a) Administer prophylactic, empiric or therapeutic antibiotics as ordered

     (b) Antifungals may be added if indicated

ACUTE LEUKEMIA

1. **Pathophysiology**

  a. Leukemia is a malignancy that affects the blood, bone marrow, lymphatic system, and spleen. There are many different types of leukemia, each based on whether the disease is acute or chronic and the type of WBC involved. Acute myelogenous leukemia (AML) is a cancer of the myeloblasts, which are granulocyte precursors (see Fig. 8.1) affecting primarily adults. Acute lymphocytic leukemia (ALL) is a cancer of the lymphocyte cell line (see Fig. 8.1) affecting primarily children. Chronic myelogenous leukemia (CML) is a cancer of mature granulocytes, and chronic lymphocytic leukemia (CLL) is a cancer of the lymphocytes. The leukemic cells themselves are nonfunctional. They crowd out the normal bone marrow cells and thereby induce pancytopenia, manifested as anemia, neutropenia, and thrombocytopenia.

  b. Patients with leukemia are usually treated on oncology wards, but complications of leukemia, including overwhelming sepsis and acute tumor lysis syndrome, bring patients to critical care units

2. **Etiology and risk factors**

  a. Leukemia results when normal genes are transformed into oncogenes. This is often caused by a gene translocation that occurs within chromosomes. The mutant gene no longer codes for normal cell replication and maturation. Instead the cell can bypass normal signals which control cell growth and can continue to produce an unlimited number of mutated cells.

  b. Risk factors for leukemia include

   i. Exposure to certain chemicals (e.g., benzene)

   ii. Exposure to certain medications (e.g., chemotherapy agents)

   iii. Radiation exposure

   iv. Chromosomal abnormalities (e.g., Down syndrome)

3. **Signs and symptoms**

  a. Symptoms: Fatigue, malaise, bone pain, headache; reports of fever, chills, night sweats

b. Signs: Pallor, petechiae, easy bruising, weight loss, fever greater than 38°C (100.4°F), flushing, lethargy, purpura, ecchymosis, hematomas, possible lymphadenopathy possible hepatomegaly, possible splenomegaly

4. **Diagnostic study findings**
   a. Laboratory
      i. Total WBC count is very high, often more than100,000/μL, with primarily immature blast cells seen on the differential. The number of normal mature WBCs is generally very low.
      ii. Low RBC and platelet counts are usually also seen because these cell lines are also crowded out of the bone marrow by leukemic cells
      iii. Chromosome abnormalities and abnormal cell morphology are associated with the various types
   b. Bone marrow biopsy is usually performed to help with the diagnosis and guide treatment
5. **Interprofessional collaboration: Nurse, physician (oncologist), advanced practice provider, pharmacist, social worker, psychologist, psychiatrist**
6. **Management of patient care**
   a. Goals of care
      i. Protection against infections
      ii. Protection against injury from bleeding
      iii. Pain management
      iv. Adequate nutrition
   b. Interventions
      i. Interventions for acute leukemia depend on patient acuity, type of WBC affected, and the maturational pathway from which the abnormal cells arise. During the course of treatment to discharge, patients with leukemia may be expected to have the following needs:
         (a) Pain management is often needed for patients with acute leukemia. Expansion of the bone marrow leads to stretching of the periosteum and persistent pain in both ALL and AML.
         (b) Nutrition assessment and management; nausea, vomiting, and diarrhea may indicate a need to manage dietary intake with supplements
         (c) Prevention of infection; because infections can be caused by the patient's own endogenous flora, daily bathing and frequent oral examinations are essential
         (d) Provide education including information on prognosis, availability of leukemia support groups, and treatment protocol and share with the family and patient before discharge.
         (e) Patient and family may need education about induction therapy and additional stages of anticipated therapy including radiation and hematopoietic stem cell transplant (HSCT).
         (f) Social service support for the patient and family may be indicated when the patient's stay is prolonged (4–8 weeks) during induction or consolidation chemotherapy; provision of therapeutic distractions from pain, alopecia, nausea and vomiting, and fatigue can be challenging
   c. Potential complications
      i. Sepsis (see Ch. 10, Sepsis and Septic Shock)
         (a) The acute leukemias are initially treated with high-dose chemotherapy, called *induction therapy*, to induce bone marrow hypoplasia and allow normal cells to repopulate the bone marrow; the patient's ability to fight off infection is reduced until this repopulation is complete.

(b) Monitor for clinical manifestations of infection and sepsis, including persistent hypotension and hypoperfusion despite adequate fluid resuscitation and IV antibiotic therapy.

> **KEY CONCEPT**
>
> Fever is an important indicator of infection in patients with leukemia and low number of functional WBCs, as other signs of infection may not be present.

---

ii. Tumor lysis syndrome

(a) Tumor cell destruction during chemotherapy creates a metabolic imbalance with rapid serum uptake of intracellular potassium, phosphorus, and nucleic acids resulting in hyperuricemia, hyperkalemia, hyperphosphatemia, and possible acute kidney injury

(b) In anticipation of the possibility of acute tumor lysis syndrome, medical management should include aggressive IV hydration, alkalinization of the urine, and administration of an agent to lower uric acid (e.g., allopurinol, rasburicase) before chemotherapy is initiated. After chemotherapy is started, blood electrolyte levels should be monitored frequently and adjustments to the plan of care rapidly implemented as indicated. Hemodialysis may be necessary to prevent acute tumor lysis syndrome even with aggressive management.

MALIGNANT PERICARDIAL EFFUSION

1. **Pathophysiology**
   a. Fluid exceeding 50 mL inside the pericardial sac constitutes a pericardial effusion. The rate at which the fluid accumulates determines the stress and related consequences produced as a result of the pressure-volume relation (PVR). The PVR is a reflection of the compliance of the heart, normally of high compliance and low PVR. As fluid accumulates, the PVR increases until the relation steeps to a degree not tolerated and tamponade. A slow effusion accumulation can be tolerated without signs of tamponade whereas a rapid accumulation of less fluid would not.

2. **Etiology and risk factors**
   a. Pericardial effusions can be seen in a variety of disease processes including cardiac disease, infectious, oncologic, autoimmune, radiation, and drug-related. For the purposes of this chapter we will focus on oncologic processes.
   b. Specific etiology of pericardial effusions can be seen secondary to metastatic disease from lung or breast cancer, lymphomas, melanoma, Hodgkin disease, radiation therapy, and more rarely a primary cardiac malignancy.

3. **Signs and symptoms**
   a. Symptoms: Many effusions can be asymptomatic if accumulated slowly, otherwise, the patient may complain of chest pain, palpitations, abdominal pain, dyspnea, tachypnea, nausea, hiccups, fatigue
   b. Signs: Tachycardia, pulsus paradoxus, electrical alternans, muffled heart sounds, elevated jugular venous pressure, relief of chest pain when sitting forward, enlarged cardiac silhouette on chest radiograph, reduced/narrow blood pressure

4. **Diagnostic and study findings**
   a. Echocardiogram is the study of choice for evaluation of pericardial effusion. This may be the quickest resource. Chest CT and cardiac magnetic resonance imaging

are options in nonemergent settings and for more detailed evaluation, possibly for cardiac sources.

5. Interprofessional collaboration: Nurse, physician (oncologist, cardiology), advanced practice provider, radiologist

6. Management of patient care
   a. Goals of care
      i. Identify distress and tamponade immediately and prepare for pericardiocentesis
      ii. Continue telemetry, maintain normal sinus rhythm
      iii. Apply oxygen if needed
      iv. Adequate pain control
   b. Interventions
      i. Echocardiogram for evaluation of size of effusion and tamponade physiology
      ii. Pericardiocentesis if in cardiac tamponade
      iii. Oxygen, telemetry
      iv. Potential cardiology and oncology consults
      v. Screening for effusion etiology: past medical history may reveal potential cause, some asymptomatic effusions represent chronicity and may be idiopathic, further imaging may be needed for potential metastasis
   c. Potential complications
      i. Progression of cardiac tamponade physiology which can result in death if untreated

HEMATOPOIETIC STEM CELL TRANSPLANTATION

1. Pathophysiology
   a. Originally referred to as bone marrow transplantation, the treatment is now called HSCT, because advances have led to the ability to obtain stem cells from peripheral and umbilical cord blood, as well as the bone marrow. This procedure is performed to reconstitute the hematologic and immune systems after patients with malignancies receive dosages of chemotherapy and radiation therapy high enough to permanently kill the bone marrow. HSCT is also used in patients with aplastic anemia in an attempt to repopulate the marrow. Harvested marrow or peripheral stem cells are infused into the patient intravenously. Through their innate homing mechanism, the cells travel to the bone marrow and reestablish normal hematopoiesis.
   b. Types of transplant
      i. In allogeneic transplant, stem cells from a human leukocyte antigen (HLA)-matched donor are used. The donor is often a family member, but may also be an unrelated donor matched through a registry.
      ii. In autologous transplant, stem cells from the patient are harvested and preserved before chemotherapy is initiated; the harvested cells are infused after treatment. Using the patient's own cells eliminates the risk of rejection and graft-versus-host disease (GVHD).
      iii. Stem cells may be harvested through bone marrow aspiration in the operating room from a compatible donor with healthy bone marrow. Alternatively, peripheral stem cells are obtained by pheresis as an outpatient procedure. Autologous cells obtained from the patient with cancer may be treated to remove any cancer cells.
      iv. Stem cells are infused into the recipient intravenously where they repopulate the bone marrow over 2 to 4 weeks

2. **Etiology and risk factors**
   a. Inadequate formation of blood cells by the bone marrow results in a severe reduction of WBCs, RBCs, and platelets. Risk for these problems can be caused by disease processes, such as aplastic anemia or to treatments, such as cancer chemotherapy.
   b. Indicators for HSCT
      i. Treatment of malignancy with high doses of chemotherapy and radiation that are toxic to the bone marrow
      ii. Genetic defect (e.g., severe combined immunodeficiency disease)
      iii. Aplastic syndromes (e.g., aplastic anemia)
3. **Signs and symptoms during transplantation**
   a. Symptoms: Malaise, fatigue, weakness, lethargy, reports of chills and night sweats, sore throat, dyspnea, shortness of breath, sinus pain, headache, confusion; pain with swallowing, urination, or defecation
   b. Signs: Cough, crackles, diarrhea, temperature exceeding 38°C (100.4°F), pallor, jaundice, petechiae, rash, weight changes, loss of integrity of skin and mucous membranes; bleeding from the oropharynx, GI tract, or genitourinary tract; hepatomegaly, tachycardia, hypotension
4. **Diagnostic study findings**
   a. Laboratory
      i. Pancytopenia: WBC count, hemoglobin level, and platelet count all will be low because of pretransplant myeloablative therapy.
      ii. Renal function and electrolytes are monitored as the procedure and possible side effects affect fluid and electrolyte imbalance.
   b. Biopsy: Definitive diagnosis of the complications of HSCT often requires a bone marrow biopsy; however, biopsy may be contraindicated because of bleeding risk
5. **Interprofessional collaboration: Nurse, physician (oncologist, infectious disease specialist), advanced practice provider, pharmacist, social worker, psychologist, psychiatrist**
6. **Management of patient care**
   a. Goals of care
      i. Absence of infection
      ii. Absence of hemorrhage related to disease or treatment
      iii. Adequate renal function
      iv. Adequate pain management
   b. Interventions
      i. Provide education to patient and family related to the HSCT process and procedures and complications.
      ii. Use guidelines from the American Society for Transplantation and Cellular Therapy (DeFilipp et al., 2019) to direct patient management.
      iii. Monitor patient closely for complications of intensive chemotherapy or radiation therapy before the HSCT.
      iv. Monitor for complications of anemia, leukopenia, and thrombocytopenia.
      v. Avoid exposure to infection through the use of neutropenic precautions.
      vi. Support the patient with nutrition, fluids, and electrolytes.
      vii. Administer blood transfusions as directed.
   c. Potential oncologic complications
      i. Pancytopenia
         (a) Conditioning chemotherapy and radiation before HSCT obliterates the patient's own marrow

(b) Interventions are directed at side effects of conditioning therapy, including profound nausea and vomiting, mucositis, capillary leak syndrome, diarrhea, and bone marrow suppression

---

KEY CONCEPT

Complications which result in hemodynamic instability or respiratory failure will prompt admission to the ICU.

---

   ii. Failure to engraft
     (a) Failure of transfused peripheral stem cells and marrow cells to take up residence within the recipient's bones
     (b) May require repeat transfusion of stem cells to prevent certain death
  iii. GVHD
     (a) Immunocompetent T lymphocytes within the donated marrow or cells mount an immune response against the HLA antigens on the host cells
     (b) Tissues affected include the skin and GI tract (especially liver)
     (c) GVHD can become chronic and lead to death
     (d) Treatment includes administration of immunosuppressive medications (e.g., tacrolimus) to suppress the transplanted T lymphocytes and antiinflammatory medications (glucocorticoids) to suppress cytokines.
  iv. Venoocclusive disease
     (a) Occlusion of the hepatic circulation occurs from clotting and phlebitis
     (b) Management is mainly supportive with fluid resuscitation and assessment of increased girth, hepatomegaly, ascites, or weight gain
   v. Sepsis (see Ch. 10, Sepsis and Septic Shock)
     (a) Pancytopenia obliterates the patient's ability to fight off infection
     (b) Prophylactic use of the antifungal medications (e.g., fluconazole) decreases the incidence of *C. albicans* infection in HSCT patients; prophylactic treatment with antiviral medications (e.g., acyclovir, ganciclovir) can decrease the incidence of reactivation of herpes simplex virus and CMV in seropositive patients

ORGAN TRANSPLANT REJECTION

1. Pathophysiology
  a. When tissue from one person is transplanted into another, the immune system of the recipient recognizes the transplanted tissue, or allograft, as foreign. Rejection occurs through various adaptive immune mechanisms:
    i. *Hyperacute rejection* occurs immediately following transplant by the presence of antidonor antibodies existing in the recipient before transplantation. An antigen-antibody reaction takes place within the blood vessels of the transplanted organ, which leads to vascular occlusion and ischemia. This can result in acute failure of the transplanted organ in the operating room or early in the postoperative period. This type of rejection is rare.
    ii. *Acute cellular rejection* involves the cloning of small sensitized cytotoxic T lymphocytes (T_c) that directly attack the allograft, resulting in acute transplant rejection. It typically occurs during the first weeks and months after transplant and is usually reversible with immunosuppressive medications.
    iii. Chronic rejection is a slow immune-mediated process that is not well controlled with immunosuppressive medications. It can result in graft failure and the need

for another transplant (e.g., chronic rejection of a transplanted kidney will mean the patient has to go back on dialysis and may be considered for a second transplant).

b. Vital organs (kidney, liver, lung, heart) are first matched according to ABO blood group compatibility.

c. HLA matching of donor to recipient before transplantation is an attempt to choose a donor whose antigens match the recipient's as closely as possible so that the recipient's immune system is not triggered to attack the allograft after the transplantation procedure. This matching may be performed before kidney transplant but is often not practical for heart, lung, and other types of solid organ transplant.

d. A panel of reactive antibodies (PRA) test is done on transplant candidates to determine whether they have antibodies that will potentially react with donor HLA antigens, leading to hyperacute rejection. High levels of antibodies may develop because of previous blood transfusions, pregnancies, or previous transplants. For these patients, it is difficult to find a compatible donor. Candidates with a high PRA may receive treatment with a monoclonal antibody. Antibodies can also be removed through plasmapheresis treatments.

2. **Etiology and risk factors: Activation of the immune response against transplanted tissue**

3. **Signs and symptoms**
   a. Symptoms: Malaise, poor appetite, myalgia, tenderness of the allograft in abdominal organs
   b. Signs: Transplant organ dysfunction (e.g., low urine output and rising creatinine in kidney recipient)

4. **Diagnostic study findings: Specific to the organ transplanted**
   a. Tissue biopsy positive for pathologic changes (e.g., endomyocardial biopsy for heart transplant). Biopsy specimens will show infiltration of T lymphocytes and organ cell necrosis.
   b. Gene expression monitoring for indicators of rejection

5. **Interprofessional collaboration: Nurse, transplant medical team, transplant surgical team, pharmacist, social worker, psychologist, psychiatrist**

6. **Management of patient care**
   a. Goals of care
      i.   No evidence of transplant rejection
      ii. No evidence of active infection
      iii. No complications from immunosuppressive medication therapy
      iv. Optimal function of transplanted organ
   b. Interventions
      i. Administer immunosuppressive medications.
         (a) Intensive immunosuppression is required in the early postoperative period when the risk of rejection is highest.
         (b) Most patients receive two or three immunosuppressive medications (e.g., tacrolimus, mycophenolate mofetil, and glucocorticoids) to provide optimal coverage and avoid toxic doses of any one medication.
         (c) Monitoring of patients includes obtaining serum trough levels of some medications (e.g., tacrolimus), especially during periods of acute illness or addition/deletion of other medications.
         (d) Immunosuppressive medications are required for the rest of the patient's life to prevent graft failure associated with rejection.

> **EXPERT TIP**
> Assuring that immunosuppressive drug therapy is optimized is important, as excessive immunosuppression will lead to infection and inadequate immunosuppression will lead to rejection.

    ii. Monitor for complications of immunosuppressive medications

      (a) All increase the risk for infection

      (b) All are associated with major side effects including hypertension and renal damage

    iii. Monitor for signs of rejection (e.g., hypotension in a cardiac transplant patient)

    iv. Promote follow-up care with providers

      (a) Survival after transplant depends on following the medical regimen

      (b) Patients typically need social, economic, and psychologic support to deal with the challenges of organ transplantation

  c. Potential complications

    i. Opportunistic infection

      (a) Transplant recipients are at risk of infections that do not usually threaten immunocompetent people

      (b) Infection can rapidly progress because of their immunosuppressed state, so monitoring for infection by the patient and providers is essential

HUMAN IMMUNODEFICIENCY VIRUS INFECTION

1. **Pathophysiology**

  a. HIV infection usually progresses in phases over a period of 8 to 12 years. During the primary infection, the symptoms may be those of a mild virus. During the latent period there are usually no clinical manifestations. After years have gone by, overt AIDS occurs with an AIDS-defining illness and a CD4+ count less than 200 cells/μL.

    i. Infection with HIV can lead to the disease known as *AIDS*. Major manifestations include opportunistic infection, certain malignancies, wasting, and damage to the central nervous system.

    ii. HIV is a retrovirus that selectively infects lymphocytes known as T-helper cells or CD4+ cells, which are key cells responsible for the adaptive immune response. Like all viruses, it has to enter a body cell to reproduce.

    iii. As a retrovirus, the genetic information is carried in ribonucleic acid (RNA) rather than deoxyribonucleic acid (DNA). The virus uses the enzyme reverse transcriptase to create DNA that can change the host cell nucleus and begin production of more HIV. The newly produced virions then enter the circulation to infect more host cells.

    iv. Over time, the viral load in the blood increases and the number of CD4+ cells decreases.

  b. Disease course

    i. The initial stage of HIV infection lasts 4 to 8 weeks. High levels of virus are in the blood. The patient often experiences generalized flu-like symptoms.

    ii. The virus then enters a latent stage in which it is inactive in the infected resting CD4 cells, replicating only when the host cell is activated for an immune response. Levels of virus are high in the lymph nodes, where CD4 cells reside, but low in the blood. T_c cells, which express CD8 and so are not infected by HIV, and B cells attempt to destroy the CD4 cells harboring the virus. However, the T_c cells and B cells are crippled without adequate T helper (T_H) support.

This latent stage lasts on average between 2 and 12 years, during which time the patient is asymptomatic. During this time, the number of CD4 cells slowly declines.

iii. During the third stage of HIV infection, the patient begins to experience opportunistic infections. Levels of CD4 cells are usually below 500/mm³ and declining, whereas levels of virus in the blood are increasing. This stage can last 2 to 3 years.

iv. Once the CD4 cell levels drop below 200/mm³, the patient is considered to have AIDS. Virus levels in the blood are high. This stage ends in death, sometimes within 1 year.

2. **Etiology and risk factors**
   a. Intimate sexual contact with infected partners
   b. Black American race
   c. Male
   d. Intravenous medication use with contaminated needles
   e. Perinatal maternal to fetal transmission; breastfeeding
   f. Occupational exposure to blood and bodily fluids (this route of disease transmission is uncommon)

3. **Signs and symptoms**
   a. The Centers for Disease Control and Prevention (CDC) defines three clinical categories of HIV/AIDS. The stage is guided by CD4 counts after the stage of 0, which lasts for 6 months after initial diagnosis, and until patient develops opportunistic infection, which is stage 3.
      i. Clinical stage 1: Patient is asymptomatic or has persistent generalized lymphadenopathy.
      ii. Clinical stage 2: Patient has unexplained weight loss and certain infections including oral lesions, recurrent respiratory infections, and fungal nail infections.
      iii. Clinical stage 3: Includes illnesses that define AIDS, such as chronic diarrhea, persistent fever, opportunistic infections, such as *Pneumocystis carini or Pneumocystis jiroveci* pneumonia *(PCP), Mycobacterium tuberculosis*, and esophageal candidiasis; and malignancies, such as Kaposi sarcoma.

4. **Diagnostic study findings**
   a. Laboratory
      i. In an infected individual, blood testing becomes positive (seroconversion) after a period of time known as the *window period*. This is usually 1 to 3 months following the infection when antibodies to HIV have developed but can be years as the virus can be present in body fluids before antibodies develop.
      ii. Tests for HIV-1, the virus that causes AIDS in the United States
         (a) Enzyme-linked immunosorbent assay (ELISA) is a screening test for the antibody
         (b) Western blot test is performed to confirm diagnosis in a positive ELISA test
         (c) Viral nucleic acid test (NAT) quantifies viral load
      iii. The CDC defines three stages of infection based on CD4+ cell counts and time from diagnosis (Table 8.6)
      iv. Cultures positive for AIDS-defining infections (e.g., *P. jiroveci, M. tuberculosis*)
   b. Radiologic: Infiltrates on chest radiograph

5. **Interprofessional collaboration: Nurse, physician (infectious disease specialist), advanced practice provider, pharmacist, social worker, psychologist, psychiatrist**

6. **Management of patient care**

TABLE 8.6	**HIV Infection Stage, Based on Age-Specific CD4+ T-Lymphocyte Count or CD4+ T-Lymphocyte Percentage of Total Lymphocytes**		
Age on Date of CD4 T-Lymphocyte Test (Cells/μL [%])			
Stage	**<1 year**	**1–5 years**	**>6 years**
1	≥1500 (≥34%)	≥1000 (≥30)	≥500 (≥26)
2	750–1499 (26%–33%)	500–999 (22%–29%)	200–499 (14%–25%)
3	<750 (<26%)	<500 (<22%)	<200 (<14%)

The stage is based primarily on the CD4+ T-lymphocyte count; the CD4+ T-lymphocyte count takes precedence over the CD4 T-lymphocyte percentage, and the percentage is considered only if the count is missing.
From Centers for Disease Control and Prevention: Terms, definitions, and calculations used in CDC HIV surveillance publications. Available at https://www.cdc.gov/hiv/statistics/surveillance/terms.html.

a. Goals of care
  i. Early identification of HIV infection
  ii. Early identification and treatment of opportunistic infections
  iii. Patient and family education related to disease progression and standard precautions
b. Interventions
  i. Patient management is based on guideline recommendations from the National Institutes of Health and other national agencies (NIH guidelines, 2020; Department of Health and Human Services, 2019).
  ii. Treatment with HIV medications that interrupt the replication of the HIV virus. Consider risk versus benefit of early administration of antiretroviral medication.
  iii. Highly active antiretroviral therapy (HAART) often consists of three or four antiretroviral agents
  iv. Prophylactic agents may be prescribed to prevent bacterial, viral, and fungal infections based on residency area and CD4 counts
  v. Education to patient and family regarding recognition of signs and symptoms of infection
  vi. Education to patient and family regarding standard precautions
  vii. Nutritional counseling: Avoid fatty foods if chronic diarrhea is present, maintain good hydration, maintain high protein consumption, encourage consumption of foods that the patient likes, assess for oral lesion, maintain good oral hygiene
  viii. Psychosocial issues: AIDS is a progressive disease for which there is no cure. When indicated, palliative care should be addressed with the patient and family.
c. Potential complications
  i. Opportunistic infection
    (a) Respiratory infections with bacterial pneumonia, PCP, and pulmonary tuberculosis are common
    (b) Other common infections include CMV, toxoplasmosis, and fungal lung infections
    (c) GI distress may result from infection of the esophagus (e.g., candidiasis) or colon (e.g., CMV).
    (d) Diarrhea is common and may be caused by protozoal infection (e.g., *Cryptosporidium*).
  ii. Neurologic disorders
    (a) These are usually late complications that affect cognitive and motor function

(b) HIV-associated asymptomatic neurocognitive impairment

(c) HIV-associated dementia

iii. Malignancy

(a) There is increased incidence of malignancy because of impaired cellular immunity

(b) Common malignancies include Kaposi sarcoma, non-Hodgkin lymphoma, cervical and anal cancer

iv. Wasting syndrome

(a) Defined as involuntary loss of 10% of body weight

(b) Associated with diarrhea, chronic weakness, and fever

(c) Treatment may include nutritional supplements and enteral nutrition

v. Metabolic dysfunction associated with HAART

(a) Lipid disorders including lipodystrophy and hyperlipidemia

(b) Insulin resistance and diabetes

EXPERT TIP

Drug therapy for HIV often results in side effects. Nurses have a key role in helping patients manage these, especially the metabolic complications associated with protease inhibitors.

ANAPHYLACTIC REACTION

1. **Pathophysiology**
   a. Although there are a number of types of hypersensitivity reactions, an anaphylactic reaction is the most severe type of allergic reaction. It is an immune-mediated reaction with a rapid onset and dramatic clinical picture.
      i. Following exposure to an allergen, preexisting IgE antibodies stimulate mast cells to release histamine, a potent vasodilator. This leads to vasodilation with increased capillary permeability and generalized edema.
      ii. Cytokines released during the reaction also cause bronchospasm and laryngeal edema.
      iii. The exaggerated and systemic reaction can quickly lead to airway obstruction, pulmonary edema, hypovolemia, severe hypotension, shock, and cardiac arrest.
   b. The patient may have previously been exposed to the specific allergen (e.g., bee sting), stimulating the production of IgE antibodies.

2. **Etiology and risk factors**
   a. Medications (e.g., penicillin, local anesthetics, contrast dye)
   b. Insect stings (e.g., bees, wasps)
   c. Foods (e.g., shellfish, nuts)
   d. Latex

3. **Signs and symptoms**
   a. Early signs and symptoms: Apprehension, restlessness, chest tightness, warm sensation over the skin, erythema, itching, urticaria, abdominal pain
   b. Severe signs and symptoms: Dyspnea, wheezing, stridor, angioedema, hypotension, tachycardia, vomiting

4. **Diagnostic study findings: Usually noncontributory to the diagnosis of anaphylaxis; however, serum tryptase level is one laboratory level that can be drawn and is typically elevated in nonfood-induced anaphylaxis**

5. **Interprofessional collaboration: Nurse, physician, advanced practice provider, pharmacist, respiratory therapist**

6. **Management of patient care**

a. Goals of care
   i. Maintain patent airway
   ii. Maintain blood pressure and tissue perfusion
b. Interventions
   i. Interventions are based on the guidelines from World Allergy Organization (Simons et al., 2015)
   ii. Identify cause and remove it (e.g., stop infusion of medication)
   iii. Stop/slow absorption of allergen (e.g., apply ice to bee sting)
   iv. Early administration of epinephrine to dilate bronchioles, constrict blood vessels, and prevent circulatory collapse
   v. Administer oxygen, antihistamine, bronchodilator, glucocorticoid
   vi. Administer IV fluid to maintain vascular volume
   vii. Continuous telemetry and pulse oximetry monitoring
c. Potential complications
   i. Airway obstruction
   ii. Circulatory collapse and cardiac arrest
d. Additional nursing considerations
   i. Patient and family education regarding identification and avoidance of allergen, wearing medical alert bracelet
   ii. Education about emergency actions, use of an epinephrine pen
   iii. Referral to allergist for ongoing management

References and bibliography information are available at http://evolve.elsevier.com/AACN/corecurriculum/.

CHAPTER 9

Gastrointestinal System

Patricia Radovich, PhD, CNS, FCCM

SYSTEMWIDE ELEMENTS

ANATOMY AND PHYSIOLOGY REVIEW

1. **Upper gastrointestinal (GI) tract (Fig. 9.1)**
   a. Mouth and accessory organs; lips, gums, and teeth, and inner structures of the cheeks, tongue, hard and soft palate, and salivary glands
      i. Chewing prepares food by softening and moving it around, mixing it with saliva, and forming a bolus. Skeletal muscles for chewing are coordinated by cranial nerves V, VII, IX, X, XI, XII.
      ii. Saliva aids in swallowing; approximately 570 mL/day of saliva is secreted. Submandibular, parotid, and sublingual salivary glands along with minor salivary glands in the oral mucosa secrete mixed saliva, which is 99% water and 1% solids, and includes electrolytes and organic protein molecules.
   b. Pharynx
      i. Extends from the cricoid cartilage to the level of the sixth cervical vertebra. Swallowing receptors are stimulated by the autonomic nervous system when a food bolus moves toward the back of the mouth. The motor impulses to swallow are transmitted via cranial nerves V, IX, X, and XII.

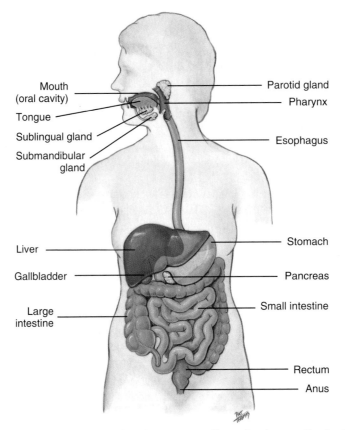

Fig. 9.1 The digestive tract and associated structures. (From Applegate, E., Applegate, E.M.S. *The anatomy and physiology learning system*, 4th ed. St. Louis, Elsevier.)

c. Esophagus
   i. Collapsible tube about 25 cm long at the level of the sixth cervical vertebra and extends through the mediastinum and diaphragm to the level of the 11th thoracic vertebra that lies posterior to the trachea and the heart. Transports food from the mouth to the stomach and prevents retrograde movement of the stomach contents.
   ii. Upper portion of the esophagus is striated skeletal muscle, which is gradually replaced by smooth muscle so that the lower third of the esophagus is totally smooth muscle
   iii. Motor and sensory impulses for swallowing and food passage derive from the vagus nerve. Lower esophagus also innervated by splanchnic and sympathetic neurons. Food moves by the strong muscular contraction of peristalsis and by gravity. In the absence of gravity, nutrients transported by muscular contractions.
   iv. Sphincters: Hypopharyngeal (proximal) prevents air from entering the esophagus during inspiration; gastroesophageal (distal) prevents gastric reflux into the esophagus
d. Blood supply
   i. Arterial supply: Celiac trunk includes the gastric, pyloric, right and left gastroepiploic arteries
   ii. Venous drainage: Gastric vein, azygous and hemizygous veins drain into the portal vein

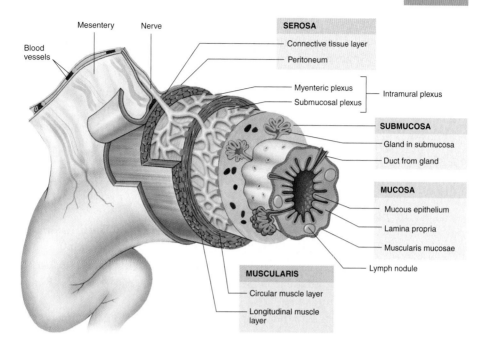

Fig. 9.2 The wall of the gastrointestinal tract is made up of four layers with a network of nerves between the layers. Shown here is a generalized diagram of a segment of the gastrointestinal tract. Note that the serosa is continuous with a fold of serous membrane called a mesentery. Note also that digestive glands may empty their product into the lumen of the gastrointestinal tract by way of ducts. (From Patton, K.T. (2022). *Anatomy and physiology*, 11th ed. St. Louis, Elsevier.)

e. Stomach
   i. Food storage reservoir and site of the start of the digestive process. Normal capacity is 1000 to 1500 mL but can hold up to 6000 mL
   ii. Layers of the stomach and intestinal wall (Fig. 9.2)
   iii. Mucosa: Cells produce mucus that lubricates and protects the inner surface. These cells are replaced every 4 to 5 days. This layer receives the majority of the blood supply of the stomach.
   iv. Epithelium: Contains the gastric, cardiac, fundic, and pyloric glands
      (a) Gastric cells (contain microvilli that monitor intragastric pH), cardiac glands (secrete alkaline mucus, a lubricant that continually bathes and protects the epithelial lining from autodigestion), fundic glands, chief cells (secrete pepsinogen, an inactive form of pepsin, in response to food ingestion; in its active form, pepsin digests proteins), parietal cells (secrete hydrochloric acid, which lowers pH and kills bacteria, and intrinsic factor, a glycoprotein necessary for vitamin B_{12} absorption)
   v. Lamina propria: Contains lymphocytes; site of gut immunologic response
   vi. Muscularis mucosae: Contains thin smooth muscle layer
   vii. Submucosa: Contains connective tissue and elastic fibers, blood vessels, nerves, lymphatic vessels, and structures responsible for secreting digestive enzymes
   viii. Circular and longitudinal smooth muscle layers: Continue the modification of food into a liquid consistency and move it along the GI tract. Movements are tonic and rhythmic, occurring every 20 seconds. Electrical activity is constantly present in the smooth muscle layers.
   ix. Serosa: Outermost layer

f. Gastric hormones
   i. Gastrin: Hormone secreted in response to distention of antrum or fundus by food. Stimulates secretion of hydrochloric acid by the parietal cells and secretion of pepsin by chief cells increasing gastric blood flow.
   ii. Histamine: Hormone secreted by mast cells in the presence of food that is critical to the regulation of gastric acid secretions
       (a) Stimulates gastric acid and pepsin secretion; initiates contraction of the gallbladder; relaxes sphincter of Oddi; increases GI motility
   iii. Gastric secretion
       (a) Approximately 1500 to 3000 mL is secreted daily and mixes with food entering the stomach
       (b) Phases of gastric secretion
           (1) Cephalic phase: Fibers of the vagus nerve stimulate the stomach to secrete gastrin (from the antrum) and hydrochloric acid
           (2) Gastric phase: Vasovagal reflexes stimulate the parasympathetic system to increase the secretion of gastrin
   iv. Gastric emptying
       (a) Is proportional to the volume of material in the stomach and depends on the character of the ingested material: Liquids, digestible solids, fats, indigestible solids
       (b) Factors accelerating gastric emptying: Large volume of liquids; anger; insulin
       (c) Factors inhibiting gastric emptying: Fat, protein, starch, sadness, duodenal hormones
   v. Vomiting
       (a) Coordinated by the vomiting center in the medulla in response to afferent impulses from various regions of the body
       (b) Stimuli that induce vomiting: Tactile stimulation to the back of the throat, increased intracranial pressure (ICP), intense pain, dizziness, anxiety
       (c) Autonomic nervous system discharge may precede vomiting: Sweating, increased heart rate, increased salivation, nausea, muscular force by the diaphragm and abdomen
   vi. Innervation
       (a) Intrinsic nervous system (intramural neurons) within the wall of the GI tract is independent of central nervous system controls
           (1) Myenteric (Auerbach's) plexus: Located between the circular and longitudinal muscles; stimulation increases muscle tone, contractions, velocity, and excitation of the digestive tract
           (2) Submucosal (Meissner's) plexus: Located between the circular and submucosal layers; influences secretions of the digestive tract; contains secretomotor and enteric vasodilator neurons
   vii. Extrinsic system: Via the central nervous system, parasympathetic system, and sympathetic system
       (a) Parasympathetic: Fibers arise from the medulla and spinal segments (e.g., vagus nerves)
           (1) Cranial segments: Transmission via the vagus nerve; innervate the stomach, pancreas, and first half of the small intestine
           (2) Sacral segments: Innervate the distal half of the large intestine, sigmoid, rectum, and anus

(3) Enhances function of the intrinsic nervous system and the secretion of acetylcholine, increases glandular secretion and muscle tone; decreases sphincter tone

(b) Sympathetic: Motor and sensory fibers arise from the thoracic and lumbar segments; distribution is via the sympathetic ganglia (e.g., celiac plexus)

    (1) Fibers run alongside blood vessels and secrete norepinephrine; inhibit GI activity by acting on smooth muscle

2. **Middle and lower GI tract: Small and large intestine**

  a. Small intestine

    i. Approximately 5 m long; extends from the pylorus to the ileocecal valve, consists of three divisions: duodenum, jejunum, ileum; primary function is absorption of nutrients

  b. Large intestine

    i. Approximately 6.5 cm in diameter and 1.5 m long; extends from terminal ileum at the ileocecal valve to the rectum

    ii. Ileocecal valve: Prevents return of feces from the cecum into the ileum

    iii. Consists of six divisions: Cecum, ascending colon, transverse colon, descending colon, sigmoid colon, and rectum

    iv. Layers of the intestinal wall (see Fig. 9.2)

      (a) Mucosa: Innermost layer; receives the majority of the blood supply; the predominant site of nutrient absorption

      (b) Epithelium: Covered with villi and microvilli that increase the surface area of the small intestine several hundred times; contain glands, crypts of Lieberkühn (intestinal glands) that secrete approximately 2 L of fluid every 24 hours and goblet cells that secrete mucus

      (c) Lamina propria: Contains lymphocytes; site of gut immunologic responsiveness

      (d) Muscularis mucosae: Contains thin smooth muscle

      (e) Submucosa: Contains loose connective tissue and elastic fibers, blood vessels, lymphatic vessels, and nerves

      (f) Muscularis: Muscle layer; function is involuntary and involved in motility

      (g) Serosa: Outermost layer; protects and suspends intestine within the abdominal cavity

      (h) Large intestinal wall contains no villi and does not secrete digestive enzymes

      (i) Epithelial surface contains cells that absorb water and electrolytes

      (j) Crypts covered by epithelial cells that produce mucus

    v. Motility: Propulsive peristatic movements that move the intestinal contents toward the anus

      (a) Small intestine: Approximately 3 to 5 hours is necessary for passage through the entire small intestine.

      (b) Large intestine: Haustral churning is the major type of movement in the colon.

      (c) Factors that enhance motility: Bacterial enterotoxins, viral infections of the gut, regional enteritis, ulcerative colitis, increased bile salts, osmotic overload, laxatives

      (d) Factors that inhibit motility: Low-bulk diet, parenteral nutrition, bed rest, dehydration, ileus, fasting, medications

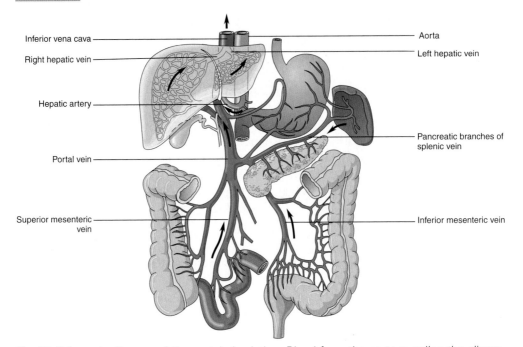

Fig. 9.3 Schematic diagram of the portal circulation. Blood from the aorta supplies the alimentary canal. Venous blood from the intestine reaches the sinusoids of the liver by way of the portal vein. Venous blood from the liver reaches the inferior vena cava by way of the hepatic veins. (From Banasik, J., Copstead, L.E. (2019). *Pathophysiology*, 6th ed. St. Louis, Elsevier.)

> vi. Poor motility causes more absorption, and the development of hard feces in the transverse colon causes constipation. Aging causes a reduction in peristalsis and decreased GI motility throughout the GI system.
> vii. Blood supply (Fig. 9.3)
> > (a) Arterial
> > > (1) Small intestine: Derived from the celiac artery (first portion of the duodenum) and the superior mesenteric arteries (remainder of the duodenum, jejunum, ileum, cecum); large intestine: superior mesenteric artery (supplies the ascending colon and part of the transverse colon), inferior mesenteric artery (feeds the transverse colon, sigmoid colon, and upper rectum), hypogastric arteries (give rise to the middle and inferior rectal and hemorrhoidal arteries), rectal arteries (arise from the internal iliac arteries, supply the distal rectum)
> > (b) Venous drainage: Splanchnic bed drains the entire GI tract.
> > > (1) Superior mesenteric vein (drains the small intestine and the ascending and transverse colon); inferior mesenteric vein (drains the sigmoid colon and rectum)
> c. Innervation: Same as for stomach
> d. Digestive enzymes
> > i. Small intestine digestive enzymes are integral function of the mucosa.
> > ii. Bile and pancreatic enzymes are secreted into the duodenum.
> > iii. In the jejunum and the ileum, food is digested and absorbed.
> > iv. Up to 3000 mL/day of digestive enzymes (e.g., lipase, amylase, maltase, and lactase); pH is approximately 7.0

e. Small intestinal hormones
  i. Secretin: Secreted by the mucosa of the duodenum in response to acidic gastric juice from the stomach and to alcohol ingestion
    (a) Augments the action of cholecystokinin (CCK); stimulates release of the alkaline component of pancreatic juice and the secretion of water, increases the bile secretion rate; decreases the motility of most of the GI tract
  ii. CCK: Secreted by the mucosa of the jejunum in response to the presence of fat, protein, and acidic contents in the intestine
    (a) Increases contractility and emptying of the gallbladder and blocks the increased gastric motility caused by gastrin; stimulates secretion of pancreatic digestive enzymes, bicarbonate, and insulin
  iii. Gastric inhibitory peptide (GIP): Secreted by the mucosa of the upper portion of the small intestine in response to the presence of carbohydrates and fat in the intestine; inhibits gastric acid secretion and motility, slowing the rate of gastric emptying
  iv. Vasoactive intestinal peptide: Secreted throughout the gut in response to acidic gastric juice in the duodenum
    (a) Main effects are similar to those of secretin, stimulates the secretion of intestinal juices to decrease the acidity of chyme and inhibits gastric secretion
  v. Somatostatin: Secreted throughout the intestine in response to vagal stimulation, ingestion of food, and release of CCK, GIP, glucagon, and secretin
    (a) Inhibits the secretion of saliva, gastric acid, pepsin, intrinsic factor, and pancreatic enzymes; gastric motility, gallbladder contraction, intestinal motility, and blood flow to the liver and intestine; the secretion of insulin and growth hormone
  vi. Serotonin: Secreted throughout the intestine in response to vagal stimulation, increased luminal pressure, and the presence of acid or fat in the duodenum; inhibits gastric acid secretion and mucin production
f. Small intestinal functions: Almost all absorption occurs in the small intestine via four mechanisms: Active transport, passive diffusion, facilitated diffusion, and nonionic transport
  i. Vitamins are absorbed primarily in the intestine by passive diffusion, except for the fat-soluble vitamins, which require bile salts for absorption, and vitamin B_{12}, which requires intrinsic factor
  ii. Water absorption: Approximately 8 L of water per day is absorbed by the small intestine
  iii. Electrolyte absorption: Most occurs in the proximal small intestine
  iv. Iron absorption: Absorbed in the ferrous form in the duodenum
    (a) Facilitated by ascorbic acid, increases in states of iron deficiency
  v. Carbohydrate absorption: Complex carbohydrates are broken down into monosaccharides or basic sugars (fructose, glucose, galactose) by specific enzymes (e.g., amylase, maltase)
  vi. Protein absorption: Protein is broken down into amino acids and small peptides; essential amino acids are lysine, phenylalanine, isoleucine, valine, methionine, leucine, threonine, and tryptophan
g. Fat absorption: Emulsification, the breaking up of fat globules into much smaller emulsion droplets aided by bile salts and phospholipids
h. Large intestinal function

    i. Absorption of water and electrolytes: Approximately 500 mL of chyme (the byproduct of digestion) enters the colon per day and, of this, 400 mL of water and electrolytes are reabsorbed.

    ii. Breakdown of cellulose by enteric bacteria

    iii. Synthesis of vitamins (folic acid, vitamin K, riboflavin, nicotinic acid) by enteric bacteria

    iv. Storage of fecal mass until it can be expelled from the body

       (a) Takes approximately 18 to 24 hours from the time food enters the colon until the intestinal contents reach the distal portion of the colon and defecation

  i. Innervation: Same as for the stomach

  j. Gut defenses

    i. The gut encounters a variety of potentially harmful substances daily; these can include natural toxins in food, insecticides, preservatives, chemical waste products, and airborne particulate matter that is swallowed.

    ii. Mechanisms exist within the GI tract to protect the integrity of the gut and thus the individual.

    iii. Fluid and cellular layers

       (a) Aqueous layer: Stationary layer immediately adjacent to the microvillus border of the enterocytes; consists of acids, digestive enzymes, and bacteria depending on the location in GI lumen

       (b) Mucosal barrier: Physical and chemical barriers that protect the wall of the gut from harmful substances. Surfaces of the stomach, intestine, biliary and pancreatic ducts, and gallbladder have cells that synthesize and release mucus.

       (c) Epithelial cells: Tight junctions between cells regulated by hormones and cytokines make them relatively impervious to large molecules and bacteria; rapid proliferation of cells minimizes the adherence of flora. The level of permeability varies within the various segments of the GI tract.

       (d) Mucus-bicarbonate barrier: Forms a layer of alkalinity between the epithelium and luminal acids that neutralizes the pH and protects against surface shear

3. Motility: Prevents bacteria in the distal small intestine from migrating proximally into the sterile parts of the upper GI system

  a. Stomach

    i. Expulsion of toxic substances as a result of stimulation of the vomiting center in the medulla, barrier against the reflux of duodenal contents back into the stomach

  b. Colon: Moves pathogens and potential carcinogens out of the body

4. Gut immunity: Necessary because the gut is a reservoir of potentially pathogenic bacteria

  a. B lymphocytes that bear surface immunoglobulin A (IgA) or synthesize secretory IgA that prevents antigens from binding to mucous cells

  b. Macrophages in the lamina propria

  c. Gut-associated lymphoid tissue in the submucosa (lamina propria or Peyer's patches) of the GI tract

  d. Glutamine is the primary fuel of the gut and maintains the gut mucosal barrier

  e. Gastric acid: Intragastric pH below 4.0 is essential; it protects the stomach from ingested bacteria and other harmful substances; prevents bacteria from entering the intestine

5. **Commensal bacteria: Natural gut flora are stable and protective in a healthy person by competing with pathogenic species for nutrients and attachment sites, and produce inhibitory substances against pathogenic species**
   a. Stomach, duodenum, and jejunum are sterile; ileum contains aerobic and anaerobic bacteria (dietary intake is a major factor in determining intestinal flora); large intestine contains large numbers of aerobic and anaerobic bacteria, and smaller numbers of yeast and fungi
6. **Impaired gut barrier function facilitates bacterial translocation, which is the egress of bacteria and/or their toxins across the mucosal barrier and into the lymphatic vessels and portal circulation**

ACCESSORY ORGANS OF DIGESTION (FIG. 9.4)

1. **Liver**
   a. Largest solid organ, weighing approximately 3 lb (1500 g), located in the right upper quadrant, beneath the diaphragm
   b. Consists of three lobes divided into eight independent segments, each of which has its own vascular inflow, outflow, and biliary drainage. Because of this division into self-contained units, each can be resected without damaging those remaining.
      i. Right lobe: Anterior (segments V and VIII) and posterior (segments VI and VII)
      ii. Left lobe: Medial (segment IV) and lateral (segments II and III); the left lobe extends across the midline into the left upper quadrant
      iii. Caudate lobe (segment I)
   c. Microscopically, the liver consists of functional units called lobules composed of portal triads in which the bile ducts, hepatocytes, and artery are located. The portal triads are then bounded by sinusoids and a central vein. A cross-section of a classic lobule or acinus is hexagonal.

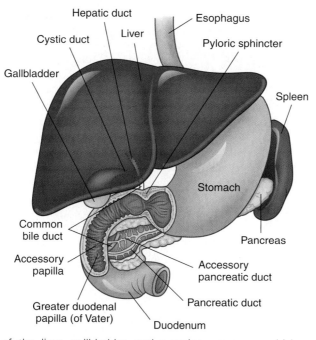

Fig. 9.4 Location of the liver, gallbladder, and exocrine pancreas, which are the accessory organs of digestion. (From McCance, K.L., Huether, S.E. (2019). *Pathophysiology: the biologic basis for disease in adults and children*, 8th ed. St. Louis, 2019, Elsevier.)

d. Blood supply (Fig. 9.5): Derived from both a vein and an artery
   i. Some 25% of cardiac output flows through the liver per minute
   ii. Portal vein (after draining the mesenteric veins and pancreatic and splenic veins) and hepatic artery (off the aorta via the celiac trunk) enter the liver at the porta hepatis or hilum (a horizontal fissure in the liver, containing blood and lymph vessels, nerves, and the hepatic ducts)
   iii. Some 75% is supplied by the portal vein; each segment receives a branch of the portal vein, and 25% is supplied by the hepatic artery, which supplies 50% of the oxygen requirements and is the main blood supply to the bile ducts
   iv. Small branches of each of these vessels enter the acinus at the portal triad (an area in the liver consisting of the portal vein, branches of the hepatic artery, and tributaries to the bile duct)
   v. Blood from both the portal vein and the hepatic artery mixes together in the hepatic sinusoids and then flows through the sinusoids to the hepatic venules (zone 3) through the central veins, branches of the hepatic vein

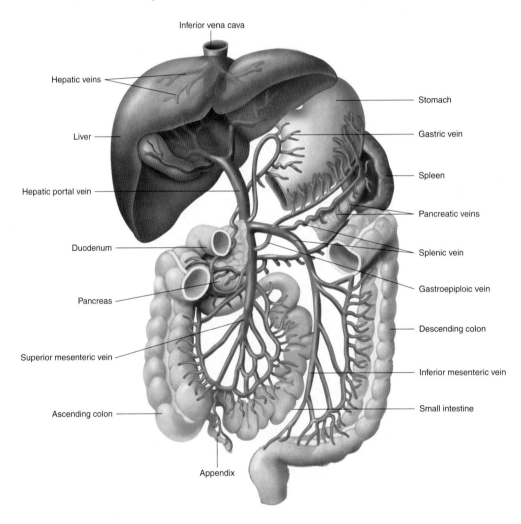

Fig. 9.5 Hepatic portal circulation. In this very unusual circulation, a vein is located between two capillary beds. The hepatic portal vein collects blood from capillaries in visceral structures located in the abdomen and empties it into the liver. Hepatic veins return blood to the inferior vena cava. (From Patton, K.T. (2020). *Anatomy and physiology*, 16th ed. St. Louis, Elsevier.)

vi. Sinusoids

   (a) Found between plates (layers) of hepatocytes; have a porous lining with fenestrations that allows nutrients in the blood plasma to wash freely over exposed surfaces (the spaces of Disse); sinusoidal lining consists of endothelial cells, Kupffer cells, perisinusoidal fat-storing cells, and pit cells.

vii. Venous drainage: Begins in the central veins in the center of the lobules; central veins empty into the hepatic veins, which empty into the inferior vena cava

2. **Biliary duct system for draining bile**

  a. Begins at the sinusoidal level as bile canaliculi, which join into ductules, intralobular bile ducts, and larger intrahepatic ducts

  b. Intrahepatic ducts come together at the porta hepatis to form the common hepatic duct, which becomes the common bile duct after joining with the cystic duct and drains into the duodenum.

  c. Blood supply: Arterial blood supply is from the cystic artery; venous drainage is via a network of small veins.

  d. Innervation: Splanchnic nerve, right branch of the vagus nerve

  e. Cystic duct attaches the gallbladder to the common hepatic duct

    i. Union of the cystic duct and the common hepatic duct forms the common bile duct; common bile duct either joins the pancreatic duct outside the duodenum or forms a common channel through the duodenal wall at the ampulla of Vater; intraduodenal segment of the common bile duct and the ampulla is the sphincter of Oddi

    ii. Presence of CCK in the blood (in response to chyme in the duodenum) facilitates delivery of bile to the duodenum, contracts the gallbladder, relaxes the sphincter of Oddi

  f. Bile is composed of water, bile salts, and bile pigments

    i. Bile salts are responsible for the absorption and emulsification of fat and fat-soluble vitamins

    ii. Bile pigments: High in cholesterol and phospholipids, give feces a brown color

    iii. Bilirubin is the major bile pigment; it is a breakdown product of hemoglobin metabolism from senescent red blood cells

    iv. Serum bilirubin

     (a) Total: Indirect bilirubin plus direct bilirubin; when total bilirubin level is elevated and the cause is unknown, indirect and direct bilirubin fractions can be measured

     (b) Indirect (unconjugated): Bilirubin bound to albumin before it binds to glucuronic acid; fat soluble. Causes of elevation of indirect bilirubin concentration in serum include the following:

      (1) Any hemolytic process (e.g., ABO mismatch in blood transfusion, β-hemolytic streptococcal infection)

      (2) Gilbert syndrome, a common disorder characterized by a mild, chronic fluctuating increase in the level of unconjugated bilirubin

      (3) Inherited deficiency of bilirubin, which results in variations of the Crigler-Najjar syndrome

    v. Diffuse hepatocellular necrosis direct (conjugated): Bilirubin bound to glucuronic acid, water soluble; concentration elevates with biliary tract obstruction (except cystic duct), diffuse biliary tract damage, acute cellular rejection after liver transplantation. Causes of elevation of direct bilirubin concentration in serum include the following:

(a) Bile duct obstruction (e.g., stones, tumor, biliary stricture after liver transplantation); cholecystitis; necrosis of the bile duct (e.g., hepatic artery thrombosis)

(1) Autoimmune diseases of biliary stasis (e.g., primary biliary cirrhosis, primary sclerosing cholangitis); inherited disorders of conjugated bilirubin excretion (e.g., Dubin-Johnson syndrome, Rotor syndrome)

g. Physiology: The liver is a metabolically complex organ with interrelated digestive, metabolic, exocrine, hematologic, and excretory functions. The many functions it performs are interwoven; each lobe is an independent functional unit, so that up to 80% of a normal, healthy liver can be destroyed and it will regenerate.

i. Digestive functions: Plays a role in the synthesis, metabolism, and transport of carbohydrates, fats, and proteins

ii. Carbohydrates: Maintains normal serum glucose levels by
(a) Glycogen storage: Approximately 900 kcal of glycogen reserves are stored in the adult liver.
(b) Glycogenesis: Conversion of excess carbohydrates to glycogen for storage in the liver as a metabolic reserve
(c) Glycogenolysis: Conversion of large stores of glycogen in muscles and liver to glucose
(d) Gluconeogenesis: Manufacture of glucose from noncarbohydrate substrate (fat, fatty acids, glycerol, amino acids)

iii. Fats
(a) Bile secretion for fat digestion plays a role in fat and lipid synthesis, metabolism, and transport
(b) Principal site of synthesis and degradation of lipids (cholesterol, phospholipids, lipoprotein): Produces approximately 1000 mg of cholesterol per day
(1) Exogenous lipoprotein metabolism
(2) Endogenous lipoprotein metabolism: Major lipoprotein synthesized by the liver is very-low-density lipoprotein (VLDL); one-third of VLDL remnants are converted to low-density lipoprotein (LDL)
(3) Direct removal of VLDL remnants; removal of 75% of LDL remnants by LDL receptors in the liver
(4) Conversion of excess carbohydrate to triglyceride, which is stored as adipose tissue
(5) Conversion of triglyceride to glycerol and fatty acids for energy
(6) Storage of triglyceride and fat-soluble vitamins (A, D, E, and K)
(7) Storage of fats, cholesterol, proteins, vitamin B_{12}, and minerals

iv. Protein
(a) Production of plasma proteins (albumin, prealbumin, transferrin, clotting factors, haptoglobin, ceruloplasmin, α1-antitrypsin, complement, α-fetoprotein)
(b) Deamination: Metabolism of amino acids
(c) Transamination: Conversion of amino acids to ammonia, conversion of ammonia to urea for urinary excretion

h. Endocrine functions: Metabolism of glucocorticoids, mineralocorticoids, hormones

i. Exocrine functions: Excretion of bile pigment, cholesterol, urea synthesis, detoxification of medications and foreign substances

j. Hematologic functions: Synthesis of bilirubin, coagulation factors

k. Excretory functions: Detoxifies and eliminates medications, hormones, and toxic substances, produces and secretes 600 to 1000 mL/day of bile, stores vitamin B_{12}, copper, and iron, filters blood via Kupffer cells (macrophages) that reside in the liver sinusoids

3. **Gallbladder: Pear-shaped saclike organ that serves as a reservoir for bile, attached to the inferior surface of the liver in the area that divides the right and left lobes (gallbladder fossa); approximately 7 to 10 cm long; holds and concentrates approximately 30 mL of bile**

4. **Pancreas: Soft, flattened gland with a lobular structure but without an external capsule 12 to 20 cm long, located in the retroperitoneal area; head lies in the C-shaped curve of the duodenum at the level of the body of L2; Body extends horizontally behind the stomach; tail is contiguous with the spleen, lying between the two layers of the peritoneum that form the lienorenal ligament at the level of the body of L1**

   a. Blood supply

      i. Arterial blood supplies from the celiac axis, which divides into the common hepatic, splenic, and left gastric arteries and the superior mesenteric artery

      ii. Venous drainage via the portal vein, which is formed by the joining together of the superior mesenteric and splenic veins

   b. Innervation

      i. Sympathetic efferent innervations via the greater, lesser, and least splanchnic nerves have an inhibitory function

      ii. Parasympathetic innervation via the vagal nerves, which stimulate exocrine secretion

   c. Duct of Wirsung: Main pancreatic duct whose terminal end, the sphincter of Oddi in the ampulla of Vater, empties into the duodenum; shares the sphincter of Oddi with the common bile duct

   d. Duct of Santorini: Accessory pancreatic duct (present in 40%–70% of persons) that lies anterior and opens into the second part of the duodenum proximal to the duct of Wirsung

   e. Pancreatic secretions: Consist of aqueous and enzymatic components

      i. Aqueous component: Ductal cells secrete water and bicarbonate; approximately 1 L of fluid per day is secreted

   f. Enzymatic component

      i. Acinar cells (part of the exocrine function of the pancreas) secrete the pancreatic enzymes

      ii. Amylase (for digestion of starches) and lipase (for digestion of fats) are secreted as active enzymes

      iii. Pancreatic proteases are secreted as inactive precursors and are converted to active enzymes in the lumen of the small intestine (for digestion of proteins)

      iv. Food in the intestine stimulates the secretion of enzymes. Changes in the proportions of various nutrients in the diet result in changes in the proportions of enzymes in the pancreatic secretions. Adaptation of the pancreatic secretions is accomplished by hormones that operate at the level of gene expression

      v. GIP and secretin increase the expression of the lipase gene

      vi. CCK increases the expression of the protease genes

      vii. In diabetic individuals, insulin regulates the expression of the amylase gene; however, how amylase expression is normally regulated in nondiabetic individuals is unknown

    viii. Certain conditions decrease pancreatic secretion: Pancreatitis, cystic fibrosis, tumors, and protein deficiency

  g. Endocrine cells found in the islets of Langerhans

    i. Alpha cells secrete glucagon, which is responsible for glycogenolysis and gluconeogenesis

    ii. Beta cells secrete insulin, which facilitates the use of glucose by tissues

    iii. Delta cells secrete somatostatin, which inhibits the secretion of insulin, glucagon, and growth hormone

    iv. Pancreatic polypeptide cells self-regulate pancreatic secretion activities and also have an effect on hepatic glycogen and GI secretions

PATIENT ASSESSMENT

1. **Nursing history**
   a. Patient health history
   b. Chief complaint
   c. History of present illness
   d. Past medical conditions (e.g., neurologic conditions, cirrhosis, diabetes), eating disorders, functional disorders or communicable diseases (e.g., viral hepatitis, jaundice)
   e. Surgical history (e.g., appendectomy, gastric bypass)
   f. Allergies
   g. Food allergies, intolerances (e.g., lactase deficiency causes lactose intolerance); medication allergies
   h. Pain: Location, duration, character, severity, alleviating and aggravating factors, relationship to changes in eating, bowel habits, or position
   i. Oral and olfactory status: Teeth, gums, tongue, pharynx, changes in taste or smell, difficulty chewing or swallowing, food patterns
   j. Nausea or vomiting: Duration, alleviating and aggravating factors, description of vomitus (undigested food, unrecognizable digested product, blood—bright red or resembling coffee grounds), timing, and relationship to pain
   k. Loss of appetite (loss of desire or interest in food), duration, association with other symptoms
   l. Dysphagia: Difficulty in swallowing, types of foods and/or liquids causing difficulty
   m. Heartburn (dyspepsia, reflux): Duration, alleviating and aggravating factors
   n. Fecal elimination: Changes in frequency of stools, diarrhea or constipation, increase in flatulence, color of stools, presence of blood (black, maroon, or bright red color); clay-colored stool—absence of bile pigment as a result of biliary obstruction or advanced cirrhosis
   o. Urinary elimination: Color of urine; dark (tea-colored) urine—acute hepatocellular necrosis or severe biliary obstruction
   p. Fatigue, weakness, easy bruising or bleeding, fever, night sweats
   q. Muscle wasting, atrophy: Wasting of the muscle over the temporal bones in the face or the muscle of the thumb
   r. Weight loss or weight gain, obesity
   s. Family history, carcinoma, liver disease, pancreatitis, peptic ulcer disease, diabetes mellitus, anemia, tuberculosis, inflammatory bowel disease: Crohn disease, ulcerative colitis, irritable bowel syndrome, obesity
   t. Social history
       i. Substance abuse: Tobacco use, alcohol use, medication use (recreational and prescription)

ii. Sexual history: Heterosexual, homosexual relationships; involvement with prostitutes

iii. Place of birth, travel history

iv. History of tattoos, piercings

u. Medication history (all medications evaluated but specifically herbal supplements, vitamins, anabolic steroids, motility agents, antacids, histamine or proton pump inhibitors, anticholinergics, antibiotics, antidiarrheals, laxatives, enemas, narcotics, sedatives, barbiturates, stimulants, antihypertensives, diuretics, anticoagulants, analgesics, nonsteroidal, steroids, chemotherapy agents)

v. Nutritional support: Indications and complications of enteral and parenteral nutritional support in the critically ill (this would include assessment of nutritional needs, management of delivery devices, and enteral and parenteral nutrition)

2. **Nursing examination of the patient**

a. Physical examination data

i. Inspection

(a) Anatomic landmarks are used to locate and describe normal and abnormal assessment findings

(1) Xiphoid process, subcostal margins, costovertebral angle

(2) Abdominal quadrants (Fig. 9.6), midline of abdomen

(3) Umbilicus, rectus abdominus muscle

(4) Anterior superior iliac spine, symphysis pubis, inguinal ligament

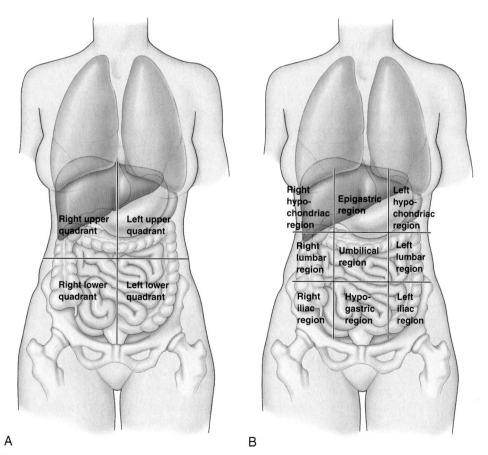

A   B

Fig. 9.6 Areas of the abdomen. **A**, Four quadrants. **B**, Nine regions. (Modified from Herlihy, B. (2022). *The human body in health and illness,* 7th ed. St. Louis, Elsevier.)

    (5) Flanks

    (6) General appearance: Physical signs of altered nutritional status (e.g., cachexia, obesity)

    (7) Oral cavity: Gingivitis, lesions (e.g., herpes simplex, *Candida albicans*, leukoplakia), ability to swallow, presence of odors (e.g., ketones, fetor, alcohol)

    (8) Abdominal profile: Evaluate with the patient lying supine on the examination table or bed

        a) Symmetry, size (girth), and contour of the abdomen from the costal margins to the symphysis pubis (flat, rounded, scaphoid, protuberant)

        b) Abdominal distention can be caused by fluid, fat, flatus, fetus, feces, malignancies, nonmalignant tumors

        c) Asymmetry can be caused by these causes, as well as by obstructions, cysts, or scoliosis

        d) Condition of umbilicus (protruding; nodular; inverted; with calculus, ecchymoses, or drainage)

        e) Caput medusa: Engorged abdominal veins around the umbilicus are seen in patients with portal hypertension or obstruction of the superior or inferior vena cava

        f) Collateral vessels that come to the skin surface and traverse the abdomen: Seen in obesity and ascites

        g) Masses, visible peristalsis or pulsations

        h) Striae, ecchymoses, hematomas, scars, wounds, stomas, hernias, engorged veins, diastasis recti, fistulas, tubes, or drains

    (9) Spider angiomas: Found above the umbilicus on the anterior and posterior thorax, head, neck, and arms

    (10) Jaundice: Evident in skin and sclerae

  ii. Auscultation: Performed in all quadrants before percussion and palpation to note location and characteristics of bowel and other sounds

    (a) Normal bowel sounds: Low-pitched, continuous gurgles heard in abdominal quadrants

    (b) Abnormal bowel sounds

        (1) Factors related to hypoactive or absent sounds: Peritonitis, paralytic ileus, anesthesia, inflammation, electrolyte imbalances, gastric or intraabdominal bleeding, pneumonia, both mechanical and nonmechanical obstruction

        (2) Factors related to hyperactive sounds: Hyperkalemia, gastroenteritis, gastric or esophageal bleeding, diarrhea, laxative use, mechanical obstruction

    (c) Bruit: Denotes increased turbulence or significant dilatation

        (1) Aortic bruit can be heard 2 to 3 cm above the umbilicus in the epigastric area and denotes partial aortic occlusion

        (2) Hepatic bruit can be heard over the liver and may indicate primary liver cancer, alcoholic hepatitis, or vascular liver metastases

        (3) Renal artery bruit can be heard to the left and/or right of midline in the epigastric areas in renal artery stenosis

        (4) Iliac artery bruit can be heard in the left and/or right inguinal areas

    (d) Venous hum or murmur heard over the liver denotes liver disease, such as alcoholic hepatitis, hemangiomas, or dilated periumbilical circulation

(e) Friction rub over the spleen denotes inflammation or infarction of the spleen

(f) Peritoneal friction rub indicates peritoneal irritation

(g) Hepatic friction rub over the liver can be heard in cases of abscess and various types of hepatitis (e.g., syphilitic)

iii. Percussion

  (a) Percussion notes or tones

  (b) Tympany is noted when percussing air-filled organs, such as the stomach; resonance is noted when striking air-filled lungs; dullness is noted over solid organs, such as the liver or spleen

  (c) Percussion to evaluate the sizes of the liver and spleen

    (1) Liver size can be estimated by percussing from the right clavicle straight down the right midclavicular line to detect changes in percussion tones

      a) Beginning at the midclavicular line below the umbilicus, percuss for the lower edge of the liver. Over the bowel, the percussion tone is tympanic and transitions to dull, which denotes the lower edge of the liver; at the level of the fifth intercostal space, percuss downward. The percussion tone transitions from the resonance of the lung tissue to dull, which denotes the upper edge of the liver.

      b) Distance between the upper and lower edges of the liver at the midclavicular line is normally about 12 cm. A span greater than 12 cm or less than 6 cm is abnormal. Gas in the colon, pregnancy, or tumors can impair accurate assessment of the liver span.

    (2) Spleen can be percussed (dull tones) only if grossly enlarged (e.g., portal hypertension) at the left midclavicular line below the left costal margin. To determine the presence of masses or abnormal fluid (ascites) and air collections:

      a) Collections can be confirmed by shifting dullness (fluid remains dependent with changes in position), fluid waves can be elicited by placing the hands on either side of the abdomen, then tapping one hand against the abdomen and feeling the wave transmitted to the opposite hand

      b) Difference between fluid and fat can be determined by placing the hands on either side of the abdomen, having an assistant place his or her hand on the midline, and then pressing downward with one hand. Transmission of fat waves will be halted by the center hand, whereas fluid waves will continue toward the opposite hand.

iv. Palpation

  (a) Light and deep palpation are done to determine the tone of the abdominal wall (relaxed, tense, rigid), areas of tenderness or pain, and the presence and characteristics of masses. Light palpation is done before deep palpation to determine areas of tenderness or resistance (guarding); observe the patient's face for nonverbal signs of discomfort.

  (b) Visceral tenderness: Dull, poorly localized (e.g., bowel obstruction)

  (c) Somatic tenderness: Sharp, well localized (e.g., late appendicitis, capsular stretching of the swollen liver)

  (d) Rebound tenderness: Occurs when palpation is suddenly withdrawn; associated with peritonitis

  (e) Contralateral tenderness: Tenderness on the side opposite palpation (e.g., early appendicitis)

(f) Referred tenderness: Tenderness in an area distant from the source (e.g., right shoulder blade pain referred from the gallbladder)

(g) Murphy's sign: Severe right upper quadrant tenderness elicited on deep palpation under the right costal margin, exacerbated by deep inspiration and associated with cholecystitis

(h) To determine liver size: Palpate at the patient's right side

(1) Right flank area is supported with the left hand and the fingertips of the right hand are slid under the right costal margin, using firm pressure

(2) Fingertips are advanced as the patient inhales deeply and the liver edge moves 1 to 3 cm downward

(3) Fingertips are held steady as the patient exhales and inhales again, and the smooth (normal) edge of the liver may be felt moving past the fingertips

(4) The liver is not normally palpated more than 1 to 2 cm below the right costal margin (in cases of alcoholic liver disease or fatty liver disease, the liver may be enlarged with the margins projecting down into the abdomen 4–5 cm)

(i) To determine spleen size: Palpate from the patient's right side

(1) Left flank area is supported with the right hand and the fingertips of the left hand are slid under the left costal margin, using firm pressure

(2) Fingertips are advanced as the patient inhales deeply and the spleen edge moves 1 to 3 cm downward

(3) Fingertips are held steady as the patient exhales and inhales again, and the smooth (normal) edge of the spleen may be felt moving past the fingertips

(4) The spleen is not normally palpable, except in cases of enlargement or inferior displacement

3. **Monitoring data (see Diagnostic studies)**

4. **Appraisal of patient characteristics: Patients in critical care units with acute GI problems have conditions that vary in complexity. During their hospitalization, their clinical status may move along the continuum of care from improvement to deterioration in a nonlinear fashion. This potential for gradual or abrupt changes in clinical condition with possibly life-altering effects creates barriers in the ability to monitor life-sustaining functions with precision. Clinical attributes of patients with acute GI disorders that the nurse needs to assess include the following: Resiliency, vulnerability, stability, complexity, resource availability, participation in care and decision-making, and predictability.**

DIAGNOSTIC STUDIES

a. Laboratory: Laboratory testing will be discussed within each specific patient health problem.

b. Radiologic

i. Abdominal flat-plate radiography: To visualize the position, size, and structure of the abdominal contents, truncal skeleton, and soft tissues of the abdominal wall. Dilated bowel loops, free air, fluid accumulations, pneumatosis, and intramural bowel gas can be identified on plain radiographic films. Patient should be placed in an upright position.

ii. Computed tomography (CT) of the abdomen: Can be done with or without intravenous (IV), oral, or rectal contrast

(a) To visualize the gallbladder, liver, pancreas, spleen, loops of the small and large intestine, extrahepatic bile ducts, and portal vein and to determine the presence of vascular problems, infection, tumors, and pancreatic pseudocyst

(b) Use of contrast-enhanced images allows for improved visualization of tumors, vascularity of masses, and differences within bowel loops

iii. Positron emission tomography (PET): Use of radioisotopes (carbon, oxygen, nitrogen, and fluorine, and some metals like copper and gallium and their decay products) to reveal physiologic function, not anatomic structure. It is used to evaluate for colorectal, liver, pancreatic, and neuroendocrine diseases.

iv. Magnetic resonance imaging (MRI)

(a) Same applications as CT with a greater potential for tissue characterization and a greater ability to diagnose and characterize diffuse liver and pancreatic disease; can also detect arterial and venous blood flow, vessel patency, bile ducts, and the presence of strictures within the ducts, however less effective than CT for evaluating disorders of the bowel because the movement of the intestine degrades MRI images

v. Ultrasonography of the abdomen: To visualize the sizes and echotextures of the gallbladder, liver, pancreas, and spleen; to determine the presence or absence of disease (fatty infiltration, cirrhosis), the cause of masses (cysts, abscesses, tumors), and the presence of foreign bodies (gallstones); to evaluate the bile ducts and accumulation of fluids; and to determine the direction of blood flow, the development of collateral vessels, and vessel patency.

vi. Upper GI series: Contrast is used to visualize the position, contours, and size of the entire upper GI tract (especially the stomach and duodenum); to detect ulcers, tumors, strictures, and obstructions. Barium swallow is used to examine swallowing, motility, and emptying in the esophagus.

vii. Small bowel follow-through: To visualize the small bowel from the ligament of Treitz to the ileocecal valve to detect ulcers, tumors, diverticula, polyps, and inflammatory bowel disease

viii. Lower GI series: Barium enema is used to visualize the position, contours, and size of the entire lower GI tract; to detect ulcers, tumors, strictures, obstructions, polyps, inflammatory bowel disease, and diverticula; and to evaluate melena after inconclusive upper GI series. Avoid barium studies if there is a suspicion of enteric perforation.

ix. Esophagogastroduodenoscopy (EGD) or upper endoscopy: Visualization and photography of the esophagus, stomach, and proximal duodenum by means of an endoscope

(a) To detect obstruction, strictures, ulcers, or tumors; to evaluate melena, hematemesis, heme-positive nasogastric drainage, dysphagia, odynophagia, dyspepsia, nausea, vomiting, or unexplained abdominal pain or to perform biopsy and obtain brush cytology and culture specimens; to place stents; to remove foreign bodies; to place feeding tubes; or to control bleeding

x. Capsule endoscopy: The patient swallows a capsule with a camera (approximately the size of a large vitamin) that provides endoscopic evaluation of the GI tract. It is commonly used to visualize the small intestine and diagnose diseases (such as Crohn disease, celiac disease, and malabsorption syndrome).

xi. Flexible sigmoidoscopy: Visualization and photography of the rectum, sigmoid colon, and descending colon up to 65 cm by means of a flexible sigmoidoscope or colonoscope

(a) To detect inflammatory disease, tumors, obstruction, strictures, and polyps; to evaluate unexplained chronic diarrhea or pain, lower GI bleeding; to perform biopsy, obtain specimens for brush cytology studies, perform polypectomy, and obtain culture specimens; to remove foreign bodies; and to control bleeding

    xii. Colonoscopy: Visualization and photography of the colon from the rectum to the ileocecal valve by means of a colonoscope

        (a) To detect polyps, strictures, obstruction, tumors, or inflammatory disease; to evaluate lower GI bleeding, unexplained chronic abdominal pain, unexplained iron-deficiency anemia, or changes in bowel patterns; to perform biopsy, obtain specimens for brush cytology studies, perform polypectomy, and obtain culture specimens; to remove foreign bodies; and to control bleeding

    xiii. Endoscopic retrograde cholangiopancreatography (ERCP): Visualization and photography of the biliary and/or pancreatic ducts by means of a flexible (fiberoptic) endoscope

        (a) To detect tumors, bile duct stones, obstruction, and pancreatitis; to evaluate jaundice, elevated levels on liver tests, and chronic unexplained abdominal pain; to perform biopsy and obtain specimens for brush cytology studies and cultures; to place stents; or to remove stones

    xiv. Angiography: Selective catheterization of the visceral arterial system and portal venous system; to reveal vessel sizes, patency, and flow rates of the vessels, as well as the direction of the blood flow

    xv. Cholangiography: During ERCP, radiopaque dye is used to enhance the radiograph and allow visualization of the gallbladder and bile ducts assessing for stricture, bile duct leaks, cholangiopathy, and so on.

c. Other testing

    i. Biopsy

    ii. Abdominal paracentesis: Withdrawal of peritoneal fluid for diagnostic purposes or symptomatic relief by means of a large-bore needle

    iii. Peritoneoscopy (laparoscopy): Examination of the structures and organs within the abdominal cavity by means of a laparoscope

    iv. Gastric lavage: Insertion of a gastric tube through the nose or mouth to examine the gastric contents or secretions for occult blood or pH

    v. Schilling's test: Vitamin B_{12} absorption test to determine whether vitamin B_{12} absorption is defective and if the cause is intrinsic factor deficiency. Oral radioactively labeled vitamin B_{12} and intrinsic factor, and intramuscular nonradioactive vitamin B_{12} are administered, and 24- to 48-hour urine excretion is measured.

    vi. Esophageal function studies (Bernstein test), an acid-perfusion test, is an attempt to reproduce the symptoms of gastroesophageal reflux. It helps differentiate esophageal pain caused by esophageal reflux from that caused by angina pectoris. If the patient suffers pain with the instillation of hydrochloric acid into the esophagus, the test is positive and indicates reflux esophagitis.

PATIENT CARE

1. **Inability to establish or maintain a patent airway**

    a. Description of problem: With acute hemorrhage or encephalopathy, there may be an inability to maintain the airway because of altered levels of consciousness or possible aspiration because of vomiting. Clinical findings may include altered rate and depth of respirations, decreased oxygen saturation, dyspnea or tachypnea, and cyanosis.

    b. Goals of care: Reestablish and maintain a patent airway

c. Interprofessional collaboration on health care team: Nurse, physician (radiologist/surgeon), advanced practice provider, respiratory care provider

2. **Fluid volume deficit**
   a. Description of problem: Associated with hemorrhage, GI fluid and blood losses, third-spacing, or sepsis. Clinical findings may include the following:
      i. Anxiety or diminished mental status, tachycardia; decreased pulse pressure, cardiac output, and cardiac index, orthostatic hypotension progressing to profound hypotension, oliguria, anuria, decreased hemoglobin level, hematocrit, and platelet count; increased international normalized ratio (INR); hematemesis or melena, elevated blood urea nitrogen (BUN), creatinine, lactate levels, and metabolic acidosis
   b. Goals of care: Restore normal circulating fluid volume
   c. Interprofessional collaboration on health care team: Nurse, physician, advanced practice provider, laboratory technician, pharmacist, blood bank personnel

3. **Electrolyte and/or acid-base imbalances**
   a. Description of problem: May be related to hemorrhage, GI losses, third-spacing, sepsis, excessive diuresis (iatrogenic or disease related), or renal failure
   b. Goals of care: Restore and maintain electrolyte balance and normalize pH
   c. Interprofessional collaboration; Nurse, physician/surgeon, advanced practice provider, pharmacist, dietician
   d. Interventions as previously discussed

4. **Alterations in GI motility**
   a. Description of problem: May be associated blunt abdominal trauma, diabetes, sepsis, endocrine disorders, medications, or genetic disorders in which the gut has lost its ability to coordinate muscular activity because of endogenous or exogenous causes.
   b. Goals of care
      i. Improvement in motility and ease of elimination
   c. Interprofessional collaboration: Nurse, physician (radiologist/surgeon), advanced practice provider, pharmacist, nutritional team
   d. Interventions
      i. Assess the following factors (diet, medications, toxic substances, immobility, infection, hemodynamic instability, neurologic conditions) that may contribute to the alteration in GI motility
      ii. In addition, assess for neurologic conditions and response to systemic conditions
      iii. Age-related changes in GI function (see Ch. 16, Older Adult Patients)

5. **Impaired nutrition**
   a. Description of problem: May be associated with inadequate intake, anorexia (intake less than the body requirements) because of nausea, vomiting, diarrhea, reduced absorption, or increased metabolic needs
   b. Goals of care
      i. Ensure that minimum daily requirements for both calories and nutrients are met
   c. Interprofessional collaboration: Nurse, physician (radiologist/surgeon), advanced practice provider, pharmacist, nutritional team
   d. Interventions
      i. Perform accurate monitoring and recording of patient weight, monitoring of intake and output, including calorie count
      ii. Assess bowel sounds and for signs of malabsorption or obstruction

   iii. Complete a comprehensive nutritional assessment, including increases in energy requirements

   iv. Administer oral and/or parenteral nutritional support and monitor for the patency of feeding tubes if used

   v. Monitor for complications of central venous catheters if used

   vi. Monitor patient response to and tolerance of the nutritional regimen (e.g., electrolyte balance, hydration, hypoglycemia, or hyperglycemia)

SPECIFIC PATIENT HEALTH PROBLEMS

ABDOMINAL TRAUMA
(See Ch. 11, Multisystem Trauma)

BOWEL INFARCTION (OBSTRUCTION, PERFORATION)

1. **Pathophysiology: Partial or complete interruption of the intestinal blood supply: Mediator release, inflammation, ischemia, and infarction of the bowel.**

2. **Etiology and risk factors**
   a. Mesenteric blood flow disrupted on either the venous or arterial sides as a result of embolism, thrombosis, or a low-flow state
   b. Arterial embolism 50%: Coronary artery disease, heart failure, valvular heart disease, atrial fibrillation, history of arterial emboli
   c. Arterial thrombosis 25%: Generalized atherosclerosis
   d. Venous thrombosis 5%: Hypercoagulable states, inflammatory conditions (e.g., pancreatitis, diverticulitis), trauma, heart failure, renal failure, portal hypertension, decompression sickness
   e. Nonocclusive ischemia 20%: Conditions resulting in low-flow states (e.g., heart failure, shock, cardiopulmonary bypass) or splanchnic vasoconstriction (e.g., vasopressors, cocaine, methamphetamine)
   f. Other risk factors: Greater than 50 years of age; medications that cause vasoconstriction (allergy medication, birth control pills); chronic hypertension; atrial fibrillation; abdominal adhesions; inflammatory bowel disease

3. **Signs and symptoms**
   a. Early signs and symptoms: Severe pain with few physical findings; mild tachycardia; vomiting; diarrhea
   b. Later signs and symptoms: Increasing abdominal tenderness, guarding; abdominal rigidity, absent bowel sounds; guaiac positive bowel movement; hemodynamic instability and shock; death

4. **Diagnostic study findings**
   a. Noninvasive study findings
      i. Laboratory studies
         (a) Elevated white blood cell count (WBC), creatinine kinase (CK), elevated lactate, potassium, amylase, lactate dehydrogenase, increasing acidosis on blood gas or chemistry panel
         (b) Kidney, ureter, bladder (KUB) abdominal x-ray: Perforated viscus, normal or free air in the abdomen. Late findings: Ileus, small bowel obstruction, edematous bowel walls, submucosal gas, thumb printing of bowel wall.
         (c) Abdominal ultrasound with Doppler: Identification of arterial occlusion
         (d) Abdominal CT scan (noncontrast): Visualization of abdominal structures to identify ischemic related changes

b. Invasive study findings
   i. Selective mesenteric angiography: Arterial or venous vascular occlusions
   ii. CT angiography: Arterial or venous occlusion, bowel edema and distention, free air
5. **Interprofessional collaboration: Nurse, physician (radiologist/surgeon), advanced practice provider, pharmacist, dietician, chaplain, palliative care provider**
6. **Management of patient care**
   a. First goal of care: Early identification of the condition
      i. Interventions: Performing clinical examination, ordering and implementing appropriate diagnostic testing, reviewing results of diagnostic tests and communicate findings, immediate consult to surgery for exploratory laparotomy
   b. Second goal of care: Anticoagulation or embolic lysis for thrombosis-related ischemia
      i. Interventions: Identification of contraindications to anticoagulation or lysis, obtain appropriate anticoagulant or antithrombotic, administer anticoagulant or antithrombotic, monitor coagulation profile
   c. Third goal of care: Restore fluid and electrolyte balance
      i. Interventions: Appropriate IV fluids, monitor renal function and serial serum lactate; respiratory, cardiovascular, renal and multiorgan dysfunction assessments
   d. Fourth goal of care: Pain management (see Ch. 20 Pain)
7. **Potential complications**
   a. Cardiac arrest because of severe acidosis
      i. Mechanism: Tissue necrosis leads to elevation in serum potassium and lactate leads to severe metabolic acidosis, which results in dysrhythmias and widening of the QRS complex
      ii. Management: Administration of glucose and insulin to reduce hyperkalemia, surgery to remove necrotic tissue, administration of bicarbonate if metabolic acidosis presents with pH less than 7.2
   b. Peritonitis and sepsis
      i. Mechanism: Perforation or compromise of the integrity of the intestinal wall leads to translocation of bacteria outside of the intestine into the abdominal cavity
      ii. Management: Administration of antibiotics, monitor for signs and symptoms of sepsis
   c. Intestinal infarction
      i. Mechanism: Occlusion of the blood supply leads to necrosis of tissue
      ii. Management: Preparation and transport to operating room for surgery
   d. Intestinal scarring
      i. Mechanism: Ischemia of the bowel tissue leads to the development of scar tissue that narrows the lumen of the intestine
      ii. Management: Monitoring and interventions as appropriate by GI provider
   e. Other interventions
      i. Consider hypercoagulable workup and long-term anticoagulation or antiplatelet therapy: Patients with arterial embolism or venous thrombosis require long-term anticoagulation with warfarin. Patients with nonocclusive ischemia may be treated with antiplatelet therapy.
      ii. Positioning: As the patient's condition and comfort dictate

   iii. Skin care: Postoperative wound care and pressure relief are required because the patient is susceptible to skin breakdown from diarrhea, fistula formation, wound drainage, dehydration, hypotension, and malnutrition.

   iv. Nutrition: Nutritional needs will be increased because of increased metabolic needs and a reduction in intake pre-/postoperatively. Cause of the condition and the caloric requirements will determine how these metabolic needs are met (enteral or parenteral route).

   v. Discharge planning: Patient may need assistance at home for dressings, IV antibiotics, wound care, parenteral or enteral nutrition, and physical therapy.

   vi. Pharmacology: Patients will be receiving a complex variety of medications postoperatively (antibiotics, insulin, narcotics, anxiolytics, vasopressors, inotropic agents, proton pump inhibitors, diuretics, cathartics).

   vii. Psychosocial issues: Family support for body image alterations, role changes, and financial issues.

   viii. Ethical issues: Living will, durable power of attorney for health care, refusal of treatment, consent for treatment

FUNCTIONAL GASTROINTESTINAL DISORDERS (OBSTRUCTION, MOTILITY [ILEUS, DIABETIC GASTROPARESIS, GERD, INFLAMMATORY BOWEL SYNDROME])

1. **Pathophysiology: Mechanical impairment or complete arrest of the passage of contents through the intestine. There is a reduction in secretory and absorptive functions of the mucosa, and the bowel wall becomes edematous and congested with intensification of the peristalsis.**

KEY CONCEPT

Inflammatory bowel disease (IBD) typically has a relapsing and remitting course.

---

2. **Etiology and risk factors**
   a. Mechanical obstruction (e.g., tumor, volvulus, intussusception) or a failure of the intestine to work properly (paralytic ileus), abdominal wall or groin hernia, inflammatory disease (e.g., Crohn disease or ulcerative colitis), prior abdominal or pelvic surgery, history of cancer (e.g., colon) or irradiation, severe constipation, or ingesting foreign objects
3. **Signs and symptoms**
   a. Severe bloating and abdominal distention, abdominal cramps around the umbilicus or epigastrium, abdominal pain, guarding, decreased appetite, hypotension. fever, nausea and vomiting, constipation or small volume diarrhea, decreased urine output, dehydration, extraintestinal manifestations (arthralgia, eye, skin, elevated liver tests)

EXPERT TIP

The relationship of pain to alterations in intake and changes in bowel pattern is very important in determining the etiology of the condition. It is also important to ask the patient about extraintestinal symptoms.

---

4. **Diagnostic study findings**
   a. Noninvasive study findings
      i. Laboratory studies
         (a) Complete blood count: Elevated WBCs, increased hematocrit, basic metabolic panel: Hypokalemia, hypernatremia, elevated BUN and creatinine

(b) Metabolic acidosis (obtain serial arterial blood gases [ABGs] and serum lactate levels)

    ii. Supine and upright abdominal x-rays: Distention of bowel loops, fluid levels, and gas in the bowel wall

    iii. Abdominal CT scan: Identifying the specific site (e.g., transition point) and severity of obstruction (partial versus complete), distention of the bowel, gas bubbles, typical "bird-beak" deformity at the site of the twist in a volvulus, and inflammatory changes

  b. Invasive study findings

    i. Colonoscopy: Direct visualization of obstruction of colon

    ii. Endoscopy: Direct visualization of obstruction of the upper portion of the small intestine

5. **Interprofessional collaboration: Nurse, physician (radiologist/surgeon), advanced practice provider, pharmacist, nutritional team**

6. **Management of patient care**

  a. First goal of care: Identification of level and source of obstruction

    i. Interventions: Ongoing clinical examination and monitoring, ordering, implementing, and review of appropriate diagnostic tests, including serial KUBs with contrast, nasogastric tube for decompression of stomach; administer oxygen and monitor saturation levels; monitoring patient with partial obstruction for 72 hours and prepare for surgery if partial obstruction not relieved

    ii. Administer special low-fiber diet in cases of partial obstruction in patients who are able to take oral intake; in a complete small bowel obstruction, the risk of strangulation is high and preparation for surgical intervention is needed; administer antibiotics for gram-negative and anaerobic organisms if appropriate, administer medications to reduce mucosal inflammation

  b. Second goal of care: Pain management (see Ch. 20 Pain)

  c. Third goal of care: Decompression and emptying of the GI contents to relieve distention and nausea

> **KEY CONCEPT**
> These patients may have several liters of liquid fecal matter within their intestines. Be prepared for frequent suction canister changes until decompression is complete.

    i. Interventions: Method of decompression, prescribe antiemetic therapy, insert a nasogastric (NG) tube for decompression and reduction of nausea and vomiting, administer antiemetics medication

  d. Fourth goal of care: Restore fluid and electrolyte balance

    i. Interventions: Cardiac monitor, IV access and ordering of appropriate fluids; monitor renal function; respiratory, cardiovascular, renal, and multiorgan dysfunction assessments

  e. Potential complications

    i. Hypovolemic shock

      (a) Mechanism: Fluid loss from emesis, bowel edema, and loss of absorptive capacity leads to dehydration

      (b) Management: IV fluid administration to rehydrate and minimize fluid losses

    ii. Gangrene

      (a) Mechanism: Distention of intestine and reduced blood flow: tissue ischemia. Unrelieved ischemia or incarcerated bowel: Necrosis and gangrene.

      (b) Management: Surgical resection of necrotic bowel; administer antibiotics

  iii. Septicemia

      (a) Mechanism: Tissue ischemia; bacterial translocation

  iv. Management: Administer antibiotics and fluids, monitor lactate

  v. Renal insufficiency

      (a) Mechanism: Reduction in mean arterial pressure, infection, hypotension, nephrotoxic medications, hepatorenal syndrome

      (b) Management: Monitor renal function, avoid nephrotoxic medications

f. Other interventions

  i. Positioning: As the patient's condition and comfort dictate

  ii. Skin care: Frequent assessments and offloading for skin breakdown prevention

  iii. Nutrition: May include nothing by mouth, enteral nutrition or parenteral nutrition with supplements specific to meet the patient caloric needs; monitoring for nutritional complications, such as delayed gastric emptying, refeeding syndrome, and obstruction.

  iv. Infection control: Decrease risk of infectious complications early identification treatment

  v. Discharge planning: Patient may need assistance at home for dressings, IV antibiotics, wound care, parenteral or enteral nutrition. Physical therapy may also be required.

  vi. Pharmacology: May include cholinergic agonists, prokinetic agents, opioid antagonists, antidiarrheals, antibiotics, biologics, and immunomodulating medications.

EXPERT TIP

Medical therapies for IBD include immunomodulating and biologic agents which act on specific cytokines involved in the inflammatory process.

---

  vii. Psychosocial issues: Anxiety related to fear of not being able to reach toilet when needed; significant variations in healing and/or depression because of long periods of disease or hospitalization

GASTROINTESTINAL INFECTIONS (*CLOSTRIDIUM DIFFICILE*)

1. **Pathophysiology: a bacterium that can cause symptoms ranging from diarrhea to life-threatening inflammation of the colon**
2. **Etiology and risk factors: commonly affect older adults in hospitals or in long-term care facilities and typically occurs after use of antibiotic medications**
3. **Signs and symptoms: Watery diarrhea 3 to 15 times a day, abdominal cramping and tenderness, tachycardia, fever, nausea, loss of appetite, dehydration, weight loss, abdominal distention, renal injury**
4. **Diagnostic findings**
   a. Noninvasive study findings
      i. Laboratory studies
         (a) Complete blood count: Elevated WBCs, increased hematocrit, basic metabolic panel: hypokalemia, hypernatremia, elevated BUN and creatinine; a stool toxin test as part of a multistep algorithm (i.e., glutamate dehydrogenase [GDH] plus toxin; GDH plus toxin, arbitrated by nucleic acid amplification test [NAAT])
         (b) Interprofessional collaboration: Nurse, physician (radiologist/surgeon), advanced practice provider, pharmacist, nutritional team, and hospital epidemiology

5. **Management of patient care**
   a. Positioning: As the patient's condition and comfort dictate
   b. Skin care: Frequent assessments and offloading for skin breakdown prevention
   c. Nutrition: Include nothing by mouth, enteral nutrition, or parenteral nutrition with supplements specific to meet the patient's caloric needs
   d. Infection control: Contact precautions pending the *C. difficile* test results then continue contact precautions for at least 48 hours after diarrhea has resolved or until discharge depending on recommendations from hospital epidemiology. Daily cleaning of rooms and terminal room cleaning with sporicidal agent.
   e. Discharge planning: Patient may need assistance at home for dressings, IV antibiotics, wound care, parenteral or enteral nutrition. Physical therapy may also be required.
   f. Pharmacology: May include antidiarrheals, antibiotics
   g. Psychosocial issues: Anxiety related to fear of not being able to reach toilet when needed and isolation

ABDOMINAL COMPARTMENT SYNDROME

1. **Pathophysiology: Persistently increased intraabdominal pressure (IAP; $\geq$12 mm Hg); diminished gut perfusion, increased pressure on the arteries, capillaries, and veins in the abdominal cavity. Intestinal wall edema: Increases the IAP.**
2. **Etiology and risk factors**
   a. Primary ACS is associated with injury or pathology of the abdominopelvic region associated with abdominal trauma. Shock, reperfusion injury and massive fluid resuscitation, and ongoing hemorrhage result in intestinal edema and elevated IAP.
   b. Secondary ACS: Sepsis, major burns, major traumatic injuries outside the abdominopelvic region, and fluid resuscitation result in secondary ACS
   c. Other conditions: Diminished abdominal wall compliance (acute respiratory failure with elevated intrathoracic pressure, abdominal surgery with primary fascial or tight closure, major trauma/burns, prone positioning). Head-of-bed elevation, central obesity/high body mass index, increased intestinal luminal contents (gastroparesis, ileus, colonic pseudoobstruction). Increased peritoneal contents (hemoperitoneum or pneumoperitoneum, ascites); capillary leak/fluid resuscitation acidosis, hypotension, hypothermia, massive transfusion, coagulopathy, massive fluid resuscitation, pancreatitis, sepsis, major burns/trauma.
3. **Signs and symptoms**
   a. Decreased preload, increase in afterload, decreased urine output. Increased peak inspiratory pressures, decreased tidal volume, decreased compliance, increased ICP, decreased cerebral perfusion pressure.
4. **Diagnostic study findings**
   a. Noninvasive study findings
      i. Laboratory studies
         (a) Complete blood count: Elevated hemoglobin and hematocrit with dehydration, elevated white count if translocation of bacteria occurs. Metabolic panel: Hypokalemic, hypochloremic metabolic alkalosis with severe emesis. Elevated BUN levels with dehydration, elevated lactate, metabolic acidosis, may signal bowel ischemia.
      ii. Ultrasound, abdominal x-rays are unreliable
   b. Invasive study findings
      i. Bladder IAP: Elevated levels greater than 12 mm Hg in adults; once over 20 mm Hg, organ damage begins to occur

    ii. Nasogastric IAP measurement in patients with bladder trauma, neurogenic bladders, outflow obstruction, and tense pelvic hematomas

5. **Interprofessional collaboration: Nurse, physician (radiologist/surgeon), advanced practice provider, pharmacist**
6. Management of patient care
   a. First goal of care: Optimize tissue oxygenation and perfusion to prevent end organ system failure
   b. Second goal of care: Optimizing perfusion at the global and regional levels and optimal fluid administration
   c. Third goal of care: Evacuation and decompression of bowel
      i. Interventions: Monitoring effectiveness of decompression and evacuation interventions, insertion of orogastric/nasogastric tubes and rectal tubes, administration of enemas as needed, administration of gastro- and coloprokinetic agents to improve motility (e.g., metoclopramide)
   d. Fourth goal of care: Correction of electrolyte abnormalities
      i. Interventions: Monitor, communicate, and correct electrolyte abnormalities (e.g., hypokalemia, hypomagnesemia, hypophosphatemia, and hypercalcemia)
   e. Fifth goal of care: Evacuation of air, blood, ascites, abscesses, and tumors
      i. Interventions: Prepare and transport patient to interventional radiology or the operating room (OR) if needed, monitor IAP, notify physician of increases in pressure or deterioration of other system functions (e.g., renal)
   f. Potential complications
      i. Hypovolemic shock
         (a) Mechanism: Fluid loss from emesis, bowel edema, and loss of absorptive capacity leads to dehydration
         (b) Management: IV fluid administration to rehydrate and minimize fluid losses
      ii. Gangrene
         (a) Mechanism: Distention of intestine, reduction in blood flow, prolonged tissue ischemia leads to necrosis and gangrene
         (b) Management: Resection of necrotic bowel; administer antibiotics
      iii. Septicemia
         (a) Mechanism: Translocation of intestinal bacteria
         (b) Management: Administer antibiotics to minimize complications, obtain lactate levels, fluid administration
      iv. Acute kidney injury (AKI)
         (a) Mechanism: Reduction in mean arterial pressure, infection, hypotension, nephrotoxic medications, hepatorenal syndrome
         (b) Management: Minimize exposure to nephrotoxic agents, support blood pressure, monitor intake and output
   g. Other interventions
      i. Positioning: As the patient's condition and comfort dictate
      ii. Pain management (see Ch. 20 Pain)
      iii. Nutrition: Consideration should be given to reducing the rate to minimal or trophic levels to maintain intestinal function and integrity. In patients where IAP is significantly elevated, enteral nutrition may be held until this is resolved.
      iv. Discharge planning: May need physical therapy, home care assistance with dressings, IV antibiotics
      v. Pharmacology: Antibiotics and pain medication

vi. Psychosocial issues: Alterations in body image, anxiety or depression related to ability to return to previous level of function

ACUTE ABDOMEN

1. **Pathophysiology: Sudden onset of abdominal pain associated with inflammation of the peritoneal cavity**
2. **Etiology and risk factors**
   a. Perforated or ruptured viscus (esophagus, stomach, liver, pancreas, gallbladder, bile duct, bowel, appendix, or diverticulum)
   b. Erosion, technical error during surgery/procedure; foreign body, trauma, or infection, perforated or ruptured blood vessel (peptic ulcer disease, abdominal aortic aneurysm, tumor, or trauma)
   c. Acute cholecystitis: Inflammation of the gallbladder wall may be associated with gallstones
   d. Bowel ischemia [see Bowel Infarction, (obstruction, perforation), Malnutrition and malabsorption]
   e. Extraabdominal cause (altered host response)
3. **Signs and symptoms**
   a. Persistent severe abdominal pain, referred pain, nausea, vomiting, reflux, or anorexia, alteration in bowel patterns, fecal odor of gastric drainage, abdominal distention; hyperactive or hypoactive bowel sounds, guarding of the abdomen, rebound tenderness, fever, pallor, tachypnea, dehydration, evidence of blunt or penetrating trauma
4. **Diagnostic study findings**
   a. Noninvasive study findings
      i. Laboratory studies
         (a) Elevated WBC count with an elevated neutrophil, basophil counts, increased numbers of bands (immature neutrophils), elevated alkaline phosphatase level, elevated serum amylase, lipase levels, low hemoglobin, hematocrit
         (b) ABG levels: Metabolic acidosis
         (c) Blood and body fluid culture results positive
      ii. Abdominal flat-plate radiography: Alteration in the position, size, or structure of abdominal contents; free air or free fluid in the abdomen
      iii. Abdominal ultrasonography: Masses (cysts, abscesses, tumors), foreign bodies (gallstones), infarction
      iv. Hepatobiliary iminodiacetic acid (HIDA) scan: (cholescintigraphy and hepatobiliary scintigraphy) problems of the liver, gallbladder, and bile ducts.
      v. Abdominal CT or MRI: Vascular problems, infection, masses, or pancreatic pseudocyst
      vi. EGD: Bleeding from peptic ulcer, esophageal tear; flexible sigmoidoscopy or colonoscopy: Lower GI ulceration, perforation, bleeding, abscess, ischemia
      vii. Abdominal paracentesis: Blood, bile, pus, urine, or feces in abdominal cavity.
   b. Invasive study findings
      i. Cholangiography: Cholangitis
      ii. ERCP: Biliary or pancreatic stones, obstruction of ducts
      iii. Arteriography: Bleeding, infarction
      iv. Peritoneoscopy (laparoscopy): Bleeding, perforation, rupture, abscess, ischemia
5. **Interprofessional collaboration: Nurse, physician, advanced practice provider, dietitian, respiratory therapist, pharmacist, radiologist or technician, consultant (e.g., hepatologist, infectious disease specialist)**

6. Management of patient care
  a. First goal of care: Restore hemodynamic equilibrium and fluid balance
    i. Interventions: Monitor input and output (I&O), hemodynamic parameters, administer IV fluids and blood products as appropriate, monitor respiratory system for effects of volume administration
  b. Second goal of care: Restore electrolyte balance
    i. Interventions: Monitor for and correct electrolyte imbalances
  c. Third goal of care: Early identification of infectious processes
    i. Interventions: Minimize potential for hospital acquired infection, monitor for changes in clinical condition indicative of escalating infectious process (e.g., physical assessment, vital signs, laboratory results, blood cultures)
  d. Fourth goal of care: Pain management (see Ch. 20, Pain)
  e. Potential complications
    i. Sepsis
      (a) Mechanism: From a localized infection to mild systemic inflammation to septic shock, resulting in cardiovascular system derangements
      (b) Management: Monitor blood pressure, vascular resistance, oxygen supply and demand, minimize myocardial workload, and optimize tissue oxygenation
    ii. Myocardial infarction
      (a) Mechanism: Increased myocardial workload reduced myocardial oxygen
      (b) Management: Monitor oxygen supply and demand, minimize myocardial workload
    iii. Dehydration
      (a) Mechanism: Hemorrhage, third-spacing, nausea, vomiting, diarrhea, intraoperative losses
      (b) Management: Administer fluids as appropriate, monitor intake and output and venous pressures
    iv. Renal insufficiency
      (a) Mechanism: Reduction in mean arterial pressure, infection, hypotension, nephrotoxic medications, hepatorenal syndrome
      (b) Management: Administer fluids as appropriate, monitor I&O and renal function
    v. Fistula formation or abscesses
      (a) Mechanism: Pancreatic enzymes or perforation of bowel
      (b) Management: Wound care to minimize fluid collections and abscesses, administration of antibiotics to prevent or minimize complications
  f. Other interventions
    i. Positioning: As the patient's condition and comfort dictate
    ii. Skin care: Postoperative wound care and pressure relief are required, as patient is susceptible to skin breakdown from diarrhea, fistula formation, wound drainage, dehydration, hypotension, and malnutrition
    iii. Pain management (see Ch. 20, Pain)
    iv. Nutrition: Initiate to meet increased metabolic demands of surgery, fever, wound healing. Etiology and the caloric requirements will determine enteral or parenteral route.
    v. Infection control: Antibiotic administration and monitoring for progression of condition
    vi. Discharge planning: Patient may need assistance at home for dressings, IV antibiotics, wound care, parenteral or enteral nutrition, and physical therapy

   vii. Pharmacology: Patients will be receiving a complex variety of medications, such as antibiotics, opioids, anxiolytics, vasopressors, inotropic agents, proton pump inhibitors, diuretics

  viii. Psychosocial issues: Patient may be anxious because of multiple interventions and condition changes. Family support for body image alterations, role changes, and financial issues

   ix. Ethical issues: Advanced directives, durable power of attorney for health care, refusal of treatment, consent for treatment

ACUTE LIVER FAILURE

1. Pathophysiology

  a. Development of hepatic encephalopathy within 8 weeks of symptoms or within 2 weeks of the onset of jaundice

---

KEY CONCEPT

Patients with encephalopathy are at increased risk for falls and should not be out of bed without assistance.

---

  b. Occurs in individuals with a history of normal liver function, massive hepatocellular necrosis, elevated serum alanine transaminase (ALT) level; prolonged coagulation and hypoglycemia can also occur, except in cases of acute fulminant liver failure caused by acetaminophen toxicity; the mortality rate is 80% to 100% without liver transplantation

2. Etiology and risk factors (Box 9.1)

BOX 9.1   **Etiology, Signs, and Symptoms of Acute Liver Failure**

ETIOLOGY OF ACUTE LIVER FAILURE

- Viral hepatitis: Acute hepatitis A and B
- Autoimmune hepatitis
- Acetaminophen toxicity: Liver failure from intentional overdose and unintentional therapeutic misadventure has a better prognosis than that resulting from other causes
- Hepatotoxic medications or substances
- Mushroom poisoning (e.g., because of *Amanita phalloides, Amanita verna,* and *Amanita venosa; Galerina autumnalis, Galerina marginata,* and *Galerina venenata; Gyromitra* species)
- Viral infections: Herpes virus family, especially in immunocompromised patients
- Acute Wilson disease, acute Budd-Chiari syndrome
- Venoocclusive disease and graft-versus-host disease after bone marrow transplantation
- Reye syndrome

SIGNS AND SYMPTOMS

- Prodromal symptoms (vague, flu-like symptoms), fever
- Jaundice
- Hyperventilation, respiratory alkalosis
- Hepatic encephalopathy (confusion): Rapid progression to hepatic coma
- Profound coagulopathy and hypoglycemia
- Hepatorenal syndrome
- Sepsis, metabolic acidosis
- Intracranial hypertension
- Hyperdynamic circulation
- Systolic ejection murmur
- Eventual cardiovascular collapse
- Liver is enlarged during the acute inflammatory stage, then becomes atrophied as hepatocellular necrosis progresses

---

Modified from Bernal, W., Wendon, J. (2013). Acute liver failure. *New England Journal of Medicine,* 369, 2525–2534; Erden, A., Esmeray, K., Karagöz, H., et al. (2013). Acute liver failure caused by mushroom poisoning: a case report and review of the literature. *International Medical Case Reports Journal,* 6, 85–90.

3. **Signs and symptoms (see Box 9.1)**
4. **Diagnostic study findings**

> **EXPERT TIP**
> Acute liver failure can progress rapidly over several hours resulting in encephalopathy. Continuous assessment and caution is required with regards to oral intake and mobility.

  a. Noninvasive study findings
     i. Laboratory
        (a) Increased levels of aspartate aminotransferase (AST), ALT, alkaline phosphatase, and gamma-glutamyl transferase (GGT). Severe elevations followed by a progression back to normal that may be misinterpreted as improvement in the patient's status but is not a favorable sign if it occurs in the setting of increasing prothrombin time (PT), INR, and bilirubin levels; indicates near-complete hepatocellular necrosis.
        (b) Increased serum bilirubin, creatinine, BUN levels, serum lactate level, serum ammonia level, and WBC count; prolonged PT and INR; levels of factors V and VII less than 20% of normal (poor prognostic sign); decreased serum glucose level, hemoglobin level, and hematocrit
        (c) Positive results on cultures of body fluids; positive results on hepatitis serologic testing or tests for autoimmune markers depending on cause; positive urine toxicology screen results; positive stool guaiac test results
  b. Chest radiograph: Bilateral infiltrates, pleural effusions or evidence of aspiration pneumonitis
  c. CT scan of the head: Normal until very late in the process
  d. Cerebral perfusion scan may show decreased or absent flow late in the process; performed before liver transplantation to rule out brain death
5. **Interprofessional collaboration (see Acute Abdomen)**
6. **Management of patient care**

> **KEY CONCEPT**
> Reduced liver function will result in prolonged half-life of medications and medication metabolites.

  a. First goal of care: Optimize liver function
     i. Interventions: Establish the etiology of the acute liver failure, collaborate with team on initiation of treatment interventions
  b. Second goal of care: Stabilize for liver transplantation if appropriate
     i. Interventions: Communication and collaboration between admitting team and transplant evaluation team, obtain laboratory studies and other evaluation studies for transplant workup, monitor vital signs, neurologic status. Monitor and replace electrolytes frequently; phosphorous depletion occurs in a regenerating or recovering liver.
  c. Third goal of care: Monitor and treat for complications
  d. Potential complications
     i. Infection or sepsis
        (a) Mechanism: Depressed immune system, breaks in the skin barrier; altered level of consciousness and risk of aspiration
        (b) Management: Aseptic line care, monitor for infection, administer antibiotics

ii. Brainstem herniation (most common cause of death in fulminant liver failure) or intracranial hemorrhage
   (a) Mechanism: Increased coagulation times increase the risk of intracranial bleeding and pulmonary hemorrhage; increased risk of hypoxia, which increases the cerebral edema
   (b) Management: Monitor ICP
iii. Renal failure
   (a) Mechanism: Progression of liver failure may lead to renal failure (hepatorenal syndrome)
   (b) Management: Administer fluids as appropriate, monitor intake and output and renal function
iv. Respiratory failure
   (a) Mechanism: Pulmonary edema, hemorrhage, pneumonia, altered mental status
   (b) Management: Monitor respiratory function, provide ventilator support as appropriate
e. Other interventions
   i. Skin care: Severe itching with the onset of jaundice; scratching with excoriations; hematoma formation
   ii. Pain management: Consultation with a hepatologist if pain medication required
   iii. Nutrition: Metabolic rate can be increased; fluid balance is a problem with renal failure. Special enteral and parenteral solutions required because of liver and renal dysfunction.
   iv. Infection control: Immobility, altered level of consciousness, invasive lines, and depressed immune system results in increased risk of infection. Consider infectious disease consult early.
   v. Discharge planning: Prolonged recovery, assistance with home care, rehabilitation, medications, office visits
   vi. Pharmacology: Complex regimen of medications, requiring alternative choices (shorter-acting medications or medications with shorter half-lives) and dosing patterns (every 12 hours instead of every 6 or 8 hours)
   vii. Psychosocial issues: Acuity of the situation will have a profound effect on the family and increase stress

GASTROINTESTINAL BLEEDING

1. **Pathophysiology**
   a. Peptic ulcer disease
      i. Both duodenal and gastric ulcers are classified as peptic ulcers; imbalance between acid and pepsin production; loss of the protective factors of bicarbonate, mucus, and cell renewal; mucosal lining of the stomach and duodenum is affected
   b. Duodenal ulcers: Oversecretion of acid
   c. Gastric ulcers: A reduction in the gastric mucosal barrier; decreased mucosal blood flow, altered cellular renewal, and reduction in mucous secretion, bacterial infection, or damaging agents
      i. The risk of gastric ulcers is increased with *Helicobacter pylori* infection
   d. Variceal bleeding: Approximately 30% of cirrhotic patients have esophageal varices; increasing to 90% after 10 years. The mortality rate is 20% at 6 weeks;

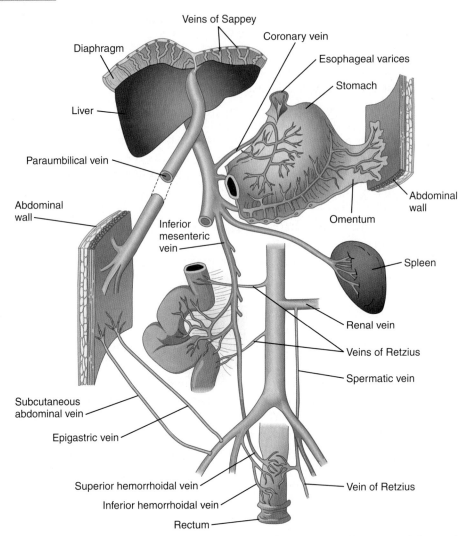

Fig. 9.7 Collateral circulation in the liver. (From Good, V.S., Kirkwood, P.L. (2018). *Advanced critical care nursing*, 2nd ed. St. Louis, 2018 Elsevier.)

bleeding ceases spontaneously in up to 40% of patients. This is most common fatal complication of cirrhosis.

   i. Portal circulation is high flow with low pressure; increased resistance (either intrahepatic or extrahepatic) to blood flow—results in spontaneous rupture and bleeding; varices in the distal esophagus and esophagogastric junction increased tendency to bleed; can also form throughout the GI tract (Fig. 9.7)

  e. Mallory-Weiss syndrome: Tear in the mucosa or submucosa at the gastroesophageal junction; longitudinal, caused by forceful or prolonged vomiting; occurring more often in those over 50 years; a history of medication or alcohol use may be present

  f. Esophagitis/gastroesophageal reflux disease (GERD): Frequent or ongoing backflow of acid resulting in chronic inflammation and tissue damage in the esophagus

  g. Stress ulcers (gastric, duodenal): Common in critically ill patients; characterized by mucosal ischemia that leads to alterations which result in the loss of protective functions

---

KEY CONCEPT

Stress ulcers develop silently and manifest with sudden GI bleeding.

    h. Causes of lower GI bleeding
- i. Crohn disease: Less common, usually caused by deep ulceration in the colon
- ii. Ulcerative colitis: Can cause exsanguination because of diffuse ulceration, colitis resulting from ischemia, radiation, chemotherapy
- iii. Diverticula: Most common cause of acute massive colonic blood loss
- iv. Intestinal polyps: Intermittent or occult bleeding
- v. Angiodysplasia (arteriovenous malformation of the mucosa): Common cause of chronic or intermittent low-grade bleeding in aged patients
- vi. Hemorrhoids

2. Etiology and risk factors
- a. Gastric ulcers associated with decreased tissue resistance; 3 to 4 times more common in men; associated with malignancy; may lead to nonhealing ulcer in stomach
- b. Duodenal ulcers associated with increased hydrochloric acid level; most frequent sites are the pylorus and the first portion of the duodenum
- c. Can occur at any age; common among young adults, seasonal trend, with higher incidence in the spring and fall
- d. Pharmacologic agents may play a role: Salicylates, indomethacin, phenylbutazone, nonsteroidal antiinflammatory medications (NSAIDs), corticosteroids, antineoplastic agents, vasopressors, reserpine
- e. Caffeine use, alcohol abuse, cigarette smoking, familial tendency
- f. Variceal bleeding is associated with portal hypertension
- g. Prehepatic (presinusoidal) factors in which the wedge hepatic venous pressure is less than the portal pressure: Portal vein thrombosis caused by the presence of cirrhosis, hepatoma, umbilical vein catheterization in infancy, or hypercoagulable state
- h. Intrahepatic (sinusoidal) factors in which the wedge hepatic venous pressure is increased and equals the portal pressure
- i. Postnecrotic cirrhosis (e.g., chronic active hepatitis and cirrhosis), alcoholic cirrhosis
- j. Posthepatic (postsinusoidal) factors in which the site of obstruction to flow is distal to the sinusoids: Hepatic vein thrombosis (e.g., Budd-Chiari syndrome), venoocclusive disease after bone marrow transplantation; diseases causing portal hypertension: splenomegaly or splenic vein thrombosis not caused by liver disease; fulminant hepatitis; cirrhosis of various causes; metastatic carcinoma; diseases of the hepatic venules, veins, or inferior vena cava; cardiac diseases (e.g., right heart failure and severe pulmonary hypertension)

3. Signs and symptoms
- a. Epigastric pain with bleeding: Heartburn; with duodenal ulcers, pain is relieved by food; stops when bleeding begins, nausea, vomiting, hematemesis or projectile hematemesis and melena, weight loss, abdominal tenderness or guarding, hyperactive bowel sounds, orthostatic hypotension; narrow pulse pressure, coagulopathy, hyperdynamic circulation, hemodynamic changes, increased minute ventilation, lethargy, malaise, pale skin and/or mucous membranes

4. Diagnostic study findings
- a. Noninvasive study findings
  - i. Laboratory studies
    - (a) Hemoglobin level, hematocrit (decreased; true extent of blood loss may not be immediately apparent), elevated BUN, prolonged PT, increased INR, decreased albumin, platelet count (may be decreased in cirrhosis), blood tests or stomach biopsy (to detect colonization by *H. pylori*), guaiac testing of nasogastric drainage and stool for occult blood

      ii. Upright chest radiography or upright and lateral abdominal radiography: Shows free air under the diaphragm with perforated, bleeding ulcers

     iii. CT: To document cirrhosis, identify the presence of collateral circulation and rule out hepatoma

     iv. Doppler ultrasonography: To evaluate patency of and flow in the portal vein and hepatic veins

  b. Invasive study findings

      i. Upper GI series: To localize an ulcer

     ii. Selective mesenteric angiography: To localize the site of bleeding when endoscopy cannot be performed

     iii. Upper GI endoscopy: To reveal the location of an ulcer, rule out other causes of bleeding

        (a) Differential diagnosis for variceal bleeding is complex and includes peptic ulcer disease, gastritis, Mallory-Weiss tear of the esophagus, and Boerhaave syndrome, among others

        (b) Definitive identification is made by endoscopic examination of the esophagus, stomach, and duodenum and/or colonoscopy

        (c) Endoscopy grade and classification of esophageal, gastric, and/or duodenal varices according to size, location, and risk factors

     iv. Superior mesenteric artery arteriography: To measure hepatic vein pressure gradient and to image the portal and hepatic venous systems

      v. Angiography: To evaluate blood flow, identify the source of bleeding; can be used to embolize a vessel

     vi. Nasogastric intubation: To obtain gastric aspirate

5. **Interprofessional collaboration: Nurse, physician /surgeon, advanced practice provider, pharmacist, and interventional radiologist**

6. **Management of patient care**

  a. First goal of care: Minimize blood loss; replenish losses

      i. Interventions: Ongoing assessment of clinical condition, type and cross for number of units anticipated, administer blood, platelets and fresh frozen plasma, monitor hemoglobin, hematocrit every 6 hours or consider a transjugular intrahepatic portosystemic shunt (TIPS)

  b. Second goal of care: Optimize hemodynamic status

      i. Interventions: Frequent clinical assessments and communication of goals of therapy, monitor vital sign trends, administer IV fluids and blood products, accurate I&O, monitor for signs of respiratory complications

  c. Third goal of care: Restore circulating blood volume

      i. Interventions: Monitor vital signs and hemodynamic status, monitor for signs/ symptoms of bleeding, administer IV fluids, blood products as appropriate, provide appropriate IV access

  d. Potential complications

      i. Hypovolemia

        (a) Mechanism: Can occur as a result of massive third-spacing of fluids or hemorrhage

        (b) Management

          (1) Third-spacing: Rapid replacement of fluids

          (2) Hemorrhaging: Administration of blood products, use of a Minnesota tube

          (3) Either third-spacing or hemorrhaging: Use of vasoactive medications; accurate and rapid recording of intake and output

    (4) GI surgery for gastric ulcers or refractory variceal bleeding, or surgical shunt construction
- ii. Aspiration
  - (a) Mechanism: Vomiting of blood or GI contents, hypotension, or encephalopathy prevents the ability to protect the airway and can result in aspiration, which may lead to bacterial pneumonia
  - (b) Management: Swallow study, decompress stomach using nasogastric tube, position patient on side
- iii. Multiorgan dysfunction syndrome
  - (a) Mechanism: Severe hypotension, reduced oxygen delivery, hypoxia
  - (b) Management: Monitor vital signs and organ function, optimize oxygen delivery
- iv. Acute respiratory distress syndrome (ARDS), respiratory failure
  - (a) Mechanism: Ventilation/perfusion (VQ) mismatch, acidosis, increased ventilatory pressures, aspiration
  - (b) Management: Ventilatory support, optimize oxygen delivery, prevent aspiratory
- v. Acute renal tubular necrosis, acute renal failure
  - (a) Mechanism: Prolonged hypotension, use of vasoactive medications or nephrotoxic antibiotics
  - (b) Management: Avoid nephrotoxic medications, optimize fluid balance, support blood pressure
- e. Other interventions
  - i. Positioning: Head of the bed raised to prevent aspiration; the patient may need to lie on the side to minimize the risk of aspiration
  - ii. Skin care: Prevention of breakdown caused by lower GI bleeding or decreased skin perfusion caused by shock, keep clean and dry
  - iii. Pain management: Pain may be sharp or dull; worsen with food consumption. Pain management is individualized depending on comorbidities (encephalopathy, renal failure).
  - iv. Aspirin and other NSAIDs should be avoided
  - v. Nutrition: Patient will be on nothing-by-mouth (NPO); the use of total parenteral nutrition (TPN) or lower elemental enteral feedings may be necessary
  - vi. Infection control: Depressed immune system increases the risk of infection if surgery is performed; risk of aspiration is significant
  - vii. Discharge planning: Recovery periods may be either short or prolonged; this may be a new diagnosis requiring increased patient and family education

GASTROINTESTINAL BARIATRIC SURGERY
(See Ch. 15, Bariatric Patients)

CHRONIC LIVER FAILURE: DECOMPENSATED CIRRHOSIS
1. **Pathophysiology**
   - a. Cirrhosis is a chronic and usually slowly progressive disease of the liver involving the diffuse formation of connective tissue (fibrosis), nodular regeneration of the liver after necrosis, and chronic inflammation
   - b. Changes are often irreversible; 10 years after diagnosis, the probability of developing decompensated cirrhosis is approximately 60%
2. **Etiology and risk factors (Box 9.2)**

BOX 9.2 Etiology, Signs, and Symptoms of Cirrhosis

ETIOLOGY AND RISK FACTORS FOR CIRRHOSIS

- Alcoholism (Laënnec cirrhosis): Development of cirrhosis preceded by a reversible stage of alcoholic hepatitis
- Postnecrotic cirrhosis
- Viral hepatitis (chronic active hepatitis B, C, F, or G)
- Medication or toxin induced (prescription medications, herbs, heavy metals)
- Autoimmune hepatitis
- Autoimmune diseases of biliary stasis (primary biliary cirrhosis, primary sclerosing cholangitis)
- Inborn errors of liver metabolism: Wilson disease (copper metabolism), hemochromatosis (iron metabolism), α1-antitrypsin deficiency
- Nonalcoholic fatty liver disease, associated with obesity, hyperlipidemia, protein-calorie malnutrition, diabetes mellitus, chronic corticosteroid use, jejunoileal bypass, short bowel syndrome
- Hepatic vein thrombosis (Budd-Chiari syndrome)
- Right-sided heart failure: Cardiac cirrhosis

SIGNS AND SYMPTOMS OF CIRRHOSIS

- Fatigue, alteration in sleep pattern: Insomnia, day-night reversal
- Pruritus
- Muscle wasting, weight loss
- Abdominal distention with ascites
- Anemia, hematomas, ecchymosis
- Clay-colored stools
- Fetor hepaticus: Musty breath, poor dentition
- Altered mental status, asterixis
- Visible stigmata of liver disease: Jaundice, temporal and upper body muscle wasting, parotid enlargement, spider angiomas, palmar erythema, leukonychia, possible clubbing of the fingers, testicular atrophy, gynecomastia in males, striae, the development of abdominal wall collaterals, caput medusae
- Umbilical hernia, incisional hernia, splenomegaly
- Hyperdynamic circulation: Increased heart rate, systolic ejection murmur
- Possible decrease in lung sounds in the bases because of pleural effusions
- Hepatic bruit (hepatoma or alcoholic hepatitis superimposed on cirrhosis)

Modified from National Institutes of Diabetes, Digestive and Kidney Diseases: Cirrhosis 2018. Available at https://www.niddk.nih.gov/health-information/liver-disease/cirrhosis/symptoms-causes.

---

3. **Signs and symptoms (see Box 9.2)**
4. **Diagnostic study findings**
   a. Noninvasive study findings
      i. Laboratory
         (a) ALT, AST, alkaline phosphatase, GGT levels: Not usually markedly elevated in advanced cirrhosis but depends on the cause of the liver disease
         (b) Bilirubin level: Elevated in advanced cirrhosis except in diseases of biliary stasis, in which it is elevated PT, INR: Prolonged PT and increased INR; the most sensitive index of synthetic liver function in a readily available laboratory test
         (c) Platelet count: May be decreased because of portal hypertension and splenomegaly early in the disease
         (d) Blood ammonia level: May be elevated (may be affected by a variety of factors not related to liver disease)
         (e) Hemoglobin level, hematocrit: Decreased BUN; creatinine levels: decreased until hepatorenal syndrome occurs
         (f) Serum sodium level: Decreased (at times critically)
         (g) Hepatitis serologic findings: Variable
         (h) Ascitic fluid: Send fluid for cell count and cultures, WBC increased absolute neutrophil count, culture results positive for a specific organism whenever paracentesis performed.

(i) CT: Liver volume decreased, spleen volume increased, possible presence of ascites or tumor, evidence of portal hypertension and collaterals, portal vein patency

(j) MRI, magnetic resonance venography, magnetic resonance arteriography, magnetic resonance cholangiopancreatography: To evaluate organs, vessels, bile ducts for abnormalities (portal vein thrombosis, liver cancer)

(k) Abdominal ultrasonography: To determine liver and spleen sizes, portal vein patency, presence of hepatoma, bile duct dilatation, presence of small amounts of ascites

  b. Invasive study findings

    i. ERCP: May show dilated bile ducts or beading (narrowing) of ducts

    ii. Upper GI endoscopy: Reveals esophageal, gastric, and/or duodenal varices

    iii. Abdominal paracentesis if ascites present: To test fluid for infection (important)

    iv. Liver biopsy: For staging of inflammation and fibrosis

5. Interprofessional collaboration: Nurse, physician, advanced practice provider, dietitian, laboratory technician, physical therapist, consultant (hepatologist, gastroenterologist, surgeon, interventional radiology)

6. Management of patient care

  a. First goal of care: Optimize remaining liver function

    i. Interventions: Collaboration in treatment goals and interventions, eliminate hepatotoxic medications, remove unnecessary IVs, urinary catheters, provide nutritional supplements, monitor liver function and administer medication as scheduled to prevent worsening portal hypertension or encephalopathy. Assess volume status and need for fluid administration, diuresis, or dialysis.

  b. Second goal of care: Stabilize decompensation

    i. Interventions: Rapid identification and intervention to prevent further decompensation, administer beta-blockers to reduce portal pressures, administer lactulose and antibiotics to minimize encephalopathy, fall precautions, antireflux precautions, monitor weight and ascites, reinforce with caregiver importance of appointments and optimize nutrition

  c. Potential complications

    i. Portal hypertension and splenomegaly

      (a) Mechanism: Increased hydrostatic pressure (>10 mm Hg) within the portal venous, which increases the resistance to blood flow into and out of the liver resulting in esophageal varices and gastroesophageal variceal bleeding; backward venous congestion via the splenic vein, results in pancytopenia (anemia, leukopenia, thrombocytopenia)

      (b) Management

        (1) Restriction on the amount of weight to be lifted (no more than 40 pounds)

        (2) Frequent monitoring for consequential pancytopenia

        (3) Use of β-blockers or scheduled endoscopic treatments

        (4) A variety of surgical shunts may be used for refractory bleeding depending on origin of bleeding and patient's candidacy for surgery

        (5) Transjugular intrahepatic portosystemic stents may be used for refractory bleeding. This procedure may be combined with embolization of portal vein collaterals once a pathway has been created by the TIPS.

    ii. Ascites

      (a) Mechanism: Caused by transudation of fluid from the liver surface as a result of portal and lymphatic hypertension and increased membrane permeability, increased hydrostatic pressure and decreased oncotic pressure in the portal venous system, a rise in hepatic sinusoidal pressure, excess hepatic lymph, and hypoalbuminemia

    (b) Management

        (1) Low-sodium diet, judicious use of diuretics

        (2) Accurate intake and output measurements

        (3) Monitoring for refractory conditions (increasing ascites with increasing creatinine level)

        (4) Transjugular intrahepatic portosystemic stents may be used for refractory ascites

  iii. Spontaneous bacterial peritonitis

    (a) Mechanism: Result of the translocation of bacteria from GI lumens to the ascitic fluid

    (b) Management

        (1) Paracentesis to verify primary versus secondary peritonitis

        (2) Administration of antibiotics and diuretic therapy

  iv. Malnutrition

    (a) Mechanism: Reduced caloric intake, reduced synthesis of albumin by the liver, increased caloric needs

    (b) Management: Nutritional supplements, enteral feedings, parenteral nutrition

  v. Hepatic encephalopathy

    (a) Mechanism

        (1) Neuropsychiatric syndrome develops; nitrogenous/toxic compounds arising from gut flora accumulate because of impaired transformation and elimination. Rule out other etiologies of altered mental status (e.g., sepsis, bleeding, toxicity from medications)

        (2) Four grades of alteration of mentation (Table 9.1)

    (b) Management

        (1) Neurologic monitoring for altered level of consciousness

        (2) Administration of lactulose to enhance GI motility

  vi. Pulmonary complications

    (a) Mechanism: The result of hypoxemia, hepatohydrothorax, increased intrapulmonary vascular shunting, and changes in intrapleural pressure and IAP (e.g., pleural effusions), hepatopulmonary syndrome (pulmonary capillary vasodilation and intrapulmonary shunts)

    (b) Management: See Ch. 3, Pulmonary System

  vii. Hepatorenal syndrome

    (a) Mechanism: "Functional" form of acute renal failure with advanced end-stage liver disease; decreased effective circulating plasma volume, release of mediators of vasoconstriction, causing a diversion of renal blood flow; consider nephrology consult

    (b) Management: Monitor I&O; dialysis

  viii. Infection or sepsis

    (a) Mechanism: Depressed immune system and breaks in the skin barrier; aspiration

    (b) Management: Administer antibiotics, minimize risk for infection

d. Other interventions

  i. Positioning

TABLE 9.1	**Clinical Assessment of Hepatic Encephalopathy**			
	Grade I	**Grade II**	**Grade III**	**Grade IV**
Level of consciousness	Awake	Decreased, but opens eyes spontaneously	Somnolent to semi-stuporous but arousable to verbal and painful stimuli; does not open eyes spontaneously	Comatose; no response to pain
Orientation	Total orientation with trivial lack of awareness then progression to disorientation	Minimal disorientation to time and place progressing to severe confusion	Complete disorientation when aroused	Coma
Intellectual functions	Mental clouding; a slowness in answering questions; impaired handwriting; subtle changes in intellectual function: impaired performance on addition takes: decrease in psychometric test scores	Amnesia for past events; impaired performance on subtraction tasks; decrease in psychometric test scores	Inability to perform computations	Coma
Behavior	Forgetfulness, restlessness, irritability, untidiness, apathy, disobedience	Subtle personality changes, inappropriate behavior, decreased inhibitions	Lethargy; bizarre behavior (e.g., unprovoked rage)	Coma
Mood	Euphoria, anxiety, depression, crying	Lethargy or apathy, paranoia	Increased apathy	Coma
Neuromuscular function	Muscular incoordination tremors, yawning, insomnia	Hypoactive reflexes, asterixis, ataxia, slurred speech	Inability to cooperate; nystagmus and Babinski's sign	Coma

HEPATIC ENCEPHALOPATHY TYPES

A. Encephalopathy associated with acute liver failure

B. Encephalopathy associated with portal-systemic bypass and/or intrinsic hepatocellular disease

C. Encephalopathy associated with cirrhosis and portal hypertension or portal systemic shunts

    Subcategory of type C

        Episodic hepatic encephalopathy subdivisions: Precipitated, spontaneous, recurrent

        Persistent hepatic encephalopathy subdivisions: Mild, severe, treatment dependent

        Minimal hepatic encephalopathy

Modified from 2014 Practice Guideline by the European Association for the Study of the Liver and the American Association for the Study of Liver Diseases.

Gastrointestinal System

9

    (a) Orthostatic hypotension: Need for slow, deliberate movements to prevent dizziness and falls

  ii. Skin care

    (a) Skin will be very dry, increase in bruising because of low platelet count and elevated coagulation factors

 iii. Pain management (see Ch. 20, Pain)

 iv. Nutrition: Ascites may cause early satiety; low zinc levels in liver disease may result in diminished taste or metallic taste; patients develop severe muscle wasting and malnutrition

    v. Infection control: Depressed immune system increases risk of infection; ascites creates the risk of peritonitis

    vi. Discharge planning: Recovery periods are short and rehospitalization frequent with decompensation. Assistance with home care, rehabilitation, medications, office visits.

    vii. Psychosocial issues: Chronicity of the situation will have a profound effect on the family unit and increase stress. Depression can occur in both the patient and primary caregiver. Refer to rehabilitation program for substance or alcohol abuse history.

CARCINOMA OF THE GASTROINTESTINAL TRACT

1. **Pathophysiology**
   a. Esophageal carcinoma: About 10% the upper third of the esophagus, 60% are in the middle third, and 30% are in the lower third
   b. Gastric neoplasms: Most common type of neoplasm is primary carcinoma beginning in the mucosal glands
      i. Malignant neoplasms: Up to 90% to 95% of stomach cancers are adenocarcinomas; other less common types are lymphomas, GI stromal tumor (GIST), or leiomyosarcomas
      ii. Gastric adenocarcinomas may be either diffuse or tubular
   c. Pancreatic neoplasms
      i. Pancreatic cancer is the fourth leading cause of cancer deaths among both male and female Americans
      ii. Most pancreatic cancers begin in the pancreatic ducts. Some 75% begin in the exocrine pancreas. Can metastasize to lymph nodes or liver.
      iii. Some 75% occur within the head or neck of the pancreas, 15% to 20% in the body of the pancreas, and 5% to 10% in the tail
   d. Neoplasms of the colon and rectum
      i. Most are caused by malignant conversion of an adenomatous (polyp) lesion and take years to develop
      ii. Most common are or adenomas; slightly more than half in the descending or distal colon; one-fourth are in the cecum and ascending colon

2. **Etiology and risk factors**
   a. Squamous cell esophageal cancer
      i. Most common type of esophageal cancer with multifactorial etiology, incidence increases over age 40 years
      ii. Precipitating factors
      iii. Excess alcohol consumption, cigarette smoking, opiate smoking; ingestion of nitrites, lye; consumption of dry rations or rough foods without adequate fluid intake; gastroesophageal reflux (persistent heartburn and acid regurgitation); trouble swallowing; Barrett esophagus; insufficient intake of vitamins A, C, E, B12, riboflavin, folic acid
   b. Gastric cancer
      i. Adenocarcinomas account for 95% of gastric cancers, affects mostly white males followed by Hispanic and Pacific Islanders over 50 years of age, and persons of lower socioeconomic status
   c. Pancreatic cancer
      i. Risk factors
         (a) Cigarette smoking: Heavy smokers are 2 to 3 times more likely to develop the disease, Black American race, male gender, age over 60 years, chronic

pancreatitis, long-standing diabetes mellitus, obesity, genetic mutation of a gene on chromosome band 9p21k

d. Colorectal cancer
   i. Risk factors
      (a) Alcohol use, acromegaly, colorectal polyps, metastatic neoplasm in other organ(s), irradiation for gynecologic cancers, diet high in animal fat, low in fiber, low in selenium, pernicious anemia
e. Neoplasms of the liver
   i. Primary liver cancer (originating within the liver) is the most common type of liver cancer. Incidence increases with age; most cases occur in individuals 50 to 85 years of age; a male predominance.
   ii. Most neoplasms originate in the parenchymal cells; sarcomas and angiosarcomas form in connective tissue
   iii. Hemangioendotheliomas are tumors of blood vessels in the liver
      (a) Commonly associated with viral cirrhosis, but all patients with cirrhosis are at risk
f. Neoplasms of the hepatobiliary tract
   i. Adenocarcinoma of the extrahepatic ducts: Increasing incidence in men between ages 50 and 80 years

3. **Signs and symptoms**
   a. Esophageal cancer
      i. Progressive dysphagia, odynophagia, weight loss over a short time, anorexia, regurgitation or vomiting, aspiration pneumonia, cough, hoarseness, pain radiating to the chest and/or back
   b. Gastric cancer
      i. Heartburn, epigastric pain, and odorous breath, belching, bloating, early satiety, postprandial fullness, dysphagia, dyspepsia, vomiting, weight loss, blood in the stool, frank bleeding, pernicious anemia
   c. Pancreatic cancer
      i. Initial symptoms are often insidious and exist for months before diagnosis: Jaundice, clay-colored stools caused by the lack of conjugated bilirubin, dark tea-colored urine caused by increased excretion of bilirubin, weight loss, pain: gnawing, visceral type radiating at times from the epigastric area to the back. Usually improves by bending or sitting forward.
   d. Colorectal cancer
      i. Left colon: Abdominal distention, pain, vomiting, constipation, cramps, bright red blood in the stool
      ii. Right colon: Pain, palpable mass in the right lower quadrant, anemia, brick-red blood in the stool
      iii. Proximal colon: Iron deficiency
      iv. Sigmoid colon: Hematochezia
      v. Rectum: Bright red blood coating the stool
      vi. Change in bowel habits: Constipation, diarrhea, smaller-diameter stools (see Liver cancer and cholangiocarcinoma)

4. **Diagnostic study findings**
   a. Noninvasive study findings
      i. Laboratory
         (a) Elevated levels of carcinoembryonic antigen, α-fetoprotein, and CA 19-9, decreased hemoglobin and glucose levels, increased red cell mass, alkaline phosphatase level, serum calcium level, positive result on stool guaiac test

    ii. Barium swallow testing, ultrasonography, bone scan, chest CT or MRI, abdominal CT or MRI

    iii. Digital rectal examination: Yields positive findings for blood

  b. Invasive study findings

    i. Upper GI studies reveal "linitis plastica" (leather bottle stomach) with gastric neoplasms

    ii. Esophagogastroduodenoscopy, sigmoidoscopy, or colonoscopy

    iii. Biopsy specimen obtained during procedure tests shows carcinoma; used for staging and classification

    iv. Metastasis evaluation: Chest radiograph, CT scan, MRI, bone scan, colonoscopy, EGD and/or PET scan for further investigation and staging

5. Interprofessional collaboration: See Acute Abdomen

6. Management of patient care

  a. First goal of care: Immediate recognition and treatment of GI bleeding and/or relief of GI obstruction (esophagus, stomach, small or large bowel, bile ducts)

    i. Interventions: Early recognition and notification of team members of signs of bleeding, monitor vital signs and laboratory results, provide patient education on signs/symptoms of bleeding, establish goal parameters for hemoglobin level, administer medications or blood products as needed

  b. Second goal of care: Prevent malnutrition through nutritional support

    i. Interventions: Dietary evaluation of patients, evaluation of dietary assessments and caloric goal setting with supplemental vitamin and minerals, provision of enteral or parenteral nutrition, surgical palliative bypass when appropriate

  c. Third goal of care: Minimize GI distress and the side effects of treatments (nausea, vomiting, diarrhea)

    i. Interventions: Evaluate potential for side effects and prescribe or implement preventive measures, administer antiemetics as needed, use nonpharmacologic measures to reduce patient stress

  d. Potential complications

    i. Surgery (single or recurrent): A variety of surgical options now exist for patients with carcinoma of the GI tract

    ii. Esophagogastrectomy

      (a) Indication: Esophageal cancer

      (b) Potential complications: Anastomotic leak, paralyzed vocal cord, chylothorax, gastroparesis

    iii. Gastric resections (gastrectomy: subtotal or total with either duodenostomy [Billroth I] or Roux-en-Y [Billroth II])

      (a) Indication: Gastric cancer

      (b) Potential complications: Anastomotic leak, evisceration, hemorrhage, cardiac failure, dysrhythmias, infection (wound or respiratory), malnutrition, ileus, hypovolemia, malnutrition, acute liver failure, or renal failure (see Ch. 6, Renal System)

    iv. Whipple (pancreaticoduodenectomy)

      (a) Indication: The presence of a malignant or premalignant neoplasm in the head of the pancreas or one of the other periampullary structures (bile duct, ampulla, or duodenum)

      (b) Potential complications: Infection, bleeding, leakage of pancreatic enzymes, delayed gastric emptying, weight loss, and diabetes

  e. Other interventions

    i. Positioning: For comfort

    ii. Skin care: Prevention of breakdown

iii. Pain management (see Ch. 20, Pain)

iv. Nutrition: Consumption of chilled foods with little odor, avoidance of greasy or spicy foods, that stimulate the release of pancreatic enzymes. High-calorie supplements or special recipes may be used. If caloric intake cannot be maintained, consider TPN or lower elemental enteral feedings.

v. Infection control: Depressed immune system increases the risk of infection

vi. Discharge planning: Home care, palliative care, or hospice care depending on the needs and wishes of the patient and family

vii. Pharmacology: Complex chemotherapy regimen and other medications for pain control, nausea, diarrhea, and GI motility. Vigilance needed for drug-drug or drug-food interactions.

viii. Psychosocial issues: Acute nature of the situation's profound effect may require crisis intervention and planning

ACUTE PANCREATITIS

1. **Pathophysiology**
   a. Overview: Inflammation of the pancreas results when activated pancreatic proteases digest pancreatic tissue itself. Pancreatic secretions build up, and trypsin accumulates and activates the other pancreatic proteases.
   b. Classification of pancreatitis
      i. Acute pancreatitis: Single episode characterized by abdominal pain and elevated levels of enzymes (amylase, lipase) with inflammation of the pancreas, which returns to normal after resolution of the episode, 80% of cases are related to biliary stones or alcohol use
      ii. Mild pancreatitis does not have other organ damage or complications, and recovery is uneventful. Severe pancreatitis is characterized by impaired pancreatic function and systemic complications; recovery prone to complications.
      iii. Recurrent chronic pancreatitis: Progressive destruction of the acinar cells as a result of persistent inflammation
   c. Other processes contribute to the initiation of pancreatitis
      i. Obstruction of the pancreatic duct, pancreatic ischemia, premature activation of zymogens (inactive digestive enzymes), leading to premature release of active pancreatic enzymes, which begin autodigestion of the pancreas
      ii. Release of cytokines (platelet-activating factor, tumor necrosis factor, interleukin-1), which damage the pancreas
      iii. Release of kinins, which creates capillary wall permeability; pancreatic and peripancreatic edema with loss of up to 6 L of fluid into the interstitial space
      iv. Release and activation of systemic inflammatory mediators (cytokines), including complement, kinins, histamine, prostaglandin, clotting factors; results in systemic effects
   d. Results in increased vascular permeability, vasodilation, vascular stasis, and microthrombosis, with significant effects on other organ systems
   e. Forms of acute pancreatitis
      i. Mild, edematous (interstitial pancreatitis): 95% of cases; 5% mortality; edematous pancreas with minimal or no necrotic damage; gross architecture is preserved
      ii. Severe, hemorrhagic (necrotizing pancreatitis): 5% of cases; mortality 10% to 50%

iii. Extensive peripancreatic tissue necrosis and hemorrhage. Necrosis of fat throughout the abdomen. Retroperitoneal hemorrhage caused by tissue necrosis or erosion of a pseudocyst into the vascular structure, vascular inflammation, and thrombus formation.

iv. Classification of chronic pancreatitis: Lithogenic (chronic calcifying stones); obstructive, inflammatory, or fibrotic; alcohol use; malnutrition; or idiopathic causes. Acinar cell injury occurs with activation of pancreatic proenzymes to their active forms, which results in autodigestion

2. **Etiology and risk factors**
   a. Alcoholism, obstruction of the pancreatic ducts; gallstones (biliary, pancreatic), structural abnormalities (duodenum-ampulla, bile ducts, pancreatic duct), tumor, inflammation, infection, edema, complication of abdominal surgery or diagnostic procedure (e.g., ERCP), abdominal trauma (blunt or penetrating, shock), medication toxicity (cyclosporine, corticosteroids, azathioprine, thiazides, sulfonamides, tetracycline, estrogens), familial hyperlipidemia, chronic hyperparathyroidism, hypercalcemia, infection (Mycoplasma, Streptococcus, Salmonella, Paramyxovirus [mumps], cytomegalovirus, echovirus, Epstein-Barr virus, coxsackie virus, hepatitis virus)

3. **Signs and symptoms**
   a. Vary from a mild, almost asymptomatic case to a fulminant condition of massive pancreatic necrosis
   b. Abdominal pain manifested in majority of cases; epigastric or right upper quadrant pain is knifelike and twisting in nature; begins suddenly and reaches the apex quickly; may radiate to all abdominal quadrants and the lumbar area; associated with nausea and vomiting, low-grade fever, diminished bowel sounds, tenderness on palpation, visceral tenderness: initial tenderness is diffuse, caused by capsular distention and release of kinins, may cause the patient to double over, with a facial expression of pain, nausea, vomiting, pallor, diaphoresis, anorexia, vomiting, diarrhea, abdominal distention, jaundice; dark, foamy urine, steatorrhea: bulky, pale, foul-smelling stools, Cullen's sign (bluish discoloration of the periumbilical area), Turner's sign (bluish discoloration of the flanks), peritoneal lavage reveals blood in the peritoneal cavity ("beef broth" tap), hypoactive or absent bowel sounds, rebound tenderness

4. **Diagnostic study findings**
   a. Noninvasive study findings
      i. Laboratory
         (a) Amylase increases 2 to 12 hours after onset of symptoms of acute pancreatitis and peaks 12 to 72 hours afterward. It may rise 5 to 10 times the normal level; returns to normal within a week. Pancreatitis is likely if the level reaches 3 times above the upper limit of normal. Lipase: Level increases in the blood within 4 to 8 hours of the beginning of an acute attack and peaks at 24 hours afterward. Lipase is both more sensitive and more specific than amylase for the diagnosis of acute pancreatitis. Lipase may rise to several times its normal level and remain elevated longer than amylase. Chronic pancreatitis: Lipase production drops to less than 10% of the normal level, steatorrhea (fatty, foul-smelling stools) develops. Amylase and lipase may be normal or decreased, even during acute attacks. Elevated urine amylase and lipase levels: With good renal function, better indexes of pancreatic damage than are serum levels. Decreased serum ionized calcium level (<2.0 mg/dL): Calcium binds to areas of fat necrosis.

Gastrointestinal System

9

      (b) Decreased serum ionized calcium level (<2.0 mg/dL): Calcium binds to areas of fat necrosis

      (c) Intermittently elevated serum glucose level: Indicates beta-cell involvement

      (d) Presence of C-reactive protein

      (e) Elevated WBC count, serum bilirubin, BUN, triglyceride levels, AST, ALT, lactate dehydrogenase, alkaline phosphatase, and trypsin levels

      (f) Decreased albumin level

      (g) Elevated or decreased hematocrit

  ii. Abdominal plain film: Presence of dilated duodenum (sentinel loop) or transverse colon

  iii. CT: Evidence of pancreatic inflammation, pseudocyst, abscess, obstruction of the pancreatic duct, peripancreatic and retroperitoneal necrosis

  iv. MRI: Similar to CT in identifying inflammation; also identifies areas of poor perfusion and debris in fluid collections

  v. Ultrasonography: Evidence of diffuse pancreatic enlargement, pseudocyst, or abscess, or presence of gallstones, bile duct dilatation

b. Invasive study findings

  i. ERCP: Not accurate for the diagnosis of acute pancreatitis but can provide evidence of biliary or pancreatic stones. Early ERCP with sphincterotomy and stone extraction may ameliorate the course of biliary pancreatitis.

5. Interprofessional collaboration: Nurse, physician, advanced practice provider, dietitian, laboratory technician, physical therapist, consultant (gastroenterologist, surgeon), pain management team

6. Management of patient care

a. First goal of care: Optimize pancreatic function

  i. Interventions: Aggressive supportive care, decrease inflammation, limit infection or superinfection, initiate nutritional support, administer antibiotics, identify and treat complications as appropriate

b. Potential complications

  i. Local complications: Wound infections and skin breakdown in the area of wounds, incisions, and fistulas

      (a) Mechanism: Pancreatic enzymes autodigest body tissues they contact, which leads to pancreatico-cutaneous fistula formation and increased skin breakdown

      (b) Management: Keep skin clean and dry, use ostomy bags or drains to minimize drainage contact with skin

  ii. Hypovolemia

      (a) Mechanism: Massive third-spacing of fluids may result in fluid collections, necrosis, pseudocysts, abscesses, fistulas, intestinal obstruction

      (b) Management: Accurate intake and output, monitor for infection, administer antibiotics

  iii. Systemic inflammatory response and sepsis

      (a) Mechanism: Result of sepsis or inflammatory condition in the setting of an abscess or necrotizing pancreatitis

      (b) Management: Monitor for infection, administer antibiotics, and support blood pressure with vasopressors and fluids, monitor lactate levels

  iv. Multiple organ dysfunction syndrome

(a) Mechanism: Organ damage as result of sepsis in the setting of an abscess or necrotizing pancreatitis

(b) Management: Monitor for organ dysfunction, provide support as appropriate

v. ARDS

(a) Mechanism: Respiratory failure in the setting of sepsis, which leads to increased VQ mismatch, decreased compliance

(b) Management: Administer oxygen, support ventilator, monitor for deterioration

vi. Acute renal tubular necrosis, acute renal failure

(a) Mechanism: Hypotension, inadequate preload, use of nephrotoxic antibiotics, vasoconstriction from vasoactive medications

(b) Management: Administer fluid and diuretics as needed, monitor for deterioration

vii. Disseminated intravascular coagulation

(a) Mechanism: Because of sepsis, hypotension, elevated cytokine levels

(b) Management: Monitor for coagulation disorders

viii. Pain

(a) Mechanism: Pancreatitis is usually described by patients as the worse pain they have ever had. This can be caused by gallstones or to the inflammation of the tissues where autodigestion is occurring.

(b) Management: Administer pain medication, monitor response to medication

c. Other interventions

i. Positioning: For patient comfort

ii. Skin care: Prevention of excoriation because of fistula drainage; keep clean and dry

iii. Nutrition: Patient will need to be on NPO status initially, sometimes for weeks, which necessitates the use of TPN or lower elemental enteral feedings; education about adequate oral care for long-term NPO patients is important.

iv. Discharge planning: Recovery periods are prolonged and rehospitalizations occur; patient will need assistance with home care, rehabilitation, medications, frequent office visits

v. Psychosocial issues: Chronicity of the illness will increase the stress on the family unit. Depression may occur in both the patient and primary caregiver.

HEPATITIS

1. **Pathophysiology: Acute inflammation of the entire liver, characterized on biopsy specimens by centrilobular necrosis and infiltration of the portal tracts by leukocytes. May be a multisystem infection involving many organs: Regional lymphadenopathy, splenomegaly, ulceration of the GI tract, acute pancreatitis, myocarditis, serum sickness, vasculitis, and nephritis.**

2. **Etiology and risk factors**

   a. Viral, medication related, or autoimmune, less acute forms can produce subacute hepatic necrosis or cholestatic liver disease, or silently progress to cirrhosis; multiple viruses cause hepatitis in humans

   b. Hepatitis A virus infection (formerly called infectious hepatitis)

   i. Fecal-oral transmission; can also be transmitted by ingestion of raw or undercooked shellfish contaminated by sewage dumped into the ocean; usually self-limiting

   c. Hepatitis B virus infection

      i. Transmission
- (a) Mother-to-neonate vertical transmission
- (b) Homosexual and heterosexual transmission
- (c) Parenteral transmission (IV medication abuse, transfusion of blood or blood products, hemodialysis, exposure to contaminated equipment, body piercings, razors)

d. Hepatitis C virus (HCV) infection (formerly called *non-A, non-B hepatitis*)
- i. Transmission
  - (a) Parenteral transmission (IV medication abuse, nasal cocaine use, transfusion of blood or blood products, hemodialysis, body piercings, razors, toothbrush sharing, acupuncture, health care exposure)
- ii. Vertical transmission: 3% to 5% in HCV RNA-positive-monoinfected mothers but can be as high as 19% in HIV-coinfected mothers.

e. Hepatitis D virus infection
- i. Transmitted parenterally and as a coinfection with hepatitis B; may lead to fulminant hepatitis

f. Hepatitis E virus infection
- i. Epidemiology and clinical course similar to those of hepatitis A; prevalent among young adults

g. All viruses in the herpesvirus family (herpes simplex, cytomegalovirus, Epstein-Barr virus, varicella-zoster virus)

h. Autoimmune hepatitis
- i. Idiopathic hepatitis characterized by chronic inflammation and plasma cells in liver tissue, autoantibodies, and increased serum globulin levels, associated with four antibodies: antinuclear antibody (ANA), antismooth muscle antibodies (ASMA), antineutrophil cytoplasmic antibodies (ANCA), antiliver kidney microsomal antibodies (anti-LKM)

i. Medication-related hepatitis
- i. Form of medication allergy in which the immune response is directed toward the liver cells, causing necrosis that affects a particular region of the liver lobule (e.g., acetaminophen causes centrilobular necrosis)
- ii. Severe reaction produces diffuse necrosis and/or cholestasis

j. Categories of hepatitis
- i. Acute hepatitis: Acute onset of inflammation, usually self-limiting
- ii. Acute fulminant hepatitis: A rare but serious complication of hepatitis resulting in rapid deterioration and acute liver failure.
- iii. Asymptomatic carrier state (viral hepatitis)
- iv. Infected person is unable to clear hepatitis antigen because of ineffective cellular immunity; carrier is able to transmit hepatitis to others but suffers no liver damage
- v. Chronic hepatitis

k. Hepatitis antigen, chronic liver inflammation, and viral replication persist for at least 6 months; progressive liver damage may develop into cirrhosis

3. **Signs and symptoms**

a. Anicteric (not jaundiced) cases: Usually asymptomatic except for flu-like symptoms; occasionally hepatomegaly, splenomegaly, and lymphadenopathy may occur

b. Icteric cases (small proportion of cases)

c. Prodromal period associated with not feeling well: Malaise, fatigue symptoms subside with the onset of jaundice; among smokers and drinkers, loss of the desire to smoke or drink; dark urine, followed by lightening of the urine, fever, nausea, vomiting, diarrhea, hepatomegaly, splenomegaly

4. **Diagnostic study findings**
   a. Noninvasive study findings
      i. Laboratory
         (a) Increased WBC count, serum total bilirubin level, ALT, AST, and, to a lesser degree, alkaline phosphatase and GGT, positive results on hepatitis serologic testing (Table 9.2), presence of autoimmune markers: ANA, ASMA, ANCA, anti-LKM
         (b) Ultrasonography may show hepatomegaly or splenomegaly, or give normal results
   b. Invasive study findings
5. **Interprofessional collaboration: Nurse, hepatologist/surgeon, nurse practitioner, nutrition team, pharmacist, chaplain, palliative care services**
6. **Management of patient care**
   a. First goal of care: Supportive care
      i. Interventions: see Pancreatitis
   b. Second goal of care: Optimize liver function and functional status
      i. Interventions: Minimize hepatoxic medications, initiate treatment for underlying condition (e.g., immunosuppression or antiviral therapy if appropriate), monitor for progression of encephalopathy, coagulopathy, or elevation of liver tests
   c. Potential complications
      i. Cirrhosis (see Chronic Liver Failure)
      ii. Ascites (see Chronic Liver Failure)
      iii. Encephalopathy (see prior coverage and Ch. 5, Neurologic System)
      iv. Increased ICP (see Ch. 5, Neurologic System)
      v. Liver failure (see Acute Liver Failure)
      vi. Infection or sepsis
      vii. Renal failure
      viii. Liver cancer (see prior coverage)
      ix. Malnutrition (see prior coverage)
   d. Other interventions
      i. Skin care: Prevention of breakdown because of pruritus caused by deposition of bile salts, dryness, itching
      ii. Pain management: Avoid acetaminophen, as well as aspirin and other NSAIDs in severe cases of hepatitis
      iii. Nutrition: If disease is severe, nutritional supplements, enteral or parenteral nutrition may be required
      iv. Discharge planning: Recovery periods occur after prolonged illness without relapse. If the disease is fulminant, the hospital course may vary from long hospitalization to liver transplantation.
      v. Pharmacology: Caution required with medications because of decreased liver function and possible renal impairment
      vi. Psychosocial issues: In the acute or chronic state, the psychosocial issues may involve body image and intimacy issues (fear of transmission); however, the acute nature of fulminant hepatitis will have a profound effect on the family unit and increase stress. If this is a new condition, there may be significant educational needs and complex treatment decisions.

TABLE 9.2 Serologic Testing for Viral Hepatitis

Serologic Test	Description and Purpose
HEPATITIS A VIRUS (HAV)	
HAV total antibody	Presence in serum confers lifelong immunity
HAV IgM	Level rises early during infection (detectable at 3–4 weeks after exposure and just before liver test values become elevated); indicates acute infection; returns to normal in approximately 6 months
HAV IgG	Level rises slowly during infection (detectable at 6–12 weeks after exposure and persists permanently)
HEPATITIS B VIRUS (HBV)	
HBsAg	HBV *surface* antigen; most commonly used marker for HBV infection; detectable within 30 days of exposure and persists up to 3 months after jaundice appears unless a carrier state develops, in which case it will persist longer; presence in serum (seropositivity) indicates active HBV infection
Anti-HBs	Antibody to HBsAg; presence in serum (seropositivity) indicates HBV immunity because of HBV infection or vaccination; detectable 4–12 weeks after HBsAg disappears
HBeAg	HBV *e* antigen; found only in sera positive for HBsAg; presence in serum (seropositivity) indicates high titer of HBV (extensive viral replication) and increased infectiousness (ongoing viral replication); detectable 4–6 weeks after exposure; persistence of this marker in blood predicts development of chronic HBV infection
HBcAg	HBV *core* antigen; not detectable in serum, detectable only in hepatocytes
Anti-HBc (total)	Antibody to HBcAg; detectable 3–12 weeks after exposure during what is referred to as the "*window phase*" (after HBsAg disappears but before antibody to HBsAg appears)
HBV DNA	HBV DNA detected by process of nucleic acid hybridization
PCR for HBV DNA	Test detects polymerase-containing virions; PCR process amplifies DNA in blood so that it is easily detected; very sensitive test
HEPATITIS C VIRUS (HCV)	
HCVAb	Antibody to HCV; presence in serum (seropositivity) is diagnostic for chronic infection only; absence (seronegativity) does not exclude the diagnosis of HCV infection; false-positive results may occur
HCV RNA	HCV RNA detected by process of nucleic acid hybridization; presence in serum is diagnostic of viremia in acute or chronic HCV hepatitis; test also used to monitor response to interferon-α therapy
HCV genotype	Test identifies six different genotypes and several subtypes of the virus; used to determine appropriate treatment options and durations
PCR for HCV RNA	Detects polymerase-containing virions; PCR process amplifies RNA in blood so that it is easily detected; very sensitive test
bDNA	Quantitative test of HCV RNA for determining amount of virus; research assay not yet licensed by the U.S. Food and Drug Administration
HEPATITIS D VIRUS (HDV; HEPATITIS DELTA VIRUS)	
HDAg (total)	HDV antigen; detectable only concurrently with HBV infection
HDV IgM	Level rises early in infection; if persistent, may indicate chronic infection
HDV IgG	Level rises slowly during infection; persists for life
HDVAb	Antibody to HDV; detectable only concurrently with HBV infection
HDV RNA	Detected by process of nucleic acid hybridization
HEPATITIS E VIRUS (HEV)	
PCR for HEV RNA	Detects polymerase-containing virions; PCR process amplifies RNA in blood so that it is easily detected; very sensitive test

From Pagana, K.D., Pagana, T.J. (2017). *Mosby's manual of diagnostic and laboratory tests*, 6th ed. St. Louis, Elsevier.

DNA, Deoxyribonucleic acid; *PCR*, polymerase chain reaction; *RNA*, ribonucleic acid.

Gastrointestinal System

9

END-STAGE GASTROINTESTINAL SYSTEM CONDITION: LIVER TRANSPLANTATION

1. **Indications: Treatment option for fulminant liver failure and end-stage liver disease, certain cases of hepatoma, and other conditions, such as polycystic liver disease and metabolic conditions. Liver disease may reoccur in the transplanted liver.**
   a. Prevalence: Currently approximately 15,194 patients await liver transplantation; however, only about 6500 are done per year. Donors may come from a donor declared brain dead, a donor with cardiac death, or a living donor: Either entire liver or split liver can be used.
2. **Etiology and risk factors: Donor and recipient are matched by blood group (ABO), age, size, CMV status, and presence of viral disease (HBV or HCV)**
3. **Signs and symptoms: Preoperatively: Jaundice, coagulopathy, encephalopathy, deterioration of liver tests, development of ascites, gastric or esophageal varices. Postoperatively: Improving liver function, resolving coagulopathy and encephalopathy.**
4. **Diagnostic study findings**
   a. Laboratory: Increased WBC count, reductions in serum total bilirubin level, ALT, AST, and, to a lesser degree, alkaline phosphatase and GGT
   b. Noninvasive study findings: CT, MRI, or ultrasonography may show hepatomegaly or splenomegaly, or give normal results; assess blood flow through portal vein and biliary flow
      i. Invasive study findings: ERCP normalization of bile flow; liver biopsy: Normal tissue or signs of rejection
5. **Interprofessional collaboration: (see Acute Abdomen) and liver transplant surgeon**
6. **Management of patient care**
   a. First goal of care: Supportive care during the early postoperative period the patient requires monitoring for primary nonfunction of the new liver, monitoring for improvement in mentation and levels of coagulation factors, rejection, side effects, levels of immunosuppression and monitoring for infection
   b. Second goal of care: Optimize liver function and functional status
      i. Interventions: Minimize hepatoxic medications, initiate treatment for underlying condition (e.g., immunosuppression or antiviral therapy if appropriate), monitor for progression of encephalopathy, coagulopathy or elevation of liver tests
   c. Potential complications:
      i. Infection: Fever higher than 101° F or associated with chills; the number of potential infectious organisms is large in the immunosuppressed population
      ii. Rejection: Dramatic or persistent increase in the results of LFTs
      iii. Surgical complications: Ischemic insult to the liver (hepatic artery problems), biliary complications
      iv. Medication toxicities or hypersensitivities: Monitor medications, immunosuppression levels, and avoid known hepatoxic medications
   d. Other interventions
      i. Skin care: Prevention of breakdown because of pruritus caused by deposition of bile salts, dryness, itching
      ii. Pain management: Discussions with the transplant team are needed to choose the best pain medication options for these patients
      iii. Nutrition: Enteral or parenteral nutrition may be required
      iv. Discharge planning: Recovery periods occur after prolonged illness, acute rehabilitation may be needed

v. Pharmacology: Caution required with medications because of decreased liver function and possible renal impairment

vi. Psychosocial issues: New family unit roles and return to employment may occur. Significant educational needs regarding initial postoperative treatments.

NUTRITIONAL SUPPORT IN THE CRITICALLY ILL PATIENT

1. **Pathophysiology: Including increased energy expenditure, stress hyperglycemia, loss of muscle mass, characterized by catabolism exceeding anabolism, eventually psychologic and behavioral problems. Malabsorption may develop in patients with chronic liver failure because of reduction in the bile-salt pool, bacterial overgrowth resulting from impaired small-bowel motility, portal hypertension or medications, such as neomycin. Carbohydrates are believed to be the preferred energy source during critical illness, as fat mobilization is impaired.**

> **EXPERT TIP**
> Many patients continue to be malnourished. It is important that the nurse collaborate with the nutrition team to ensure recommendations are communicated to providers.

2. **Etiology and risk factors: Hospitalization, surgery, trauma, burns, sepsis, multiorgan dysfunction, GI disorders, chronic disease, malignancies, psychologic disorders, alcohol and medication abuse, older age, strictures in the throat or esophagus, stroke, and degenerative neurologic disorders, pain, nausea, weakness, and altered mood or mental status, dissatisfaction with food choices and dietary restrictions**

3. **Signs and symptoms: Poor intake, weight loss, wounds, infection**

4. **Diagnostic study findings**

   a. Noninvasive study findings

      i. Laboratory tests

         (a) Albumin, transferrin, prealbumin and retinol-binding protein (RBP), C-reactive protein (CRP), ceruloplasmin, calcium, magnesium, phosphate, comprehensive metabolic panel, osmolality, vitamin levels

      ii. Nutrition screening should occur within the first 24 hours of admission including weight and height, recent weight change, oral intake

      iii. Assessment of calorie, protein, vitamin, mineral, electrolyte, and fluid needs and the route of nutrition support

      iv. Dietary and fluid intake, anthropometry, caloric expenditure, swallow screen

      v. Physical examination for nutrient deficiencies, the detection of the presence of edema, dehydration, fluid balance, vital signs, pressure ulcers

   b. Invasive study findings: Patient diagnosis and condition dependent

5. **Interprofessional collaboration: Nurse, physician/surgeon, nurse practitioner, nutrition team, pharmacist, chaplain, social worker, palliative care services.**

6. **Management of patient care**

   a. First goal of care: Nutrition support therapy in the form of early enteral nutrition (EN) to be initiated within 24 to 48 hours in the critically ill patient who is unable to maintain nutritional intake

      i. Interventions: Verify feeding tube placement before use, prefer use of EN over parenteral nutrition (PN) in critically ill patients who require nutrition support therapy; GI contractility factors should be evaluated when initiating EN, overt signs of contractility should not be required before initiation of EN; in the setting of hemodynamic compromise or instability, EN should be withheld until the patient is fully resuscitated and/or stable; initiation/reinitiation of EN may be considered with caution in patients undergoing withdrawal of vasopressor support. Level of feeding, by postpyloric enteral access device placement in patients deemed to be at high risk for aspiration.

   (a) Enhanced Recovery After Surgery (ERAS) is the implementation of a multimodal perioperative plan of care that involves perioperative management after colorectal surgery, vascular surgery, thoracic surgery, and radical cystectomy. The goal is to modify the physiologic and psychologic responses to major surgery. Preoperative: Reduction in time without nutrition, elimination of mechanical bowel preparation, nutritional screening, carbohydrate loading.

> **KEY CONCEPT**
> The ERAS is an evolving program and as more research is done more areas of surgical practice may be included.

   (b) Postoperative: Gum chewing, early enteral feeding, mobilization

  ii. ARDS and those expected to have a duration of mechanical ventilation ≥72 hours, either trophic or full nutrition by EN is appropriate

  iii. High nutrition risk or severely malnourished should be advanced toward goal as quickly as tolerated over 24 to 48 hours while monitoring for refeeding syndrome. Efforts to provide more than 80% of estimated or calculated goal energy and protein within 48 to 72 hours should be made to achieve the clinical benefit of EN over the first week of hospitalization.

  iv. To reduce risk of aspiration and ventilator-associated pneumonia (VAP), for all intubated intensive care unit (ICU) patients receiving EN, the head of the bed should be elevated 30 to 45 degrees and use of chlorhexidine mouthwash twice a day should be considered.

  v. Low or high nutrition risk, use of supplemental PN should be considered after 7 to 10 days if unable to meet more than 60% of energy and protein requirements by the enteral route alone; as tolerance to EN improves, the amount of PN energy should be reduced and finally discontinued when the patient is receiving more than 60% of target energy requirements from EN.

  b. Second goal of care: Managing delivery devices

  c. Interprofessional interventions

   i. Assess contraindications and risk for aspiration

   ii. Interventions

    (a) No aspiration risk or gastric problems if a nasogastric tube can be used; if there is aspiration risk or delayed gastric emptying, use a nasoduodenal or nasojejunal tube.

    (b) If enteral feeding is needed for more than 4 weeks with no aspiration risk or gastric problems, consider a gastrostomy tube.

    (c) When enteral feeding is needed for more than 4 weeks with the risk for aspiration or delayed gastric emptying, consider jejunostomy or combined gastrostomy-jejunostomy.

    (d) Assess for complications: Sinusitis, dysphasia, migration, dislodgement, tube occlusion, pulmonary aspiration, esopharyngeal discomfort, erosion of the nasal septum

  d. Third goal of care: Reduce incidence of unintentional underfeeding (i.e., a lower actual caloric and protein intake than the amount prescribed)

i. Interprofessional interventions: Patients should be monitored daily for tolerance of EN. Inappropriate cessation of EN should be avoided. Ordering a feeding status of NPO for the patient surrounding the time of diagnostic tests or procedures should be minimized to limit propagation of ileus and to prevent inadequate nutrient delivery.

(a) Monitor electrolyte abnormalities hypophosphatemia, hypokalemia, and hypomagnesemia; observe for refeeding syndrome in those at increased risk (body mass index <16 kg/m^2; unintentional weight loss >15% in the past 3 to 6 months; little or no nutritional intake for >5 days; history of misuse or use of medications, including insulin, chemotherapy, antacids, or diuretics; low levels of potassium, phosphate, magnesium)

(b) Observe for hypercapnia in patients on mechanical ventilation, azotemia, hyperglycemia, hypertriglyceridemia, elevated liver tests, hypertonic dehydration, and metabolic acidosis. ICU patients with AKI or AKI and acute/chronic liver disease should be placed on a standard enteral formulation, and standard ICU recommendations for protein (1.2–2 g/kg actual body weight per day) and energy (25–30 kcal/kg/day) provision should be followed.

References and bibliography information are available at http://evolve.elsevier.com/AACN/corecurriculum/.

CHAPTER

10

Sepsis and Septic Shock

Diane McLaughlin, DNP, AGACNP-BC, CCRN

CROSSWALK

- **Quality and Safety in Nursing Education (QSEN):** Patient-centered care, Teamwork and collaboration, Evidence-based practice, Informatics
- **National Patient Safety Goals:** Use medicines safely, Prevents infection, Identify patient safety risks
- **American Nurses Association (ANA) standards for Professional Nursing Practice:** Standard 1. Assessment, Standard 2. Diagnosis, Standard 3. Outcomes Identification, Standard 4. Planning, Standard 5. Implementation, Standard 6. Evaluation, Standard 9. Communication, Standard 10. Collaboration, Standard 11. Leadership, Standard 12. Education, Standard 13. Evidence-based practice and research, Standard 14. Quality of practice, Standard 16. Resource utilization, Standard 17. Environmental health
- **AACN standards for Progressive and Critical Care Nursing Practice:** Standard 1. Quality of practice, Standard 2. Professional practice evaluation, Standard 3. Education, Standard 4. Communication, Standard 6. Collaboration, Standard 7. Evidence-based practice/research/clinical inquiry, Standard 8. Resource utilization, Standard 9. Leadership, Standard 10. Environmental health
- **AACN Healthy Work Environment (HWE):** Skilled communication, True collaboration, Effective decision-making
- **PCCN content:** Multisystem- Healthcare-acquired infections, Infectious diseases, Sepsis, Shock states, Wounds
- **CCRN content:** Integument—Wounds, Multisystem- Healthcare-acquired infections, Infectious diseases, Multiorgan dysfunction, Sepsis and septic shock

SYSTEMWIDE ELEMENTS

ANATOMY AND PHYSIOLOGY REVIEW

1. **Review of key concepts**
   a. The definition of sepsis has continued to evolve since its first published definition in 1991. In 2001 the definition was refined, as systemic inflammatory response syndrome (SIRS) was found to be overly sensitive and nonspecific. Over the decade, a series of studies continued to shape the definition of sepsis. In 2016, the Third International Consensus (SEP 3) refined the definitions for Sepsis and Septic Shock and included new clinical criteria (Sequential Organ Failure Assessment [SOFA]). In 2021, the Surviving Sepsis Campaign: International Guidelines for Management of Sepsis and Septic Shock (2021) made additional recommendations. Further changes are anticipated in the future as concepts, diagnosis, and treatment strategies are studied.
      i. *Sepsis:* A syndrome characterized by pathogen factors and host factors (e.g., age, gender, medications, comorbidities) that evolves over time to include a

dysregulated host response and life-threatening organ dysfunction caused by infection

    ii. *Septic shock:* Sepsis-induced state with hypotension requiring vasopressor support, despite adequate volume resuscitation along with perfusion abnormalities, including a serum lactate greater than 2 mmol/mL (18 mg/dL)

    iii. *SIRS:* A systemic inflammatory response to a variety of severe clinical insults (such as pancreatitis, ischemia or reperfusion, multiple trauma and tissue injury, hemorrhagic shock, and immune-mediated organ injury) in the absence of infection. Response is manifested by two or more of the following four criteria (although 10%–15% of all sepsis patients may have one or fewer SIRS):

      (a) Temperature above 38.3° C (100.9° F) or below 36° C (96.8° F)

      (b) Heart rate above 90 beats/minute

      (c) Respiratory rate (RR) above 20 breaths/minute or arterial partial pressure of carbon dioxide ($PaCO_2$) below 32 mm Hg

      (d) White blood cell (WBC) count above $12,000/mm^3$ or below $4000/mm^3$, or more than 10% immature (band) forms

    iv. *Infection:* Microbial phenomenon characterized by an inflammatory response to the presence of microorganisms or the invasion of normally sterile host tissue by organisms without a dysregulated host response or organ dysfunction

    v. *Bacteremia:* Presence of viable bacteria in the blood

b. Surviving Sepsis Campaign: International Guidelines for Management of Sepsis and Septic Shock (2021)

    i. The quick Sequential Organ Failure Assessment (qSOFA) is no longer recommended as a single screening tool sepsis (SSC, 2021).

    ii. Treatment guidelines have been refined with revised recommendations from Sep-3 (2016).

    iii. Hospitals and health systems are encouraged to use a sepsis performance improvement program as routine care.

    iv. Patients should be screened using screening tools such as qSOFA, SIRS, NEWS, and MEWS for sepsis and septic shock (SSC, 2021).

    v. *Nonintensive care unit (non-ICU) settings:* Use the Quick Sequential Organ Failure Assessment (qSOFA). A qSOFA score of 2 or more criteria present in patients with suspected infection meets the criteria for *sepsis* and is predictive of increased in-hospital mortality, prolonged ICU stay, and identifying patients at risk:

      (a) Altered mental status

      (b) RR 22 or more per minute

      (c) Systolic blood pressure (BP) 100 or less mm Hg

    vi. *ICU Setting:* Use the SOFA (Table 10.1). An acute change of the SOFA score of 2 or more points present in patients with suspected infection meets the criteria for *sepsis*:

      (a) This predictive tool evaluates dysfunction in the respiratory, renal, hepatic, cardiovascular, hematologic, and neurologic systems.

      (b) The SOFA score is a reliable outcome predictor for organ failure. The number of failed organs correlates with ICU and overall hospital mortality.

        (1) One failed organ: mortality rate of 11%

        (2) Two failed organs: mortality rate of 33%

        (3) Three failed organs: mortality rate of 51%

        (4) More than three failed organs: mortality rate of 79% or higher

TABLE 10.1 Sequential Organ Failure Assessment

Organ System and Assessment	SCORE				
	0	1	2	3	4
RESPIRATORY					
PaO_2/FiO_2 (mm Hg)	>400	≤400	≤300	≤200[a]	≤100[a]
RENAL					
Creatinine level (mg/dL) or urine output	<1.2	1.2–1.9	2.0–3.4	3.5–4.9 or <500 mL/day	≥5.0 or <200 mL/day
HEPATIC					
Bilirubin level (mg/dL)	<1.2	1.2–1.9	2.0–5.9	6.0–11.9	≥12.0
CARDIOVASCULAR					
Hypotension	No hypotension	MAP <70 mm Hg	Dopamine ≤5 or dobutamine (any dose)[b]	Dopamine >5 or epinephrine ≤0.1 or norepinephrine ≤0.1[b]	Dopamine >15 or epinephrine >0.1 or norepinephrine >0.1[b]
COAGULATION					
Platelet count (×1000/mm³)	>150	≤150	≤100	≤50	≤20
NEUROLOGIC					
Glasgow Coma Scale score	15	13–14	10–12	6–9	<6

FiO₂, Fraction of inspired oxygen; *PaO₂*, arterial partial pressure of oxygen.
[a]With ventilatory support.
[b]Adrenergic agents administered for at least 1 hour (doses given are in mcg/kg/min).
From Bansal, V., Doucet, J. (2015). Multiple organ dysfunction syndrome. *Scientific American Surgery*, 6, 1–20.

    vii. Criteria for *septic shock*, suggesting a more advanced disease state than *sepsis* and predictive of worsened morbidity and mortality, includes meeting criteria for *sepsis* plus:

      (a) Vasopressor requirement to maintain mean arterial pressure (MAP) 65 mm Hg or more despite adequate fluid resuscitation AND

      (b) Serum lactate level over 2 mmol/L (>18 mg/dL)

KEY CONCEPTS
- Sepsis and septic shock are time-sensitive conditions.
- Delays in recognition and treatment of sepsis are associated with increased mortality.
- Routine screening and a process for systematic and timely recognition and treatment are recommended for optimal survival.
- Sepsis bundles of care and their use have been associated with decreased mortality rates. Mortality improves with each additional bundle compliance element achieved.

---

2. **Epidemiology**
   a. Sepsis is the leading cause of death in United States hospitals. Half of patients who die in U.S. hospitals have sepsis.
     i. Sepsis develops in more than 1.5 million people in the United States each year. It is diagnosed in more than 30 million people worldwide.
     ii. Some 80% of cases begin before hospitalization.
     iii. This rate is increasing at a rate of 10% each year.
     iv. More than 250,000 people in the United States die of sepsis each year; globally this number is closer to 6 million deaths.
     v. Some 10% of ICU admissions are caused by septic shock and carry a death rate of greater than 50%.

b. Sepsis is the most expensive condition treated in the United States.

c. Sepsis caused by gram-negative organisms carries a higher mortality rate compared with gram-positive sepsis.

d. Gram-positive bacteria are responsible for approximately 47% of infections resulting in sepsis. Gram-negative bacteria account for approximately 62%. A mix of gram-positive and gram-negative organisms occurs in 15% of infections. Fungal pathogens account for 19% of the infections.

e. Septic shock carries a mortality rate of 40% or higher.

f. Health care costs of severe sepsis exceed $20 billion annually of total U.S. hospital costs.

3. **Cellular pathophysiology**

a. Physiologic insult, such as infection, traumatic injury, surgical incision, burn injury, or pancreatitis, incites development of a proinflammatory state characterized by the expression of multiple mediators in an effort to limit damage from the insult (Fig. 10.1).

b. When phagocytic cells destroy bacteria, a cascade of events follows. The sequence of events may vary depending on whether gram-negative or gram-positive organisms are involved.

c. All gram-negative bacteria have a common group of molecules in the outer membrane, referred to as lipopolysaccharide (LPS) or endotoxin.

d. Components of the gram-positive bacteria cell wall, such as lipoteichoic acid or peptidoglycan, bind to receptors to stimulate cytokine release; bacterial components stimulate the coagulation and complement cascades.

e. Regardless of the inciting pathogen, the cytokines involved in the massive inflammatory reaction known as SIRS may lead to multiple organ dysfunction and are similar to those released in septic shock.

f. Consequences of cytokine production

 i. Systemic vasodilation resulting in decreased afterload and hypotension

 ii. Increased capillary permeability resulting in decreased preload, third-spacing, and interstitial edema

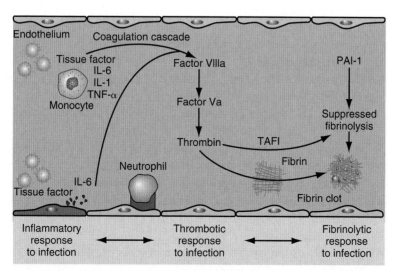

Fig. 10.1 Inflammation, coagulation, and impaired fibrinolysis in sepsis. *IL,* Interleukin; *PAI,* plasminogen activator inhibitor; *TAFI,* thrombin activatable fibrinolysis inhibitor; *TNF,* tumor necrosis factor. (From Ahrens, T., Vollman, K. (2003). Severe sepsis management: are we doing enough? *Critical Care Nurse,* 23(5), 2–16.)

    iii. Relative hypovolemia associated with volume redistribution to interstitium from the vascular space because of loss of endothelium function and increased capillary leak

    iv. Decreased tissue oxygen extraction

    v. Platelet aggregation, fibrin deposits, and activation of a clotting cascade, leading to microcirculatory coagulation, maldistribution of blood flow, and tissue hypoxia

    vi. Multiorgan dysfunction

g. Cytokine regulation (Table 10.2)

    i. Proinflammatory cytokine production and inflammatory processes are normally strongly repressed by the antiinflammatory compensatory response mechanisms.

    ii. SIRS and sepsis develop when homeostasis is disrupted and are associated with overproduction of proinflammatory cytokines.

h. Cytokine cascade: Triggering actions of LPS are not fully understood; bacterial products stimulate the production of cytokines by macrophages and monocytes (see Table 10.2)

    i. Cytokine release begins with the release of tumor necrosis factor-α (TNF-α), followed by the release of interleukin (IL)-1 and IL-6.

    ii. TNF-α and IL-1 cause a variety of physiologic effects; interferon-γ released from natural killer cells, in response to TNF and bacterial products, amplifies the functions of IL-1 and TNF-α.

      (a) Increased temperature set point, which causes fever or may cause hypothermia

      (b) Decreased systemic vascular resistance and increased capillary permeability

      (c) Increased release of leukocytes from the bone marrow

    iii. IL-6 is released from T cells and monocytes after tissue injury and may inhibit the release of other cytokines (TNF-α, IL-1); IL-6 stimulates the liver to release chemical mediators known as *acute-phase proteins* (e.g., C-reactive protein [CRP]).

      (a) CRP levels increase in tissue-damaging infections

        (1) CRP binds to the C-polysaccharide cell wall complement found in bacteria and fungi.

        (2) Complement system is activated following the binding of CRP to the cell wall component, which leads to a complement-mediated increase in phagocytosis.

        (3) Increased serum concentrations of CRP are associated with sepsis and death.

      (b) Procalcitonin is also an amino acid peptide precursor that increases in the presence of bacterial infection and proinflammatory cytokines.

        (1) Levels peak approximately 6 hours after the onset of infection.

        (2) Levels decrease as infection resolves.

        (3) Levels correlate proportionately to severity of infection.

    iv. Effects of cytokines are mediated at target tissues by nitric oxide, arachidonic acid metabolites (prostaglandins, eicosanoids, platelet-activating factor), and lipoxygenase derivatives.

    v. TNF-α and IL-1 stimulate the production of other cytokines, which leads to a cascade effect with complex amplification and modulation (upregulation and downregulation).

TABLE 10.2 Response to Cytokine and Mediator Release in Systemic Inflammatory Response Syndrome

Cytokine/Mediator/ Precursor	Release	Response
ARACHIDONIC ACID METABOLITES		
Arachidonic acid is one of the nutritional essential fatty acids of the body; present in the cell membrane; represents one of key fatty acids in phospholipids	Arachidonic acid gives rise to mediators during interactions with three enzymes: cyclooxygenase and peroxidase (cyclooxygenase pathway) and lipoxygenase (lipoxygenase pathway)	See prostaglandins, thromboxane A_2, and leukotrienes
	Arachidonic acid gives rise to eicosanoids (physiologically active compounds known as *prostaglandins, thromboxanes*, and *leukotrienes*)	
BRADYKININ		
Vasoactive peptide generated by the contact (kallikrein-kinin) system	Bacterial product	Vasodilation, hypotension, increased vessel permeability
	Product of the Hageman factor (factor XII), clotting factor XI, prekallikrein, and high-molecular-weight kininogen	
Proinflammatory		
	TNF-α and IL-1 activate Hageman factor, which stimulates release	
HISTAMINE		
Vasoactive amine	C5a of complement cascade binds to mast cells and triggers release	Increased vessel permeability of postcapillary venules
Proinflammatory	Also released from basophil granules	Pulmonary vasoconstriction
		Vasodilation of capillaries and venules
INTERLEUKINS		
Generic term for cytokines produced by leukocytes; name derived from function: Communicates (inter) among white blood cells (leukins); affect the growth and differentiation of immune system cells		
IL-1		
Proinflammatory	Bacterial products stimulate the release of IL-1 from macrophages, monocytes, lymphocytes, neutrophils, and endothelial cells	Production of other cytokines (TNF-α, IL-6, IL-8, PAF, leukotrienes, thromboxane, prostaglandins)
	Similar to TNF-α; has a synergistic effect	Activation of T and B cells with B-cell growth and immunoglobulin production
	Increases in concentration as a "second wave" to TNF-α	
		Vasodilation, hypotension
		Increased vessel permeability
		Fever, sleep, anorexia
		Myocardial depression, hypercoagulability, and ACTH release

TABLE 10.2 Response to Cytokine and Mediator Release in Systemic Inflammatory Response Syndrome—cont'd

Cytokine/Mediator/Precursor	Release	Response
IL-6		
Proinflammatory and antiinflammatory	Released early in sepsis by activated T cells, antigen-presenting cells, monocytes, and macrophages in the presence of bacterial antigens, TNF-α, and IL-1	Fever Cortisol production Decreased IL-1 and TNF-α production Activation of T and B cells; B-cell growth and immunoglobulin production Hepatic synthesis of acute-phase proteins, such as C-reactive protein
IL-8 (NEUTROPHIL-ACTIVATING FACTOR)		
Proinflammatory	Produced under the influence of TNF-α and IL-1 by macrophages and endothelial cells C5a, bacterial products, IL-1, and TNF-α stimulate the production of IL-8	May be involved in mediating local organ dysfunction Chemoattraction for neutrophils and T cells to participate in inflammatory response; stimulation of cell oxidative burst, degranulation, and release of proteases Tissue damage, cell aggregation Increased vessel permeability
IL-10		
Antiinflammatory	Released by T cells, B cells, and macrophages Produced late in the activation process; stimulated by LPS (endotoxin)	Inhibition of the release of TNF-α and IL-1 from activated T lymphocytes Deactivation of macrophages by suppression of the production of reactive oxygen intermediates Promotion of B-cell production of immunoglobulins
INTERFERONS		
IFN-α		
Antiviral cytokine Proinflammatory Soluble factor that interferes with viral replication when applied to uninfected cells	Released from white blood cells to target uninfected cells	Chills and fever Sickness symptoms: Fatigue, myalgia T-cell proliferation Antiviral effect
IFN-β		
Antiviral cytokine Proinflammatory Soluble factor that interferes with viral replication when applied to uninfected cells	Released from fibroblasts to target uninfected cells	T-cell proliferation Antiviral effect

Continued

TABLE 10.2 Response to Cytokine and Mediator Release in Systemic Inflammatory Response Syndrome—cont'd

Cytokine/Mediator/ Precursor	Release	Response
IFN-γ		
Antiviral cytokine Proinflammatory	Released from natural killer cells and T cells in response to TNF-α and IL-1 Targets unaffected cells, macrophages, proliferating B cells, and inflammatory cells	Enhanced release and amplified actions of TNF-α and IL-1 Increased number of TNF-α receptors on macrophages, which makes them more sensitive to TNF-α effects Antiviral effect Differentiation of immunoglobulin synthesis Activation of natural killer cells
LEUKOTRIENES		
Metabolites of arachidonic acid Proinflammatory	PLA$_2$ is an enzyme secreted during shock and in response to TNF-α, IL-1, IL-8, and complement PLA$_2$ triggers the release of fatty acids, such as arachidonic acid, from many body cells, which leads to the production of leukotrienes Leukotrienes are produced from neutrophils, monocytes, and eosinophils	Tissue inflammation, vessel damage, and increased permeability of vessels, which occur as a result of the production of superoxide PMN accumulation and activation because of chemotactic properties Renal, pulmonary, and coronary vasoconstriction Reduced cardiac contractility
MONOCYTE CHEMOATTRACTANT PROTEIN-1		
Amino acid polypeptide Chemotactic agent Proinflammatory	Bacterial products, activated complement, and cytokines activate PMNs, monocytes, and endothelial cells to produce MCP-1	Attraction and activation of monocytes and macrophages because of its chemotactic properties Oxidative burst from cells, which increases metabolism and degranulation Release of proteases with resultant vessel damage and increased vessel permeability
NITRIC OXIDE		
Free radical molecule Molecule synthesized by NOS, thought to be endothelium-derived relaxant factor Proinflammatory	Two forms of NOS: (1) an inducible form (iNOS), whose production is stimulated by LPS and cytokines; (2) a constitutive (or endothelial) form (cNOS), normally produced in the vascular endothelium cNOS is continuously produced by the endothelium near vascular smooth muscle cells and inhibits leukocyte and platelet adhesion iNOS is released from many body cells in response to LPS, cytokines, and activated mediators	Smooth muscle relaxation, vasodilation, hypotension (**Note:** iNOS has a greater potential to produce pathologic hypotension than does cNOS) Depressed myocardial function Mitochondrial respiration inhibition Increased capillary permeability Increased leukocyte adhesion

Sepsis and Septic Shock

10

TABLE 10.2 **Response to Cytokine and Mediator Release in Systemic Inflammatory Response Syndrome—cont'd**

Cytokine/Mediator/Precursor	Release	Response
PLATELET-ACTIVATING FACTOR		
Lipophilic organic mediator Phospholipid produced by a variety of cells, including activated mast cells, platelets, endothelium, basophils, and leukocytes Proinflammatory	PLA_2 enzymes, found in most cells, are secreted during shock and in response to LPS, TNF-α, IL-1, IL-8, complement, and other cytokines PLA_2 triggers the release of lipid mediators, including PAF, from many body cells	Activation of neutrophils and eosinophils Inflammation of many body tissues: nerves, GI tract, cartilage, and blood vessels Increased permeability of vessels; decreased myocardial contractility; vasodilation; hypotension; bronchoconstriction Platelet aggregation Prostaglandin synthesis
PROSTAGLANDINS		
Metabolites of arachidonic acid produced in the cyclooxygenase pathway	PLA_2 enzymes are found in most cells and are secreted during shock in response to TNF-α, IL-1, IL-6 and complement; PLA_2 causes the release of arachidonic acid from the cell membrane, which leads to the production of prostaglandins; several types are produced: PGD_2, PGE_2, and PGI_2 prostacyclin	Chemoattraction Vasodilation Fever PGD_2 is produced by connective tissue mast cells and leads to vasodilation and bronchial constriction PGI_2 inhibits platelet aggregation PGE_2 inhibits T-cell and B-cell proliferation, inhibits immunoglobulin synthesis
THROMBOXANE A$_2$		
Metabolite of arachidonic acid produced in the cyclooxygenase pathway Proinflammatory	PLA_2 enzymes, found in most cells, are secreted during shock and in response to LPS (endotoxins), TNF-α, IL-1, IL-6, PAF, and complement PLA_2 causes release of arachidonic acid from the cell membrane, which leads to the production of thromboxane A_2 Thromboxane A_2 is synthesized by platelets	Inflammation Platelet aggregation; increased WBC adherence Increased vascular permeability Vasoconstriction in the pulmonary circulation
TUMOR NECROSIS FACTOR-α		
Polypeptide secretory product of the monocyte-macrophage system Proinflammatory	Released from activated macrophages in response to endotoxins, IL-1, and IL-2 Plasma levels rise immediately after administration of endotoxin, before fever or stress hormone levels increase	Increased formation of oxygen radicals; injury to lungs, GI tract, and kidney injury Recruitment and activation of neutrophils, macrophages, lymphocytes Increased cytokine production (IL-1, IL-6, IL-8, PAF); mediation and replication of all effects of LPS; stimulation of arachidonic acid metabolism and production of leukotrienes, thromboxane, prostaglandins, and further production of TNF-α

Continued

TABLE 10.2 Response to Cytokine and Mediator Release in Systemic Inflammatory Response Syndrome—cont'd

Cytokine/Mediator/ Precursor	Release	Response
		Initial hyperglycemia followed by hypoglycemia; hypotension, metabolic acidosis, coagulopathy
		Fever, increased oxygen consumption, sleep, anorexia
		Increased capillary permeability, vasodilation, microvascular constriction, noncardiac pulmonary edema
		Activation of the coagulation cascade
		Activation of NOS to produce nitric oxide
		TNF-β also produced with similar effects

ACTH, Adrenocorticotropic hormone; *GI*, gastrointestinal; *IFN*, interferon; *IL*, interleukin; *LPS*, lipopolysaccharide (endotoxin); *MCP-1*, monocyte chemoattractant protein-1; *NOS*, nitric oxide synthase; *PAF*, platelet-activating factor; *PG*, prostaglandin; *PLA$_2$*, phospholipase A$_2$; *PMNs*, polymorphonuclear cells; *TNF*, tumor necrosis factor; *WBC*, white blood cell.

From Hotchkiss, R., Monneret, G., Payen, D. (2013). Immunosuppression in sepsis: a novel understanding of the disorder and a new therapeutic approach. *Lancet Infectious Disease*, 13(3), 260–268; Hotchkiss, R., Monneret, G., Payen, D. (2013). Sepsis-induced immunosuppression: from cellular dysfunctions to immunotherapy. *Nature Reviews. Immunology*, 13, 862–874.

(a) IL-8 induces chemotaxis of activated polymorphonuclear leukocytes and acts as an inflammatory mediator, which leads to tissue damage.

(b) TNF-α and IL-1 activate the coagulation cascade
  (1) Bacterial products, TNF-α, and IL-1 induce intravascular coagulation and fibrin deposits
  (2) Thromboplastin (factor III) and factor VIII activate the extrinsic coagulation pathway
  (3) Factor XII (Hageman factor) activates the intrinsic coagulation pathway

(c) TNF-α and IL-1 activate the complement cascade by factor XII and bacterial products
  (1) C5a component (one of more than 20 proteins involved in the complement cascade) is a vasoactive anaphylatoxin that binds to macrophages and monocytes.
  (2) Complement stimulates an oxidative burst.
  (3) Complement causes the release of oxygen radicals and proteases that damage cells, particularly type II pneumonocytes in the lungs.
  (4) Complement enhances adherence of neutrophils, platelets, and thrombus to the endothelium with degranulation (emptying out granules with digestive substances) and aggregation (clumping), which leads to microvasculature damage.
  (5) C5a binds to mast cells, basophils, and platelets; causes the release of histamine, serotonin, prostaglandins, and leukotrienes; and results in vessel dilation, increased blood flow, increased capillary permeability, and increased plasma leakage.
  (6) C5a leads to the release of more TNF-α, IL-1, and IL-8.

(d) TNF-α and IL-1 activate the kinin cascade with the production of bradykinin.
  (1) Potent vasodilation
  (2) Increased vascular permeability

4. **Role of bacterial translocation**
  a. Theory in humans describes the passage of microbes, such as normal bacterial flora of the gut or of microbial products across an injured intestinal mucosal wall from the gut lumen to the mesenteric lymph nodes, other organs, and bloodstream, and may be a major contributor to the development of the septic cascade.
  b. Common enteric organisms:
    i. *Enterococcus*
    ii. *Escherichia coli*
    iii. *Klebsiella pneumoniae*
    iv. *Streptococcus spp.*
    v. *Bacteroides fragilis*
  c. Conditions thought to increase gut permeability and microbial translocation:
    i. Mucosal ischemia and mucosal hypoperfusion caused by shock or mesenteric vasoconstriction from intense sympathetic nervous system (SNS) stimulation
    ii. Also associated with total parenteral nutrition, thermal injury, glucocorticoid administration, and endotoxin release
  d. Other conditions that contribute to microbial translocation include obstructive jaundice, burns, endotoxemia, hemorrhage, immunosuppression, malnutrition, ischemia, reperfusion injury, total parenteral nutrition, and antibiotic therapy

5. **Etiology**
  a. Most common sites of origin of bacteremia and sepsis
    i. Pneumonia (36%–42% of all cases)
    ii. Infection of unknown source (20%–21% of all cases)
    iii. Urinary tract infection (10%–18% of all cases)
    iv. Intraabdominal infection (8% of all cases)
    v. Skin and soft tissue (7%–9% of all cases)
    vi. Intravascular catheters (1% of all cases)
  b. Most common organisms in hospitalized patients:
    i. Gram-negative aerobes
      (a) *E. coli*
      (b) *Klebsiella* and *Citrobacter* species
      (c) *Pseudomonas aeruginosa*
  c. Gram-positive organisms are becoming more common because of association with use of intravascular catheters and invasive devices
  d. Most common aerobic organisms are the following:
    i. *Staphylococcus aureus*
    ii. *Pseudomonas* species
    iii. *Enterobacteriaceae*
    iv. *Streptococcus pneumoniae*
    v. *Klebsiella* species
    vi. Other common organisms
      (a) Methicillin-resistant *S. aureus* (MRSA)
      (b) Vanc-resistant enterococcus
      (c) *Enterococcus*

(d) *Streptococcus epidermidis*

e. Other organisms

   i. Viral

     (a) COVID 19 is a virus and should not to be utilized for Sepsis Guidelines and SEP 1 CMS guidelines. It is not responsive to antibiotics. Virus and fungal infections are not included in the CMS guidelines. (SSI, 2021).

   ii. Fungal

   iii. Parasitic

   iv. Anaerobic organisms: *Clostridium, Bacteroides fragilis*

f. Multidrug resistant organisms (MDRO)

   i. Definition

     (a) Pathogens, predominantly bacteria, which cannot be killed by conventional antibiotics. These bacteria have developed a resistance over time because of antibiotic overuse. Fewer antibiotics are available to treat MDROs.

   ii. Types

     (a) MRSA is one of the most common in health care organizations

     (b) Vancomycin-resistant *enterococci* (VRE)

     (c) *C. diff* (*Clostridium difficile*)

     (d) Carbapenem resistant *Enterobacteriaceae* (CRE)

     (e) Acinetobacter

   iii. Patient's natural flora altered, predisposing patient for a resistant form of an organism

   iv. Associated with increased morbidity, mortality, length of stay, and cost

6. **Risk factors**

a. Predisposing factors for the development of bacteremia or sepsis

   i. Extremes of age: Older adult (age >65 years old) and children

   ii. Male gender

   iii. Black race

   iv. Severe burn injury, recent trauma, recent surgical procedures, and invasive procedures

   v. Chronic health conditions:

     (a) Chronic obstructive pulmonary disease

     (b) Chronic kidney disease

     (c) Liver disease

     (d) Diabetes

   vi. Immunosuppression:

     (a) Infection with human immunodeficiency virus (HIV)

     (b) Chemotherapy

     (c) Corticosteroids

     (d) Bone marrow suppression

   vii. Malignancy

   viii. Malnutrition and total parenteral nutrition

   ix. Social and recreational factors:

     (a) Alcohol use and abuse

     (b) Abuse of other medications

     (c) Decreased socioeconomic status

   x. Long-term care facility residence

   xi. Prolonged ICU length of stay

ASSESSMENT

1. **History**
   a. Patient health history
      i. Significant past medical and surgical history, with a review of all major systems and the identification of recent invasive procedures, prior hospitalization, and recent travel history
      ii. History of chronic disease: Diabetes mellitus; alcoholism; pulmonary, liver, heart disease; renal failure, cancer
      iii. Acute illness: Trauma, burns, cholelithiasis, intestinal obstruction, pancreatitis, appendicitis, peritonitis, diverticulitis
      iv. Wounds, indwelling catheters, or any suspected source of infection
   b. Family health history
      i. Chronic disease or infections
   c. Social history
      i. Significant others
      ii. Ability of the patient and significant others to manage stress
      iii. Financial obligations of the patient and significant others
      iv. Parenting responsibilities of the patient
      v. Smoker, illicit drug use, sexual activity
   d. Medication history
      i. Medications with immunosuppressive properties (chemotherapeutic medications, corticosteroids)
      ii. Antibiotics
   e. Nutritional history
      i. Causes of primary malnutrition
         (a) Anorexia nervosa
         (b) Alcohol abuse
      ii. Secondary malnutrition
         (a) Iatrogenic malnutrition
         (b) Surgical malnutrition
2. **Physical examination**
   a. Physical examination data
      i. Inspection: Clinical presentation may vary, depending on the patient's underlying health and organ function
         (a) Acute distress with anxiety, restlessness, confusion, disorientation, and somnolence progressing to unresponsiveness
         (b) Flushed, warm, dry skin or pale, cold, mottled skin (particularly in the older adult or progressive shock state); decreased capillary refill; shaking chills and shivering in some patients
         (c) Tachypnea and dyspnea
         (d) Decreased urinary output; significant edema or positive fluid balance
         (e) Petechiae, purpura
         (f) Redness, swelling, or drainage, especially on or near invasive lines, catheters, or wounds
      ii. Palpation
         (a) Tachycardia with rapid, weak, and thready peripheral pulses. Initially, pulses may be bounding and rapid.
         (b) Warm skin (older adult may present with cool skin rather than hyperthermia)
         (c) Abdominal distension

(d) Cap Refill is recommended as an adjunct for measuring perfusion with fluid resuscitation (SSC, 2021).
iii. Percussion
(a) Dullness over areas of consolidation
iv. Auscultation
(a) Pulmonary crackles from interstitial pulmonary edema; wheezing without a history of bronchospastic airway disease
(b) Absence of bowel sounds; may progress to paralytic ileus
b. Monitoring data
i. Monitor for potential signs and symptoms of infection
(a) Core temperature: Above 38.3° C (100.9° F) or below 36° C (96.8° F)
(b) Heart rate above 90 beats/minute
(c) RR higher than 20 breaths/minute
(d) Pain, redness, swelling, or drainage noted on the skin, catheter insertions sites, or wounds/incisional lines
ii. Hemodynamic variables
(a) Cardiac index may be initially increased and then decreased in sepsis; may be low in older adult patients and those with underlying cardiac disorders
(b) Oxygen delivery and consumption: Variable, but often elevated in early stage of sepsis, then decreased as septic shock progresses; oxygen extraction below 20% of oxygen delivery (normally 20%–25%)
(1) Experts suggest that the designations of "warm shock" and "cold shock" be abandoned and that the extent of tissue perfusion be used to determine the extent of shock (e.g., central venous sample [$ScvO_2$], serum lactate and base deficit values).
(2) If hemodynamic variables (such as oxygen delivery and consumption) are not available, lactate levels or base deficit can be used (see Diagnostic Studies).
(c) Pain (See Ch. 20, Pain)

KEY CONCEPT
Elevated lactate *alone* is not an indicator of sepsis or septic shock, rather anaerobic metabolism, hypoperfusion and tissue hypoxia from a variety of reasons.

---

c. Appraisal of patient characteristics: Patients with acute or life-threatening infectious disease processes enter critical care units with a wide range of clinical characteristics. During their stay, their clinical status may slowly or abruptly improve or deteriorate. Changes in the patient's condition may involve one or all life-sustaining functions, and functions can be easy or nearly impossible to monitor with precision. Examples of clinical attributes that the nurse should assess when caring for a patient with sepsis and septic shock are the following: Resiliency, vulnerability, stability, complexity, resource availability, participation in care and decision-making, and predictability.
3. **Diagnostic criteria for sepsis**
a. Laboratory investigations: Blood cultures and antibiotic sensitivities
i. Identify causative organisms; blood culture results are positive in only 33% of septic patients for uncertain reasons (bacteremia may be intermittent)
b. Urine, sputum, and wound cultures to correlate with blood cultures

---

KEY CONCEPT
Positive blood cultures are helpful for individualizing treatment; however, they are not a prerequisite for diagnosis. Up to 33% of sepsis patients have negative blood cultures.

---

c. Inflammatory variables
   i. WBC count above 12,000/mm^3 or below 4000/mm^3, or more than 10% immature (band) forms
   ii. Plasma CRP more than two standard deviations above the normal
   iii. Plasma procalcitonin more than two standard deviations above the normal
d. Organ dysfunction variables
   i. Altered mental status
      (a) Arterial hypoxemia (partial pressure of oxygen [PaO$_2$]/fraction of inspired oxygen [Fio$_2$] <300)
      (b) Acute oliguria (urine output <0.5 mL/kg/h for at least 2 hours despite fluid resuscitation
      (c) Increase in creatinine over 0.5 md/dL
      (d) Coagulation abnormalities (international normalized ratio [INR]>1.5 or activated partial thromboplastin time [aPTT] >60 seconds)
      (e) Ileus
      (f) Thrombocytopenia (platelet count <100,000 µL)
      (g) Hyperbilirubinemia (plasma total bilirubin >4 mg/dL or 70 µmol/L.
e. Hyperglycemia (plasma glucose >140 mg/dL)
   i. Tissue perfusion variable
      (a) Hyperlactatemia (>1 mmol/L)

> **EXPERT TIP**
> Critical hypoperfusion, is evidenced by a lactate level of greater than 4 mmol/L because of sepsis in the presence of a normal BP.

PATIENT CARE

1. **Prevention**
   a. Routine sepsis screening
      i. Early identification of infection is the first step
   b. Use of sepsis screening tools and order sets for patients with suspected sepsis
   c. Performance improvement efforts, national performance measures (e.g., Centers for Medicaid and Medicare [CMS] Sepsis measures), bundle compliance, and sharing of quality data should be used to improve patient outcomes
      i. Viral and fungal infections are not included in the CMS Guidelines (SSI, 2021).
   d. Source control: Assist with treatments to limit the nidus of infection
      i. Removal of necrotic tissue or infected devices
      ii. Débridement of burned tissue
      iii. Drainage of abscesses
   e. Monitor compliance with unit infection prevention and control procedures:
      i. Hand washing
      ii. National Patient Safety Goals 2020 for The Joint Commission can be found online at: https://www.jointcommission.org/-/media/tjc/documents/standards/national-patient-safety-goals/2020-hap-npsg-goals-final.pdf
      iii. Screen for MRSA on ICU admission
      iv. Isolation, usually standard precautions and contact isolation until culture negative according to institutional policy
      v. Environmental cleaning precautions, including decontamination of equipment
      vi. Frequent dressing changes
      vii. Wound isolation
      viii. Optimal management of invasive lines and catheters
         (a) Frequent catheter and tubing changes

(b) Removal when no longer necessary
f. Use of and compliance with infection control bundles
g. Ventilator associated pneumonia (VAP) bundle
   i. Associated with endotracheal intubation longer than 48 hours (aspiration of pharyngeal secretions, contaminated respiratory equipment)
   ii. Consists of a multipronged approach:
      (a) Avoiding intubation if possible
      (b) Hand hygiene
      (c) Assess readiness for extubation daily
      (d) Minimize sedation (use agents other than benzodiazepines, daily sedation interruption)
      (e) Provide early exercise and mobilization
      (f) Minimize pooling of secretions above endotracheal tube cuff
      (g) Elevate head of bed 30 to 45 degrees
      (h) Maintain and change ventilator circuit
      (i) Decontamination of the oropharynx (e.g., frequent oral care, suctioning, use of oral chlorhexidine gluconate)
h. Prevention of hospital acquired pneumonia
i. Central line–associated bloodstream infection (CLABSI) bundle
   i. Hand hygiene
   ii. Full barrier precautions
   iii. Personal protective equipment during insertion
   iv. Chlorhexidine skin antisepsis
   v. Optimal catheter site selection (such as avoiding the femoral site when possible)
   vi. Sterile dressing, use of chlorhexidine impregnant patch at insertion site
   vii. Daily review of line necessity
j. Compliance with catheter-associated urinary tract infection (CAUTI) bundle
   i. Aseptic insertion for appropriate conditions only
   ii. Hand hygiene
   iii. Proper securement of the catheter
   iv. Maintenance of tubing free of kinks or dependent loops
   v. Maintaining collection bag below the level of the bladder at all times
   vi. Daily review of catheter necessity
k. Long-standing antibiotic overuse is a key risk factor for MDROs
   i. Consider antibiotic stewardship program
   ii. Conduct periodic risk assessments for acquisition and transmission
   iii. Staff, patient, family, and provider education, including protocols for communication and readmission
   iv. Partnership with laboratory and infection prevention team members to aid in the identification, surveillance, prevention of transmission, and epidemiologic trends
2. **Management of infection and exaggerated inflammatory process**
   a. Description of problem
      i. Exaggerated, hyperresponsive, or "malignant" inflammation
      ii. Inadequate primary defenses
         (a) Broken skin, traumatized tissues
      iii. Inadequate secondary defenses
         (a) Immunosuppression
         (b) Invasive procedures
         (c) Malnutrition

> ### BOX 10.1   Sepsis Resuscitation Goals/Endpoints
>
> - Use dynamic measures of volume assessment and reassessment, such as passive leg raise, rather than central venous pressure
> - Use lactate guided resuscitation
> - Obtain mean arterial pressure >65 mm Hg in most patients, but consider 80 to 85 mm Hg in those with chronic hypertension

From Singer, M., Deutschman, C., Warren Seymour, C., et al. (2016). The third international consensus definitions for sepsis and septic shock (Sepsis-3). *Journal of the American Medical Association*, 315, 801–810.

> ### BOX 10.2   Surviving Sepsis Campaign Hour-1 Bundle
>
> - Measure lactate level; remeasure if elevated
> - Obtain blood cultures before administering antibiotics
> - Administer broad-spectrum antibiotics
> - Begin rapid administration of 30 mL/kg crystalloid for hypotension or lactate level ≥4 mmol/L
> - Apply vasopressors if hypotensive during or after fluid resuscitation to maintain mean arterial pressure ≥65 mm Hg

From Singer, M., Deutschman, C., Warren Seymour, C., et al. (2016). The third international consensus definitions for sepsis and septic shock (Sepsis-3). *Journal of the American Medical Association*, 315, 801–810.

---

     iv. Defining characteristics: See definition of SIRS

  b. Goals of care and resuscitation endpoints suggesting return to hemodynamic stability (Box 10.1)

  c. Interprofessional collaboration: Nurse, physician, advanced practice provider, respiratory therapist, physical therapist, pharmacist, dietitian, and nursing leader as appropriate

  d. Interventions (Box 10.2)

     i. Administer antimicrobial agents as soon as possible

       (a) Within 1 hour of presentation

          (1) In septic shock, mortality increases by 7% to 8% for every hour of antibiotic delay

       (b) Use of prolonged beta-lactam antibiotics for maintenance-6-8 hrs (after initial bolus) over conventional bolus infusion is now recommended (SSI, 2021).

     ii. Monitor antibiotic levels, particularly aminoglycoside levels, for renal and ototoxic effects

    iii. Monitor for reaction to antibiotics

       (a) Superinfection or opportunistic infection: Infection with organisms, such as *Candida albicans* is usually controlled by normal body flora

       (b) Allergy: Rash and anaphylactic shock

       (c) Resistance: Reemergence of symptoms of fever, purulence, and increased WBC count

     iv. Monitor hemodynamic parameters (see Boxes 10.1 and 10.2)

     v. Be prepared to administer fluid resuscitation (see Box 10.2)

       (a) Initial 30 mL/kg crystalloid fluid challenge if hypotensive or serum lactate over 4 mmol/L (or >36 mg/dL). Repeat lactate following fluid resuscitation.

          (1) Balanced crystalloids, such as lactated Ringer's or plasmalyte, is probably preferred

> **EXPERT TIP**
> Serum lactate is prognostic and a severity of illness indicator. The higher the lactate level is in sepsis, the less likely the patient is to survive.

> **KEY CONCEPT**
> Intravenous fluid administration utilizing a pressure bag typically infuses 1 liter of crystalloid in 15 to 20 minutes.

    vi. Administer vasoactive medications as needed if fluid resuscitation fails to maintain BP and organ perfusion
      (a) Combined inotropic agent and vasopressor may be used
        (1) First choice: Norepinephrine, titrated to target MAP over 65 mm Hg
        (2) Vasopressin is often used as a norepinephrine sparing agent if high doses are required
    vii. Protocol-based standard care involves optimizing cardiac preload, afterload, and contractility to balance oxygen delivery with cellular requirements and demand.
      (a) Patient monitoring with arterial line and central venous oxygen saturation ($ScVO_2$) may be necessary
      (b) Goal of patient therapy: See Box 10.1
    viii. Treat possible adrenal insufficiency with corticosteroids
      (a) For adults with severe sepsis and ongoing requirements for vasopressive therapy, using IV corticosteroids within 4 hrs of initiation of vasopressors is recommended (SSI, 2021).
        (1) It is no longer recommended to check cortisol level nor adrenocorticotropic hormone (ACTH) test results before initiating corticosteroid therapy.
        (2) Effects of corticosteroids
          a) Decrease inflammatory response
          b) Improve vessel reactivity to vasopressor agents
          c) Decrease the time the patient requires vasopressors
          d) Improve patient outcome
        (3) Dosage: Hydrocortisone (Solucortef) 100 mg IV bolus followed by 200 to 300 mg IV daily in divided doses may be given and then tapered appropriately when vasopressors are no longer required.
    ix. Vitamin C is no longer recommended for adults with severe sepsis (SSI, 2021).
    x. Optimize oxygen delivery and utilization; minimize oxygen demand
    xi. Manage pain, anxiety, and restlessness with medications and nursing interventions
  e. Maintain strong rapport with the family and provide frequent updates and education because the course of this disease is often unpredictable

3. **Management of maldistribution of blood flow (renal, cerebral, cardiopulmonary, gastrointestinal, peripheral)**
  a. Description of problem
    i. Hypodynamic state with decreased cardiac output and index is a common initial presentation. Septic shock can transition from a hypodynamic state in the early stages to hyperdynamic in the late stages.
    ii. Inability of the tissues to use oxygen; $ScVO_2$ above 80% as late signs of organ dysfunction manifest; oxygen extraction ratio below 20%
    iii. Excessive microvascular coagulation, microthrombin formation and impaired fibrinolysis, platelet aggregation, and consumption of clotting factors

    iv. Decreased systemic vascular resistance and hypotension (systolic BP <90 mm Hg)

    v. Changes in sensorium (restlessness, anxiety, and disorientation progressing to unresponsiveness)

  b. Goals of care (see Box 10.1)

  c. Interprofessional collaboration: Nurse, physician, advanced practice provider, respiratory therapist, physical therapist, pharmacist, dietitian, and nursing leader as appropriate

  d. Interventions (see Management of Infection and Exaggerated Inflammatory Process)

4. Management of oxygenation and ventilation (See Ch. 3, Pulmonary System)

  a. For adults with sepsis-induced hypoxemic respiratory failure SSI, 2021, suggests the use of high-flow nasal cannula (HFNC) over noninvasive ventilation (NIV).

  b. For adults with sepsis-induced severe ARDS we suggest VV ECMO when conventional mechanical ventilation fails in an experienced center (SSI, 2021).

  c. For adults with sepsis-induced moderate-severe ARDS we suggest using intermittent NMBA boluses over continuous infusions (up to 48 hrs) (SSI, 2021).

5. Management of thermoregulation

  a. Description of problem

    i. Related to the body's response to infection and the inflammatory process

    ii. Core temperature below 36° C (96.8° F) or above 38.3° C (100.9° F)

    iii. Flushed, warm skin or pale, cool skin

    iv. Increased or decreased metabolic rate

  b. Goals of care

    i. Establish normothermia

    ii. Skin is warm and dry

  c. Interprofessional collaboration: Nurse, patient care technician, physician, advanced practice provider, respiratory therapist, physical therapist, pharmacist, dietitian, and nursing leader as appropriate.

  d. Interventions

    i. Monitor core temperature hourly

    ii. After the source of increased or decreased temperature is identified, maintain normothermia by the use of antipyretic medication as prescribed

      (a) Acetaminophen (Tylenol)

      (b) Nonsteroidal antiinflammatory drugs

    iii. Surface cooling

      (a) Strategies:

        (1) Use tepid baths

        (2) Cooling blankets

        (3) Ice packs

        (4) Commercially offered cooling blankets

    iv. Invasive cooling

      (a) Strategies

        (1) Esophageal cooling

        (2) Cooling IV catheters

        (3) Administration of cooled IV fluids

    v. Monitor core temperature at all times to reduce the risk of hypothermia

    vi. Avoid too rapid of temperature shifts, as can cause fluid and electrolyte shifts and cardiac arrhythmias

    vii. Manage shivering that may occur

      (a) Surface counterwarming

    (1) Warm blankets
    (2) Commercially offered heating blankets
    (3) Socks, mittens
   (b) Administer medications to treat shivering
    (1) Buspirone (Buspar)
    (2) Magnesium
    (3) Meperidine (Demerol)

6. Management of the catabolic state resulting in malnutrition
 a. Description of problem
  i. Increased body temperature
  ii. Increased body metabolism
  iii. Decreased intake or processing of nutrients
  iv. Loss of body weight and muscle mass
 b. Treatment goals
  i. Body weight as appropriate for gender and body frame
  ii. Nitrogen balance is positive
  iii. Muscle mass is adequate
 c. Interprofessional collaboration: See Management of Infection and Exaggerated Inflammatory Process
 d. Interventions: (see Ch. 9 Gastrointestinal System)
  i. Initiate enteral feedings within 24 to 48 hours to limit gastrointestinal microbial translocation.
   (a) Avoid bolus feeds as can cause postprandial hypotension
  ii. Initiate trophic feeding (10–20 kcal/h or up to 500 kcal/day) for the initial phase of sepsis
   (a) Advance as tolerated after 24 to 48 hours to more than 80% of target energy goal over the first week of ICU stay
  iii. A protocolized approach to enteral feeding and blood glucose management should be considered.
   (a) Target blood glucose range of 110 to 180 mg/dL for the general ICU population
   (b) Ranges for specific patient populations (postcardiovascular surgery, head trauma, etc.) may differ.
   (c) Both hyperglycemia and hypoglycemia may be associated with a poor prognosis.
  iv. Provide family/significant others with distinct goals for nutritional support.
  v. Obtain metabolic care to determine true nutritional needs.

7. Long-term Outcomes and Goals of Care (SSI, 2021).
 a. For adults with sepsis or severe sepsis SSI 2021 suggests discussing goals of care and prognosis within 72 hours.
 b. Suggests integrating principles of palliative care into the treatment plan.
 c. Screening for economic, social support (housing, nutrition, financial and spiritual) and to make referrals to meet those needs.
 d. Families be included in shared decision-making post-ICU and hospital discharge.
 e. For adults with sepsis and severe sepsis who have new impairments we recommend discharge plans to include follow-up.
 f. Assessment and follow-up for physical, cognitive, and emotional problems after hospital discharge.

References and bibliography information are available at http://evolve.elsevier.com/AACN/corecurriculum/.

Multisystem Trauma

Renee M. Holleran, FNP-BC, PhD, CCRN (Alumnus), CEN, CFRN, CTRN (Retired), FAEN

CROSSWALK

- **Quality and Safety in Nursing Education (QSEN):** Patient-centered care, Teamwork and collaboration, Evidence-based practice, Quality improvement, Safety, Informatics
- **National Patient Safety Goals:** Identifies patients correctly, Improve staff communication, Use medicines safely, Use alarms safely, Prevent infection, Identify patient safety risks, Prevent mistakes in surgery
- **American Nurses Association (ANA) standards for Professional Nursing Practice:** Standard 1. Assessment, Standard 2. Diagnosis, Standard 3. Outcomes identification, Standard 4. Planning, Standard 5. Implementation, Standard 6. Evaluation, Standard 7. Ethics, Standard 9. Communication, Standard 10. Collaboration, Standard 11. Leadership, Standard 12. Education, Standard 13. Evidence-based practice and research, Standard 14. Quality of practice, Standard 15. Professional practice evaluation, Standard 16. Resource utilization, Standard 17. Environmental health
- **AACN Scope and Standards for Progressive and Critical Care Nursing Practice:** Standard 1. Quality of practice, Standard 2. Professional practice evaluation, Standard 3. Education, Standard 4. Communication, Standard 5. Ethics, Standard 6. Collaboration, Standard 7. Evidence-based practice/research/clinical inquiry, Standard 8. Resource utilization, Standard 9. Leadership, Standard 10. Environmental health
- **AACN Standards for Establishing and Sustaining Healthy Work Environments (HWE):** Skilled communication, True collaboration, Effective decision-making
- **PCCN content:** None
- **CCRN content:** Cardiovascular—Cardiac trauma, Respiratory—Thoracic trauma, Gastrointestinal—Acute abdominal trauma, Renal and Genitourinary—Acute genitourinary trauma, Neurologic—Acute spinal cord injury, Traumatic brain injury, Multisystem—Trauma

SYSTEMWIDE ELEMENTS

TRAUMA CONCEPTS AND PHYSIOLOGY REVIEW

1. **Definitions**
   a. Injury: Physical harm or damage to the body resulting from an exchange, usually acute, of mechanical, chemical, thermal, or other environmental energy that exceeds the body's tolerance
   b. Unintentional injury: Accidental harm or damage to the body resulting from sudden, unplanned traumatic events, such as motor vehicle crashes, burns, drowning, exposure to poisons, falls, explosions, electrical accidents, or firearm injuries
   c. Intentional injury: Harm or damage to the body resulting from planned or premeditated injurious acts, for example, assaults (beatings, gunshot wounds, stab wounds), homicides, and suicides

   d. Trauma systems: An organized system developed to provide care for injured patients. Levels of trauma care have been developed along with standards as to how these levels can be achieved (American Trauma Society, n.d.).

      i. Level I trauma center: Tertiary care system and the center of the care system. The facility must be accessible and allow for an efficient transfer process. Must have adequate personnel and resources for complex injuries, as well as provide leadership, education, research, and system planning related to the care and prevention of trauma.

      ii. Level II trauma center: Should be able to provide initial definitive care for the injured patient, except for complex specialized injuries. When there is not a level I in a service area, the level II center must be able to provide the leadership and education as a level I center.

      iii. Level III trauma center: These centers can provide prompt assessment, resuscitation, emergency operations, and stabilization of an injured patient and arrange for transfer and transport if needed. They should participate in larger regional trauma systems.

      iv. Level IV trauma center: These centers provide advanced trauma life support before patient transfer to a higher level of care. These centers are in remote areas where no higher level of care is available.

      v. Level V trauma center: Provides initial evaluation, stabilization, and diagnostic capabilities and prepares patients for transfer to higher levels of care. Should have advanced trauma life support (ATLS) educated staff and trauma nurses; may provide surgery and critical care; need to have agreements for patient transfer to a higher level of care

2. Etiology and risk factors

   a. Factors associated with trauma

      i. Physical

         (a) Age: Older adult and very young are at risk

            (1) Patients older than 65 years of age fare worse after trauma than younger patients

               a) Injury is more severe because of increased body fragility, blunted compensatory mechanisms, and the presence of underlying organ dysfunction, with decreased organ reserve

               b) Risk for trauma is higher because of poor vision, weak lower extremities, unsteady gait, and impaired balance, use of multiple medications

            (2) Very young (<5 years) have higher mortality rates than children aged 6 to 14 years

         (b) Gender and the incidence of trauma: More males than females are injured between the ages 1 to 46 years

            (1) Pregnancy affects injury severity and outcome (see Ch. 17, High-Risk Obstetric Patients)

            (2) Females more at risk for domestic violence

         (c) Ethnicity

            (1) Poisoning, motor vehicle traffic, and falls are the most common cause of mortality across all races and ethnicities in the United States

            (2) Increased death from homicides seen more in Black American males between the ages of 15 and 34 years

(d) Type of injury: Blunt versus penetrating

(e) Preinjury health status: Preexisting organ dysfunction or conditions, such as diabetes mellitus, chronic obstructive pulmonary disease, atherosclerotic heart disease, hypertension, and cystic kidney disease increase susceptibility to injury and impair the response to injury

ii. Environmental factors: Speed limits, legal drinking age, mandatory helmet laws, availability of guns, residence near water, residence in cold climates

(a) Unintentional injury rates are highest in rural areas

(b) Intentional injury rates are highest in urban areas

iii. Socioeconomic factors: Working in a high-risk occupation (construction, heavy industry), living in a high-crime area, living in a poorly maintained home, and membership in a gang; the lower the income, the higher the death rate in Black Americans and White Americans

iv. Psychologic-neurologic factors: Risk-taking behaviors, antisocial behavior, mental illness, depression, poor judgment, and previous head injury

v. Use of alcohol and other medications that lead to impairment: Approximately half of all trauma patients have a history of alcohol or substance use; use of alcohol and other medications places the patient at risk for injury

(a) Decreased level of alertness; impaired motor function, coordination, and balance; increased reaction time

(b) Impaired judgment, perception, and cognitive ability; increased risk-taking behavior and feeling of invulnerability among adolescents; increased violent behavior; reduced inhibitions

(c) Increased physiologic fragility; injury may be severe, and recovery may be slower

vi. Social and economic burden of trauma

(a) Trauma affects all ages and sexes, and, because of this, the effect of life years lost is equal to the life years lost from cancer, heart disease, and human immunodeficiency virus (HIV) combined

(b) The economic burden of trauma is in the billions of dollars annually in healthcare costs and lost productivity

b. Mechanisms of injury

i. Blunt injury: Trauma that occurs when a surface of the body has impact with a blunt object. Common mechanisms include objects (stationary or those in movement). Common causes are motor vehicle crashes and falls. Caused by a combination of forces:

(a) Acceleration: Change in the rate of velocity or speed of a moving body; as velocity increases, so does tissue damage

(b) Deceleration: Decrease in the velocity of a moving object; acceleration-deceleration forces are a common cause of blunt injury

(c) Shearing: Structures slip relative to each other because of forces across a plane

(d) Crushing and compression: Squeezing, stretching, or inward pressure; hollow organs (stomach, bowel, urinary bladder) are less likely to rupture (except in a seat belt injury) than are solid organs (liver, spleen), which are less compressible

ii. Penetrating injury: Trauma that occurs from foreign objects that enter into tissue, causing direct damage from entry or indirect damage because of the tissue deformation associated with energy transference into the surrounding tissues

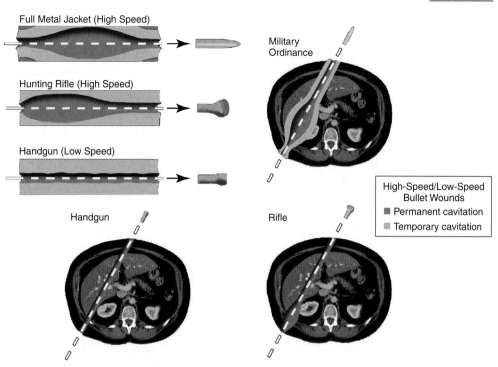

FIG. 11.1 Mass and velocity determine a bullet's energy, which transfers into living tissue and results in cavitation. The highest energy bullets form the largest cavities and have the greatest potential for tissue injury. The cavity formed is either temporary or permanent. The temporary cavity reverses following the passage of the bullet. However, the stretch effects from the temporary cavity may result in tissue injury. Given identical bullet trajectories, the high-energy military ordinance bullet creates a larger cavity that would be expected to cause much more right renal damage. (From Hanna, T.N., Shuaib, W., Han, T., et al. (2015). Firearms, bullets, and wound ballistics: an imaging primer. *Injury, 46,* 1183–1424.)

(a) Gunshot wounds
   (1) Energy of a bullet is dissipated into the tissues. When the bullet enters the body, a permanent cavity is formed that distorts, stretches, and compresses the surrounding tissues (Fig. 11.1).
   (2) Blast effect (muzzle blast): Cavity from a gunshot wound produces damage to structures not in the direct path of the bullet.
   (3) High-velocity bullets cause extensive cavitation and significant tissue destruction. Low-velocity bullets have limited cavitation potential and result in less tissue destruction.
   (4) Extent of the injury is proportional to the amount of kinetic energy lost by the object:

$$K = \left[\text{mass} \times \left(V1^2 - V2^2 \right) \right] \big/ 2$$

   where K = kinetic energy, V1 = impact velocity, and V2 = velocity after impact
   (5) Tissue yaw: Amount of tumbling and movement of the nose of the object; the more yaw, the more damage (see Fig. 11.1)
(b) Stab wounds: Follow a more predictable pattern than gunshot wounds and may involve less tissue destruction unless vital organs or vessels are lacerated

      (c) Impalement: Usually a low-velocity penetrating injury that occurs in motor vehicle crashes, with falls, and after being hit by falling or flying objects

      (d) Avulsion and degloving: Tearing away of tissue, which results in full-thickness skin loss; occurs when the skin is sliced by a sharp object or when a person is thrown from a moving vehicle

3. Prevalence

  a. Injury remains the leading cause of death in people aged 1 to 44 years

  b. Injury is the third leading cause of death for all age groups

  c. Causes of injury include poisoning, motor vehicle traffic deaths, falls, firearm injuries, drowning, and burns

  d. In 2018 approximately 167,128 deaths resulted from injury which included all age groups

  e. Approximately 67,000 intentional deaths (particularly suicides and homicides) occur each year

  f. In 2018 there were 2,530,238 poisonings reported in the United States

  g. In 2018 the Centers for Disease Control and Prevention (CDC) statistics reported 67,367 deaths from overdoses, many related to opioids

4. Pathophysiology of the response to injury

  a. Stress response

    i. Initial stress response, known as the "ebb phase," is initiated by tissue injury, acute blood loss, shock, hypoxia, acidosis, and hypothermia, as well as feelings of pain, anxiety, and fear.

    ii. Sympathetic nervous system (SNS): Afferent nerve signals reach the brain following the presentation of stimuli. Stimulation of the splanchnic nerves occurs, which leads to the release of epinephrine, norepinephrine, cortisol, and growth hormone into the circulation.

      (a) Increase in heart rate and contractility, vasoconstriction, and blood pressure (BP)

      (b) Increase in minute ventilation

      (c) Prolonged and excessive stimulation leads to severe and uneven arteriolar vasoconstriction, reduced microcirculatory blood flow, and impaired delivery of oxygen and nutrients to tissues

        (1) In the absence of hypovolemia, redistribution of intravascular volume from the venous capacitance vessels leads to increased central blood volume and increased intraluminal capillary pressure

        (2) Loss of intravascular volume because of increased capillary permeability leads to intravascular hypovolemia, hypoperfusion, and edema

      (d) Following restoration of the fluid balance, the body develops a hyperdynamic state or "flow phase" to compensate for oxygen debt

        (1) This phase may last for weeks; the degree and duration of the hypermetabolic response depend on the injured tissue mass, loss of barriers to infection, degree of malnutrition, age, gender, and preinjury health status

        (2) Inability to achieve and maintain a hyperdynamic state (high cardiac index, oxygen delivery, and oxygen consumption) is associated with higher mortality rates

    iii. Hypothalamic-pituitary-adrenal secretions: Adrenal secretion of corticosteroids is regulated by both the hypothalamus and pituitary

      (a) Stimuli: Fear, pain, hypotension, hypovolemia, tissue injury

      (b) Effects of corticosteroid secretion: Sodium retention, insulin resistance, hyperglycemia, gluconeogenesis, lipolysis, protein catabolism, ketogenesis, and enhancement of the catabolic effects of tumor necrosis factor (TNF)-α, interleukin-1 (IL-1), and IL-6

   iv. Protein synthesis is modified to enhance immune function

      (a) Increase in the synthesis of acute-phase proteins (e.g., C-reactive protein [CRP])

      (b) Decrease in the synthesis of other proteins (e.g., albumin, skeletal muscle, and transferrin)

      (c) These physiologic effects occur in an effort to increase energy, which is needed to heal massive tissue injury

   v. Antidiuretic hormone (ADH) release: Loss of blood volume is sensed by atrial receptors, and hypotension is sensed by pressure receptors in the carotid sinus, aortic arch, and pulmonary artery

      (a) Receptors communicate with neurons in the hypothalamus, which synapse with cells in the posterior pituitary gland

      (b) Posterior pituitary gland releases ADH, which leads to vasoconstriction and water retention

   vi. Renin-angiotensin release: Renin is released from the juxtaglomerular cells when renal blood flow is diminished or when they are stimulated by the SNS. Renin catalyzes a reaction that leads to vasoconstriction, aldosterone stimulation, and decreased sodium and water excretion.

   vii. Endogenous opioids: Released from the pituitary gland as part of an initial stress response to decrease pain, inhibit feedback of pituitary activation, decrease adrenocorticotropic hormone (ACTH) release, and increase insulin release; may decrease immune response

   viii. Coagulopathy: From excessive bleeding, massive blood transfusions, hypothermia, and inflammatory response

   ix. Locally produced mediators

      (a) Endothelial disruption leads to activation of Hageman factor (factor XII), which activates other systems

        (1) Coagulation cascade, leading to clotting and fibrinolysis

        (2) Complement cascade, initiating inflammation, and increased capillary permeability

        (3) Kinin and plasmin systems

      (b) Activation of arachidonic acid metabolism leads to activation of other mediators

        (1) Prostaglandins: Vasoconstriction and platelet aggregation

        (2) Leukotrienes: Mediator of vascular tone and inflammation

        (3) Platelet-activating factor: Stimulates platelet and neutrophil activation, which leads to microvascular thrombosis at the site of injury

        (4) Activation of cytokine cascades: TNF-α, IL-1, IL-6, and IL-8

      (c) Oxygen radicals: Released from ischemic tissues on reperfusion and activated by localized circulating immune effector cells, which leads to further tissue injury

b. Psychologic response (varies with the circumstances): Fear, withdrawal, anger, hostility, anxiety, depression, regression, intrusion or avoidance, and hyperarousal

c. Metabolic derangements

   i. Edema: Prolonged trauma and stress lead to an influx of sodium and water from the intravascular space into the interstitial space, which results in intravascular fluid volume deficit and interstitial edema; increased capillary permeability from circulating mediators increases edema

ii. Increased cardiac output (CO): Heart rate and contractility increase as a result of the stress response; when bleeding is controlled and the fluid volume is replaced, hyperdynamic circulation occurs; the patient may not exhibit the response of tachycardia in the presence of certain medications (e.g., β-adrenergic and calcium channel blockers)

iii. Impaired oxygen transport: Altered microcirculation because of vasoconstriction at the tissue level leads to decreased tissue perfusion

iv. Hypermetabolism: Oxygen consumption increases to supranormal levels 10% to 25% above the baseline. Extent of the increase depends on the severity of the injury.

v. Altered protein metabolism: Total body catabolism is increased, particularly within the skeletal muscles, which results in a loss of lean body mass. Hepatic synthesis of proteins increases. Growth hormone induces potent anabolic effects to incorporate amino acids into proteins.

vi. Altered glucose metabolism: Glucose level increases because of stress hormones; insulin resistance occurs; glycogen stores are converted to glucose

vii. Altered fat metabolism: Lipids in the form of stored fuel are broken down into fatty acids for energy.

viii. Leukocytosis: Increased number of granulocytes, which occurs even without infection; increased degranulation

ASSESSMENT

1. **History**
   a. Source: Patient, family, partner, significant other, prehospital personnel, or bystander
   b. Mechanism of injury
      i. Motor vehicle crashes
         (a) Restrained, unrestrained, or airbag; helmet use (motorcycle)
         (b) Driver or passenger; location in vehicle; ejection from the vehicle
         (c) Type of vehicle; speed of the vehicle
         (d) Direction and force of the collision, rollover crash, time of extraction
      ii. Falls
         (a) Setting and context (e.g., slipping on ice, falling from a balcony during a party)
         (b) Angle and height of the fall; the risk for serious injury is increased for falls from a height above 10 feet; type of impact surface; landing position
      iii. Gunshot wound
         (a) Type of weapon (rifle, handgun, shotgun); caliber of the weapon
         (b) Velocity of the bullet; range at which the weapon was fired; position of the assailant
         (c) Intentional or unintentional
         (d) If self-inflicted, hand dominance
         (e) Estimated depth of penetration; entry site; angle of entry/exit site; angle of exit
      iv. Stab wound
         (a) Type of weapon; size and length of blade
         (b) Intentional or unintentional

   (c) If self-inflicted, hand dominance

   (d) Estimated depth of penetration; entry site; angle of entry

   c. Description of the event

   i. Location and time

   ii. People involved and their disposition

   iii. Context (e.g., during an argument, while at a party, during work, or while driving home)

   d. Alcohol and substance use involvement

   e. Past health history: AMPLE

   i. *A:* Allergies

   ii. *M:* Medications

   (a) Prescription and over-the-counter (OTC) medications

   (b) Herbal and natural substances

   (c) Tetanus immunization

   iii. *P:* Past illnesses (medical and surgical), pregnancies

   iv. *L:* Last meal (time, quantity, type)

   v. *E:* Events preceding the injury, environment and exposure

   f. Social history

   i. Partner, spouse, housemates, roommates, significant others, contact person, dependents, children, parents, guardians

   ii. Education; occupation; financial considerations, ability to maintain income, and insurance coverage

   iii. Religion/spiritual beliefs

   g. Other

   i. Height, weight

   ii. Last menstrual period, potential for pregnancy

2. **Physical examination (primary and secondary surveys)**

   a. Physical examination data

   i. Primary survey: Rapid assessment (30 seconds to 2 minutes) that simultaneously identifies and manages life-threatening injuries: ABCDEFG (Emergency Nurses Association, 2020). It begins with an Across the Room Observation. This assessment includes what the patient looks like upon arrival in the trauma room and their overall physiologic stability including presence of uncontrolled hemorrhage.

   (a) *A:* Alertness and Airway—level of consciousness, ability to maintain a patent airway. Note: While protecting the cervical spine, manual stabilization or a cervical collar is mandatory during airway assessments and interventions.

   (1) Assessment of Alertness

   a) A: Alert: Interactive, able to keep airway clear

   b) V: Responds to verbal stimuli

   c) P: Responds to pain, pressure to specific areas

   d) U: Unresponsive. Be sure to check if patient has a pulse.

   (2) Assessment: Airway is open

   a) Patient speaks or makes appropriate sounds

   b) No foreign material visible in the mouth

   c) Look, listen, and feel for exhaled breath

   (3) If the airway is obstructed, expect some of the following signs:

   a) Inability to speak or make sounds

   b) Substernal and intercostal retractions

    c) No air exchange

    d) Stridor (inspiratory, expiratory)

    e) Nasal flaring (children, infants)

    f) Restlessness and confusion, progressing rapidly to unresponsiveness

(4) Emergency interventions during the primary survey. Note: Maintain alignment of the cervical spine at all times:

    a) Chin lift or jaw thrust

    b) Suction

    c) Airway management

        1) Oropharyngeal airway

        2) Nasopharyngeal airway

        3) Laryngeal mask airway

        4) Laryngeal tube airway

        5) Endotracheal intubation

    d) Cricothyroidotomy: When other means of airway maintenance are not possible or are contraindicated

(b) *B: Breathing and ventilation*—maintain adequate breathing.

(1) Assessment: Spontaneous, regular respirations of at least 10 breaths/minute with equal, bilateral chest expansion and audible breath sounds

(2) If breathing is compromised, expect:

    a) Respiratory rate (RR) less than 10 or more than 29 breaths/minute (adults)

    b) Difficult or labored breathing; intercostal or substernal retractions, accessory muscle use

    c) Decreased or absent breath sounds

    d) Asymmetric or paradoxical chest expansion

    e) Changes in color (pallor, duskiness, cyanosis)

    f) Tracheal deviation

    g) Restlessness, confusion, anxiety, and disorientation, progressing to unresponsiveness

(3) Emergency interventions during the primary survey

    a) Assist ventilations with bag-valve-mask and oxygen therapy

    b) Other options as needed in emergencies

        1) Needle or tube thoracostomy

        2) Covering of sucking chest wounds with a three-sided occlusive dressing

        3) Intubation and mechanical ventilation

        4) Chest tube insertion

(c) *C: Circulation:* maintain adequate circulation

EXPERT TIP

In early shock, circulatory compromise may have few clinical signs especially if the patient is young and in good health. On the other hand, in an already compromised patient, only a small amount of blood loss may bring on severe stress response. ATLS ® 10ᵗʰ edition notes that changes in pulse pressure and base deficit are more sensitive measures of the level of shock the patient is suffering and the need for resuscitation.

(1) Assessment levels of hemorrhagic shock:
    a) Class I
        1) Blood loss of 15% or less
        2) Pulse pressure normal
        3) Base deficit: 0 to 2 mEq/L
    b) Class II (Mild)
        1) 15% to 30% blood loss
        2) Pulse pressure decreased
        3) Normal to elevated heart rate
        4) Base deficit -2 to -6 mEq/L
    c) Class III (Moderate)
        1) 31% to 40% blood loss
        2) Increased heart rate
        3) Decreased BP
        4) Pulse pressure decreased
        5) Base deficit -6 to -10 mEq/L
    d) Class IV (Severe)
        1) Greater than 40% blood loss
        2) Increased heart rate
        3) Decrease BP
        4) Pulse pressure decreased
        5) Base deficit -10 mEq/L or less

(2) Emergency interventions during the primary survey
    a) Control of hemorrhage with external pressure dressings, stabilization of the pelvis, damage control surgery
    b) Insertion of short large-bore peripheral catheters; intraosseous needles can be used if no other access is available, wound packing, application of combat application tourniquet, application of a pelvic binder, application traction splints, eFAST Exam
    c) Fluid resuscitation with crystalloids for burns and dehydration. Patients with blood loss require fluids that can carry oxygen. The source of the bleeding must be located and managed before any aggressive resuscitation. Permissive hypotension (the BP is allowed to remain lower than normal) may be helpful until the bleeding is stopped. A target BP must be identified to prevent bleeding from continuing, restarting, or the development of coagulopathy. However, the patient with a traumatic brain injury (TBI) needs a cerebral perfusion pressure of at 50 to 70 mm Hg. Strongly consider blood products following repeated/sustained BP less than 90 mm Hg
    d) Massive transfusion protocols should be in place. Transfusion should be used to maintain the hemoglobin level between 7 and 9 g/dL.
    e) Patients who are on anticoagulants, such as warfarin may require fresh frozen plasma to reverse existing coagulopathy. Vitamin K and prothrombin complex concentrate may also be used as reversal agents. However, the potential for a cerebrovascular accident or a pulmonary embolus from a preexisting condition, such as atrial fibrillation must be weighed against the risk of continued bleeding when reversing coagulation agents.

(d) *D:* Disability: Monitor the level of consciousness
  (1) Assessment: Brief neurologic evaluation including calculate Glasgow Coma Scale (GCS), pupils, seizure activity and identifying lateralizing signs, such a Babinski response. Observe for trending of GCS.
  (2) If mental status is compromised, expect:
    a) Decreased alertness; unresponsiveness to verbal and tactile stimulation
    b) Pupils unequal in size or responsiveness; fixed and dilated pupils
    c) Ipsilateral or bilateral deficits in motor response; extremity rigidity
  (3) Emergency interventions during the primary survey
    a) Maintain and protect the airway; maintain breathing and circulation
    b) Initiate emergency measures to control increased intracranial pressure (ICP; see Ch. 5, Neurologic System)
    c) Protect the patient from self-harm
    d) Check blood sugar
    e) Rule out sources of intoxication, such as alcohol
    f) Consider naloxone administration if history of opioid use
    g) Head/spine radiograph, CT scan, remove backboard as soon as possible, remove helmet

---

EXPERT TIP

Assessing GCS, eye opening to pressure rather than pain and three sites for physical simulation, such as trapezius, fingertip pressure, and suborbital notch pressure. Changes to the verbal component has replaced the words inappropriate or incomprehensible to words and sound and motor assessment has replaced the word withdrawal with normal and abnormal flexion.

(e) *E:* Exposure and environmental control
  (1) Assessment: Remove all of the patient's clothing. Be careful not to cause any additional injury to the patient or the staff from glass or other potential toxic sources, such as fuel.
  (2) Inspect the patient for uncontrolled bleeding and additional injuries.
  (3) Emergency interventions during the primary survey
    a) Manage any obvious hemorrhage or injury
    b) Always be aware that clothing may be evidence, especially in incidents that result from violence, such as a gunshot wound. Clothing should be stored in appropriate containers, for example, paper bags and labeled with the patient's identifying information. Maintain chain of custody.
    c) Maintain the patient's body temperature
      1) Increase resuscitation room temperature
      2) Warming devices, such as forced air radiant warming lights
      3) Covering the patient with warm blankets
      4) Administering warm fluids
(f) *F:* Full set of vital signs, family presence
  (1) Measure full set of vital signs including BP, pulse rate, RR, and temperature.
  (2) Assess the family's understanding of the patient's condition, facilitate visiting and support of the patient, and use the family to assist in meeting the patient's emotional and spiritual needs.
  (3) Include family in End-of-Life Decisions when indicated

(g) *G:* Get monitoring devices and give comfort adjuncts using the LMNOP mnemonic (Emergency Nurses Association, 2020)

    (1) L: Lactic acid: An elevated lactic acid level can be associated with poor tissue perfusion; Arterial blood gases (ABGs): An abnormal base deficit can also indicate poor tissue perfusion

    (2) M: Monitor cardiac rhythm, which may indicate signs of injury, such as a cardiac tamponade

    (3) N: Consider the insertion of a nasogastric or orogastric tube to prevent vomiting, which could put the patient at risk for aspiration

    (4) O: Oxygen and ventilation assessment by using a pulse oximetry and/or end-tidal carbon dioxide ($ETCO_2$) to assess tissue perfusion

    (5) P: Pain assessment and management

(h) Reevaluation: Obtain a portable radiograph of chest and pelvis in the resuscitation area.

    (1) Consider the need for patient transfer and initiate this process by the most appropriate transport vehicle and transport team.

ii. Secondary survey: *H* through *J* mnemonic; complete head-to-toe physical examination begun as soon as the primary survey and emergency life-saving interventions are accomplished. *Note:* Ongoing trauma resuscitation continues during the secondary survey as needed (Emergency Nurses Association, 2020).

(a) *H:* History and head-to-toe assessment

    (1) Mnemonic MIST

       a) MOI: Mechanism of injury

       b) Injuries sustained

       c) Signs and symptoms seen in the field

       d) Treatment provided in the field

    (2) Patient history if the patient and/or family can provide it

       a) Allergies and tetanus status

       b) Medications

       c) Past medical history

       d) Last oral intake

       e) Events and environmental factors related to the injury

(b) *H:* Head-to-toe assessment

    (1) Abrasions, ecchymosis, swelling, and skin lacerations may indicate involvement of underlying structures or mechanism of injury. *Note:* Absence of external injury does not rule out the possibility of severe underlying injury.

    (2) Unusual drainage may indicate injury to internal structures.

       a) Otorrhea, rhinorrhea, and blood from the nose or ears may indicate a basilar skull fracture.

    (3) Blood at the urinary meatus may indicate a lower urinary tract injury or a pelvic fracture.

    (4) Inspect for protruding bone fragments or viscera.

    (5) Note a deformity or dislocation of the extremities.

    (6) Locate the entry and exit wounds of penetrating injuries. Do not remove impaled objects until a surgeon is present and ready for an operative procedure (or the injury may be worsened).

> **EXPERT TIP**
> A tertiary survey should be completed on all trauma patients after admission. This may occur hours, days, or weeks later. Injuries can be missed during the initial evaluation, especially when the patient has been severely injured.

    iii. Palpation: Abnormal findings
      (a) Skull depressions and deformities; facial deformity
      (b) Deformity or abnormal movement of the bony thorax; presence of subcutaneous emphysema
      (c) Abdominal guarding, tenderness, and rigidity
      (d) Pelvic fractures: Palpate for instability over the iliac crests and the symphysis pubis
      (e) Deformities and point tenderness of extremities and spine
      (f) Absence of peripheral pulses
    iv. Percussion: Note dullness over blood-filled collections or internal hematomas
    v. Auscultation of the heart and lungs for adventitious sounds and of the gastrointestinal tract for hypoactivity or hyperactivity
  b. Appraisal of patient characteristics: Patients who have suffered a traumatic episode enter critical care units with a wide range of clinical characteristics. During their stay, their clinical status may slowly or abruptly improve or deteriorate. Changes in the patient's condition may involve one or all life-sustaining functions, and functions can be easy or nearly impossible to monitor with precision. Examples of clinical attributes that the nurse should assess when caring for a trauma patient include the following: Resiliency, vulnerability, stability, complexity, resource availability, participation in care and decision-making, and predictability.

PATIENT CARE

1. **Impaired oxygenation and ventilation (see Ch. 3, Pulmonary System)**
  a. Additional interventions
    i. Maintain cervical spine protection during airway management until cervical spine injury is ruled out
    ii. Nasotracheal intubation is not recommended for the patient who has facial or basilar skull fractures (to avoid possible penetration of cribriform plate and iatrogenic brain injury)
    iii. Suspect airway compromise in intoxicated patients
2. **Intravascular volume depletion (see Ch. 4, Cardiovascular System)**
  a. Additional interventions
    i. Warm all fluids to body temperature, if possible, to prevent hypothermia
    ii. Use short, large-bore peripheral intravenous (IV) catheters or large-bore trauma catheters at multiple sites for rapid volume resuscitation
      (a) Avoid stopcocks, which slow infusion
      (b) Avoid long lengths of tubing, which increase resistance to flow
    iii. Administer pressurized fluids rapidly using a rapid volume infuser or pressure bag
    iv. Monitor for hypocalcemia and coagulopathy if multiple blood transfusions are needed
    v. Anticipate the need for immediate transfer to the operating room in cases of intravascular volume depletion and hemodynamic instability
      (a) Definitive operative repair versus damage-control surgery

(1) Extensive, definitive surgical repair may result in complications (triad of death) and poor patient outcomes

    a) Hypothermia

    b) Acidosis

    c) Coagulopathy

(2) To reduce these complications and the resultant mortality, damage control surgery or a staged laparotomy has been implemented; sacrifices the completeness of immediate repair. Repair accomplished in three stages:

    a) First stage: Operative repair of life-threatening injuries only

    b) Second stage: Patient transport to the intensive care unit (ICU) for aggressive rewarming, ongoing resuscitation, and attainment of hemodynamic stability

    c) Third stage: Within 24 to 48 hours after the initial operation, the patient returns to the operating room for definitive repair of intraabdominal injuries

  (b) Use of the three-stage approach has improved patient outcomes and allows for the stabilization of hemodynamics, correction of coagulopathy, rewarming, and optimization of pulmonary function

3. **Altered thermoregulation (see Hypothermia)**

4. **Infection and exaggerated inflammatory process (see Ch. 8, Hematologic and Immune Systems)**

5. **Impaired fibrinolysis system (see Ch. 8, Hematologic and Immune Systems)**

6. **Pain (see Ch. 20, Pain)**

7. **Catabolic state resulting in malnutrition (see Ch. 10, Sepsis and Septic Shock; Ch. 9, Gastrointestinal System)**

8. **Posttraumatic stress disorder (see Ch. 2, Psychosocial Aspects of Critical Care)**

9. **Diagnostic studies**

  a. Laboratory

    i. Complete blood count (CBC): Reflects the amount of blood lost but may take more than 2 hours to show a decrease in hematocrit with slow bleeding

     (a) Marked drop in hemoglobin level and hematocrit after fluid resuscitation with crystalloids because of dilution and mobilization of fluid during the recovery phase

     (b) Leukocytosis with a "shift to the left," which reflects the release of immature cells in response to either trauma or infection

     (c) Platelets: Need to be replaced to stem additional bleeding if below 50,000/mm^3

    ii. Blood typing and cross-matching: To determine the presence of antigens to ensure compatible blood transfusions

    iii. Blood chemistry panel: To determine levels of glucose (usually elevated from stress response and decreased peripheral utilization of insulin), magnesium (may be decreased from loss in urine), and ionized calcium (often decreased because of the use of citrate in blood transfusions)

     (a) Baseline levels of blood urea nitrogen (BUN) and creatinine, and liver function tests to determine the response to injury

     (b) Baseline electrolyte levels

    iv. Arterial lactate levels: To determine the adequacy of tissue oxygen extraction and to warn of impending organ failure

    v. Arterial and venous blood gas levels: To determine the adequacy of ventilation, oxygen delivery, and oxygen consumption

      (a) Acidosis may be seen with tissue perfusion deficits; hypoxemia may be seen with hypoventilation

      (b) Arterial oxygenation may be monitored noninvasively with pulse oximetry

      (c) Base deficit may occur because of perfusion deficits and metabolic acidosis

    vi. Urine and blood medication screening

      (a) Blood alcohol concentration

      (b) Routine urine medication screen for commonly abused substances in the given community

    vii. Urinalysis: To determine the presence of blood, bacteria, ketones, glucose, myoglobin, and bilirubin

    viii. Other blood studies: Amylase and coagulation studies

    ix. Pregnancy test: Should be performed for females of childbearing age

  b. Radiologic

    i. Radiographic studies are used to locate fractures, abnormal air or fluid collections, and foreign objects, such as bullets.

      (a) Indicate the position of major organs

      (b) In multiple traumas, views of the cervical spine, chest, pelvis, and extremities may be performed.

    ii. Focused Assessment with Sonography for Trauma (FAST) is a noninvasive ultrasonographic study of four abdominal compartments (subxiphoid, left upper, right upper, and suprapubic region) to detect intraabdominal injuries and cardiac tamponade; it is not intended to replace CT.

    iii. CT: Detects the presence of soft tissue injury, hematomas, fractures, and tissue swelling; definitive examination when FAST results are equivocal.

    iv. Intravenous pyelography, cystography, and retrograde urethrography: For renal or lower urinary tract injury

    v. Magnetic resonance imaging (MRI), angiography, ultrasonography, echocardiography

  c. Electrocardiography (ECG)

  d. Diagnostic peritoneal lavage (DPL) may be used to determine the extent of an abdominal injury or bleeding. Use of DPL may be helpful in patients with blunt trauma with an unstable condition when a solid or hollow organ injury is suspected. DPL has largely been replaced by sophisticated imaging techniques, but may be used in patients who are too unstable to be evaluated by CT.

10. Inspect posterior services

  a. Posterior of the patient is inspected after the patient has been evaluated and cleared of spinal and pelvic injuries. If injuries are present, logrolling may be contraindicated.

    i. Designate a team leader who is positioned at the patient's head

    ii. Team members are positioned at one side of the patient to maintain the torso, hips, and lower extremities

    iii. Maintain vertebral column when turning the patient

    iv. When possible, avoid turning patient on the injured side

    v. Inspect for additional injuries; a digital rectal examination is no longer recommended

    vi. Remove the spinal board if not already done

     vii. Consider using alternative methods if available including lift-and-slide; 6 plus lift-and-slide; straddle lift-and-slide; and mechanical devices, such as scoop stretchers.

11. **Keep reevaluating**
    a. Primary survey
    b. Vital signs
    c. Patient's level of pain
    d. Unidentified injuries

HEAD AND SPINAL TRAUMA

1. **Epidemiology**
   a. The most recent statistics related to traumatic brain injury (TBI) has reported approximately 2.8 million people sustain a TBI each year. About 50,000 die and 282,000 are hospitalized. Patients who have head trauma are also at risk of suffering a spinal cord injury (SCI).

> **KEY CONCEPT**
> It is important to remember that injury to the spinal cord can impair respiratory function.

2. **Pathophysiology of TBI**
   a. Blunt or penetrating trauma to the head and neck can result in TBI and/or SCI.
   b. TBI can be differentiated into primary injury (direct or focal injury to brain tissue and vasculature that occurs at the time of impact) and secondary injury
   c. Secondary injury (a cascade of intracellular molecular and biochemical events initiated by the primary insult) occurs over hours to days, worsening the initial injury. Brain cells are more vulnerable to these insults in the first few hours and days after injury; their occurrence increases morbidity and mortality. Numerous systemic or intracranial complications can initiate or exacerbate secondary brain injury.
      i. Molecular and biochemical mechanisms associated with secondary brain injury
         (a) Injury depolarizes brain cells and halts aerobic metabolism, which quickly leads to energy depletion
         (b) Ionic fluxes occur (e.g., Na^+, water, Ca^{++} moves into cells and K^+ moves out); disruption of calcium homeostasis is thought to trigger numerous pathologic events
         (c) Proteases (e.g., calpains) and lipases are activated and break down cytoskeletal proteins and lipids
         (d) Phospholipases are activated; these break down membranes and lead to free fatty acid accumulation
         (e) Production of toxic eicosanoids (e.g., thromboxane, leukotrienes, prostaglandins) may be triggered
         (f) Conversion to anaerobic metabolism produces acidosis and increased lactate
         (g) Release of excitatory neurotransmitters (e.g., glutamate, aspartate) increases the accumulation of intracellular Ca^{++}
         (h) Excessive free oxygen radicals are produced that damage cell membranes by lipid peroxidation
         (i) Nitric oxide also mediates cell damage related to excitotoxicity and intracellular hypercalcemia

(j) Other mechanisms contribute to delayed cell death after TBI. These may include apoptosis (genetically regulated cell self-destruction) and inflammatory processes.

d. Intracranial insults that can cause secondary brain injury

    i. Intracranial hypertension and factors that elevate ICP (e.g., intracranial hemorrhage or infection, hydrocephalus, brain edema [usually peaks 3–5 days after TBI], cerebral hyperemia)

    ii. Seizures: Increase cerebral metabolic needs and ICP

    iii. Cerebral vasospasm, loss of cerebral autoregulation, cerebral ischemia

e. Systemic insults that can cause secondary brain injury

    i. Hypotension (systolic BP <90 mm Hg) is associated with doubled mortality rate in patients with severe TBI

    ii. Hypoxia (PaO_2 <60 mm Hg) reduces cerebral oxygenation and causes cerebral vasodilation, which increases ICP

    iii. Hypercapnia causes cerebral vasodilation, which increases ICP; hypocapnia causes vasoconstriction, which contributes to cerebral ischemia

    iv. Hyperthermia increases cerebral metabolic demands

    v. Both hyperglycemia and hypoglycemia have adverse effects

    vi. Acute hypoosmolality can cause cerebral edema

    vii. Electrolyte disorders, particularly sodium imbalance, can lead to cellular swelling or dehydration

    viii. Systemic inflammatory disorders, anemia, acid-base imbalances have detrimental effects

    ix. Coagulopathy contributes to intracranial hemorrhage

f. Types of head injury (Box 11.1)

3. **Pathophysiology of spinal trauma**

a. Primary injury to the spine can result from blunt or penetrating trauma directly to the spinal cord, spinal column, or surrounding structures, which can result in fractures, dislocation, and/or subluxation. Stretching, torn, or strained ligaments may also cause significant injury. Damage to the cord may result in a contusion, cord transection, or incomplete cord transection (Tables 11.1 and 11.2). Secondary injury to the spinal cord follows the same path as the molecular, chemical, and inflammatory changes discussed in TBI. Neurogenic shock can occur when the cord has been damaged around T6 or higher. Because of disruption of sympathetic regulation, peripheral vascular resistance is lost and there is generalized vasodilation. Blood is pooled in the area below the level of the injury.

EXPERT TIP

Damage to the cord at C3 to C5 can cause loss of phrenic nerve function, and the diaphragm can be paralyzed.

---

    i. Signs and symptoms of neurogenic shock

      (a) Bradycardia

      (b) Hypotension

      (c) Warm, normal skin color

4. **Spinal shock occurs when there is disruption in transmission of impulses in the spinal cord at the level of injury.**

a. Signs and symptoms of spinal shock

    i. Transient loss of reflexes below the level of injury

BOX 11.1   Types of Head Injuries

SKULL FRACTURES
- Amount of damage is determined by characteristics (shape, weight, mass), velocity, and momentum of impacting object, direction of force, and thickness of skull at point of contact.
- Types:
  Linear: Simple break or crack with no displacement of bone. Concern if fracture occurs over a major vascular channel (e.g., temporal region over middle meningeal artery) because laceration can cause intracranial bleeding.
  Depressed: Depression of inner table more than one-half thickness of skull; may cause brain contusion, laceration, or hemorrhage.
  Open (compound): Associated with open scalp laceration; increased risk of infection.
  Basilar: At base of skull, most commonly affects anterior and middle fossae; accounts for about 20% of all skull fractures. Most commonly arise from linear fracture that extends to skull base. Potential complications include dural tear (allows CSF leakage, increases risk of infection), cerebrovascular injury (e.g., internal carotid artery) producing hemorrhage, vessel thrombosis, aneurysm formation or fistula creation, and cranial nerve damage.

FOCAL BRAIN INJURY
- Contusion: Bruising of brain tissue with associated hemorrhage and edema. Progressive edema formation can create mass effect, increased intracranial pressure (ICP), and brain herniation. Can occur anywhere in brain but most often in frontal and temporal lobes where cranial walls, bony projections of skull base, and dural folds restrict movement. Temporal lobe contusions, because of their precarious location near tentorium, warrant special attention because expansion of lesion can cause herniation onto brainstem without warning of ICP elevation. Coup contusions occur at point of impact; contrecoup contusions occur at opposite pole from impact.
- Epidural hematoma (EDH): Blood accumulation beneath skull and above dura; most often from arterial source. Most commonly associated with temporal bone fracture that lacerates middle meningeal artery. EDH compresses brain yet is associated with little underlying primary brain injury.
- Subdural hematoma (SDH): Blood accumulation beneath dura, usually because of venous bleeding from torn bridging veins. As SDH expands it compresses brain and increases ICP. Categorized into three groups according to timing of presentation:
  Acute: Often associated with more underlying primary brain injury than EDH; poor prognosis.
  Subacute: Prognosis better than that of acute SDH because of less severe underlying brain injury and lower likelihood of progressing to brainstem compression.
  Chronic: SDH accumulates slowly, likely because of small rebleeds; over 2–4 days blood congeals and thickens. After about 2 weeks, clot breaks down and eventually becomes xanthochromic fluid encased by membranes. SDH eventually reabsorbs or becomes calcified.
- Intracerebral hematoma (ICH): Hemorrhage into brain parenchyma produced by shearing and tensile stresses within brain tissue that result in rupture of intracerebral vessels. Frequently occurs in white matter of frontal and temporal regions, less commonly deep in hemispheres or cerebellum. May be single or multiple, often associated with other intracranial lesions and penetrating injuries. Hypertensive bleed or aneurysm rupture should be ruled out as source if single ICH is present.
- Subarachnoid hemorrhage (SAH): Bleeding into subarachnoid space. Commonly seen with severe traumatic brain injury; may predispose to hydrocephalus and cerebral vasospasm.
- Intraventricular hemorrhage (IVH): Bleeding into ventricles; may be associated with extension of SAH or ICH.

DIFFUSE BRAIN INJURY
- Most often caused by acceleration-deceleration and rotational forces that create tension, stretching, and shearing of nerve fibers with subsequent failure of conduction.
- Location, amount, and severity of axonal dysfunction determine clinical severity of injury:
  Concussion: Temporary neurologic dysfunction because of transient conduction impedance.
  Diffuse axonal injury (DAI): Diffuse white matter shearing associated with severe widespread mechanical disruption of axons and neuronal pathways primarily in hemispheres, corpus callosum, diencephalon, and brainstem. Severe DAI often associated with deep intracerebral contusions and diffuse cerebral edema that can raise ICP. It is thought that all head trauma involves varying degrees of histopathologic changes consistent with diffuse axonal disruption with a continuum of clinical responses. Severe DAI has a high mortality; survivors can have profound neurologic deficits.

Modified from Air and Surface Transport Nurses (2018). Transport nurse advanced trauma course (TAPC). Author. Retrieved from https://astna.rtolms.com/Custom/Pages/Curriculum/Default.aspx#c2573/369.

TABLE 11.1 Incomplete Spinal Cord Injury Syndromes

Incomplete Spinal Cord Injury Syndrome	Associated Type of Spinal Cord Injury	Clinical Presentation
Central cord syndrome	Injury and edema in the center of the spinal cord	Greater motor loss in the upper extremities than in the lower limbs; varying sensory loss
Brown-Séquard syndrome	Hemisection of the cord causes injury	Ipsilateral loss of motor, position, and vibratory sense; contralateral loss of pain and temperature perception at and below the spinal cord injury
Anterior cord syndrome	Disruption of the blood supply to the anterior two-thirds of the spinal cord resulting in cord ischemia	Loss of motor function and pain and temperature sensation below the level of the lesion, with sparing of proprioception, vibration, and light touch sensations
Posterior column syndrome (rare)	Posterior column injury	Loss of vibration and position sense
Cauda equina syndrome	Cauda equina (lumbosacral nerve roots distal to the spinal cord)	Variable presentation, asymmetric weakness to complete paralysis of the lower extremities. Severe pain, radicular or loss of sensation. Loss of bowel, bladder, and sexual function.

From Coplin, W. (2015). Traumatic spinal cord injury. In J.C. Hemphill, A.A. Rabenstein, O.B. Samuels, editors, *The practice of neurocritical care* (pp 163–178), Wisconsin, Neurocritical Care Society.

TABLE 11.2 Level of Spinal Cord Injury and Associated Motor and Respiratory Muscle Function Loss

Level of Spinal Cord Injury	Motor and Respiratory Muscle Function Loss
C1–C4	Quadriplegia with loss of spontaneous respiratory function
C4, C5	Quadriplegia with possible phrenic nerve involvement
C5, C6	Quadriplegia with gross arm movements; phrenic nerve intact, providing for diaphragmatic breathing
C6, C7	Quadriplegia with biceps intact, diaphragmatic breathing
C7, C8	Quadriplegia with triceps, biceps, and wrist extension intact with some function of intrinsic hand muscles; diaphragmatic breathing
T1–T12	Paraplegia with varying loss of intercostal and abdominal muscle function
Below L1	Cauda equina injury; variable motor and sensory loss in the lower extremities, can cause dysfunction of bowel and bladder

From Coplin, W. (2015). Traumatic spinal cord injury. In J.C. Hemphill, A.A. Rabenstein, O.B. Samuels, editors, *The practice of neurocritical care* (pp 163–178), Wisconsin, Neurocritical Care Society.

      ii. Loss of bowel and bladder function
      iii. Motor loss below level of the injury
  5. Potential complications of spinal cord injuries (Box 11.2)
  6. Etiology and risk factors
    a. An estimated 2.5 million Americans sustain TBIs each year; 280,000 survive and require hospitalization; approximately 5.3 million Americans are living with a disability from suffering a TBI, and approximately 50,000 die of TBI.
    b. Approximately 12,500 new cases of SCI occur annually in the United States.
      i. Males more commonly sustain both TBI and SCI injuries

BOX 11.2 Potential Complications of Spinal Cord Injury

HYPOVENTILATION AND INEFFECTIVE COUGH

Mechanism

- Spinal cord injury (SCI) above T12 can paralyze muscles involved in respiration (see Table 11.2), reducing maximal inspiratory force and forced vital capacity.
- Functional muscles for respiration may fatigue, which reduces effectiveness of spontaneous ventilation.
- Paralysis of abdominal and intercostal muscles leads to ineffective cough.
- Ineffective cough, decreased vital capacity, and immobility increase risk for atelectasis; together with endotracheal intubation and possible aspiration, increase likelihood of pneumonia.

Management

- Monitor respiratory status, including pulmonary function test results (e.g., vital capacity, tidal volume, negative inspiratory force) and respiratory gas exchange (e.g., pulse oximetry, arterial blood gas [ABG] levels, end-tidal CO_2), to detect respiratory muscle fatigue and onset of pulmonary complications. Notify physician of respiratory deterioration.
- Noninvasive positive pressure ventilation or intubation and mechanical positive pressure ventilation may be used for inadequate spontaneous ventilation or gas exchange.
- Aggressive pulmonary hygiene (i.e., chest physical therapy, suctioning) should be instituted; bronchoscopy may be used to remove secretions and open airways when routine hygiene maneuvers are ineffective.
- Once patient is stable and able to participate in care, provide manually assisted coughs. An insufflator-exsufflator cough machine may also be used to help clear secretions.
- Apply abdominal binder below costal margin in quadriplegic patients with no abdominal distension; helps to better position diaphragm and improve lung volumes.
- Have patient perform frequent incentive spirometry; teach family to encourage its use.
- Involve physical therapist in respiratory strengthening exercises.

NEUROGENIC SHOCK

Mechanism

- SCI at or above T6 (usually complete lesions) causes disconnection of sympathetic nervous system from higher control centers, which results in loss of vascular tone and cardiac accelerator response.
- Vasodilatation results, decreasing venous return and causing hypotension.
- Loss of cardiac accelerator response can lead to bradycardia and possibly junctional rhythm or ventricular escape beats.
- Because vagal nerve remains intact, profound bradycardia and cardiac arrest can occur, sometimes aggravated by fast position changes or suctioning.

Management

- Use hemodynamic parameters and indicators of tissue perfusion to guide fluid replacement and use of inotropic and vasoactive agents. Maintain blood pressure in desired range and ensure adequate tissue perfusion.
- Continuously monitor electrocardiogram; treat symptomatic bradycardia with atropine; pacemaker may be required. Prevent bradycardia by oxygenating well before and after suctioning and avoiding rapid position changes.

POIKILOTHERMIA OR ALTERATION IN THERMOREGULATION

Mechanism

- Disconnection of sympathetic nervous system from hypothalamic control center causes inability to regulate body temperature, which tends to drift toward ambient room temperature.

Management

- Monitor body temperature frequently.
- Warm or cool patient to maintain normothermia; take precautions to prevent hypothermia and hyperthermia.

ADYNAMIC ILEUS

Mechanism

- Thought to be triggered by disruption of autonomic innervation to the gastrointestinal tract. Causes abdominal distention, which can interfere with diaphragmatic excursion and increase risk for vomiting and aspiration.

Continued

BOX 11.2   **Potential Complications of Spinal Cord Injury—cont'd**

Management
- Inspect abdomen for distention; place gastric tube to decompress bowel.

GASTROINTESTINAL MUCOSAL EROSION AND BLEEDING

See Ch. 9, Gastrointestinal Bleeding

URINE RETENTION

Mechanism
- During spinal shock and after injury to sacral plexus, bladder is atonic and retains urine; may lead to reflux, stone formation, and renal deterioration, and increases risk for urinary tract infection. Manifests with bladder distention and no urine output.

Management
- Indwelling urinary catheter is necessary when spinal shock and hemodynamic instability are present. Once those conditions resolve and fluid intake is limited to 2000–2400 mL/day or less, intermittent catheterization should be initiated. Keep urine output at less than 500 mL per catheterization. If patient is able, teach self-catheterization. Monitor patient for urinary tract infection.

WEAKNESS OR PARALYSIS IN ONE OR MORE EXTREMITIES

See Weakness or Paralysis of One or More Extremities under Patient Care.

Modified from Air and Surface Transport Nurses (2018). Transport nurse advanced trauma course (TAPC). Author. Retrieved from https://astna.rtolms.com/Custom/Pages/Curriculum/Default.aspx#c2573/369.

---

    ii. Peak incidence is seen at 15 to 24 years of age; high rate also seen in those over age 75 years

  c. Common causes

    i. Transportation-related crashes involving motor or recreational vehicles, pedestrians, and/or bicycles

    ii. Violence: Mostly from firearms or assaults

    iii. Falls: Most common cause of visits related to TBI across all age groups, highest hospitalization rates were for patients over the age of 65 years

    iv. Falls second common cause of SCI

    v. Industrial accidents

    vi. Sports and leisure activities

  d. Factors that increase the risk for injury

    i. Alcohol and medication use impairs gross and fine motor skills, reaction time, and judgment and can confound diagnosis by altering level of consciousness (LOC)

    ii. Misuse of or failure to use safety devices (e.g., restraining devices, such as seat belts or cycling helmets)

    iii. Medical conditions that cause seizures or reduce LOC, visual acuity, or neuromuscular control; medications that cause dizziness; medication interactions; multiple medications

---

EXPERT TIP

Alcohol and drug use impair gross and fine motor skills, reaction time, and judgment, and can confound diagnosis by altering the assessment.

e. Mechanisms of injury for TBI
   i. Skull deformation: Delivery of force directly to the head distorts the skull contour, causing contusion, laceration, and/or hemorrhage beneath the site of contact.
   ii. Acceleration-deceleration: Head is thrust quickly forward then backward, which causes straight linear movement of the skull and brain. The brain moves slower than the skull, so the brain is injured as it impacts the sides and rubs against the rough projections of the skull. Compression, tension, and shearing may also injure brain tissue.
   iii. Rotation: Acceleration or deceleration causes the brain to move in a nonlinear, twisting path. Compressive, stretching, shearing, and tensile strains cause brain and vascular injury, particularly in areas where tissues of different density interface (e.g., gray and white matter, fibrous and cerebral tissue). Rate, extent, and direction of angular acceleration determine the extent of injury.
   iv. Penetrating injuries: Object penetrates the scalp and skull and enters the brain, where it can cause brain contusion, laceration, and/or hemorrhage with subsequent edema and necrosis. Severity of the injury is determined by the velocity, size, shape, direction, and action of the object within the skull, as well as the areas affected. Increases the risk for intracranial infection and posttraumatic seizures.
      (a) Gunshot wounds: Constitute the leading cause of TBI deaths; the mortality rate for such wounds is above 90% in the United States. Two-thirds of firearm-related TBIs are self-inflicted.
         (1) Local parenchymal destruction occurs along the bullet track. Shock waves are transmitted throughout the intracranial vault; a temporary cavity (which may be much larger than missile diameter) forms along the primary bullet track, then collapses within milliseconds, which causes local and remote brain injury.
         (2) If the bullet has insufficient energy to exit the skull, it may ricochet off the inner skull or a dural barrier (e.g., the falx), creating a second and occasionally, a third track. Bullet course is highly variable.
         (3) Death results from damage to vital brain structures, extensive tissue destruction, and intracranial hypertension because of cerebral edema and hemorrhage
      (b) Stab wounds: Penetrating object can lacerate the brain parenchyma, cranial nerves, and/or blood vessels
f. Mechanism of injury for SCI
   i. Axial loading: Application of force to the top of the head, which can result in TBI and vertebral body fractures

---

EXPERT TIP

Injury between T1 and T11 may result in damage to the intercostal muscles, which will lead to hypoventilation and hypoxia. Injury between T7 and T12 can result in loss of abdominal muscles that support breathing.

---

   ii. Flexion: Excessive anterior movement of the head onto the chest, can result in tearing or straining, tearing of interspinous ligaments, disruption of capsular ligaments around facet joints, fracture of posterior elements of the vertebral column, disruption of posterior ligaments, often result in unstable injuries

   iii. Extension: Excessive posterior movement of the head and neck, tearing of anterior longitudinal ligament, separation of vertebral bodies, disc rupture, and avulsion of upper vertebral body from disc

   iv. Rotation: Excessive rotation of head, torso, and neck; can occur with flexion and extension injuries. Unilateral facet dislocation.

   v. Penetrating: Direct damage to the spinal cord, symptoms depend on level of injury, but can include respiratory arrest leading to death

7. **Signs and symptoms (Box 11.3)**
8. **Diagnostic study findings**
   a. Laboratory: Abnormal coagulation parameters. Massive brain tissue damage can activate clotting, which results in consumptive coagulopathy.
   b. Medication screen: Alcohol or medications, such as hallucinogens, which can alter mental status and interfere with obtaining an adequate neurologic examination
   c. Blood sugar: Hypoglycemia can alter mental status
   d. Radiologic for TBI
      i. CT scan: Noncontrast CT (NCCT) is recommended for initial screening examination for moderate to severe TBI. Defines intracranial hematomas, contusions, and occasionally diffuse axonal injury (DAI). Cerebral edema may be seen. Detects shift of intracranial contents, as well as effacement of ventricles and basilar cisterns.
        (a) Epidural hematoma (EDH): Appears lens shaped
        (b) Subdural hematoma (SDH): Crescent-shaped and covers most of the hemisphere
        (c) Intracerebral hematoma (ICH): Area of hyperdensity within the parenchyma
        (d) Contusions: Heterogeneous areas of hemorrhage and edema
        (e) DAI: Suspected if there are small hemorrhages in the deep white matter, corpus callosum, or brainstem; diffuse cerebral edema may be seen; normal in mild cases
      ii. MRI: Not recommended as the primary evaluation study because of difficulties managing the patient and availability. Indicated when NCCT is read as normal, but patient continues to have persistent unexplained neurologic findings. MRI is used for the accurate diagnosis of DAI.
   e. Radiologic recommendations for spinal injuries
      i. CT: To identify bony injuries
      ii. MRI: To identify soft tissue and ligamentous injuries
      iii. NEXUS criteria to differentiate patients who may safely have their cervical spine cleared without radiologic examination:
        (a) Patient does not have midline tenderness *and* patient does not have any mental status changes resulting from trauma, alcohol, or medications *and*
        (b) No focal neurologic deficit at any time since the injury
        (c) Patient has no other distracting painful injuries, such as fractured ribs. Distracting painful injuries include but are not limited to any long bone fractures, visceral injuries requiring surgical consult, large lacerations, degloving or crush injuries, large burns, or any other injury producing acute functional impairment.
        (d) Remove the cervical collar and have the patient demonstrate range of motion.

BOX 11.3 Signs and Symptoms of Head Trauma

SCALP LACERATIONS

- Often associated with significant bleeding.

DEPRESSED SKULL FRACTURES

- Disruption in skull contour; neurologic presentation depends on location and extent of brain injury.

BASILAR SKULL FRACTURES

Cerebrospinal Fluid Leak

- Cerebrospinal fluid (CSF) rhinorrhea (nasal drainage) seen with anterior fossa fracture with dural tear.
- CSF otorrhea (ear drainage) seen in petrous bone fractures with dural tear and tympanic membrane rupture. If tympanic membrane is intact, CSF can course through Eustachian tube into nasopharynx and present as CSF rhinorrhea.
- Suspect CSF leakage in patients who complain of postnasal drip or salty or sweet taste, or when halo sign (yellowish or clear circle of drainage surrounding blood stain) appears on bed linens or dressings.
- Most CSF leaks occur immediately after injury but may be delayed; most heal spontaneously in 5–7 days.

Cranial Nerve Injuries

Fracture site and orientation determine which cranial nerves are damaged:

- Cranial nerve (CN) I: Associated with anterior fossa fractures.
- CN V and VI, and particularly CN VII and VIII: Associated with middle fossa fractures
- CN IX, X, XI, and XII: May occur with fractures of posterior fossa involving occipital condyle (rare)

HEMOTYMPANUM, BATTLE SIGN, AND RACCOON EYES

- Hemotympanum and Battle sign (ecchymosis over mastoid bone) indicate middle fossa fracture.
- Hearing is decreased if CSF is behind tympanic membrane or if tympanic membrane ruptures.
- "Raccoon eyes" (bilateral periorbital ecchymosis) seen in anterior fossa fractures.

TRAUMATIC BRAIN INJURY

Severity

Severity of head injury is based on Glasgow Coma Scale (GCS) score determined after initial resuscitation; considered reliable predictor of outcome; probability of poor outcome increases as GCS score decreases:

- Mild head injury: GCS score of 13–15
- Moderate head injury: GCS score of 9–12
- Severe head injury: GCS score of 3–8 or deterioration to GCS score of 8 or lower.

Distinguishing Types of Brain Injury

Some types of traumatic brain injury are difficult to distinguish based on clinical presentation alone because multiple kinds of injury often coexist. Neurologic status can deteriorate with time if areas of intracranial hemorrhage and edema expand, intracranial pressure (ICP) rises, or other secondary insults occur. Focal neurologic deficits seen with small localized lesions.

Contusions

- Presentation depends on size and location.
- Focal deficits may progress to signs associated with increased ICP if hemorrhage and edema expand.

Intracranial Hematomas/Hemorrhage

Clinical course varies, depending on location, rate, volume of accumulation, and presence of other intracranial injuries. It is not possible to differentiate type of hematoma based on clinical presentation.

Epidural Hematoma

In as few as one-third of patients, there is a brief period of unconsciousness followed by a lucid interval and then progressive deterioration of neurologic status. An epidural hematoma (EDH) can collect rapidly, and patient's condition can deteriorate precipitously. Irritability and agitation can quickly

Continued

BOX 11.3 Signs and Symptoms of Head Trauma—cont'd

progress to coma and hemiparesis or hemiplegia to decorticate or decerebrate posturing. Pupil abnormalities (e.g., unilateral fixed and dilated pupil) are often seen. Other symptoms may include headache (usually focal), vomiting, and possibly seizures and late vital sign changes. Posterior fossa EDH, which may have delayed onset, can cause nausea, vomiting, headache, stiff neck, and cardiovascular and respiratory instability.

Subdural Hematoma

Acute: Signs of neurologic deterioration evident within 48 hours. Most patients arrive in coma or deteriorate within hours of injury; in less severe cases, patient may be conscious or have a lucid period. Other signs of expanding mass lesion (motor deficits, pupil changes, CN dysfunction, eventually vital sign changes) often seen.

Subacute: Signs of neurologic deterioration and increased ICP are delayed 2–14 days after injury.

Chronic: Signs do not develop for 2 weeks or longer after low-impact head injury. Usually occurs in patients with brain atrophy (e.g., older adult, chronic alcoholics). Clinical presentation may include headache, nausea, vomiting, gait disturbance, progressive decline in level of consciousness, seizures, and eventually motor dysfunction and pupil abnormalities.

Intracerebral Hematoma

- Similar to contusions.

Subarachnoid Hemorrhage

See Signs and Symptoms in Intracranial Aneurysms under Specific Patient Health Problems.

Concussion

- Mild concussion causes brief period of confusion without loss of consciousness. Retrograde or posttraumatic amnesia may occur. Repeated mild concussions can have cumulative effects.
- Classic concussion associated with brief loss of consciousness with disorientation and retrograde and posttraumatic amnesia.
- Patient may have persistent complaints of neurologic sequelae, such as headaches, visual disturbance, memory problems (particularly short term), short attention span, information-processing problems, behavioral disorders, and dizziness—referred to as postconcussion syndrome. No anatomic evidence of injury is noted on computed tomographic scan.

Diffuse Axonal Injury

- Classified based on clinical presentation and duration of coma, which has an immediate onset:
  Mild: Coma lasts 6–24 hours, with persistent mild to moderate cognitive and neurologic deficits common after emergence from coma. Transient decorticate or decerebrate posturing noted in about one-third of patients, but all follow commands within 24 hours.
  Moderate: Coma lasts more than 24 hours, with mild to severe cognitive, behavioral, memory, and intellectual deficits persisting after emergence from coma. Most patients move purposefully or withdraw, but some exhibit transient decorticate or decerebrate posturing; no prominent signs of brainstem dysfunction.
  Severe: Coma lasts days to months. Severe cerebral and neurologic dysfunction is evident (e.g., decorticate and decerebrate posturing). Autonomic dysfunction (e.g., elevated BP, heart rate, and temperature; profuse sweating) seen with diencephalic involvement. Severe residual neurologic deficits are common.

Modified from Air and Surface Transport Nurses (2018). Transport nurse advanced trauma course (TAPC). Author. Retrieved from Halliwell, K. (2018). Transport Professional Advanced Trauma Course Provider Manual and Advanced Skills Guide. Air & Surface Transport Nurses Association (Publisher).

9. **Goals of care**
   a. Secondary brain injury is prevented by maintaining adequate cerebral perfusion pressure (CPP; between 50 and 70 mm Hg) and oxygenation, avoiding brain ischemia, and preventing systemic and neurologic complications.
   b. Secondary SCI is prevented by maintaining appropriate immobilization, maintaining adequate oxygenation, managing hypotension depending on the cause

of the hypotension, avoiding spinal cord ischemia, and preventing systemic and neurologic complications.

    c. Recovery of neurologic function is optimized.

    d. Systemic complications associated with brain and SCI and neurologic dysfunction (e.g., pulmonary aspiration, fluid and electrolyte imbalance, malnutrition, skin breakdown, contractures, gastrointestinal erosion, deep vein thrombosis) are prevented (see Box 11.2).

10. **Interprofessional collaboration (see Ch. 5, Increased Intracranial Pressure)**

11. **Management of patient care (Boxes 11.4 and 11.5)**

    a. Anticipated patient trajectory: Numerous factors influence clinical course and outcome, including the type, location, severity, and extent of the primary injury; the occurrence, frequency, severity, and duration of factors causing secondary brain injury; age; preexisting disease; and associated injuries. Other specific needs for patients with acute severe TBI include the following:

        i. Positioning (see Ch. 5, Increased Intracranial Pressure)

           (a) Continuous immobilization with semirigid cervical collar, maintain head and neck alignment until cervical spine injury is ruled out. Positioning for patient care should be limited to using a Four-Person Logroll. However, as noted earlier other methods or devices may be used. Care should be taken to prevent pressure injuries.

           (b) When a portion of the cranium is removed (e.g., for skull fracture repair, decompressive craniectomy), position the head so there is no compression of the unprotected brain. Once intracranial monitoring devices are removed, apply a protective helmet as indicated.

        ii. Skin care (see Ch. 5, Increased Intracranial Pressure)

        iii. Pain management: TBI and associated injuries likely to require analgesia (see Ch. 5, Increased Intracranial Pressure)

        iv. Nutrition: Maintain normoglycemia. Metabolic expenditure and nitrogen excretion increase after TBI. Nonparalyzed TBI patients should receive

---

BOX 11.4 Recommended Treatment Sequence for Initial Management of Severe Traumatic Brain Injury

1. Perform Primary and Secondary Survey with appropriate critical interventions, as well as evaluation and emergency diagnostic or therapeutic procedures as indicated.
2. Perform the following interventions:
   - Endotracheal intubation
   - Fluid resuscitation
   - Supplemental oxygen administration
   - Sedation and possibly administration of a short-acting paralytic agent
3. If there is evidence of brain herniation or neurologic deterioration, consider hyperventilation and, if patient is adequately hydrated, bolus administration of mannitol.
4. Take the patient for a computed tomographic (CT) scan of the head.
5. If there is evidence of a surgically treatable lesion on CT scan, move the patient to the operating room for intervention (e.g., removal of a space-occupying lesion).
6. Once operative intervention is complete or if no surgically treatable lesion is present, move the patient to an intensive care unit and monitor and manage intracranial pressure and cerebral perfusion pressure.

From Capizzi, A., Verduzco-Gutierrez, M. (2020). Traumatic brain injury: an overview of epidemiology, pathophysiology, and medical management. *Medical Clinics of North America*, 104, 213–238; Galvagno, S., Nahmias, J., Young, D. (2019). Advanced trauma life support® update: management and applications for adults and special populations. *Anesthesiology Clinics*, 37, 13–32; Brain Trauma Foundation. *Guidelines for the management of severe traumatic brain injury*, 4th ed, 2016. Accessed from https://braintrauma.org/uploads/03/12/Guidelines_for_Management_of_Severe_TBI_4th_Edition.pdf.

BOX 11.5 **Treatment Pathway for Patients With Severe Traumatic Brain Injury**

1. Insert intracranial pressure (ICP) monitor and maintain ICP at less than 20 mm Hg and cerebral perfusion pressure between 50 and 70 mm Hg.
2. Initially treat increasing ICP with general maneuvers, such as proper positioning, pain control, sedation, seizure prophylaxis, body temperature control, adequate oxygenation, ventilation and volume resuscitation, and possibly pharmacologic management (sedation and neuromuscular blockade). Consider therapeutic cooling to 34°–35°C, although this procedure remains controversial.
3. Support mean arterial pressure (MAP) to maintain cerebral perfusion pressure 50–70 mm Hg
4. Maintain normovolemia with fluids; if patient does not respond to fluids, use vasopressors/inotropes to maintain MAP.
5. With increasing ICP, use osmotic therapy (mannitol or hypertonic saline).
6. Seizure management should be initiated if seizures occur. The evidence does not support prophylactic anticonvulsants.
7. Resistant intracranial hypertension:
   - High-dose barbiturate coma
   - Hyperventilation to a $PaCO_2$ of less than 35 mm Hg, preferably while monitoring effect on cerebral oxygenation or cerebral blood flow
   - Decompressive craniectomy
8. Emerging therapies
   - Medications: Magnesium, corticosteroids, progesterone, glutamate scavengers, and stem cell therapy
   - Monitoring: Pupilometer, near-infrared spectroscopy with ultrasound Doppler monitor cerebral blood flow and cerebral oxygen, electroencephalography to monitor altered mental status, Bispectral Index Monitoring for patient in pentobarbital coma, and invasive brain temperature monitoring.

From Brain Trauma Foundation. *Guidelines for the management of severe traumatic brain injury*, 4th ed, 2016. Accessed from https://braintrauma.org/uploads/03/12/Guidelines_for_Management_of_Severe_TBI_4th_Edition.pdf.

---

nutrition that supplies 140% of their resting metabolic expenditure; paralyzed patients, 100% with 15% of caloric replacement as proteins. When possible, use the enteral route for nutrition. Full caloric replacement should be achieved within 7 days after TBI. (See Dysphagia under Patient Care.)

   v. Infection control (see Ch. 5, Increased Intracranial Pressure)

     (a) Ensure adequate debridement and irrigation of contaminated scalp wound before closure

     (b) If cerebrospinal fluid (CSF) leak is suspected or confirmed, take precautions to prevent intracranial infection

       (1) Do not put anything into the patient's nose or ears, including tissue, dressings, packing, suction catheters, nasogastric tubes, or nasal cannula

       (2) Place a dry, sterile dressing loosely over the patient's ear or as a mustache dressing to absorb drainage. Note the character and amount of drainage.

       (3) Encourage closure of a dural tear

         a) Instruct the patient not to blow the nose

         b) Prevent the patient from engaging in the Valsalva maneuver or vigorous coughing to avoid further tearing of the dura and increased CSF flow

         c) Maintain a lumbar drain or ventriculostomy to drain CSF

         d) Surgical closure may be required

       (4) Use of prophylactic antibiotics remains controversial

     (c) Administer prescribed prophylactic broad-spectrum antibiotics after penetrating TBI

   vi. Transport (see Ch. 5, Increased Intracranial Pressure)

vii. Discharge planning (see Ch. 5, Increased Intracranial Pressure)

viii. Pharmacology (see Ch. 5, Increased Intracranial Pressure)

    (a) Provide supplemental oxygen; increased fraction of inspired oxygen (FiO_2) may be used for brief periods if the brain tissue oxygen ($PbrO_2$) level is low

    (b) Administer prescribed fluids. Typically, isotonic solutions are used, and glucose-containing or hypotonic solutions are avoided. Fluid needs should be based on hemodynamic and clinical assessment parameters. Avoid fluid overload, which can exacerbate cerebral edema and respiratory failure.

    (c) Blood and other fluid loss from associated injuries can require large volume and blood product repletion. Hematocrit at or above 30% can help optimize cerebral oxygen delivery. Fresh frozen plasma, platelets, and/or cryoprecipitate may be used to correct coagulopathy.

    (d) Once euvolemia is assured, vasoactive and inotropic agents may be used to support BP so that a CPP between 50 to 70 mm Hg is maintained. Be cautious in the administration of sedatives and diuretics to prevent hypotension.

    (e) Interventions directed at brain injury management need not be instituted until after airway, breathing, and circulation are established unless brain herniation or neurologic deterioration not associated with an extracranial cause is evident. In the latter case, an IV mannitol bolus may be given if the patient is adequately hydrated.

    (f) Administer anticonvulsants as prescribed

ix. Psychosocial issues (see Ch. 5, Increased Intracranial Pressure)

x. Treatments (see Ch. 5, Increased Intracranial Pressure): Recommended sequence of pharmacologic, noninvasive, and invasive treatments for initial TBI management and treatment of intracranial hypertension are described in Boxes 11.3 and 11.4.

    (a) Noninvasive

        (1) Control blood loss from scalp laceration via direct compression followed eventually by surgical repair

        (2) Maintain normothermia as described under Increased Intracranial Pressure. Therapeutic hypothermia may reduce ICP and risk of death or poor neurologic outcome in severe TBI, but clinical evidence insufficient to recommend routine use.

        (3) Hyperventilation: Can be used during initial resuscitation if the patient demonstrates neurologic deterioration or brain herniation. In the absence of increased ICP, prolonged partial pressure of carbon dioxide ($PaCO_2$) reductions to less than or equal to 30 mm Hg and, in first 24 hours after TBI, chronic prophylactic reductions to 30 mm Hg or less should be avoided because cerebral perfusion can be compromised. Brief periods of hyperventilation may be necessary for patients with neurologic deterioration or for longer if ICP elevations are refractory to other therapy. If necessary, first lower $PaCO_2$ to 30 to 35 mm Hg; if ICP remains refractory to intervention, then consider reduction to below 30 mm Hg (see Boxes 11.3 and 11.4). Cerebral blood flow (CBF) or oxygenation monitoring recommended if $PaCO_2$ is less than 30 mm Hg to detect brain ischemia.

    (b) Invasive

        (1) Patients with severe TBI require intubation and ventilatory support

        (2) Repair scalp lacerations within 24 to 48 hours

(3) Remove space-occupying lesions (e.g., hematoma) as soon as possible

(4) Unilateral or bilateral decompressive craniectomy (e.g., removal of cranium, opening of dura) allows room for the edematous brain to control refractory ICP elevations

xi. Ethical issues (see Ch. 5, Increased Intracranial Pressure)

b. Potential complications (See health problems described under Patient Care)

i. Increased ICP and related complications

(a) Mechanism: Development of cerebral edema, hyperemia, intracranial hemorrhage, venous outflow obstruction, and posttraumatic hydrocephalus can all increase intracranial volume, which results in intracranial hypertension

(b) Management (see Increased Intracranial Pressure)

(c) ICP monitoring is recommended, an abnormal CT scan with a GCS 8 or less

ii. Vasospasm: Most common in patients with severe TBI who have subarachnoid hemorrhage (SAH; see Ch. 5, complications under Intracranial Aneurysms)

iii. Seizures (see Ch. 5, Seizures)

(a) Mechanism: Epileptogenic focus created at the time of injury. Early seizures occur within the first 7 days after TBI; late seizures occur at least 7 days following injury. Severity of the TBI directly correlates with the risk for seizures. Other risk factors for late seizures include penetrating head injury, brain contusion, depressed skull fracture, intracranial hemorrhage, prolonged unconsciousness, and early seizures.

(b) Management: Treat seizures when they occur with medications. Prophylactic seizure treatment is no longer recommended.

iv. Intracranial infection (see Ch. 5, Bacterial Meningitis and Viral Encephalitis)

v. The American Academy Neurology recommends that patients with TBI, especially with disorders of consciousness be transferred to centers that can provide a multidisciplinary approach to TBI. (https://www.aan.com/Search/Search?SearchValue=Traumatic+Brain+Injury+Management+Guidelines)

THORACIC TRAUMA: PULMONARY AND CARDIAC

PULMONARY TRAUMA

1. **Pathophysiology**

a. Depends on the type and extent of injury. Trauma to the chest or lungs may interfere with any of the components involved in inspiration, gas exchange, and expiration.

b. Blunt injuries: Chest wall damage must be evaluated in conjunction with the accompanying intrathoracic and intraabdominal visceral injuries. Injuries seen with blunt trauma include the following:

i. Visceral injuries without chest wall damage

(a) Pneumothorax, hemothorax

(b) Lung contusion

(c) Diaphragmatic injury

(d) Myocardial contusion, aortic rupture, pericardial tears

(e) Rupture of the trachea or bronchus

ii. Soft tissue injuries: Possibly a sign of severe underlying damage

(a) Cutaneous abrasion

      (b) Ecchymosis

      (c) Laceration of superficial layers

      (d) Burns

      (e) Hematoma

   iii. Fracture of the sternum: Occurs either as a result of direct impact or as the indirect result of overflexion of the trunk

   iv. Rib fractures as a result of overflexion or straightening. Rib fractures can be unifocal or multifocal. Lateral aspects of fourth to ninth ribs most commonly injured. Multiple fractures (the fracture of two or more adjacent ribs in two or more places) result in chest wall instability or flail chest and are often complicated by injuries to the soft tissues and pleura.

    v. Separation or dislocation of ribs or cartilage from a blow to the anterior chest

   vi. Lower rib fractures often associated with abdominal organ injuries.

  c. Penetrating injuries

    i. Pleural cavity, as well as the chest wall has been entered. Damage to deeper structures is a serious consequence.

   ii. Extent of injury and the organs injured generally can be predicted by the course of the wound and the nature of the penetrating instrument. High-velocity projectiles do more damage than is apparent from the surface.

   iii. Injuries seen with penetrating trauma:

      (a) Open sucking chest wounds with air entering the pleural space during inspiration

      (b) Hemothorax, hemopneumothorax, or chylothorax

      (c) Combined thoracoabdominal injuries (esophageal, diaphragmatic, or abdominal viscus injuries)

      (d) Damage to the trachea and large airways

      (e) Wounds of the heart or great vessels

2. Etiology and risk factors

  a. Blunt trauma: Automobile crashes, falls, assaults, explosions

  b. Penetrating trauma: Automobile crashes; falls; assaults; explosions; injury by bullets, knives, shell fragments, free-flying objects; industrial accidents

3. Signs and symptoms

  a. Chief complaint varies with the specific injury. Tachypnea, dyspnea, pain, and respiratory distress may occur with any injury. Other symptoms vary with the type of trauma.

  b. Fractures of the ribs, sternochondral junction, or sternum: Pain accentuated by chest wall movement, deep inspiration, or touch

  c. Flail chest: Dyspnea and localized pain

  d. Trauma to the lung parenchyma, trachea, or bronchi: Hemoptysis, respiratory distress

  e. Contusion of the heart: Angina

  f. Rupture of the aorta and major vessels: Dyspnea and backache, intense pain in the chest or back unaffected by respirations; rapid exsanguination may occur

  g. Open sucking chest wound: If the opening in the chest wall is smaller than the diameter of the trachea, the patient may have minimal subjective symptoms. If the opening is larger, more air enters the pleural space, which collapses the lung, impairs ventilation and gas exchange, and results in dyspnea.

  h. Skin: Ecchymosis, hematomas, abrasions, burns, and lacerations

  i. Increased work of breathing: Use of accessory muscles, intercostal retractions

    j. Shallow respirations (seen with pain from rib fractures); tachypnea often accompanies pain and apprehension

    k. Chest wall asymmetry seen with tension pneumothorax or hemothorax. In flail chest, chest wall movement is paradoxical (sinks on inspiration and flails out on expiration)

    l. Subcutaneous emphysema: May be palpable in pneumothorax or rupture of the trachea or bronchus

    m. Position of the trachea may be displaced—toward the injured side in pneumothorax, toward the contralateral side in hemothorax, or tension pneumothorax

    n. Ipsilateral tympany or hyperresonance in pneumothorax and tension pneumothorax

    o. In rupture of the diaphragm, the left hemidiaphragm is usually involved, which results in dullness (from fluid-filled bowel) or tympany (from gas-filled bowel) heard over the left chest

    p. Dullness to percussion with hemothorax, hemopneumothorax, or parenchymal hemorrhage

    q. Reduced breath sounds heard in any condition in which there are shallow respirations; diminished or absent breath sounds heard in pneumothorax, tension pneumothorax, flail chest, hemothorax, or hemopneumothorax; bronchial breath sounds heard with parenchymal hemorrhage

    r. Bowel sounds may be heard in the chest with rupture of the diaphragm

  4. Diagnostic study findings

    a. Radiologic

      i. Chest radiography is performed for all injuries if the patient is stable

        (a) Visualizes rib fractures, parenchymal hemorrhage, hemothorax, or hemopneumothorax

        (b) Pneumothorax: Expiratory chest films are often used in the diagnosis

        (c) Tension pneumothorax: Shows a shift in the mediastinum to the unaffected side in addition to pneumothorax

        (d) Rupture of the diaphragm: Shows bowel loops in the thorax

        (e) Rupture of the aorta or major vessels: Revealed by a widening of the mediastinum

      ii. CT or CT angiogram (CTA) of the chest is indicated with severe mechanisms of injury, abnormal chest radiographs, altered mental status, distracting injuries, or clinically suspected thoracic injuries.

      iii. MRI and transesophageal echocardiography (TEE) may be indicated in suspected cardiac trauma

    b. ECG: To evaluate for cardiac injury, in which tachycardia, dysrhythmias, and electrocardiographic changes may be found

    c. Transthoracic echo may be useful to evaluate for structural abnormalities, effusion, and valve dysfunction.

    d. Bronchoscopy: May confirm a diagnosis of rupture of the trachea or bronchus

  5. Goals of care

    a. Maintain patent airway

    b. ABG levels and pulmonary parameters are restored to and maintained within acceptable limits for the patient

    c. Chest wall integrity and stability are restored

    d. Integrity of the pleural space is reestablished

    e. Chest pain and dyspnea are minimized

  6. Interprofessional collaboration (see Ch. 3, Acute Respiratory Failure)

7. **Management of patient care**
   a. Anticipated patient trajectory
      i. Positioning: Keep the head of the bed elevated 30 to 45 degrees to optimize ventilation and prevent aspiration; provide symptomatic treatment for uncomplicated rib fractures to ensure the ability to cough and deep breathe.
      ii. Skin care: Clean and remove debris from wounds; reinforce dressings as necessary; provide wound care around chest tubes and at other invasive sites.
      iii. Pain management: May require the use of epidural or specific nerve blocks to manage pain related to fractured ribs to assist with ventilation to prevent complications from inadequate ventilation.
      iv. Nutrition: Provide adequate nutrition to promote healing.
      v. Infection control: See Acute Respiratory Failure. Patient with a history of penetrating trauma with "dirty" or contaminated instruments and/or multiple wounds may be especially at risk.
      vi. Transport (see Ch. 18, Patient Transport)
      vii. Discharge planning: Evaluate the need for rehabilitation on discharge; anticipate home care equipment needs
      viii. Pharmacology: Antibiotics as needed, sedatives and pain medication
      ix. Psychosocial issues: Unanticipated nature of the trauma may increase the difficulty of the patient and family in adjusting to the patient's current circumstances (see Ch. 2, Psychosocial Aspects of Critical Care).
      x. Treatments
         (a) Intubation, mechanical ventilation, suctioning, O_2 therapy, O_2 delivery devices (see Ch. 3, Acute Respiratory Failure)
         (b) Provide nutrition
         (c) Perform suctioning as needed to stimulate cough and clear the airways of blood and secretions
         (d) Intrapleural chest tubes drainage system management
         (e) Assist with emergency decompression of tension pneumothorax through insertion of a large-bore needle into the second anterior intercostal space or insertion of a chest tube
   b. Potential complications
      i. Hospital-associated infection via aspiration, urinary tract infection, wound contamination (see Ch. 3, Acute Respiratory Failure and Chronic Obstructive Pulmonary Disease)
      ii. Blunt thoracic aortic injury. ATLS® -10 recommends that if there are no contraindications, a beta-blocker may be administered to lower the heart rate and decrease the risk of a rupture.

CARDIAC TRAUMA

Trauma to the heart can occur from penetrating injuries (e.g., knife, gunshot wounds) or nonpenetrating injuries [deceleration, myocardial contusions from falls, motor vehicle crashes, crush injuries and direct impact to the chest (e.g., being struck by an animal)]. Injury may be to the pericardium, a single chamber, two or more chambers, the great vessels, and/or the coronary arteries. A majority of patients who sustained significant blunt chest trauma have other injuries including TBI, lungs, and spinal column.

1. **Pathophysiology**
   a. Penetrating cardiac trauma: High prehospital mortality
      i. Open wound hemorrhages into the pericardial space. Hypovolemic shock may be present as a result of the hemorrhaging. Most stab wounds to the heart result in tamponade.

  ii. Gunshot wounds cause cellular damage to adjacent areas of the myocardium
   (a) Myocardial damage is usually extensive, with profuse bleeding
   (b) Most commonly affects the right ventricle (RV); often more than one chamber involved

 b. Nonpenetrating or blunt trauma
  i. Deceleration injury is caused by:
   (a) Sternal compression
   (b) Impingement of the heart between the sternum and spinal column
   (c) Rupture or dissection of the aorta at the ligamentum arteriosum, where it is anchored
  ii. Blunt aortic trauma creates a shearing force within the vessel
   (a) Causes laceration
   (b) Intimal tear may cause dissections
   (c) Hemorrhage, cardiac tamponade, and subsequent shock are the most pressing events
   (d) With cardiac tamponade: Decreased ventricular (diastolic) filling volume leads to hypovolemia, hypotension, and death
  iii. Myocardial contusion: Direct damage to the myocardium causes temporary or permanent myocardial dysfunction
   (a) RV is the chamber most commonly injured, because of its anatomic position (behind the sternum). Second in frequency is the left ventricle (LV).
   (b) If significant pulmonary contusion and adult respiratory distress syndrome have occurred, pulmonary hypertension results, causing the right chambers to fail.
  iv. Electrical injuries: Tissue damage because of the conversion of electrical energy into thermal energy
   (a) Autonomic nervous system emits a large amount of catecholamines
   (b) Myocytes may be stunned, injured, or damaged, which decreases contractility and CO

2. Etiology and risk factors
 a. Penetrating trauma
  i. Gunshot wounds, knives, ice picks, low-velocity shrapnel, flying objects
  ii. Fractures of ribs and sternum (rare cause)
 b. Nonpenetrating or blunt trauma
  i. Motor vehicle crashes
  ii. Falls
  iii. Physical crushing assaults, direct blows to the chest by the fist or objects, such as a steering wheel or baseball
  iv. Kicks from large animals
  v. Blasts, electrical injuries, lightning strikes
  vi. Commotio cordis: Sudden cardiac arrest in young patients, usually athletes from blunt force trauma to the chest
 c. Iatrogenic trauma: Cardiopulmonary resuscitation (CPR), endomyocardial biopsy, pericardiocentesis

3. Signs and symptoms
 a. History of blunt or penetrating trauma to the chest
 b. Open wounds to the chest
 c. Chest pain
 d. ECG changes consistent with ST elevation, T wave elevation

e. Physical examination
i. Hypotension
ii. Cardiac arrhythmia
iii. Most common valve ruptured is the aortic. Observe for signs and symptoms of acute aortic insufficiency—cardiogenic shock, chest pain, dyspnea.
iv. Urinary output absent or decreased (aortic rupture)
v. Myocardial contusion: May produce subtle signs of chest pain, similar to those of myocardial infarction (MI)
vi. Inspect patients for associated injuries: Head, neck, chest, abdomen
vii. Jugular venous pressure: Increased with tamponade
viii. Pulses may be decreased in the legs
ix. Discrepancy between pulses in the upper extremities; no femoral pulses (suspect blunt trauma in high-speed automobile crashes, truncal deceleration—sternal, first rib injuries)
x. Isolated upper body hypertension (blunt trauma to the aorta)
xi. New holosystolic murmurs heard with a ruptured ventricular septum, diastolic murmur with aortic insufficiency
xii. Pericardial rub: Heard in contusions and pericardial tamponade

4. **Diagnostic study findings**
a. ECG: If troponin levels are abnormal, need to monitor the patient closely for at least 24 hours
i. Sinus tachycardia, atrial flutter or fibrillation, premature ventricular contractions, ventricular tachycardia, ventricular fibrillation, pulseless electrical activity (PEA)
ii. Prolonged QTc interval
iii. Low voltage, electrical alternans (in pericardial effusions)
iv. Right bundle branch block (ruptured ventricular septum)
v. Right precordial ECG lead V_4R: To check for signs of RV injury
vi. Infarct patterns with coronary artery lacerations
vii. ST elevations (pericarditis, coronary lacerations)
b. Radiologic
i. Chest radiograph: Rib and sternal fractures, enlarged heart or mediastinum, pneumothorax, hemothorax
c. Ultrasound echocardiography: Helps detect lesions in valves and septum, pericardial effusions, tamponade; evaluates LV function
d. CTA of coronary arteries with contrast, MRI heart function and morphology without contrast
e. TEE: Potential for additionally diagnosing aortic dissections
f. Ultrasound pericardiocentesis: For treatment of tamponade

5. **Goals of care**
a. Oxygenation is adequate
b. Hemodynamics are stable
c. BP is normal
d. Sinus rhythm is maintained, and the patient is free of ectopy and arrhythmias

6. **Interprofessional collaboration (see Ch. 4, Chronic Stable Angina Pectoris); also, emergency medical service personnel, intensive care personnel, rehabilitation services personnel**

7. **Management of patient care**
a. Anticipated patient trajectory: Rapid transport to a trauma center, if nearby, affords the patient the best chance of survival

i. Psychosocial issues: Many patients do not survive. Families need help identifying community resources (counseling, spiritual support, social services) for grieving and loss.

ii. Treatments

(a) Perform rapid assessment of airway, breathing, circulation, need for cervical immobilization

(b) Perform CPR as needed: Cardiac resuscitation may be refractory to CPR and defibrillation because of mechanism of injury

(c) Ensure adequate oxygenation: Use pulse oximetry, check ABG results, evaluate the need for intubation or mechanical ventilation (there is a high risk of hypoxemia)

(d) Listen to breath sounds: Check for tension pneumothorax

(e) Monitor continuously for adequate pulse, BP, and hemodynamics

(f) Closely observe for arrhythmias, PEA

(g) Ensure adequate access. Central line and arterial line are often indicated

(h) Prepare the patient for emergency procedures

(1) Pericardiocentesis: For tamponade

(2) Chest tube insertion: For tension pneumothorax, hemopneumothorax or significant pneumothorax. ATLS® -10 recommends that placement of a smaller size chest tube 28 F to 32 F.

(3) Emergency thoracotomy: At bedside or in the emergency department, if the patient is in extremis (bridge to the operating room)

(4) Emergency surgery in the operating room for repair of ventricles, valves

(5) Fasciotomies, debridement in cases of electrical burns

(i) Treat contusion similarly to MI with rest, close monitoring, oxygenation, maintenance of fluid balance, treatment of arrhythmias

b. Potential complications

i. Hypovolemia

(a) Mechanism: Because of hemorrhage, hypovolemic shock, insensible fluid loss with burns; decreased contractility, which severely lowers CO

(b) Management

(1) Monitor vital signs continuously, particularly BP, temperature, heart rate

(2) Watch for changes in mental status

(3) Closely watch hemodynamics: central venous pressure, pulmonary artery occlusion pressure, MAP

(4) Elevate the lower extremities to increase preload, if necessary

(5) Weigh daily; maintain strict intake and output measurements

(6) Maintain adequate IV access

(7) Administer volume expanders as ordered, including blood, crystalloids, colloids

(8) Observe the condition of the skin: Color, turgor, temperature, and refill

(9) Monitor laboratory values for abnormalities

ii. Sudden death and arrhythmias (see Ch. 4, Cardiac Rhythm Disorders)

iii. Infection

(a) Mechanism: Foreign body, trauma, surgery

(b) Management

(1) Monitor for elevated temperature, localized pain, swelling, redness at trauma site

(2) Check temperature often; report if it exceeds parameters (e.g., $\geq 38.3°$ C [101° F])

(3) Check laboratory results (e.g., leukocyte count elevated). Monitor culture reports.

(4) Frequently monitor invasive line and wound sites

(5) Keep wounds clean; change dressings per unit standards

(6) Administer antibiotics as ordered to maintain therapeutic blood levels

(7) Maintain blood and body fluid precautions, good hand-washing technique

(8) Maintain aseptic technique for bedside procedures

(9) Monitor daily assessment of necessity of invasive lines, IV lines, and urinary catheter

    iv. Other potential complications include the following:

      (a) Traumatic pericarditis, tamponade because of blunt or penetrating trauma

      (b) Embolization is a potential problem when bullets or fragments remain in chambers

      (c) Coronary artery lacerations cause tamponade, MI, shock, severe hemorrhage, and death

      (d) Late complications with contusions and lacerations: Myocardial fibrosis can cause akinesia, hypokinesia, LV aneurysms, heart failure

      (e) Electrical injuries can cause cardiac arrest, MI, hypertension (because of increased peripheral vasospasm)

ABDOMINAL TRAUMA

1. **Anatomy of the abdomen and pelvis**
   a. Abdominal organs
      i. Liver, spleen, gallbladder, pancreas, stomach, bowel (small and large), abdominal aorta
   b. Pelvis and pelvic organs
      i. Bladder, ureters, and urethra
      ii. Reproductive organs: Uterus, ovaries, scrotum, testes
      iii. Kidneys
      iv. Femoral arteries
      v. Aorta
2. **Pathophysiology**
   a. Injuries occurring from the nipple line to the inguinal crease increase the risk of abdominal trauma and often involve injury to multiple organs. Thoracic injuries increase the risk of abdominal injury, including blunt and penetrating injuries to the diaphragm.
   b. Pelvic fractures may involve injures to abdominal organs.
   c. Because of vasculature of the abdominal organs, especially the solid organs, such as the liver and spleen and the vasculature of the pelvis, the patient with severe injury is at risk of hemorrhage. Mortality from pelvic trauma hemorrhage can range from 14% to 60%.
   d. Liver is the most commonly injured organ in the body regardless of the cause of the trauma.
3. **Etiology and risk factors**
   a. Penetrating abdominal and pelvic trauma
      i. Injury with a sharp metal or wooden object; impalement on a sharp object, gunshot wound

    ii. Gunshot wounds: Visceral injury possible, even when the bullet does not penetrate the abdomen; caused by blast effect; caliber of bullet important

  b. Blunt abdominal and pelvic trauma

    i. Moving vehicular crashes: Damage can occur with and without seat belt

    ii. Acceleration-deceleration injuries in passengers and pedestrians, ejection from a vehicle, falls

    iii. Physical violence: Punch, kick, use of a blunt object, rape, sports injury, crush injury

4. Signs and symptoms

  a. Pallor, hypotension, diminished or absent femoral pulses

  b. Respiratory difficulty, diminished or absent breath sounds

  c. Increased abdominal girth, entrance and exit wounds, impalement by foreign object

  d. Abdominal tenderness, pain with guarding, rebound tenderness. Severe pain with any movement.

  e. Dullness on percussion suggests fluid in the abdomen; hyperresonance indicates a perforated viscus

  f. Marbled appearance of the abdomen

  g. Cullen's sign: Bluish discoloration of the periumbilical area

  h. Turner's sign: Bluish discoloration of the flanks

  i. Coopernail's sign: Bruising of the scrotum or labia, indication of pelvic injury

  j. Referred pain: Pain radiating to the left shoulder (Kehr's sign) is likely a splenic injury; referred pain to the testicle may indicate a duodenal injury.

  k. Positive FAST examination

  l. Peritoneal lavage: Reveals blood ("beef broth" tap), urine, bile, or feces in the peritoneal cavity (this test is no longer routinely performed, but in some areas of the world, it is still useful when a FAST examination is not available.)

EXPERT TIP
Always begin palpation of the injured abdomen away from the area of pain to get a better evaluation.

---

5. Diagnostic study findings

  a. Laboratory

    i. Serum

      (a) Hemoglobin and hematocrit

      (b) Type and screen or crossmatch depending on the patient's status

      (c) Coagulation studies

      (d) Lactate level

      (e) Base deficit

      (f) Electrolytes

      (g) Liver function studies

      (h) Urine pregnancy tests in females of reproductive age

      (i) Stool analysis for presence of blood

    ii. Urine

      (a) Volume: May be diminished if significant renal damage, obstruction, or hypovolemia present

      (b) Urinalysis: Erythrocytes and protein may be present, but renal trauma can still exist without this response

      (c) Hematuria: Gross or microscopic; negative findings allow the exclusion of a penetrating genitourinary injury with 90% confidence

b. Radiologic
 i. FAST examination
 ii. Pelvic radiograph
 iii. CT of chest and abdomen with contrast
 iv. Contrast studies: Urethrography, cystography, IV pyelogram, and GI contrast studies
 c. Surgical exploration: Usually indicated for all hematomas; allows the immediate repair of major lacerations and evaluation of bowel/organ integrity

6. **Goals of care**
 a. Hemostasis is reestablished by the replacement of fluid and blood volume. Surgery or interventional radiology may be required to manage uncontrolled hemorrhage.
 b. Vital signs are stable, and ABG levels are acceptable
 c. Organ function is reestablished and maintained
 d. Stabilization of the pelvic fracture as indicated by injury
 i. Application of a pelvic stabilization device
 ii. Interventional radiology for hemorrhage management
 iii. Preperitoneal packing: Involves a midline incision from the umbilicus to pubic symphysis and packing is placed in selected areas of the pelvis to manage hemorrhage.

7. **Interprofessional collaboration (see Ch. 6, Electrolyte Imbalances)**

8. **Management of patient care**
 a. Anticipated patient trajectory: Clinical course of abdominal and pelvic trauma patients is affected by the nature and extent of concurrent injury to one or more organ systems, complications, comorbidities, rehabilitative potential, and degree of support from patients' families or significant others. Patients with abdominal and pelvic trauma may be expected to have needs in the following areas:
 i. Skin care: Wound management
 (a) Control bleeding
 (b) Determine fluid volume loss
 (c) Provide wound care as warranted; apply sterile dressings
 (d) Observe for signs of infection—redness, swelling, pus, complaints of pain, numbness or coolness; with evidence of infection, consider topical or IV antibiotic
 ii. Pain management
 (a) Assess and document objective and subjective complaints of pain
 (b) Collaborate with the physician and pain management team to establish pharmacologic and nonpharmacologic approaches for pain relief
 (c) Evaluate the effectiveness of pain control, including patient expression of relief
 iii. Nutrition
 (a) Identify the route for nutritional supplements and fluid replacement
 (b) Provide adequate calories, protein, vitamins, minerals, and nutrients to promote wound healing and protein sparing, and prevent rhabdomyolysis
 iv. Infection control
 (a) Consider the need for tetanus toxoid
 (b) Obtain a urine sample for culture and sensitivity testing upon emergency department admission
 (c) Administer antibiotics as ordered
 (d) Use an aseptic and sterile technique as appropriate (e.g., in wound care)

v. Transport: High-risk situations requiring consideration for early transfer include the following:

(a) Open pelvic injury with or without renal injury

(b) Pelvic ring injury: Unstable fracture

(c) Pelvic fracture associated with shock and uncontrolled hemorrhage

vi. Discharge planning

(a) Rehabilitation (e.g., at a facility or with support at home)

(b) Family or significant other support system

(c) Wound care: Nature and frequency

(d) Pain management

vii. Psychosocial issues

(a) Traumatic stress syndrome; provide posttraumatic stress support, if warranted

(b) Implement measures to reduce anxiety, stress, and fear in the patient and family

viii. Treatment: Surgical intervention may be necessary

b. Potential complications

i. Hemorrhage

(a) Mechanism: Intraabdominal and bladder injuries are associated with a high risk of major blood loss because of the sites of major vascular channels

(b) Management: (see Ch. 4, Cardiovascular System)

ii. Extravasation of urine

(a) Mechanism: Puncture, tear, or laceration to the kidney, ureter, bladder, and/or urethra

(b) Management

(1) Early recognition

(2) Urinary catheterization

a) Increased resistance during catheter insertion warrants radiologic examination; catheters should never be forced, because obstruction suggests trauma or hematoma

b) Extravasated urine contributes to infection (e.g., peritonitis); temperature must be monitored closely

c) Adequate hydration should be provided to sustain urine output

d) Patency of the catheter should be maintained; constant irrigation may be prescribed

(3) Surgical intervention (when indicated)

(4) Effective pain management

iii. Systemic complications

(a) Other early complications

(1) Ileus

(2) Sepsis, shock

(3) Impairment or loss of renal function

(b) Late complications may include

(1) Intraabdominal hypertension (see Ch. 9, Gastrointestinal System)

References and bibliography information are available at http://evolve.elsevier.com/AACN/corecurriculum/.

Burns

Karah Cripe Sickler, RN, DNP, AG-ACNP-BC

SYSTEMWIDE ELEMENTS

ANATOMY AND PHYSIOLOGY REVIEW

1. **Definitions**
   a. Burn: Tissue injury caused by the coagulation of cellular proteins as a result of heat produced by thermal, chemical, electrical, or radiation energy; degree of coagulation depends on the following:
      i. Temperature of the injuring agent
      ii. Duration of exposure to the injuring agent
      iii. Area exposed to the injuring agent
      iv. Special considerations: The young and the older adult may experience more severe burns because their skin is thinner and more vulnerable
   b. Extent of thermal injury: Total surface area of the injured tissue (Fig. 12.1)
   c. Depth of thermal injury: Extent of the injury through the layers (thicknesses) of skin (Fig. 12.2)
      i. Zone of hyperemia
         (a) Outer zone of minimal injury; heals rapidly
         (b) Tissue is red (hyperemic) but blanches and refills with pressure
         (c) No cell death

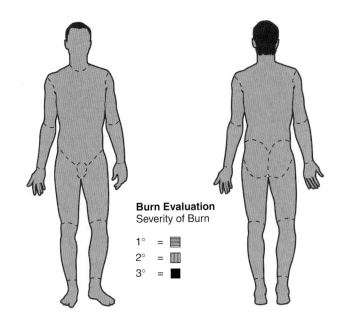

Burn Evaluation
Severity of Burn

1° = ▤
2° = ▥
3° = ■

Lund and Browder chart								
AREA	**AGE–YEARS**					% 2º	% 3º	% TOTAL
	0–1	1–4	5–9	10–15	ADULT			
Head	19	17	13	10	7			
Neck	2	2	2	2	2			
Ant. Trunk	13	17	13	13	13			
Post. Trunk	13	13	13	13	13			
R. Buttock	2½	2½	2½	2½	2½			
L. Buttock	2½	2½	2½	2½	2½			
Genitalia	1	1	1	1	1			
R.U. Arm	4	4	4	4	4			
L.U. Arm	4	4	4	4	4			
R.L. Arm	3	3	3	3	3			
L.L. Arm	3	3	3	3	3			
R. Hand	2½	2½	2½	2½	2½			
L. Hand	2½	2½	2½	2½	2½			
R. Thigh	5½	6½	8½	8½	9½			
L. Thigh	5½	6½	8½	8½	9½			
R. Leg	5	5	5½	6	7			
L. Leg	5	5	5½	6	7			
R. Foot	3½	3½	3½	3½	3½			
L. Foot	3½	3½	3½	3½	3½			
					Total			

FIG. 12.1 The Lund and Browder chart is used to assess and graphically document size and depth of the burn wound. (From Carlson, K.K. (2009). *AACN advanced critical care nursing*, St. Louis, Elsevier.)

ii. Zone of stasis
   (a) Represents cellular damage of variable degree caused by the decreased blood flow
      (1) Middle zone of injury, the cells of which can either recover or become necrotic over the initial 24 hours following injury; burn resuscitation is aimed at decreasing the expansion of this area
   (b) Tissue is red but does not blanch with pressure

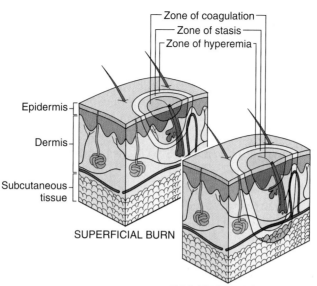

Zone of coagulation
Zone of stasis
Zone of hyperemia

Epidermis

Dermis

Subcutaneous tissue

SUPERFICIAL BURN

FULL-THICKNESS BURN

FIG. 12.2 Concentric zones of hyperemia, stasis, and coagulation within a burn.

        (c) Recovery depends on adequate resuscitation to correct hypovolemia, restore blood flow, and prevent hypervolemia

   iii. Zone of coagulation

        (a) Area of injury where the temperature reached at least 45° C (113° F)

        (b) Characterized by protein coagulation and cell death

        (c) Tissue is black, gray, or khaki to white and does not blanch with pressure

        (d) There is irreversible tissue loss in this area

2. Epidemiology

  a. Third leading cause of death from unintentional injury for group 5 to 9 years of age. No greater than the fifth leading cause of death by unintentional injury for any other age group.

  b. In the United States, there are approximately 1.2 million burn injuries per year

    i. 75% are mild and are treated outpatient

    ii. Approximately 50,000 per year require admission to major burn center

  c. Infection is a major cause of morbidity and mortality

  d. Pneumonia is especially common and can often be fatal in burn patients

  e. 300 children aged 0 to 19 years are treated for burns in emergency rooms every day in the United States

    i. Of these, two children die every day from severe burns

    ii. Young children (<4 years old) are most likely burnt by scalding

  f. Aging process makes older adults less able to respond to conventional therapy. Underlying organ dysfunction leads to a diminished compensatory response to burn injury and greater potential to develop multiple organ dysfunction syndrome (MODS).

3. Gender demographics in relation to burns

  a. Males are more commonly involved in serious burn injuries.

4. Cellular pathophysiology: Cellular injury occurs when tissues are exposed to an energy source (thermal, chemical, electrical, radiation); responses are both local and systemic

a. Local response: Coagulation of cellular proteins, which leads to irreversible cell injury with local production of complement, histamine, and oxygen free radicals
   i. Activation of complement (particularly C5a) and histamine release lead to increased vascular permeability
   ii. Creation of oxygen free radicals (by-products formed during oxidative processes; independent molecules with positive or negative charges), such as superoxide or hydroxyl, produce tissue injury
      (a) Attach to electrons from cell lipids and proteins to alter the integrity of the cell membrane and endothelium in the microvascular circulation, which leads to edema
         (1) Pulmonary vascular injury, pulmonary interstitial edema, and intraalveolar hemorrhage
         (2) Red blood cell (RBC) lysis and intravascular hemolysis
      (b) Alter the structure of deoxyribonucleic acid (DNA) and prevent the repair of the genetic code; may lead to total cell destruction
b. Systemic response: Initiation of systemic inflammation with the release of mediators
   i. Burn injury causes the release of vasoactive substances, such as histamine, prostaglandins, interleukins, arachidonic acid metabolites, bradykinin, and serotonin
   ii. Stress hormones are produced: Release of cortisol, glucagon, and epinephrine
c. Consequences of local and systemic responses

KEY CONCEPT
Fluid shifts related to burn injury are substantial and may oftentimes be much more severe than the outer injury indicates.

---

   i. Fluid shifts from blood into the interstitial and intracellular spaces as the injured tissue releases mediators that cause increased vascular permeability
      (a) Systemic response occurs when the burn covers 20% or more of the total body surface area (TBSA)
      (b) Sodium-rich fluid and plasma proteins are lost into the interstitium; most evident in the first 12 hours after injury
         (1) Decreased capillary oncotic pressure
         (2) Increased interstitial oncotic pressure
      (c) Tissue edema is often associated with airway instability, respiratory failure, limb ischemia, progression of burn injury, and compartment syndromes (increased pressure within an anatomic compartment that compromises the perfusion, viability, and function of the associated tissues)
      (d) Usually leads to hemoconcentration, increased hematocrit, and increased blood viscosity
   ii. Decreased intravascular volume; decreased blood flow to the skin, kidneys, and the gastrointestinal tract
      (a) Compensatory increase in systemic vascular resistance
      (b) Decreased cardiac output (CO)
      (c) Further decrease in organ perfusion
   iii. Uncorrected response
      (a) Hypovolemic shock (see Ch. 4, Cardiovascular System)
      (b) Anaerobic metabolism: Metabolic acidosis develops; decreased adenosine triphosphate (ATP) to fuel the sodium-potassium pump, which results

in increased intracellular sodium and water, and decreased intracellular potassium, magnesium, and phosphate
  (c) Hyperkalemia from cellular lysis and as a complication of metabolic acidosis
  (d) Delayed resuscitation increases the risk for the development of abdominal compartment syndrome; patient presentation consists of abdominal distension, declining urine output, hypotension, and decreasing pulmonary compliance

> **EXPERT TIP**
> Time from burn injury to fluid resuscitation should be treated as a perfusion goal analogous to the time goals seen in acute myocardial infarction (MI) and stroke. Prompt fluid resuscitation may improve patient outcomes.

  iv. Burn injuries initially have decreased metabolism, followed by a hypermetabolic response: Increased oxygen consumption, negative nitrogen and potassium balance, excessive muscle wasting, glucose intolerance, hyperinsulinemia, insulin resistance, sodium retention, and peripheral leukocytosis
  (a) Burn hypermetabolism puts patients at risk for increased morbidity and mortality
  (b) Hypermetabolic response can last up to 3 years postinjury
  v. Specific changes in organ systems other than the skin
  (a) Immune: Inflammatory response, immune dysfunction
  (b) Neurologic: Mental status changes (agitation, confusion, coma) may occur in the presence of hypoxia or hypovolemia
  (c) Cardiovascular
    (1) Initial: Reduced heart rate, cardiac output, and contractility. Blood pressure (BP) can be a relatively insensitive indicator of moderate fluid changes because catecholamine release raises BP and thereby masks the signs of inadequate organ and tissue perfusion.

> **KEY CONCEPT**
> In the initial response to burns, many factors, such as heart rate (HR), stroke volume, and urine output along with BP should be considered to accurately assess responsiveness to fluid resuscitation.

    (2) 48 to 72 hours postinjury: Increased CO, and thus myocardial oxygen demand, from hypermetabolism. HR increases up to 160% of normal heart rate.
  (d) Pulmonary
    (1) Pulmonary hypertension; vascular and perivascular inflammation
    (2) Microvascular leak with interstitial pulmonary edema and ventilation-perfusion mismatch
    (3) Changes with smoke inhalation
      a) Air, smoke, and steam can cause a thermal injury to the pulmonary mucosa
      b) Increased airway edema, neutrophil adhesion, bronchospasm
      c) Procoagulable and decreased antithrombin: high risk for pulmonary emboli
      d) Cast formation in airway because of leakage of exudate into bronchi

> **KEY CONCEPT**
> Inhalation injuries require an increased amount of volume during fluid resuscitation because of the surface area of the pulmonary vasculature.

    d. Gastrointestinal/nutritional (See Ch. 9; see Impaired Nutrition and Malnutrition)
        i. Delayed peristalsis and possible development of ileus because of sympathetic nervous system response
      ii. Decreased albumin production
     iii. Alteration in nutrient metabolism
          (a) Carbohydrate: Excess glucose can lead to hypertriglyceridemia, hyperglycemia, lactic acidemia
          (b) Lipid: Increased lipolysis, leading to hepatic steatosis if excessive lipid
     iv. Protein: Increase proteolysis, muscle wasting leading to azotemia
    e. Renal/fluids and electrolytes
        i. Decreased renal perfusion and ischemic injury
      ii. Myoglobinuria from muscle damage, leading to obstructed renal tubules
     iii. Renal failure can occur in up to 30% of all burn patients with an associated mortality rate of greater than 50%. Fluid creep: Overresuscitation of the burn patient either by excess fluid or fluid administered much more rapidly than formula dictates.
          (a) Associated with higher mortality, abdominal compartment syndrome, acute respiratory distress syndrome (ARDS)
          (b) Can be mitigated by appropriate burn size calculation, use of colloid as adjunct, titration of fluids to urine output

5. Classification of burn injury
    a. American Burn Association classification (Table 12.1)

TABLE 12.1 American Burn Association Burn Classification

Degree of Injury	Partial Thickness		Full Thickness	Considerations
	Adults	Children	Adults and Children	
Minor	<15%	<10%	<2%	Does not include burns to special areas, such as eyes, ears, face, hands, feet, or perineum
				Does not include people at high risk (people at extremes of age, those with inhalation injury or electrical injury, those with complex injuries, those with chronic illnesses)
Moderate	15%–25%	10%–20%	<10%	Can be treated on an outpatient basis
				Excludes special area burns as earlier
				Excludes high-risk patients as earlier
				Can be treated on an outpatient or inpatient basis, depending on severity and location
Major	>25%	>20%	>10%	Includes special area burns as earlier
				Includes high-risk patients as earlier
				Should be treated at specialized burn unit or burn center

Data from Johnson, J.Y. (2001). Burns. In P.L. Swearingen, J.H. Keen editors: *Manual of critical care nursing: nursing interventions and collaborative management*, 4th ed, St. Louis, Mosby.

b. Classification by depth
   i. Superficial (formerly first-degree) burns
      (a) Skin layer: Epidermal
      (b) Appearance: Dry, pink to red, blanches
      (c) Discomfort: Painful
      (d) Healing: 3 to 6 days without scarring
   ii. Superficial partial thickness (formerly superficial second degree)
      (a) Skin layer: Papillary dermis
      (b) Appearance: Blisters, red, moist, weeps, blanches
      (c) Discomfort: Severely painful when touched
      (d) Healing: 7 to 21 days; scarring rare but possible
   iii. Deep partial-thickness (formerly deep second-degree) burns
      (a) Skin layer: Reticular dermis
      (b) Appearance: Blisters, waxy or wet, decreased blanching
      (c) Discomfort: Decreased sensation to touch, painful only with deep pressure
      (d) Healing: Variable time, may require surgical excision/ grafting, likely scarring
   iv. Full-thickness (formerly third-degree) burns
      (a) Skin layer: Epidermis and dermis, all skin appendages involved
      (b) Appearance: Waxy white to leathery, dry, inelastic, not blanchable
      (c) Discomfort: Absent pain sensation superficially, deep pressure causes pain, area surrounding burn is painful
      (d) Healing: Variable time, will require early surgical excision and skin grafting, scarring and functional limitations may occur
   v. Fourth-degree burns
      (a) Skin layer: All layers of skin plus the fascia, muscle, and/or bone
      (b) Appearance: As earlier for full-thickness burns but may have exposed fascial, muscle, or bone
      (c) Discomfort: Pain only to very deep pressure in area of burn otherwise painless, area surrounding burn very painful
      (d) Healing: Will only heal with surgical intervention, time variable for healing

6. **Etiology and risk factors**
   a. Factors associated with burns
      i. Physical factors
         (a) Age: Incidence highest in the older adult patient and in children younger than 2 years of age; children 2 to 5 years of age are also at risk
            (1) Older adult (>65 years of age) may have poor vision, are at risk for overmedication, may have poor living conditions, or may smoke while using oxygen
            (2) Very young patients (<5 years of age) lack an understanding of the consequences of their behavior, such as playing with fire or matches, or understanding concepts, such as boiling water on stove
         (b) Type of burn: Thermal, electrical, chemical, radiation
         (c) Preburn health status: Preexisting organ dysfunction or conditions (e.g., diabetes mellitus, chronic obstructive lung disease, heart failure, hypertension, renal insufficiency or failure) impair compensatory responses to burns
      ii. Environmental factors
         (a) Presence of fire escapes, smoke alarms, sprinkler systems, firewalls, fire extinguishers

(b) Compliance with federal regulations on combustible and flammable products (nightclothes, plastic in airplanes)

   iii. Socioeconomic factors

      (a) Working in a high-risk occupation: Firefighters, construction workers, roofers, chemical workers, paving contractors, electricians, or electrical line workers

      (b) Living in a poorly maintained home

      (c) Low socioeconomic status

   iv. Personality and psychologic factors: Risk-taking behaviors, antisocial behavior, mental illness, depression, poor judgment, inadequate childcare, geriatric abuse or neglect

      (a) Burns are sometimes associated with physical abuse (cigarette burns, burns from curling irons, scalding)

      (b) Burns may occur when young children are inadequately supervised

         (1) Playing with matches or lighters

         (2) Setting off fireworks

         (3) Kitchen accidents: Boiling water, stoves

         (4) Bathroom accidents: Hot water in a bathtub

      (c) Burn may be a suicide gesture or attempt

      (d) Burn may be a result of drug use or manufacturing (i.e., methamphetamines)

   v. Alcohol and other medications of abuse (see Ch. 11 Multisystem Trauma): People who use alcohol often smoke; intoxication increases the risk for burns

   vi. Temporal factors

      (a) Most deaths from house fires occur during the winter owing to fireplace use and heaters

      (b) Injuries from fireworks and barbecue grills occur during the summer

      (c) The majority of burn injuries with a known place of occurrence are reported to have occurred in the home

  b. Causes

   i. Thermal: Contact with flames or hot objects

      (a) House fires are responsible for 75% of all burn deaths, but most of these deaths are caused by smoke inhalation or carbon monoxide poisoning

         (1) In patients under 60 years old with a TBSA of 0.1% to 19.9%, the presence of inhalation injury increased mortality 16-fold

         (2) Only 5% of all burn victims have a thermal injury from house fires

      (b) Clothing ignition: Contact with flames

         (1) Responsible for 5% of all burn deaths (up to 75% in the older adult population)

         (2) Second leading cause of hospitalization, but rates are decreasing because of legislation requiring nonflammable clothing

   ii. Scalds: Contact with hot liquids or steam

      (a) Responsible for 3% of all burn deaths and 30% of burn hospital admissions

      (b) Often caused by hot water in bathtubs and showers and spillage of hot coffee

      (c) Children under age 4 years are most often affected

      (d) Older adults are susceptible because of fragile, thin skin

   iii. Chemical: Contact with caustic or toxic chemicals, leading to coagulation of tissue protein, precipitation of chemical compounds in cells, cellular dehydration, and protoplasmic poisoning

      (a) Home: Cleaning agents

      (b) Industry: Explosions and contact with chemicals

    (c) Chemical agents
        (1) Oxidizing agents: Cause tissue oxidation (e.g., potassium permanganate)
        (2) Corrosive agents: Cause tissue denaturation (loss of normal properties of cellular proteins, e.g., phenol, lye, white phosphorus)
        (3) Desiccants: Cause severe cellular dehydration (e.g., sulfuric acid)
        (4) Vesicants: Cause blistering (e.g., dimethyl sulfoxide, poisonous gases used in warfare)
        (5) Protoplasmic poisons: Cause cellular coagulation (e.g., acetic acid, tannic acid, oxalic acid)
        (6) Management
           a) Remove chemical from body contact, brush off chemical powders
           b) Flush chemical from wound with large amounts of saline or water for at least 15 minutes; flush eyes for 30 minutes
           c) Remove all clothing and discard
           d) Do not rub skin, blot, or brush off with a washcloth
           e) Cover all burned areas with dry sterile dressings until appropriate burn care is instituted
           f) Do not use neutralizing agents! Can worsen burns
  iv. Electrical: Contact with an electrical current or flash caused by electrical arcing. Important considerations:
    (a) Amperage—amount of electronic current
    (b) Voltage—measure of flow of current
    (c) Duration of contact—longer contact causes more injury
    (d) Surface area of contact—greater surface area causes greater injury
    (e) Direct damage to tissues and nerves
    (f) Injury may be much deeper than the entrance or exit wound may show
    (g) Cause approximately 1000 deaths per year
    (h) Cardiac injuries and dysrhythmias are a main concern

KEY CONCEPT
Electrical injury should always be equated with myocardial injury until proven otherwise.

    (i) Injuries: Over 1000 volts are associated with a greater degree of deep tissue injury
    (j) Most common in summer: Lightning; electrocution in homes, on farms, or in industrial locations
    (k) Household: Hair dryers and wall sockets
    (l) Industrial: Electrical transmission lines
    (m) Tissue reaction:
        (1) Coagulation necrosis, direct damage to nerves and vessels, tissue anoxia and cell death, asphyxiation caused by tetany of muscles of respiration or respiratory arrest, long bone or vertebral fractures from tetanic contractions of muscles, muscle destruction
    (n) Findings
        (1) White charred skin, leathery skin, odor of burned skin, decreased or absent pain, cardiac dysrhythmias, entrance and exit wounds, contractions of skeletal muscles, changes in vision, seizure activity, paralysis, signs of multitrauma may be present

      (o) Management
         (1) Patient should only be removed by trained professionals
         (2) Turn off electrical source
         (3) Initiate basic life support
         (4) Administer humidified oxygen
         (5) Monitor cardiac rhythm
         (6) Cover entry and exit wounds with dry sterile dressing
         (7) Increase urine output goals, monitor for fluid creep, myoglobinuria, and rhabdomyolysis
    v. Radiation: Exposure to ionizing radiation (alpha and beta particles, gamma rays, x-rays), either inadvertent or caused by a catastrophic disaster or accident
      (a) Long-term biologic effect, which results in chronic health concerns
      (b) Intracellular destruction of DNA, loss of genetic information
      (c) Acute injury symptoms similar to the early symptoms of thermal injury (pain, swelling, redness, tissue ischemia); several weeks may pass before symptoms appear
      (d) Management typically requires a burn center with appropriate training

ASSESSMENT

1. **History**
    a. Complete description of the burn injury
      i. Time: Delay of treatment may result in a minor or moderate burn becoming a major injury
      ii. Location: Closed-space injuries are related to smoke inhalation
      iii. Context or situation: Falling asleep while smoking; pulling boiling water off a stove; occupational exposure
      iv. Burning agent, temperature of agent, length of exposure; determine whether an odor or visible airborne substance was present, as well as the quality and intensity of the odor or visible substance
      v. Actions of witnesses
    b. Suspicion of physical abuse: If abuse is suspected, obtain in-depth information. Factors that raise suspicion include the following:
      i. Delay in seeking treatment
      ii. Burns not consistent with the reported history
      iii. Bruising at different stages of healing
      iv. Reports of the burn differ among household members
      v. History of previous injury
    c. Past medical and surgical health history, with particular emphasis on organ malfunction: Heart failure, hypertension, chronic obstructive pulmonary disease, diabetes mellitus, and renal failure, and so on.
      i. A shock state postburn can precipitate further end organ malfunction
    d. Substance use and abuse: Detailed history of smoking, use of alcohol, and other medications of abuse
    e. Family and social history: Household members and relationships; household and childcare responsibilities; occupation, education, and job status; financial situation and insurance coverage; religion

KEY CONCEPT

An assessment of family and support structure dynamics is key, as it can significantly affect discharge care.

    i. A burn injury may be accompanied by an extended hospitalization with multiple surgical procedures. This may place stress on the patient and family, causing anxiety, depression, and feelings of hopelessness (see Ch. 2, Psychosocial Aspects of High Acuity and Critical Care).

  f. Allergies and current medications

2. Physical examination

  a. Physical examination data

    i. Primary survey: Rapid assessment (30 seconds to 2 minutes) that simultaneously identifies and manages life-threatening injuries

      (a) ABCDEF: *A*irway; *B*reathing; *C*irculation; and *D*isability; *E*xposure, evaluation, and emergency, life-saving interventions; and *F*luid resuscitation

      (b) Airway

        (1) The goal of airway management in the burn is early intubation for patients with suspected smoke inhalation, soot in the oropharynx, dysphagia, singed facial hair, oral edema or burns, facial burns, respiratory distress, upper airway trauma, altered mentation, hypercarbia or hypoxia, or hemodynamic instability

      (c) Breathing

        (1) An initial chest x-ray should be taken to rule out nonsymptomatic inhalation injury

      (d) Circulation

        (1) The initial goal is to establish at least two large-bore intravenous (IV) catheters, preferably through nonburned tissue. Peripheral IV access is initially more expeditious and safer.

      (e) Disability

        (1) Assess the patient's overall cognitive function (Glasgow Coma Scale [GCS], pupils equal, round, reactive to light and accommodation [PERRLA], blood glucose level to verify)

      (f) Exposure

        (1) Remove clothing to stop further injury and inspect all skin surfaces

        (2) Cover the patient with dry sterile dressings to prevent heat loss; wet dressings compromise an already impaired temperature regulation, and the lower temperature further complicates resuscitation efforts

        (3) Hypothermia exacerbates peripheral hypoperfusion, further decreases CO, and can cause coagulopathies

      (g) Fluid

        (1) Begin fluid resuscitation via the Parkland Formula or Modified Parkland Formula (Table 12.2)

    ii. Burn-specific secondary survey: This survey complements the trauma secondary survey (see Ch. 11 Multisystem Trauma) and includes a complete head-to-toe assessment to identify accompanying traumatic injuries, such as fractures, internal hemorrhage, and head injury; details of this survey include neurologic, otolaryngologic, chest, cardiac, abdomen, genitourinary, and

TABLE 12.2 Phases of Burn Care Management

Phase	Goals	Management Considerations
EMERGENT		

Resuscitative phase: Lasts 48–72 hours after injury or until diuresis takes place	Maintain airway, breathing, and circulation
	
	Maintain excretory function
	
	Preserve joint function and mobility
	
	Prevent complications
	
	Preserve self-concept
		1. Endotracheal intubation and mechanical ventilation if needed
		
		2. Fluid resuscitation (formulas vary)
		
		  a. Standard formula is usually a balanced salt solution, such as lactated Ringer's solution or normal saline: $4\,mL \times kg \times (\%\ burn \times 100)$ equals volume per 24 hours; 50% is given in first 8 hours, 25% in second 8 hours, and 25% in third 8 hours
		
		  b. Electrolyte replacement based on laboratory results
		
		3. Intravenous medication for pain and anxiety management
		
		4. Wound care and ongoing debridement
		
		  a. Wash burn surface with mild soap; rinse; apply appropriate topical antimicrobial (silver sulfadiazine, aqueous 0.5% silver nitrate, and 5% or 11.1% mafenide acetate cream); cover wounds with sterile dry sheets
		
		  b. Immerse minor burns in normal saline solution at 55° C (31° F)
		
		5. Nutritional support (often enteral by nasoduodenal route)

ACUTE/WOUND COVERAGE		
Acute phase: Characterized by eschar separation; lasts until spontaneous healing of burn wound occurs or until grafts are in place (variable time period lasting weeks to months)	Perform early excision of eschar and grafting Provide wound coverage; may use allograft if autograft is not available Prevent complications (sepsis, cardiovascular collapse)	1. Maintenance of hydration and electrolyte balance (monitor for decreased potassium and sodium) 2. Wound cleansing with bedside shower or shower tables 3. Ongoing debridement followed by topical application of antimicrobial agents (silver sulfadiazine, mafenide acetate, silver nitrate) 4. Skin grafting 5. Ongoing pain management, emotional support, nutritional support, occupational and physical therapy
CONVALESCENT/REHABILITATIVE		
Time period for inpatient rehabilitation	Promote return (functionally and cosmetically) to usual roles and responsibilities Support patient in adapting emotionally to burn injury Encourage maximum function of body parts	Ongoing pain management, emotional support, nutritional support, occupational and physical therapy, speech therapy if needed

extremity assessments, and radiography and laboratory studies (discussed later); usually takes place in an intensive care or burn unit. *Note:* Ongoing resuscitation continues during the secondary survey as needed.

(a) Neurologic: Assess for significant anoxic or carbon monoxide injury, address pain and anxiety; a decreased loss of consciousness may also be related to medications, alcohol, hypoxia, or hypotension

(b) Otolaryngologic and ophthalmologic: Evaluate the external ear and cornea for injury; fluorescein staining may be needed to detect subtle eye injury

(c) Chest: Ensure adequate oxygenation and ventilation; treat bronchospasm with bronchodilators; if circumferential chest burns are present, an escharotomy may be required to adequately ventilate; suspect inhalation injury if one or more of the following are present: Odor of smoke, burns of the intraoral cavity, cough, hoarseness, expiratory wheezes, chest pain, shortness of breath, singed nasal hair, circumoral burns, and blackened, carbonaceous sputum

(d) Abdomen: Evaluate for concern for abdominal compartment syndrome, bladder pressure monitoring may be warranted; hallmarks of compartment syndrome are the inability to ventilate and decreasing urine output despite aggressive resuscitation (see Ch. 9 Gastrointestinal System)

(e) Genitourinary: Evaluate for burns of the genitals, urinary catheter insertion should be considered early if burns are present to genitals as insertion may not be possible once edema ensues, considerations include attention to the foreskin following catheter insertion to prevent the development of paraphimosis with edema of the soft tissue

(f) Extremities: Monitoring of perfusion is paramount; early identification of the loss of perfusion, sensation, and/or movement is vital to detecting compartment syndrome

   (1) The definitive treatment to manage early loss of perfusion to extremities is bedside escharatomy

(g) Miscellaneous: Determine the presence of electrical or chemical injury, ascertain tetanus immune status, and evaluate whether abuse is a possibility

iii. Inspection of the burn: See classification by depth (see Table 12.1)

(a) Location: Severity is increased for burns on the hands, face, eyes, ears, feet, and genitalia

   (1) Studies have shown that, in patients with perineal burns, mortality can be as high as 25% to 50%

(b) Appearance: Color, consistency, and changes in vessels

(c) Depth: Severity depends on the intensity and duration of the exposure

(d) Extent: Percentage of the body surface area involved; severity depends on the intensity and duration of exposure

(e) Considerations

   (1) Check for current entry and exit sites for electrical burns. There may be small entry and exit sites but large areas of injury lying underneath the skin ("iceberg effect"). Internal damage may not be evident for hours or days.

   (2) Monitor for increased swelling and edema, which may lead to airway obstruction or compartment syndrome

   (3) Depth and severity of a burn may not be evident until several days after the initial injury

Burns

12

   iv. Inspection, palpation, percussion, and auscultation of body systems to monitor for multisystem effects of an injury and inflammatory response (see Ch. 11 Multisystem Trauma)
- b. Physiologic monitoring data
  - i. Vital signs: Widely variable depending on the catecholamine stress response, burn severity, and medication therapy
    - (a) Serial measurement of vital signs: Essential to monitor the response to burns and to interventions
    - (b) Respiratory rate
      - (1) Typical following major burns: Tachypnea
      - (2) Absence of tachypnea following a major burn indicates central nervous system suppression (because of alcohol or other medications of abuse) or injury, airway obstruction, and restricted chest excursion from injured skin
        - a) Monitor for edema of neck and airway
        - b) Monitor for circumferential eschar formation around the neck or chest
        - c) Monitor for signs of obstruction: Stridor, hoarseness, restlessness, behavior changes, and decreased level of consciousness
    - (c) Heart rate
      - (1) Typical following burn: Tachycardia
        - a) Well-conditioned athletes and patients taking β-adrenergic or calcium channel blockers have lower heart rates
        - b) Electrical burns may lead to dysrhythmias (ventricular fibrillation, asystole)
        - c) Cardiac injuries and dysrhythmias can occur regardless of the voltage
        - d) All patients with an electrical injury should have an initial electrocardiogram to rule out cardiac injury
        - e) Patient may have decreased or absent peripheral pulses or delayed capillary refill
    - (d) Blood pressure
      - (1) Goal: Systolic BP above 90 mm Hg
      - (2) Typical following burns: Variable, depending on fluid loss and the patient's age, but hypotension often present
      - (3) CO is often decreased in the first 24 hours postinjury
      - (4) Young adults may maintain BP in spite of significant fluid losses
      - (5) Older adults have less compensatory mechanisms and less tolerance for fluid deficits
      - (6) Alcohol intoxication may lead to either hypotension or hypertension
    - (e) Temperature
      - (1) Goal temperature: Above 37° C (98.6° F)
      - (2) Typical following burns: Decreased core temperature of 35° to 37° C (95°–98.6° F) because of exposure or loss of heat from open wounds
      - (3) Hyperthermia may develop because of increased tissue metabolism and infection
    - (f) Pain (see Ch. 20 Pain)
      - (1) Patients should be continually assessed for pain
    - (g) Hemodynamics and urinary output: In General, urine output is more commonly used to determine the success of fluid resuscitation

(1) Goal: 0.5 to 1.0 mL/kg/h for adults

(2) Typical following burns: Decreased urine output

c. Appraisal of patient characteristics: Patients with acute or life-threatening burns enter critical care units with a wide range of clinical characteristics. During their stay, their clinical status may slowly or abruptly improve or deteriorate. Changes in the patient's condition may involve one or all life-sustaining functions, and functions can be easy or nearly impossible to monitor with precision. Examples of clinical attributes that the nurse should assess when caring for a patient with an acute burn injury are the following: Resiliency, vulnerability, stability, complexity, resource availability, participation in care and decision-making, and predictability.

3. **Diagnostic studies**

a. Expected laboratory values after burns

 i. Arterial blood gas (ABG)

(a) Respiratory alkalosis with an arterial partial pressure of carbon dioxide ($PaCO_2$) below 35 mm Hg may occur early because of tachypnea

(b) For patients with carbon monoxide poisoning, a decrease in measured arterial partial pressure of oxygen (PaO_2) will not be seen, but a marked decrease in directly measured arterial oxygen saturation (SaO_2) will be seen

(c) Metabolic acidemia with a pH below 7.34 occurs after major burns

(1) pH usually returns to normal with the correction of fluid deficit and the correction of low CO states

(2) Base deficit is typical

(d) In severe burns and inhalation injuries, a progressive increase in the fraction of inspired oxygen is needed to maintain PaO_2 and SaO_2

(e) Patients with inhalation injury are at a much higher risk of developing reactive airway disease, ARDS, and pneumonia

 ii. Carboxyhemoglobin (COHb) level: More than 10% is diagnostic of carbon monoxide poisoning. Absence of COHb does not rule out inhalation injury; severe poisoning is consistent with levels of 20% to 40% and levels between 30% and 70% are associated with coma and death.

(a) Hemoglobin has a 200 times higher affinity for carbon monoxide than oxygen

 iii. Complete blood count (CBC) and differential

(a) Postburn period is associated with leukocytosis (increased white blood cell count, as high as 30,000/mm³; usually resolves in 48 hours)

(b) Leukopenia may occur as a side effect of topical treatment with silver sulfadiazine or because of systemic inflammatory responses

(c) Local heat may lead to RBC destruction; however, usually increased hematocrit because of hemoconcentration and "third-spacing" occurs

(d) Thrombocytopenia may occur during the first 72 hours as a result of dilution and some microvascular thromboses

 iv. Nutritional parameters

(a) Serum glucose levels: Elevated from the stress response

(b) Total protein and albumin levels: Decreased because of protein loss from increased vascular permeability

 v. Electrolyte levels

(a) Hyperkalemia caused by tissue destruction, RBC hemolysis, and increased intracellular sodium concentration from osmotic changes

(b) Sodium imbalance

     (1) Hypernatremia resulting from intravascular fluid loss and hemoconcentration

     (2) Hyponatremia resulting from sodium loss and hemodilution

  vi. Coagulation studies: Elevations in prothrombin time (PT) and partial thromboplastin time (PTT) during the first 3 days after burn injury because of the leakage of clotting factors from the intravascular space

  vii. Blood alcohol level and medication toxic screen to identify

     (a) Circumstances of the burn injury

     (b) Risk of withdrawal

     (c) Complications of substance use

  viii. Blood urea nitrogen level is often elevated because of increased tissue and RBC destruction and dehydration; creatinine level is normal unless acute renal failure is occurring

  ix. Wound specimen cultures and wound biopsy as ordered to isolate infectious source

 b. Radiologic

  i. Chest radiograph may be normal early in the patient's course; bilateral patchy infiltrates suggest developing pneumonitis

  ii. The pathophysiology of the burn injury causes increased blood flow and fluid shift into the interstitial and alveolar space, thus exacerbating lung injury postburn

  iii. Helical computed tomography (CT) may be useful for patients with possible blunt injuries of the head, neck, chest, abdomen, or pelvis

 c. Laryngoscopy (with upper airway involvement) and/or bronchoscopy (with lower airway involvement) may be necessary in suspected cases of inhalation injury

 d. Bronchoscopy

  i. Bronchoscopy should be used with suspected inhalation injury

  ii. Sooty, gray mucosa, hoarseness, stridor, or respiratory distress may be the first signs of inhalation injury

PATIENT CARE

1. Potential for airway compromise (see Ch. 3, Pulmonary System)

KEY CONCEPT

Maintaining a patent airway is the main focus for a burn patient in the immediate resuscitative phase.

---

 a. Description of problem: Secretions and obstruction from airway edema

 b. Goals of care: Maintain airway patency

 c. Interprofessional collaboration: Nursing, physician, burn surgeon, advanced practice providers, respiratory therapy

 d. Interventions

  i. Monitor for carbonaceous sputum, hoarseness, and stridor

  ii. Maintain the airway with an oral or nasal airway or jaw lift and chin thrust

  iii. Maintain head of bed greater than 45 degrees if head burn to prevent worsening of swelling

---

EXPERT TIP

Keep the patient's head in a neutral position until the cervical spine has been determined to be without injury, or maintain intubation as needed.

---

2. **Impaired oxygenation and ventilation (see Ch. 3, Pulmonary System)**
   a. Description of problem: Inflammatory process, decreased lung expansion, tracheobronchial obstruction, and alveolar-capillary membrane changes
   b. Goals of care: Maintain adequate oxygenation and ventilation, use low-tidal volume ventilator management to prevent further lung injury
   c. Interprofessional collaboration: Nursing, physician, burn surgeon, advanced practice providers, respiratory therapy
   d. Interventions
      i. Institute low-volume mechanical ventilation (5–7 mL/kg)
      ii. Institute IV pain control measures rapidly
      iii. Avoid overly aggressive fluid resuscitation, which can lead to increasing pulmonary and peripheral edema
      iv. Monitor for the formation of inelastic eschar on the upper chest and neck, which impedes adequate respiratory excursion
      v. Monitor intraabdominal pressures if intraabdominal hypertension is suspected in the presence of decreasing pulmonary compliance
      vi. When assessing respiratory symptoms, patient complaints of headache are often seen in carbon monoxide poisoning; dizziness, weakness, nausea, vomiting, and decreased mentation may be associated with more severe poisoning
      vii. Nebulizers with combination of bronchodilators, heparin, and acetylcysteine
      viii. Consider frequent bronchoscopy with inhalation injury until sloughing/soot cleared

3. **Intravascular volume depletion**
   a. Description of problem: Decreased intravascular volume related to fluid loss through damaged tissue and systemic inflammatory response to burn injury
   b. Goals of care: Maintain intravascular volume, correct fluid shifts, metabolic acidosis, and electrolyte abnormalities through fluid resuscitation
   c. Interprofessional collaboration: Nursing, physician, burn surgeon, advanced practice providers, respiratory therapy.
   d. Interventions (see Table 12.2)
      i. Control any bleeding with pressure.
      ii. Use large-bore peripheral catheters or central venous catheters to initiate rapid fluid resuscitation.
         (a) It is recommended that vascular access be obtained through nonburned tissue, but if needed, it can be accessed through burned tissue.
         (b) Frequently assess vascular access for infiltration, especially in resuscitative phase as edema rapidly progresses.
      iii. Use an accepted formula to calculate fluid replacement needs
         (a) Do not overresuscitate with fluids.
         (b) Overresuscitation can lead to complications, such as pulmonary edema, compartment syndromes, and third-spacing.
         (c) Parkland formula:

$4 \times$ weight (kg) $\times$ (% burn $\times$ 100) = the total volume delivered over 24 hours; 50% to be given over the first 8 hours and the remaining 50% to be given over the following 16 hours

         (d) Modified Brooke:

$2 \times$ weight (kg) $\times$ (% burn $\times$ 100) = the total volume delivered over 24 hours; 50% to be given over the first 8 hours and the remaining 50% to be given over the remaining 16 hours

(e) The beginning of the resuscitation time frame begins upon patient arrival to the emergency department

(f) Use hourly urinary output values to guide fluid replacement, with a goal of at least 0.5 to 1.0 mL/kg/h for adults

(g) Be sure to account for prehospital fluid

4. **Infection and exaggerated inflammatory process**
   a. Description of problem: Loss of protective skin barrier, inadequate primary defenses, exaggerated inflammatory response
   b. Goals of care: Patient will remain free of infection
   c. Interprofessional collaboration: Nursing, physician, burn surgeon, advanced practice providers, respiratory therapy, pharmacists
   d. Interventions
      i. Administer tetanus toxoid as prescribed
      ii. Initial debridement and excision of all nonviable tissue is recommended as soon as possible
      iii. Wounds should be cleansed with antibacterial soap
      iv. Antimicrobial topical therapy, such as silver sulfadiazine or mafenide acetate should be used
      v. Strict infection control practices, such as reverse isolation are recommended

5. **Altered thermoregulation**
   a. Description of problem: Loss of skin tissue decreases thermoregulatory ability
   b. Goals of care: Patient will maintain normothermia
   c. Interprofessional collaboration: Nursing, physician, burn surgeon, advanced practice providers, respiratory therapy
   d. Interventions
      i. Do not cover large burns with saline-soaked dressings, which lowers core temperature
      ii. If the patient is hypothermic, rewarm the patient and maintain and warm ambient temperature
      iii. Minimize personnel traffic in and out of the patient's room

6. **Catabolic state resulting in malnutrition and hyperglycemia (also see Ch. 9 Gastrointestinal System)**
   a. Description of problem: Hypermetabolic state related to thermal injury
   b. Goals of care: Maintain normothermia, decrease catabolic tissue destruction, and maintain blood glucose control
   c. Interprofessional collaboration: Nursing, physician, burn surgeon, advanced practice providers, respiratory therapy, dietician
   d. Interventions
      i. Initiate glycemic control with intensive insulin therapy
      ii. Utilization of insulin therapy for glycemic control will have different goals based on institution; however, glycemic control is associated with improved wound healing, reduced infections, antiinflammatory effects, and possibly reduced mortality
      iii. Maintain normothermia through the control of ambient room temperature and controlling exposure of burned tissue
      iv. Initiate enteral feeding as soon as possible after injury

7. **Altered tissue perfusion (peripheral)**
   a. Description of problem: Altered tissue perfusion relation to peripheral vascular constriction via mechanical (burn edema) or inflammatory (burn shock response or sepsis)

   b. Goals of care: Patient will maintain adequate peripheral perfusion

   c. Interprofessional collaboration: Nursing, physician, burn surgeon, advanced practice providers

   d. Interventions

     i. Remove constricting jewelry to limit tissue hypoperfusion

     ii. Monitor for the need of escharotomy (incision is made through an encircling eschar to release constricted tissue) or fasciotomy

       (a) Check peripheral pulses hourly and as needed, with a Doppler ultrasonographic examination if necessary

       (b) Notify the physician if capillary refill time is longer than 3 seconds or if numbness and tingling of the extremities or dusky extremities are present

     iii. Keep extremities above the level of the heart.

8. **Common side effects of topical burn medications**

   a. Description of problem: Common topical medications used for treating burns can cause specific side effects that the nurse must be aware of

   b. Goals of care: Assess the patient for signs and symptoms of common side effects that happen with topical burn medications

     i. Silvadene (silver sulfadiazine): Leukopenia, thrombocytopenia

     ii. Sulfamylon (mafenide acetate): Can cause pain upon application, can also cause metabolic acidosis and myelosuppression

     iii. Silver nitrate: Can cause pain on application and discoloration of the skin

9. **Altered patient and family coping (see Ch. 2, Psychosocial Aspects of High Acuity and Critical Care)**

References and bibliography information are available at http://evolve.elsevier.com/AACN/corecurriculum/.

CHAPTER 13

Hypothermia

Carrol Graves, MSN, RN, CCRN, CNL

CROSSWALK

- **Quality and Safety in Nursing Education (QSEN):** Patient-centered care, Teamwork and collaboration, Evidence-based practice, Safety
- **National Patient Safety Goals:** Use medicines safely, Use alarms safely, Prevent infection, Identify patient safety risks
- **American Nurses Association (ANA) standards for Professional Nursing Practice:** Standard 1. Assessment, Standard 2. Diagnosis, Standard 3. Outcomes identification, Standard 4. Planning, Standard 5. Implementation, Standard 6. Evaluation, Standard 9. Communication, Standard 10. Collaboration, Standard 12. Education, Standard 13. Evidence-based practice and research, Standard 14. Quality of practice, Standard 16. Resource utilization
- **AACN Scope and Standards for Progressive and Critical Care Nursing Practice:** Standard 4. Communication, Standard 6. Collaboration, Standard 7. Evidence-based practice/research/clinical inquiry, Standard 8. Resource utilization, Standard 10. Environmental health
- **AACN Standards for Establishing and Sustaining Healthy Work Environments (HWE):** Skilled communication, True collaboration, Effective decision-making
- **PCCN content:** None
- **CCRN content:** Multisystem—Thermoregulation

SYSTEMWIDE ELEMENTS

ANATOMY AND PHYSIOLOGY REVIEW

1. **Temperature regulation definitions**
   a. Normothermia: Core temperature (peripheral artery [PA] catheter, esophageal, urinary bladder), 37°C ± 0.5°C (98.6°F ± 0.9°F).

> **EXPERT TIP**
> PA catheter, esophageal probe, rectal and bladder probe temperature reflect core temperature. Esophageal is preferred method of temperature monitoring as rectal and bladder probe can lag.

   b. Hypothermia: Core temperature (PA catheter, esophageal, urinary bladder) below 35°C (95°F).
   c. Body temperature is regulated by the hypothalamus as it receives input from the central and thermal receptors.
      i. Temperature regulation is from a stimulus-feedback system that signals the autonomic reflexes to control cooling responses if there is excess heat or the generation of heat through shivering if temperature falls.
      ii. Heat production is initiated by the hypothalamus and endocrine systems. Thyrotropin-stimulating hormone-releasing hormone stimulates the release

of thyroid stimulating hormone which stimulates the release of thyroxine (T4). T4 acts on the adrenal medulla to release epinephrine which causes vasoconstriction, stimulates glycolysis, and increases the metabolic rate.

(a) Increased heat production by metabolic systems via shivering

d. Heat production is increased by shivering, triggered by the skin cooling

e. Shivering increases metabolism, ventilation, cardiac output (CO), and mean arterial pressure (MAP). These dynamics continue to increase until approximately 32°C (89.6°F), at which point they begin to decrease with further decreases in temperature.

f. At temperatures lower than 32°C (98.6°F), shivering is ineffective, and rewarming requires the addition of exogenous heat.

g. Shivering may cease below a core temperature of approximately 33.3°C (92°F). At this point, metabolism decreases with further decreases in core temperature.

    i. Preventing further heat loss via vasoconstriction

2. **Physiology of hypothermia**

a. At temperatures less than 30°C (86°F), CO decreases and bradycardia generally occurs

b. Electrical conduction abnormalities below 30°C (86°F) lead to dysrhythmias, such as premature atrial and ventricular contractions, atrial fibrillation, and ventricular fibrillation.

c. Coagulopathies: Impaired platelet function, decreased enzymatic activity of clotting factors, inhibits fibrinogen synthesis, increased clotting time, derangements in thromboelastograph

d. Cerebral activity begins to decrease at a core temperature of approximately 33°C to 34°C (91.4°F–93.2°F) and continues to decrease with further decreases in temperature. Decreases in the temperature of the brain leads to irritability, confusion, apathy, poor decision-making, lethargy, somnolence and coma, and decreases cerebral oxygen requirements.

e. Stress from cold decreases circulating blood volume as a result of a combination of factors: Cold-induced diuresis, extravascular plasma shift, and inadequate fluid intake

f. Less oxygen is released from oxyhemoglobin to the tissues in hypothermia because of a shift in the oxygen dissociation curve.

g. Below 28°C (82.4°F), most patients are unconscious and not shivering.

h. Once the body temperature falls below 25°C (77°F), the myocardium is prone to ventricular fibrillation caused by acidosis, hypocarbia, and hypoxia; hypoventilation and respiratory acidosis are caused by decreased ventilator response to carbon dioxide.

i. Mechanisms of heat loss (Table 13.1)

3. **Etiology and risk factors**

a. Predisposing factors

    i. Environmental: Skin exposure, wet clothing, low ambient temperature, and air movement

    ii. Extremes of age: Infancy (<2 years), advanced age (≥65 years). The generation of heat in the older adult decreases with the decrease in metabolism and muscle activity; the body's natural insulation is decreased with thinner skin; some medications exacerbate the older adult's susceptibility to cold.

    iii. Disease states that decrease metabolism: Hypothyroidism, hypoadrenalism, malnutrition, hypoglycemia, circulatory shock, water intoxication

    iv. Cutaneous disruptions: Wounds, burns, severe psoriasis, exfoliative dermatitis

TABLE 13.1	**Mechanisms of Heat Loss**		
Mechanisms of Heat Loss	**Definition**	**Affected By**	**Methods to Increase Heat**
Radiation	Heat transfer between two objects, through air or space, without direct contact	• Vasodilation and vasoconstriction depend on the amount of skin exposed to the environment • Heat loss limited by clothing and warming of the environment	• Warming lights • Warm environment • Temperature of the room
Conduction	Heat transfer from warmer to cooler objects by direct contact	• Wet clothes/gown	• Warm blankets • Circulating water blanket • Cardiopulmonary bypass • Arteriovenous rewarming
Convection	Heat transfer to or from a gas or liquid in motion	• Temperature of fluids, infusions and medications • Temperature of oxygen delivered	• Forced air warming devices
Evaporation	Loss of heat accompanied by water loss from skin to the surrounding air	• Heat loss is decreased if the skin is covered • Heat loss is increased with open wounds, wet skin, and tachypnea	• Head, feet, and hand covering • Clothing • Warm, humid oxygen

From Dow, J., Giesbrecht, G.G., Danzl, D.F., et al. (2019). Wilderness Medical Society practice guidelines for the out-of-hospital evaluation and treatment of accidental hypothermia. *Wilderness Environmental Medicine*, 30(4S), S47–S69.

    v. Hospital-associated causes: Exposure during an examination or wound care (especially if patient has large wounds), fluid resuscitation, blood transfusion, immobilization, and surgery

    vi. Socioeconomic factors
- (a) Effective home heating system
- (b) Ability to purchase clothes
- (c) Adequate physical care for elderly and children

    vii. Medications and other substances: Alcohol, phenothiazines, hypnotics, anxiolytics, antidepressants, narcotics, neuromuscular blocking agents, anesthesia, and oral hypoglycemics

  b. Types of hypothermia

    i. Accidental or spontaneous hypothermia: Caused by accident or insult, such as cold exposure. Examples: Outdoor accidents, cold water immersion, sleeping outdoors in winter, multiple trauma leading to exposure to cold environmental conditions, falls, and immobilization indoors.

    ii. Primary hypothermia: Associated with an inherent defect of central nervous system control of thermoregulation. Examples: Diencephalic epilepsy, cerebrovascular accidents, head injuries, neoplasms, and degenerative diseases.

    iii. Secondary hypothermia: Associated with an underlying disease process, multiple trauma, mental illness, a severe infection, and medication or substance use or abuse; can also be a type of accidental hypothermia

      (a) Diseases: Hypothyroidism, hypopituitarism, malnutrition, myocardial infarction, vascular insufficiency, pancreatitis, uremia, and carcinoma

    (b) Multiple trauma: Hypovolemic shock, burns, acute spinal cord transection, and near-drowning, large burns/open wounds

    (c) Mental illness: Dementia, self-neglect

    (d) Infection: Bacterial, viral, parasitic, fungal

    (e) Medication and substance use as mentioned previously

  iv. Induced therapeutic hypothermia, also called target temperature management (TTM): Used as a method of treatment

  v. Indications: All adult patients with return of spontaneous circulation (ROSC) after cardiac arrest who are comatose (does not follow commands) should have TTM.

EXPERT TIP

TTM should begin as soon as ROSC is obtained to improve neurologic outcome.

    (a) Exclusion criteria may include terminal conditions, do-not-resuscitate status, or those whose resuscitation has lasted more than 1 hour.

    (b) Induction-target temperature between 32°C (89.6°F) and 36°C (96.8°F), generally at a rate of 1°C/h, with target temperature reached in approximately 4 hours (if preinduction temperature is 37°C [98.6°F]).

    (c) Maintenance: Lasting 24 hours while avoiding large deviations in fluctuation from goal temperature.

    (d) Rewarming: Slowly rewarm at 0.2°C to 0.5°C/h until physiologic temperature of 36.5°C to 37°C (97.7°F–98.6°F) is achieved.

    (e) Complications: Bradycardia, decreased CO, elevated clotting times, electrolyte imbalances, overcooling, vasoconstriction, shivering (increases oxygen consumption and metabolic rate), cold diuresis (caused by peripheral vasoconstriction and increased venous return)

    (f) Shiver management

        (1) Nonpharmacologic: Cover head, hands, and feet

        (2) Pharmacologic: Use of nonsteroidal antiinflammatory drugs, analgesics, sedatives, opiates, and neuromuscular blockade, magnesium sulfate

---

EXPERT TIP

Management of shivering promotes effective temperature management.

    (g) Postrewarming: Maintain normothermia for 72 hours

    (h) Actively prevent fever after TTM. Fever after rewarming is associated with worse neurologic injury

    (i) Nursing care with targeted temperature management

        (1) Eye care

        (2) Venous thromboembolism prophylaxis (early mobilization, sequential compression devices, compression stockings, chemical prophylaxis)

        (3) Bundles of care to prevent hospital-acquired infections

        (4) Maintain skin integrity

        (5) Nutrition and hydration management

        (6) Prevention of fever

        (7) A written protocol that outlines the process including monitoring (electrocardiogram [ECG], urine output, blood pressure [BP]) and clinical interventions should be used

    vi. Acute brain injuries: Improves neurologic outcomes

        (a) Possible indications: Ischemic stroke when outside the goal time for thrombolytic therapy; increased intracranial pressure; hypoxic encephalopathy in hanging injury cases; traumatic brain injury

        (b) Physiology

           (1) Following ischemic insult and reperfusion of the brain, TTM acts by decreasing glutamate, glycerol, lactate, and pyruvate concentrations in the infarct area where tissue is at risk; these excitotoxic substances overstimulate neurons in the area of ischemic damage.

           (2) TTM decreases the adhesion of neutrophils in the ischemic tissue.

           (3) Decrease in temperature by 1°C (1.8°F) results in a 6% to 7% decrease in cerebral metabolic rate.

           (4) Oxygen supply to ischemic areas of the brain improves when blood flow increases subsequent to reduction of metabolic rate.

           (5) Two additional potential benefits (mechanisms for these changes are unknown)

              a) Intracranial pressure is decreased with TTM

              b) May act as an anticonvulsant

4. Effect of hypothermia on medications

  a. Metabolized and excreted at lower rates

  b. Protein binding is increased

  c. Lower doses are required to achieve the same efficacy in treatment outcomes. Medications given to hypothermic patients may have toxic levels when the patient is rewarmed.

KEY CONCEPT

Hypothermia reduces the clearance of some drugs commonly used in the intensive care setting.

---

5. Methods of cooling/rewarming (Table 13.2)

TABLE 13.2   Methods of Cooling/Rewarming After Target Temperature Management

Device	Method of Warming	Considerations
Traditional warming device, hydrogel or external wraps	Warmed or cooled fluids circulate through channels in a thermal blanket, pad, or upper body/thigh wrap	Temperature is controlled through a feedback loop system with a core temperature measurement device, from the patient, attached to the console and automatically regulates the water temperature according to the set target temperature
Forced air device	Device blows cool or warm air through a disposable blanket that is placed in direct contact with the patient	
Intravascular warming/cooling device	Central venous catheter with temperature-controlled saline solution balloons or distal metallic heat transfer elements that cool or warm the blood as it flows by the catheter	Catheter is attached to a console. Temperature is controlled through a feedback loop system with a core temperature measurement device, from the patient, attached to the console and automatically regulates the pressure, temperature, and flow rate of the circulating saline according to the set target temperature

From Vaity, C., Al-Subaie, N., & Cecconi, M. (2015). Cooling techniques for targeted temperature management post-cardiac arrest. *Critical Care* 19, 103.

ASSESSMENT

1. **History**
   a. Patient health history
      i. Current history of exposure or trauma, including the length of time of exposure and ambient or outdoor temperature
      ii. Significant past medical and surgical history, with a review of all major systems and of past traumatic injuries
         (a) New masses
         (b) Infectious signs and symptoms
         (c) Sleep patterns
   b. Relevant family history
   c. Social history
      i. Living situation: Older adults who live alone on limited incomes are at high risk for hypothermia during the winter or after falling
      ii. Alcohol use: Daily and weekly patterns
      iii. Outdoor activities, hobbies, and occupations
      iv. Relationships with significant others
      v. Nutrition, daily patterns of eating, and ability to afford adequate nutrition
      vi. Financial difficulties: Ability to afford clothing, medications, heating
   d. Medication history: Prescribed and over-the-counter medications, particularly phenothiazines, hypnotics, anxiolytics, antidepressants, steroid use, thyroid medications; any changes in medication doses
2. **Physical examination**
   a. Physical examination data
      i. Inspection
         (a) Respiratory: Assess the patency of the airway and breathing. Expect tachypnea and hyperventilation progressing to bradypnea, hypoventilation, and apnea; the more severe the hypothermia, the more depressed the respiratory drive and the higher the risk for inadequate maintenance of the airway and breathing
         (b) Circulatory: Pallor
         (c) Neurologic: Confusion, anxiety, and apathy progressing to a decreased level of consciousness, pupil dilation, and coma
         (d) Musculoskeletal: Increased preshivering muscle tone progressing to shivering and then rigidity
         (e) Renal: Cold-induced diuresis progressing to oliguria
         (f) Skin: Piloerection;
         (g) Hematologic: Prolonged bleeding, difficulty clotting, bruising
         (h) Terminal burrowing behavior: Paradoxical reaction of severely hypothermic patients who undress and find a position of protection because of vasodilation and feelings of warmth
            (1) Final mechanism of protection, with slowly developing lethal hypothermia
            (2) Autonomous process of the brainstem; triggered in final, lethal hypothermia
      ii. Auscultation
         (a) Circulatory: Rapid heart rate progressing to slow and then absent heart sounds; hypertension progressing to hypotension and an absence of BP
         (b) Respiratory: Decreased airflow, diminished or absent breath sounds, and crackles and gurgles from pulmonary congestion and pulmonary edema

   (c) Gastrointestinal: Diminished bowel sounds progressing to absent bowel sounds
  iii. Palpation
   (a) Circulatory: Weak, rapid pulses progressing to a slow or absent pulse, diminished capillary blanching, and cold skin
   (b) Gastrointestinal: Distention from paralytic ileus
   (c) Musculoskeletal: As shivering diminishes at lower temperatures, hyporeflexia occurs, followed by rigidity and finally peripheral areflexia
  iv. Percussion
   (a) Gastrointestinal: Increased tympany accompanied by upper abdominal distention indicates paralytic ileus
   (b) Respiratory: With severe hypothermia, dullness may indicate lung congestion and pulmonary edema
 b. Monitoring data
  i. Vital signs
   (a) Temperature: Axillary and tympanic methods are inadequate for core temperature measurement.

KEY CONCEPT

Whichever temperature monitoring method is chosen, it should be used consistently to enhance precision.

---

   (1) Electronic or digital: Measures oral, rectal, or axillary
   (2) Thermistors in catheters or probes measure:
    a) Rectal: May reflect a falsely low temperature if the probe is in cold feces or when the lower extremities are frozen
    b) Esophageal: Probe should be inserted 24 cm (9.5) inches below the larynx. Increases risk of aspiration.
    c) Bladder: May be falsely elevated with peritoneal lavage and falsely decreased in cold diuresis
    d) Pulmonary artery
   (3) Infrared: Measures tympanic or temporal artery
   (b) 34.5°C to 36.5°C (94.1°F–97.7°F) is usually accompanied by
    (1) Tachycardia
    (2) Increased BP and CO
    (3) Increased respirations
   (c) 32°C to 34.5°C (89.6°F–94.5°F) is associated with
    (1) Bradycardia
    (2) Hypotension
    (3) Decreased CO
   (d) Under 32°C (89.6°F) is associated with
    (1) Ventricular dysrhythmias
    (2) Asystole
    (3) Apnea
    (4) See Table 13.3 for additional data
 c. Appraisal of patient characteristics: Patients with acute or life-threatening hypothermia enter critical care units with a wide range of clinical characteristics. During their stay, their clinical status may slowly or abruptly improve or deteriorate. Changes in the patient's condition may involve one or all life-sustaining functions, and functions can be easy or nearly impossible to monitor with precision. Examples

TABLE 13.3 **Clinical Symptoms Associated With Hypothermia**	
Temperature	**Signs and Symptoms**
35°C (95°F)	• Shivering • Numbness • Dusky skin color
34°C (93.2°F)	• Severe shivering • Loss of finger movement • Cyanosis • Moderate confusion • Sleepy • Moderate to severe decreased reflexes • Progressive loss of shivering • Bradycardia • Shallow respirations • Possibly unresponsive as temperature nears 32°C
32°C (89.6°F)	• Hallucinations • Delirium • Sleepiness progressing to coma • Shivering has ceased • Minimal to absent reflexes • Oxygen utilization is decreased significantly • Metabolism is decreased by 35%–50%
31°C (87.8°F)	• Rarely conscious • Reflexes absent • Extremely shallow respirations • Profound bradycardia • Potential electrical conduction abnormalities
28°C (82.4°F)	• Respirations progress to apnea • Severe rhythm disturbances • Patient appears dead
24°C–26°C (75.2°F–78.8°F)	• Myocardium prone to ventricular fibrillation caused by acidosis, hypocarbia, hypoxia, hypoventilation, and respiratory acidosis • Death from electrical conduction abnormalities or respiratory arrest

From Dow, J., Giesbrecht, G.G., Danzl, D.F., et al. (2019). Wilderness Medical Society practice guidelines for the out-of-hospital evaluation and treatment of accidental hypothermia. *Wilderness Environmental Medicine*, 30(4S), S47–S69.

of clinical attributes that the nurse should assess when caring for a patient with hypothermia include the following: Resiliency, vulnerability, stability, complexity, resource availability, participation in care and decision-making, and predictability.

3. **Diagnostic studies**
   a. Laboratory data
      i. Coagulopathies: Impaired platelet function, decreased enzymatic activity of clotting factors, inhibits fibrinogen synthesis, increased clotting time, derangements in thromboelastograph
      ii. Hypokalemia
      iii. Thrombocytopenia

    iv. Hyperglycemia (because of insulin resistance)

    v. Hypomagnesaemia

    vi. Metabolic and respiratory acidosis

    vii. Leukopenia

    viii. Hematocrit increases 2% with each 1°C decrease in temperature

    ix. ECG: Prolonged PR, QT, and QRS segment; depressed ST segment; inverted T waves; Osborn (J waves) waves; atrial fibrillation; atrioventricular blocks

    x. Elevated troponins

> **EXPERT TIP**
> Hypothermia causes electrolytes to shift intracellularly. These shifts may cause cardiac arrhythmias.

PATIENT CARE

1. Hypothermia

  a. Description of problem: Decrease in body temperature, core temperature below 35°C (95°F)

  b. Goals of care: Core temperature is 37°C (98.6°F) within 24 hours

  c. Interprofessional collaboration: Nursing, physician, intensivist, advanced practice providers, respiratory therapy, case manager, dietician, pharmacist.

  d. Interventions

    i. Institute passive rewarming (relies on endogenous heat generation and ambient temperature to increase the core body temperature slowly at a rate of 0.5°C to 2°C/hour [0.9°F–3.6°F] until normothermia is restored

      (a) Remove the patient from a cold environment

      (b) Remove wet clothing

      (c) Increase the ambient room temperature

      (d) Decrease the airflow in the room

      (e) Cover the patient with blankets; cover the patient's head

      (f) Passive rewarming is reserved for relatively healthy, mildly hypothermic (temperature >32°C [89.6°F]) and hemodynamically stable patients

    ii. Institute active rewarming using both external and internal methods for moderate to severe hypothermia (see Table 13.2)

    iii. Monitor for decrease in core temperature of up to 2°C (3.6°F) after active rewarming is discontinued. Occurs when blood circulates to peripheral tissues, recools, and returns to the body's core.

    iv. Monitor for rewarming shock (vascular collapse because of decreased CO, hypotension, cardiac dysrhythmias); consequence of warming the periphery before the core

      (a) When the periphery is warmed before the core, cold, hyperkalemic, lactate-rich blood is shunted to the core of the body, which leads to shock

      (b) Limit rewarming to 2°C (3.6°F)/hour to decrease the risk of rewarming shock

    v. Monitor acidosis and electrolyte imbalances. Correct acidosis. Use caution when replacing electrolytes because of shifts when rewarming.

    vi. Teach preventive strategies to at-risk patients and staff caring for them

      (a) Limit exposure to cold temperatures

      (b) Maximize body coverage

      (c) Monitor the intake of cold or room-temperature fluids

2. **Altered oxygenation and ventilation (see Ch. 3, Pulmonary System)**
   a. Description of problem: Inadequate airway related to hypoventilation, bradypnea, or apnea. Inability to protect airway because of decreased loss of consciousness (LOC)
   b. Goals of care: Maintain adequate airway and ventilation
   c. Interprofessional collaboration: Nurse, physician, intensivist, advanced practice provider, respiratory therapist, dietician, pharmacist.
   d. Interventions
      i. Monitor respirations; a respiratory rate of 4 breaths/min or more may be sufficient for a hypothermic patient with adequate airway protection
      ii. Monitor LOC for ability to protect airway
      iii. Administer warm (42°C–46°C [107.6°F–114.8°F]) humidified oxygen as an adjunct to other warming methods. Heated, humidified oxygen is not effective as a sole source of rewarming.
      iv. Rapid sequence intubation with paralysis may not be effective or necessary if the paralytic used is not able to overcome the trismus caused by profound hypothermia. Fiberoptic intubation or cricothyroidotomy may be needed to place an endotracheal tube. Supraglottic devices may provide a better option.
      v. Avoid hyperventilating the patient if an advanced airway is in place. Adjust ventilation to keep arterial partial pressure of carbon dioxide within the normal range.
      vi. Avoid overinflation of the cuff of the airway device with cold air. The cuff will expand as the victim rewarms.

3. **Altered hemodynamics (see Ch. 4, Cardiovascular System)**
   a. Description of problem: Depending on the patient's temperature, hemodynamic instability may include anything from asystole to bradycardia. Hypothermic patients may have a cold diuresis that, as the patient warms and vasodilates, they become hemodynamically unstable because of hypovolemia.
   b. Goals of care: Patient remains hemodynamically stable with a pulse
   c. Interprofessional collaboration: Nurse, physician, intensivist, advanced practice provider, respiratory therapist, pharmacist
   d. Additional interventions
      i. Prevent stimulation of an irritable myocardium, which may lead to lethal ventricular dysrhythmias.
      ii. Because of an irritable myocardium, central venous access lines that contact the heart should be avoided. Internal jugular and subclavian central lines that extend into the right atrium are contraindicated because of the risk of inducing ventricular fibrillation. Femoral vein or intraosseous access allows central venous access without inducing dysrhythmias.
      iii. Hypothermia initially activates the sympathetic nervous system leading to tachycardia, vasoconstriction, and shivering. Rewarming results in hypotension because of vasodilation.
      iv. Move and maintain the patient in a horizontal position to avoid aggravating hypotension and to prevent orthostasis
      v. Initiate cardiopulmonary resuscitation (CPR) when appropriate.
         (a) Before initiating CPR, palpate for a carotid pulse for 1 minute because the presence of a pulse may be difficult to detect in hypothermic patients
         (b) Attempt defibrillation once if the patient's temperature is below 30°C (86°F); if unsuccessful, wait until patient temperature exceeds 30°C (86°F), then attempt defibrillation again.

      (c) Note there is no temperature cutoff for performing CPR in accidental hypothermia.

    vi. Resuscitation with intravenous (IV) fluids as appropriate

      (a) Consider using IV fluids other than lactated Ringer's solution to support circulation because the hypothermic liver may have trouble metabolizing the lactate in the solution

      (b) Administer potassium-containing solutions cautiously to prevent hyperkalemia as patient is rewarmed

      (c) As rewarming and losing vasoconstriction, ensure fluid status is euvolemic and BP will decrease with increase in intravascular space

    vii. Use IV vasoactive medications cautiously because toxicities may occur during rewarming. Increase the interval between medication doses to twice the interval recommended by the American Heart Association's Advanced Cardiac Life Support standards. The American Heart Association does not address medication doses or intervals in the hypothermic patient. Note the following:

      (a) Bradycardic dysrhythmias may be atropine resistant; slow heart rates are usually not corrected with medications or pacemakers unless the rhythm persists after rewarming.

      (b) As long as the temperature is below 30°C (86°F), after one defibrillation, medications are withheld until the patient's temperature exceeds 30°C (86°F).

      (c) In hypothermic patients, bretylium tosylate is more effective in the treatment of ventricular arrhythmias. Lidocaine is generally ineffective, and procainamide is associated with the increased incidence of ventricular fibrillation.

      (d) Amiodarone HCL is less effective in hypothermia and has the risk of inducing torsades de pointes.

    viii. Strict input and output: May have a cold diuresis that precipitates hypovolemia as the patient vasodilates during the warming process

4. Altered state of consciousness (see Ch. 3, Pulmonary System; Ch. 5, Neurologic System)

  a. Description of problem: At a temperature of 34°C (93.2°F), patients begin to experience confusion. As the patient's temperature continues to decrease, confusion increases, and patients may hallucinate and exhibit increasing signs of delirium. By the time the patient's temperature reaches 31°C (87.8°F), they are rarely conscious. With temperatures as low as 28°C (82.4°F), patients may appear dead.

  b. Goals of care

    i. Temperature returns to 37°C (98.6°F) within 24 hours

    ii. Patient returns to baseline neurologic status

  c. Interprofessional collaboration: Nurse, physician, intensivists, advanced practice provider, neurologist

  d. Additional interventions

    i. Monitor ability to protect airway

      (a) Decreased mental status that accompanies hypothermia may result in airway obstruction from the patient's tongue.

      (b) Endotracheal intubation can be managed safely in most hypothermic patients without inducing cardiac dysrhythmias.

      (c) Use care during airway management to immobilize the cervical spine until cervical spine injury, which may accompany hypothermia, is ruled out.

    ii. Assess the patient's baseline LOC and neurologic status. Changes may occur as a result of hypothermia or as a result of the condition causing hypothermia.

5. **Altered skin integrity**
   a. Description of problem: Skin that is cold is susceptible to injury from pressure or heat
   b. Goals of care: Temperature returns to 37°C (98.6°F) without skin impairment from rewarming process or pressure-related breakdown
   c. Interprofessional collaboration: Nurse, physician, wound care team
   d. Interventions
      i. Avoid localized pressure to cold skin
      ii. Do not apply heat directly to the skin
      iii. Do not use small chemical heat packs as they do not provide enough heat to affect core temperature, and they create the risk of thermal burns
      iv. Monitor skin integrity frequently. If gel pads or wraps are used for rewarming, monitor skin under these devices.

6. **Alcohol and drug intoxication**
   a. Description of problem: Core temperature below 35°C (95°F) with evidence of hypotension and alcohol or drug intoxication
   b. Goals of care
      i. Temperature returns to 37°C (98.6°F) within 24 hours
      ii. Patient experiences no symptoms of alcohol or substance withdrawal
   c. Interprofessional collaboration: Nurse, physician, intensivists, advanced practice provider, psychiatrist, or substance abuse specialist
   d. Interventions
      i. Institute rewarming techniques described previously
      ii. Monitor blood alcohol concentration to determine the degree of alcohol intoxication. Blood alcohol concentration of 100 mg/dL or higher indicates legal intoxication in most states.
         (a) Alcohol impairs thermoregulation by diminishing shivering, decreasing cold perception, and suppressing the hypothalamus
         (b) Monitor for hypotension related to depression of the vasomotor center and vasodilation
         (c) Malnourished or alcoholic patients should receive thiamine intravenously during rewarming to limit the risk of neurologic impairment from thiamine deficiency
         (d) Institute alcohol and substance abuse assessment and appropriate therapeutic strategies to limit substance use and abuse in the future

References and bibliography information are available at http://evolve.elsevier.com/AACN/corecurriculum/.

Hypothermia

13

SYSTEMWIDE ELEMENTS

ANATOMY AND PHYSIOLOGIC REVIEW

1. **Definitions**
   a. Toxicology: Study of adverse effects of chemicals on living organisms
   b. Toxicant: A toxic substance in the environment
   c. Toxin: A poison or venom of plant or animal origin, including from microorganisms
   d. Poison: A substance that can cause illness or death in a living organism
   e. Absorption: Extent and rate of substance movement from outside the body to an intravascular compartment (blood). Factors affecting absorption include the following:
      i. Route: Percutaneous injection (subcutaneous, intravenous, intramuscular), ingestion, inhalation, insufflation, transdermal, mucosal
      ii. Chemical characteristics of the toxin: Solubility in water and lipids, molecular weight, dissolution rate
      iii. Physiologic conditions: Presence of adsorbent substances, gastric emptying time, intestinal motility, spontaneous vomiting, tissue perfusion, metabolic rate, and organ function

f. Distribution: The way in which a substance disseminates throughout the body. Factors affecting distribution include the following:
   i. Tissue perfusion
   ii. Physical size of the person
   iii. pH of the drug or toxin
   iv. Protein and tissue binding capacity
   v. Lipid solubility

g. Clearance: Measurement of the body's ability to eliminate a substance from blood or plasma over time
   i. Expressed as the volume of blood or plasma completely cleared of a drug per unit of time
   ii. Elimination results from several processes
      (a) Metabolism of the drug into a form that can be excreted via the liver and kidneys
      (b) Excretion of the drug in urine, feces, and perspiration, as well as respiratory elimination
      (c) Chelation: Combining of metallic ions with molecular ring structures so that the ion is held by chemical bonds from each of the participating rings
      (d) Binding to activated charcoal
      (e) Extracorporeal drug removal through processes, such as hemodialysis and hemoperfusion (Table 14.1)

2. **Epidemiology**
   a. In 2018, the 55 U.S. poison control centers reported approximately 2.1 million human poison exposures, 77% of which were unintentional.
   b. In 2017, 84% of exposures were nontoxic, minimally toxic, or had a minor effect.
   c. Intentional exposures are significantly more likely to result in fatality.

TABLE 14.1 **Hemodialysis and Hemoperfusion**

Technique	Characteristics	Toxic Compounds
HEMODIALYSIS		
Toxic compounds diffuse down the concentration gradient through semipermeable membrane from blood into dialysis solution	Low molecular weight	Acetaminophen
	Water soluble	Ethylene glycol
	Low volume of distribution	Lithium
	Poor protein binding	Methanol
	Low body clearance	Salicylate
		Ethanol
HEMOPERFUSION		
Blood is pumped through a cartridge containing activated charcoal and/or carbon, which absorbs toxin	High molecular weight	Carbamazepine
	Low volume of distribution	Phenobarbital
	Not limited by protein binding (as is hemodialysis)	Phenytoin
	Low body clearance	Theophylline

From Decker, B.S., Goldfarb, D.S., Dargan, P.I., et al. (2015). Extracorporeal treatment for lithium poisoning: systematic review and recommendations from the EXTRIP workgroup. *Clinical Journal of the American Society of Nephrology*, 10, 875–887; Ornillo, C., Harbord, N. (2019). Fundaments of toxicology—approach to the poisoned patient. *Advances in Chronic Kidney Disease*, 27(1), 5–10; Roberts, D.M., Yates, C., Megarbane, B., et al. (2015). Recommendations for the role of extracorporeal treatments in the management of acute methanol poisoning: a systematic review and consensus statement. *Critical Care Medicine*, 43(2), 461–472.

d. In 2018, 79.3% of poison exposures were by ingestion, 6.8% by dermal, 6.1% by inhalation, 4% by ocular, 1.8% by bite/sting, and 0.9% by parental.

3. **Physiologic response to poisons**
   a. If the concentration of a chemical in tissues does not exceed a critical level, the effects of poison ingestion are usually reversible
   b. Local toxicity: Effects that occur at the site of first contact between a biologic system and a toxicant
   c. Systemic toxicity: Effects that occur after the absorption and distribution of a toxicant
      i. Most toxins affect one or two organs predominantly, but a target organ for toxicity is not always the place where a substance accumulates
      ii. The central nervous system is involved most frequently, followed by the cardiovascular system, blood and hematopoietic organs and tissues (bone marrow, spleen, tonsils, lymph nodes), visceral organs (liver, kidney, lung), and skin
      iii. Muscle and bone are least often affected
   d. Physiologic effect of a toxicant depends on the particular nature of the poison (Table 14.2)

4. **Etiology and risk factors**
   a. Common substances
      i. Local community trends dictate the epidemiology of intentional toxicant ingestion by substance abusers.
         (a) Prescription medications: Barbiturates, benzodiazepines, sleep medications, opioids, amphetamines, methylphenidate, anabolic steroids
         (b) Nonprescription medications: Acetaminophen, dextromethorphan, loperamide
      ii. Illicit drugs: Heroin, cocaine, methamphetamine, lysergic acid diethylamide, MDMA, Kratom, synthetic cannabinoids, synthetic cathinones (bath salts). The legality of marijuana use is state dependent, but it continues to be a commonly abused substance. Commonly abused designer drugs, or club drugs, are listed in Table 14.3. Most are analogs of phenylethylamine, fentanyl, meperidine, and phencyclidine.
      iii. Analgesics, sedatives/hypnotics/antipsychotics, antidepressants, and cardiovascular drugs were most frequently implicated in adult poisonings in 2018.
   b. Factors associated with poisoning
      i. Life-span considerations
         (a) Children under the age of 6 years account for almost half (47.7%) of all poisonings but have a low incidence of associated death.
         (b) Adults 19 years of age and older account for the majority of poison fatalities.
      ii. Gender
         (a) Males under the age of 13 years have a higher incidence of poisoning exposures than females.
         (b) Female adolescents and adults have a higher incidence of poisoning exposures than males.
      iii. Routes of exposure

> **KEY CONCEPT**
> Substances are most rapidly adsorbed through the intravenous and inhalation routes.

TABLE 14.2 Symptoms and Treatments for Commonly Ingested Toxic Substances

Substance	Therapeutic Level	Vital Signs	Symptoms	Medication Treatment
Acetaminophen	10–20 mcg/mL	Normal (early), hypotension may be present	Anorexia, nausea, vomiting, diaphoresis, and malaise, may have right upper quadrant abdominal pain and tenderness, bleeding	N-acetylcysteine (NAC) (Mucomyst); loading: 140 mg/kg PO; maintenance: 70 mg/kg PO every 4 hours; Give activated charcoal if less than 4 hours since ingestion Use NAC if levels are toxic even if ingestion was more than 24 hours earlier Repeat dose if patient vomits within 1 hour If vomiting persists, consider nasogastric decompression and may administer metoclopramide
Amphetamines	None	Hypotension, tachycardia; hyperthermia, tachypnea	Mydriasis, diaphoresis, dry mucous membranes; hyperactivity, agitation, psychosis, paranoia, headache, hyperreactive reflexes, tremors, seizures, flushed skin	May give activated charcoal for oral ingestion. Administer benzodiazepines (for agitation or seizures), external cooling (for hyperthermia), IV hydration (to replace fluid losses and prevent myoglobin damage in renal tubules), consider beta-blocker for tachyarrhythmia. Hemodialysis may be necessary for patients with acute renal failure, acidosis, and hyperkalemia
Anticholinergics	Varies by compound	Hyperthermia, labile blood pressure, tachycardia	Hallucinogenic toxidrome: Hallucinations, psychosis, panic, mydriasis Variable, ranging from anxiety, agitation, confusion, hyperactivity, seizures, and delirium to lethargy, decreased mental status, and coma	None
Arsenic	<5 mcg/L	Hypotension and tachycardia	Nausea, vomiting, abdominal pain, excessive salivation, watery diarrhea, dehydration	Chelation therapy. Support circulation with crystalloids and pressor agents as needed Administer blood if GI hemorrhage occurs Monitor for seizure activity Orogastric lavage may be necessary; initiate hemodialysis for renal dysfunction and clearance of arsenic
Barbiturates	10–25 mcg/mL	Hypothermia, hypotension, and bradypnea progressing to apnea; bradycardia	Stupor and coma, confusion, slurred speech, apnea; ataxia, decreased reflexes, coma	Administer sodium bicarbonate to enhance elimination of phenobarbital only Orogastric lavage may be necessary

Continued

TABLE 14.2 **Symptoms and Treatments for Commonly Ingested Toxic Substances—cont'd**

Substance	Therapeutic Level	Vital Signs	Symptoms	Medication Treatment
Benzodiazepines	300–400 ng/mL	Hypotension and bradypnea progressing to apnea	Stupor and coma, confusion, slurred speech, apnea: weakness, headache, and vertigo; diminished or absent bowel sounds, nausea, diarrhea, decreased reflexes	Flumazenil; use caution in patients with seizure or potential for seizure Orogastric lavage may be necessary
Carbamazepine	6–12 mcg/mL	Hypotension, hypothermia, bradypnea, tachycardia	CNS stimulation, hallucinations, seizures, mydriasis, nystagmus	Hemoperfusion Orogastric lavage may be necessary May need whole bowel irrigation if medication is enteric coated Give cathartics Monitor for seizures
Cocaine	None	Hypertension, tachycardia; hyperthermia, tachypnea to apnea	Vasoconstriction; mydriasis; hyperthermia, tachycardia, and hypertension; headache; abdominal pain and nausea; euphoria; increased energy, alertness; insomnia, restlessness; anxiety; panic attacks, paranoia, psychosis; arrhythmia, heart attack; stroke; seizure, coma	Administer high-flow oxygen Monitor ECG continuously Whole bowel irrigation may be necessary for body packers Administer benzodiazepines (for agitation) and vasodilators (for hypertension); may administer beta-blockers (for ventricular dysrhythmias) Provide cooling for hyperthermia Monitor for seizures Suspect cyanide poisoning with any serious smoke inhalation injury Administer 100% oxygen Administer crystalloids and vasopressors for hypotension Give sodium bicarbonate to correct acidosis Orogastric lavage may be necessary

Continued

Cyclic antidepressants	Varies by compound	Lethargy, confusion, dizziness, somnolence, seizures, coma	Administer sodium bicarbonate to prevent and treat dysrhythmias and hospital protocols to treat ventricular arrhythmias
			Monitor ECG continuously
			Administer sodium bicarbonate, and consider hyperventilation to keep pH at 7.50–7.55
			Correct hypotension with crystalloids and vasopressors if needed; avoid dopamine, which may increase dysrhythmias and may not correct hypotension because catecholamine stores have been depleted by overdose
Cyanide	<1 mcg/mL	Smell of bitter almonds, anxiety, agitation, lethargy, headache, seizures, abdominal pain, vomiting, cherry-red skin color or cyanosis	Hydroxocobalamin is more frequently used than cyanide kits (Cyanokit), supportive therapy
Digitalis glycosides	0.8–2 ng/mL	Hypotension, bradycardia, or tachycardia	Activated charcoal may be necessary, continuous ECG monitoring, may need blood pressure support if hypotensive
			Digoxin immune fab (Digibind)
Ethanol	None	Bradycardia or tachycardia; hypertension or hypotension; hypothermia; tachypnea leading to apnea	Never assume that decreased mental status is a reflection of intoxication alone, because alcohol intoxication is often associated with traumatic injuries
		Stupor and coma, confusion, slurred speech, apnea; agitation, released inhibitions progressing to depressed mental status, nausea, vomiting, ataxia, poor motor coordination	Consider magnesium and potassium administration to counteract electrolyte depletion
			Administer multivitamins with folate (for nutrition) benzodiazepines (for withdrawal symptoms)
			Hemodialysis

Continued

TABLE 14.2 Symptoms and Treatments for Commonly Ingested Toxic Substances—cont'd

Substance	Therapeutic Level	Vital Signs	Symptoms	Medication Treatment
Ethylene glycol (antifreeze)	None	Hypertension, tachycardia, tachypnea	Decreased mental status, lethargy, seizures, slurred speech, coma, abdominal pain, nausea, vomiting	Administer ethanol 100–150 mg/dL IV to prevent formation of toxic metabolites by competitive inhibition; maintain blood alcohol level of 100–150 mg/dL Maintain normal pH with sodium bicarbonate administration Consider hemodialysis as an option Administer benzodiazepines for prevention of seizures Hemodialysis
Iron	<100 mcg/dL	Hypotension, tachycardia	Five stages of iron poisoning: Stage I—GI symptoms; stage II—GI symptoms improve; stage III—shock and acidosis; stage IV—hepatic necrosis; stage V—bowel obstruction	Chelation therapy, supportive treatment
Isoniazid (INH)	3–5 mcg/mL 1–2 hours after dose	Tachycardia, hypotension, and hyperthermia	Nausea, vomiting, dizziness, ataxia, hyperreflexia, slurred speech; hallucinations, seizures, coma, oliguria	Control seizures with pyridoxine 1 g for every gram of INH ingested (give 1 g over 2–3 minutes) along with diazepam and lorazepam
Isopropyl alcohol (rubbing alcohol)	None	Hypotension, bradypnea, and hypothermia	Ataxia, areflexia, dizziness, headache, muscle weakness, abdominal pain and cramping, gastritis, hematemesis, poor peripheral tissue perfusion	Provide supportive treatment, with attention to cardiorespiratory problems May consider hemodialysis for patients with high levels (400–500 mg/dL)
Lead	<10 mcg/dL	Hypertension and tachycardia	Anorexia, constipation, abdominal pain, vomiting, lethargy, fatigue, hyperactivity, ataxia, seizures, coma, numbness and tingling of extremities	Chelation therapy, supportive treatment
Lithium	0.6–1.2 mEq/L	Hypotension (late)	Weakness, fatigue, tremor, muscle twitching, ataxia, slurred speech, confusion, restlessness, hyperreflexia, stupor, coma, diuresis, dehydration, diarrhea	Orogastric lavage may be necessary May consider hemodialysis for renal failure Monitor for seizures Hemodialysis

Continued

Mercury	<10 mcg/L	Hypotension (late), tachypnea (inhaled mercury)	Tremor, ataxia, paresthesia, tunnel vision, dyspnea, increased salivation, diarrhea, abdominal pain	Chelation therapy, supportive treatment
Methanol (antifreeze)	None	Hypotension, tachypnea, temperature variations	Visual disturbances, blindness, blurred vision, dimmed vision, inebriation, headache, dizziness, seizures, coma, nausea, vomiting, abdominal pain	Hemodialysis
Opioids	None	Hypotension, bradycardia, hypothermia, bradypnea	Stupor and coma, confusion, slurred speech, apnea; narcotic toxidrome: Altered mental status, miosis, decreased bowel sounds; seizures, ataxia, nausea, vomiting, hyporeflexia	Naloxone 2 mg (may be repeated) if opioid dependence is suspected, give 0.1–0.2 mg naloxone, (may be repeated) Position patient to limit risk of aspiration Continuous airway and respiratory assessment
Phencyclidine (PCP)	None	Hypertension, tachycardia, tachypnea, hyperthermia	Mydriasis, diaphoresis, dry mucous membranes; range of neurologic behaviors: From calm and unresponsive to excited, paranoid behavior; tremor; hyperactivity; myoclonic or dystonic movements; blank stare, dysconjugate gaze, nystagmus, blurred vision, miosis	Treat hypertension, benzodiazepines (for agitation); IV hydration, control hyperthermia
Phenothiazines	Variable	Hypotension, tachycardia, temperature variations	Memory deficits, confusion, dizziness, lethargy progressing to coma, decreased bowel sounds, miosis or mydriasis	Orogastric lavage may be necessary Continuous ECG monitoring

Continued

TABLE 14.2 Symptoms and Treatments for Commonly Ingested Toxic Substances—cont'd

Substance	Therapeutic Level	Vital Signs	Symptoms	Medication Treatment
Salicylates	15–30 mg/dL	Tachycardia; hyperthermia, tachypnea	Metabolic acidosis; tinnitus, diminished hearing, vertigo, agitation, hyperactivity, stupor, coma, increased bleeding tendencies, diaphoresis, nausea, vomiting	Orogastric lavage may be necessary Provide treatment for hyperthermia if necessary Provide alkalization of urine with sodium bicarbonate Implement hemodialysis for acute renal failure Monitor for and treat hypokalemia Hemodialysis
Sedatives	Variable	Hypotension, hypothermia, bradypnea progressing to apnea, bradycardia	Stupor and coma, confusion, slurred speech, apnea; ataxia, incoordination, paradoxical excitement	Orogastric lavage may be necessary, monitor for hypothermia, hypercapnia
Theophylline	8–20 mcg/mL	Hypotension, tachycardia; tachypnea	Tremor, hyperactivity, confusion, restlessness, agitation, seizures, nausea, vomiting	Implement hemodialysis for acute renal failure Orogastric lavage may be necessary Continuous ECG monitoring Hemoperfusion

CNS, Central nervous system; *ECG,* electrocardiogram; *GI,* gastrointestinal; *IV,* intravenous; *PO,* per mouth.

From Dart, R.C., Bronstein, A.C., Spyker, D.A., et al. (2015). Poisoning in the United States: 2012 Emergency Medicine Report of the National Poison Data System. *Annals of Emergency Medicine,* 65(4), 416–422; National Institute on Drug Abuse: Commonly abused drugs charts, Bethesda, Maryland, 2019, National Institute on Drug Abuse. Retrieved from: https://d14rmgtrwzf5a.cloudfront.net/sites/default/files/nida_commonlyuseddrugs_final_printready.pdf; Rech, M., Donahey, E., Cappiello, D., et al. (2015). New drugs of abuse, *Pharmacotherapy,* 35(2), 189–197.

TABLE 14.3 **Designer Drugs**

Street Name	Characteristics	Treatment
AMPHETAMINES		
Serenity, Tranquility, Peace	Euphoria, sympathetic nervous system stimulation, hallucinations	Treatment is supportive. Benzodiazepines for agitation
Ecstasy, "E," Adam, XTC	Euphoria, empathy Nausea, anorexia, anxiety Insomnia, sympathetic nervous system stimulation Enhanced pleasure, heightened sexuality, expanded consciousness, extraversion	Treatment is supportive
Love drug	Relaxation, sensory distortion Agitation, hallucinations	None
FENTANYL		
China white	Signs of opioid toxicity (decreased respiratory efforts) Lethargy to coma	Administration of naloxone Precautions for withdrawal
GHB		
G, Georgia Home Boy, Goop, Grievous Bodily Harm, Liquid Ecstasy, Liquid X, Soap, Scoop	Euphoria, drowsiness, confusion, memory loss, hallucinations, aggressive behavior, vomiting, unconsciousness, seizures, bradycardia, hypothermia, coma, death	Benzodiazepines for agitation/ treatment of seizures
KETAMINE		
Cat Valium, K, Special K, Vitamin K	Memory problems, dreamlike states, hallucinations; sedation; confusion and problems speaking; problems moving, to the point of being immobile; hypertension, respiratory depression, death	None
MEPERIDINE		
New heroin, synthetic heroin	Euphoria similar to that produced by heroin	Treatment is supportive
SYNTHETIC CATHENONES		
Khat, Bath Salts, Meow Meow, MCAT, Ivory wave, Bubbles, Vanilla Sky, Cloud 9, Explosion, White Lightening	Euphoria, increased energy, empathy, alertness, and increased libido Sympathomimetic toxidrome: Agitation, hallucinations, tachycardia, hypertension, mydriasis, tremor, rhabdomyolysis, electrolyte abnormalities, renal failure, seizures	Treatment is supportive Benzodiazepines for agitation/ treatment of seizures. Reverse electrolyte abnormalities and treat hypertension per protocols
SYNTHETIC CANNABINOIDS		
Spice (including variants, such as Spice Gold, Spice Diamond, Spice Silver) K2, Krypton, Aztec Fire, Bombay Blue, Fake Weed, Yukatan Fire	Euphoria and alteration in mood and sensorium Anxiety, paranoia, hallucinations, psychosis, seizures, tachycardia, hypertension	Treatment is supportive Benzodiazepines for agitation and seizures. Gastrointestinal decontamination may be necessary
SALVIA		
Diners Sage, Mystic Sage, Sally D, Magic Mint	Hallucinations and altered sense of self, flushed sensation, tachycardia	Treatment is supportive Benzodiazepines for agitation

14 Toxin Exposure

TABLE 14.3 **Designer Drugs—cont'd**		
Street Name	**Characteristics**	**Treatment**
DESOMORPHINE		
Krokodil, Crocodile, Zoombie Drug	Analgesic effects 10 times that of morphine and stronger than heroin IV usage causes extreme damage to vasculature, muscle, and tissue leading to necrosis and gangrene at injection sites	Treatment is supportive. Consider naloxone administration. May require psychiatric treatment

From Desomorphine (Dihydrodesoxymorphine; dihydrodesoxymorphine-D; Street Name: Krokodil, Crocodil.) http://www.deadiversion.usdoj.gov/drug_chem_info/desomorphine.pdf.; National Institute on Drug Abuse. http://www.drugabuse.gov/drugs-abuse/commonly-abused-drugs-charts.; Weaver, M.F., Hopper, J.A., Gunderson, E.W. (2015). Designer drugs 2015: assessment and management. *Addiction Science and Clinical Practice*, 10(8), 1–9.

    (a) Inhalation: Exposure through the respiratory tract, typically a gas inhalation
    (b) Intravenous: Injection directly into the vascular system via a superficial vein
    (c) Subdermal: Injection under the dermis of the skin ("skin-popping")
    (d) Transdermal: Absorption through direct contact with skin
    (e) Transmucosal: Absorption through a mucous membrane
    (f) Ingestion: Exposure to a substance by swallowing

EXPERT TIP

Ingested substances are subject to the "first-pass effect" of the liver. Therefore the oral bioavailability of many substances may be reduced.

---

    (1) "Body packing": Swallowing of containers, condoms, balloons, or plastic bags filled with illegal drugs for the purpose of smuggling.
        a) This practice is more dangerous when a person ingests drugs in an unplanned and hurried manner to conceal evidence ("body stuffing"). Deaths have occurred in body stuffers when a package reaches the alkaline milieu of the small intestine and the contents burst, causing cardiopulmonary arrest.
  iv. Environmental factors
    (a) Greater than 90% of poison exposures occur in a home
    (b) Approximately 2% of poison exposures occur in the workplace
    (c) Less than 2% of poison exposures occur at school
 c. The majority of unintentional poison exposures are undefined or related to one of the following causes:
  i. Environmental: Any passive, nonoccupational exposure resulting from the contamination of air, water, or soil
  ii. Occupational: Exposure that occurs as a direct result of being in the workplace
  iii. Therapeutic error: Unintentional deviation from a proper therapeutic regimen that results in use of the wrong dosage, wrong substance, or incorrect route
  iv. Unintentional misuse: Improper or incorrect use of nonpharmaceutical substances
  v. Bite or sting: Animal or insect bites and stings
  vi. Food poisoning: Suspected or confirmed ingestion of contaminated food

ASSESSMENT

1. **History**
   a. History of present illness
      i. May be obtained directly from patient, family, friend, partner, significant other, prehospital personnel, or bystander.
      ii. The history of present illness or patient's complete medical history may be incomplete if the patient presents with altered mental status and bystander knowledge is limited. Search electronic medical records for historical information.

EXPERT TIP

Consider hypo- or hyperthermia if patient was found in extreme temperatures. For patients with hypo- or hyperthermia, do not forget to consider other causes, such as sepsis.

---

   iii. Description of the event
      (a) Location of person at time of ingestion/exposure

EXPERT TIP

A pill bottle may be misleading as the container label may not represent the quantity, dose, or actual medication contained in the bottle. Loose pills may be identified by the imprint code.

      (b) Substance(s) involved
      (c) Timing of exposure
      (d) Intent of exposure
      (e) Cumulative amount of ingestion/exposure
         (1) Determine if exposure is repeated, acute, or chronic
      (f) Route of exposure
      (g) Type of container of the substance and labeling
      (h) Estimation of amount of substance ingested
      (i) Patient's symptoms after ingestion/exposure (if witnessed)
      (j) Any applied home first aid or prehospital treatment
      (k) Body packing or body stuffing: If the patient was confronted by police for illegal substance use or transport, suspect hurried substance ingestion.
   iv. Pattern of alcohol and substance use
      (a) Suspect polysubstance abuse in known drug abusers
      (b) Attempt to obtain reports of substance use patterns from the patient or electronic medical records, first responders, friends, and family members
   b. Past health history

KEY CONCEPT

The pneumonic "SAMPLE" is helpful in remembering the elements of a complete health history:

Situation

Allergies

Medications

Past illnesses

Last oral intake

Events preceding ingestion/exposure

Toxin Exposure

14

    i. Allergies
    ii. Medications
      (a) Prescription and over-the-counter drugs
      (b) Herbal and natural substances
    iii. Past illnesses (medical and surgical)
    iv. Last meal (time, quantity, type)
    v. Events preceding ingestion/exposure
    vi. Psychiatric history or known mental illness
    vii. Tetanus immunization for parenteral exposures

  c. Social history
    i. Living situation, including type of domicile and current occupants
    ii. Occupation
    iii. Current and previous substance abuse, alcohol intake, tobacco use, marijuana use, use of vaping products

  d. Other
    i. Estimated height and weight
    ii. Gynecologic history and potential for pregnancy

KEY CONCEPT

If patient history is limited, obtaining a detailed physical examination is the most important element in determining appropriate patient management.

---

2. Physical examination
  a. Initial assessment
    i. Determine the patency of the airway, adequacy of respirations and circulatory status.
    ii. Obtain a complete set of vital signs, including temperature and accurate respiratory rate.
      (a) Note: vital signs are widely variable, depending on the toxic compound (see Table 14.2).

KEY CONCEPT

The Glasgow Coma Scale is a standardized tool used to assess level of consciousness. It helps to determine a baseline mental status and establish a trend.

---

    iii. Observe the general appearance of the patient.
    iv. Assess the gross neurologic status of the patient.
      (a) Level of consciousness
      (b) Pupil size and response
    v. Remove the patient's clothes and inspect for occult trauma, wounds and needlesticks, or medicine patches.

  b. Detailed assessment
    i. Complete physical examination to include breath sounds, bowel sounds, skin temperature, mucous membranes, and muscle tone.
    ii. Complete neurologic examination, including tremors, quality of speech, motor exam, coordination, and reflexes.
    iii. Observe for the presence of toxidromes.

  c. Continued monitoring
    i. Perform serial physical examinations to establish a trend of deteriorating or improving status.

    ii. Frequent assessment of vital signs should occur every 15 minutes if unstable, every hour if stable.

   iii. Continuous cardiac monitoring with pulse oximetry.

   iv. Appraisal of patient characteristics: Patients with acute or life-threatening toxin exposure enter critical care units with a wide range of clinical characteristics. During their stay, their clinical status may slowly or abruptly improve or deteriorate. Changes in the patient's condition may involve one or all life-sustaining functions, and functions can be easy or nearly impossible to monitor with precision. Examples of clinical attributes that the nurse should assess when caring for a patient with a toxin exposure are the following: Resiliency, vulnerability, stability, complexity, resource availability, participation in care and decision-making, and predictability.

EXPERT TIP

If the patient presents as a known substance abuser with the presence of a classic toxidrome, is clinically stable, has normal vital signs, has no significant comorbidities and is able to provide a history, no diagnostic workup may be necessary.

---

3. **Diagnostic studies**
   a. Laboratory studies (as indicated)
     i. Point-of-care blood glucose
       (a) Mandatory on all patients with altered mental status!

KEY CONCEPT

For all suspected drug or toxicant exposures at a level that could cause potential harm, via any route, call Poison Control at 1–800-222–1222. The poison control centers are staffed by toxicologists who will guide your workup and management of the patient.

---

     ii. Complete blood count (CBC)
    iii. Basic metabolic profile (BMP)
    iv. Liver function tests
     v. Blood alcohol level (BAL)
       (a) *Note:* BAL does not necessarily correlate with patient's clinical level of intoxication, especially if they are a chronic abuser.
    vi. Drug levels
       (a) Aspirin and acetaminophen for all suspected overdoses
       (b) Other drug-specific levels depending on suspected substance (lithium, valproic acid, etc.)
   vii. Urine drug screen (UDS)
       (a) *Note:* UDS is notoriously misleading. Substances are often detectable long after the clinical effects have subsided, and many substances are not detected on routine laboratory drug testing.

EXPERT TIP

In many cases of toxicant exposure or overdose, the diagnosis is made based on the history and physical examination. The diagnostics help to assess the severity of illness and guide the subsequent management of the patient.

---

   viii. Prothrombin time (PT)/international normalized ratio (INR), partial thromboplastin time (PTT) for substances with anticoagulant effects

ix. Arterial blood gas (ABG) or venous blood gas to assess acidosis

x. Carboxyhemoglobin levels for possible carbon monoxide exposure

xi. Serum or urine human chorionic gonadotropin to screen for pregnancy

xii. *Note:* Serial laboratory studies may be necessary for abnormal tests. The recommended time interval for repeat tests and length of monitoring is guided by the recommendations of the Poison Control Center.

b. Additional diagnostic studies

   i. Chest x-ray

      (a) Assess pulmonary edema for suspected inhalation injuries

   ii. Electrocardiogram (ECG)

      (a) Many toxicants can cause prolonged QT intervals or arrhythmias

   iii. Head computed tomography (CT) without contrast

      (a) If signs of traumatic injury or if occult trauma may be possible

      (b) For patients with altered mental status that does not improve during the time a toxicant is expected to metabolize

PATIENT CARE

1. **Potential for compromised airway (see Ch. 3, Pulmonary System for airway assessment)**

   a. Description of problem: Unable to protect airway because of decreased loss of consciousness (LOC). Airway edema because of toxic inhalation or ingestion.

   b. Goals of care: Maintain adequate airway and ventilation

   c. Interprofessional collaboration: Nurse, emergency medicine physician, advanced practice provider, respiratory therapist, pharmacist, social worker (as needed), psychiatrist, case manager

   d. Nursing interventions

      i. Determine patency of airway; gag reflex present or absent

      ii. Use caution when intubating a potential overdose patient. Gag reflex may be absent. Aspiration is a risk. Ensure the capability for suctioning is present.

2. **Impaired oxygenation and ventilation (see Ch. 3, Pulmonary System)**

   a. Description of problem: Inadequate breathing related to hypoventilation, bradypnea, or apnea. Inhalation injuries may cause pulmonary edema and impair oxygen exchange in alveoli.

   b. Goals of care: Maintain adequate airway and ventilation

   c. Interprofessional collaboration: Nurse, emergency medicine physician, advanced practice provider, respiratory therapist, pharmacist, social worker (as needed), psychiatrist, case manager

   d. Nursing interventions

KEY CONCEPT

100% oxygen may be considered an antidote for carbon monoxide poisoning while awaiting carboxyhemoglobin results. Do not rely on arterial partial pressure of oxygen (PaO_2) or arterial oxygen saturation (SaO_2) determinations to assess carbon monoxide poisoning.

---

   i. Assess respirations and oxygen saturation.

   ii. Initiate supplemental oxygen to treat hypoxia.

   iii. If respirations are inadequate, open the airway and assist ventilation via bag-valve mask.

> **EXPERT TIP**
>
> In the setting of carbon monoxide toxicity, carbon monoxide binds to hemoglobin, which produces a compound known as carboxyhemoglobin. This decreases the oxygen-carrying capacity of the blood and inhibits the transport, delivery, and utilization of oxygen by the body. The affinity between hemoglobin and carbon monoxide is approximately 230 times stronger than the affinity between hemoglobin and oxygen; therefore hemoglobin binds to carbon monoxide in preference to oxygen. On ABG, PaO_2 will be normal but acidosis may be present. The oxygen saturation is often normal as well.

3. **Cardiac dysrhythmias and hemodynamic compromise (see Ch. 4, Cardiovascular System)**
   a. Description of the problem: The systemic effects of various toxic exposures may predispose the patient to alterations in heart rate, blood pressure, and temperature regulation.
   b. Goals of care: Patient remains hemodynamically stable
   c. Interprofessional collaboration: Nurse, emergency medicine physician, advanced practice provider, respiratory therapist, pharmacist, social worker (as needed), psychiatrist, case manager
   d. Interventions
      i. Monitor cardiac rhythm and obtain 12-lead ECG
      ii. Manage hypotension with fluid resuscitation using intravenous (IV) crystalloids and/or medications per protocol or Poison Control recommendations
4. **Altered state of consciousness (see Ch. 5, Neurologic System)**
   a. Description of the problem: Various toxicants may pass through the blood-brain barrier and have direct effects on neurologic functioning. The clinical effects depend on the mechanism of action of the toxicant. Alterations in LOC may also be a result of metabolic or electrolyte disturbance, or hypoperfusion of the central nervous system.
   b. Goals of care
      i. Patient returns to baseline neurologic status
   c. Interprofessional collaboration: Nurse, emergency medicine physician, advanced practice provider, respiratory therapist, pharmacist, social worker (as needed), psychiatrist, case manager
   d. Additional nursing interventions
      i. Frequent neurologic checks to monitor mental status
      ii. Monitor the airway status and consider intubation for significant alteration in LOC
      iii. Provide for patient safety (e.g., fall precautions, seizure precautions, 1:1 monitoring)
5. **Altered temperature regulation (see Hypothermia)**
   a. Description of problem: The systemic effects of various toxic exposures may predispose the patient to either hypothermia or hyperthermia.
   b. Goals of care: Return of core temperature to within a normal temperature range of 36.1°C to 37.2°C (97°F–99°F).
   c. Interprofessional collaboration: Nursing, physician, intensivist, advanced practice providers, respiratory therapy, case manager
   d. Additional nursing interventions
      i. Monitor core temperature and manage hypothermia and hyperthermia per protocols.

    ii. Institute passive rewarming (relies on endogenous heat generation and ambient temperature to increase the core body temperature slowly at a rate of 0.5°C to 2°C/h [0.9°F–3.6°F] until normothermia is restored).

    iii. Initiate active rewarming for moderate (28°C–32°C) or severe (20°C–28°C) hypothermia (warm IV fluids, warming blanket).

    iv. Patients with hyperthermia may need IV fluid resuscitation and passive or active cooling measures. Body temperatures above 104°F are considered life-threatening.

6. Nausea, vomiting, diarrhea

  a. Description of the problem: Patient may experience uncontrolled vomiting or diarrhea because of toxic exposure. This may cause complications such as aspiration, hypotension, or severe electrolyte disturbance.

  b. Goals of care

    i. Prevention of aspiration

    ii. Decrease incidence of hypovolemia and electrolyte disturbance related to vomiting and diarrhea

  c. Interprofessional collaboration: Nurse, emergency medicine physician, advanced practice provider, respiratory therapist, pharmacist, social worker (as needed), psychiatrist, case manager

  d. Additional nursing interventions

    i. Administer antiemetic medication per protocols.

    ii. Administer crystalloid IV fluids to replace lost volume per protocols.

    iii. Ensure aspiration precautions are followed (e.g., if no head/neck injury patient may need to be placed on their side).

INTERVENTIONS FOR INGESTION OF TOXIC SUBSTANCE (FIG. 14.1)

1. Interventions for the comatose patient

  a. Airway stabilization is top priority (see previous discussion).

  b. In all comatose adult and adolescent patients, anticipate giving the following drugs if necessary:

    i. Naloxone 2 mg IV, intramuscular, intranasal, or endotracheal, to antagonize opioids at the mu receptor.

      (a) Administer routinely to patients with respiratory rates below 12 breaths per minute

      (b) Use smaller doses (0.1 or 0.2 mg) for opioid-dependent patients who are not apneic to avoid withdrawal symptoms

      (c) Half-life is 30 minutes, which is significantly shorter than some formulations of opioids; after this time, symptoms may recur, indicative of the possible need for further dosages or continuous infusion

      (d) If no response, consider other causes of respiratory depression

    ii. Endocrine metabolic agent

      (a) If the blood glucose level can be determined rapidly, administer hypertonic dextrose only to patients with a blood glucose level below 60 mg/dL.

      (b) Administer 50% dextrose in water 100 mL IV (50 g dextrose or D5W) to rule out hypoglycemia as a cause for unresponsiveness (except in patients known to be hyperglycemic).

      (c) If the glucose level cannot be determined rapidly, consider hypertonic dextrose for patients with altered level of consciousness and a nonfocal neurologic examination.

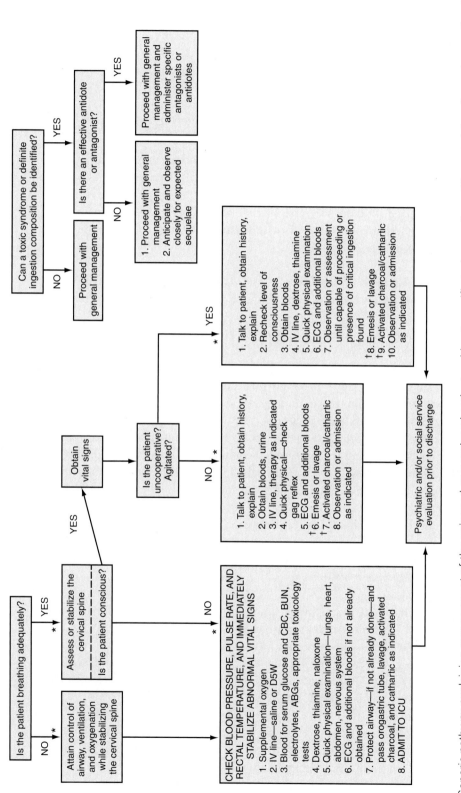

Fig. 14.1 Generic pathway explaining management of the poisoned or overdosed patients without specific toxic symptoms. The *asterisks* refer to the smaller algorithm, which reminds the clinician to consider antidotal intervention when appropriate throughout toxicologic care. †If indicated. *ABG*, Arterial blood gas; *BUN*, blood urea nitrogen; *CBC*, complete blood count; *D5W*, 5% dextrose in water; *ECG*, electrocardiogram; *ICU*, intensive care unit; *IV*, intravenous. (From American College of Surgeons. (2018). *Advanced trauma life support for doctors, student course manual*, 10th ed. Chicago.)

14 Toxin Exposure

(d) Hypoglycemia may result from exposure to insulin, oral hypoglycemic agents, ethanol (alcohol), and salicylates.

> **EXPERT TIP**
>
> The liver is able to carry a stored version of glucose called glycogen, which it can convert into glucose for release into the bloodstream. Ethanol (alcohol) can inhibit this ability of the liver to release glucose when the body needs it, causing hypoglycemia.
>
> Salicylate-induced hypoglycemia is thought to be caused by several mechanisms: Increasing insulin secretion in those with type 2 diabetes, increasing insulin sensitivity, and inhibiting renal excretion.

   iii. Do not administer physostigmine, analeptics (amphetamines, caffeine), or flumazenil routinely until the toxicant is identified and use of these drugs is warranted.

   iv. Provide an antidote (see Table 14.2): If no antidote is available, maintain vital functions, remove the toxic substance, and limit the absorption of any remaining substance.

GENERAL MANAGEMENT STRATEGIES FOR GASTRIC DECONTAMINATION

1. **Gastric lavage: Rarely indicated and should not be done without consultation with a toxicologist.**
   a. May be beneficial in cases of ingestion of a life-threatening intoxicant within 1 to 2 hours of presentation.
   b. Advance a large (36 Fr–40 Fr) orogastric tube and confirm placement by chest x-ray.
   c. Place patient in left lateral position with head of bed down 20 degrees.
   d. Instill 250 mL of room temperature fluid and remove by gravity or suction.
   e. Repeat as needed until fluid is clear.
   f. Do not use in cases of ingestion of a caustic agent (chemical injury, including ingestion of acetic acid [permanent wave solution], ammonia [cleaning agents], phosphorus [matches, fireworks], benzalkonium chloride [detergents], oxalic acid [disinfectants, bleach], formaldehyde, iodine [antiseptics], and sulfuric acid [batteries, drain cleaners]).
   g. Examine for splash injuries to skin or eyes
   h. Do not give emetics
2. **Administration of activated charcoal: May be administered alone or after gastric lavage produces a clear effluent.**
   a. Indications
      i. Depends on the route, timing, amount and nature of the toxin.
      ii. Should be administered in consultation with a toxicologist.
      iii. Most beneficial if given within 1 to 2 hours of ingestion.
      iv. Can be given orally only in patients who are awake and alert and have a patent airway. Otherwise, airway should be secured and activated charcoal administered via a gastric tube.
   b. Considerations
      i. The first dose may be given with a cathartic; premixed solutions are available; do not use multiple-dose cathartics.
         (a) Magnesium citrate, magnesium sulfate, sorbitol
         (b) Contraindications to cathartic use: Trivial toxin ingestion in children, ileus, diarrhea, abdominal trauma, intestinal obstruction, renal failure
   c. Dose: 1 g/kg of body weight in children, and 25 to 50 g in adults
   d. Administer orally or via gastric tube

e. May be given in multiple doses every 1 to 4 hours, but do not repeat the cathartic dose; discontinue after the first charcoal stool

f. Adsorption begins 1 minute after administration

g. Effective in overdose of digitalis, phenobarbital, carbamazepine, phenytoin, theophylline, salicylate, propoxyphene, cyclic antidepressants, isoniazid, amphetamines, cocaine, amitriptyline, phenylbutazone

h. Ineffective in overdose of ethanol (alcohol), hydrocarbons, caustic agents, corrosives, iron, or lithium

    i. Side effects: Diarrhea, constipation, vomiting, aspiration, intestinal obstruction, reduction of therapeutic levels of prescribed drugs

3. **Emetics**

a. Indications: Ipecac is no longer used routinely as a poison treatment intervention in the home or emergency department, but use may be considered within 60 minutes of ingestion in an alert patient with a protected airway. The administration of syrup of ipecac should occur only if poison control personnel or an emergency department physician recommends it.

4. **Whole-bowel irrigation: Polyethylene glycol and electrolytes for oral solution**

a. Indications: Ingestion of sustained-release drugs, slowly dissolving agents (iron tablets, paint chips), drugs with high morbidity (lithium, potassium), and vials or drug packets (cocaine, heroin) for smuggling purposes

b. Clears the entire gastrointestinal tract without inducing emesis or causing a fluid and electrolyte disturbance

c. Dose: 1 to 2 L/h orally or by nasogastric tube until rectal effluent is clear

d. Contraindications: Ileus, obstruction, perforation, gastrointestinal bleeding, ingestion of quickly absorbing drugs or liquids, parenterally administered drugs, or caustic agents

5. **Hemodialysis, hemoperfusion, and hemofiltration (see Table 14.1)**

a. Hemodialysis is usually performed for 4 to 6 hours in poisoned patients when indicated

b. Hemodialysis also corrects metabolic acid-base disturbances, hyperkalemia, and fluid overload

c. Hemoperfusion clears the blood of substances that bind to plasma proteins

d. Hemofiltration can remove larger molecules, such as aminoglycoside antibiotics

    i. Can be used after the other two techniques to prevent a rebound of toxin levels

    ii. Administration of diuretics is not indicated and does not enhance clearance of toxins.

TREATMENT FOR BODY STUFFING/BODY PACKING

1. **If the patient becomes symptomatic while in police custody, suspect body stuffing unless proven otherwise.**
2. **Treatment should be guided by the poison control center; some possibilities include metoclopramide, oral activated charcoal, polyethylene glycol and electrolyte solutions, whole bowel irrigation, and surgical intervention.**

ADDITIONAL INTERVENTIONS FOR THE PURPOSEFUL INGESTION

1. **Make appropriate referrals to a social worker or behavioral health specialist**
2. **Monitor the environment for items that could be used for self-inflicted injury**
3. **Implement suicide precautions if appropriate**

Toxin Exposure

14

ENVENOMATION

1. **Spider bites**
   a. Brown recluse (southern United States)
      i. Clinical presentation
         (a) Initial bite is usually painless. Within 24 hours may develop into a papular lesion that may become necrotic over the next 3 to 4 days. May take weeks to heal.
         (b) If the spider was not identified, consider alternate causes of necrotic lesions.
         (c) Approximately 10% of patients may develop systemic symptoms including fever, vomiting, hemolysis, myalgias, and malaise.
      ii. Patient care
         (a) Primarily supportive: Wound care, analgesics
         (b) Tetanus, diphtheria, pertussis (TDAP)
         (c) Antibiotics if infection is suspected
         (d) Hospitalization for patients with systemic symptoms
         (e) Surgery for wounds larger than 2 cm, 2 to 3 weeks after the bite
         (f) No antivenom available in the United States
   b. Black widow (found all over the world, but in the United States, it is mainly in the rural south)
      i. Clinical presentation
         (a) Immediate pinprick sensation that spreads throughout the extremity
         (b) Target-shaped area of erythema develops within 1 hour
         (c) Diffuse muscle spasm—trunk, back, abdomen
         (d) Severe pain that waxes and wanes
         (e) Hypertension, tachycardia, headache, nausea, vomiting, diaphoresis. May progress to respiratory failure, shock, and coma.
         (f) Systemic symptom onset within 12 hours, may last several days
      ii. Patient care
         (a) Wound care
         (b) TDAP
         (c) Antibiotics if infection is suspected
         (d) Supportive care: IV crystalloids, analgesics, antiemetics, benzodiazepines for hypertension and spasms
         (e) Antivenom may alleviate symptoms but has not been proven to improve mortality rates, which are very low.
2. **Snake bites**
   a. Epidemiology
      i. Average of 4735 venomous snake bites occur annually in the United States.
      ii. Most occur in males over the age of 19 years.
      iii. Deaths are rare—approximately five to six deaths per year.
         (a) In general, occurs in children, elderly, or when there is a delay in administration of antivenom
         (b) Deaths are primarily caused by crotalid bites

KEY CONCEPT

Consult poison control for all snake bites except in very mild cases for direction in managing the patient.

b. Crotalids
   i. Examples
      (a) Rattlesnakes (southwestern United States, Florida)
      (b) Cottonmouths (eastern and southern United States)
      (c) Copperheads (eastern and southern United States)
   ii. Clinical presentation
      (a) Tissue toxicity
         (1) Causes local vascular and tissue damage and an inflammatory cascade causing pain, swelling, and erythema
         (2) May be myotoxic, causing rhabdomyolysis
         (3) Local effects occur within 30 to 60 minutes
         (4) Variable severity. Over time the patient may develop ecchymosis, bullae, and tissue necrosis
      (b) Hematologic toxicity
         (1) Coagulopathy may be early or delayed
            a) Elevated PT
            b) Thrombocytopenia
            c) Hypofibrinogenemia
         (2) Hemorrhage is rare but may occur
      (c) Neurotoxicity
         (1) Rare, except in bites from the Mojave rattlesnake
         (2) Prevents release of acetylcholine, producing cranial nerve abnormalities, weakness, or paralysis
      (d) Systemic toxicity
         (1) Nausea, vomiting, diaphoresis, perioral paresthesias are common
         (2) Hypotension, tachycardia, respiratory distress, angioedema, cardiovascular collapse, confusion are rare
c. Elapids
   i. Examples
      (a) Arizona coral snake (Arizona, New Mexico)
      (b) Eastern coral snake (southern United States)
      (c) Texas coral snake (Louisiana, Arkansas, Texas)
   ii. Clinical presentation
      (a) Little or no tissue damage
      (b) Blockade of postsynaptic acetylcholine causing ptosis, cranial nerve palsies, dysarthria, dysphagia
      (c) Severe cases may lead to respiratory paralysis and death
      (d) Symptom onset 6 to 12 hours
d. Patient care
   i. Nursing interventions
      (a) Assess airway, breathing, and circulation. Consider early intubation for bites to the head, neck, or face because of the risk of airway obstruction from swelling
      (b) Provide wound care and elevate the affected extremity
      (c) Monitor the extremity for progressive tissue damage, compartment syndrome and adequate distal tissue perfusion
      (d) IV access
      (e) Cardiac monitoring
   ii. Diagnostics
      (a) CBC, BMP, PT-INR, fibrinogen, creatine kinase

iii. Pharmacologic interventions
  (a) IV crystalloid bolus or infusion for hypotension
  (b) Analgesics
  (c) TDAP
  (d) Prophylactic antibiotics are not indicated
  (e) Blood products are not indicated to treat coagulopathy
  (f) Antivenom
    (1) Indications: Progressive tissue damage, significant hematologic toxicity, systemic or neurotoxic symptoms.
      a) Crotalids: Crotalidae polyvalent immune FAB or crotalidae immune F(ab)$_2$
      b) Initial dose is four to six vials, mixed with saline and infused over 1 hour. Repeat dose until local progression halts, hematologic parameters improve, and neurologic/systemic symptoms improve.
      c) Contraindication: Known allergy
    (2) Elapids
      a) North American Coral Snake Antivenin (NACSA)
      b) One-time dose of three to five vials IV

References and bibliography information are available at http://evolve.elsevier.com/AACN/corecurriculum/.

Bariatric Patients

Angela Benefield, DNP, RN, AGCNS-BC, CCRN-CSC-CMC

CROSSWALK

- **Quality and Safety in Nursing Education (QSEN):** Patient-centered care, Teamwork and collaboration, Evidence-based practice, Quality improvement, Safety, Informatics
- **National Patient Safety Goals:** Improve staff communication, Use medicines safely, Prevent infection, Identify patient safety risks, Prevent mistakes in surgery
- **American Nurses Association (ANA) standards for Professional Nursing Practice:** Standard 1. Assessment, Standard 2. Diagnosis, Standard 3. Outcomes identification, Standard 4. Planning, Standard 5. Implementation, Standard 6. Evaluation, Standard 7. Ethics, Standard 8. Culturally congruent practice, Standard 9. Communication, Standard 10. Collaboration, Standard 12. Education, Standard 13. Evidence-based practice and research, Standard 14. Quality of practice, Standard 15. Professional practice evaluation, Standard 16. Resource utilization, Standard 17. Environmental health
- **AACN Scope and Standards for Progressive and Critical Care Nursing Practice:** Standard 1. Quality of practice, Standard 2. Professional practice evaluation, Standard 3. Education, Standard 4. Communication, Standard 5. Ethics, Standard 6. Collaboration, Standard 7. Evidence-based practice/research/clinical inquiry, Standard 8. Resource utilization, Standard 9. Leadership, Standard 10. Environmental health
- **AACN Scope and Standards for Progressive and Critical Care Nursing Practice (HWE):** Skilled communication, True collaboration, Effective decision-making, Appropriate staffing, Authentic leadership
- **PCCN content:** None
- **CCRN content:** Multisystem—Bariatric conditions

SYSTEMWIDE ELEMENTS

ANATOMY AND PHYSIOLOGY REVIEW

1. **Definitions**
   a. Obesity, also known as *adiposity*, is defined as a chronic, progressive, and multifactorial, disease characterized by an increase in body fat. The dysfunction in adipose and abnormal fat tissues results in many metabolic, biomechanical, and psychosocial health disturbances (Obesity medical Association, 2020).
   b. Overweight: Excess body weight compared with established standards. The World Health Organization classifies overweight as a body mass index (BMI) of $25 \, kg/m^2$ or higher and obesity as BMI of $30 \, kg/m^2$ or higher. Excess weight may come from muscle, bone, fat, and/or water.
   c. Obesity refers to an abnormal proportion of body fat.
   d. Individual may be overweight without being obese (e.g., body builder); however, many people are both.
   e. Lifelong, progressive, life-threatening, genetics-related, multifactorial disease. Excess fat storage with multiple comorbidities.

f. Obesity may lead to adipocyte and/or adipose tissue endocrine and immune dysfunctions, which contributes to metabolic disease known currently as adiposopathy or "sick fat" disease.

g. Bariatrics (from the Greek *baros* for "weight"): Healthcare related to the treatment of obesity and associated conditions.

2. **Etiology: Complex and multifaceted**
   a. Causes may include social, neurobehavioral behavioral, genetic, metabolic, biochemical, cultural, psychosocial, and iatrogenic factors, such as concomitant prescribed medications (e.g., hormonal therapy and glucocorticoids), and hypothalamic surgery
   b. Diet, appetite control, ethnicity, and sedentary lifestyle are contributing factors

3. **Prevalence**
   a. More than one-third of U.S. adults (39.8%) and 18.5% of youth are obese. Approximately 93.3 million are affected. The prevalence of obesity is higher among middle-aged adults (42.8%) than among younger adults (35.7%) (Centers for Disease and Control Prevention [CDC], 2017).
   b. According to World Health Organization (WHO, 2020), 2016 data show more than 1.9 billion adults, 18 years and older, were overweight. Of these over 650 million were obese. Worldwide epidemic in both developed and developing countries.

4. **Pathophysiology of obesity: Physiologic sequelae of excess body fat adversely affect most body systems (Table 15.1)**
   a. The adipocyte is increasingly found to be a complex and metabolically active cell. Recent literature views the adipocyte as an active endocrine gland producing several peptides and metabolites that may be relevant to the control of body weight; several neurologic and gut hormones are currently being studied.
   b. Many of the adipocytokines and peptides released by adipocytes are proinflammatory and play a role in blood coagulation. Others are involved in insulin sensitivity and appetite regulation (e.g., Leptin, which signals satiety to the hypothalamus). However, the function of many cytokines remains unknown or unclear.
   c. The stomach mucosa in individuals with adiposity secretes higher levels of the hormone Ghrelin, which increases appetite.
   d. A current area of active research focuses on the cues for the differentiation of preadipocytes to adipocytes. The recognition that this process occurs in white and brown adipose tissue, even in adults, has increased its potential importance in the development of obesity and the relapse to obesity after weight loss.

ASSESSMENT

1. **History: Clinical significance to acute and critical care nursing**
   a. Obesity is directly and indirectly associated with a wide spectrum of serious health disorders that may accompany, underlie, and complicate the reason for admission (see Table 15.1).

EXPERT TIP

Patients with obesity experience a vast host of emotional and psychologic burden because of societal prejudice, stigma, and biases. Words, such as *fat* and *morbid obesity* are perceived by patients with obesity as more undesirable and stigmatizing than terms such as *BMI and weight*. Adopting "People First" language when discussing obesity (e.g., *Patient with obesity* rather than *obese or morbidly obese patient*) and providing weight sensitivity training and are essential to minimize stigmatization and to provide ethical, and culturally competent patient-centered care.

TABLE 15.1	**Pathophysiology and Potential Health Problems Associated With Obesity**	
System	**Major Pathophysiologic Sequelae**	**Potential Health Problems**
Pulmonary	Limited diaphragmatic excursion leads to ↓ vital capacity, functional residual capacity, total lung capacity	↑ Respiratory rate, shallow breaths; ↑ Risk of atelectasis
	↓ Alveolar ventilation, shunting	Ventilation/perfusion mismatching
	↓ Expiratory reserve volume	Hypoxemia, respiratory acidosis
	↓ Thoracic and pulmonary compliance	Difficulty weaning from ventilator
	↑ Work of breathing	Obstructive sleep apnea
	Alveolar collapse	Obesity hypoventilation syndrome
	Small airway closure, asthma	↑ Risk of pneumonia, aspiration
	↑ Respiratory drive, chronic CO_2 retention	↑ Risk of airway compromise
	Risk for central or obstructive sleep apnea	
	Risk for difficult intubation	
Cardiovascular	Possible chronic hypoxemia, polycythemia, and pulmonary hypertension because of sleep apnea	↑ Risk of right and left heart failure for BMI >30 kg/m²
		Systemic arterial hypertension
		Myocardial infarct, stroke
	↑ Left ventricular mass, hypertrophy dilatation	Chronic venous insufficiency, deep vein thrombosis, pulmonary embolism
	↑ Total blood volume because of accumulated adipose tissue, which increases stroke volume and cardiac output	↑ Risk of dysrhythmia (atrial fibrillation); ↑ afterload
		ECG morphology changes
	↑ Cardiac deconditioning	Over- or underestimation of BP measurement because of inappropriate BP cuff size
Endocrine	↑ Metabolic requirements of excess adipose tissue	Type 2 diabetes mellitus; need for monitoring and managing serum glucose levels
	↑ Insulin resistance	Hyperlipidemia
	Stress of critical illness may deplete protein rather than glucose stores	Gallbladder disease, gallstones
Gastrointestinal	↑ Intraabdominal pressure	↑ Gastroesophageal reflux
	↑ Gastric volumes	↑ Risk of aspiration pneumonia (enteral feeding route preferred)
	↑ Nutritional requirements affected by mobilization of protein rather than lipid stores for ↑ energy needs	↑ Constipation
		↑ Pancreatitis
	Hypermetabolism associated with critical illness may lead to malnutrition and depleted protein reserves	↑ Risk for fatty liver disease
Immune	Protein-energy malnutrition that may coexist with obesity can impair cell-mediated immunity, phagocyte function, complement system, and antibody concentrations	↑ Impaired healing, wound infection
		↑ Skin breakdown, pressure and deep tissue injury
		↑ Risk for some types of cancers
	Obesity is associated with an impaired immune response	↓ Resistance
		↓ Phagocytosis
Musculoskeletal	↑ Joint trauma because of weight bearing	Osteoarthritis of hips, hands, back, knees
	Impaired, low, or no mobility	Rheumatoid arthritis
	↑ Pain with movement	Decreased functional status because of cardiopulmonary impairment
	↑ Disuse atrophy of musculature	

Continued

TABLE 15.1	Pathophysiology and Potential Health Problems Associated With Obesity—cont'd	
System	**Major Pathophysiologic Sequelae**	**Potential Health Problems**
Genitourinary	↑ Intraabdominal pressure ↑ Estrogen levels	↑ Risk of abdominal compartment syndrome ↑ Stress incontinence ↑ Menstrual disturbance, ↓ Fertility
Psychosocial	Possible low self-esteem, negative body image because of social stigma of obesity ↑ Perceived or actual social rejection or lack of compassionate care from healthcare providers ↑ Anxiety, self-induced social isolation	Depression Social isolation because of stigma Lack of cooperation with or participation in care Possible limited support system Delays in seeking treatment due to perception of provider bias

BP, Blood pressure; *BMI*, body mass index; *ECG*, electrocardiogram.

From the Obesity Medicine Association, 2020; Hamdy, O., Uwaifo, G. (2020). Obesity practice essential. *Medscape.*

   b. When obese patients are hospitalized, they pose several additional challenges to healthcare facilities and staff
      i. Increased risk for all complications related to immobility (e.g., skin breakdown, cardiac deconditioning, atelectasis, deep venous thrombosis, muscle atrophy, urinary stasis, constipation, bone demineralization)
     ii. Likelihood of longer length of stay than nonobese
    iii. Vulnerability to care issues is unique to this population
      (a) Technical difficulties with common procedures, such as endotracheal intubation, weaning from mechanical ventilation, accurate blood pressure measurement because of improper cuff size, positioning, weighing, and ambulation
      (b) Challenges in establishing vascular access, managing fluid balance, and determining nutritional requirements
      (c) Altered pharmacokinetics and medication dosing is challenging in patients with obesity because of a large volume of distribution for lipophilic medications, increased clearance of hydrophilic medications, and a decrease in lean body mass and tissue water, which leads to possible underdosing or overdosing

> **EXPERT TIP**
> Interprofessional collaboration/consultation with pharmacist is essential to ensure appropriate dosing of medication in the bariatric population.

      (d) Inability to perform some diagnostic tests because of size or weight
      (e) Lack of availability of equipment, supplies, or additional staff that optimal care might suggest
      (f) Opioid analgesics and sedatives management may present respiratory challenge in patients with obesity because of obstructive sleep apnea (OSA) and hypoventilation
      (g) Care provider bias and inadequate communication skills may influence care delivered and patient's participation in care delivery

2. **Physical examination: Screening measures**
   a. BMI: Ratio of weight (in kilograms) to the square of height (in meters)

> **KEY CONCEPT**
> BMI alone does not reflect excess adiposity. Waist circumference provides additional risk information not accounted for by BMI.

   i. Most common and widely accepted means of gauging and expressing the degree of excess weight
   ii. Caution needed when interpreting BMI in children and in adults with edema, ascites, pregnancy, or highly developed muscles because elevated BMI does not accurately reflect excess adiposity in such cases
   iii. BMI classifications are based on risk of cardiovascular disease. The recommended classifications for BMI adopted by the National Institutes of Health (NIH) and WHO 2019 for Caucasian, Hispanic, and African American individuals are:
       (a) Normal weight BMI $\geq$18.5 to 24.9 kg/m^2
       (b) Preobesity BMI $\geq$25.0 to 29.9 kg/m^2
       (c) Obesity class I BMI $\geq$30.0 to 34.9 kg/m^2
       (d) Obesity class II BMI 35 to 39.9 kg/m^2
       (e) Obesity class III BMI$\geq$40 kg/m^2
   iv. The current BMI cutoffs underestimate risk in the Asian and South Asian population. Thus, guidelines for Asians: Overweight is a BMI between 22 kg/m^2 to 25 kg/m^2 in different Asian populations and, for high risk, it varies from 26 kg/m^2 to 31 kg/m^2.
   b. Waist circumference
   i. Waist circumference is a measurement of abdominal obesity. It also provides cardiometabolic risk information that is not accounted for by BMI alone.
   ii. Patients with abdominal obesity (also called *central adiposity, visceral, android, or male-type obesity*) are at increased risk for heart disease, stroke, diabetes, hypertension, dyslipidemia (also known as *metabolic syndrome*), and nonalcoholic fatty liver disease.
   iii. Waist circumference is used with BMI for identifying adults at increased risk for morbidity and mortality, particularly in the BMI range 25 kg/m^2 to 35 kg/m^2. A waist circumference of 40 inches or more (102 cm) for men and 35 inches or more (88 cm) for women is considered elevated and indicative of increased cardiometabolic risk, morbidity, and mortality.
   iv. There is ethnic variability in values that predict increased risk. In Asian females, a waist circumference greater than 80 cm and in Asian males a value over 90 cm is considered abnormal.
   c. Appraisal of patient characteristics: Bariatric patients enter critical care units with a wide range of clinical characteristics. During their stay, their clinical status may slowly or abruptly improve or deteriorate. Changes in the patient's condition may involve one or all life-sustaining functions, and functions can be easy or nearly impossible to monitor with precision. Examples of clinical attributes that the nurse should assess when caring for bariatric patients include the following: Resiliency, vulnerability, stability, complexity, resource availability, participation in care and decision-making, and predictability.

PATIENT CARE

1. Pulmonary complications

EXPERT TIP

Patients with adiposity are at higher risk for pulmonary complications. Patient positioning in reverse Trendelenburg's position improves respiratory mechanics.

---

  a. Obesity hypoventilation syndrome (OHS); also known as Pickwickian syndrome

     i. Definition: Oxygenation decreases as BMI increases, likely because of elevated intraabdominal and chest wall pressures in which mass and weight compress the thoracic cavity and limit diaphragmatic excursion. Chronic CO_2 retention leads to hypercapnia, respiratory acidosis, and dependence on hypoxia for ventilatory drive.

     ii. Related to OSA, characterized by drowsiness, narcosis, daytime napping, difficulty sleeping at night, fatigue, hypersomnolence, depression, right heart failure, and further weight gain

     iii. Incidence of respiratory complications has a direct relationship to BMI, especially among those over 350 lb.

     iv. Risk factors include male gender, middle age, mild sedation, and a BMI over $30 \, kg/m^2$; 90% of OSA patients develop OHS.

     v. Intervention: Screen and assess for OSA using a validated method; use noninvasive positive-pressure ventilation in patients with OSA; mechanical ventilation and difficult airway cart must be readily available.

EXPERT TIP

Some bariatric patients are at high risk for difficult airway management and intubation. Use of noninvasive ventilation and presence of difficult airway cart must be readily available.

---

  b. Respiratory failure

     i. Obese patients are at risk for respiratory failure because of their high oxygen consumption and dysfunctions in pulmonary mechanics (see Table 15.1) for common health problems

     ii. Interventions

EXPERT TIP

In mechanically ventilated patients with obesity, the use of tidal volume (V_T) based on ideal body weight, low V_T, moderate to high positive end-expiratory pressure, and noninvasive ventilation in preoxygenation before intubation and after extubation improves oxygenation and reduces atelectasis.

     (a) Mechanical ventilation initiated with a V_T of 6 to 8 mL/kg in patients with respiratory failure, based on ideal (not actual) body weight, then titrated to the patient's ventilator mechanics; use of moderate-higher positive end-expiratory pressure levels improves oxygenation and decreases atelectasis

     (b) Placement in reverse Trendelenburg's position at 45 degrees and ramp positioning during anesthesia are recommended to improve respiratory mechanics, maximize lung function, and increase successful ventilation or weaning. Supine position leads to decreased compliance and increased airway resistance.

    iii. Evidence suggests obese patients may be at risk for difficult intubation, compromised airway, and severe life-threatening complications related to intubation, which may occur 20-fold more often in the intensive care unit (ICU). The use of fiberoptic scope may be necessary if provider cannot visualize the larynx and airway landmarks to insert the endotracheal tube.

        (a) Assess risk factors for difficult airway placement (e.g., obesity, short or thick neck, facial edema, swollen tongue, protruding maxillary incisors, restricted jaw or neck movement, and receding mandible)

        (b) Pulmonary embolism (PE; see Ch. 3, Pulmonary System)

           (1) Risk factors in obesity include prolonged immobility, venous stasis, polycythemia, increased intraabdominal pressure (can increase pressure on deep veins), and venous thrombosis (incidence is twice as high in obesity)

           (2) Bariatric surgery is associated with increased incidence of PE

           (3) Interventions (see Ch. 3, Pulmonary System)

2. Cardiovascular disease

    a. Obesity risk factors include hypertension, insulin resistance and diabetes mellitus, dyslipidemia prothrombotic factors, and central obesity (see Table 15.1) for cardiovascular consequences of obesity

    b. Interprofessional collaboration between patient, nurse, physician, surgeon, advanced practice provider, respiratory therapy, case manager, pharmacist, dietician, and wound specialist is paramount to achieve optimal outcomes

3. Potential skin integrity complications: Pressure injuries

KEY CONCEPT

Meticulous skin assessment, pressure injury prevention, and wound and ostomy consultation are essential in the bariatric population. Close attention to pressure caused by prolonged positioning, tubes, and devices, and ongoing risk assessment and implantation of skin protection strategies are paramount in preventing skin alteration and pressure injuries.

---

    a. Contributing factors include moisture, dehydration, and malnutrition result from pressure, friction, and/or shear; often related to insufficient frequency of and/or ineffective repositioning of the very obese patient, as well as the presence of multiple overlapping skin folds that can foster the growth of bacteria or yeast

    b. Patients with obesity are at risk for atypical pressure injuries caused by pressure within skin folds related to positioning during surgery, tubes, catheters, devices, or an ill-fitting bed, chair or wheelchair

      i. Pressure within skin folds can be enough to cause skin breakdown; tubes, tracheostomies, and catheters burrow into skin folds and further erode the skin surface

      ii. Pressure from side rails or armrests not designed to accommodate a larger person can cause pressure ulcers on the patient's hips

     iii. Interventions

        (a) Use equipment properly sized for the patient

        (b) Implement measures to reduce pressure and skin breakdown; place and secure tubes and monitor cables so the patient does not rest on them; reposition patient and tubing at least every 2 hours

        (c) Reposition the abdominal panniculus to prevent ulceration beneath it; alert patients can help lift the panniculus; dependent or unconscious patients can be turned onto the side to aid the nurse in lifting it

(d) Assess and manage tracheostomy; use absorbent dressings to soak drainage and protect surrounding skin; tracheostomy ties should be longer and wider to prevent trauma within skin folds

(e) Consult the wound nurse for proper bariatric surfaces; use appropriate lifts to reposition, and use pressure reduction aids to offload vulnerable pressure areas; precautions must be taken to prevent friction and shear by using appropriate bed surface, and meticulous frequent skin integrity monitoring

(f) Assess nutritional and physical activity status. Interdisciplinary collaboration with dietitians, and physical therapy is essential component of care delivery in acute and critical care

4. **Other potential complications related to obesity (see Table 15.1)**

CARE OF THE BARIATRIC SURGERY PATIENT

1. **Pathophysiology**
   a. Surgical procedures result in weight loss by restricting the amount of food the stomach can hold, causing malabsorption of nutrients, or by a combination of both gastric restriction and malabsorption. Bariatric procedures also often cause hormonal changes.
   b. The most common bariatric surgery procedures are gastric bypass, sleeve gastrectomy, adjustable gastric band, and biliopancreatic diversion with duodenal switch

2. **Indications for bariatric surgery**
   a. Class III: BMI $\geq 40\,kg/m^2$, or more than 100 pounds overweight. BMI $\geq 35\,kg/m^2$ and at least two obesity-related comorbidities (e.g., type 2 diabetes, hypertension, OSA and other respiratory disorders, nonalcoholic fatty liver disease, osteoarthritis, or heart disease)
   b. Inability to achieve a healthy weight loss sustained for a time period with prior weight loss efforts

3. **Potential surgical complications**
   a. Restrictive procedure complications may include gastric perforation or tearing, esophagitis, gastritis, peritonitis, band too tight, stricture with gastrointestinal obstructive symptoms (e.g., dysphagia), slippage, partial or complete bowel obstruction, and cardiac dysrhythmia.
   b. Malabsorptive procedure complications can include gastric, duodenal, or distal anastomosis leaks, fistula formation, peritonitis, sepsis, incisional hernia, wound infection, diarrhea, and abdominal cramping.
   c. Diagnostic study findings
      i. Noninvasive study findings
         (a) Laboratory studies: Vitamin and mineral, albumin, decreased transferrin levels
         (b) Chest x-ray can identify dilated esophagus; slippage of band can be identified by drinking a dye and using x-ray to observe it
      ii. Invasive study findings: Endoscopy provides visualization of esophagus and stomach
   d. Mechanism and recognition of complications
      i. Bleeding: Mechanisms include anastomotic ulceration or *Helicobacter pylori* infection

(a) Recognition and management: Coffee ground or bright red emesis or melena. Endoscopic diagnosis and treatment using proton pump inhibitors with/without antibiotics.

ii. Nausea and vomiting

(a) Mechanism: Associated with inappropriate diet and nonadherence with a gastroplasty diet

(b) Recognition and management: History, endoscopic diagnosis. Education and reeducation regarding diet.

iii. Bowel obstruction

(a) Mechanism: In lap band, dislodgement of band restricting flow. In gastric bypass, when the Roux limb passes through the transverse mesocolon or at the mesenteric defect at the jejunojejunostomy results in a mechanical obstruction.

(b) Recognition and management: Cramping, periumbilical pain with or without nausea, and vomiting. Diagnostic radiographic studies may be normal. If symptoms persist or become severe, surgical exploration is indicated to rule out internal hernia.

iv. Dumping syndrome

(a) Mechanism: Vasomotor and gastrointestinal symptoms, which can be attributed to rapid gastric emptying or rapid exposure of the small intestine to nutrients.

(b) Recognition and management: Clinical history and glucose tolerance testing. Managed through dietary measures. Patients are instructed to take smaller, more frequent meals (up to six per day) and to avoid drinking with meals or the first 2 hours postprandially.

RELATED BARIATRIC CARE ISSUES

1. Safe patient-handling issues

> ### KEY CONCEPT
> Appropriate staffing, proper training, and maintaining competencies on use of specialized bariatric equipment and lifts are critical for nurse and patient safety and injury prevention.

  a. Potential for physical injury

    i. Increasing incidence, cost, and number of back injury claims associated with patient care. More than half of strains and sprains are attributed to manual lifting and among the most frequent causes of nursing-related injuries.

    ii. Lack of appropriate equipment and/or inadequate staffing at the facility: Nursing care is often delayed and becomes increasingly more complicated and problematic as the size and weight of the patient population increase.

  b. Attitudes toward patients with adiposity may include and communicate a negative bias

    i. As with other conditions, obesity is best discussed using "people-first" language

2. Bariatric equipment issues

  a. Standard hospital equipment, such as chairs or bed frames, may pose safety risks for bariatric patients and their caregivers. Equipment, such as heavy-duty walkers (for patients weighing 300–1000 lb.) and heavy-duty beds, lifts, wheelchairs, transfer and repositioning aids can make care easier and safer by reducing work-related back injuries among caregivers and lowering the risk of patient injury.

3. **Policy issues**

   a. Policy makers, insurance carriers, healthcare facilities, and clinicians all need to use standardized measurements and definitions when developing policies, procedures, and protocols for critically ill bariatric patients. Documentation of BMI, OSA screening in medical records, and appropriate referrals are essential to improving patient outcomes and preventing adverse events.

References and bibliography information are available at http://evolve.elsevier.com/AACN/ corecurriculum/.

Older Adult Patients

Jenny G. Alderden, PhD, APRN, CCRN, CCNS

AGE-RELATED BIOLOGIC AND BEHAVIORAL DIFFERENCES

1. Biologic and behavioral differences between older and younger adults require modification of nursing care.
2. Age-related changes derive from three sources, according to Sloane's rule of thirds:
   a. One-third are related to disease processes more common in older adults.
   b. One-third are related to disuse and inactivity, which increases with age.
   c. One-third result from the aging process and occur in virtually all people who live long enough. These changes aggravate diseases and the changes associated with disuse.
3. Table 16.1 summarizes normal age-related changes and implications for nursing care.

AGE-RELATED CHANGES IN MEDICATION ACTION AND CLINICAL IMPLICATIONS

1. The prevalence of adverse drug reactions (ADRs) increases with age. Patients aged 65 years and older are twice as likely to be hospitalized for ADR-related problems compared with their younger counterparts.
2. Polypharmacy is the use of multiple medications by a patient. Although polypharmacy most commonly refers to prescribed medications, over-the-counter medications and herbal/supplements necessitate consideration.

TABLE 16.1 **Normal Changes With Aging**

Organ/ Function	Normal Age-Related Changes	Implications for Nursing
NEUROSENSORY		
Vision	Decrease in peripheral vision, color discrimination, pupil size and response time, tear production, lens accommodation Yellowing and opacifying of lens Thinning and yellowing of conjunctiva	• Increase lighting levels • Eliminate glare • Avoid blue-green contrasts in written materials • Increase time to accommodate darkness and close vision • Provide artificial tears as needed • Provide access to reading glasses
Hearing	Ossification of middle ear structures Degeneration of cerumen glands, tympanic membrane, cochlea, otic nerve Loss of speech discrimination, especially sibilant consonants Possible increased confusion because of poor hearing	• Remove accumulated wax intensifying hearing loss • Minimize background noise impairing speech discrimination • Assume position to promote lip reading (face in the light, hands away from the mouth) • Ensure hearing aid is functional and used
Taste and smell	Degeneration of taste buds Increased threshold for taste Smell declines more than any other sense	• Use the patient's preferred seasoning to help increase food intake • Use of cinnamon can increase the sweetness of food making it more desirable
Proprioception, balance, and gait	Slowed kinesthetic reflexes and increased postural sway, which increase fall risk Altered gait patterns Decreased deep tendon reflexes	• Provide handrails and assistive devices • Ensure an uncluttered environment • Provide prosthetics for other senses (hearing and vision) • Recommend balance training
Sleep patterns	Low sleep efficiency (time asleep/time in bed), more awakenings, less stage 4 sleep	• Be aware that daytime sleepiness may increase fall risk • Investigate insomnia for treatable causes
Tactile	Skin changes and nerve loss decrease tactile sensitivity, especially of fingertips, palms, and lower body	• Use caution with heating pads, ice, pressure, and immobility because damage may occur without the awareness of the patient
PSYCHOEMOTIONAL		
Cognition	Decrease in neurons, brain mass, and levels of certain neurotransmitters Slowed central processing, depression, decreased vocabulary, benign forgetfulness (not dementia)	• Present stimuli individually and at a slow pace • Allow time for response • Regularly assess cognition and depression with standardized measurement tools • Provide environmental cues for memory
CARDIORESPIRATORY		
Heart	Increased mass (causes benign fourth heart sound) Decreased coronary blood flow, contractility, cardiac output, stroke volume, cardiac reserve, pulse rate	• Adjust assessment to accommodate altered response patterns: Heart rate slower to accelerate and slower to return to baseline • Pulse is less responsive to fever, blood loss, anxiety

TABLE 16.1 **Normal Changes With Aging** —cont'd

Organ/ Function	Normal Age-Related Changes	Implications for Nursing
Lungs	Weaker chest wall muscles and increased anterior-posterior diameter Decreased chest compliance, chemoreceptor response, expiratory flow, vital capacity, cough response, ventilation at lung bases	• Consider susceptibility to hypoxia and pneumonia in assessments
Vasculature	Decreased baroreflex, elasticity, blood flow Increased circulation time, systolic hypertension, atherosclerosis	• Do not decrease blood pressure rapidly, as this can compromise blood flow to brain and vital organs • Do not draw blood from a sclerosed vein
GENITOURINARY		
Kidneys	Decline in all aspects of renal function; decreased renal reserve Function may decline markedly with stress Because of decreased muscle mass, serum creatinine is poor indicator of renal function	• Use measured or age-adjusted calculated estimate of creatinine clearance to determine renal function • Ensure adequate hydration
Micturition	Prostatic hypertrophy in males Decreased perineal muscle tone and spastic detrusor, which may cause urgency or incontinence in women	• Consider obstruction as a reason for low urine output, especially in males taking anticholinergic medications • Assess for incontinence history and provide pads as needed
GASTROINTESTINAL		
Secretions	Decreased saliva, hydrochloric acid digestive enzymes Impaired vitamin and nutrient absorption	• Elevate head after meals to promote esophageal emptying • Provide frequent, small meals • Provide multivitamin therapy with B vitamins and fat-soluble vitamins (A, D, E, K) • Recognize higher risk for infections
Motility and sphincters	Slowed peristalsis, which increases constipation Decreased tone of internal anal sphincter, which may lead to fecal incontinence	• Provide dietary bulk and fluids to reduce constipation • Respond rapidly to toileting requests
MUSCULOSKELETAL		
Bones	Decrease of 1 to 3 inches from maximum height Bones smaller, more fragile	• Reported height may overestimate actual height, so measure height for body mass index or dosage calculations • Use hip protectors to reduce fracture risk
Muscle and soft tissue	Decreased muscle mass (reduces strength, balance, and glucose tolerance) and subcutaneous fat (impairs temperature control) Crosslinking of cartilage, which increases stiffness	• Implement measures to decrease fall risk • Provide warm environment because of cold sensitivity • Basal temperature is lower, so "normal" temperature may represent fever

Older Adult Patients

16

Continued

TABLE 16.1	**Normal Changes With Aging—cont'd**	
Organ/ Function	**Normal Age-Related Changes**	**Implications for Nursing**
OTHER		
Endocrine	Increased insulin concentration; decreased insulin receptor sensitivity	• Assess for evidence of decreased glucose tolerance
Integumentary	Slow cell replacement, loss of elasticity, dryness, thinning of skin Decreased subcutaneous fat and nerve density	• Avoid bathing with drying soaps • Handle extremities with palms (not fingertips) because tissue is friable
Immunologic	Decreased T-cell function and cell-mediated immunity Decreased antibody response to foreign antigens, but increased autoimmune response	• Ensure vaccinations are current
Hematologic	Slight decrease in hemoglobin level, iron level, hematocrit, T-cell count, white cell count Slight increase in erythrocyte sedimentation rate	• If changes are more than slight, evaluate for treatable conditions
Blood chemistry	Slight decreases in levels of albumin, B_{12}, thyroid hormones Slight increase in creatinine, potassium, cholesterol levels	• If changes are more than slight, evaluate for treatable conditions

From Kaeberlein, M.R., Martin, G.M. (2016). *Handbook of the biology of aging*, 8th ed. London, Academic Press; Kane, J., Ouslander, J. (2013). *Essentials of clinical geriatrics*, 7th ed. New York, McGraw Hill; Reuben, D.B., Herr, K.A., Pacala, J.T., et al. (2015). *Geriatrics at your fingertips*, 17th ed. New York, American Geriatrics Society.

KEY CONCEPT
Polypharmacy increases the risk of drug interactions and adverse medication events.

---

3. **The primary reason older people have more adverse medication events is caused by higher occurrence of diseases and therefore increased medications, but age-related changes in medication pharmacokinetics also contribute.**
   a. Age-related changes in medication pharmacokinetics:
      i. Medication absorption shows few age-related changes, although decreased gastric acid alters the dissolution of some medications (e.g., enteric-coated tablets dissolve faster and may cause irritation).
      ii. Body composition alters the distribution of medications:
         (a) Greater fat mass increases the storage and half-life of lipid-soluble medication (e.g., benzodiazepines).
         (b) Decreases in total body water lead to higher concentrations of hydrophilic medications (e.g., digoxin, aminoglycosides, such as gentamicin, theophylline).
         (c) Decreased serum albumin increases unbound (active) medication concentration in protein-bound medications like warfarin, nonsteroidal antiinflammatory drugs ([NSAIDs]; naproxen, ibuprofen), furosemide, phenytoin, amiodarone, and midazolam.
      iii. Metabolism of high-clearance medications (avidly metabolized and undergo first-pass metabolism), such as morphine and metoprolol, decreases because of decreased liver blood flow.

(a) If a medication reference indicates that the medication undergoes first-pass metabolism, the amount of an oral dose reaching the systemic circulation is increased.

(b) Reduced hepatic blood flow leads to high serum concentrations of high clearance medications regardless of route of administration.

iv. Excretion of medications eliminated unchanged (heparin, gentamicin) or as active metabolites (morphine and meperidine) by the kidneys is impaired with aging.

(a) Adjust according to the dosage in the package insert or medication reference for the estimated creatinine clearance or glomerular filtration rate: http://www.merckmanuals.com/professional/geriatrics/drug-therapy-in-the-elderly/pharmacokinetics-in-the-elderly

v. Polypharmacy is the concurrent use of multiple medications and increases the risk of medication interactions and adverse medication reactions. The most significant medication interactions include the following:

(a) Medications decreasing gastric acid production (e.g., H2-blockers, proton pump inhibitors, antacids) may alter the absorption of oral medication.

(b) Concurrent use of two medications highly bound ($\geq$90%) to plasma albumin, such as warfarin, NSAIDs, furosemide, phenytoin, amiodarone, and midazolam, may increase the effect of both medications, especially if age or disease impairs medication elimination.

(c) Concomitant use of medications inducing or inhibiting cytochrome P450 superfamily of mixed-function oxidases (CYP) and other enzyme systems can influence each medication's metabolism. Examples include theophylline, warfarin, midazolam, and simvastatin. An overall decrease in CYP activity occurs with aging.

(d) Medications whose output is affected by urine pH (e.g., quinidine, amphetamines, ephedrine, phenobarbital) or that undergo tubular secretion (e.g., probenecid, cimetidine, omeprazole) can interact with and contribute to the toxicity of medications like methotrexate, procainamide, acyclovir, nitrofurantoin, and cisplatin.

vi. Assess for medication interactions with a frequently updated reference source, such as http://www.drugs.com/drug_interactions.php.

4. **Nonadherence to the medication regimen and prescribing error, in addition to physiologic and pharmacologic factors, also contributes to adverse medication reactions.**

a. Drug regime complexity is associated with nonadherence among older people.

b. Recommendations to reduce errors in medication adherence include assisting the patient in maintaining accurate medication lists, informing patients of the generic and brand names of medications, and using medication administration times as opportunities for teaching.

5. **Potentially inappropriate medications are medications associated with harm among older people.**

> **EXPERT TIP**
> Medication lists should be reviewed at every care transition, including admission, discharge, or transfer to identify any medication changes, duplicates, or omissions.

a. The Beers Criteria identifies potentially inappropriate medications, including over-the-counter medications, and may be accessed online at the American Geriatrics

Society website: http://geriatricscareonline.org/ProductAbstract/american-geriatrics-society-updated-beers-criteria-for-potentiallyinappropriate-medication-use-in-older-adults/CL001.

   b. Medications with anticholinergic activity are associated with adverse events among older people, including falls, constipation, urine retention, cognitive changes, tachycardia, pneumonia, and blurred vision. Anticholinergic medications are common in the following medication classes: Antiemetic, antihistamine, tricyclic antidepressant, antiarrhythmic, urinary antispasmodic, and antiparkinsonian agents.

      i. Despite these risks, nearly half (48%) of older people in nursing homes are prescribed one or more medications with anticholinergic effects.

      ii. Validated tools are available to assess for medications with anticholinergic activity. Specific medication examples include digoxin, diphenhydramine, and amitriptyline.

6. **Supplements and herbal medications may interact with prescribed or over-the-counter medications. https://www.webmd.com/interaction-checker/default.htm**

   a. Examples of supplement-medication interactions include risk for bleeding because of ginkgo biloba extract taken with warfarin and risk of serotonin syndrome in older adults taking St. John's wort with serotonin-reuptake inhibitors.

7. **Underutilization of appropriate medication is also a concern among older people.**

   a. START (Screening Tool to Alert doctors to the Right Treatment) is a set of 34 validated criteria developed by a consensus process involving experts in geriatric pharmacotherapy, aiming to identify potential prescribing omissions in older hospitalized patients.

   b. Utilizing strategies only seeking to limit the overall number of drugs prescribed to older adults may cause harm.

THE FOUR MS OF AGE-FRIENDLY HEALTH CARE

1. **Age-Friendly Health Systems are health systems constructed to provide high-quality care to older adults by reliably aligning with the "four Ms": What Matters, Medication, Mentation, and Mobility. Table 16.2 identifies key actions required for delivering Age-Friendly care.**

> **KEY CONCEPT**
> The 4 Ms of Age-Friendly Health Care, What **M**atters, **M**edication, **M**entation, and **M**obility, provide a framework for delivering consistently high-quality care to hospitalized older adults

   a. What **M**atters refers to the clinician's responsibility to know and align care with the older person's specific preferences and goals.

      i. Care preferences and goals will be different for individual patients and may change over time.

      ii. Assessing What Matters and aligning care is an ongoing process.

      iii. If appropriate, include the patient's family or other people important to the patient in discussions about What Matters.

   b. **M**edication emphasizes avoiding harm associated with medication use.

      i. As described earlier, issues of concern include consistent review for high-risk medication use, addressing drug-drug interactions (including over-the-counter and herbal medicines), and potential for underprescribing.

      ii. Review and reconcile medications at admission, discharge, and with every transition in care (including transitions between units within the same hospital).

TABLE 16.2 The Four Ms of Age-Friendly Health Care

Goals of Care	Assessment	Intervention
WHAT <u>M</u>ATTERS: KNOW AND ALIGN CARE WITH THE OLDER PERSON'S PREFERENCES AND GOALS		
Know what matters to each patient	Ask the older adult what matters: "What matters to you?"	• Document what matters in the electronic health record
Align the care plan with what matters	Ensure the plan of care reflects what matters to the patient. If medical care is inconsistent with the patient's stated wishes, work with the patient and family to promote consistency between the medical plan of care and what matters to the patient	• Ensure the entire interdisciplinary care team is aware of what matters • Communicate by discussing the patient's priorities (not just disease processes) in medical decision-making • Whiteboards may be converted to "what matters" boards including information about what matters to the person (goals, food preferences, leisure activities, what soothes them, etc.) • The palliative care team can clarify goals of care and share decision making to ensure medical care aligns with what matters to the patient
Ensure advance directives are in place, as applicable, aligning with what matters	Ask the patient if he or she has an advance directive and, if the patient has one, ensure it is on file	• If appropriate, assist the patient in obtaining an advance directive. A referral to social work or another discipline may be needed.
Promote comfort	Ask the older person what would make him or her more comfortable	• Ensure older people have their adaptive equipment (glasses, hearing aids) • Ensure sufficient oral hydration, and provide preferred foods if possible • If a patient on a specialty diet (e.g., cardiac diet) and dislikes the food or undereats, it may be necessary to liberalize the patient's diet to promote adequate intake and comfort
<u>M</u>EDICATION: AVOID HARM ASSOCIATED WITH MEDICATION USE		
Minimize high-risk medication use	Evaluate the use of high-risk medications using the BEERS criteria (described earlier), or another validated tool	• Determine whether high-risk medications are needed on a case-by-case basis • If possible, replace high-risk medications with nonpharmacologic interventions (preferred for medications used to treat behavioral symptoms) or less risky medications
Conduct discharge medication teaching throughout the hospital stay	Assess patient's understanding of their current outpatient medication regimen	• Use medication administration as teaching time, ensuring patients understand the "why, when, and how much" of their outpatient medications • Ensure patients understand medication side effects, and what to do if a side effect occurs (e.g., "If you are dizzy, call the clinic") • If patients have difficulty taking medications before discharging to home, consider a consultation to evaluate the need for home healthcare services
Conduct medication reconciliation at admission, and at all transfers, including between units within the same hospital, and discharge	Review the medication list to identify any medication changes, duplicates, or omissions	• If any inconsistencies are noted, work with the prescribing providers to rectify the discrepancy. This is particularly critical to cases where multiple providers prescribe. • It may be necessary to evaluate potential drug-drug interactions. Consider a pharmacy consult for patients with multiple prescribed medications, particularly if the medications are prescribed by multiple people.

Older Adult Patients

16

Continued

TABLE 16.2 The Four Ms of Age-Friendly Health Care—cont'd

Goals of Care	Assessment	Intervention
MENTATION: PREVENT, TREAT, AND MANAGE DELIRIUM, DEPRESSION, AND DEMENTIA		
Assess delirium every 12 hours • Delirium is a disturbance in attention and awareness that develops over hours to days and additional disturbance in cognition where the disturbances are not better explained by another condition • Delirium may also include psychomotor changes, such as hypoactivity, hyperactivity, and impaired sleep architecture • Emotional states, including fear, depression, or euphoria, may accompany delirium	The Confusion Assessment Method (CAM)-ICU tool is validated for the identification of delirium in the ICU among older patients. Individuals with depression, dementia, and other psychiatric diagnosis are susceptible to delirium. When in doubt, assume the patient has delirium	• Document delirium status in the electronic health record. Notify the rest of the care team if a patient develops new-onset delirium
If a patient develops delirium, goals of care include: 1. Treat the underlying condition 2. Prevent complications including loss of functional ability (which may be irreversible among older adults), aspiration, or skin breakdown 3. Maintain adequate hydration and nutrition 4. Treat pain and discomfort. Pain can cause or exacerbate delirium. 5. Manage agitation, if present, to maintain safety 6. Support a normal sleep-wake cycle 7. Environmental manipulation to promote cognitive engagement and avoid sensory overstimulation	Targeted testing for potentially reversible causes of delirium—including electrolyte disturbances, medication toxicity or withdrawal, fecal impaction, or infection—may be indicated	• Early and aggressive mobility for prevention of functional decline • A swallow study may be indicated to evaluate the risk of aspiration • Skincare including continence support and frequent redistribution of pressure • Preserve the patient's normal sleep-wake cycle, including appropriate environmental stimulation during the day and protection of sleep at night • Consider the implementation of, at minimum, a 4-hour "no wake zone" at night • Promote cognitive stimulation during the day, such as visits from friends, books on tape, or music. However, avoid sensory overstimulation • Promote orientation to date and time with clocks, windows with outside views, calendars, and verbal cues • The presence of a patient care attendant or family member at the bedside may reassure the individual and will also provide opportunities for cognitive stimulation • Ensure glasses and hearing aids are used during waking hours to avoid sensory disorientation • Avoid the use of restraints because they are associated with prolonged delirium and worse outcomes • Avoid medications implicated in worsening delirium: benzodiazepines, opioids, dihydropyridines, and antihistamines

TABLE 16.2 **The Four Ms of Age-Friendly Health Care—cont'd**

Goals of Care	Assessment	Intervention
Recognize dementia and provide safety and comfort to individuals with dementia	A variety of available validated tools assess for the presence of dementia	• Individuals with dementia experience higher risk for delirium. See delirium in the previous text for interventions to prevent or treat delirium. • Evaluate home safety, including driving safety for patients who still drive • Understand and respond to behaviors: • Problem solve the meaning of the behavior. (Is the person uncomfortable, or do they feel threatened?) • Encourage mobility to promote function and comfort • Help the person engage in pleasurable activities, like listening to preferred music • Distract, reassure, and comfort the person • Do not challenge or confront the person
Screen for, and treat, depression. Specific goals of care include: 1. Ameliorate depressive symptoms 2. Maintain safety	Depression among older people is often poorly recognized and inadequately treated. Depression is not a normal consequence of aging. Untreated depression is linked to poor health outcomes and increased risk for subsequent development of dementia. Assess for depression using a standardized scale	• Assess for and treat sleep alterations • Assess and treat pain • Assess for suicide risk and implement safety measures as indicated • Assess for the use of medications or substances with depressive effects (benzodiazepines, CNS depressants, alcohol) • Recognize social isolation as a risk factor for depression and incorporate resources supporting social connections within care planning and discharge planning
Assess and treat pain (see Ch. 20, Pain)	Conduct frequent pain assessment while the patient is awake. Cognitively impaired older adults can report whether they have pain. For nonverbal individuals, use a validated nonverbal pain assessment scale	• Pain management principles are the same as other age groups • Because of age-related changes in pharmacokinetics, older adults do not tolerate some analgesics • Avoid medications with active metabolites, such as morphine and meperidine. Codeine and tramadol require activation by the liver, which may be impaired by age-related changes. • Nonsteroidal antiinflammatory medications (NSAIDs), such as ibuprofen carry a risk of gastrointestinal adverse effects with prolonged or regular use. Cyclooxygenase-2 inhibitors carry a gastrointestinal and cardiovascular risk. • Regular dosages of acetaminophen are preferred for osteoarthritis, but the total dose should not exceed 4 g/day. Some older adults have experienced hepatic damage at 3 g/day, so the minimum effective daily dose should be used. • Avoid long-acting opioids because of potentially adverse effects • Monitor for constipation, nausea, or dizziness while receiving pain medications

Older Adult Patients

16

Continued

TABLE 16.2   The Four Ms of Age-Friendly Health Care—cont'd

Goals of Care	Assessment	Intervention
Facilitate restorative sleep	Sleep-related problems are common among older adults. It is necessary to distinguish between normal aging-related sleep changes and sleep changes from a disease process. People with dementia or depression exhibit poor quality sleep compared with age-matched controls.	• Evaluate for obstructive sleep apnea, which is more common among older people • Obstructive sleep apnea is associated with cardiac abnormalities and changes in cognition • Preserve the patient's normal sleep-wake cycle. Provide stimulation during the day and a restful atmosphere for sleep at night. • Consider the implementation of, at minimum, a 4-hour "no wake zone" at night • Use caution in administering sleeping medications. Older people have a high risk of adverse effects, including cognitive impairment and balance problems from sleep medication.
MOBILITY: ENSURE OLDER PEOPLE MOVE SAFELY AND MAINTAIN FUNCTIONAL STATUS		
Screen for mobility limitations	Use a validated tool, such as the Timed Up and Go (TUG), if possible. Assess for pain with mobility, impairments in gait, and effects of medications that can impair mobility (e.g., dizziness, orthostatic hypotension). Consider a physical therapy consultation for a mobility assessment	• Screen mobility status upon admission and an ongoing basis, and document the results • Share results of the mobility screening with the interdisciplinary team, particularly physical and occupational therapy • Develop a patient-centered plan of care aiming to promote mobility
Promote safe mobility	Track the amount of time patients spend seated, standing, and walking, observing how often these events occur	• Consider a physical therapy consult to develop a personalized mobility plan • If patients are unable to get out of bed, facilitate in-bed exercises aimed at improving muscle strength • Use safety equipment, such as gait belts or other devices to minimize risk for falls • Minimize the use of "tethers" if possible (tethers include monitor leads, catheters, or other devices impeding mobility) • Encourage patients to set a mobility goal based on what matters to them • Facilitate opportunities for patients to participate in several "mobility events" throughout the day based on their functional status and goals • Include ongoing mobility in discharge planning, and ensure patients have a safe home environment for mobility (e.g., access to needed equipment—such as walkers and grab bars—and the absence of fall risks like loose rugs)

CNS, Central nervous system; *ICU,* intensive care unit.

From Institute for Health Care Improvement (IHI): *Age friendly health systems: Guide to using the 4M's in the care of older adults,* 2019. Available at http://www.ihi.org/Engage/Initiatives/Age-Friendly-Health-Systems/Documents/IHIAgeFriendlyHealthSystems_GuidetoUsing4MsCare.pdf.

   c. **M**entation encompasses preventing, treating, and managing delirium, depression, and dementia.

      i. Screen for depression using a validated tool.

      ii. Depression is treatable and *not* a normal part of aging.

        (a) Screen for delirium using a validated tool, such as the Confusion Assessment Method (CAM)-ICU.

      iii. Individuals with dementia experience higher risk for both depression and delirium.

   d. **M**obility entails ensuring older adults move safely and maintain the functional status necessary to do what **M**atters.

      i. Mobility, a component of overall function, is defined as a person's ability to move or be moved.

      ii. Declines in mobility are common during hospitalization, with a 5% to 10% loss of muscle strength for each week spent in bed.

      iii. Mobility loss is associated with more time on the ventilator, morbidity, mortality, and increased likelihood of discharge to a nursing home.

      iv. Promoting mobility results in a shorter length of stay and quicker recovery after surgery.

      v. Basic mobility is better than nothing: A progressive model starting with exercises in bed resulted in muscle strength gains among older patients.

      vi. In implementing a mobility program, the risk of falling should be balanced against the competing risk of deconditioning and loss of functional status.

2. **Examples of programs consistent with the principles of Age-Friendly Health Systems include the geriatric resource nurse model "Nurses Improving Care for Health System Elders" (NICHE), the "Acute Care for the Elderly" (ACE) interprofessional team model, and the "Hospitalized Elder Life Program" (HELP), a multicomponent program aimed at preventing functional and cognitive decline during hospitalization.**

References and bibliography information are available at http://evolve.elsevier.com/AACN/corecurriculum/.

High-Risk Obstetric Patients

Jennifer T.N. Treacy, MSN, APRN, FNP

CROSSWALK

- **Quality and Safety in Nursing Education (QSEN):** Patient-centered care, Teamwork and collaboration, Evidence-based practice, Quality improvement, Safety
- **National Patient Safety Goals:** Identify patients correctly, Improve staff communication, Use medicines safely, Use alarms safely, Prevent infection, Identify patient safety risks, Prevent mistakes in surgery
- **American Nurses Association (ANA) Standards for Professional Nursing Practice:** Standard 1. Assessment, Standard 2. Diagnosis, Standard 3. Outcomes identification, Standard 4. Planning, Standard 5. Implementation, Standard 6. Evaluation, Standard 9. Communication, Standard 10. Collaboration, Standard 12. Education, Standard 13. Evidence-based practice and research, Standard 14. Quality of practice, Standard 16. Resource utilization, Standard 17. Environmental health
- **AACN Scope and Standards for Progressive and Critical Care Nursing Practice:** Standard 1. Quality of practice, Standard 3. Education, Standard 4. Communication, Standard 6. Collaboration, Standard 7. Evidence-based practice/research/clinical inquiry, Standard 8. Resource utilization, Standard 10. Environmental health
- **AACN Standards for Establishing and Sustaining Healthy Work Environments (HWE):** Skilled communication, True collaboration, Effective decision-making
- **PCCN content:** None
- **CCRN content:** Multisystem—Life-threatening maternal/fetal complications

SYSTEMWIDE ELEMENTS

ANATOMY AND PHYSIOLOGY REVIEW

1. **Physiologic changes in pregnancy**
   a. This group of patients is usually in good health and is made up of younger ages than the typical high-acuity patient. Nursing and medical management can be a challenge because of fetal viability concerns and alterations in maternal physiology and diseases specific to pregnancy.
   b. Box 17.1 defines some common obstetric abbreviations that may be encountered in obstetric patients' charts. Tables 17.1 and 17.2 summarize some of the most significant physiologic changes that nurses and providers need to keep in mind when providing care to these patients in high-acuity settings.

BOX 17.1   Glossary of Obstetric Terms

EDC	estimated date of confinement (same as EDD)
EDD	estimated date of delivery
EFM	external fetal monitoring
EGA	estimated gestational age
FHR	fetal heart rate
G	gravida (number of pregnancies)
+ GFM	gross fetal movement present
IBOW	intact bag of waters
IUP	intrauterine pregnancy
LMP	last menstrual period
P	parity (number of viable gestation births, includes stillbirths)
PIH	pregnancy-induced hypertension (also known as preeclampsia, with or without severe features)
PROM	premature rupture of membranes (before the onset of labor)
PPROM	preterm premature rupture of membranes (before 37 completed weeks of gestation)
ROM	rupture of membranes
US	ultrasonography

This list of common obstetric abbreviations can aid in interpreting the patient's chart and prenatal record.

From Sibai, B.H. (2016). Hypertension. In S.G. Gabbe, J.R. Niebyl, J.L. Simpson, et al, *Obstetrics: normal and problem pregnancies*, 7th ed. Philadelphia, Elsevier.

TABLE 17.1   Physiologic Changes in Pregnancy

System	Changes
Cardiovascular	Between 10th and 12th weeks of pregnancy, blood volume starts to rise, peaking at 40%–50% above baseline at 32nd–34th weeks, then declining slightly by 40th week. Systemic vascular resistance decreases, which causes blood to pool in lower extremities and often results in orthostatic hypotension. These are earliest and most significant changes in maternal physiology.
	Midpregnancy, systolic blood pressure falls 3–5 mm Hg, as diastolic declines 5–10 mm Hg
	During last half of pregnancy, decrease in colloid osmotic pressure shifts fluid into the extravascular space, which causes lower-extremity edema
	Between 14th and 20th weeks, pulse slowly rises 10–15 beats/min to a new rate that persists to term
	Cardiac output increases by 30%–50%
Pulmonary	Diaphragm may rise up to 4 cm, by late pregnancy, because of the enlarging uterus. After 24th week, thoracic breathing replaces abdominal breathing and mild dyspnea is common. Higher estrogen levels cause nasal mucosa to swell, which makes nasal stuffiness and nosebleeds common.
	As oxygen requirements increase, rising estrogen levels relax costal ligaments so the chest can expand. This permits deeper breathing, which allows minute respiratory volume to increase by 26%, while respiratory rate increases only about 2 breaths/min. This hyperventilation decreases alveolar CO_2 concentration and is reflected in arterial blood gas levels as compensated respiratory alkalosis (pH, 7.40–7.45; partial pressure of oxygen [PaO_2], 100–110 mm Hg; arterial partial pressure of carbon dioxide [$PaCO_2$], 25–30 mm Hg; bicarbonate [HCO_3] level, 17–22 mEq/L). The alkalotic state facilitates the diffusion of nutrients to and wastes from the fetus through the placenta.
Renal	The primary change is the dilation and enlargement of the kidneys and urinary system. To compensate for the drop in alveolar CO_2 concentration, the kidneys excrete additional HCO_3. During the second trimester, renal plasma flow and glomerular filtration rate (GFR) increase 35% and 50%, respectively, but both drop late in pregnancy. In response to hormonal changes, an enlarging uterus, and increased blood volume, ureters dilate and elongate, which leads to urinary stasis.

Continued

High-Risk Obstetric Patients

17

TABLE 17.1	Physiologic Changes in Pregnancy—cont'd
System	Changes
	Because of the increased GFR, serum levels of blood urea nitrogen, creatinine, and uric acid are lower, and patients may require higher or more frequent doses of some medications to maintain therapeutic levels.
Gastrointestinal	There is displacement of the stomach and intestines because of the enlarging uterus. Progesterone relaxes smooth muscle, which causes progressive gastric reflux as the uterus enlarges. Intestinal transit time increases, which allows better absorption of nutrients but also causes constipation.
Reproductive	The uterus enlarges to about 20 times its normal size to hold the fetus, placenta, and amniotic fluid. After the 12th week of pregnancy, it grows out of the pelvis and into the abdominal cavity.
	After 16 weeks, the supine position may cause the uterus to compress the vena cava and iliac veins, which decreases blood flow to the uterus and lower extremities; the left lateral position is recommended.
Hematologic	The largest change is a marked increase in plasma volume, red cell volume, and coagulation factors. Hemoglobin level and hematocrit are slightly lower in the second trimester (the "physiologic anemia" of pregnancy) because of a rise in plasma that is disproportionate to that of red blood cells. A hemoglobin level of 10–11 g/dL and a hematocrit of 32%–39% are considered normal during this time.
	Because white blood cell (WBC) levels respond to physiologic stress, WBC counts rise to between 10,000 and 12,000/mm^3 during pregnancy and up to 25,000/mm^3 during labor. Platelet counts stay within the normal range. Platelet counts below 130,000/mm^3 might indicate disseminated intravascular coagulation, and platelet counts below 100,000/mm^3 could signal HELLP syndrome, an extension of pregnancy-induced hypertension characterized by hemolysis, elevated liver enzyme levels, and lowered platelet counts.

HELLP, hemolysis, elevated liver enzymes and *low platelets*. From Brown, H. (2016). *Physiology in pregnancy*. In *Merck Manual*. Retrieved from http://www.merckmanuals.com/professional/gynecology-and-obstetrics/approach-to-the-pregnant-woman-and-prenatal-care/physiology-of-pregnancy.

TABLE 17.2	Comparison of Hemodynamic Profiles in Pregnant and Nonpregnant Women	
Hemodynamic Parameter	Pregnant	Nonpregnant
Cardiac output (L/min)	6.2	4.3
Central venous pressure (mm Hg)	3.7	3.6
Colloid osmotic pressure (mm Hg)	18	20.8
Heart rate (beats/min)	83	71
Left ventricular stroke index (mL/beat)	48	41
Mean arterial pressure (mm Hg)	90	86
Pulmonary capillary wedge pressure (mm Hg)	7.5	6.3
Pulmonary vascular resistance (dyne/s/cm^{-5})	78	119
Systemic vascular resistance (dyne/s/cm^{-5})	1210	1530

From Galan, H., Goetzl, L. (2016). Normal values in pregnancy. In S.G. Gabbe, J.R. Niebyl, J.L. Simpson, et al, *Obstetrics: normal and problem pregnancies*, 7th ed. Philadelphia, Elsevier; Clark, S.L., Cotton, D.B., Lee, W., et al. (1989). Central hemodynamic assessment of normal term pregnancy. *American Journal of Obstetrics and Gynecology*, 161, 1439; Spatling, L., Fallenstein, F., Huch, A., et al. (1992). The variability of cardiopulmonary adaptation to pregnancy at rest and during exercise. *British Journal of Obstetrics and Gynaecology*, 99(8):1.

SPECIFIC PATIENT HEALTH PROBLEMS

POSTPARTUM HEMORRHAGE

1. **Definition**
   a. Subjective assessment of blood loss greater than standard norms, a 10% to 15% decline in hematocrit, and need for blood transfusion. Postpartum hemorrhage (PPH) can also be defined as blood loss of more than 500 mL at vaginal birth and greater than 1000 mL at cesarean birth.
2. **Pathophysiology**
   a. Pregnant patients adapt more effectively to blood loss because of increased red blood cell (RBC) mass, plasma volume, and cardiac output
   b. Early during hemorrhage, the body compensates with a rise in the systemic vascular resistance to maintain blood pressure and perfusion of vital organs. As bleeding continues, vasoconstriction is no longer effective, which results in drops in blood pressure, cardiac output, and end organ perfusion. Table 17.3 classifies the physiologic responses that occur at various stages of PPH.
3. **Etiology and risk factors: PPH is one of the leading causes of maternal morbidity and mortality, contributing to 30% of obstetric deaths. Over half of these occur within 24 hours of birth and may complicate up to 5% of all births. Management requires understanding of normal delivery blood loss, the physiologic response to and common causes of PPH, and appropriate interventions.**
   a. Assess patient risk factors in four categories:
      i. History: Previous PPH, leiomyomata, previous cesarean delivery or uterine procedure
      ii. Fetal: Multifetal gestation, polyhydramnios, large-for-gestational age
      iii. Maternal: Gestational hypertension, anemia, *H*emolysis, *e*levated *l*iver enzymes, and *l*ow *p*latelet count (HELLP) syndrome, vaginal birth after cesarean section, prolonged labor, induction or augmentation, prolonged third stage of labor, episiotomy
      iv. Placental/uterine issues: Abruption or previa, retained placenta, chorioamnionitis, inversion or subinvolution of the uterus, instrumentation during delivery
   b. Distinguished by the timing of the hemorrhage (identifying the source is crucial for effective management)
   c. Early/primary postpartum hemorrhage (within 24 hours of delivery)
      i. Uterine atony

TABLE 17.3 Postpartum Hemorrhage Classification and Physiologic Response

Hemorrhage Class	Acute Blood Loss (mL)	% Lost	Physiologic Response
1	900	15	Asymptomatic
2	1200–1500	20	Tachycardia, tachypnea, narrowed pulse pressure, orthostatic hypotension
3	1800–2100	30–35	Worsening tachycardia, worsening tachypnea, hypotension, cool extremities
4	>2400	40	Shock, oliguria, or anuria

From Francois, K., Foley, M. (2016). Antepartum and postpartum hemorrhage. In S.G. Gabbe, J.R. Niebyl, J.L. Simpson, et al, *Obstetrics: normal and problem pregnancies*, 7th ed. Philadelphia, Elsevier; Modified from Baker, R.J. (1977). Evaluation and management of critically ill patients. *Obstetrics and Gynecology Annual*, 6, 295; Bonnar, J. (2000). Massive obstetric haemorrhage. *Bailliere's Best Practice and Research. Clinical Obstetrics and Gynaecology*, 14, 1.

      ii. Lower genital tract lacerations and episiotomy

     iii. Lower urinary tract lacerations

     iv. Retained placental fragments

      v. Uterine rupture

     vi. Operative delivery

  d. Late/secondary postpartum hemorrhage (24 hours to 6 weeks after delivery)

      i. Infection

     ii. Retained placental fragments

4. **Interprofessional collaboration: Nurse, physician (obstetrician, anesthesiologist), advanced practice provider (including certified nurse midwife), respiratory therapist**

5. **Management of patient care (see Ch. 4, Cardiovascular System for hemorrhagic shock interventions):**

  a. Draw blood for cross-matching and baseline laboratory values: Hemoglobin level, hematocrit, platelet count, fibrinogen level, prothrombin time, partial thromboplastin time

  b. Estimate the volume of blood loss

  c. Identify the cause of the hemorrhage

> **EXPERT TIP**
> Uterus fundus may be firm but lower segment is dilated.

      i. Uterine atony: Boggy, large uterus, clots, bleeding

     ii. Lacerations: Firm uterus, bright-red blood, steady stream of unclotted blood

    iii. Hematoma: Firm uterus, bright-red blood, extreme perineal-pelvic pain, unexplained tachycardia

     iv. Retained placental fragments: Placenta not delivered intact, uterus remains large, absence of pain, bright-red blood

  d. Assess the fundus: Determine the level of firmness and the placement of the fundus

  e. Include estimates of the amount of lochia in intake and output assessments

  f. Administer prescribed uterotonic medications (Table 17.4), which are the basis of medication therapy for postpartum hemorrhage

  g. Obstetric team involvement in appropriate surgical interventions related to PPH management

  h. Care of the mother-infant dyad at appropriate time to promote bonding

HYPERTENSIVE DISORDERS OF PREGNANCY

1. **Definitions**

  a. Classification of hypertensive states in pregnancy

      i. Gestational hypertension

     ii. Preeclampsia-eclampsia

    iii. Chronic hypertension (of any cause that predates pregnancy)

    iv. Chronic hypertension with superimposed preeclampsia (chronic hypertension in association with preeclampsia)

> **EXPERT TIP**
> Increased risk of developing cardiovascular disease and chronic hypertension in the future.

  b. Gestational hypertension: Occurs after 20 weeks' gestation or within the first 24 hours postpartum. Some 50% will go on to develop preeclampsia.

TABLE 17.4	**Medications for Postpartum Hemorrhage-Uterotonic Therapy**				
Medication	**Dose**	**Route**	**Dosing Frequency**	**Side Effects**	**Con-traindications**
Oxytocin (Pitocin)	10–80 units in 1000 mL of crystalloid solution	First line: IV Second line: IM or IU	Continuous	Nausea, emesis, water intoxication	None
Methylergonovine (Methergine)	0.2 mg	First line: IM Second line: IU/PO	Every 2–4 hours	Hypertension, hypotension, nausea, emesis	Hypertension, preeclampsia
Prostaglandin $F_{2\ alpha}$ (Hemabate)	0.25 mg	First line: IM Second line: IU	Every 15–90 minutes, 8 doses maximum	Nausea, emesis, diarrhea, flushing, chills	Active cardiac, pulmonary, renal, or hepatic disease
Prostaglandin E_2 (Dinoprostone)	20 mg	PR	Every 2 hours	Nausea, emesis, diarrhea, flushing, headache	Hypotension
Misoprostol (Cytotec)	200–1000 mcg	First line: PR Second line: PO/SL	Single dose	Nausea, emesis, diarrhea, fever, chills	None

IM, Intramuscular; *IU*, intrauterine; *IV*, intravenous; *PO*, per mouth; *PR*, per rectum; *SL*, sublingual.

From ACOG: Committee opinion. (2017). Emergent therapy for acute-onset, severe hypertension during pregnancy and the postpartum period. *Obstetrics & Gynecology*, 129(4), e90–e95; Brown, C.M., Garovic, V.D. (2014). Drug treatment of hypertension in pregnancy. *Drugs*, 74(3), 283–296; Mustafa, R., et al. (2012). A comprehensive of hypertension in pregnancy. *Journal of Pregnancy*, 2012, Article ID 105918.

    i. Mild: Systolic less than 160 mm Hg or diastolic less than 110 mm Hg, plus proteinuria less than 1+ on dipstick and less than 5 g in 24 hours

    ii. Severe: Systolic more than 160 mm Hg or diastolic more than 110 mm Hg, plus proteinuria of more than 5 g in 24 hours

  c. Preeclampsia (previously called *pregnancy-induced hypertension* [PIH]): Usually occurs after 20 weeks' gestation with or without severe features

    i. Blood pressure of more than 140 mm Hg systolic or more than 90 mm Hg diastolic with proteinuria of 0.3 g protein or higher in a 24-hour urine specimen

    ii. Severe: Hypertension (>160 mm Hg systolic and >110 mm Hg diastolic) on two occasions at least 6 hours apart while on bed rest, worsening proteinuria with other symptoms including headache, visual changes, epigastric or right upper quadrant pain, and shortness of breath. May also include thrombocytopenia, pulmonary edema, and oliguria (<500 mL in 24 hours).

2. **Pathophysiology**

  a. Characterized by vasoconstriction, hemoconcentration, and possible ischemic changes in the placenta, kidney, liver, and brain

  b. Intense vasoconstriction because of dysfunction of the normal interactions of vasodilatory and vasoconstrictive substances

  c. Thrombocytopenia: Platelet count lower than 100,000/mm³

  d. Decreased renal perfusion and reduced glomerular filtration rate

---

BOX 17.2 **Most Common Risk Factors for Preeclampsia**

- Nulliparity or pregnancy of new genetic makeup (same mother, different father)
- Multifetal gestation
- Preeclampsia in a previous pregnancy
- Preexisting medical conditions (e.g., pregestational diabetes, vascular disease, chronic hypertension, or renal disease)
- Maternal age >35 years or older
- Maternal weight <100 lb or obesity before pregnancy
- Black American race
- Family history of pregnancy-induced hypertension
- Antiphospholipid syndrome

From Sibai, B.H. (2016). Preeclampsia and hypertensive disorders. In S.G. Gabbe, J.R. Niebyl, J.L. Simpson, et al, *Obstetrics: normal and problem pregnancies*, 7th ed. Philadelphia, Elsevier.

---

   e. Hepatic system: Mildly elevated liver enzyme levels, subcapsular hematomas, or hepatic rupture
   f. Central nervous system (CNS): Eclamptic convulsions
   g. HELLP syndrome
3. **Intrauterine growth restriction may also be seen. Preeclampsia with severe features is usually an indication for delivery regardless of gestational age or fetal maturity. Careful expectant management may be considered to allow time for delivery of corticosteroids to promote fetal lung maturity.**
4. **Etiologic and risk factors: Hypertensive disorders, the most common medical complications of pregnancy, affect 5% to 10% of pregnancies. About 30% of cases are caused by chronic hypertension, and 70% are caused by gestational hypertension or preeclampsia. Spectrum of the disorder ranges from mildly elevated blood pressure with minimal clinical significance to severe hypertension and multiorgan dysfunction. Specific causes of preeclampsia are unknown (Box 17.2 lists common risk factors).**
5. **Interprofessional collaboration: Nurse, obstetric nurse, physician including maternal fetal medicine (MFM), anesthesiology and neonatology, advanced practice provider**
6. **Management of patient care: Systematic assessments are critical to patient management; frequency is dictated by the patient's condition and response to therapy (Table 17.5)**
   a. History: Medical history, past pregnancies, current pregnancy
   b. Physical examination
      i. Frequent monitoring for signs of cardiac decompensation (see Ch. 4, Cardiovascular System), pulmonary edema (see Ch. 3, Pulmonary System), and renal failure (see Ch. 6, Renal System)
      ii. Hourly monitoring (deep tendon reflexes, clonus, and level of consciousness) for signs of increasing CNS irritability, increasing intracranial pressure, and magnesium sulfate toxicity
      iii. If the patient is antepartum, examination for fetal status and signs of placental abruption or decreased uteroplacental perfusion
         (a) Assess for uterine activity, hypertonicity, hypercontractility
         (b) Assess fetal movements, baseline fetal heart rate, and variability
   c. Psychosocial and family assessment
   d. Laboratory tests

TABLE 17.5 Selected Alphabetical Pharmacotherapy Commonly Used for Preeclampsia (With Severe Features)

Drug	Dose	Indication	Maternal/Fetal Side Effects	Notes
Calcium gluconate	1 g prefilled unit, given slow IV push	Antagonist for magnesium sulfate	Maternal cardiac dysrhythmias if not given slowly	Used for treatment of $MgSO_4$ toxicity
Hydralazine	5–10 mg IV bolus q 20 min to total dose of 30–40 mg	Antihypertensive	Maternal: Rebound hypertension, tachycardia, headache. Fetal: Tachycardia, uteroplacental insufficiency, fetal distress	Primary or secondary medication
Labetalol	Increase dosing: 20, 40, 80 mg every 10–15 minutes to a total dose of 300 mg or infusion 1–2 mg/min	Antihypertensive	Maternal: Contraindicated in first-degree heart block and asthma. Decreases uterine vascular resistance. Fetal: Increased uteroplacental perfusion, Fetal and neonatal bradycardias, hypotension, and hypoglycemia	Secondary
Magnesium sulfate ($MgSO_4$)	Loading dose 4–6 g IV over 15–30 min; maintenance dose 2–3 g/IV infusion	Anticonvulsant	Maternal: CNS depression, flushing, nausea, vomiting, headache, respiratory depression, cardiac arrest	Primary. Requires close monitoring of maternal and fetal vital signs
Nifedipine	10–30 mg PO repeat in 45 minutes if needed	Antihypertensive	Maternal: Rebound hypertension, effects of medication can be exacerbated if given following magnesium sulfate, fetal safety has not been established	Tertiary. Medication may interfere with labor progress
Nitroglycerin	Initial infusion is titrated according to response, begin at 5 mcg/min and increase by doubling dose every 5 minutes	Antihypertensive	Maternal: Hypotension, tachycardia, pallor, nausea and vomiting, sweating, headache	Use with caution. Fetal response dependent on maternal dose

Continued

TABLE 17.5   Selected Alphabetical Pharmacotherapy Commonly Used for Preeclampsia (With Severe Features)—cont'd

Drug	Dose	Indication	Maternal/Fetal Side Effects	Notes
Sodium nitroprusside (in severe hypertensive emergency refractory to other medications)	Individualized dosing: Dosage varies considerably between patients, hence the need for individual titration. In adults not receiving other hypotensive agents, the average dosage of sodium nitroprusside is 3 mcg/kg per minute. The initial dose is normally within the range of 0.5–1.5 mcg/kg per minute, but can then be adjusted in a stepwise fashion, e.g., in increments of 0.5 mcg/kg per minute every 5 minutes, to fall between 0.5–8 mcg/kg per minute. In hypertensive patients receiving concomitant antihypertensive medication, smaller doses might be required	Antihypertensive	Use only in life-threatening emergencies	Use with caution; concern exists related to potential lethal complications from cyanide toxicity in both mother and fetus
Methyldopa	0.5–3 gm PO in 2 divided doses	Antihypertensive	Maternal: Decreased mental alertness, impaired sleep, sense of fatigue and depression, xerostomia	Primary for initial management, considered safe in pregnancy, category B

CNS, Central nervous system; *IV*, intravenous; *PO*, per mouth

From ACOG Practice Bulletin No. 203. (2019). Chronic hypertension in pregnancy. *Obstetrics & Gynecology*, 133(1), e26–e50; Lim, K-H. (2016). Preeclampsia.http://emedicine.medscape.com/article/1476919-overview; Mustafa, R., et al. (2012). A comprehensive of hypertension in pregnancy. *Journal of Pregnancy*, 2012, Article ID 105918.

TABLE 17.6 **Comparison of HELLP Syndrome and Disseminated Intravascular Coagulation**

	HELLP Syndrome	Disseminated Intravascular Coagulation
Signs and symptoms	Nausea with or without vomiting Epigastric pain or pain in right upper abdominal quadrant Hypertension varying from mild to severe Malaise	Obvious signs of bleeding, such as hematuria or hematoma development at venipuncture sites, hemorrhage in the conjunctiva, and petechiae
Laboratory blood values	Increased aminotransferase, bilirubin, hemoglobin levels, and increased hematocrit Decreased platelet count	Elevated levels of fibrin degradation products, prothrombin time, and stimulated partial thromboplastin time
Treatment	Delivery of the fetus if the outcome of the mother or fetus is endangered Platelet administration if the cell count is <20,000/mm³ Monitoring of liver function Observation for organ systems dysfunction	Volume blood and clotting factor replacement Removal of the underlying precipitating factor to reverse the DIC dysfunction

HELLP, Hemolysis, elevated liver enzymes, and low platelet count.

From Sibai, B.H. (2016). Hypertension. In S.G. Gabbe, J.R. Niebyl, J.L. Simpson, et al, *Obstetrics: normal and problem pregnancies*, 7th ed. Philadelphia, Elsevier.

    i. Monitor RBC count, platelet count, hemoglobin level, hematocrit, coagulation profile (for hemolysis); assess for coagulation defects (increased factor VIII activity, platelet aggregation), decreased oxygen-carrying capacity, hemoconcentration, or thrombocytopenia

    ii. Measure serum creatinine, uric acid, blood urea nitrogen (BUN), and alkaline phosphatase levels

    iii. Order liver function tests to check for elevated lactate dehydrogenase, serum glutamic-oxaloacetic transaminase, and serum glutamic-pyruvic transaminase levels

e. Other interventions (Table 17.6)

    i. Only definitive treatment for preeclampsia with severe features is delivery of fetus regardless of gestational age

    ii. Goal is to end the pregnancy with the fewest adverse effects to the mother and fetus

    iii. Additional management decisions may include the use of an arterial and/or pulmonary artery line for patients with severe preeclampsia in the following situations:

        (a) Oliguria unresponsive to fluid challenge

        (b) Pulmonary edema

        (c) Hypertensive crisis refractory to conventional therapy

        (d) Cerebral edema

        (e) Disseminated intravascular coagulation (DIC)

        (f) Multisystem organ failure

iv. Nursing care requires accurate and astute patient assessments, strict regulation of input and output, urinary catheterization with urometer, and comprehensive knowledge of pharmacologic therapies, management regimens, and possible complications

HEMOLYSIS, ELEVATED LIVER ENZYMES, LOW PLATELET COUNT SYNDROME

1. **Definition**
   a. Symptoms of HELLP syndrome (three characteristic abnormalities): Hemolysis, elevated liver enzymes, low platelet count (blood pressure may be normal)

> **EXPERT TIP**
> Diagnosed most often in the third trimester.

2. **Pathophysiology**
   a. Chronic vasoconstriction that occurs in preeclampsia causes fibrin deposits in hepatic sinusoids, which obstruct hepatic blood flow and alter liver function.
   b. Liver swells, stretching Glisson's capsule and producing epigastric and right upper abdominal quadrant pain.
   c. Hemorrhagic periportal necrosis, subcapsular hemorrhages, and spontaneous liver rupture may occur in extreme cases. Serum liver enzyme levels rise, with aspartate aminotransferase values of 60 IU or higher (normal ≥35 IU). Jaundice and acute hepatic failure may occur.
   d. Maternal hypoglycemia is a serious prognostic indicator.
   e. Patients with severe HELLP syndrome (all three abnormalities) are at greater risk for developing DIC than patients with partial HELLP syndrome (one or two clotting abnormalities). Despite treatment, the syndrome can escalate into DIC because the production of many clotting factors is increased in pregnancy (see Table 17.6). With DIC, the clinical picture is hemorrhage and shock (see Ch. 8, Hematologic and Immune Systems).
3. **Etiology and risk factors**
   a. Occurs in 15% to 20% of patients with severe preeclampsia or eclampsia; is also an indication for delivery to avoid jeopardizing the patient's health
4. **Interprofessional collaboration: Nurse, obstetric nurse, physician including MFM, anesthesiology and neonatology, advanced practice provider, respiratory therapist, chaplain**
5. **Management of patient care**
   a. Patients who progress from HELLP to DIC need transfusions of fresh frozen plasma, platelets, cryoprecipitate, and packed RBCs. Hypotension is treated with vasopressors (e.g., dopamine). Until the patient's condition is stabilized, the patient requires close monitoring in the intensive care unit (ICU).
   b. Critical care nurses need to know what the signs and symptoms of worsening condition are and how to handle complications
      i. Focus on maintaining adequate organ perfusion and watch for signs of fluid overload, bleeding, and thrombosis
      ii. Administer volume replacement based on the patient's hemodynamic profile (see Table 17.2)
      iii. Monitor blood pressure every 5 to 15 minutes while titrating vasopressors; keep mean arterial pressure greater than 60 mm Hg

iv. Regularly assess peripheral pulses, perfusion, and heart rate and rhythm; check intravenous (IV) and puncture sites for bleeding

v. Administer supplemental oxygen; assess breath sounds at least every 30 minutes; respiratory difficulty could indicate fluid overload or acute respiratory distress syndrome (ARDS)

vi. Monitor arterial blood gas concentrations and lactate, electrolyte, BUN, and creatinine levels

vii. Watch for signs of acute tubular necrosis (e.g., decreased urinary output, increased BUN and creatinine levels, electrolyte abnormalities, metabolic acidosis)

viii. Check urine output hourly until stable, then check every 2 hours

ix. Assess vaginal discharge, bleeding at incision sites, and level of consciousness hourly while the patient's condition is unstable and every 2 hours once stable

x. Assess bowel sounds every 2 hours and monitor the patient for signs of returning gut motility. Initiate an oral diet as tolerated.

xi. Continue to monitor deep tendon reflexes; watch for clonus and signs of CNS irritability. Seizures can occur up to 48 hours after delivery, so maintain seizure precautions.

AMNIOTIC FLUID EMBOLISM

1. **Definition**
   a. A rare, sudden, and sometimes fatal complication around the time of birth

> **EXPERT TIP**
> May also occur within 30 minutes postpartum.

2. **Pathophysiology**
   a. Amniotic fluid is normally contained within the uterus, sealed off from the maternal circulation by the amniotic sac. An amniotic fluid embolism (AFE) occurs when this barrier is broken and, possibly under a pressure gradient, amniotic fluid enters the maternal venous system via the endocervical veins, placental site (if the placenta is separated), or uterine trauma site. Release of amniotic fluid containing vasoactive substances leads to pulmonary arterial spasm. Pulmonary hypertension, pulmonary capillary injury, hypoxia, hypotension, and cor pulmonale with left ventricular failure may result.

3. **Etiology and risk factors**
   a. Predisposing factors for AFE include placental abruption, uterine overdistension, fetal death, trauma, tumultuous or oxytocin-stimulated labor, multiparity, advanced maternal age, and rupture of membranes, cesarean deliveries, and instrument assisted vaginal deliveries

4. **Interprofessional collaboration: Nurse, physician including obstetrician and anesthesiologist, advanced practice provider, social work, chaplain**

5. **Management of patient care: AFE is clinically a biphasic process with the initial alterations involving central hemodynamics and oxygenation, with a distinct sequence:**
   a. Respiratory: Severe cyanosis, restlessness, dyspnea, tachypnea, pink frothy sputum, and respiratory distress
   b. Cardiovascular: Hypotension, shock, and dysrhythmias, but no chest pain and eventually cardiovascular collapse

    c. Hemorrhage

    d. CNS: Extreme anxiety, apprehension, and convulsions leading to coma

6. **Other interventions**

    a. Once a presumptive diagnosis is made, supportive measures must be initiated

    b. With cardiac arrest, resuscitation follows standard advanced cardiac life support (ACLS) protocols for obstetric patients (https://cpr.heart.org/-/media/cpr-files/cpr-guidelines-files/algorithms/algorithmacls_ca_in_pregnancy_inhospital_200612.pdf?la=en)

    c. AFE should be managed in the ICU. Nurses in high-acuity settings without obstetric expertise may become anxious when caring for pregnant patients; however, the initial priorities of care are the same as for any emergency: Maintenance of the airway, breathing, and circulation. The major difference in obstetric emergencies is the need to care for two patients.

    d. Continuous fetal monitoring for signs of compromise should be performed by an obstetric nurse with expertise in electronic fetal monitoring

    e. To ensure optimal uterine perfusion, the mother's hips should be displaced 30 degrees to the left (which prevents the gravid uterus from compressing the inferior vena cava and decreasing venous return)

    f. Oxygenation

        i. Consider high flow nasal cannula (HFNC) or oxygen 8 to 10 L/min at a concentration of 100%

        ii. If a more aggressive approach is needed, provide endotracheal intubation and mechanical ventilation using a high fraction of inspired oxygen (FIo_2) (>60%) and positive end-expiratory pressure (typically started at 5 cm H_2O with 2- to 3-cm increments) until arterial partial pressure of oxygen (PaO_2) is satisfactory

    g. Goal is to maintain PaO_2 above 60 mm Hg and arterial oxygen saturation at 90% or higher

    h. Circulation

        i. Position flat or in slight Trendelenburg position to improve venous return and CNS perfusion

        ii. Provide fluid therapy, pharmacologic agents, electrocardiographic (ECG) monitoring to detect and treat arrhythmias

        iii. Volume replacement with isotonic crystalloids is first-line therapy for maintaining blood pressure and avoiding overhydration in those predisposed to pulmonary edema

        iv. Maintain systolic blood pressure at 90 mm Hg or higher and acceptable organ perfusion (urinary output ≥25 mL/h)

    i. Fetal considerations: In many instances, AFE does not occur until after delivery. When AFE occurs before or during delivery, the fetus is in grave danger from the outset because of maternal cardiopulmonary crisis. Therefore as soon as the mother's condition is stabilized, delivery of a viable infant should be expedited. If resuscitation of the mother is futile, emergency bedside cesarean delivery may be necessary to save the infant.

ACUTE FATTY LIVER OF PREGNANCY

1. **Pathophysiology**

    a. During pregnancy with acute fatty liver of pregnancy (AFLP), there is a buildup of lipids in the liver, kidneys, and pancreas, as well as the bone marrow and brain. This can lead to excessive fat buildup, particularly in the liver, leading to organ failure. Initial symptoms may include persistent nausea and vomiting. This can lead to malaise, anorexia, abdominal pain, and jaundice. In severe cases, hypertension, proteinuria, and edema may be seen making it difficult to differentiate from preeclampsia.

2. **Etiology**
   a. This is the most common cause of liver failure in pregnancy. It is rare (1 in 10,000 pregnancies), but maternal mortality is high at 18%. It is most often seen in the third trimester and may worsen immediately postpartum.

3. **Risk factors include multiple gestation, preeclampsia, and AFLD with a preceding pregnancy**

4. **Interprofessional collaboration: Nurse, obstetric nurse, physician including obstetrician and anesthesiologist, advanced practice provider, respiratory therapist, social worker, chaplain**

5. **Management of patient care**
   a. Interventions
      i. Control of hypertension
      ii. Monitoring of fluctuating glucose levels
      iii. Management of coagulation abnormalities
   b. Laboratory tests include: Serum aminotransferase, bilirubin, prothrombin, creatinine, and fibrinogen
      i. Management of pulmonary edema or ARDS
      ii. Management of hepatic encephalopathy
      iii. Intubation and antibiotic therapy
      iv. Intensive supportive care and prompt delivery
      v. Infants should be assessed for defects in fatty acid oxidation

SPECIAL CONSIDERATIONS

TRAUMA

1. **Pathophysiology**
   a. Major physiologic changes in pregnancy potentially alter the signs and symptoms of injury, as well as the patterns and severity of injury

> **KEY CONCEPT**
> When caring for the pregnant trauma patient, maternal resuscitation is the first priority.

   b. Blunt force trauma may cause placental abruption (separation of the placenta from the uterine wall) or uterine rupture with risks of fetal injury and death. The most common mechanisms of injury are motor vehicle crashes, assaults, and falls.
   c. In early pregnancy, the uterus is endopelvic and protected by the bony pelvis. Maternal pelvic fractures can also lead to fetal trauma (including skull fracture and bleeding).
   d. Morbidity and mortality of penetrating injury vary based on the timeliness of the pregnancy.
      i. The early gravid uterus is muscular and can absorb a great amount of energy
      ii. As the uterus increases in size, other abdominal organs may be protected, and so the risk of maternal injuries to visceral organs is relatively low.
      iii. The increasing gravid uterus displaces the intestines upward and places the mother at risk of an intestinal injury. These injuries can place the mother at risk of serious injury, infections, and death.

      iv. Maternal outcomes from penetrating injuries to the uterus are generally good depending on where the injury occurs, but the fetus has poor outcomes, especially with gunshot wounds to the abdomen.

  e. Severe trauma may cause shock and death.

  f. Pregnant trauma patients who sustained injury are at greater risk for the development of DIC.

2. **Etiology and risk factors**
   a. Trauma is one of the leading causes of maternal and fetal morbidity and mortality during pregnancy in the United States.
   b. The majority of cases are caused by motor vehicle accidents, intimate partner violence (IPV), and falls (with fall risk increasing significantly in the third trimester because of changes in body mechanics). Other types of trauma in pregnancy include: Burns, accidental poisoning, toxic exposure, homicide, and suicide.

KEY CONCEPT

IPV can occur in all ages, demographics, and ethnicities.

---

  c. Unrestrained patients have a higher risk of premature delivery and fetal death.

3. **Interprofessional collaboration: Nurse, obstetric nurse, physician (trauma surgeon, obstetrician, anesthesiologist), advanced practice provider, respiratory therapist, chaplain**

4. **Management of patient care: see Ch. 11, Multisystem Trauma**
   a. The primary trauma survey should be completed with the goal of maternal resuscitation and stabilization. Initial maternal resuscitation plans are the same for the nonpregnant patient. The focus of care is to save the mother, which will help save the child.
   b. Indications of potential harm to the pregnancy in the injured pregnant patient:
       i. Vaginal bleeding: Placental abruption or previa
       ii. Ruptured membranes: Prolapsed cord
       iii. Bulging perineum
       iv. Contractions: Early or imminent labor
       v. Abnormal fetal heart tones
       vi. Kleihauer-Betke test: Identifies fetal blood in the maternal circulation
   c. The patient should be placed in the left lateral position to promote blood return to the placenta (and fetus).
   d. Abdominal examination is critical in the obstetric patient to determine maternal and fetal injuries.
   e. A brief fetal assessment should be performed before the maternal secondary survey including heart sounds. Once the mother is stable, a fetal ultrasound should be performed.
   f. If the mother is Rh–negative with a history of abdominal trauma, she should receive one dose of Rho(D) immune globulin (RHOgam) within 72 hours of the injury.
   g. Perimortem cesarean section may need to be considered if the mother's condition is threatened by the fetus or the fetus is threatened by the loss of the mother's vital signs.

5. **Diagnostic testing: see Ch. 11, Multisystem Trauma**
   a. The use of radiographic examinations should be performed in the injured pregnant patient when indicated. Limit the number of radiographic studies; shield the abdomen with a lead apron when the abdomen is not being examined; ensure that

someone is monitoring the number of radiographs that are being ordered while in the critical care unit.
   b. Fetal monitoring should be performed in pregnancies beyond 20 to 24 weeks gestation.
   c. Fetal assessments should include ultrasound evaluations by trained providers.

CARDIOPULMONARY CONCERNS IN PREGNANT PATIENTS

1. **Pregnancy-related changes can affect the ability to effectively provide cardiopulmonary (CPR) to the patient**

> **EXPERT TIP**
> Fetus will only tolerate maternal acidosis for a short interval. Resuscitative measures should continue through operative delivery to promote fetal circulation.

   a. The patient should be placed in the left lateral position to promote blood return to the placenta (and fetus)
2. **There is a higher risk of aspiration because of delays of gastric emptying**
3. **Therapies and medications according the ACLS guidelines should be provided, including defibrillation (see Ch. 4, Cardiovascular System)**

References and bibliography information are available at http://evolve.elsevier.com/AACN/corecurriculum/.

Patient Transport

Renee M. Holleran, FNP-BC, PhD, CCRN (Alumnus), CEN, CFRN, CTRN (Retired), FAEN

CROSSWALK

- **Quality and Safety in Nursing Education (QSEN):** Patient-centered care, Teamwork and collaboration, Evidence-based practice, Quality improvement, Safety, Informatics
- **National Patient Safety Goals:** Identify patients correctly, Improve staff communication, Use medicines safely, Use alarms safely, Prevent infection, Identify patient safety risks, Prevent mistakes in surgery
- **American Nurses Association (ANA) Standards for Professional Nursing Practice:** Standard 1. Assessment, Standard 2. Diagnosis, Standard 3. Outcomes identification, Standard 4. Planning, Standard 5. Implementation, Standard 6. Evaluation, Standard 9. Communication, Standard 10. Collaboration, Standard 11. Leadership, Standard 12. Education, Standard 13. Evidence-based practice and research, Standard 14. Quality of practice, Standard 16. Resource utilization, Standard 17. Environmental health
- **AACN Standards for Progressive and Critical Care Nursing Practice:** Standard 1. Quality of practice, Standard 2. Professional practice evaluation, Standard 3. Education, Standard 4. Communication, Standard 5. Ethics, Standard 6. Collaboration, Standard 7. Evidence-based practice/research/clinical inquiry, Standard 8. Resource utilization, Standard 9. Leadership, Standard 10. Environmental health
- **AACN Standards for Establishing and Sustaining Healthy Work Environments (HWE):** Skilled communication, True collaboration, Effective decision-making, Appropriate staffing, Meaningful recognition, Authentic leadership
- **PCCN content:** None
- **CCRN content:** None

1. Definitions
    a. *Inter*facility critical care transport involves the delivery of a critically ill or injured patient from a scene or from one clinical facility to another to a higher level of care or definitive care
    b. *Intra*facility critical care transport involves the transfer of a critically ill or injured patient from one diagnostic, treatment, or inpatient area within the hospital to another, for example, radiology

> **EXPERT TIP**
> Considerations before transport:
>
> - Is the transport necessary?
> - Could the test be performed at the patient's bedside?
> - Is the transport needed for a lifesaving intervention?
> - Collaborate the transport with stakeholders so the patient will not have to wait at the destination
> - Determine appropriate level of competent care/needed clinician(s)
> - Does the destination have the appropriate equipment to assure the patient's continued care and safety?
> - Has an optimal route for the transport been determined?

MEMBERS OF THE TRANSPORT TEAM

1. **Interfacility transport team**
   a. There are several levels of care delivered by the transport team. The team must provide the level of care that is required by the patient. Federal guidelines, along with local and state regulations, dictate the level of care transport teams may provide.

> **KEY CONCEPT**
> A Commission on Accreditation of Medical Transport Systems (CAMTS)-accredited transport program should be selected for patient transport. The level of education, certification, competencies, and equipment that are required to deliver appropriate and safe care during the transport process will be provided.

   b. Levels of care of transport teams (Table 18.1)
2. **Intrafacility transport team**
   a. Team members should be able to anticipate, assess, and intervene effectively if the patient experiences problems during transport. Staff competent in managing unstable patients and in interpreting and intervening appropriately should be present. The level of care provided should be consistent with in-hospital care. Ensure appropriate certifications of staff based on the type of patients being transported (e.g., advanced cardiovascular life support [ACLS], Pediatric Advanced Life Support [PALS], or Neonatal Resuscitation Program [NRP]) (see Ch. 1, Professional Caring and Ethical Practice).
   b. Every team member should have critical care, emergency, trauma, or transport certification and/or experience.

INDICATIONS FOR TRANSPORT

1. **Interfacility: General indications for transport include the following:**
   a. Illness or injury are beyond the scope of care at the referring facility
   b. Diagnostic test, procedure, or treatment is not available at the referring facility
   c. State or local regulations dictate that a particular type of patient (e.g., pediatric or trauma patient) must be cared for at a specific facility
   d. Patient or family requests the transfer and transport
2. **Intrafacility**
   a. Transfer to perform a required diagnostic test or therapeutic procedure that is beyond the scope of care within the unit (e.g., computed tomography, magnetic resonance imaging, cardiac catheterization)

TABLE 18.1 Levels of Care of the Transport Team

Level of Care	Care Delivered	Description of Team
Basic Life Support	Capable of delivering prehospital basic life support	Minimum of one medical personnel, Emergency Medical Technician (EMT) required (paramedic preferred)
Advanced Life Support	Capable of delivering prehospital advanced life support	A minimal of two medical personnel. The vehicle operator may be the second team member for surface transports. One member must be a national registered or state certified/licensed paramedic. The other team member may be an EMT or paramedic.
Emergency Critical Care	Capable of delivering out-of-hospital care during the acute resuscitation phase before definitive care is provided (e.g., comparable to emergency department stabilization or a critical care unit (CCU) transfer to more definitive care	One team member is a registered nurse (RN), the second can be a primary care provider, a resident, staff physician, or paramedic with the appropriate experience and competencies to manage the patient who requires transport
Critical Care	Capable of delivering out-of-hospital care comparable to tertiary intensive care unit (ICU) care during interfacility transport to a higher level or specialty care ICU	A minimum of two transport team members are required: (1) a critical care RN and (2) a paramedic. Additional team members may be present depending on the scope of care, for example, a respiratory therapist, advanced practice provider, physician, or perfusionist
Specialty Care	Neonatal, pediatric, or high-risk obstetric transports	A minimum of two transport team members—(1) a nurse or physician and (2) a respiratory therapist or a critical care paramedic—should be present

From Semonin Holleran, R., Wolfe, A., Frakes, M. (2018). *Patient transport principles and practice.* St. Louis, Elsevier.

b. Transfer to another critical care unit or to a monitored bed

c. Transfer to an operative suite

MODES OF INTERFACILITY TRANSPORT

1. **Determine the need and method of transport**
   a. Evaluate the patient to identify the illness or injury that requires transport. Anticipate the most serious problem that may occur during transport.
   b. Determine the type of medical care required by the patient both at the scene of the injury or the referring facility.
   c. Is the transport time critical? If no, then determine what mode of transportation is available. If the transport is time-critical, consider how long it will take a transport vehicle to get to the patient and how long it will take patient to arrive to a receiving facility.
   d. Consider specific logistics related to transport including available resources, ground traffic, accessibility, and weather

2. **Air transport (rotor wing and fixed wing)**
   a. Advantages
      i. Time saving—can usually deliver the patient "door to door"
      ii. Air medical transport teams are generally proficient in advanced and critical care life support
      iii. Aircraft (especially rotary-wing aircraft) are able to access environments that ground vehicles cannot
   b. Disadvantages
      i. Physiologic effect of flight stressors, such as altitude and noise

ii. Weather restrictions

iii. Space and weight limitations

iv. Fear of flying

3. **Ground transport**

a. Advantages

i. Ground vehicles can travel in inclement weather

ii. Space allows for more personnel and equipment

iii. More readily available

b. Disadvantages

i. Time constraints

ii. Traffic and road conditions can impede transport

iii. Motion sickness

iv. Increased risk of patient complications during long transports

v. Long transports may contribute to increased transport team fatigue

RISKS AND STRESSES OF TRANSPORT

1. **All types of patient transport**

a. Physiologic instability during transport (e.g., inadequate stabilization of the patient's airway, breathing, and circulation; unstable cardiac rhythm)

b. Potential for further injury or death with transport

c. Inadequate patient assessment and/or monitoring during transport

d. Lack of equipment, medications, or supplies required for care or resuscitation

e. Equipment that malfunctions or is ill suited to the patient's age, condition, or size

f. Rapid, disorganized transport because of lack of a team leader or ineffective leadership

g. Inadequately trained transport personnel

h. Unavailability or lack of readiness of treatment area personnel to perform the procedure

2. **Interfacility transport**

a. Risks of transport

i. Possibility of transport vehicle accidents

ii. Long distances between treatment areas

iii. Loss of the effects of pain management, sedation, or anesthesia during the transport

iv. Delayed patient arrival because of mechanical failure of the transport vehicle, traffic problems, or bad weather

v. Safety hazard for transport team related to combative patient

b. Stresses of air transport

i. Barometric pressure changes

(a) May cause dysbarism (body gas expansion) and barotrauma (tissue damage)

(b) Trapped gases may affect the following:

(1) Patient condition (e.g., gas expansion may lead to tension pneumothorax or cause abdominal pain)

(2) Equipment (e.g., high altitude may slow intravenous [IV] flow rate)

ii. Hypoxia: Decreased oxygen at high altitude

(a) Hypoxic hypoxia because of reduced fraction of inspired oxygen (Fio_2) or some condition that interferes with the diffusion of oxygen from the alveoli into the systemic circulation

(b) Hypemic hypoxia because of reduced oxygen-carrying capacity caused by conditions, such as anemia, blood loss, or carbon monoxide poisoning

(c) Stagnant hypoxia—caused by conditions, such as shock, acute myocardial infarction, or heart failure, which slow the transport of oxygen to tissues

(d) Histotoxic hypoxia because of interference with the tissue utilization of available oxygen caused by agents, such as alcohol or narcotics, or poisons, such as cyanide

c. Stresses of air and ground transport

　i. Noise: Can range from 100 to 120 dB

　　(a) May come from sources, such as rotor blades, engines, sirens, or cabin noises from equipment or loud voice communications

　　(b) May make it difficult to hear physiologic sounds (heart, breath, Korotkoff sounds) and equipment alarms, and to communicate verbally with the patient

　ii. Temperature: Thermal changes (heat or cold) related to the following:

　　(a) External factors

　　　(1) Ambient temperature outside the transport vehicle

　　　(2) Vehicle's inability to maintain a comfortable environment

　　　(3) Altitude—temperature decreases as altitude and barometric pressure increase

　　(b) Internal factors: Patient may not be able to maintain body temperature because of illness, injury, or medications, particularly neuromuscular blocking agents (NMBAs)

　iii. Vibration

　　(a) Sources vary with the mode of transport

　　　(1) Ground: Road conditions, condition of the transport vehicle

　　　(2) Fixed-wing aircraft: Air turbulence, especially at lower altitudes

　　　(3) Rotary-wing aircraft: Transition from main or tail rotors

　　(b) Can cause symptoms of mild startle reaction, including increased heart, respiratory, and metabolic rates

　iv. Motion (acceleration, turning or banking, gravitational forces, visual field motion)

　　(a) May lead to motion sickness, vomiting, disorientation, fear

　　(b) Sunlight flickering through the main rotors of rotary-wing aircraft can cause flicker vertigo, nausea, disorientation; covering the eyes may help prevent this

3. Intrafacility transport

a. Insufficient number of staff accompanying the patient

b. Inadequate transport team staff mix to meet the patient's needs during transport

c. Unanticipated delays related to elevator, battery, or electrical power failure

d. Lack of communication between the originating and receiving areas regarding the transport

e. Lack of preplanning patient oxygen requirements

f. Red flags to consider when considering an intrafacility transport

　i. High ventilator use requirements that are difficult to maintain

　ii. Pressure limiting sedation

　iii. High-frequency oscillatory ventilation

　iv. Noninvasive ventilators that cannot be battery powered (e.g., oxygen, bilevel/continuous positive airway pressure)

　v. More than two chest tubes

vi. Chest tubes that require constant suction
vii. Dependence on an intraaortic balloon pump (IABP) or to another cardiopulmonary perfusion device
viii. Continued bleeding during ongoing resuscitation
ix. Patient with an open abdomen or viscera
x. Patient requiring continuous renal replacement therapy
xi. Unstable spinal injury

> **EXPERT TIP**
> Many patient and logistical conditions should be considered before departure to ensure a safe and uneventful transport.

OVERRIDING PRIORITIES IN PATIENT TRANSPORT

1. **Paramount determinants in decisions regarding patient transfer and transport**
   a. Health, well-being, and safety of the patient require the following:
      i. Securing of the patient for transport
      ii. Securing of all equipment and supplies
      iii. Chemical or physical restraint of the patient when indicated to avoid harm to self or others
   b. Health, well-being, and safety of the transport team require the following:
      i. Physical restraint of team members during takeoffs, landings, and ground vehicle movement
      ii. Discussion of Crew Resource Management
      iii. Training to ensure competence of all transport team members
      iv. Training of all who use the transport service
         (a) Method for setting up a landing zone
         (b) Safety at the helicopter pad and in approaching aircraft, ground vehicle safety (e.g., securing loose articles and wearing hearing protection)
         (c) Hot versus cold loading
2. **Safety of the patient and transport team may require refusal to transport because of**
   a. Weather restrictions-poor visualization of landing area, ice, winds
   b. Maintenance issues: Scheduled or unscheduled maintenance, or unsafe maintenance of an aircraft or ground vehicle (e.g., vehicles not properly inspected according to the manufacturer's recommendations or state or federal regulations)
   c. "Program shopping": One program or facility refuses the transport because of weather and the referring entity attempts to find another program to undertake the transport despite unsafe transport conditions

PREPARATION FOR TRANSPORT

1. **Select the appropriate transport service. Determined by the needs of the patient:**
   a. Basic life support team
   b. Advanced life support team
   c. Emergency critical care transport team
   d. Critical care
   e. Specialty care (e.g., neonatal, pediatric, perfusion, respiratory care)
2. **Select the equipment for transport. Desired attributes:**
   a. Indicated by the patient's illness or injury

   b. Adapted for the transport setting
   c. Able to be safely restrained and viewed by the transport team in the transport vehicle
   d. Lightweight and portable
   e. Redundant, multifunction (e.g., noninvasive and invasive blood pressure monitoring, end-tidal CO_2, and pulse oximetry)
   f. Easy to clean and maintain
   g. Sufficient battery life for transport with backup power source
   h. Sufficient oxygen or blended for transport
   i. Able to withstand the stresses of transport, including vibration, temperature changes, accidental dropping, use by multiple persons

3. **Secure equipment and supplies for transport**
   a. Suggested items for inclusion:
      i. Monitor, automated external defibrillator (AED), defibrillator, external pacemaker
      ii. Pulse oximeter and end-tidal CO_2 monitor
      iii. Advanced airway equipment (age appropriate)
      iv. Transport ventilator and/or bag-valve device
      v. Portable suction devices
      vi. Adequate portable oxygen
      vii. Emergency medications (for ACLS, PALS, NRP, NMBA, sedation, analgesia)
      viii. Adequate amount of medications for the transport
      ix. IV supplies: Fluids, needles, start kits (in case IV is lost during transport), infusion pumps
      x. Any other devices or medications the patient may require depending on the patient's illness or injury
   b. Ensure that the equipment and supplies are adequate to last for transport to the diagnostic or treatment area, for completion of the procedure, and, when warranted, for the return of the patient to the unit. This requires preplanning and, at times, calculations (e.g., oxygen usage).

4. **Assess and prepare the patient for transport**
   a. Airway
      i. Rapid primary survey with immediate interventions to secure and maintain a patent airway
      ii. Assessment of the patency of any in-place airway device, such as an endotracheal tube
   b. Ventilation (breathing)
      i. Determine if altitude may place the patient at risk (e.g., a patient with thoracic trauma may need a chest tube for transport)
      ii. Ventilator-dependent patient should trial the transport team's equipment before transfer to the air or ground vehicle
      iii. Provide oxygen administration for all patients during transport

---

EXPERT TIP

There is conflicting evidence in the literature for mandatory oxygen during transport. Oxygen administration should be based upon local protocols, with a goal of maintaining oxygen saturation greater than 94% in nonchronic obstructive pulmonary disease patients is appropriate, as higher levels may be harmful. Many patients who do not require oxygen at the initial facility may be transported on room air.

c. Circulation
  i. Control of bleeding
  ii. Establishment and maintenance of venous access
  iii. Insertion of other invasive lines as indicated
  iv. Anticipation of IV fluid and medication needs
  v. Securing of the necessary circulatory support equipment (e.g., IABP, left ventricular assist device, extracorporeal membrane oxygen machine)
d. Gastric function
  i. Altitude can increase the risk of vomiting; consider a gastric tube to prevent aspiration
  ii. Motion can cause nausea and vomiting; administer prophylactic antiemetics, as prescribed or per protocol
e. Splinting: To prevent further injury and enhance patient comfort
f. Pain
  i. Estimate the patient's probable needs for analgesia and sedation
  ii. Determine whether the patient has received an NMBA; closely monitor the need for analgesia and/or sedation
g. Wound care: Perform an initial appraisal; reinforce dressings for transport if indicated
h. Safety: Assess the potential of the patient to harm self or the transport team; restrain if necessary

5. **Notify the receiving unit or procedure area**
  a. Time the unit or area should expect the patient to arrive
  b. Equipment that will be required by the patient upon arrival
  c. Equipment that will be required to maintain the patient during the procedure

6. **Prepare the family for interfacility transport**
  a. Allow the family to see the patient before transport
  b. Explain to the family why transfer is required
  c. Identify who will be caring for their family member during transport
  d. Provide directions to the receiving facility or unit within the facility
  e. Remind the family to follow all traffic laws while in transit to the receiving facility
  f. Obtain family contact information to pass on to receiving facility

7. **Other interventions recommended before intrafacility transport**
  a. Suction the endotracheal tube or other airway device, as indicated
  b. Attach the patient to the transport ventilator; assess tolerance before leaving the unit
  c. Ensure the patency and flow rate of IV sites and medications
  d. Assess the patient's neurologic status
  e. Administer sedatives, analgesics, and any other medications that may be required during the transport. Remember that movement can cause the patient severe pain and anxiety
  f. Ensure that patients who require monitoring equipment will continue to be monitored during transport whenever possible (e.g., via wireless or battery-powered equipment)
  g. Explain the need for transport to the patient and family
  h. Ensure that adequate personnel are available to move the patient
  i. If there is a procedure nurse, notify the nurse with a report that includes patient diagnosis, current medications and treatments, and planned interventions or procedures

PATIENT CARE DURING TRANSPORT

1. **Patient access: Position team members so they can assess and manage the patient**
2. **Management of care: Divide into three phases (pre-, during, and posttransport)**
   a. Pretransport:
      i. Why is transport required?
      ii. Proper identification of the patient
      iii. Complete any required questionnaires before procedures
      iv. Receiving department has all of the equipment needed by the patient, has been notified, and is expecting the patient
      v. Transport route is clear
      vi. Airway equipment, including suction device, is readily accessible
      vii. Check function of all IV lines, ensure they are visible; at least one is accessible for medication administration
      viii. All intake and output (urinary, gastric, chest tube, other) are monitored and documented
      ix. Check function of all tubes and drainage systems; secure to reduce the possibility of dislodgement
   b. During transport:
      i. Check and plug in all transport monitors and place equipment within the transport team's line of sight. Use visible alarms.
      ii. If the patient requires chemical or physical restraint for safe transport, ensure that the patient receives adequate sedation, analgesia, and environmental control.
      iii. Monitor the patient's response to fluids, medications, or procedures performed during transport.
      iv. Team needs to keep in mind that movement, noise, temperature changes, and fear can increase the patient's oxygen demand and pain and make its management more challenging.
      v. Check vital signs every 5 minutes in the unstable patient, and every 15 minutes in the stable patient.
   c. Posttransport:
      i. Restart any stopped interventions and medications, for example, enteral feedings
      ii. Clean any used equipment
      iii. Restock any used supplies and check any equipment used
      iv. Document any instances that may have occurred during the transport
3. **Documentation of care**
   a. Interfacility transport
      i. Continuity of care requires maintaining a complete and accurate record of care from the referring facility to the transport team to the receiving facility
      ii. Information needed by the receiving facility includes the following, for example:
         (a) Patient's name, age, chief complaint or admitting diagnoses, interventions provided, and the patient's response
         (b) Reason(s) for transport, the patient's status during transport
   b. Intrafacility transport
      i. Indications and authorization for transport
      ii. Preparation and baseline vital signs, assessment before transport
      iii. Patient care during transport

LEGAL AND ETHICAL ISSUES RELATED TO TRANSPORT

1. **Emergency Medical Treatment and Active Labor Act (EMTALA)**
   a. Screen all patients who come to an emergency department to determine whether a medical emergency is present
   b. Stabilize patient with a medical emergency within the capabilities of the emergency department
   c. If the patient requires transportation for care, the receiving hospital must accept the patient if bed and personnel are available
   d. Referring hospital must send or transfer all copies of medical records, diagnostic studies, informed consent documents, and provider transfer certifications
   e. Transport patient by qualified personnel, with appropriate equipment, and via the most suitable mode of transport

> **KEY CONCEPT**
> Referring facility is responsible for assuring appropriate level of care during transport.

2. **Consent for transport**
   a. Explanation of the need for transport
   b. Explanation of the risks and benefits of transport
   c. Signed transfer form should be obtained when possible
3. **Written policies and procedures**
   a. Must include the indications for transport, facilities to which patients may be referred, and procedure for preparing patients for transfer and transport
   b. Should specify whether a family member may or may not accompany the transport team (this may differ among agencies/programs)
4. **Documentation**
   a. Quality improvement parameters
   b. Regulations of the Health Insurance Portability and Accountability Act (HIPAA): Appropriate use of patient information to improve care
5. **Decision to transport or not to transport**
   a. No-transport decisions: Transport team needs established policies for "no transport" or the ability to consult with medical direction when making this decision
   b. Family consultation: When possible, the patient's family should be included in decisions not to transport
   c. Cardiopulmonary arrest
      i. Assess patients who have had a cardiopulmonary arrest to determine the benefits of transport, because the effectiveness of cardiopulmonary resuscitation (CPR) can be compromised during transport
      ii. In addition, the transport team may be at risk while performing CPR during transport, by sustaining needlesticks when administering medications during CPR, and by exposure to blood or body fluids during CPR
   d. Advance directives or a Physician Order for Life Sustaining Treatment (POLST)
   e. Do-not-resuscitate orders (DNR)
   f. Refusal of transport by the patient, family, or others

References and bibliography information are available at http://evolve.elsevier.com/AACN/corecurriculum/.

Patient Transport

18

Mary Beth Flynn Makic, PhD, RN, CCNS, CCRN-K, FAAN, FNAP, FCNS and
Catrina Cullen, RN, BSN, CCRN

- **Quality and Safety in Nursing Education (QSEN):** Patient-centered care, Teamwork and collaboration, Evidence-based practice, Quality improvement, Safety
- **National Patient Safety Goals:** Identify patients correctly, Improve staff communication, Use medicines safely, Use alarms safely, Identify patient safety risks, Prevent mistakes in surgery
- **American Nurses Association (ANA) Standards for Professional Nursing Practice:** Standard 1. Assessment, Standard 2. Diagnosis, Standard 3. Outcomes identification, Standard 4. Planning, Standard 5. Implementation, Standard 6. Evaluation, Standard 9. Communication, Standard 10. Collaboration, Standard 11. Leadership, Standard 12. Education, Standard 13. Evidence-based practice and research, Standard 14. Quality of practice, Standard 15. Professional practice evaluation, Standard 16. Resource utilization, Standard 17. Environmental health
- **AACN Standards for Progressive and Critical Care Nursing Practice:** Standard 1. Quality of practice, Standard 2. Professional practice evaluation, Standard 3. Education, Standard 4. Communication, Standard 6. Collaboration, Standard 7. Evidence-based practice/research/clinical inquiry, Standard 8. Resource utilization, Standard 9. Leadership, Standard 10. Environmental health
- **AACN Standards for Establishing and Sustaining Healthy Work Environments (HWE):** Skilled communication, True collaboration, Effective decision-making, Appropriate staffing
- **PCCN content:** Multisystem—Pain, Behavioral/Psychosocial—Substance abuse
- **CCRN content:** Multisystem—Pain, acute and chronic, PICS

SYSTEMWIDE ELEMENTS

CONSIDERATIONS BEFORE SEDATION

1. Pain must be treated first, before sedation, as pain may often be the cause of agitation and delirium (see Ch. 2, Psychosocial Aspects of Critical Care, Ch. 20, Pain and PADIS guidelines: https://www.sccm.org/ICULiberation/Guidelines).
2. Determine whether intermittent or continuous sedation is required. Many studies recommend intermittent sedation to prevent complications that may be related to sedation.
3. Pharmacologic properties of sedating medications, dose dependent, alter the patient's responsiveness, airway reflexes, effectiveness of ventilation, and/or cardiovascular function.
4. Before administering sedating medications, perform a brief history and physical examination, asking about previous experiences with sedation.
5. Obtain patient history concerning chronic pain, opioid use, anxiolytic agent use, antipsychotic agent use, use of over-the-counter analgesics, and illicit substance use.

6. Inquire about gastric reflux disease or symptoms of dysphagia.
7. Inquire about a history of respiratory disease (e.g., asthma, chronic obstructive pulmonary disease [COPD]), obstructive sleep apnea (OSA), or chronic snoring.
8. Assess the patient's blood pressure, heart rate, respiratory rate (unprotected airway versus protected airway).
    a. Sedating agents may lower the patients' blood pressure and heart rate and depress respirations.
    b. Intravenous (IV) fluids may be required to support the patient's blood pressure.
    c. Close monitoring of the patient is necessary for changes in vital signs related to sedation medication administration.
9. Administer sedating medications in reduced dosages for the sedation-naive patient.
10. Patients with a history of, or current chronic use of sedation medications, substance abuse, addiction, and/or dependence may require higher doses of sedating agents to achieve clinical sedation.
    a. Tolerance to sedating medications may require higher and/or more frequent dosage administration in patients with a history of chronic sedation medication use.
11. Indications for sedation in the intensive care unit (ICU)
    a. Pain: Defined as "an unpleasant sensory and emotional experience associated with actual or potential tissue damage or described in terms of such damage." (Devlin et al, 2018).
    b. Anxiety: Feelings of nervousness, apprehension, restlessness, panic, or fear; tachycardia, tachypnea, and diaphoresis, trembling, and fatigue are common physical symptoms.
    c. Agitation: An unpleasant state of extreme arousal, excitement, tense, confused, irritable or irrational behavior; increased muscle tone, tachycardia, tachypnea, and diaphoresis are common physical symptoms (see Ch. 2, Psychosocial Aspects of Critical Care).
    d. Delirium: Syndrome characterized by the acute onset of cerebral dysfunction with a change or fluctuating baseline of mental status, inattention, and/or disorganized thinking (see Ch. 2, Psychosocial Aspects of Critical Care)
    e. Posttraumatic stress disorder (PTSD): Mental health condition triggered by a traumatic event. Symptoms include flashbacks, nightmares, anxiety, difficulty coping, uncontrollable thoughts of the event (Diagnostic and Statistical Manual of Mental Disorders [DSM-5], 2013) (see Ch. 2, Psychosocial Aspects of Critical Care).
    f. Postintensive care syndrome (PICS): Condition that encompasses new or worsening impairments in the patient's physical, cognitive, or psychologic status arising after critical illness and persisting beyond the acute hospitalization
    g. Pain: Somatic symptom of discomfort of varying intensity (e.g., sharp, dull, intermittent, constant) from injuries, surgery, trauma, procedures, preexisting conditions, and so on. Assess for and treat pain in addition to sedation needs to meet therapeutic care goals for the patient.
12. Patient Airway Assessment
    a. Protected airway: Ensure endotracheal tube is secured and mechanical ventilation is meeting the patient's oxygenation and ventilation requirements.
    b. Unprotected airway: Assess patient's respiratory rate, respiratory effort, and absence of snoring.
13. Institutional Policy for Nurse Administered Sedation
    a. Review hospital policy for sedation practice, including what level of provider can administer sedation, and monitoring requirements.

19 Sedation

b. Follow the hospital policy for frequency of assessing the patient's level of sedation using a valid and reliable tool.

PRACTICE CONSIDERATIONS DURING ADMINISTRATION OF SEDATION

1. **Assessment of the patient's level of anxiety, agitation, and sedation and response to sedative medication.**
   a. Altered response to medications may be caused by underlying medical conditions
   b. Altered response to medications may be caused by lack of prior exposure (naive patient) and/or tolerance to sedating medication
   c. Delayed emergence
      i. Overdose of sedative caused by individual variability or drug interaction
      ii. Delayed elimination caused by comorbidities, advanced age, liver or kidney dysfunction
   d. Withdrawal symptoms: May cause agitation or confusion
      i. From medications the patient was previously taking
      ii. From sudden cessation of sedative or opioid use, which can cause a return of agitation; early symptoms of opioid or sedative withdrawal include tachycardia, fever, salivation, restlessness and irritability, yawning, nausea, vomiting, and diarrhea
   e. Drug interactions of sedatives with other medications the patient is receiving

---

EXPERT TIP

Initiate and titrate sedation slowly and with low-dose increments, until desired sedation and patient comfort are achieved, to avoid unintentional oversedation. Review the patient metabolic laboratory results and review drug metabolism information for each agent before administering sedation agents.

---

2. **Sedation management considerations**
   a. Effects of undersedation
      i. Anxiety, agitation, irritability, increased metabolic demand
      ii. Tachycardia, hypertension, dysrhythmias, fever
      iii. Wound disruption, patient injury
      iv. Recall or awareness
      v. Need for neuromuscular blockade agents (NMBA)
   b. Effects of oversedation
      i. Delayed emergence, delirium
      ii. Delayed weaning from ventilator
      iii. Complications of immobility: Pressure-related injury, venous stasis, muscle atrophy, decreased gastric motility, atelectasis, and pneumonia. See PADIS Guidelines for assessments and interventions (Devlin et al, 2018).
      iv. Prolonged ICU and/or hospital length of stay, increased tests and costs
3. **Plan for patient comfort**
   a. Overall plan
      i. Establish treatment goals daily
      ii. Maintain light levels of sedation rather than deeper levels of sedation unless clinically contraindicated
      iii. Use daily sedation interruption or weaning protocol. See ABCDEF Bundle (www.iculiberation.org) from the Society of Critical Care Medicine, PADIS Guidelines (https://www.sccm.org/ICULiberation/Guidelines),
      iv. Use valid and reliable objective tools to assess sedation and pain

   v. Choose the right medication or combination of medications; reevaluate the need for sedation

   vi. Observe and treat signs and symptoms of withdrawal

b. Pain management

   i. Before administering sedating medications, assess and rule out the need for analgesia, and treat reversible physiologic causes of pain (see Ch. 20, Pain).

   ii. Routinely assess the patient for pain using valid and reliable objective assessment scales.

     (a) If the patient can verbally communicate, ask the patient to report severity of pain using a pain scale and attributing factors (e.g., aggravating and alleviating)

     (b) For nonverbal patients and mechanically ventilated patients, use behavioral pain assessment tools (e.g., Behavioral Pain Scale; Critical-Care Pain Observation Tool).

     (c) Vital signs should not be used as a primary assessment of pain, when possible

     (d) Consider preemptive analgesia to alleviate pain before procedures especially in the care of patients requiring NMBAs

   iii. Opioid analgesic medications used to treat pain may also cause sedation and respiratory depression.

   iv. Opioids: Provide analgesia and anxiolysis

     (a) Recommended for IV use in the critically ill: Fentanyl, hydromorphone, morphine

     (b) Scheduled doses or continuous infusion preferred over "as needed." Patient-controlled analgesia can be used if the patient is able to understand and operate the equipment.

     (c) Nonsteroidal antiinflammatory drugs (NSAIDs) and/or acetaminophen may be used as adjuncts to opioid agents. Assess kidney function with NSAIDs and hepatic function with acetaminophen.

     (d) Naloxone is an opioid antagonist that can be administered to reverse overdose and excessive adverse effects of opioid agents

       (1) Naloxone causes a catecholamine release that may precipitate adverse cardiovascular effects in older patients or patients with cardiovascular disease

   v. For known or suspected opioid overdose (full reversal)

     (a) Adults: 0.4 to 2 mg IV, intramuscularly (IM), or subcutaneously every 2 to 3 minutes as needed up to a total dose of 10 mg. For patients with chronic opioid addiction, use smaller doses and titrate slowly to minimize cardiovascular adverse effects and withdrawal symptoms (Clinical Pharmacology Online, 2021).

     (b) For respiratory depression associated with therapeutic opioid use (e.g., postoperative)

       (1) Adults: 0.1 to 0.2 mg IV at 2- to 3-minute intervals until the desired response is obtained. Additional doses may be necessary at 1- to 2-hour intervals depending on patient response, as well as the dosage and duration of action of the opiate agonist (Clinical Pharmacology Online, 2021).

EXPERT TIP

The assessment and treatment of pain can reduce sedation requirements during procedures.

TABLE 19.1 Sedation Assessment Scales for Adult Patients	
Sedation-Agitation Scale	**Richmond Agitation-Sedation Scale**
1 Unarousable (minimal or no response to noxious stimuli, does not communicate or follow commands)	-5 Unarousable (no response to voice or physical stimulation)
2 Very sedated (arouses to physical stimuli but does not communicate or follow commands, may move spontaneously)	-4 Deep sedation (no response to voice, but any movement to physical stimulation)
3 Sedated (difficult to arouse, awakens to verbal stimuli or gentle shaking but drifts off again, follows simple commands)	-3 Moderate sedation (any movement, but no eye contact to voice)
4 Calm and cooperative (calm, awakens easily, follows commands)	-2 Light sedation (brief, <10 s awakening with eye contact to voice)
5 Agitated (anxious or mildly agitated, attempts to sit up, calms down to verbal instructions)	-1 Drowsy (not fully alert, but has sustained, >10 s awakening with eye contact to voice)
6 Very agitated (does not calm, despite frequent verbal reminding of limits; requires physical restraints; bites endotracheal tube)	0 Alert and calm
7 Dangerous agitation (pulling at endotracheal tube, trying to remove catheter, climbing over bed rail, striking at staff, thrashing from side to side)	1 Restless (anxious or apprehensive but movements are not aggressive or vigorous)
	2 Agitated (frequent nonpurposeful movement or patient-ventilator dyssynchrony)
	3 Very agitated (pulls on or removes tubes or catheters or shows aggressive behavior toward staff)
	4 Combative (overly combative or violent, immediate danger to staff)

From Devlin, J.W., Skrobik, Y., Needham, D.M., et al. (2018). Clinical practice guidelines for the prevention and management of pain, agitation/sedation, delirium, immobility, and sleep disruption in adult patients in the ICU. *Critical Care Medicine*, 46(9), e825-e873.

4. **Assessment of sedation**
   a. Establish a sedation goal and ensure that it is regularly redefined and documented
   b. Use a sedation interruption or weaning protocol to standardize care
   c. Use a validated behavioral sedation assessment scale
   d. Sedation scales do not assess anxiety or pain. Remember to assess for PADIS.
   e. Sedation scales (Table 19.1)
      i. Richmond Agitation-Sedation Scale (RASS)
      ii. Sedation-Agitation Scale (SAS)
      iii. RASS and SAS have been found to be the most valid and reliable sedation assessment tools measuring the quality and depth of sedation in adult ICU patients.
   f. Additional objective assessments to measure the level of sedation
      i. Monitor vital signs: Blood pressure, continuous heart rate monitoring, respiratory rate, and effort. Vital sign changes alone are not adequately specific or sensitive to safely evaluate sedation effectiveness.
      ii. Monitor oxygenation using continuous pulse oximetry (SpO_2)
      iii. Capnography (e.g., end-tidal carbon dioxide [$EtCO_2$] monitoring) assists with real-time measurement of ventilation effectiveness and will show signs of respiratory compromise before signs of hypoxemia (e.g., decrease in SpO_2) are detected.

iv. Objective brain function measures (e.g., Bispectral index monitor [BIS], Narcotrend Index [NI], auditory evoked potentials [AEP])

   (a) These devices are not recommended to assess depth of sedation in noncomatose adult patients or those not receiving NMBAs

   (b) For patients receiving NMBAs, objective brain function measures may be used in addition to subjective behavioral sedation assessments

> **EXPERT TIP**
>
> Changes in pulse oximetry readings are delayed compared to real-time changes in ventilation effectiveness that can be more quickly detected using $EtCO_2$ monitoring.

5. **Pharmacology**

   a. Sedation agent dosage and use change dynamically with practice. Current pharmacy resources and/or consultation with a clinical pharmacist should occur during establishment of the plan for sedation with all patients.

   b. Sedation agents may be administered via a continuous infusion or intermittent dosing based on the individualized sedation goals set for the patient

      i. Collaborating with clinical pharmacists and following sedation protocols with daily sedation interruption reduces adverse complications caused by prolonged use of sedation or oversedation. Protocols that may be used include ABCDEF Bundle (www.iculiberation.org) from the Society of Critical Care Medicine, PADIS Guidelines (https://www.sccm.org/ICULiberation/Guidelines), and Vanderbilt Critical Illness, Brain Dysfunction and Survivorship (CIBS) Center (www.icudelirium.org).

      ii. Continuous infusion of sedation agents may result in unpredictable accumulation of the sedating agents

      iii. Behavioral sedation assessment tools, physiologic response to sedation, and sedation goals need to be continually assessed when administering sedation medications

   c. Benzodiazepines: Produce amnesia, hypnosis, and anxiolysis, but not analgesia; not recommended as the primary sedation agent for most adult patients. Delayed emergence from sedation with benzodiazepine medications can occur with prolonged use. All benzodiazepine medications are metabolized by the liver, so drug clearance is reduced in patients with hepatic dysfunction. Main adverse effects are respiratory depression and hypotension.

      i. Midazolam

         (a) Recommended for short-term use. Prolonged use may cause unpredictable awakening when infusions continue longer than 48 hours.

         (b) Midazolam may be used for rapid sedation of acutely agitated patients

         (c) Onset of action after IV administration is dose-dependent. An initial loading dose of 0.01 to 0.05 mg/kg IV, which can be repeated at 10- to 15-minute intervals until adequate sedation is achieved. Onset of action should be 3 to 5 minutes for sedation, with duration of action 20 to 80 minutes; elimination half-life, 1 to 5 hours (Clinical Pharmacology Online, 2021).

         (d) Continuous maintenance IV infusion dosing for midazolam range is 0.02 to 0.1 mg/kg/h. Dose should be titrated to the desired level of sedation and incorporate the daily awakening trial.

         (e) Use caution with older patients for whom delayed emergence can occur.

    ii. Lorazepam
      (a) May be used for intermittent IV sedation
      (b) Initial dose ranges for intermittent sedation from 0.02 to 0.06 mg/kg every 2 to 6 hours. Onset of action after IV dose, 15 to 20 minutes; half-life, 8 to 15 hours; not recommended for continuous infusion (IBM Micromedex, 2021).
      (c) Slower clearance and delayed emergence from sedation may occur.
      (d) Elimination and half-life are increased in patients with renal failure, causing prolonged clinical effects of the drug.
   iii. Flumazenil
      (a) Benzodiazepine antagonist is used to reverse benzodiazepine-induced sedation, but the agent has limited efficacy in reversing respiratory depression.
      (b) Consider giving naloxone before flumazenil if an opioid agent was also given with the benzodiazepine agent and oversedation with respiratory depression must be treated.
      (c) Use caution when using flumazenil in patients with chronic benzodiazepine use or history of high-dose tricyclic antidepressants because the drug may induce seizures or withdrawal.
      (d) Initial dose of flumazenil is 0.2 mg IV over 30 seconds. An additional dose of 0.3 to 0.5 mg may be repeated at 1-minute intervals; maximum cumulative dose is 3 mg (Clinical Pharmacology Online, 2021).
  d. Propofol: Produces sedation, hypnosis, anxiolysis, as well as providing amnesic and antiemetic effects, but no analgesia effects. Amnestic effects with light sedation are less than that produced by benzodiazepine agents.
    i. Approved for sedation of intubated adults on mechanical ventilation in the ICU
    ii. Rapid onset of action (10–50 seconds); short duration of action 3 to 10 minutes once discontinued; half-life, 3 to 12 hours with short-term use; half-life is longer with long-term infusion use. Typical initial IV bolus dose is 5 mcg/kg, followed by infusion depending on age and patient comorbidities. Continuous infusion rates of 5 to 50 mcg/kg/min are typical. Dose and rate of infusion should be individualized.
   iii. Preferred sedative when rapid awakening and frequent neurologic assessments are important
   iv. Has negative inotropic and chronotropic properties and inhibits sympathetic tone, which may result in decreased blood pressure and reduced cardiac output
    v. Pain on injection is reported
   vi. Respiratory depression is dose dependent. Close continuous respiratory monitoring or protected airway is required during administration.
   vii. Can elevate triglyceride levels; monitor after 2 days of infusion. Propofol-related infusion syndrome (PRIS) is a rare condition that may occur in patients with long duration or receiving high doses of propofol.
  viii. Add total caloric intake from lipids contained in medication in nutritional support orders
   ix. No reversal agent. Duration of action is under 15 minutes. Stop infusion and support patient cardiovascular and respiratory system if oversedation from propofol is suspected.

e. α$_2$-Agonists: Provide hypnosis, anxiolysis, and analgesia, but no amnesia. Minimal respiratory depression.
  i. Clonidine
    (a) Blocks sympathetic nervous system to produce effects
    (b) Transient increase in blood pressure is seen after IV dosing that may be followed by reduction in heart rate and blood pressure
    (c) Following IV administration onset of action is 5 to 10 minutes with duration of action 5 to 8 hours. Half-life is highly variable, 6 to 24 hours, and is prolonged in patients with compromised renal function.
    (d) Enables use of lower dosages of opiates to achieve comfort
    (e) Excessive sedation from clonidine may be treated with naloxone therapy and IV fluids to support blood pressure
  ii. Dexmedetomidine
    (a) Selective α$_2$-agonist that inhibits the release of norepinephrine
    (b) Has sedative and analgesic effects without causing respiratory depression
    (c) Recommended IV loading dose is 1 mcg/kg over 10 minutes to minimize cardiovascular side effects followed by a continuous infusion of 0.2 to 0.7 mcg/kg/h. Onset of action is 5 to 10 minutes and half-life is approximately 2 hours. Titration of infusion should not occur more frequently than every 30 minutes, which reduces the incidence of hypotension.
    (d) May produce transient elevations in blood pressure followed by bradycardia and hypotension
    (e) No reversal agent. Duration of action is under 10 minutes. Stop infusion and support patient cardiovascular and respiratory system if oversedation is suspected.
f. Ketamine: Provides dissociative sedation and mild analgesia
  i. Has analgesic properties at lower doses that may augment analgesic agents used concomitantly
  ii. Psychometric side effects include possible hallucinations; other side effects include vomiting, increased blood pressure and heart rate, and rarely laryngospasm
  iii. Initial dose IV is 1 to 2 mg/kg with an onset of action within 30 seconds and duration of action is 5 to 10 minutes; a repeat dose of 0.5 to 1 mg/kg every 5 to 10 minutes as needed. Prolonged effect may occur in older adult patients.
  iv. Dosage should be reduced if patient is also receiving propofol (Diprivan).
  v. Hypersalivation may be an adverse reaction that may be treated with glycopyrrolate or atropine and oral suctioning.
6. **Nonpharmacologic methods to decrease anxiety**
  a. Frequently reorient the patient
  b. Use cards with phrases or picture boards to aid communication with intubated patients unable to speak
  c. Provide soft lighting, pictures, or familiar items from home
  d. Provide music therapy, massage, therapeutic touch, animal-assisted interventions open visitation
  e. Establish sleep–wake cycles; provide for periods of uninterrupted sleep; open window curtains and turn on lights during daylight hours; close curtains and dim lights during nighttime hours.
  f. Engage patient in care decisions
  g. Encourage mobility; sitting in bed, out of bed to a chair, walking short distances, and so on.

> **EXPERT TIP**
> Goals for sedation need to be clearly understood. The nurse should complete a thorough assessment of the patient's risk associated with administration of sedatives and analgesic agents. If oversedation occurs and reversal agents and support interventions are required, continue to monitor the patient for a minimum of 90 minutes or until the patient returns to presedation baseline assessment parameters.

7. **Delirium**
   a. Characterized by acute onset and fluctuating course of inattention accompanied by either a change in cognition or a perceptual disturbance. (see Ch. 2, Psychosocial Aspects of Critical Care)
   b. Assessment of delirium
      i. Clinical history and assessment
         (a) Emergence delirium is associated with postanesthesia recovery
      ii. Depth of sedation and duration of receiving sedation medications
      iii. Assessment: Confusion Assessment Method (CAM) and CAM for the ICU (CAM-ICU)
         (a) Bedside scale that involves observation for the onset of changes in mental status or level of consciousness, inattention, disorganized thinking
         (b) Can be completed in 2 minutes
         (c) Can be completed with intubated patients
         (d) Should be completed routinely in ICU patients

8. **Other considerations**
   a. Sleep promotion is essential for patients in high-acuity settings to reduce delirium and immune dysfunction
   b. Sedative agent dose should be titrated with the end point defined and administration interrupted daily to reassess the patient and minimize the effects of prolonged sedative use
   c. Withdrawal effects can occur if opioids, benzodiazepines, or propofol are used for longer than 7 days
   d. Use of sedation guidelines, an algorithm, or a protocol is recommended to reduce oversedation

9. **Competency of the nurse administering sedatives (these requirements are equally applicable to nurses administering procedural sedation)**
   a. Knowledge of sedatives and analgesics agent pharmacology and safe administration practices
   b. Knowledge of sedation and analgesic reversal agents and indications for use
   c. Possession of the following competencies (Synergy Model—nursing competencies based on patient needs):
      i. Evaluates physical and psychosocial needs of the patient
      ii. Knowledge of the relevant anatomy, physiology, and recognition and management of cardiac dysrhythmias, cardiopulmonary resuscitation, and advanced cardiovascular life support procedures
      iii. Ability to assess hemodynamic changes in blood pressure, heart rate, preload and afterload
      iv. Ability to apply principles of respiratory physiology and oxygen transport and uptake, and to use oxygen delivery devices to maintain and/or restore a patent airway (e.g., nasal cannula, simple mask, ambu-bag, noninvasive mechanical ventilation, mechanical ventilation). Assesses ventilation effectiveness and use of capnography. Knows principles of airway management to include use of oral airway, jaw thrust maneuver, and suctioning techniques.

v. Ability to anticipate and recognize all of the following potential complications and to institute nursing interventions in accordance with existing orders, protocols, or guidelines:

  (a) Pulmonary: Respiratory depression, hypoxemia, hypercapnia, respiratory obstruction, laryngospasm, bronchospasm, increased neck circumference, presence of facial hair that may limit ability to obtain seal with oxygen face mask delivery devices

  (b) Cardiovascular: Cardiac dysrhythmias, hypertension, and hypotension

  (c) Allergic reaction

vi. Knowledge of organizational policies and the legal implications for nurses administering sedatives and analgesics.

KEY CONCEPT

Essential elements of safe sedation practice require a thorough assessment of the patient before administering sedative and analgesic agents (be familiar with your facility policies). Assess and treat pain, as well as addressing sedation goals. Judiciously administer sedation agents especially to patients at risk for adverse events, such as the older patient. Closely monitor the patient during and after sedation agent administration. Manage sedation to achieve care goals, as oversedation and prolonged sedation can adversely affect the patient's long-term recovery outcomes.

SPECIFIC PATIENT HEALTH PROBLEMS

PROCEDURAL SEDATION AND ANALGESIA FOR THE PATIENT IN HIGH ACUITY SETTINGS

1. **Definitions (Table 19.2)**

  a. *Minimal sedation (anxiolysis):* Drug-induced state in which patients respond normally to verbal commands. Although cognitive function and physical

TABLE 19.2 Continuum of Depth of Sedation

	Minimal Sedation (Anxiolysis)	Moderate Sedation (Conscious)	Deep Sedation	Dissociative Sedation
Responsiveness	Normal response to verbal stimulation	Purposeful response to verbal stimulation or light tactile stimulation	Purposeful response following repeated or painful stimulation	Purposeful response to verbal stimulation or light tactile stimulation
Airway	Unaffected	No intervention required	Intervention may be required	No intervention required
Spontaneous ventilation	Unaffected	Adequate	May be inadequate	Adequate
Cardiovascular function	Unaffected	Usually maintained	May be impaired	Usually maintained
Suggested monitoring by nurses	Continuous: cardiac monitoring, blood pressure, SpO_2, and $EtCO_2$	Continuous: cardiac monitoring, blood pressure, SpO_2, and $EtCO_2$	NA	Continuous: cardiac monitoring, blood pressure, SpO_2, and $EtCO_2$

EtCO$_2$, End-tidal carbon dioxide; *SpO$_2$,* pulse oximetry.
Modified from American Society of Anesthesiologists Continuum of Depth of Sedation: Definitions of general anesthesia and levels of sedation/analgesia. Revised October 29, 2019. http://www.asahq.org/~/media/Sites/ASAHQ/Files/Public/Resources/standards-guidelines/continuum-of-depth-of-sedation-definition-of-general-anesthesia-and-levels-of-sedation-analgesia.pdf.

19 Sedation

coordination may be impaired, airway reflexes and ventilatory and cardiovascular functions are unaffected.

b. *Moderate (conscious) sedation:* Drug-induced depression of consciousness in which the patient gives a purposeful response to verbal commands alone or to verbal commands accompanied by light tactile stimulation. No interventions are required to maintain the patient's airway, and spontaneous ventilation is adequate. Cardiovascular function is usually maintained.

c. *Deep sedation/analgesia:* Drug-induced depression of consciousness in which the patient cannot be easily aroused but responds purposefully following repeated or painful stimulation. The ability to independently maintain ventilatory function may be impaired. Assistance may be required to maintain a patent airway and spontaneous ventilation may be inadequate, but cardiovascular function is usually maintained.

d. *Dissociative sedation:* Drug-induced trance-like cataleptic state characterized by significant analgesia and amnesia without compromise of protective airway reflexes, spontaneous breathing, and cardiopulmonary stability

e. *Procedural sedation and analgesia (PSA):* Administration of sedative and analgesic agents to alter state of consciousness that allows the patient to tolerate an unpleasant or painful procedure while maintaining spontaneous breathing and cardiopulmonary stability. The intent of sedation, not necessarily the agent used, that determines treatment to relieve anxiety or to facilitate a procedure with sedation.

f. *Palliative sedation:* Sedation provided for end-of-life care to patients with intractable pain.

2. **Moderate sedation and analgesia for procedures**

a. Intent for procedure should be understood and sedation goals determined.

b. Informed consent should be obtained.

c. Continuous monitoring equipment (i.e., heart rate, blood pressure, SpO_2, $EtCO_2$) and emergency equipment to include suctioning equipment should be immediately available during the procedure.

d. Qualified, competent staff should provide care for patients undergoing procedures requiring sedation; staff should be adequately trained to rescue patients who reach a deeper level of sedation than intended.

3. **Indications and contraindications for procedural sedation and analgesia (PSA)**

a. PSA is indicated for patients needing moderate sedation for painful, invasive, manipulative, or constraining procedures.

b. Patients with significant comorbid conditions, advanced age, dehydration, history of respiratory diseases (e.g., COPD, OSA, central sleep apnea), or obesity are at increased risk of adverse events with PSA.

c. Patients with a history of substance abuse, addiction, or dependence may require higher doses of sedation agents or more frequent incremental dosing because of tolerance.

d. Procedural sedation is not appropriate for managing pain or anxiety in the terminally ill nor for seizure management.

e. To reduce the risk of adverse events in older patients initiate sedation more slowly, with lower dosing of sedation and analgesic agents

4. **Practice considerations**

a. Individual state board of nursing (SBN) position statements have specific position statements on the issue of sedation and analgesia. Know your SBN's ruling on nonanesthesiologist-administered sedation.

b. National position statements
  i. American Nurses Association position statement: Available at https://www.nursingworld.org/practice-policy/nursing-excellence/official-position-statements/id/procedural-sedation-consensus-statement/
  ii. The Joint Commission: Permission to administer moderate sedation. Available at: https://www.jointcommission.org/en/standards/standard-faqs/critical-access-hospital/medical-staff-ms/000001366/
  iii. Centers for Medicare and Medicaid Services. Revised hospital anesthesia services interpretive guidelines: State operations manual, appendix A. January 14, 2011. Available at: https://www.cms.gov/Medicare/Provider-Enrollment-and-Certification/SurveyCertificationGenInfo/downloads/SCLetter11_10.pdf
  iv. American Society of Anesthesiologists (ASA): Practice Guidelines for Moderate Procedural Sedation and Analgesia 2018. Available at: https://anesthesiology.pubs.asahq.org/article.aspx?articleid=2670190 or https://www.asahq.org/standards-and-guidelines
  v. American Association of Nurse Anesthetists (AANA): Registered nurses engaged in the administration of sedation and analgesia. Available at https://www.aana.com/docs/default-source/practice-aana-com-web-documents-(all)/non-anesthesia-provider-procedural-sedation-and-analgesia.pdf?sfvrsn=670049b1_4
  vi. Position statements on the use of propofol for moderate sedation has been addressed by some nursing specialty practices and SBNs.
    (a) Some SBNs specifically say it is not within the registered nurse (RN)'s scope of practice; others say it is within the scope of practice; others have not addressed the issue.
    (b) American Society of Anesthesiologist and American Association of Nurse Anesthetists have a joint statement on the safe use of propofol. Available at: http://www.asahq.org/~/media/sites/asahq/files/public/resources/standards-guidelines/statement-on-safe-use-of-propofol.pdf.
    (c) Society for Gastroenterology Nurses and Associates provides resources and links to SBN statements on nonanesthesiologist administration of propofol. Available at: https://www.sgna.org/Practice-Resources/GI-Nurse-Sedation/NAPS-CAPS
    (d) Evidence continues to mount showing safety in nonanesthesia provider-administered propofol.
    (e) Propofol administration to patients with protected airway and on mechanical ventilation should not be confused with administration of propofol for PSA in a nonintubated patient.
    (f) Know the position of your SBN and hospital policy and procedure.

KEY CONCEPT
Know the healthcare organization's policy on nurse administered sedation where you practice. Also review your state board practice guidelines.

---

5. **Preprocedural assessment**
  a. History
    i. Review of systems noting comorbid disease: Systemic disease (e.g., lupus), renal and/or hepatic impairment, cardiovascular disease, diabetes mellitus, respiratory disease (e.g., COPD, asthma)
    ii. Adverse experience with sedation, analgesia, or general anesthesia

     iii. History of smoking, alcohol use, prescription, and illicit drug use

     iv. History of chronic pain or chronic use of opioids and/or anxiolytic medication

     v. History of obstructive airway disorder or condition associated with increased risk in maintaining the airway: Snoring, stridor, OSA, obesity

     vi. Current medications, including over-the-counter or herbal products; drug and food allergies

     vii. Time of last oral intake

  b. Physical examination—focused on the heart and lungs

     i. Physical airway examination

       (a) Obesity (body mass index >35 kg/m^2)

       (b) Short neck or limited extension of the neck

       (c) Small mouth opening, dental appliances, nonvisible uvula, micrognathia, trismus, large tongue, significant malocclusion

     ii. Baseline vital signs, heart rhythm, oxygen saturation, respiratory rate and depth, and EtCO$_2$

     iii. Pregnancy status if the patient is a female of childbearing age

     iv. Pain assessment

     v. Confirmation of the individual as the correct patient using two methods of identification

  c. Preprocedural preparation

     i. Provide education to the patient and family or significant other

     ii. Review chart for presence of informed consent. Healthcare provider obtaining patient consent should discuss the benefits, risks, and limitations of, as well as alternatives for, sedation and analgesia.

     iii. Start an IV line

     iv. Complete a preprocedure check with healthcare team immediately before starting PSA, verify that the patient and the procedure are the correct ones

     v. Obtain baseline vital signs, heart rhythm, oxygenation, and ventilation (EtCO$_2$)

     vi. Perform a time out before starting sedation and procedure with all team members

6. Intraprocedural monitoring of patients

  a. Basic assessments

     i. Pain

     ii. Level of consciousness. Talk with the patient intermittently to assess level of sedation and patient ability to provide purposeful responses (e.g., minimal to moderate sedation is maintained).

     iii. Ventilation and oxygenation: Respiratory rate, bilateral ventilation (using a stethoscope), oxygen saturation and EtCO$_2$

     iv. Heart rate and rhythm: Electrocardiogram monitor

     v. Blood pressure: Continuous blood pressure monitor

     vi. Vital signs: Documentation at least every 5 minutes during the procedure

     vii. Report significant variations to the provider immediately (i.e., abnormal vital signs, nasal flaring, grunting, retractions, wheezing, dyspnea, apnea, flaccid muscle tone, increasing difficulty or inability to arouse the patient)

  b. Other nursing responsibilities

     i. Monitor the response to medications

     ii. Monitor the IV site, fluids administered, and urine output

     iii. Position the patient with the head of bed elevated at least 30 degrees if not contraindicated for the procedure

     iv. Ensure the patient's dignity, privacy, and comfort

     v. Act as patient liaison with the provider

   c. The nurse responsible for patient monitoring should have no other duties that would take them from the patient's bedside.

7. **Postprocedural monitoring of patients**

   a. Practice guidelines for postprocedure care are similar to those for patients who recover in the postanesthesia care unit.

   b. Continued observation and monitoring (using a validated sedation and pain assessment scale and objective measurements) are required until the patient has recovered from the sedation-analgesia; then care is resumed as before.

8. **Emergency equipment**

   a. Supplemental oxygen, oxygen delivery device, bag-valve mask device, suction apparatus, appropriately sized airways, positive pressure device, intubation equipment, reversal medication in room where sedation is performed

   b. Defibrillator immediately available

9. **Pharmacology for procedures (see also Pharmacology under General Consideration)**

   a. Benzodiazepines: Midazolam, lorazepam

   b. Opioids: Fentanyl, morphine, hydromorphone

   c. Other agents: Propofol, ketamine, dexmedetomidine

   d. Reversal agents: Naloxone, flumazenil

   e. Medication administration: Titrate all medications to effect (decreases risks and increases patient comfort). Administer smaller dosages to older patients and sedation/analgesia naive patients.

10. **Special conditions**

   a. Patients at increased risk for developing complications (e.g., patients at extremes of age; those with significant cardiac, pulmonary, hepatic, or renal disease; pregnant patients; those with a history or current substance abuse (prescription medications, illicit medication, alcohol) may need preprocedural consultation with an appropriate specialist.

   b. For severely compromised or medically unstable patients, an anesthesia or certified critical care intensivist provider may need to administer sedation.

   c. Activate a rapid response or medical emergency team if patient becomes compromised during sedation and/or procedure.

EXPERT TIP

Evaluate the time of day and availability of additional resources that may be needed during a PSA. If resources are limited, evaluate the ability to delay the procedure and associated PSA to ensure optimal patient safety and care.

References and bibliography information are available at http://evolve.elsevier.com/AACN/corecurriculum/.

Tonya Sawyer-McGee, BSN, MSN, MBA, RN, DNP, ACNP-BC

CROSSWALK

- **Quality and Safety in Nursing Education (QSEN):** Patient-centered care, Teamwork and collaboration, Evidence-based practice, Quality improvement, Safety
- **National Patient Safety Goals:** Identify patients correctly, Improve staff communication, Use medicines safely, Identify patient safety risks
- **American Nurses Association (ANA) Standards for Professional Nursing Practice:** Standard 1. Assessment, Standard 2. Diagnosis, Standard 3. Outcomes identification, Standard 4. Planning, Standard 5. Implementation, Standard 6. Evaluation, Standard 7. Ethics, Standard 8. Culturally congruent practice, Standard 9. Communication, Standard 10. Collaboration, Standard 12. Education, Standard 13. Evidence-based practice and research, Standard 14. Quality of practice, Standard 16. Resource utilization, Standard 17. Environmental health
- **AACN Standards for Progressive and Critical Care Nursing Practice:** Standard 1. Quality of practice, Standard 2. Professional practice evaluation, Standard 3. Education, Standard 4. Communication, Standard 5. Ethics, Standard 6. Collaboration, Standard 7. Evidence-based practice/research/clinical inquiry, Standard 8. Resource utilization, Standard 10. Environmental health
- **AACN Standards for Establishing and Sustaining Healthy Work Environments (HWE):** Skilled communication, True collaboration, Effective decision-making
- **PCCN content:** Multisystem—Pain, Behavioral/Psychosocial—Substance abuse
- **CCRN content:** Multisystem—Pain, acute and chronic

SYSTEMWIDE ELEMENTS

ANATOMY AND PHYSIOLOGY REVIEW

1. **Description and definition**
   a. "An unpleasant sensory and emotional experience associated with actual or potential tissue damage, or described in terms of such damage" (Devlin et al., 2018).
   b. May mask other symptoms, such as depression, anxiety, or insomnia.
   c. Pain is complex and from different sources (e.g., visceral, somatic, and neuropathic) (Devlin et al., 2018).
   d. Pain is "whatever the experiencing person says it is, existing whenever the experiencing person says it does" (McCaffery, 1968).
   e. Nurses need to consider the dimensions of pain: Physiologic, sensory, behavioral, cognitive, sociocultural, and spiritual
      i. Physiologic: Anatomic structure and physiologic functioning
      ii. Sensory: Quality and severity of pain
      iii. Behavioral: Verbal and nonverbal response to pain
      iv. Cognitive: Beliefs, thoughts, motivation, and attitudes related to pain
      v. Sociocultural: Social cultural norms and beliefs regarding pain
      vi. Spiritual: religious, spiritual practices or preferences related to pain

> ### KEY CONCEPT
> Pain is subjective, can be acute or chronic, and is based on an individual's perception of pain, and can occur in any body region and is composed of several dimensions nurses should consider when assessing and managing pain.

2. **Etiology**
   a. Caused by different disease processes that may have varied or similar pain characteristics (Kishner, Paulk, Schraga, Loffe, & Cho, 2019).
   b. Surgical events (e.g., incisions; presence of drains, tubes, orthopedic hardware)
   c. Traumatic injuries (e.g., fractures, lacerations)
   d. Medical conditions (e.g., pancreatitis, ulcerative colitis, migraine, coronary artery disease)
   e. Psychologic conditions (e.g., anxiety, depression), which can increase pain perception, prolong the pain experience, and lower the pain threshold
   f. Routine daily patient care procedures (e.g., turning; suctioning; placement or removal of catheters, tubes, or drains; paracentesis)
   g. Immobility
   h. Preexisting chronic pain conditions and preexisting cognitive conditions
   i. Musculoskeletal conditions (e.g., low back pain/neck fibromyalgia)

3. **Classifications**
   a. Acute
      i. Lasts days to 1 month
      ii. Can be somatic (on skin or soft tissues below skin), visceral (inside organs), or referred (pain away from original source of tissue damage)
   b. Subacute
      i. Lasts 1 to 3 months after initial insult (Hooten et al., 2017)
   c. Chronic
      i. Pain 3 months or greater
      ii. Usually no cure and can be intermittent or continuous in nature
      iii. May need specialized treatment from a specialist for management (Hooten et al., 2017)
   d. Categories
      i. Visceral
         (a) Pain caused by a lesion or disease involving the thoracic, abdominal, or pelvic viscera; pain is poorly localized and can cause referred pain to distant areas of the body. Quality can be described as aching, deep, or colicky.
      ii. Musculoskeletal
         (a) Caused by a lesion or disease of the musculoskeletal system including muscles, ligaments, tendons, cartilaginous structures and joints
      iii. Neuropathic
         (a) Caused by a lesion or disease of the central or peripheral somatosensory nervous system (e.g., peripheral neuropathy)
      iv. Inflammatory
         (a) Caused by an inflammatory process with infiltration of immune cells that cause tissue damage (e.g., broken bone; infected joint)

4. **Pain considerations**
   a. The 2018 PADIS Guidelines (Devlin et al., 2018) recommend a protocol-based pain assessment and management approach.

20 Pain

> **KEY CONCEPT**
> Pain is influenced by many factors and can have a negative impact on a patient's quality of life (QOL). Often *treat pain first (after determining the cause),* then determine if sedation is needed.

b. Many high-acuity patients experience continuous pain related to their condition or treatments. Pain assessment, management, and treatment are a priority.

c. In high-acuity patient populations, pain is often undertreated and represents one of patients' greatest worries, further exacerbating the pain experience.

d. Factors that influence the response to pain include demographics, such as age, sex, culture, beliefs, mood, previous pain experiences, current diagnosis and situation, sleep deprivation, amount of perceived control over the situation, and psychosocial support.

   i. Other factors that influence pain include the following in Table 20.1 based on 2018 PADIS guidelines.

e. Negative effects of pain on one's QOL can include suffering, fear, agitation, anxiety, depression, demoralization, and hopelessness.

f. Despite advances in pain management, the critically ill are at high risk for undertreatment of pain, including minor procedures and daily care events.

g. Efforts should be made to obtain information regarding a patient's precritical illness state to improve pain control.

h. Pain intensity is best maintained at a level that allows the patient an opportunity to heal with the minimum amount of discomfort.

i. Barriers and misconceptions can hinder effective pain management, including the clinician's personal values, belief experiences, sociocultural levels, reluctance of patients to report pain, and confusion about addiction, tolerance, and physical dependence with regard to pain medications.

5. **Pathophysiology**

> **KEY CONCEPT**
> Understanding the pathophysiology of pain will contribute to improved identification and treatment of pain.

a. Because of a noxious stimulus, which may damage tissue and cause pain

b. Three parts of the nervous system are involved in the sensation and perception of pain: afferent, nociception (e.g., cerebral cortex, diencephalon, midbrain, brainstem), and efferent.

   i. Sensations leading to type of nociception depend on type of tissue involvement.

     (a) Skin: Noxious stimuli are commonly thermal, mechanical (e.g., a cut), and chemical (e.g., exogenous allergens)

     (b) Joints: Noxious stimuli usually from mechanical stress (e.g., excessive joint force such as twisting) and chemical inflammation

     (c) Visceral organs: Mechanical distension, chemical irritants, and traction are common causes

     (d) Muscles: Strenuous mechanical exertion (e.g., overstretching) and chemical modalities are most common (Chen, Kandle, Murray, et al. 2020).

   ii. Afferent pathways occur from the peripheral nervous system (PNS) to the central nervous system (CNS)

TABLE 20.1	**Factors That Influence Pain**
Assessment	• Behavior
	• Patient self-report of pain
	• Physiologic
	• Proxy reporters
Protocol-based assessment and management	• Analgesia initially
	• Then, analgosedation
Multimodal analgesia to ↓ use of opioids	• Types: acetaminophen, NSAIDS, nefopam, neuropathic meds used for analgesia, lidocaine, etc.
Procedural analgesia	• Opioid vs. no use
	• Low vs. high-dose opioid
	• Nitrous oxide
	• NSAIDS (gel vs. systemic)
	• Local analgesia
	• Isoflurane
Nonpharmacologic analgesia	• Massage
	• Cold therapy
	• Relaxation/meditation techniques
	• Music

NSAID, Nonsteroidal antiinflammatory drug.
Modified from Devlin, J., Skrobik, Y., Gélinas, C., et al. (2018). Clinical practice guidelines for the prevention and management of pain, agitation/sedation, delirium, immobility, and sleep disruption in adult patients in the ICU. *Critical Care Medicine*, 46(9), e825–e873.

    iii. Nociception: Nociceptor nerve endings in afferent PNS that respond to stimuli (chemical, mechanical, thermal); detect damage to tissues. Involves the following four process:

      (a) Transduction: Begins with tissue damage from chemical, mechanical, thermal stimuli activating nociceptor, sufficient amounts of noxious stimulation activates the action potential sodium-potassium pump, converting noxious stimuli to an impulse (e.g., bumping your arm). Substances released from traumatized tissue: Prostaglandins, bradykinin, serotonin, substance P, and histamine.

      (b) Transmission: Electrical energy sent from periphery to spinal cord detecting source of pain.

      (c) Perception: Pain stimulus reaches the brain and patient's awareness of pain experience.

      (d) Modulation: Release of chemicals (e.g., endorphins, serotonin) to reduce pain transmission signal

    iv. Efferent pathways are those where motor neurons carry nerve impulses away from the central nervous system during pain responses

---

KEY CONCEPT

Perceptions of pain can be afferent or efferent. Pain perception occurs in the cortical structures of the brain and involves four processes: Transduction, transmission, perception, and modulation.

---

6. **Pathophysiologic effects and manifestations of acute pain (Table 20.2)**
   a. Amplifies the body's stress response

Pain

20

TABLE 20.2	Summary of Pathophysiologic Effects and Manifestations of Acute Pain	
Pathophysiologic Effects	**Manifestations**
↑ body's stress response	Recent, <3 months, lasting days to weeks
Delays patient recovery	Sharp, dull, radiating, shooting, tingling, fluctuates in intensity and varies by location
Contributes to metabolic and endocrine abnormalities	May cause increased blood pressure, grimacing, tachycardia, pallor

Modified from Devlin, J., Skrobik, Y., Gélinas, C., et al. (2018). Clinical practice guidelines for the prevention and management of pain, agitation/sedation, delirium, immobility, and sleep disruption in adult patients in the ICU. *Critical Care Medicine*, 46(9), e825–e873.

    b. Causes endocrine and metabolic abnormalities

    c. Impedes a patient's recovery

    d. Acute pain can become refractory; permanent changes can occur in pain pathways after even a brief exposure to severe, unrelieved acute pain and transition to chronic pain that outlasts the healing period

7. **Neuropathic pain**

    a. Radicular: Radiates from a compressed or inflamed nerve root (e.g., back pain radiating to foot)

    b. Radiculopathy: Occurs with radicular nerve pain and causes problems with reflexes, weakness of muscles, or numbness; can exist with or without radicular pain (Kishner et al., 2018)

       i. Chronic malignant pain often treated with opioids as main treatment of choice for various conditions (e.g., amputation chronic obstructive pulmonary disease [COPD], heart failure, organ failure, cancer, human immunodeficiency virus/acquired immunodeficiency virus)

      ii. Somatic pain: Defined localized pain, patients are able to pinpoint, nerve endings in bone, muscle, and skin. Quality can depend on injury, mechanism, and location.

    c. Neuropathic pain: Stimuli abnormally processed by the nervous system. Complex chronic pain state involving damaged/dysfunctional nerve fibers versus stimulation of usual pain pathways and pain receptors. Can involve afferent or efferent, CNS or PNS involvement (phantom limb pain, postmastectomy syndrome, postthoracotomy syndrome, nerve compression/plexopathies, polyneuropathy, metabolic neuropathies, diabetic neuropathy, postherpetic neuralgia, mononeuropathies, e.g., carpal tunnel syndrome, radiculopathy).

    d. Disorders of sensation symptoms: Dysesthesias typically lasting long after resolution or caused by PNS and CNS remodeling

       i. Hyperesthesia: Increased sensitivity to stimulation (feeling)

      ii. Hypoesthesia: Decreased sensitivity to stimulation (feeling)

     iii. Hyperalgesia: Increased response to stimulation (pain)

     iv. Hypoalgesia: Decreased response to stimulation (pain)

      v. Allodynia: Painful response to a stimulus not usually associated with pain

8. **Other terms relevant to pain**

    a. Addiction: Chronic, neurophysiologic disease. Persistent pattern of compulsive and dysfunctional opioid use characterized by an impaired control over drug use, continued use despite harm, use for effect other than pain relief, and craving.

KEY CONCEPT
Patients with addictive disease are at high risk for undertreatment of pain and have the right to receive quality pain management. Nurses should be knowledgeable on titration of opioids and benzodiazepines based on assessment findings (e.g., pain, side effects, mood).

b. Pain threshold: Duration or intensity of pain that a person is willing to endure
c. Pain tolerance: Point at which an increasing intensity of a stimulus is felt as painful
d. Tolerance: State of adaptation characterized by the need for increasing or more frequent doses of medication to maintain an effect. Does not, in and of itself, imply addiction.
e. Pseudoaddiction: Not a diagnosis; a situation created by undertreatment of pain. Behaviors may mimic those of addiction but cease with effective pain control.
f. Physical dependence: Physiologic state of reliance on an opioid, evidenced by withdrawal symptoms if the opioid is abruptly stopped or an opioid antagonist is given. Does not, in and of itself, imply addiction.

KEY CONCEPT
Nurses need to recognize the signs and symptoms of opioid withdrawal which include: lacrimation, rhinorrhea, pupil dilation, yawning, tremor, gooseflesh, insomnia, diarrhea, vomiting, irritability, elevated blood pressure, muscle cramps, and dysphoria.

BACKGROUND
1. **The big picture: Balancing current evidence, guidelines, standards, and performance measures while providing safe patient and family-centered care**
2. **Increased scrutiny on treatment, indication, efficacy, prescribing of opioid medications, and link to increased heroin use, while may not necessarily affect use in acute pain management, may affect discharge planning, patient education, transitions, and long-term management of pain. This impacts not only the outpatient healthcare system but also the inpatient healthcare system. All levels of the healthcare team should be aware of the implications for their patients and how to effectively use interventions for all types of pain, both pharmacologic and nonpharmacologic.**
3. **Ethical standards**
   a. Treatment of pain is an ethical obligation
   b. Unrelieved pain leaves patients vulnerable to other issues unrelated to their pain (e.g., self-esteem, depression, anxiety)
   c. Clinicians should maintain and respect ethical principles of integrity, autonomy, equity, nonmaleficence, and beneficence
4. **The Joint Commission (2018) pain management standards include:**
   a. The following should be addressed in organizations' policies:
      i. Organizational leadership role
      ii. Medical staff involvement in pain management care
      iii. Provision of care related to treatment and services
      iv. Performance improvement for data reporting related to treatment of pain

Additional statements on pain management from The Joint Commission are found at https://www.jointcommission.org/joint_commission_statement_on_pain_management/

(a) The hospital conducts a comprehensive pain assessment that is consistent with its scope of care, treatment, and services and the patient's condition. This standard allows organizations to set their own policies regarding which patients should have pain assessed based on the population served, and the services delivered.

(b) The hospital uses methods to assess pain that are consistent with the patient's age, condition, and ability to understand.

(c) The hospital reassesses and responds to the patient's pain, based on its reassessment criteria.

(d) The hospital either treats the patient's pain or refers the patient for treatment. *Note:* Treatment strategies for pain may include pharmacologic and nonpharmacologic approaches. Strategies should reflect a patient-centered approach and consider the patient's current presentation, the healthcare providers' clinical judgment, and the risks and benefits associated with the strategies, including potential risk of dependency, addiction, and abuse.

b. Patient-centered approach that takes into consideration the unique patient needs, values, and current presentation

5. **Modified World Health Organization (WHO) (2019) Analgesic Ladder (Fig. 20.1)**

a. "The unreasonable failure to treat pain is viewed as an unethical breach of human rights"

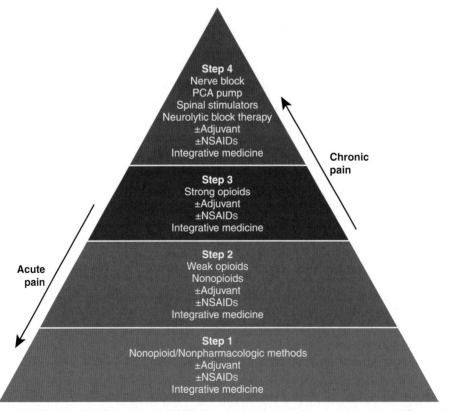

Fig. 20.1 WHO Pain Relief Ladder. *NSAID,* Nonsteroidal antiinflammatory drug; *PCA,* patient controlled analgesia. (Modified from Yang, J., Bauer, B.A., Wahner-Roedler, D.L., et al. (2020). The modified WHO analgesic ladder: is it appropriate for chronic non-cancer pain? *Journal of Pain Research*, 13, 411–417.)

b. Original ladder consisted of 3 steps:
   i. First step (mild pain): Nonopioid analgesics, such as nonsteroidal antiinflammatory drugs (NSAIDs) or acetaminophen with or without adjuvants to be used
   ii. Second step (moderate pain): Use weak opioids (e.g., hydrocodone, codeine, tramadol) with or without nonopioid analgesics, and with or without adjuvants
   iii. Third step (severe and persistent pain): Use of potent opioids (morphine, methadone, fentanyl, oxycodone, buprenorphine, tapentadol, hydromorphone, oxymorphone) with or without nonopioid analgesics, and with or without adjuvants (Anekar & Castella, 2020).
c. WHO analgesic ladder for adults revised in 2019 after public comments and includes an additional step in management of chronic noncancer pain: Evidence-based best practice guideline for cancer pain management that strongly influences noncancer pain strategies.
   i. Fourth step "Essential to have adequate knowledge about pain, assess its degree in a patient through proper evaluation, and to prescribe appropriate medications."
d. Opioid rotation should be adopted to improve analgesia and reduce side effects and patients should receive education about the uses and side effects of drugs to avoid misuse or abuse (Anekar & Castella, 2020).

KEY CONCEPT

Summary of 2019 WHO Pain Relief Ladder:

If pain occurs, there should be prompt oral administration of medications in the following order incorporating integrative medicine therapies along the way and including additional step in this sequence:
1. Nonpharmacologic methods
2. Nonopioids ± adjuvant analgesic
3. Weak opioids
4. Strong opioids

Opioid administration should only be when the benefits outweigh the risks to reduce risk of dependence. Nurses should make sure they understand the providers' directions regarding the drug, its dosage, and side effects to provide the optimum amount of medication.

---

6. **U.S. Food and Drug Administration (FDA)**
   a. 2016 safety announcement for entire class of opioid pain medicines
      i. May interact with antidepressants and migraine medicines to cause a serotonin syndrome
      ii. May cause adrenal insufficiency affecting stress response
7. **Centers for Disease Control and Prevention (CDC)**
   a. Guidelines for prescribing opioids for chronic pain
      i. Not intended for patients in active cancer treatment, palliative care, end-of-life care
   b. Recommendations in opioid use during perioperative period
      i. Develop a coordinated time-limited treatment plan for managing postoperative pain, including responsible prescriber
      ii. Avoid escalating the opioid dose before surgery
      iii. Do not discharge a patient with more than 2 weeks supply of opioid. Continued opioid therapy will require appropriate reevaluation by the surgeon.
      iv. Taper off opioids added for surgery as surgical healing takes place

v. Major surgeries should be able to be tapered to preoperative doses or lower by 6 weeks

vi. For some minor surgeries, it may be appropriate to discharge patients on acetaminophen, NSAIDs only, or with a very limited supply of short-acting opioids (e.g., 2–3 days)

8. **The American College of Critical Care Medicine (ACCM): Guidelines for the Management of Pain, Agitation/Sedation, Delirium, Immobility & Sleep Disruption (Devin et al., 2018)**

a. Summary of pain statements and recommendations

i. Pain is common and poorly treated

ii. Routine monitoring and preemptive treatment for all patients

iii. Use validated tools: Behavioral Pain Scale (BPS) and Critical Care Pain Observation Tool (CPOT), both validated for French- and English-speaking intensive care unit (ICU) patients. Not validated in brain-injured patients (Tables 20.3 and 20.4). CPOT and the BPS remain the most robust scales for assessing pain in critically ill adults unable to self-report their pain.

iv. For critically ill patients who can communicate effectively, self-reported pain scale using the 0 to 10 numeric rating scale is the most valid tool

v. Vital signs are not a primary assessment tool or indicator of pain in critically ill but may be a cue to further assess patients.

vi. Consider using family as proxy reporters to help report patient pain.

vii. Use opioid at lowest for procedural pain management in critically ill patients.

viii. Use nonopioids to decrease the amount or wean off of opioid and decrease side effects.

ix. Thoracic epidural analgesia for abdominal aortic aneurysm, traumatic rib fractures

x. Care bundles for pain, agitation, and delirium should be integrated, multidisciplinary, and work synergistically in the ICU (Fig. 20.2 and see Ch. 2, Psychosocial Aspects of Critical Care).

TABLE 20.3 Behavioral Pain Scale

SCORE RANGES FROM 3 (NO PAIN) TO 12 (MAXIMUM PAIN)

Facial expression	Relaxed	1
	Partially tightened (e.g., brow lowering)	2
	Fully tightened (e.g., brow lowering)	3
	Grimacing	4
Upper limb movement	No movement	1
	Partially bent	2
	Fully bent with finger flexion	3
	Permanently retracted	4
Compliance with mechanical ventilation	Tolerating movement	1
	Coughing but tolerating ventilation for most of the time	2
	Fighting ventilator	3
	Unable to control ventilation	4

From Gomarverdi, S., Segdighie, L., Seifrabiei, M., et al. (2019). Comparison of two pain scales: Behavioral pain scale and critical-care pain observation tool during invasive and noninvasive procedures in intensive care unit-admitted patients. *Iranian Journal of Nursing & Midwifery Research*, 24(2), 151–155.

TABLE 20.4   Critical Care Pain Observation Tool

SCORE RANGES FROM 0 (NO PAIN) TO 8 (MAXIMUM PAIN)

Facial expression	No muscular tension observed	Relaxed, neutral	0
	Presence of frowning, brow lowering, orbit tightening, and levator contraction	Tense	1
	All of the previous facial movements plus eyelid tightly closed	Grimacing	2
Body movements	Does not move at all (does not necessarily mean absence of pain)	Absence of movements	0
	Slow, cautious movements, touching or rubbing the pain site, seeking attention through movements	Protection	1
	Pulling tube, attempting to sit up, moving limbs/thrashing, not following commands, striking at staff, trying to climb out of bed	Restlessness	2
Muscle tension Evaluation by passive flexion and extension of upper extremities	No resistance to passive movements	Relaxed	0
	Resistance to passive movements	Tense, rigid	1
	Strong resistance to passive movements, inability to complete them	Very tense or rigid	2
Compliance with the ventilator (intubated patients)	Alarms not activated, easy ventilation	Tolerating ventilator or movement	0
	Alarms stop spontaneously	Coughing but tolerating	1
	Asynchrony: Blocking ventilation, alarms frequently activated	Fighting ventilator	2
OR			
Vocalization (extubated patients)	Talking in normal tone or no sound	Talking in normal tone or no sound	0
	Sighing, moaning	Sighing, moaning	1
	Crying out, sobbing	Crying out, sobbing	2

From Gomarverdi, S., Segdighie, L., Seifrabiei, M., et al. (2019). Comparison of two pain scales: Behavioral pain scale and critical-care pain observation tool during invasive and noninvasive procedures in intensive care unit-admitted patients. *Iranian Journal of Nursing & Midwifery Research*, 24(2), 151–155.

ASSESSMENT

> **KEY CONCEPT**
> Obtain a detailed pain assessment, history, and focused physical examination as the patient improves to ensure an accurate diagnosis of pain. Consider using family members as proxy reporters for the assessment of pain.

1. **Assessment considerations**
   a. When patients are unable to self-report pain, behavioral indicators may be used. Caregiver report is also helpful, as family/friends may better recognize discomfort in their loved one.
   b. Typical pain indicators may be absent despite the presence of severe pain, because of individual or cultural pain expressions, which may lead to undertreatment of pain.
   c. When conditions known to be painful exist, assume that pain is present and proceed with appropriate treatment.

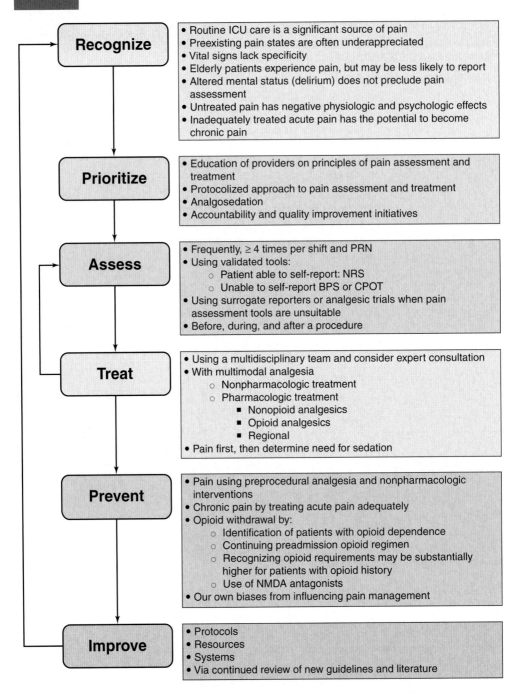

Recognize
- Routine ICU care is a significant source of pain
- Preexisting pain states are often underappreciated
- Vital signs lack specificity
- Elderly patients experience pain, but may be less likely to report
- Altered mental status (delirium) does not preclude pain assessment
- Untreated pain has negative physiologic and psychologic effects
- Inadequately treated acute pain has the potential to become chronic pain

Prioritize
- Education of providers on principles of pain assessment and treatment
- Protocolized approach to pain assessment and treatment
- Analgosedation
- Accountability and quality improvement initiatives

Assess
- Frequently, ≥ 4 times per shift and PRN
- Using validated tools:
  ○ Patient able to self-report: NRS
  ○ Unable to self-report BPS or CPOT
- Using surrogate reporters or analgesic trials when pain assessment tools are unsuitable
- Before, during, and after a procedure

Treat
- Using a multidisciplinary team and consider expert consultation
- With multimodal analgesia
  ○ Nonpharmacologic treatment
  ○ Pharmacologic treatment
    ■ Nonopioid analgesics
    ■ Opioid analgesics
    ■ Regional
- Pain first, then determine need for sedation

Prevent
- Pain using preprocedural analgesia and nonpharmacologic interventions
- Chronic pain by treating acute pain adequately
- Opioid withdrawal by:
  ○ Identification of patients with opioid dependence
  ○ Continuing preadmission opioid regimen
  ○ Recognizing opioid requirements may be substantially higher for patients with opioid history
  ○ Use of NMDA antagonists
- Our own biases from influencing pain management

Improve
- Protocols
- Resources
- Systems
- Via continued review of new guidelines and literature

Fig. 20.2 Flowchart describing the best practices when managing pain in the intensive care unit (*ICU*). *BPS*, Behavioral Pain Scale; *CPOT*, Critical Care Pain Observation Tool; *NMDA*, N-methyl-D-aspartate; *NRS*, Numerical Rating Scale; *PRN, pro re nata* (as needed). (From Sigakis, M.J.G., Bittner, E.A. (2015). Ten myths and misconceptions regarding pain management in the ICU. *Critical Care Medicine*, 43, 2468–2478; Modified from Barr, J., Fraser, G.L., Puntillo, K., et al. (2013). American College of Critical Care Medicine: Clinical practice guidelines for the management of pain, agitation, and delirium in adult patients in the intensive care unit. *Critical Care Medicine*, 41, 263–306.)

   d. Decrease in or elimination of a pain behavior following an analgesia intervention can indicate a reduction in pain but does not eliminate or reduce ongoing need for reassessment.
2. **Pain description and history**
   a. Patients pain physiology classification
   b. Intensity (0–10) mild, moderate, severe
   c. Types of tissue involved
   d. Syndromes (e.g., cancer, migraine, fibromyalgia, phantom pain)
   e. Special considerations (e.g., psychologic state, age, gender, culture)

KEY CONCEPT

Ongoing and timely assessments appropriate to the critically ill patient can identify ineffective and effective pain management and contribute to necessary revision of the analgesic plan based on patient needs.

---

   f. Location and radiation
   g. Intensity and severity
   h. Character or quality
   i. Timing and time course
   j. Alleviating and aggravating factors
   k. Patient history, relevant medical history, risk factors, and preexisting conditions that affect pain
   l. Associated factors and symptoms
   m. Effect on life and function
   n. Identify the underlying cause
   o. Previously effective methods of coping with and relieving pain
   p. Vital signs as an indicator of pain has challenges and limitation and should not be used as sole measure of patient's pain but to provide additional assessment data
3. **Frequency of pain assessment and reassessment**

KEY CONCEPT

- Always include pain intensity, quality, location, pain-related complications, and adverse effects of treatment whenever possible.
- Reassessment after intervention has taken effect is essential and should include these questions:
  - How much relief was obtained and how long did it last?
  - Were there any adverse effects?
  - Increase assessment frequency during times of inadequately controlled pain.

---

   a. No defined time frame, but best practice suggests 4 times or more per shift and as needed to meet the needs of the patient
   b. Assess prior, during, and after procedures; anticipate painful events/care/procedures
   c. Use of proxy report from family, surrogate, or a pain medication trial when pain assessment tools do not provide a valid response is considered best practice
   d. Cultural and generational differences may influence how often a patient requests pain medication despite being in pain
4. **Initial and ongoing assessment/screening of risk of abuse should occur (Opioid Risk Tool, CAGE-AID Questionnaire)**
5. **Appraisal of patient characteristics: Patients with pain enter critical care units with a wide range of clinical characteristics. During their stay, their clinical status may**

slowly or abruptly improve or deteriorate. Changes in the patient's condition may involve one or all life-sustaining functions, and functions can be easy or nearly impossible to monitor with precision. Examples of clinical attributes that the nurse should assess when caring for a patient in pain include the following: Resiliency, vulnerability, stability, complexity, resource availability, participation in care and decision-making, and predictability.

6. **Let the patient know you believe that the pain is real and is not in his or her head.**
   a. Ask and encourage the patient to take an active role in the management of his or her pain.
   b. Research shows that patients who take an active role in their treatment experience less pain-related disabilities

7. **Diagnostic studies**
   a. Used to help accurately identify the causes; however, the absence of positive study findings should not be used to deny the existence of pain
   b. Imaging studies to determine etiology or underlying pathology
   c. Blood work to identify organ dysfunction(s)
   d. Electromyography (EMG) tests to identify myopathies, some neuropathies
   e. Nerve blocks to distinguish source or types of pain

8. **Physical examination**
   a. A comprehensive history and physical examination should be performed
   b. Use of the clinical opioid withdrawal scale (COWS) is useful for assessing opioid withdrawal https://www.drugabuse.gov/sites/default/files/ClinicalOpiateWithdrawalScale.pdf
   c. Monitor for opioid withdrawal: Withdrawal is characterized by myalgias, arthralgias, anxiety, gastrointestinal complaints (diarrhea, emesis), chills, diaphoresis, opioid craving, piloerection, dilated pupils, rhinorrhea, yawning, tachycardia, hypertension, and sleep disruption.
      i. Opioid hyperalgesia: The physical examination is nonlocalizing
      ii. Opioid tolerance: Patients who are chronically exposed to opioids may have an unremarkable examination despite being on opioids. If anything, they demonstrate miosis and mild psychomotor slowing, including slowed speech (Hooten et al., 2017).
   d. Assess for the presence of delirium (see Ch. 2, Psychosocial Aspects of High Acuity and Critical Care)
   e. Observe for behaviors often associated with pain in nonverbal and verbal patients (Table 20.5)
   f. Patients who are sedated or chemically paralyzed, comatose, or sedated for painful procedures cannot exhibit pain behaviors. A full pain assessment, and the assumption that, if a condition, treatment, or procedure is known to be painful, then it should be assumed the patient has some level of pain.

KEY CONCEPT

Acknowledge of the patient's pain and proper assessment and data collection are pertinent for proper pain management.

---

9. **Pain assessment tool for competent noncritical care patients**
   a. Numerical rating scales (NRSs) use numbers to rate pain.
   b. Visual analog scales (VASs) typically ask a patient to mark a place on a scale that aligns with their level of pain.

TABLE 20.5 Common Behaviors Associated With Pain in Nonverbal Patients

Category	Behavioral Examples	Comment
Facial expressions	Frowning, grimacing, distorted expression, rapid blinking	Grimacing, frowning, and wincing may represent involuntary responses to acute pain and are felt to be valid indicators of acute pain, even in sedated patients. Some medical conditions (e.g., Parkinson disease, stroke, chemical paralysis) may result in distorted or absent facial expressions apart from pain Eye signals may also be used to indicate pain
Body movement	Restlessness, splinting, guarding, shaking, flailing, fidgeting, rigidity or tenseness, arching, clenching of fists, holding or rubbing of affected area, resistance to movement or care procedures, slow or cautious or no movement, repositioning, rocking, withdrawing	Some patients who are unable to verbally communicate may seek attention to their pain through gestures
Verbalizations	Calling out, sighing, moaning, asking for help, verbal, yelling, groaning, crying, verbal outbursts, such as "stop"	Patients with verbalizations may benefit from using analgesics as a first line
Changes in interpersonal interactions	Aggressive, disruptive, resisting care, withdrawn	Other conditions other than pain can cause changes in interpersonal interactions, such as changes in acid-base balance (e.g., hypoxia, hypercarbia, sepsis)
Changes in activity patterns	Sleep and appetite changes, sudden cessation of common routines	Some changes in activity patterns could also be related to mobility issues, medical restrictions, etc.
Change in mental status	Increased confusion, irritability, distress, crying, other psychotic type behaviors	Other conditions besides pain can lead to agitation (e.g., hypoxia, hypercarbia, sepsis) Pain behaviors are influenced by many factors (e.g., culture, duration of pain, coping skills)

Modified from article by Venable, E., Lee, H., Lee, I. (2018). *Pain assessment in persons with cognitive impairment,* https://emedicine.medscape.com/article/2113960-overview#a2.

   c. Categorical scales use words as the primary communication tool and may also incorporate numbers, colors, or relative location to communicate pain.

10. **Validated patient pain assessment tools for use with the critically ill**
   a. Self-report using NRS (1–10) is preferred for assessment of pain
   b. CPOT (see Table 20.4)
   c. BPS (see Table 20.3)
   d. Adult nonverbal pain scale (NVPS)
   e. Family/caregivers as proxy reporters involvement to inform healthcare team of usual pain-related behaviors and baseline information

11. **Monitoring data**
   a. Patient Satisfaction/Experience Pain Scores using varied pain tools appropriate for setting

PATIENT CARE

1. **Pain agent dosages and use change dynamically with practice. Current pharmacy resources and/or consultation with a clinical pharmacist should occur during establishment of the plan for sedation with all patients.**

    a. Goals of pain management
- i. Shared goal setting, plan should be individualized and appropriate for each patient
- ii. Reduction of pain intensity with achievement of optimal analgesia with the fewest adverse effects
- iii. Enhancement of physical functioning: Patient is able to comfortably perform or participate in activities necessary for recovery
- iv. Improvement of sleep and psychologic functioning
- v. Reduction of healthcare utilization (e.g., length of stay or readmission)
- vi. Promotion of return to work/school and/or role within the family/society
- vii. Improvement of health-related quality of life

    b. Treatment considerations
- i. Consider the various types of pain and multidimensional nature of pain
- ii. Use combinations of nonpharmacologic and pharmacologic methods
- iii. Nonpharmacologic approaches to pain management
  - (a) Used to supplement analgesic medications
  - (b) May make pain more tolerable for undetermined intervals
  - (c) Use combinations of physical and psychologic strategies, where appropriate. Interventions can include:
    - (1) Clinician therapeutic voice, active listening, and empathy
    - (2) Patient-family education and counseling
    - (3) Cutaneous stimulation approach to pain

EXPERT TIP

Cutaneous stimulation approach to pain:
- May apply at pain site or distal, proximal, or contralateral to pain
- Avoid both heat and cold over radiation therapy sites
- Skin must be protected to avoid tissue damage
- Cold often more effective and longer lasting than heat
- Must be removed and reapplied intermittently
- Assess sensation to touch frequently

---

        a) Superficial heat and cold
- 1) Mechanism of action: Activation of large myelinated primary afferent fibers may modify response of spinal cord to noxious stimuli and decrease muscle spasm and sensitivity to pain. Heat may increase elastic properties of muscles. Cold may cause local numbing.
- 2) Indication: Joint and muscle pain, spasm, and stiffness (e.g., from surgery, trauma, arthritis, and acute low back pain). Heat preferred for thrombophlebitis. Cold preferred for acute trauma. Avoid cold in peripheral vascular disease.

        b) Massage
- 1) Mechanism of action: May inhibit transmission of painful stimuli and relaxes muscles
- 2) Indication: Stress, anxiety, muscle tension, spasm, pain, immobility
- 3) May be acceptable form of touch to convey care and concern, family can be involved

    c) Neuromuscular electrical stimulation (NMES) or transcutaneous electrical nerve stimulation (TENS): Commonly used by physiotherapists for pain relief, stimulation of denervated muscles, disused muscles, and wound healing
       1) Mechanism of action: May inhibit transmission of painful stimuli
       2) Indications: Acute surgical, musculoskeletal, neuropathic pain
       3) Modality should be avoided in patients with pacemakers

  (d) Physical approach to pain: Relieves muscle tension, keeps joints and ligaments flexible. Multiple benefits to systems that improve patient outcomes: Decrease wound and skin breakdown, loss of consciousness, and duration of mechanical ventilation. Functional strategies include:
    (1) Early mobilization
    (2) Therapeutic exercise
    (3) Physical therapy and occupational therapy
    (4) Repositioning
    (5) Immobilization

  (e) Cognitive-behavioral approach to pain: Interferes with neural perception of pain in the brain. Refocuses or directs attention away from painful stimuli, creating central modulation of pain. Reduces stress and anxiety and increases sense of control. Use with mild to moderate pain of brief duration, procedural pain.
    (1) Education
    (2) Coping strategies
    (3) Relaxation
       a) Recommended for procedural pain management in critically ill adults
    (4) Distraction
    (5) Television, reading, visiting, humor
    (6) Music and art
    (7) Animal-assisted interventions
    (8) Prayer, meditation, and affirmations
    (9) Computer-assisted interventions, smartphones, information, and communication technologies

iv. Complementary and alternative medicine (CAM) modalities
  (a) Mainly used in chronic pain conditions but also used in acute pain. Careful consideration of individual clinical situations is necessary.
  (b) Consider use at every pain control attempt
  (c) Overlap exists between CAM and other nonpharmacologic approaches
    (1) Biofeedback
    (2) Hypnosis
    (3) Aromatherapy
    (4) Yoga
    (5) Therapeutic touch and reflexology
    (6) Acupuncture

v. Interprofessional collaboration for pain control and prevention

> **KEY CONCEPT**
> Interprofessional approach should include:
> * Education of healthcare team at every level
> * Systematic approach to pain measurement using validated tools in the ICU: BPS, CPOT
> * Patients should be routinely assessed and reassessed
> * Preemptive analgesia and/or nonpharmacologic interventions
> * ICU interprofessional rounding and collaboration

    vi. Nurses play a pivotal role in coordinating care and achieving effective pain management for patients

    vii. Other disciplines represented can include anesthesiology, advanced practice providers, clinical nurse specialists, physicians, physical medicine and rehabilitation, neurosurgery, interventional radiology, physical therapy, pain management services, palliative care, pharmacy, psychology, care management, and social and chaplain services

    viii. Barriers and misconceptions regarding pain can obstruct effective pain management, including the clinician's, the patient's, and family member's personal values and beliefs, and confusion about addiction, tolerance, and physical dependence with regard to pain medications. Additional common barriers include: Communication, neurocognitive changes, triage of patient's clinical and physical findings, and cultural differences.

    ix. Pharmacologic methods

       (a) Choice of an analgesic depends on many factors (e.g., clinical judgment, patient history, type and severity of pain, patient response to interventions)

       (b) Optimal use requires the understanding of a medication's pharmacokinetics (e.g., time to onset, peak effect, duration of action) and pharmacodynamics (e.g., mechanism of action, metabolism, and excretion), short-acting, long-acting, and continuous, with or without basal rates

       (c) Medication route

          (1) Oral

          (2) Parenteral (intravenous [IV], subcutaneous [SC], intramuscular [IM])

          (3) Epidural (intrathecal)

          (4) Transdermal/SC

          (5) Transmucosal (e.g., buccal, intranasal, rectal)

       (d) Duration of action varies by medication, dosage, route, and clinical state of patient

          (1) Most parenteral, immediate-release, and short-acting (oral) formulations can last up to 3 to 4 hours

          (2) Controlled-release formulations last 8 to 12 hours; should be given "around the clock" (ATC), not as needed

          (3) Oral extended-release formulations last 12 to 24 hours

          (4) Transdermal patches last 48 to 96 hours

          (5) Multimodal or balanced analgesia combines analgesic regimens and opioids/nonopioids to reduce the likelihood of adverse effects from a single agent

(e) Nonopioid analgesics
  (1) NSAIDS
    a) Block synthesis of prostaglandins (e.g., cyclooxygenase [COX]-1 and COX-2) to decrease inflammation. Used for low to moderate pain control (e.g., menstrual pain, tension headache, gout).
    b) Include medications, such as aspirin, ibuprofen, naproxen, etodolac, meloxicam, etc.
    c) Not recommended to use COX-1–selective NSAID as an adjunct to opioid therapy for pain management in critically ill adults
  (2) Glucocorticoids
    a) Regulated by adrenal glands
    b) Reduce pain from inflammation by blocking the intracellular conversion of phospholipids to arachidonic acid, inhibiting the production of prostaglandins and leukotrienes
  (3) Acetaminophen
    a) Has analgesic and antipyretic properties, often first line for pain problems, such as osteoarthritis (OA)
    b) No proven antiinflammatory effect, scientists have speculated it blocks COX-3 in CNS compared with PNS
    c) Can cause liver toxicity in doses over 4 grams daily
    d) Recommend use as adjuvant therapy to an opioid
  (4) Nefopam
    a) Nonopioid analgesic that inhibits dopamine, noradrenaline, and serotonin recapture in both the spinal and supraspinal spaces.
    b) Recommended to use either as an adjunct or replacement for an opioid to reduce opioid use and their safety concerns for pain management in critically ill adults
  (5) Antidepressants
    a) Effect may be related to inhibition of the reuptake of serotonin and norepinephrine in pain inhibitory pathways, as well as a peripheral mechanism involving β2-adrenergic receptors
    b) Tricyclic antidepressants (e.g., amitriptyline) and serotonin-norepinephrine (noradrenaline) reuptake inhibitors (e.g., duloxetine) commonly used, especially for neuropathic pain
  (6) Neuropathic pain medications
    a) Provide analgesic effect by lowering neurotransmitter release or reducing neuronal firing
    b) Examples include gabapentin, carbamazepine, or pregabalin
    c) Used for over several decades for nonnarcotic pain management and relief
    d) Recommended for use after cardiovascular surgery for patients in ICU
  (7) Topical analgesics
    a) Applied topically
    b) Medications, such as lidocaine or capsaicin work by blocking nerve signals that send the feeling of pain from the site of injury to the brain
    c) Creates a temporary loss of feeling to the area where it is applied
    d) Examples, such as capsaicin appear to deplete local neurons of substance P, required in the transmission of nociceptive input

e) IV lidocaine not recommended as adjunct to opioid therapy for pain management

(8) Volatile anesthetics

a) Traditionally used for general anesthesia

b) Rapid onset and recovery and has demonstrated cardioprotective effects, such as preserved mitochondrial oxygen consumption

c) Recommend not using inhaled volatile anesthetics for procedural pain management in critically ill adults

(9) Antispasmodics and muscle relaxants

a) Interrupts signaling to neurons in the CNS to decrease muscle tone and cause relaxation

b) Can cause sedation

(f) Nonpharmacologic therapies

(1) Cybertherapy/hypnosis

a) Low recommendation on offering cybertherapy (VR) or hypnosis for pain management in critically ill adults

b) Many factors (i.e., resources, ICU environment, extensive training, and patient acceptability) make this option difficult to implement.

(2) TENS applied to skin through patches delivers electrical impulse affecting peripheral nerves to decrease pain sensation; commonly used in nerve-related pain and applied several times daily for 10 to 30 minutes.

(3) Massage

a) Can be used to relieve tension of muscles surrounding a site of pain

b) Recommend massage for pain management in critically ill adults with proper training of nursing staff or designated healthcare staff

(4) Music

a) Listening to music for 10- to 45-minute increments can be helpful to relieve both nonprocedural and procedural pain in critically ill adults

(5) Acupuncture/acupressure

a) Can cause the release of inhibitory neurotransmitters, such as norepinephrine and serotonin to enhance the descending inhibitory pain pathway through pressure to areas of pain

(6) Cognitive behavioral therapy

a) Reduces pain by modifying maladaptive behaviors, physical sensations, and catastrophic thinking

b) Form of psychotherapy popular for use with chronic pain

c) Maladaptive cognitions can help maintain behavioral problems and symptoms of emotional distress

d) Can improve quality of life for individuals with depression, anxiety, fibromyalgia, arthralgia, etc.

(7) CAM

a) May involve cultural practices or use of herbal medications for pain relief (i.e., tai chi, yoga, devil's claw)

b) Medical cannabis/tetrahydrocannabinol (THC)

1) Many states have approved medical cannabis for use for pain relief and other medical conditions like fibromyalgia/seizures; THC/cannabidiol (CBD)

TABLE 20.6 **Classification of Opioids by Synthetic Process**		
Naturally Occurring Compounds	**Semisynthetic Compounds**	**Synthetic Compounds**
Morphine	Diamorphine (heroin)	Pethidine
Codeine	Dihydromorphone	Fentanyl
Thebaine	Buprenorphine	Methadone
Papaverine	Oxycodone	Alfentanil
		Remifentanil
		Tapentadol

Modified from Devlin, J., Skrobik, Y., Gélinas, C., et al. (2018). Clinical practice guidelines for the prevention and management of pain, agitation/sedation, delirium, immobility, and sleep disruption in adult patients in the ICU. *Critical Care Medicine*, 46(9), e825–e873.

      (8) Therapeutic heat/cold
        a) Application direct to the site of pain can reduce pain response and sensation
        b) Cold therapy for procedural pain management in critically ill adults is recommended especially for acute pain
  (g) Opioids
      (1) Classification types
        a) Naturally-occurring: Codeine, morphine
        b) Synthetic: Meperidine, fentanyl, methadone, tramadol, tapentadol
        c) Semisynthetic: Hydrocodone, hydromorphone, oxycodone, oxymorphone, buprenorphine (ICSI, 2017) (Table 20.6)
      (2) Basic pharmacology
        a) Opioids are classified according to their effect at opioid receptors to block pain. Can be agonists, partial agonists and antagonists.
          1) Agonist: Interacts with receptor to produce maximum analgesic effect
          2) Antagonist: Bind to receptor to produce no effect
          3) Partial agonist: Bind to opioid receptor but produce only partial analgesic response
      (3) Properties of opioid receptors
        a) Mu (Mu1, Mu2)
        b) Mu1: Supraspinal analgesia, bradycardia, sedation
        c) Mu2: Respiratory depression, euphoria, physical dependence
        d) Delta: Spinal analgesia, respiratory depression
        e) Kappa: Spinal analgesia, respiratory depression, sedation

EXPERT TIP
Opioids block the release of neurotransmitters at the opioid receptor sites.

  (h) Three broad categories of analgesics are used in pain management
      (1) Nonopioids
        a) Overview: When possible, consider scheduling medication to reduce narcotic use and side effects. Reduce dosages in the older adults and in those with renal or hepatic insufficiency (includes NSAIDs and acetaminophen).

b) Indications: Acute and chronic pain related to many causes, including surgery, trauma, arthritis, and cancer. May be effective for relief of mild pain when used alone. Both acetaminophen and NSAIDs have analgesic and antipyretic effects; NSAIDs are also effective for inflammatory pain.

c) Mechanism of action: NSAIDs have both peripheral and central actions. Nonselective NSAIDs inhibit two isoforms of COX (COX-1 and COX-2). Inhibition of COX-1, normally found in tissues (e.g., platelets, gastrointestinal [GI] tract, kidneys), results in the adverse effects of NSAIDs. Inhibition of COX-2 decreases inflammation by inhibiting prostaglandin formation.

d) Benefits: Nonopioids provide analgesia without the sedative and respiratory adverse effects of opioids, so their concurrent use allows lower opioid dosages to be given without reducing analgesia (known as *"opioid dose-sparing"* effect). Short- and moderate-duration–acting NSAIDs (e.g., naproxen, ibuprofen) are preferred for most patients.

e) Adverse effects (AEs): NSAIDs:
   1) Inhibition of platelet aggregation
   2) Adverse GI effects (e.g., ulcerations, bleeding)
   3) Renal insufficiency and acute renal failure
   4) CNS dysfunction (e.g., decreased attention span, headache)
   5) Hypersensitivity
      i) Acetaminophen: Can cause severe hepatotoxicity in patients with chronic alcoholism or liver disease and in fasting patients

(i) Opioids (Table 20.7)
   (1) Overview: Foundation of effective pain management in acutely ill patients, procedural pain
   (2) Indications: Moderate to severe acute and cancer pain, some chronic pain syndromes, and procedural pain
   (3) Adverse effects: Sedation, respiratory depression, nausea, vomiting, mental clouding, pruritus, hypotension and urinary retention usually occur with initiation of opioid therapy; however, tolerance develops, usually within a matter of days. Most adverse effects are dose related.

(j) Adjuvants: Medications that are analgesic under some conditions with a primary indication other than pain (Table 20.8)

(k) Procedural/interventional

(l) Injections

(m) Neuromodulation and neuroablation

(n) Brain and spinal cord stimulation

(o) Bolus, continuous, patient-controlled analgesia (PCA)

(p) Peripheral nerve blocks (regional)

(q) Continuous nerve blocks; average duration can be up to 3 days

PATIENT EDUCATION

1. **Continuum care education**
   a. Appropriate use of pain scales or other methods to be used to assess pain
   b. Effective pain management concepts and options (e.g., pain medications and the difference between tolerance, physical dependence, and psychologic dependence)
   c. Promote safety, comfort, and quality of life

TABLE 20.7 Opioid Analgesic

Medication	Dosing	Onset and Duration	Comments
Fentanyl (IV)	• Loading dose: 1–2 mcg/kg • Intermittent dose: • Maintenance dose: 0.35–1.5 mcg/kg every 30–60 minutes • IV infusion: 0.7–10 mcg/kg/h infusion (50–700 mcg/h) • IV infusion with as needed intermittent bolus dosing	Onset: Less than 1–2 minutes Duration: 30–60 minutes for intermittent dose	• Half-life: 2–4 hours • Metabolic pathway: Hepatic, CYP3A4/5 substrate • Accumulates in hepatic impairment • Minimal or no histamine release • Less hypotension than morphine because of minimal histamine release
PCA Fentanyl	Concentration 10 mcg/mL Loading dose 5–20 mcg	Demand dose: 5–20 mcg Lock-out interval: 4–10 min	Max in 4 hours 300 mcg
Hydromorphone (IV, PO)	• Loading dose: 0.5–2 mg • IV intermittent: 0.2–1 mg every 1–2 hours • IV infusion: 0.5–3 mg/h infusion • PO: 7.5 mg	Onset: 5–15 min Duration: 4–5 hours	• Half-life: 2–3 hours • Metabolic pathway: Glucuronidation (Non-CYP), nephrotoxic • Accumulates in hepatic and/or renal impairment; slow titration is needed
PCA Hydromorphone	Concentration: 0.2 mg/mL Loading dose: 0.05–0.4 mg	Demand dose: 0.05–0.4 mg Lock-out interval: 5–10 min	Max in 4 hours 6 mg
Morphine (IV, PO)	• Loading dose: 2–10 mg • IV intermittent: 2–10 mg every 1–2 hours • IV infusion: 0.07–0.5 mg/kg/h infusion • PO: 30 mg	Onset: 5–10 min Duration: 4–5 hours	• Half-life: 3–4 hours • Metabolic pathway: Glucuronidation (Non-CYP) • Good alternative for patients on medications that alter CYP3A4 metabolism and will with fentanyl • Accumulates in hepatic and/or renal impairment; slow titration is needed • Preload reduction and myocardial depression; this may be a desirable effect, may also be undesirable • Histamine release and vagal vasodilation leading to hypotension, and bradycardia

Continued

TABLE 20.7   **Opioid Analgesic—cont'd**

Medication	Dosing	Onset and Duration	Comments
PCA Morphine	Concentration: 1 mg/mL Initial loading: 1 mg	Demand dose: 0.5–2.5 mg Lock-out interval: 5–10 minutes	Max in 4 hours 30 mg
Remifentanil	• Loading dose: Optional: 1.5 mcg/kg • IV infusion: 0.5–15 mcg/kg/h infusion (using ideal body weight); Max 0.2–0.4 mcg/kg/min	Onset: 1–3 minutes Duration: 5–10 minutes	• Very short acting, quick reversal when stopped • Metabolism: Hydrolysis by plasma esterase • Does not accumulate in hepatic and/or renal impairment • Advantage over longer-acting opioids in neurologic assessment and multiorgan failure

Medication tables are not meant to be all-inclusive but to point out common medication dose and usage based on recent guideline recommendations and do not replace the use of approved pharmacy resources that are updated frequently.

IV, Intravenous; *PCA,* patient controlled analgesia; *PO,* per mouth.

From Devlin, J., Skrobik, Y., Gélinas, C., et al. (2018). Clinical practice guidelines for the prevention and management of pain, agitation/sedation, delirium, immobility, and sleep disruption in adult patients in the ICU. *Critical Care Medicine, 46*(9). e825–e873; Lexicomp. (2020). *Drug information handbook: a clinically relevant resource for all healthcare professionals,* 25th ed. Hudson, OH: Lexi-Comp, Inc.; Clinical Pharmacology Online, Elsevier. Available at: https://www.clinicalkey.com/pharmacology/. Accessed January 15, 2021; Clinical Pharmacology Online. Elsevier. Available at: https://www.clinicalkey.com/pharmacology/. Accessed January 15, 2021.

TABLE 20.8 Adjuvant Medications Commonly Used to Treat Pain

Medication	Indication and Mechanism of Action	Adverse Effects	Comments
Anticonvulsants: gabapentin, pregabalin, carbamazepine	Use to treat neuropathic pain (e.g., diabetic or postherpetic neuropathy) Cell membrane stabilizer, decreases ectopic neuron firing, calcium channel	Sedation, mental clouding, dizziness, gastrointestinal upset	• Pain management in ICU patients who have had cardiovascular surgery • Gabapentin (widely used) usually dosed, starting dose 100–300 mg 3 times a day; titrate slowly up to a max of 3600 mg/day until symptoms resolve or adverse effects occur • Reduce dose in renal insufficiency • Avoid or stop use if decrease LOC
Acetaminophen (IV/PR/PO)	Usually first-line agent in mild to moderate nociceptive pain Mechanism of action remains unclear; it is historically categorized along with NSAIDs because it inhibits the cyclooxygenase (COX) pathways	Adverse effects of acetaminophen administered may include the following: Hepatotoxicity Skin rash, hypersensitivity reactions Nephrotoxicity (elevations in BUN, creatinine) Hematologic: Anemia, leukopenia, neutropenia, pancytopenia Decreased serum bicarbonate Decreased levels of sodium and calcium Hyperammonemia Hyperchloremia Hyperuricemia Increased serum glucose Increased bilirubin and alkaline phosphatase	• Used as adjunct to opioid to decrease pain and opioid use in critically ill patients • Caution is necessary for patients with renal or hepatic impairment or patients with alcoholic liver disease, glucose 6 phosphate dehydrogenase deficiency, or severe hypovolemia • Avoid or stop if increase LFTs
Nefopam	Primary unknown but thought to increase the inhibiting tone of serotonergic and noradrenergic/norepinephrinergic descending pathways by inhibiting the synaptic uptake of dopamine, noradrenaline/norepinephrine, and serotonin	Diaphoresis, nausea, sedation	***Not available in North America Stop or avoid use if risk of increased heart rate Anticholinergic effects (urinary retention, seizure, delirium, glaucoma) If administered, administer alone as an alternate therapy to opioids

Continued

TABLE 20.8 Adjuvant Medications Commonly Used to Treat Pain—cont'd

Medication	Indication and Mechanism of Action	Adverse Effects	Comments
Low-dose ketamine	N-methyl-D-aspartate (NMDA) receptors, opioid receptors, monoaminergic receptors, muscarinic receptors, and voltage sensitive Ca ion channel receptor antagonist with analgesic and anesthetic effects	Severe allergic reaction (anaphylaxis) Cardiac arrhythmia Depressed cough reflex Muscle twitching Increased salivation Muscle spasms High blood pressure (hypertension) Fast or slow heart rate Seizures Visual hallucinations Vivid dreams Double vision Low blood pressure (hypotension)	• 0.5 mg/kg IVP × 1; 1–2 mcg/kg/min as adjunct to opioid therapy when trying to reduce opioid use in postsurgery cardiovascular ICU patients • Stop or avoid if decrease LOC

BUN, Blood urea nitrogen; *ICU*, intensive care unit; *IV*, intravenous; *IVP*, intravenous pyelogram; *LFTs*, liver function tests; *LOC*, loss of consciousness; *NSAID*, nonsteroidal antiinflammatory drug; *PO*, per mouth; *PR*, as needed.

From Devlin, J., Skrobik, Y., Gélinas, C., et al. (2018). Clinical practice guidelines for the prevention and management of pain, agitation/sedation, delirium, immobility, and sleep disruption in adult patients in the ICU. *Critical Care Medicine*, 46(9), e825–e873; Lexicomp. (2020). *Drug information handbook: a clinically relevant resource for all healthcare professionals*, ed 25. Hudson, OH: Lexi-Comp, Inc; Clinical Pharmacology Online. Elsevier. Available at: https://www.clinicalkey.com/pharmacology/. Accessed January 15, 2021.

2. **Acute education**
   a. Pain management as an important part of patient care
   b. Responsibility of the patient to report ineffective pain relief and concerns regarding the pain management plan
   c. Patient/family/caregiver education
   d. Discharge planning
   e. Use of appropriate pain scales and methods to be used to assess pain
   f. Develop patient specific goals, which include pain relief and functional ability
   g. Transition to oral medications, with the lowest side effect profile
   h. Responsibility of the patient to report ineffective pain relief and concerns regarding the pain management plan
   i. Management of pain medication adverse effects (e.g., constipation)

SPECIFIC CLINICAL PROBLEMS RELATED TO PAIN THERAPY

1. **Respiratory comprise the most serious of related problems**
   a. Pathophysiology
      i. Overall decrease in respiratory function generally because of sedation
      ii. Decreased respiratory rate and lung excursion
   b. Patients at risk

> **KEY CONCEPT**
> Avoid respiratory compromise, sedation, constipation, and GI adverse effects by starting with low doses, evaluate frequently, and slowly increase doses of pain medication.

      i. Age over 55 years
      ii. Preexisting pulmonary disease (e.g., COPD)
      iii. Breathing difficulty at baseline
      iv. Known or suspected sleep-disordered breathing
      v. Obstructive sleep apnea
      vi. Oral or airway abnormalities
      vii. Comorbidities (systemic, renal, or hepatic)
      viii. Preoperative anesthesia risk
   c. Signs and symptoms
      i. Overt signs and symptoms tend to be late findings
      ii. Low end-tidal volumes (mechanically ventilated)
      iii. Low respiratory rate
      iv. Shallow breathing
      v. Depressed vital signs
      vi. Agitation and delirium (see Ch. 2, Psychosocial Aspects of High Acuity and Critical Care)
   d. Diagnostic study finding: Chest x-ray—Atelectasis
   e. Noninvasive study findings: End-tidal carbon dioxide, pulse oximetry (SPO_2) monitoring may be a late sign of respiratory depression
   f. Invasive study findings: Increased arterial partial pressure of carbon dioxide ($PaCO_2$) levels, decreased arterial partial pressure of oxygen (PaO_2) levels
2. **Oversedation (see Ch. 19, Sedation)**
   a. Pathophysiology: Side effect of most pain medications and interventions, CNS depressant, opioid receptor modulation
   b. Complications include but are not limited to: Decreased mobility, deconditioning, skin breakdown from immobility, constipation, atelectasis, and respiratory depression

> **KEY CONCEPT**
> Think critically; anticipate and recognize tipping points and complications that can create multisystem chains of events throughout body.

   c. All patients at risk
   d. Reversal agents
      i. Naloxone: Opiate antagonist competitively binds to the opioid receptors
        (a) Complications of naloxone
          (1) Development of pulmonary edema and hypertension
          (2) Patient may renarcotize as the half-life of naloxone is about 20 minutes and the half-life of most narcotics is greater than 20 minutes
      ii. Flumazenil: Reversal of benzodiazepine effects
        (a) Complications of flumazenil
          (1) Risk of seizures
3. **Constipation/other GI effects**
   a. Pathophysiology: Slowed GI motility
   b. Treat with aggressive bowel regimen when on opioids
4. **Uncontrolled pain**
   a. Treat with increased opioid dosing and add pain adjunct
   b. Consider scheduled opioid dosing around the clock at a lower dose to minimize side effect of peaks and troughs
   c. Hyperalgesia: Increased pain despite escalating doses with uncontrolled side effect
   d. Treat with opioid rotation, consider specialty consultation

SPECIFIC PATIENT HEALTH PROBLEMS

1. **Key pain issues and concerns by topic**
   a. Opioid-tolerant patients
      i. Two types of opioid-tolerant patients
        (a) Chronic pain patients who tolerate opioids
        (b) Patient opioid use because of addiction
      ii. Recognize signs of drug-seeking and relief-seeking behaviors
      iii. Prevention of transition of acute pain to chronic pain
      iv. High risk of undertreatment of pain or pain treatment being withheld
      v. Accept the patient's self-report of pain
      vi. May need higher doses for effective pain relief
      vii. Risk of respiratory depression is less in this population but still exists
      viii. Opiate agonist, such as methadone treat addiction, not pain
      ix. Understand the difference between addiction and pseudoaddiction
      x. Withdrawal risk and effect on critical illness
      xi. Psychosocial misconceptions, false beliefs, behaviors, and stereotyping by patient and healthcare team
   b. Older adult with or without dementia (see Ch. 16, Older Adult Patients)

> **KEY CONCEPT**
> Older adults and pain management:
> - Challenge in identifying pain in persons with dementia
> - Effect of untreated pain is deterioration of physical, cognitive, and functional ability
> - Untreated pain can lead to an increase in behavioral and physiological symptoms of dementia

      i. Underidentification of pain and undertreatment of pain

     ii. Delirium related to pain and/or pain medications

    iii. Chronic pain

    iv. Substance abuse, polypharmacy, and additive effects of pain and sedation

     v. Withdrawal

    vi. Reduced clearance of medications by liver and kidney

   vii. Decreased sensory of pain leading to injury (e.g., skin breakdown, infection, untreated chest pain)

c. Diabetic patient (see Ch. 7, Endocrine System)

      i. Neuropathy treated along with acute pain treatment with multimodality focus

     ii. Risk of skin breakdown and impaired healing

    iii. Reduced or heightened pain

d. Sickle cell crisis (see Ch. 8, Hematologic and Immune Systems)

      i. Specific pain needs and guidelines

     ii. Risk of undertreatment

    iii. Alterations in opioid metabolism

    iv. Neuropathic pain

     v. Pain can decrease fluid intake and contribute to hypoventilation, which can heighten pain

e. Bariatric patient (see Ch. 15, Bariatric Patients)

      i. Obstructive sleep apnea

     ii. Medication dosing

    iii. Gastrointestinal motility

f. Pulmonary patient (see Ch. 3, Pulmonary System)

      i. Thoracic surgery

        (a) Epidural analgesia and paravertebral block

        (b) Intercostal and intrapleural blocks

     ii. Mechanically ventilated patient

g. Cardiology patient (see Ch. 4, Cardiovascular System)

      i. Chest pain

     ii. Open heart surgery

h. Neurologic patient (see Ch. 5, Neurologic System)

      i. Neurogenic, neuropathic, central pain, and chronic pain issues

     ii. Identification of pain in nonverbal patients and patients with altered cognition

    iii. Treatment of pain

        (a) Effect of sedation and level of consciousness

        (b) Identification of changes in neurologic status

i. Burn patients (see Ch. 12, Burns)

      i. Specific pain needs, treatments, and guidelines

     ii. Physiologic changes contribute to pharmacokinetics and pharmacodynamics, creating inconsistent responses to medications

j. Trauma patient (see Ch. 11, Multisystem Trauma)

      i. Transport of trauma patients and pain control consideration (see Ch. 18, Patient Transport)

     ii. Under- and overtreatment of pain

    iii. Specific pain needs, treatments, and guidelines

k. Palliative and end of life (see Ch. 21, Palliative and End-of-Life Care)

      i. Specific pain needs, treatments, and guidelines

References and bibliography information are available at http://evolve.elsevier.com/AACN/corecurriculum/.

Pain

20

Palliative and End-of-Life Care

Clareen Wiencek, PhD, RN, ACNP, ACHPN, FAAN

CROSSWALK

- **Quality and Safety in Nursing Education (QSEN):** Patient-centered care, Teamwork and collaboration, Evidence-based practice, Quality improvement, Safety, Informatics
- **National Patient Safety Goals:** Identify patients correctly, Improve staff communication, Use medicines safely, Prevent infection, Identify patient safety risks
- **American Nurses Association (ANA) Standards for Professional Nursing Practice:** Standard 1. Assessment, Standard 2. Diagnosis, Standard 3. Outcomes identification, Standard 4. Planning, Standard 5. Implementation, Standard 6. Evaluation, Standard 7. Ethics, Standard 8. Culturally congruent practice, Standard 9. Communication, Standard 10. Collaboration, Standard 11. Leadership, Standard 12. Education, Standard 13. Evidence-based practice and research, Standard 14. Quality of practice, Standard 16. Resource utilization, Standard 17. Environmental health
- **AACN Scope and Standards for Progressive and Critical Care Nursing Practice:** Standard 1. Quality of practice, Standard 3. Education, Standard 4. Communication, Standard 5. Ethics, Standard 6. Collaboration, Standard 7. Evidence-based practice/research/clinical inquiry, Standard 8. Resource utilization, Standard 9. Leadership, Standard 10. Environmental health
- **AACN Standards for Establishing and Sustaining Healthy Work Environments (HWE):** Skilled communication, True collaboration, Effective decision-making, Meaningful recognition
- **PCCN content:** Multisystem—End-of-Life
- **CCRN content:** Multisystem—End-of-Life

SYSTEMWIDE ELEMENTS

CONCEPT REVIEW

1. **Descriptions**
   a. The terms *palliative care, hospice,* and *end-of-life care* are often used synonymously. The care provided is similar, but the time frame in which the care is provided, and the reimbursement mechanisms vary. Similarities include:
      i. Patient- and family-centered care
      ii. Care is provided by an interprofessional team
      iii. Advance care planning
      iv. Care is in accordance with the patient and family wishes/goals of care
      v. Quality of life is optimized
      vi. Care is holistic
      vii. Communication expertise
      viii. Organized and structured system of care

b. Palliative care (PC): Can be initiated anytime within the course of disease or life-threatening illness; however, it is most beneficial when initiated early. PC is appropriate at any age and any stage in a serious illness, and it can be provided along with curative treatment.

> **KEY CONCEPT**
> PC can be initiated at any age and any stage in a serious illness. It may also be provided along with curative treatment. PC can also be provided in the outpatient, acute, and critical care settings.

    c. Hospice: A specific type of PC provided to individuals with a life expectancy measured in months, not years. Hospice teams provide patients and families with expert medical care, emotional, and spiritual support, focusing on improving patient and family quality of life. The patient must meet the criteria to receive hospice under the Medicare or Medicaid hospice benefit, despite source of insurance.
        i. In the setting of terminal illness, disease-modifying therapies may no longer be beneficial and cause more harm than good
        ii. Grief and bereavement services are provided to the family
    d. End-of-life care (EOLC): Supports the needs of those patients, and their families, who are imminently facing death

2. **Background**
    a. Etiology
        i. Annually, more than 5 million patients are admitted to the intensive care unit (ICU), and an average of 55,000 ICU patients are being cared for daily across the United States.
        ii. Some 20% of dying patients experience an ICU stay within 3 days of their death.
        iii. The Center to Advance Palliative Care (CAPC, 2020) reports that in 2019, 72% of hospitals with more than 50 beds and 94% of hospitals with more than 300 beds report a PC team. This is an increase from 67% in 2015 and only 7% in 2001.

3. **The changing U.S. populace and need for PC, hospice, and EOLC**
    a. By 2035, it is estimated that 78 million Americans will be over the age of 65 years and that 81% of this demographic will be living with multiple chronic conditions.
    b. Currently, 90 million Americans live with chronic illnesses in the United States, and, despite our best efforts, 70% will die of their condition.
    c. By 2030, chronic and life-limiting illnesses, such as dementia and cancer are also expected to rise by 45% within this aging population.
    d. There are an increasing number of patients with chronic conditions requiring complex care who frequently are functionally dependent, requiring institutionalized care. In 2019 at least 12 million adults and over 400,000 children live with a serious illness.
    e. In addition, the United States has an increasingly diverse population that requires culturally congruent care, particularly in regard to healthcare beliefs and the dying process.
    f. PC and EOLC is needed to meet the demands of our changing population, to assure our aging and chronically ill patients receive the care they deserve.

4. **Who will benefit from PC**
    a. Persons of all ages throughout the life span
    b. Those living with persistent, progressive, or recurring medical conditions
        i. This includes patients who require long-term supportive care
        ii. Patients with developmental or intellectual disabilities
        iii. Patients with life-limiting illnesses

Palliative and
End-of-Life Care

21

BOX 21.1   **Benefits of Palliative Care**

- Improved quality of life
- Improved symptom management
- Improved mood
- Improved satisfaction (patients, families, and providers)
- Improved survival
- Increase in advanced care planning
- Improved healthcare resource utilization
- Improved patient and family support
- Decreased hospital readmission rates
- Decreased costs of care

From Hartjes, T. (2015). Making the case for palliative care in critical care. *Critical Care Nursing Clinics of North America*, 27(3), 289–295.

    c. In the National Consensus Project, 2018, vulnerable and underserved populations were mentioned as a special population (e.g., homeless, migrant workers, veterans, prisoners, older adults, and persons with mental illness)

5. Benefits of PC (Box 21.1)

    a. PC can be offered in conjunction with disease-modifying therapy, such as ICU care, surgery, or chemotherapy, whether or not cure is possible

    b. PC provides biopsychosocial support to the patient, to relieve symptoms, support the family, and improve quality of life.

6. Models of PC and hospice (Table 21.1)

    a. Seriously ill and injured patients, families, and communities should receive quality PC in all care settings. This is achieved by the delivery of primary palliative nursing by every nurse, regardless of setting. In 2017 the American Nurses Association in collaboration with multiple nursing organizations called for nurses to lead and transform the delivery of PC: This call to action encourages every nurse to provide primary PC at the bedside. If a formal PC consult is required, it would be provided by certified advanced practice nurses and physicians in a consulting role congruent with the 2015 National Academy of Medicine (formerly the Institute of Medicine) report that defined primary and specialist PC.

    b. Primary: An integrative approach that incorporates PC principles into the daily practice of the unit and the providers. Care is patient- and family-centered. Examples include:

        i. Effective and timely communication between patients, their families, and ICU providers

        ii. Education of patients and families, who are included in decision-making processes

        iii. Basic discussions of prognosis, goals of treatment, and code status

        iv. Ensuring the alignment of treatment plans with patients' goals

        v. Management of pain and common symptoms that are not complex or requiring specialist level PC

        vi. Initiating discussion of social and spiritual support

        vii. Considerations for transitions of care postdischarge

    c. Specialist or consultative: This approach includes an interprofessional team, which is external to the critical care setting, and who has special knowledge, experience and preferably certification in PC. The implementation of this approach is varied. Management includes:

        i. Refractory pain or complex symptoms

        ii. Complex physiologic or existential distress

TABLE 21.1 **Palliative Models of Care**		
Integrative/Primary Palliative Care	**Consultative/Specialist Palliative Care**	**Combination Approach**
• In this model, the basic PC needs of ICU patients are integrated into daily practice by the ICU staff • Staff training in PC • Weekly interprofessional ICU team rounds for patients who stay longer than 5 days • Use of PC protocols or bundles are used • Allows PC to be tailored to meet the needs of individual units (e.g., ICUs often operate under a "closed" model) • Communication between team members and patient/family is timely • Assures alignment of care and patient goals	• Interprofessional team that is external to the ICU with an expertise in PC • Roles include communicating prognosis, treatment options, and assessing and working with patients and families to establish patient-centered goals of care • Consultative models avoid overburdening ICU staff, who frequently struggle to find time for family meetings and goals of care discussions during busy shifts • Must have hospital infrastructure and support to implement • Works well with an "open" ICU model	• Ideally, consultative and integrative PC should be combined in the ICU to provide the greatest improvements in symptom control and communication with family members • This can be achieved by including a specialist PC team on daily/weekly ICU rounds, which studies show increases the use of PC in the ICU and decreases overall ICU LOS without increasing mortality • Nurses can facilitate and document these weekly rounds, as well as serve as advocates and navigators of the healthcare system for the patient and family

ICU, Intensive care unit; *LOS,* length of stay; *PC,* palliative care

From Hartjes, T., Meece, L., Horgas, A. (2014). Implementing palliative care in the ICU: providing patient and family centered care. *Nursing Critical Care,* 9(4), 17–22; Hartjes, T. (2015). Predicting which patients will benefit from palliative care: use of bundles, triggers and protocols. *Critical Care Nursing Clinics of North America,* 27(3), 307–314.

     iii. Assistance with conflict resolution regarding goals or methods of treatment
     iv. Assistance in addressing cases of near futility
     v. Assisting patients as they transition between hospital units to ensure care continuity
  d. The Medicare Hospice Benefit affords patients four levels of care to meet their clinical needs: Routine home care, general inpatient care (GIP), continuous home care, and inpatient respite care. Payment covers all aspects of the patient's care related to the terminal illness, including all services delivered by the interdisciplinary team, medication, medical equipment, and supplies. Routine home care is the most common. However, GIP is provided in a Medicare certified hospital or nursing facility for pain control or other acute symptom management and requires 24-hour care by a registered nurse (RN).

7. **PC and EOLC quality standards and metrics**
  a. National Consensus Project for Quality Palliative Care (NCP): Leaders from across the United States met to discuss the standardization of PC with the goal of improving quality of care. The 4th edition was published in 2018.
     i. Eight domains of practice are necessary to provide quality PC:
       (a) Domain 1: Structure and Processes of Care
       (b) Domain 2: Physical Aspects of Care
       (c) Domain 3: Psychologic and Psychiatric Aspects
       (d) Domain 4: Social Aspects of Care
       (e) Domain 5: Spiritual, Religious, and Existential Aspects of Care

      (f) Domain 6: Cultural Aspects of Care

      (g) Domain 7: Care of the Patient Nearing the End of Life

      (h) Domain 8: Ethical and Legal Aspects of Care

   ii. The National Academy of Medicine (formerly the Institute of Medicine) has identified six aims for quality healthcare, and this has been incorporated into the NCP guidelines previously discussed. They include care that is:

      (a) Timely

      (b) Patient-centered

      (c) Beneficial and effective

      (d) Accessible and equal

      (e) Knowledgeable (based on evidenced-based practice)

      (f) Efficient

   iii. The Joint Commission uses the NCP Guidelines for Quality Palliative Care as a basis for recommended standards of care and advanced certification.

   iv. The National Quality Forum has identified 14 quality measures to be evaluated by PC, hospice, and EOLC programs, as well as 38 preferred practices to ensure quality, outlined within the eight domains of practice (National Consensus Project, 2018).

   v. The American Academy of Hospice and Palliative Medicine and Hospice and Palliative Nursing Association recommendations, "Measuring What Matters Top 10"

      (a) These quality measures use the National Consensus Project for quality PC previously discussed. They include:

         (1) Comprehensive assessment

         (2) Screening for physical symptoms

         (3) Pain treatment

         (4) Dyspnea screening and management

         (5) Discussion of emotional or psychologic needs

         (6) Discussion of emotional/religious concerns

         (7) Documentation of a healthcare surrogate

         (8) Treatment preferences

         (9) Care consistency with documented preferences

         (10) Global measure for quality of care

   vi. The guidelines do not discuss care specific to the ICU. The Center to Advance Palliative Care (CAPC) and the National Institutes of Health created the following tools to assist in the development and implementation of PC in critical care (CAPC, 2020):

      (a) Improving PC in the ICU project (IPAL-ICU)

      (b) Improving PC in the emergency department (ED) project (IPAL-ED)

 b. Certification and credentialing of PC programs, staff, and facilities will improve quality of services provided

 c. Education and continuous training of all team members

   i. In 2015 the IOM described the importance of PC and hospice education for all healthcare providers

   ii. Many medical and nursing schools are incorporating communication and PC content into their curricula. This will enable providers to discuss advance care planning, deliver "bad news" when needed, and create treatment plans with the patient's and family's goals of care in mind.

> **BOX 21.2   Examples of Screening Criteria for Palliative Care Consults**
>
> - Life-limiting or life-threatening condition
> - The "surprise question": Would you be surprised if the patient died within 12 months? If the answer is "No," then the patient may benefit from PC
> - Frequent admissions for same condition
> - Current hospice patient or diagnosis with less than 6 months to live
> - Difficult-to-control physical or psychologic symptoms
> - Prolonged ICU admission >10 days
> - Awaiting, or deemed ineligible for, solid-organ transplantation
> - Patient/family/surrogate emotional, spiritual, or relational distress
> - Multisystem organ failure or artificial life support therapy in place
> - Patient has undergone any type of palliative surgery
> - Withdrawal of treatment is being considered
> - Disagreement of goals of care within family and/or treatment team

ICU, Intensive care unit; *PC*, palliative care.
From Hartjes, T., Meece, L., Horgas, A. (2014). Implementing palliative care in the ICU: providing patient and family centered care. *Nursing Critical Care*, 9(4), 17–22; Hartjes, T. (2015). Predicting which patients will benefit from palliative care: use of bundles, triggers and protocols. *Critical Care Nursing Clinics of North America*, 27(3), 307–314. Implementing ICU Screening Criteria for Unmet Palliative Care Needs. A Guide for ICU and Palliative Care Staff A Technical Assistance Monograph from the IPAL-ICU Project 2013.

ASSESSMENT FOR PALLIATIVE CARE, HOSPICE, OR END-OF-LIFE CARE SERVICES

1. **Assessments should be completed on admission to the hospital and be ongoing (daily and with a change in condition) to appropriately identify high-acuity patients who may benefit from PC services (Box 21.2).**
   a. It is suggested that individualized screening criteria be created for each facility to "trigger" timely PC interventions or consults
   b. Triggers can be objective, or with patient- or disease-specific criteria
      i. A retrospective review of ICU admissions across the United States determined up to 20% met one or more primary triggers for PC. Of those patients requiring a PC consult, 85% were captured by five triggers.
      ii. It is important to capture patients and families in need early in their disease process or admission.
      iii. It is equally important to not overwhelm the consultative team with referrals; thus use of integrative/primary PC strategies is important, and the consultative team can assist with difficult-to-manage patients (difficult to control symptom management, complex communication, emotional or social concerns).
   c. Appraisal of patient characteristics: Patients with significant life-limiting illnesses or who are at end-of-life enter critical care units with a wide range of clinical characteristics. During their stay, their clinical status may slowly or abruptly improve or deteriorate. Changes in the patient's condition may involve one or all life-sustaining functions, and functions can be easy or nearly impossible to monitor with precision. Examples of clinical attributes that the nurse should assess when caring for these patients include the following: Resiliency, vulnerability, stability, complexity, resource availability, participation in care and decision-making, and predictability.

PATIENT CARE

1. **PC strategies can be integrated into the usual and daily care in the high-acuity setting:**
   a. Identification of medical decision maker
   b. Determination of advance directive status

    c. Investigation of resuscitation preference

    d. Distribution of family information leaflet

    e. Regular pain assessment

    f. Optimal pain management

    g. Offer of social work support

    h. Offer of spiritual support

    i. Interprofessional family meeting

2. **PC bundles: The care and communication PC bundle can be instituted and incorporates the nine strategies previously discussed based upon hospital admission day:**

> **KEY CONCEPT**
>
> High-acuity patient care settings are familiar with the concept of bundled care. These series of independent best-practice interventions, when provided together, can improve quality of care and good patient outcomes.

    a. Day 1: Identify decision maker, complete advance directives, determine code status, assess and manage reoccurring pain, and provide information leaflets (see Ch. 1 Professional Caring and Ethical Practice)

    b. Day 3: Visits by the social worker and chaplain

    c. Day 5 or sooner: Conduct a meeting between the family and the interprofessional PC team

      i. Forming the plan of care

      ii. Confirm understanding of medical opinion by patient and family

        (a) Disease-related

        (b) Treatment options

        (c) Prognosis

      iii. Understanding of the patient/family's wishes, goals, and values

        (a) Support patient and family in decision-making

      iv. Create the best plan in often difficult situations

      v. Communication pearls

        (a) The mnemonic "SPIKES" may be used to ensure a consistent and structured approach before the meeting. S-setting, P-perception, I-invitation or information, K-knowledge, E-empathy, S-summary or strategize

        (b) Think of the family conference as a procedure; it is just as important as any other aspect of care

        (c) Provide chunks of information and then check to assure they understand

        (d) Expect interruptions

        (e) 80–20 rule (listen 80%, speak 20%)

        (f) Nodding by the patient or family does not mean they understand what is being discussed

        (g) Restate and confirm decisions

3. **The use of protocols provides a standardized approach to care and are common in the high-acuity setting. Examples include algorithms, clinical pathways, and order sets.**

    a. Protocols and order sets that can facilitate and standardize PC include:

      i. Pain management

      ii. Sedation management

      iii. Compassionate extubation

      iv. Withdrawal of artificial support sedation orders

4. **Common patient care problems encountered in PC and EOLC**
   a. PC focuses on the relief of symptoms, such as pain, dyspnea, fatigue, constipation, nausea, loss of appetite, anorexia, dysphagia, depression, delirium, and difficulty sleeping
5. **Goals of symptom management**
   a. Achievement of optimal symptom management with the fewest adverse effects
   b. Frequent pain assessment, treatment, and reduction of pain intensity
   c. Enhancement of physical functioning
   d. Improvement of psychologic and spiritual functioning
   e. Reduction of unwanted and unnecessary healthcare utilization (e.g., length of stay or readmission)
   f. Promotion of return to work/school and/or role within the family/society
   g. Improvement of health-related quality of life
6. **Interprofessional collaboration: Nurse, physician, advanced care provider, social worker, chaplain, respiratory therapy, physical therapy, clinical pharmacist, psychology, pain management specialist, case manager, hospice staff**
   a. Team members address all domains
   b. All have a shared responsibility for the patient
   c. Nurses play a pivotal role in coordinating care and achieving symptom management
7. **Treatment considerations**
   a. Management plan is individualized
   b. Use combinations of pharmacologic and nonpharmacologic methods to treat symptoms (see Ch. 20, Pain)
   c. Integrative medicine and complementary and alternative medicines (CAM): These approaches create healing environments that support patient, family, and providers. Can be used to manage physical symptoms, distress, and improve coping skills.
      i. Physical environment strategies
         (a) Stimulus modulation (e.g., reduce sleep disruption with use of eye masks, turning off artificial lights, decreasing noise and movement)
         (b) Essential oils
      ii. Nondrug modalities for symptom management
         (a) Acupuncture and acupressure
         (b) Art therapy
         (c) Pet therapy
      iii. Massage
      iv. Mind-body practices (e.g., hypnosis, guided imagery, yoga)
      v. Homeopathy (e.g., *Pulsatilla*, as well as *Carbo-Veg* could be given to ease respiratory discomfort, *Cuprum* for cramps, spasms and jerking, *Rhus-Tox* for restlessness)
      vi. Biofield therapy (e.g., reiki, healing touch, qigong)
      vii. Therapeutic music
      viii. Spiritual support
      ix. Mindful use of language (relationships and conversations)

TRANSITIONING GOALS OF CARE TO END-OF-LIFE (BOX 21.3)

1. **Five aspects of quality EOLC include:**
   a. Pain and symptom management
   b. Avoid prolongation of the dying process
   c. Sense of self-control
   d. Relief of burden on the family
   e. Strengthened relationships with loved ones

BOX 21.3 **Proposed Core Components for Quality End-of-Life Care**

- Frequent assessment of physical, emotional, social, and spiritual well-being
- Identification and management of emotional distress
- Availability of specialist palliative care in complex situations or transfer to inpatient palliative/hospice unit if available
- Referral to hospice for prognosis of ≤6 months
- Access to coordinated care services 24 hours a day
- Primary palliative care for management of simple pain and common symptoms
- Provision of specialist palliative care for refractory pain and complex or refractory symptoms
- Patient and family counseling
- Family caregiver support
- Consideration to social needs
- Consideration of religious and spiritual needs
- Consistent assessment and revision of care plan and goals of care

From Hartjes, T. (2015). Predicting which patients will benefit from palliative care: use of bundles, triggers and protocols. *Critical Care Nursing Clinics of North America*, 27(3), 307–314.

---

2. **Dying trajectories**
   a. Individuals with terminal illness, such as cancer, will generally maintain function until months just before death, when a steady decline in activities of daily living (ADLs) will be noted.
   b. Frailty: Slow, steady decline of aging that typically includes decrease in ADLs and weight loss requiring caregiver assistance
   c. Organ failure may seem to worsen, followed by intermediate recovery to a level below the baseline. The extent of decline is often difficult to predict.
3. **The dying process: Education of family regarding the normal dying process is essential; thorough documentation of family education is recommended (see Ch. 2, Psychosocial Aspects of Critical Care).**
   a. Patients demonstrate detachment from the physical world with less desire to talk and increased periods of sleep. Use periods of lucidity to assure communication with the family and loved ones.
4. **Loss of appetite**
   a. As death nears, individuals may lose the desire to eat or drink, or experience difficulty swallowing.
   b. Provide comfort with mouth care to include ice chips and sponge-tipped applicators, as well as comfort feeds when possible, reassuring family this is a natural process and artificial nutrition and hydration can often cause more discomfort in the dying stage.
5. **Change in bowel and bladder function**
   a. Keep areas clean and dry, and support with comfort and stool softeners if needed.
6. **Changes in breathing, congestion, and swallowing, often called "death rattle" or noisy breathing**
   a. Support the individual by wiping the mouth and maintaining the head of bed elevated as indicated.
   b. Educate the family and provide gentle background music if appropriate.
   c. Pharmacologic treatment with drying agents, such as glycopyrrolate (Robinul) and atropine may be helpful in reducing secretions.
7. **Changes in skin, temperature, and color**
   a. Intermittent feelings of hot and cold, with cool, dusky extremities is seen.
   b. Treatment includes education; maintain comfort and support as possible.

8. **Confusion, restlessness, and agitation; terminal delirium**
   a. Visual and auditory hallucination experiences may be present. Care includes support of the patient and family and treatment of terminal delirium.
   b. Use a gentle voice, reassuring touch, comfort, and pharmacologic measures as indicated.
9. **Closure: Encourage significant others to say goodbye and "permit" death (see Ch. 2, Psychosocial Aspects of Critical Care)**
   a. Although not easy, many patients want permission from loved ones to die knowing they will be okay, to say goodbyes and have closure, legacy, and a peaceful death
10. **Being present at the moment of death**
   a. Some individuals need private time to die; saying goodbye and leaving the room may make it easier for the individual to let go.

ADDITIONAL CONSIDERATIONS (SEE CH. 2, PSYCHOSOCIAL ASPECTS OF CRITICAL CARE)

1. **Counseling of patient and family**
   a. Patients may experience emotional distress from disease, symptoms, prognosis, demoralization, loss of function, difficulty coping, financial difficulty, and family dynamics
   b. Family members experience similar distress. Bereavement services can be offered to loved ones from the hospital or local hospice services to reduce complicated grief and posttraumatic stress syndrome (PTSD) associated with death in an ICU setting.
2. **Family caregiver support**
   a. Assess if caregivers wish to participate in care of the patient and/or the extent to which they are providing care for the patient
   b. Determine if caregivers need assistance
   c. Provide assistance and facilitate respite time
3. **Provide attention to the patient's social, spiritual, and cultural needs**
4. **Terminal delirium (see Ch. 2, Psychosocial Aspects of Critical Care)**
   a. Delirium occurs in up to 70% of actively dying patients
   b. This often occurs as the result of reduced oxygen, dehydration, progression of their disease or from pain medications, and occurs when the patient is near death. This condition seems distressing to the patient and may also be upsetting to the family. This may contribute to distress, complex grief, and PTSD in family if not diagnosed and managed.
   c. Educate and support family to understand the causes
   d. Provide a quiet and supportive environment (dim lights, speak softly, introduce yourself, prevent hasty movements)
5. **Palliative sedation (see Ch. 19 Sedation and Ch. 20, Pain)**
   a. Palliative sedation may be used at the end-of-life to relieve suffering that cannot be adequately treated with other therapies. It is rarely used as most patients' symptoms can be appropriately managed with PC consultation.
   b. May be used to treat refractory delirium, pain, or dyspnea and is only considered when patients or surrogate decision makers have given informed consent and there is consensus among staff and expert consultants about the appropriateness of the therapy.

References and bibliography information are available at http://evolve.elsevier.com/AACN/corecurriculum/.

Palliative and End-of-Life Care

21

Jan Odom-Forren, PhD, RN, CPAN, FASPAN, FAAN and
Denise O'Brien, DNP, RN, ACNS-BC, CPAN, CAPA, FASPAN, FCNS, FAAN

CROSSWALK

- **Quality and Safety in Nursing Education (QSEN):** Patient-centered care, Teamwork and collaboration, Evidence-based practice, Quality improvement, Safety
- **National Patient Safety Goals:** Identify patients correctly, Improve staff communication, Use medicines safely, Use alarms safely, Prevent infection, Identify patient safety risks, Prevent mistakes in surgery
- **American Nurses Association (ANA) Standards for Professional Nursing Practice:** Standard 1. Assessment, Standard 2. Diagnosis, Standard 3. Outcomes identification, Standard 4. Planning, Standard 5. Implementation, Standard 6. Evaluation, Standard 9. Communication, Standard 10. Collaboration, Standard 12. Education, Standard 13. Evidence-based practice and research, Standard 14. Quality of practice, Standard 16. Resource utilization, Standard 17. Environmental health
- **AACN Standards for Progressive and Critical Care Nursing Practice:** Standard 1. Quality of practice, Standard 3. Education, Standard 4. Communication, Standard 6. Collaboration, Standard 7. Evidence-based practice/research/clinical inquiry, Standard 8. Resource utilization, Standard 10. Environmental health
- **AACN Standards for Establishing and Sustaining Healthy Work Environments (HWE):** Skilled communication, True collaboration, Effective decision-making
- **PCCN content:** None
- **CCRN content:** None

SYSTEMWIDE ELEMENTS

ANATOMY AND PHYSIOLOGY REVIEW

1. **Concept Review**
   a. Perioperative care: Refers to the three phases of a surgical or diagnostic procedure: preoperative phase, intraoperative phase, and the postoperative "recovery" phase. The goal: To complete an assessment and evaluation of the patient before the administration of anesthesia/sedation to: (1) prepare patient for the operative/diagnostic procedure, and (2) determine postprocedure monitoring and care needs; to promote safe, effective, quality care.
      i. Evaluate patient's health status to determine if specific preoperative assessments, evaluations, or tests are needed to reduce patient risk
         (a) Patients with complex health histories should be evaluated at least one week before the surgery
      ii. Minimize delays and cancellation on the day of surgery/procedure
      iii. Educate patient/family regarding all phases of care (e.g., fasting, home medication management, anesthesia, surgery, disposition after surgery, expected recovery)

    iv. Encourage preventative strategies to reduce the risk of unintended sequela (e.g., smoking cessation, optimize comorbid conditions)

    v. Discharge planning

KEY CONCEPT

Discharge planning should be before surgery.

ASSESSMENT

1. **History**
   a. Identify present illness or condition which necessitates surgical/diagnostic procedure
   b. Determine past medical and surgical history in an organized and systematic manner.
      i. Identify chronic illnesses that may affect the outcome of the surgery (e.g., diabetes or asthma)
      ii. Identify past surgical history and previous surgical experiences that may impact current surgical plan (e.g., nausea and vomiting, pain control).
   c. Anesthetic history of the patient and family (e.g., family history of diseases, such as malignant hyperthermia, atypical plasma cholinesterase, or glycogen storage disease) which would impact anesthetic choices
   d. Complete medication history (include all prescription, over-the-counter, herbals and complimentary and alterative medications)
      i. Include adverse drug effects, food or drug allergies and reactions
         (a) Develop plan to manage home medications pre- and postoperatively
      ii. Sensitivities, such as latex allergy
   e. Identify mobility and sensory limitations of the patient (e.g., use of walker, wheelchair and need for visual aids, hearing aids)
   f. Identify family/caregiver support: To assist with operative consent, postoperative transportation support for recovery at home
   g. Obtain legal documents (e.g., advanced directive, code status, and power of attorney paperwork)
   h. Provide preoperative education regarding:
      i. Medications: Review and provide instructions for continuing/discontinuing preoperatively
      ii. Preoperative fasting/nothing by mouth (NPO) status: Specific diet requirements or restrictions, bowel preps, fasting of solids or liquids
      iii. Preoperative education: Fasting, medications, activity, pain relief, reinforcement of postoperative expectations
2. **Physical examination**
   a. Physical examination data
      i. Complete a history and physical examination
      ii. Airway assessment by anesthesia provider

EXPERT TIP

The airway assessment is completed by the anesthesia provider. However, the bedside nurse should ask about and/or review the airway assessment to determine ease of intubation preoperatively or if the patient may be a difficult reintubation.

Perioperative Care

22

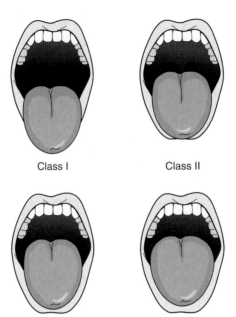

Class I   Class II

Class III   Class IV

Fig. 22.1 Mallampati classification. (From Phillips, N., Hornacky, A. (2021). *Berry & Kohn's operating room technique*, 14th ed. St. Louis: Elsevier.)

(a) Mallampati classification (Fig. 22.1)

> **EXPERT TIP**
> When considering the Mallampati classification, class 1 is expected to be an easier intubation and classes 3 and 4 a difficult intubation

      (b) Thyromental distance is the straight line with neck extended and mouth closed—from prominence of thyroid cartilage and bony point of lower mandibular border. Less than 7 cm (the width of 3 adult fingers) is associated with difficult intubation.

      (c) Mouth opening, neck range of motion, mandibular protrusion

   iii. Cognitive ability and mental status: Prior neurologic/behavioral issues

   iv. Musculoskeletal: For example, arthritis, missing limbs, ability to walk, mobility aids needed

   v. Skin assessment: Intact skin or identification of current wounds and other skin issues. Older patients can have very fragile skin and require extra care to prevent skin injury.

  b. Monitoring data

   i. Preoperative testing should be based upon patient's history, physical examination, type of surgical/diagnostic procedure, and type of anesthesia required. Testing can include (particularly for patients who will transfer to intensive care unit [ICU] after surgery):

      (a) Blood type and screen, crossmatch

      (b) Pregnancy testing: All females of childbearing age

      (c) Cardiac testing: Will depend on patient condition, electrocardiograms (ECGs), echocardiogram, stress testing

      (d) Other laboratory tests determined by examination

c. Appraisal of patient characteristics

    i. Many hospitalized patients require surgery during their illness. However, each patient and family are unique and bring a unique set of characteristics to the care situation. Examples of clinical attributes that the nurse should assess when caring for a patient with an acute respiratory disorder are the following: resiliency, vulnerability, stability, complexity, resource availability, desire for participation in care and preferred decision-making model, and predictability.

PATIENT CARE

1. **Preoperative care: Goal is to identify and reduce risks associated with the surgical/ diagnostic procedure and anesthesia and to return patient to their desirable level of function quickly.**

    a. Anesthesia evaluation (Table 22.1)

    b. Is operative procedure emergent or an elective surgery?

    c. NPO and fasting status: When was last food and drink taken?

    d. Consent: Surgeon consents patient. May have been done prior at the office.

    e. Nurse's role: Does the patient understand the procedure to be performed and the associated risks and benefits?

    f. Surgical history and physical: Updated within 30 days, if necessary, during preprocedural visit.

KEY CONCEPT

Although it is the surgeon's responsibility to ensure the patient is ready for the operating room, bedside nurses will frequently review all paperwork at the preoperative visit or if hospitalized the night before surgery.

---

    g. Some patient populations pose an increased perioperative risk and may require more extensive evaluation or testing preoperatively, examples include:

      i. Advanced age: Frailty, cognitive dysfunction, history of falls

      ii. Cardiovascular disease: Hypertension, heart failure, valvular heart disease, arrhythmias, coronary artery disease, cardiac implantable electronic devices

      iii. Cerebrovascular disease: Seizures, stroke, transient ischemic attacks

      iv. Neurologic disease: Abnormal behavior, speech, orientation or gait; abnormal muscle strength, fine motor movements. Preexisting neurologic deficits.

      v. Pulmonary disease: Asthma, pulmonary congestion, chronic obstructive pulmonary disease (COPD), pulmonary fibrosis

      vi. Obstructive sleep apnea: Can result in postoperative complications including cardiac arrhythmias, myocardial injury, and sudden death. If patient will not be ventilated in ICU, may bring own continuous positive airway pressure (CPAP) machine or use unit CPAP machine to prevent obstruction.

      vii. Renal disease/liver disease: Is there an atrioventricular shunt for dialysis, how extensive is the disease? Anesthesia provider determines which medications to use based upon whether a medication is metabolized in the liver and/or excreted by the kidneys.

      viii. Endocrine disease: Diabetes, thyroid disease, adrenal disorders, pituitary abnormalities

      ix. Anemia: If preoperative anemia is caused by iron deficiency, iron therapy may be started by oral or intravenous (IV) routes depending on the severity and type of surgical/diagnostic procedure. Iron supplementation in the setting of anemia reduces the need for red blood cells during surgery.

TABLE 22.1	**Current Definitions and American Society of Anesthesiologist-Approved Examples**	

American Society of Anesthesiologists Physical Status Classification	Definition	Adult Examples, Including, but Not Limited to:
ASA 1	A normal healthy patient	Healthy, nonsmoking, no or minimal alcohol use
ASA II	A patient with mild systemic disease	Mild diseases only without substantive functional limitations. Examples include (but not limited to): current smoker, social alcohol drinker, pregnancy, obesity (30 <BMI <40 kg/m^2), well-controlled DM/HTN, mild lung disease
ASA III	A patient with severe systemic disease	Substantive functional limitations; one or more moderate to severe diseases
		Examples include (but not limited to): poorly controlled DM or HTN, COPD, morbid obesity (BMI $\geq$40 kg/m^2), active hepatitis, alcohol dependence or abuse, implanted pacemaker, moderate reduction of ejection fraction, ESRD undergoing regularly scheduled dialysis, premature infant PCA <60 weeks, history (>3 months) of MI, CVA, TIA, or CAD/stents
ASA IV	A patient with severe systemic disease that is a constant threat to life	Examples include (but not limited to): recent (<3 months) MI, CVA, TIA, or CAD/stents, ongoing cardiac ischemia or severe valve dysfunction, severe reduction of ejection fraction, sepsis, DIC, ARDS, or ESRD not undergoing regularly scheduled dialysis
ASA V	A moribund patient who is not expected to survive without the operation	Examples include (but not limited to): ruptured abdominal/thoracic aneurysm, massive trauma, intracranial bleed with mass effect, ischemic bowel in the face of significant cardiac pathology or multiple organ/system dysfunction
ASA VI	A declared brain-dead patient whose organs are being removed for donor purposes	

ARDS, Acute respiratory distress syndrome; *BMI*, body mass index; *CAD*, coronary artery disease; *COPD*, chronic obstructive pulmonary disease; *CVA*, cardiovascular accident; *DIC*, disseminated intravascular coagulation; *DM*, diabetes mellitus; *ESRD*, end-stage renal disease; *HTN*, hypertension; *MI*, myocardial infarction; *PCA*, postconceptional age; *TIA*, transient ischemic attack. Modified from American Society of Anesthesiologists: ASA physical status classification systems, 2020. Retrieved from https://www.asahq.org/standards-and-guidelines/asa-physical-status-classification-system.

    x. Malnutrition: If patient is not taking in an adequate amount of nutrition, nutritional support should begin 7 to 10 days before surgery and can result in decreased postoperative complications.

    xi. Thromboembolic disorders (venous thromboembolism [VTE], deep venous thrombosis [DVT], pulmonary embolism): Is the patient on an anticoagulant, or is there a history of thromboembolism? Sequential compression devices and/or anticoagulants are used postoperative to prevent emboli formation. Prevention method and medications are based upon underlying condition.

    xii. Obesity: Associated with diabetes mellitus, hypertension, and cardiovascular disease. Patients with a body mass index (BMI) of over 35 kg/m^2 are at risk for wound infections, pulmonary complications, DVTs, and gastric reflux.

xiii. Tobacco use: Patients who smoke have almost 6 times the number of pulmonary complications, for example, pneumonia and atelectasis. Patients should be encouraged to stop smoking at least 12 to 48 hours before surgery which helps to reduce the effects of nicotine and carbon monoxide. Nicotine replacement therapy and behavioral support can be offered at this time as long as a replacement does not compromise the integrity of the surgery/procedure. There are times when nicotine replacement is avoided (e.g., pregnancy, breastfeeding, heart attack in the past 2 months, ongoing angina, peptic ulcer disease, arrhythmia, or uncontrolled blood pressure).

xiv. Alcohol misuse: Information regarding alcohol consumption is important. Chronic alcohol abuse can cause tolerance, dependence, and multisystem organ dysfunction. Postoperative morbidity and mortality rates are increased in alcoholic patients because of poor wound healing, infection, bleeding, pneumonia, and further hepatic decline. Delirium tremens (DTs) can occur in patients who misuse alcohol and undergo a surgical procedure. Identification and quantification of alcohol use are paramount to preventing postoperative complications. In addition to patient history, alcohol withdrawal scales are commonly used to identify the level of withdrawal so that the effect may be mitigated. Common scales include the Clinical Institute Withdrawal Assessment for Alcohol (CIWA) and CIWA-Ar and the Minnesota Detoxification scale (mMINDS).

h. Risk

i. The Revised Cardiac Risk Index (RCRI) is an instrument that estimates a patient's risk of perioperative cardiac complications.

ii. Assess Respiratory Risk in Surgical Patients in Catalonia (ARISCAT) consists of seven independent risk factors for perioperative pulmonary complications.

iii. The stroke risk index consists of seven risk factors for quick assessment of perioperative stroke.

i. Preoperative medications: Medication reconciliation should be completed before surgery that includes a list of medications, doses, and when they were last taken by the patient.

j. Surgical site infection reduction strategies

i. Appropriate use of prophylactic antibiotics: Administered within 1 hour preoperatively

ii. Appropriate hair removal: Hair clippers only if needed, no razors

iii. Controlled postoperative glucose in cardiac patients: Serum glucose levels below 200 mg/dL, collected at or closest to 6:00 AM on each of the first two postoperative days: possible insulin drip in ICU.

iv. Postoperative normothermia in colorectal surgery: Does not pertain to those patients for whom therapeutic hypothermia is being used (e.g., hypothermic cardioplegia). Normothermia should be considered for all postoperative patients.

k. Initiation/implementation of enhanced recovery after surgery protocols or clinical pathways begin preoperatively

i. Prerehabilitation—opportunity to enhance functional capacity with change interventions; physical activity, exercise, diet and nutrition, smoking and alcohol cessations strategies—depends on amount of time before surgery

---

KEY CONCEPT

Prehabilitation is a physical and/or lifestyle preparation designed to improve recovery time following surgery.

    ii. Minimal fasting: Only 2 hours before surgery; carb loading showing promise to reduce insulin resistance, minimize nitrogen and protein loss, and maintain muscle strength to accelerate recovery.

> **EXPERT TIP**
> The recommendation for fasting may vary based upon the patient population, surgery type, other patient specific variables. However, you may find many facilities still fast past midnight before the day of surgery.

2. **Intraoperative care: Goal is to promote safe anesthesia care and prevent risks associated with anesthesia, surgical/diagnostic procedure.**
   a. Anesthesia: Sedation and anesthesia are on a continuum from awake to minimal sedation, moderate sedation, deep sedation and anesthesia (Table 22.2). See Ch. 19 for more information on sedation. Anesthesia consists of general anesthesia and central neuroaxial anesthesia (spinal or epidural). Local anesthesia may be used as an adjunct. See Table 22.3 for common medications used during the perioperative period.
      i. General anesthesia: Drug-induced loss of consciousness. Patients are unarousable even with pain, typically unable to maintain ventilation, require assistance with their airway, and cardiovascular function can be impaired. Can be IV or inhalation or a combination of both.
         (a) IV technique: Usually uses an induction agent, such as propofol, as well as oxygen and nitrous oxide, an anxiolytic (benzodiazepine), an opioid analgesic, and a muscle relaxant.
         (b) Inhalation technique: May use propofol for induction or may use the inhalation agent plus oxygen and nitrous oxide for induction. The surgery may be completed using only inhalation anesthesia. Muscle relaxants are used if necessary.
         (c) Balanced anesthesia: Describes anesthesia that uses both the IV technique and inhalation agents.
         (d) Total intravenous anesthesia (TIVA): Typically used for procedures outside the operating room (OR). Also used in conjunction with Enhanced Recovery After Surgery (ERAS) protocols because TIVA is short acting.
      ii. Central neuroaxial and peripheral anesthesia: Loss of sensation in a specific area or region of the body. Common regional anesthesia broadly includes spinal, epidural, caudal, and major peripheral nerve blocks.
         (a) Epidural: Local anesthetic is dosed through a catheter placed in the epidural space with a needle. The spinal roots outside the subarachnoid space are blocked in an epidural but requires a larger dose of local anesthetics to diffuse through barriers, such as the dura. The epidural space is vascular and has a higher risk of toxicity than a spinal. The epidural catheter can be placed in the thoracic or lumbar region as appropriate for creating a pain block to the surgical area.
         (b) Spinal: Blocks the spinal roots in the subarachnoid space. Spinal anesthesia only requires a small dose of local anesthesia that is placed into the subarachnoid space with a needle. It is a one-time injection that does now allow for more dosing. A spinal can only be placed in the lower lumbar region.
         (c) Peripheral nerve blocks (PNB): Can be used as the sole anesthetic, with a neuroaxial block, with general anesthesia or for postoperative pain management. Some PNBs may be placed with use of ultrasound.

TABLE 22.2 Most Common Anesthetic Pharmacologic Choices Over the Continuum

Awake, Conscious	Minimal Sedation	Awake/Minimal/Moderate Sedation	Moderate Sedation/Deep Sedation	General Anesthesia
None Oxygen	Anxiolytics Benzodiazepines • Oral route Nitrous oxide	Topical Anesthesia • EMLA • LMX4 Local Anesthesia • At site of procedure Regional Anesthesia • Bier block • Peripheral nerve block • Upper extremity, e.g., intrascalene block, supraclavicular • Lower extremity, e.g., femoral block, popliteal block • Abdominal, e.g., Quadratus Lumborum, Transverse Abdominus Plane • Central Neuraxial block, e.g., spinal, epidural	Anticholinergics • Atropine • Scopolamine • Glycopyrrolate Benzodiazepines • Midazolam • Lorazepam Benzodiazepine antagonist • Flumazenil IV opioids • Morphine • Dilaudid • Alfentanil • Fentanyl • Remifentanil • Sufentanil Opioid antagonist • Naloxone Alpha$_2$ Agonist • Dexmedetomidine Dissociative • Ketamine	Sedatives/hypnotics • Etomidate • Propofol Inhalation • Isoflurane • Desflurane • Sevoflurane Depolarizing muscle relaxant • Succinylcholine Nondepolarizing muscle relaxant • Atracurium • Cisatracurium • Pancuronium • Rocuronium • Vecuronium Nondepolarizing muscle relaxant reversals • Neostigmine • Sugammadex Anticholinergics • Atropine • Glycopyrrolate

EMLA, Eutectic mixture of local anesthetics; *IV,* intravenous; *LMX4,* lidocaine 4%.
Modified from Brown, C. (2021). Anesthesia, moderate sedation/analgesia. In L. Schick, P.E. Windle. *Perianesthesia nursing core curriculum,* ed 4. St. Louis: Elsevier.

TABLE 22.3 **Commonly Used Perioperative Anesthetic Gases and Medications**

	Common Usage	Advantages	Disadvantages	Comments
INHALATION GASES				
Air	Maintenance with O_2; laser surgery near airway	Less support of combustion than N_2O	No anesthetic qualities	Can use as supplemental assist for Fio_2 control for fire prevention (Miller, 2015)
Oxygen (O_2)	Essential for life	Can slightly ↑ O_2 available to tissues in low cardiac output states	Can cause retinopathy in premature infants	Concentrations should be at minimum to avoid hypoxia with lasers in surgery of head, neck, and pulmonary areas (Apfelbaum et al., 2013)
Nitrous oxide (N_2O)	Maintenance; frequently for induction	Rapid induction and recovery; additive effects to other anesthetics, more analgesia than other inhalation agents	No relaxation; can depress myocardium; expands within closed spaces	Hypoxia if overdose given; ↑ uptake of other volatile agents, only nonhalogenated agent used today
Desflurane (Suprane)	Maintenance in surgical procedures	Rapid emergence; good relaxation; lowest 0.02% biotransformation to metabolites	May cause transient ↑ HR and ↓ BP; airway irritation; requires heated vaporizer	Rapid recovery phase; no need for high gas flows
Isoflurane (Forane)	Maintenance	Good relaxation; maintains cardiac output; 0.2% metabolized; inexpensive	Reduced SVR, ↑ respiratory depression; slightly irritating odor	Pungent odor; airway irritant; trigger for malignant hyperthermia
Sevoflurane (Ultane)	Induction and maintenance	Rapid induction and emergence when compared to isoflurane; good relaxation; ≈5% metabolized	Caution using sevoflurane with fresh gas flows below 1 L/min for procedures lasting longer than 1 hour; is nephrotoxic in rats; effect in humans unknown	Rapid uptake and elimination; nonpungent; excellent for inhalation induction
OPIOID ANALGESICS				
Morphine sulfate	Perioperative pain; premedication	Inexpensive; duration of action 4–5 hours; euphoria; good cardiovascular stability	Nausea and vomiting; histamine release; postural ↓ BP (↓ SVR); caution with renal failure patients	Used intrathecally and epidurally for postoperative pain; elimination half-life 2–3 hours
Alfentanil (Alfenta)	Surgical analgesia	Duration of action 0.5–1 hour; used as bolus or infusion	Possible truncal rigidity	Potency: 750 mcg = 10 mg IV morphine sulfate; elimination half-life 1.6 hours

Continued

TABLE 22.3	**Commonly Used Perioperative Anesthetic Gases and Medications—cont'd**			
	Common Usage	Advantages	Disadvantages	Comments
Fentanyl (Sublimaze)	Surgical analgesia; epidural infusion for postoperative analgesia; add to spinal anesthesia or block	Good cardiovascular stability; duration of action 0.5–1 hour	Possible truncal rigidity	Most commonly used opioid; potency: 100 mcg = 10 mg morphine sulfate; elimination half-life 3.6 hours
Remifentanil (Ultiva)	0.25–1 mcg/kg/min infusion for surgical analgesia	Easily titratable; metabolized by blood and tissue esterases; short duration; good cardiovascular stability	Requires mixing; increased cost	Potency: 25 mcg = 10 mg morphine sulfate; 20–30 × potency of alfentanil; elimination half-life 3–10 minutes
Sufentanil (Sufenta)	Surgical analgesia	Good cardiovascular stability; duration of action 0.5 hour; prolonged analgesia	Prolonged respiratory depression	Potency: 15 mcg = 10 mg morphine sulfate; elimination half-life 2.7 hours
Hydromorphone (Dilaudid)	Surgical and postoperative pain relief	Long duration of action 3–5 hours; can switch to PO form for postoperative pain management; high ceiling effect limited only by increased adverse side effects	Caution with seizure history and biliary tract surgery; addiction potential, not approved for epidural or intrathecal use in United States	Not metabolized by cytochrome P-450 enzyme pathway, which reduces its drug–drug interaction
Morphine liposomal (DepoDur)	For epidural use only	Single dose provides analgesia for up to 48 h; decreased requirements for supplemental opioids	Potential for respiratory depression; avoid other epidural medications ~48 hours	10–15 mg epidural, one dose for lower abdominal or major lower limb surgery; 10 mg post C-section delivery
DEPOLARIZING MUSCLE RELAXANTS				
Succinylcholine (Anectine, Quelicin)	Intubation; short procedures	Rapid onset; short duration	Requires refrigeration; may cause fasciculations, postoperative myalgias, and dysrhythmias; ↑ serum K+ with burns, tissue trauma, paralysis, and muscle diseases; slight histamine release	Prolonged muscle relaxation with serum cholinesterase deficiency and certain antibiotics; trigger agent for malignant hyperthermia
NONDEPOLARIZING MUSCLE RELAXANTS: INTERMEDIATE ONSET AND DURATION				
Atracurium (Tracrium)	Intubation; maintenance of relaxation	Minimal cardiovascular or cumulative effects; good with renal failure	Requires refrigeration; slight histamine release	Breakdown by Hofmann elimination and ester hydrolysis
Cisatracurium (Nimbex)	Intubation; maintenance of relaxation	Similar to atracurium	No histamine release	Similar to atracurium

Continued

TABLE 22.3 Commonly Used Perioperative Anesthetic Gases and Medications—cont'd

	Common Usage	Advantages	Disadvantages	Comments
Rocuronium (Zemuron)	Intubation; maintenance of relaxation	Rapid onset, dose dependent; elimination via kidney and liver	Vagolytic; may increase HR	Duration similar to atracurium and vecuronium
Vecuronium (Norcuron)	Intubation; maintenance of relaxation	No significant cardiovascular or cumulative effects; no histamine release	Requires mixing	Mostly eliminated in bile, some in urine
NONDEPOLARIZING MUSCLE RELAXANTS: LONGER ONSET AND DURATION				
Pancuronium (Pavulon)	Maintenance of relaxation	Increased duration	May cause ↑ HR and ↑ BP	Mostly renal elimination
INTRAVENOUS ANESTHETICS				
Etomidate (Amidate)	Induction	Minimal effects on cardiovascular system; rapid acting, smooth induction and recovery	May cause pain with injection and myoclonus with induction dose	Administer through large vein to decrease pain and thrombophlebitis on injection
Diazepam (Valium)	Amnesia; hypnotic; preoperative medication	Good sedation	Prolonged duration	Residual effects for 20–90 hours; alcohol and other CNS depressants potentiate effects
Ketamine (Ketalar)	Induction, occasional maintenance (IV or IM)	Short acting; fast onset IV; patient maintains airway; good in small children and burn patients, hypovolemic shock; bronchospastic disease	Large doses may cause hallucinations and respiratory depression; not indicated in patients with increased ICP	Increased use with subanesthetic doses; often used in trauma procedures
Midazolam (Versed)	Hypnotic; anxiolytic; sedation; often used as adjunct to induction	Excellent amnestic; water soluble (no pain with IV injection); short acting	CNS depression along with respiratory depression	Often used for anterograde amnesia for stressful procedures; insertion of invasive monitors or regional anesthesia
Propofol (Diprivan)	Induction and maintenance; sedation with regional anesthesia or MAC	Rapid onset; awakening in 5–10 minutes, even after prolonged infusion	May cause pain when injected; lipid based: can support bacterial growth if aseptic technique is compromised	Short elimination half-life (34–64 minutes); patients >80 years of age can require only 50% of dose for equal level of sedation
Sodium methohexital (Brevital sodium)	Induction	Ultrashort-acting barbiturate; low cardiac toxicity; minimal anticonvulsant properties	May cause hiccups; less amnestic effects than benzodiazepines; central respiratory system depressant	Can be given rectally

Continued

TABLE 22.3	**Commonly Used Perioperative Anesthetic Gases and Medications—cont'd**			
	Common Usage	**Advantages**	**Disadvantages**	**Comments**
LOCAL ANESTHETICS				
Bupivacaine (Marcaine, Sensorcaine)	Epidural, spinal, or local infiltration; good wound infiltration	Good relaxation; long acting; can constrict blood vessels to reduce bleeding at site	Overdose can cause cardiac collapse	Epidural or caudal: 25–150 mg depending on degree of motor block desired; duration: 3–6 hours
Chloroprocaine (Nesacaine)	Epidural anesthesia	Ultrashort acting; good relaxation	May cause neurotoxicity	Maximum dose 11 mg/kg not to exceed 800 mg; with epinephrine 14 mg/kg, maximum dose 1000 mg
Lidocaine (Xylocaine)	Epidural, spinal, peripheral IV anesthesia, and local infiltration anesthesia	Short acting; good relaxation; low toxicity	Overdose can cause convulsions; possible transient neurologic changes with spinal anesthesia	Also used for ventricular dysrhythmias; maximum dose 4.5 mg/kg; duration 60–120 minutes
Ropivacaine (Naropin)	Local infiltration anesthesia, peripheral nerve block, epidural	Long duration; less cardiotoxic than bupivacaine	Hypotension and bradycardia are prominent adverse effects when ropivacaine is used epidurally, particularly with concentrations of ropivacaine over 0.5%	200–300 mg single doses for duration up to 5 hours achieved by various regional techniques, both minor and major nerve blocks
Tetracaine (Pontocaine)	Spinal anesthesia	Long acting; good relaxation	Not appropriate for short procedures because of the long duration of action	Dose 5–20 mg (epinephrine rarely used); duration 60–180 minutes for SAB
ANTICHOLINERGICS				
Atropine	Blocks effects of acetylcholine; ↓ vagal tone; reverse muscle relaxants; treat sinus bradycardia	↑ HR; suppresses salivation, bronchial and gastric secretions	Depresses sweating; may cause dry mouth, flushing, dizziness, CNS symptoms	Quite selective at muscarinic receptors in smooth and cardiac muscle and exocrine glands
Glycopyrrolate (Robinul)	Similar to atropine	Slightly ↑ HR; does not cross blood-brain barrier; can increase gastric pH more than atropine	Prolonged duration of effects	Lower incidence of dysrhythmias than atropine
CHOLINERGIC AGENT				
Neostigmine (Prostigmine)	Reverses effects of nondepolarizing neuromuscular blocking agents	Prevents breakdown of acetylcholine by inhibiting acetylcholinesterase	The need to wait until evidence of spontaneous recovery (TOF ratio of >0.9) before administering	Given with either atropine or glycopyrrolate

Continued

TABLE 22.3 **Commonly Used Perioperative Anesthetic Gases and Medications—cont'd**

	Common Usage	Advantages	Disadvantages	Comments
OTHER				
Sugammadex (Bridion)	First SRBA to antagonize a muscle relaxant's effects	Rapidly terminates the neuromuscular block of rocuronium, and vecuronium by forming a complex with rocuronium or vecuronium in plasma to reduce the amount of drug available to bind at the neuromuscular junction	No effect on succinylcholine or benzylisoquinolinium relaxants, can affect hormone-based oral contraceptives; recommend alternative contraceptive method if used on female patients of child-bearing age for 7 days; not recommended for severe renal impairment or dialysis	If need to reestablish muscle relaxation arises after administration of sugammadex, then using a benzylisoquinolinium or succinylcholine is recommended; cases of marked bradycardia have been observed, some resulting in cardiac arrest, monitor hemodynamic changes
Dexmedeto-midine (Precedex)	Selective α_2-agonist; sedation in the ICU	Produces centrally mediated sympatholytic, sedative, and analgesic effects; hemodynamic stability, potentiates anesthetics, reduces anesthetic requirements, preserved drive	Limited amnestic effect; avoid as sole anesthetic agent with patients in which neuromuscular blockade is used; risk of bradycardia; use with caution in patients with heart block	Even at high doses does not produce general anesthesia, but is a valuable sedative in a number of settings

BP, Blood pressure; *CNS*, central nervous system; *CSF*, cerebrospinal fluid; *HR*, heart rate; *ICP*, intracranial pressure; *ICU*, intensive care unit; *IM*, intramuscular; *IV*, intravenous; *MAC*, monitored anesthesia care; *MH*, malignant hyperthermia; *PO*, oral; *SRBA*, selective relaxant binding agent; *SVR*, systemic vascular resistance, *TOF*, train-of-four.
Modified from Clinical Pharmacology Online, 2021, Elsevier. Retrieved from https://www.clinicalkey.com/pharmacology/; IBM Micromedex, 2021, IBM Corporation. Retrieved from www.micromedexsolutions.com; Nagelhout, J.J., Elisha, S. (2018). *Nurse anesthesia*, ed 6. St. Louis: Elsevier; Miller, R.D. (2015). *Miller's anesthesia*, ed 8. Philadelphia: Elsevier; Apfelbaum, J.L., et al. (2013). Practice advisory for the prevention and management of operating room fires: an updated report by the American Society of Anesthesiologists Task Force on Operating Room Fires, *Anesthesiology*, 118(2), 271–290.

    (d) Caudal: Used for surgical anesthesia in children and chronic pain management in adults. A needle is inserted through the sacral hiatus to access the sacral epidural space.

   iii. Monitored anesthesia care (MAC): Surgical site is infiltrated with local anesthesia and performed by the surgeon. The anesthesia provider supplements with sedation and analgesia and monitors the patient during the procedure. MAC may be used with some critically ill patients who cannot tolerate general anesthesia or for procedures, such as gastroenterology procedures in a gastrointestinal (GI) suite.

  b. Complications associated with anesthetic agents/techniques

    i. Hypersensitivity reactions: During surgery and postoperatively, the patient is exposed to multiple drugs and other agents that can cause a hypersensitivity reaction.

     (a) A type 1 hypersensitivity reaction occurs quickly, usually 15 to 30 minutes after exposure. When histamine, the principal mediator, binds to the

H_1 receptor site, symptoms, such as bronchoconstriction, vasodilation, increased vascular permeability, urticaria, pruritis, and increased mucus production occur.

(1) These reactions vary from mild to fatal. Progression to anaphylaxis can occur quickly with symptoms of angioedema, systemic vasodilation, hypotension, bronchospasm, and dysrhythmias.

(b) First-line treatment for anaphylaxis is epinephrine with dosage based on severity and patient history. If the patient is on beta-blockers, other vasoactive drugs can be given (e.g., norepinephrine, ephedrine, methoxamine) phenylephrine, and dopamine.

(c) Second-line treatments for less severe reactions may include: antihistamines, cromolyn sodium, and bronchodilators.

ii. Malignant hyperthermia (MH): Potentially fatal, inherited disorder that is caused by an acceleration of metabolism in skeletal muscle. MH is typically a familial autosomal dominant trait. There is greater risk of MH occurrence in males than females and those of a younger age (children <15 years of age account for greater than half of the occurrences). It occurs in all ethnicities but typically takes three exposures to anesthesia before manifesting. The best prediction of potential issue is history of familial reaction.

EXPERT TIP

MH typically occurs with the initiation of the anesthetic agent, however it can present postoperatively as well.

(a) MH occurs when a susceptible individual is administered inhalational anesthetics (except for nitrous oxide) and/or the depolarizing muscle relaxant, succinylcholine.

(b) The signs of MH include muscle rigidity, tachycardia, hyperthermia, rhabdomyolysis, increased blood acidity, hyperkalemia, and increased end-tidal carbon dioxide ($EtCO_2$).

(c) An MH crisis can occur in the OR, the postanesthesia care unit (PACU), or the ICU typically within an hour of trigger exposure. The first, hallmark signs of impending crisis are typically tachycardia, elevated CO_2, and masseter muscle rigidity; signs that often have delayed recognition in intubated patients who are waking up as they are expected findings when arousing from anesthesia.

(d) Immediate treatment with the drug dantrolene sodium usually reverses the signs of MH although the patient may require redosing. The underlying defect is abnormally increased levels of cell calcium in the skeletal muscle. Some evidence exists that susceptible patients can also develop MH with exercise or with exposure to heat. Mortality is extremely high when dantrolene is not available for treatment.

(e) Dosage of dantrolene for an MH crisis is 2.5 mL/kg. There are two formulations of dantrolene: one that was approved in 1979 (Dantrium) and one approved in 2014 (Ryanodex). During an episode of MH, the nurse must know which dantrolene is on hand. For example, the 1979 formulation requires 60 mL sterile water with no bacteriostatic agent while the 2014 formulation requires 5 mL of the same. As many as 36 vials of the 1979 formulation may be required for a patient in an MH crisis versus 3 vials of the 2014 formulation.

(f) All anesthesia departments have at least one mobile MH kit with equipment and medication needed to treat it quickly.

> **EXPERT TIP**
> Nurses in the ICU who care for postoperative patients should familiarize themselves with the MH kit and equipment.

(g) There is an organization, the Malignant Hyperthermia Association of the United States that is an excellent resource (www.mhaus.org). The priority is the administration of dantrolene sodium during a crisis but MHAUS has a 24-hour hotline that is available for further support.

(h) The goal is treatment with dantrolene sodium. However, other supportive measures are taken to relieve symptoms simultaneously with treatments, such as cooling, ventilation with 100% oxygen to decrease $EtCO_2$, insertion of a urinary catheter, or administration of bicarbonate (as appropriate based on the arterial blood gas [ABG]). The ICU may experience an MH crisis with a postoperative patient or maintain the care of a patient who experienced MH in the OR PACU. Patients who experience an MH crisis are advised to discuss the occurrence with blood relatives as their relatives are considered susceptible to it as well unless ruled out by testing. Testing is via muscle biopsy for the "gold standard" in vitro contracture test which investigates the muscle fiber contraction when exposed to caffeine or halothane.

iii. Local anesthetic systemic toxicity (LAST): Rare, but life-threatening, event is a complication of regional anesthesia. It typically results from the absorption of a large amount of local anesthetics from either a block that has required a large amount of local anesthesia or the unintentional administration of a local anesthetic into the vascular system.

(a) The most common characteristic of LAST is disturbance of the central nervous system, because of cerebral neurotoxicity.

(1) The proper dosage of local anesthetic is the lowest dose that can accomplish the duration and coverage of analgesia or anesthesia required. Prevention of LAST is a priority.

(2) Early signs can include confusion, perioral numbness, audiovisual disturbances, and decreased level of consciousness, progressing to seizures.

(3) Some of the LAST cases will progress to include cardiovascular symptoms including dysrhythmias, hypotension, and eventually cardiac arrest. LAST most commonly occurs immediately after the injection of local anesthetic, but delayed presentation may also occur. When LAST does occur, immediate management is required. As with most emergencies, airway, oxygenation, and ventilation of the patient should be maintained.

(4) After management of the patient's airway, 20% IVs lipid emulsion therapy should be administered as quickly as possible. Seizures should be managed with benzodiazepines, and advanced cardiovascular life support (ACLS) protocols followed for arrhythmias or cardiac arrest, with the exception of nonuse of lidocaine for arrhythmias.

iv. Pseudocholinesterase deficiency: Neuromuscular blocking agent, succinylcholine, is hydrolyzed quickly by plasma pseudocholinesterase, an enzyme in the liver. Patients with low pseudocholinesterase have a prolonged response to succinylcholine.

(a) The deficiency can be acquired which can occur with liver disease, severe anemia, or some drugs, such as quinidine, propranolol, and phospholine eye drops.

(b) Atypical pseudocholinesterase is inherited. Patients with an atypical presentation have been known to remain apneic for as long as 48 hours after a dose of succinylcholine and need mechanical ventilation and ICU care.

(c) The patient should be tested for absolute pseudocholinesterase activity and the dibucaine and fluoride numbers to ascertain the deficiency.

> **KEY CONCEPT**
> An important factor to keep in mind is that these patients may be paralyzed because of pseudocho-linesterase deficiency, but aware of their surroundings. Sedation may be ordered.

c. Plan of care/ongoing concerns: Before discharge from the OR, the following are discussed with the anesthesia provider and surgeon:

   i. Disposition: Does the patient go to PACU or straight to ICU (Fig. 22.2)? Dispo typically depends on hospital policy and surgeon/anesthesia preference.

    (a) PACU areas in larger hospitals routinely care for patients that are then discharged to ICUs

    (b) In some hospitals, ICU patients go directly back to ICU

   ii. Pressure injury associated with operative procedures: Preoperative nurse conducts a skin assessment before surgery and the OR nurse conducts a subsequent skin assessment before transfer out of the OR based on position of the patient during surgery.

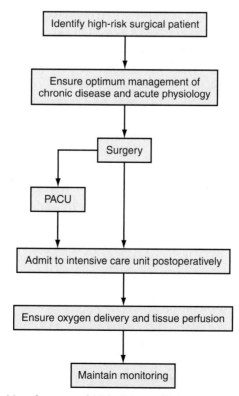

Fig. 22.2 Suggested algorithm for care of high-risk surgical patient. *PACU*, Postanesthesia care unit. (Modified from Lees, N., Hamilton, M., Rhodes, A. (2009). Clinical review: Goal-directed therapy in high risk surgical patients, *Critical Care*, 13:231.)

> **KEY CONCEPT**
> The receiving nurse should also complete a skin assessment.

    iii. Postoperative pain management: Surgical team writes orders for postoperative pain management when the patient transfers to the ICU. If the patient goes to PACU first, the anesthesia provider is responsible for pain management/orders for the PACU nurses, while they are there.

3. **Postoperative/postanesthesia care: Goal is to return the patient to hemodynamic stability and baseline or improved physiologic functioning, recognizing and treating potential complications.**

INITIAL ARRIVAL IN POSTANESTHESIA CARE UNIT OR INTENSIVE CARE UNIT

1. **Handoff: Before accepting care for a patient, a structured verbal communication occurs between the anesthesia provider and the receiving nurse. It includes a review of pertinent patient information, including history and allergies as they pertain to postoperative care, anesthesia management during the case with medications administered, from the anesthesiologist, and details of the surgical surgical/ diagnostic procedure including blood loss, from a member of the surgical or interventional team.**
   a. The nurse, upon completion of the handoff, indicates readiness to accept the transfer of care and releases the anesthesia care provider to leave the patient bedside.
   b. Various tools may be used to facilitate the process: Checklist either on paper or in electronic health record, paper or electronic summary document, badge "buddies" with list of required items, etc.

2. **Required handoff elements: Content from preoperative and intraoperative phases are combined with initial postoperative assessment elements to provide a brief, overview of patient condition and status. Any concerns or provider call parameters are discussed at the time of handoff from the operative and anesthesia team to the receiving nurse caring for the patient (Table 22.4).**

3. **Initial assessment: Quick head-to-toe survey of the patient, focusing on airway, oxygenation, and ventilation including breath sounds, respiratory rate, depth, effort; hemodynamic status: cardiac rate, rhythm, blood pressure, perfusion; temperature; pain and comfort—self-assessment of pain is the goal, if able to self-report, using a standardized pain assessment scale; sedation level, level of consciousness, stroke screen (vocalization, facial symmetry), movement/strength of extremities; status of dressings/drains/incisions; skin—color, temperature, any signs of injury**

ONGOING POSTANESTHESIA CARE—EMERGENCE FROM ANESTHESIA

1. **Respiratory function**
   a. Awareness of preexisting conditions, for example, pulmonary disease, thoracic or upper abdominal procedures, smoking history, obstructive sleep apnea, and so on, and how they will impact the postoperative period.
   b. Improving gas exchange by optimizing oxygenation and ventilation. Recent opioid and sedative administration may increase the need for oxygenation and ventilatory support in the immediate postanesthesia period. Supplemental oxygen may be needed, dependent on oxygen saturation and $EtCO_2$ levels measured by capnography.
   c. Ongoing respiratory evaluation and assessments include airway status, respiratory rate, depth, effort and ventilator settings, as well as response to respiratory/ ventilatory support. The respiratory assessment may also include advanced

TABLE 22.4	**Common Elements of Perioperative Handover Report**	
Preoperative	**Operative**	**Postoperative**
Patient history—pertinent medical conditions	Procedure performed Positioning during procedure (supine, prone, lateral, etc.)	Vital signs including blood pressure, heart rate/rhythm, respiratory rate, oxygen saturation, temperature
Allergies	Complications (procedural, anesthesia related)	Airway/ventilation status (presence of airway adjuncts)
Medications (before admission/preoperative)	Airway management (e.g., ease of intubation, attempts)	Neurologic status (level of consciousness, movement of extremities, stroke assessment)
Results of physical examination	Anesthesia/medications/reversal	Vascular access, fluid replacement
Fasting status	Estimated blood loss, intake (fluids given, blood products); urinary/ other output	Pain assessment/management plan

From Association of Perioperative Registered Nurses. *Guidelines for Perioperative Practice.* 2020. AORN, Denver, CO.

monitoring with a pulmonary artery catheter for systemic venous oxygenation (SVO_2) and pulmonary artery pressures (PAP).

    d. A "stir-up" or respiratory regimen is initiated which includes activities aimed at minimizing complications, such as atelectasis and venous stasis. Activities include deep breathing, coughing, repositioning, mobilization, and pain management.

2. Cardiovascular function

    a. Focus on maintaining adequate cardiac output

    b. Assessments include:

        i. Overall condition including skin color, temperature, and sensation; observe operative sites for bleeding

        ii. Frequent vital signs (VS), such as blood pressure (measured directly or indirectly), and heart rate. Depending on the surgery, VS may include arterial pressures, cardiac output (CO), and cardiac index (CI).

        iii. Peripheral pulse assessment with capillary refill time

        iv. Cardiac rhythm monitoring (including ST changes) and pacemaker function (including internal, transvenous, or epicardial pacemakers)

    c. Assessment may also include advanced hemodynamic monitoring as indicated by the patient's history, current status, and operative procedure

3. Neurologic function

    a. Establish baseline neurologic function during handoff and continue to monitor for alterations in neurologic functioning during emergence from anesthesia

    b. Patient may remain intentionally sedated with the use of ongoing medication delivery. Most patients emerge from anesthesia rapidly and in a predictable manner. However, some are combative, emotional, or just take longer to return to full consciousness.

    c. Elements of assessment include level of consciousness and sedation level, response to commands, pupillary response, and purposeful extremity movement

    d. Assessment may include use of the Glasgow Coma Scale and/or the Richmond Agitation Sedation Scale (RASS).

    e. Selective cranial nerve assessment may be ordered, dependent on patient history and procedure

    f. Risk of stroke is increased following general anesthesia; assess facial symmetry, speech (if able to verbalize), muscle strength and movement; any deviation should be reported immediately and evaluated

4. **Thermoregulation**
   a. Temperature assessment is completed upon arrival to the unit and periodically, typically hourly during initial recovery from anesthesia
   b. Method of assessment (e.g., oral, axillary, bladder, esophageal, temporal artery, rectal) varies depending on patient age, status, and institutional standards
   c. Patients may experience shivering following anesthesia, commonly known as "rigors," in the absence of hypothermia; initial treatment may include warm blankets and low dose IV meperidine

5. **Fluid/electrolyte balance**
   a. Vascular access is maintained during the immediate postanesthesia phase to continue infusions and administer medications, as well as allow for prompt treatment if there were an emergency.
   b. Fluids may be titrated to maintain cardiac output and adequate perfusion
   c. Monitoring of electrolytes, especially potassium, calcium, and magnesium may help minimize hemodynamic instability and cardiac dysfunction.
   d. Most common electrolyte imbalances include hypokalemia (from fluid resuscitation, nasogastric losses), hyperkalemia (from tissue catabolism or acidosis), hypocalcemia (from alkalosis, hemodilution), hypomagnesemia (from GI or urinary losses)
   e. Glucose monitoring and management should follow recommended practices and institutional guidelines
   f. Hyperglycemia may occur in postoperative patients related to hypermetabolic stress response, which increases glucose production and causes insulin resistance. It is often treated with insulin administered either via a subcutaneous (acute floor) or IV route (ICU). The goal is to maintain a normal blood glucose level while the body is recovering from surgery.

6. **Psychosocial status**
   a. Patients may emerge from anesthesia calmly or mildly agitated.
   b. Frequent reassurance, beginning when the patient arrives in the PACU/ICU, helps reorient the patient to time, place and situation; calmly stated, simple instructions may reduce patient anxiety and fear; touch or handholding may also help soothe the patient during emergence
   c. Knowledge of the patient's preoperative state (e.g., calm, anxious, agitated, crying, sedated) may guide the nurse's responses to the patient's emergence behavior

7. **Comfort management**
   a. Pain (see Ch. 20, Pain)
      i. Acute postoperative pain is assessed and reassessed as the patient is emerging from anesthesia; standard pain assessment tools are used based on patient age, population, cognitive ability, and sedation level
      ii. Previous history will guide postoperative management, for example, history of chronic pain, level of pain tolerance; patient is opiate naïve or tolerant, past response to painful experiences
      iii. In general, pain is treated aggressively to minimize hemodynamic effects of severe pain in the immediate postoperative phase of care
      iv. Treatment includes opioids (fentanyl, morphine, hydromorphone), local anesthetics, nonsteroidal antiinflammatories (IV Tylenol, ketorolac, ibuprofen), and subanesthetic ketamine infusions
      v. Nonpharmacologic complementary therapies are also beneficial, including cold therapy, heat therapy, massage, music, positioning, and others.
      vi. Pain assessment includes monitoring for pain response and side effects (sedation, respiratory depression, hemodynamic instability)

b. Postoperative nausea and vomiting are common and are best treated aggressively to avoid adverse sequelae.

8. **Skin integrity and mobility**
   a. Skin assessment is completed upon arrival to the PACU/ICU, with emphasis on pressure points associated with patient's intraoperative position, especially sacrum, heels, occiput, scapula if supine. The forehead, chin, clavicle, breasts, iliac crest, anterior thigh, anterior lower leg if prone during the procedure
   b. Risk factors for perioperative skin injury include advanced age, low BMI, hypotension, diabetes, renal insufficiency, sepsis, vascular disease, prolonged cumulative operative times (greater than 180 minutes), use of vasopressors and steroids
   c. Early initiation of mobility activities (repositioning, head of bed elevation, active or passive range of motion, use of pressure reduction surfaces) promotes skin integrity, minimizes injury and promotes patient comfort

SPECIFIC PATIENT HEALTH PROBLEMS

1. **Respiratory: Most commonly occurring complications in the PACU are respiratory complications**
   a. Upper airway: Airway obstruction
      i. Most commonly because of tongue falling back and obstructing upper airway; swelling or edema of the airway, airway injury, hemorrhage, obstructive sleep apnea, neurologic injury or muscular weakness
      ii. Obstruction is managed with chin lift/jaw thrust. If the patient is still sedated, consider oral or nasopharyngeal airway; stimulate patient to breathe deeply and awaken; may need positive pressure ventilation with bag-valve-mask (BVM) device; tracheal intubation with ventilation if unable to resolve

2. **Subglottic edema**
   a. More commonly seen in young children, may be caused by traumatic intubation, coughing while tube in place, tube movement, head or neck procedures, longer operative procedures
   b. Signs/symptoms include crowing respirations, stridor, rocking chest wall respiratory attempts
   c. Treat with supplemental humidified oxygen, nebulized mist treatment with racemic epinephrine
   d. Extended observation as rebound edema can occur

3. **Laryngospasm**
   a. Involuntary partial or complete closure of the vocal cords; may be caused by secretions, stimulation, or irritation of the laryngeal reflexes during emergence
   b. Signs/symptoms include wheezing, reduce compliance, stridor (if partial), paroxysmal chest or abdominal movements, absence of ventilation (if complete)
   c. Treat with airway maneuvers, positive pressure ventilation with BVM, possible neuromuscular blocking agent (e.g., succinylcholine) if not resolving

4. **Bronchospasm**
   a. May result from preexisting asthma, allergy or anaphylaxis, chronic pulmonary disease, histamine release, mucus plugging, aspiration, pulmonary edema, foreign body aspiration
   b. Signs/symptoms include cough, expiratory wheezing, dyspnea, use of accessory muscles, tachypnea
   c. Treat with removal of identified cause, oxygen administration, inhaled bronchodilators, epinephrine, ventilatory support

5. **Hypoxemia**
   a. May be caused by low inspired concentration of oxygen, hypoventilation, ventilation-perfusion mismatches, increased intrapulmonary right to left shunt, pneumothorax, diffuse airway collapse, pulmonary edema, pulmonary embolism
   b. Treatment includes identifying and correcting the cause, stimulation of the patient, supplemental oxygen (including high-flow nasal cannula), and/or CPAP. If unable to maintain oxygen levels, intubation with or without the addition of positive end-expiratory pressure (PEEP) may be required

6. **Hypoventilation**
   a. Patients with residual or inadequately reversed anesthetic agents (not all are reversible), sedatives, opioids, neuromuscular blocking agents on board may experience hypoventilation. It is also common in patients with upper abdominal or thoracic incisions, or in those with neuromuscular diseases.
   b. Signs/symptoms include decreased, shallow respirations, increased $EtCO_2$ levels, increased partial pressure of carbon dioxide ($PaCO_2$)
   c. Treatment includes identifying and managing cause of hypoventilation, supplemental oxygen, verbal and tactile stimulation, deep breathing, and repositioning; opioids and sedatives should be given cautiously; oxygen saturation and $EtCO_2$ levels monitored continuously

7. **Atelectasis**
   a. Common surgical occurrence occurs when alveoli collapse, resulting in hypoxemia because of ventilation-perfusion mismatch and increased pulmonary shunting
   b. Auscultated breath sounds may be diminished; rales or crackles may be heard
   c. Treatment includes coughing and deep breathing exercises, use of incentive spirometry

8. **Aspiration**
   a. Uncommon, increased risk in trauma patients (unknown last intake, possible full stomach), patients with gastroesophageal reflux disease, patients who are obese, older patients, laboring women, nonresponsive patients emerging from anesthesia with airway adjuncts in place and supine positioning
   b. Signs/symptoms include unexplained tachypnea and tachycardia, cough, bronchospasm, hypoxemia, atelectasis, interstitial edema, hemorrhage, and acute respiratory distress syndrome
   c. Prevention preferred: Premedicate at-risk patients with histamine blockers, nonparticulate antacids, and anticholinergic agents
   d. Recovery position: Side-lying, head of bed 30 degrees to minimize aspiration of saliva, vomitus, secretions
   e. Treat suspected aspiration by correcting hypoxemia, maintaining hemodynamic stability; patient may require reintubation, suctioning, mechanical ventilation, and antibiotic treatment.

9. **Pulmonary edema**
   a. Cardiogenic
      i. Associated with fluid overload, congestive heart failure, or acute pulmonary injury
      ii. Characterized by elevated pulmonary artery occlusive pressure, greater than 18 mm Hg, distended neck veins (jugular venous distension), and peripheral edema
      iii. Signs/symptoms include hypoxemia, crackles (rales), decreased pulmonary compliance on ventilator

    iv. Treatment includes identification of the cause and administration of diuretics. Fluid restriction may be ordered; respiratory support may include intubation and mechanical ventilation and PEEP

  b. Noncardiogenic pulmonary edema (NCPE) (also known as negative pressure pulmonary edema)

    i. Caused by increased capillary permeability and changes in pressure gradients within the pulmonary capillaries and vasculature

    ii. Results in acute hypoxia secondary to a rapid deterioration in respiratory status

    iii. Signs/symptoms include hypoxemia, decreased oxygen saturation levels, tachypnea, frothy sputum

    iv. Increase vigilance in patients who have experienced laryngospasm, upper airway obstruction (e.g., tongue relaxation, biting on endotracheal tube), incomplete neuromuscular blockade reversal, or a significant period of hypoxia

    v. Manage with supplemental oxygen, positive airway pressure (CPAP in spontaneously breathing patient, PEEP if intubated), hemodynamic support and continued observation may be required

10. Pulmonary embolism

  a. Patients at risk include those who are obese, immobile, undergoing long bone or pelvic procedures, have a history of congestive heart failure or malignancy

  b. Signs/symptoms include tachypnea, pleuritic chest pain, hemoptysis, breathlessness, and a sense of impending doom

  c. Treatment is supportive

  d. Prevention includes pharmacologic prophylaxis, mechanical devices (intermittent or sequential compression sleeves/pumps)

11. Pneumothorax

  a. May occur spontaneously, associated with inadvertent puncture with operative/ interventional procedure or upper extremity peripheral nerve block

  b. Signs/symptoms include diminished or absent breath sounds on affected side, tracheal displacement/deviation, mediastinal shift

  c. Treatment may include chest tube placement if patient is symptomatic and/or pneumothorax is greater than 20% of lung

12. Decreased CO

  a. Poor perfusion is the primary manifestation of cardiovascular dysfunction; may be a residual effect of anesthetic agents and adjuncts.

    i. Signs/symptoms include tachycardia, hypotension, decreased peripheral perfusion (cool extremities, capillary refill >3 seconds)

    ii. Treatment includes fluid resuscitation, identification, and management of cause if likely other than anesthetic effects

  b. Myocardial dysfunction

    i. May be caused by pathology, physiology, or anesthetic effects

    ii. Especially concerning in presence of preexisting myocardial disease

    iii. Stress of surgical/diagnostic procedure, actions of anesthetic agents may increase risk of myocardial ischemia

    iv. Continuous cardiac monitoring is essential to identify myocardial changes in the postoperative phase of care; if the patient is awake and complaining of chest pain, evaluation is needed to determine the origin (may be related to surgical procedure, other physiologic or pathologic cause); manage following standard protocols

c. Dysrhythmias
   i. Commonly occur in the postanesthesia phase of care
   ii. Include sinus tachycardia (most common), sinus bradycardia, premature ventricular contractions, supraventricular tachydysrhythmias, ventricular tachycardia
   iii. May be caused by circulatory instability, preexisting cardiac disease, increased vagal tone, medications, pain, electrolyte imbalances, hypoxemia
   iv. Treatment determined by cause and hemodynamic effects of dysrhythmia; implement standard protocols to manage, including ACLS algorithms as needed

d. Hypotension
   i. Most common cause is intravascular volume depletion as a result of inadequate replacement of blood loss, third space volume loss, insensible loss, and increased urinary output. May also be a result of reduced myocardial contractility from anesthetic agent effects, myocardial ischemia, dysrhythmias. Hypotension may also result from reduced afterload (low systemic vascular resistance) associated with sepsis, hyperthermia, sympathectomy or larger arteriovenous shunts (chronic liver failure)
   ii. Prompt treatment is needed to avoid ischemic organ damage from prolonged hypotension; identify and manage cause; administer fluids, initiate vasopressors, consider additional monitoring modalities (central lines). Goal is to maintain a mean arterial blood pressure (MAP) over 60 mm Hg to ensure perfusion of the body organs.

e. Hypertension
   i. May be preexisting and untreated; if treated, medications may have been held preoperatively, resulting in hypertension intraoperatively and/or postoperatively
   ii. In PACU/ICU, most common cause may be fluid overload, increased sympathetic nervous system activity, or preexisting hypertension
   iii. Aggressive treatment is indicated to avoid cardiovascular and neurologic consequences
   iv. Increased sympathetic nervous system activity results from the surgical stress, pain, anxiety, bowel or bladder distention, or hypothermia
   v. Treatment includes identifying and managing the cause; also vasodilators, beta-blockers, and calcium channel blockers may be administered if the cause is unidentified or is unsuccessful

13. **Bleeding/hemorrhage/coagulopathy**
    a. Bleeding is typically minimal following surgical/diagnostic procedures; hemorrhage can occur if hemostasis is inadequate or coagulopathies exist
    b. Management requires immediate response by the nurse; typically, pressure is applied, if possible, fluid resuscitation initiated, and the patient prepared for immediate return to the operating room for intervention to stop the bleeding. Adjunct therapies include reversal of anticoagulation agents, administration of blood products or fresh frozen plasma (FFP) and maintaining normothermia.

14. **Thermoregulation**
    a. Hypothermia
       i. Use of active warming therapies intraoperatively have decreased the incidence of postoperative hypothermia
       ii. Identified when the core temperature is less than 36° C; signs/symptoms include shivering, restlessness, discomfort, peripheral vasoconstriction

    iii. Without treatment, patients may experience delayed medication metabolism and elimination, myocardial ischemia, hypertension, residual effects from neuromuscular blocking agents

    iv. Treatment includes active rewarming, supplemental oxygen, and ventilatory support as needed

  b. Hyperthermia

    i. Core temperature greater than 38° C

    ii. May be the result blood transfusion reaction, warm environment, medication-induced fever, overcorrected hypothermia, sepsis

    iii. Treatment includes identifying and managing the cause of hyperthermia

    iv. Malignant hyperthermia (see Intraoperative section)

15. Neurologic

  a. Emergence excitement/agitation/delirium (Fig. 22.3)

    i. More common in children, may range from minor agitation to combative delirium threatening the safety of the patient and caregivers

    ii. Associated with multiple causative factors (see Fig. 22.3)

    iii. May see restlessness, disorientation, crying, moaning, irrational talking, inappropriate behavior

    iv. In more severe agitation or delirium, patient may become violent, thrashing, and screaming

    v. Assess the patient's oxygenation and ventilation; check for bladder distension (time of last know void, volume of fluids administered), pain, and possible alcohol withdrawal

    vi. Treatment if symptomatic; maintain safe patient environment, protecting the patient and caregivers from injury

  b. Delayed emergence

    i. Patient does not awaken as anticipated following an anesthetic administration

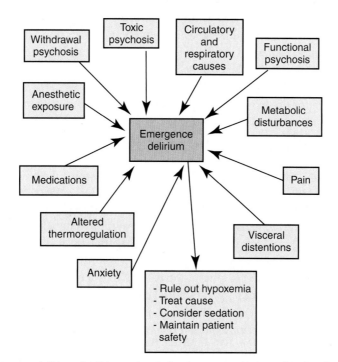

Fig. 22.3 Emergence delirium in the postanesthesia care unit: contributing factors and treatment. (From Nagelhout, J.J., Elisha, S. (2018). *Nurse anesthesia*, ed. 6, St. Louis: Elsevier.)

ii. Review possible causes including metabolic (e.g., electrolyte imbalance—hypoglycemia, hypothermia), neurologic (e.g., anoxic injury, stroke), anesthetic drug effects (e.g., medication error—overdose)

iii. Monitor and continue to evaluate to identify cause and possible treatment

c. Cerebrovascular accident/stroke

i. Rare occurrence associated with general anesthesia

ii. Evaluate patient upon arrival to PACU/ICU and on an ongoing basis (e.g., hourly), screening for stroke symptoms

iii. Positive screen necessitates evaluation, potential treatment to avoid permanent sequelae

16. **GI**

a. Postoperative ileus

i Patients undergoing abdominal surgical procedures will develop some degree of transient GI motility impairment, typically resolving within 72 hours with supportive treatment

ii. Causes are multifactorial and include interruption of GI continuity or bowel manipulation, anesthetic and analgesic medications, fluid overload, immobility, electrolyte imbalance (especially hypokalemia), intraabdominal hematoma or severe infection/sepsis, diabetes, pancreatitis, severe pain, cardiopulmonary failure

iii. Prevention strategies include minimally invasive surgical techniques, ERAS protocols which include preoperative carbohydrate loading, alvimopan (Entereg) administered preoperatively before the administration of opioids, intraoperative fluid restriction, epidural use, transversus abdominis plane block, and postoperative chewing gum

iv. Management include cautious IV fluid replacement, electrolyte replacement, ambulation, nasogastric tube placement, if bowel rest is necessary

17. **Other surgical problems and complications**

a. Specific surgical care assessment and monitoring requirements for various surgical/diagnostic procedures may be found in Chapters 3 to 5, Section II Chapters and Chapters 11, Multisystem Trauma, Chapter 15, Bariatric Patients and Chapter 17, High-Risk Obstetric Patients

18. **Discharge preparation**

a. Preparation for discharge begins preoperatively, before the patient arrival for operative/interventional procedure

i. Planning includes availability of caregivers, living arrangements (type of home, accessibility, need for assistive/adaptive devices to manage in-home care), possible need for rehabilitation (types of available facilities, patient and family preferences)

ii. Patient education includes procedural information, expectations, training, and demonstration of assistive devices (e.g., crutch training, use of a walker)

iii. Prehabilitation plan including diet, exercise, psychologic and spiritual support (e.g., use of meditation, prayer, guided imagery to reduce anxiety, prepare mentally for the procedure)

b. Discharge preparation continues upon patient arrival on the day of the procedure, including verification of preparation and caregiver availability as planned

c. Patient and caregivers informed throughout preparation phase and perioperative phase regarding status and expected outcomes

References and bibliography information are available at http://evolve.elsevier.com/AACN/corecurriculum/.

Index

Note: Page numbers followed by "*f*" indicate figures, "*t*" indicate tables, and "*b*" indicate boxes.